Fat-Soluble Vitamins				Minerals						
Vitamins A (µg RE)[d]	Vitamins D (µg)[e]	Vitamins E (mg α-TE)[f]	Vitamins K (µg)	Calcium (mg)	Phosphorus (mg)	Magnesium (mg)	Iron (mg)	Zinc (mg)	Iodine (µg)	Selenium (µg)
375	7.5	3	5	400	300	40	6	5	40	10
375	10	4	10	600	500	60	10	5	50	15
400	10	6	15	800	800	80	10	10	70	20
500	10	7	20	800	800	120	10	10	90	20
700	10	7	30	800	800	170	10	10	120	30
1000	10	10	45	1200	1200	270	12	15	150	40
1000	10	10	65	1200	1200	400	12	15	150	50
1000	10	10	70	1200	1200	350	10	15	150	70
1000	5	10	80	800	800	350	10	15	150	70
1000	5	10	80	800	800	350	10	15	150	70
800	10	8	45	1200	1200	280	15	12	150	45
800	10	8	55	1200	1200	300	15	12	150	50
800	10	8	60	1200	1200	280	15	12	150	55
800	5	8	65	800	800	280	15	12	150	55
800	5	8	65	800	800	280	10	12	150	55
800	10	10	65	1200	1200	320	30	15	175	65
1300	10	12	65	1200	1200	355	15	19	200	75
1200	10	11	65	1200	1200	340	15	16	200	75

1 Niacin equivalent (NE) = 1 mg of niacin or 60 mg of dietary tryptophan.

Retinol equivalents (REs) = 1 µg retinol or 6 µg ß-carotene.

As cholecalciferol. 10 µg cholecalciferol = 400 international units (IUs) of vitamin D.

α-Tocopherol equivalents (TEs). 1 mg d-α tocopherol = 1 α-TE.

Estimated Sodium, Chloride, and Potassium Minimum Requirements of Healthy Persons

Age	Weight (kg)	Sodium (mg)[a,b]	Chloride (mg)[a,b]	Potassium (mg)[c]
Months				
0-5	4.5	120	180	500
6-11	8.9	200	300	700
Years				
1	11.0	225	350	1,000
2-5	16.0	300	500	1,400
6-9	25.0	400	600	1,600
10-18	50.0	500	750	2,000
>18[d]	70.0	500	750	2,000

[a]No allowance has been included for large, prolonged losses from the skin through sweat.
[b]There is no evidence that higher intakes confer any health benefit.
[c]Desirable intakes of potassium may considerably exceed these values (~13,500 mg for adults).
[d]No allowance included for growth. Values for those below 18 years assume a growth rate at 50th percentile reported by the National Center for Health Statistics and averaged for males and females.

Estimated Safe and Adequate Daily Dietary Intakes of Selected Vitamins and Minerals[a]

		Vitamins		Trace Elements[b]				
Category	Age (years)	Biotin (μg)	Pantothenic Acid (mg)	Copper (mg)	Manganese (mg)	Fluoride (μg)	Chromium (μg)	Molybdenum (mg)
Infants	0-0.5	10	2	0.4-0.6	0.3-0.6	0.1-0.5	10-40	15-30
	0.5-1	15	3	0.6-0.7	0.6-1.0	0.2-1.0	20-60	20-40
Children and adolescents	1-3	20	3	0.7-1.0	1.0-1.5	0.5-1.5	20-80	25-50
	4-6	25	3-4	1.0-1.5	1.5-2.0	1.0-2.5	30-120	30-75
	7-10	30	4-5	1.0-2.0	2.0-3.0	1.5-2.5	50-200	50-150
	11+	30-100	4-7	1.5-2.5	2.0-5.0	1.5-2.5	50-200	75-250
Adults		30-100	4-7	1.5-3.0	2.0-5.0	1.5-4.0	50-200	75-250

[a]Because there is less information on which to base allowances, these figures are not given in the main table of RDA and are provided here in the form of ranges of recommended intakes.
[b]Since the toxic levels for many trace elements may be only several times usual intakes, the upper levels for the trace elements given in this table should not be habitually exceeded.

HUMAN NUTRITION

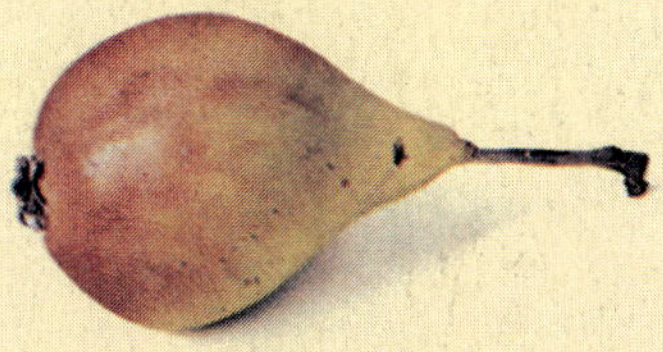

Helen A. Guthrie, Ph.D., R.D.

The Pennsylvania State University

Mary Frances Picciano, Ph.D.

The Pennsylvania State University

With the assistance of

Andrew Scott, Ph.D.

with *255* illustrations

Mosby

St. Louis Baltimore Boston Carlsbad Chicago Naples New York
Philadelphia Portland London Madrid Mexico City Singapore
Sydney Tokyo Toronto Wiesbaden

HUMAN NUTRITION

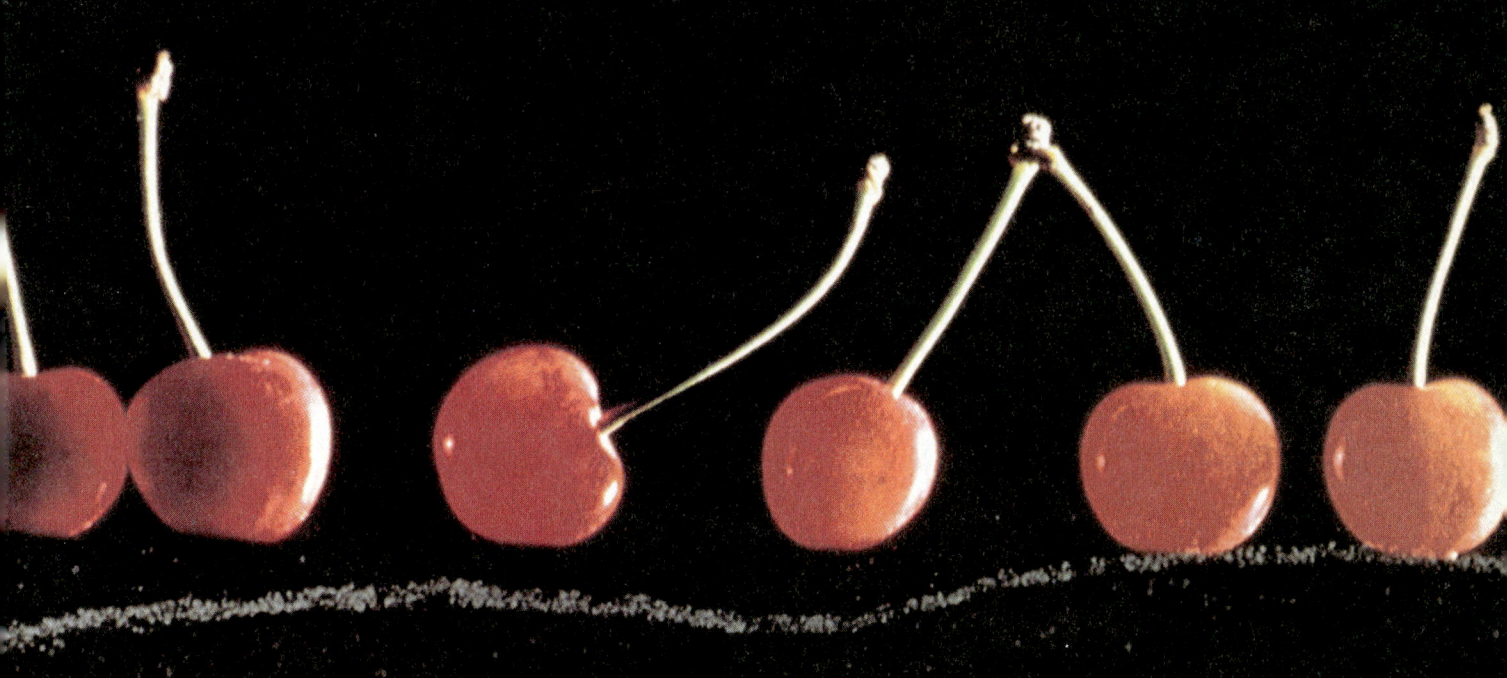

Mosby
Dedicated to Publishing Excellence

A Times Mirror
Company

Publisher: James M. Smith
Acquisitions Editor: Vicki Malinee
Managing Editor: Terry Eynon
Project Manager: Patricia Tannian
Senior Production Editor: Suzanne C. Fannin
Manufacturing Supervisor: Theresa Fuchs
Design: Gail Morey Hudson
William Seabright and Associates
William Seabright
Donald Kye
Cover Illustration: Shoji Yoshida/The Image Bank

Printed in the United States of America
Composition by Carlisle Communications, Ltd.
Printing/binding by Von Hoffmann Press, Inc.

Mosby–Year Book, Inc.
11830 Westline Industrial Drive
St. Louis, Missouri 63146

Guthrie, Helen Andrews.
Human nutrition / Helen A. Guthrie, Mary Frances Picciano with the assistance of Andrew Scott.
p. cm.
Includes bibliographical references and index.
ISBN 0-8151-4043-6
1. Nutrition. I. Picciano, Mary Frances.
II. Scott, Andrew, 1955- . III. Title.
TX354.G79 1995
613.2--dc20 94-38703
CIP

95 96 97 98 99/9 8 7 6 5 4 3 2 1

CONTENTS IN BRIEF

DETAILED TABLE OF CONTENTS

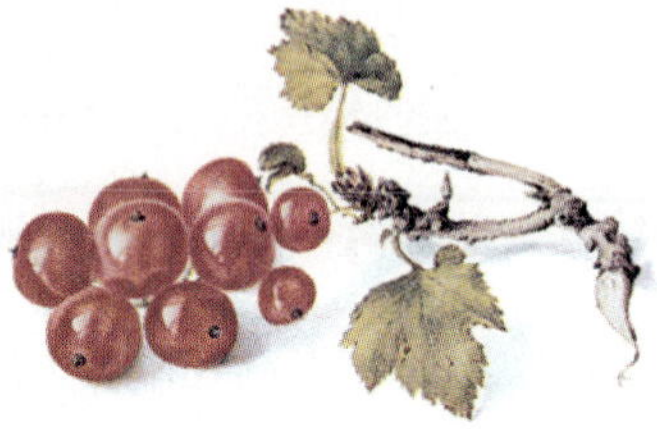

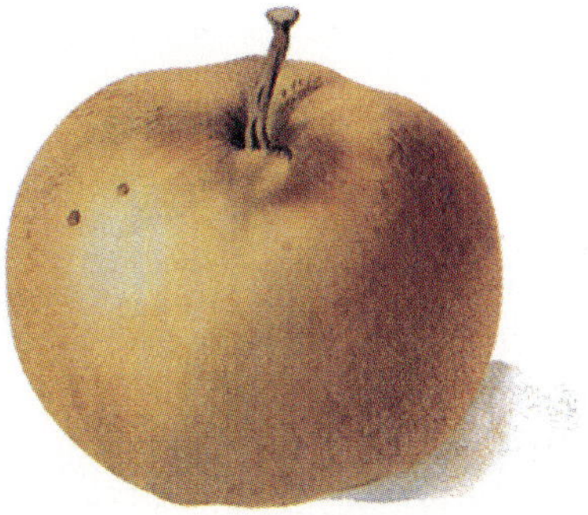

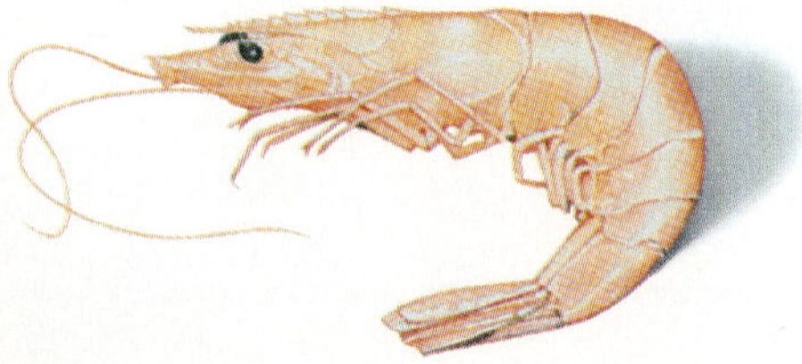

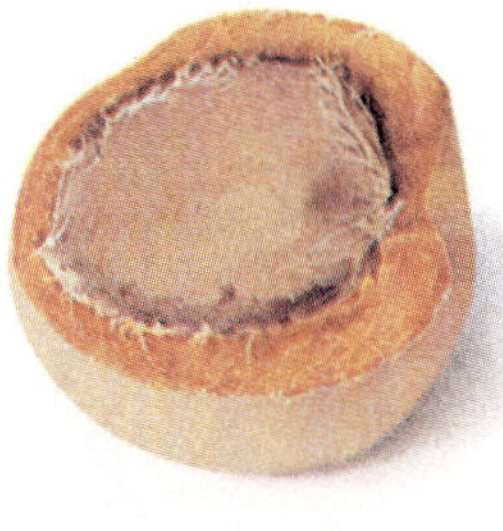

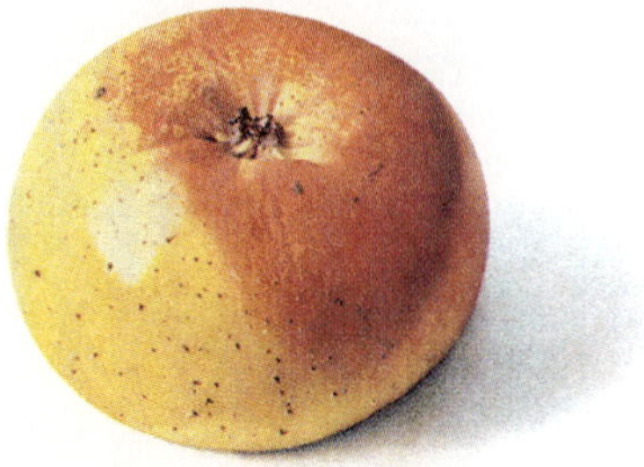

APPENDIXES A-1

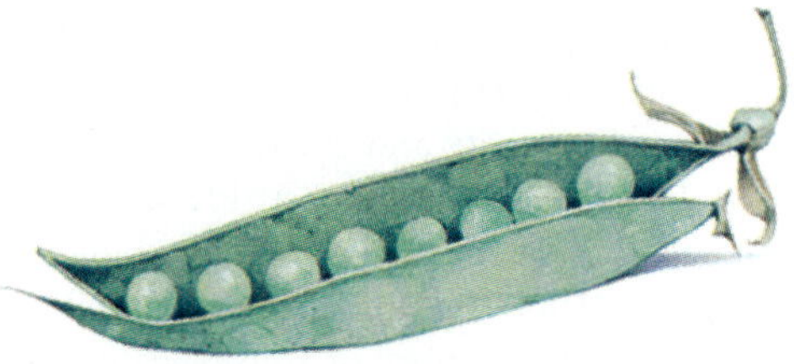

PREFACE

Almost three decades have passed since the first edition of Guthrie's *Introductory Nutrition* appeared. The science of nutrition has undergone many transitions during the seven editions of that text, as have the needs of both instructors and students. In this new text we sought to maintain those successful familiar elements that characterized previous editions and at the same time to respond to the needs of modern students for an accurate and engaging summary and interpretation of the field of nutrition.

APPROACH

Human Nutrition provides a comprehensive, sound, and thoroughly updated account of nutrition principles and their application for students engaged in their first systematic study of nutrition. We sought advice from experienced and successful teachers using a variety of creative approaches to address the needs of modern students. We also incorporated valuable recommendations provided in critical reviews by recognized experts in nutrition and applied normal nutrition. The material is presented in a user-friendly, easily readable, and attractive format with care taken so that complex and intricate relationships are neither distorted nor oversimplified. Dr. Andrew Scott provided invaluable assistance to ensure that the writing style was fresh and interesting while keeping the content scientifically accurate.

AUDIENCE

Students on campuses today are an exceedingly diverse group, representing many ethnic and racial backgrounds, with varying levels of maturity and a variable range of life experiences. We have presented the basic life science concepts on which an understanding of nutrition builds in a manner relevant for the student who wishes solely to become a well-informed consumer or who plans to pursue a career in nutrition or the related health sciences. The students of today face many new challenges and are constantly bombarded with nutrition information in print and in electronic media and from entrepreneurs who wish to capitalize on the current awareness of nutrition and its relationship to health and wellness. This text is designed to provide the student with the basic competence to interpret these ever-changing and increasingly complex messages and to make well-informed decisions that will shape their lives and their careers.

NEW FEATURES

Human Nutrition incorporates many new features to capture student interest and enhance learning.

Design

A modern, full-color design and almost 300 new illustrations and photographs provide visual appeal. The larger type and page size add to the ease of readability.

Illustrations

Formulas for nutrients are presented in relevant chapters, and metabolic and synthetic pathways are introduced throughout the text for students with a background in the life sciences and the intellectual curiosity to explore their application to nutrition. At the same time, students without that expertise are introduced to the basic processes and concepts in clear, nonthreatening prose.

Expanded Content

- A new chapter on food safety is included. The successful application of nutrition requires a knowledge not only of the types and combinations of foods needed to furnish required nutrients, but also of proper food handling and preparation techniques to ensure quality and safety.
- The text also addresses a number of nutrition topics that receive or are likely to receive popular attention as they relate to the maintenance of health and prevention of disability such as trans fatty acids, omega-3 fatty acids, carotenoids, synthetic lipids, artificial sweeteners, pseudovitamins, vitamin-related compounds, and biotechnology.
- The chapter on trace minerals is expanded to reflect recent advances in the field and to include many conditionally essential minerals and representative food values.

Overviews

Three overview sections summarize the principles of digestion, absorption, and excretion and distinguishing features of vitamins and minerals. These overviews help students review their understanding of the material they learned previously or provide conceptual framework for uninitiated students.

Personalized Learning And Critical Analysis

A new end-of-chapter section of personal diet activities directs students to apply material and analyze and evaluate aspects of their own diet. Dr. Michael Kelley from San Diego State University provided invaluable assistance in the development of these activities.

Issues And Opinions Boxes
The Issues and Opinions box at the end of each chapter contains timely and often controversial aspects of nutrition that are related to topics discussed in the text. In many cases the topics highlighted in this section are too tentative to include in the textual material and/or are receiving wide media attention.

Latest Findings From Dietary Surveys
Data from the most recent national survey, National Health and Nutrition Examination Survey (NHANES) III on nutrient intakes of various segments of the population, are used throughout the text and summarized in Appendix K.

Documentation
Each chapter contains references for important core concepts and/or recent scientific findings on various topics, which enable the student and instructor to explore and evaluate original resources.

PEDAGOGICAL AIDS

In addition to the new pedagogical features mentioned above, this edition contains a number of proven and successful learning aids to assist student learning.

Chapter Summaries
These "By Now You Should Know" sections are a series of summary statements that emphasize key concepts and applications of the principles of the topics discussed.

Study Questions
Questions at the end of each chapter allow students to evaluate their understanding of the material and direct them to sections for further study or analysis.

Additional Readings
Suggested readings at the end of the chapter allow students to delve more deeply into topics of interest. We were careful to include only those references that are easily accessible in many libraries. Occasionally we included one or two classic references for students who wish to obtain a historical account of the topic under discussion, but primarily the listing contains the most recent and relevant articles on the subject.

Glossary
The glossary contains definitions of all key terms found in bold print throughout the text and many italicized terms. With over 1000 entries, the glossary reflects the comprehensive nature of the text and enhances its overall usefulness.

Appendixes
Human Nutrition contains 12 appendixes that are valuable resources for the student.

A. **Chemistry and Life.** This summarizes important principles of chemistry as they apply to nutrition and all life processes.

B. **Daily Values.** Values established by the FDA as standards for nutrient labeling purposes.

C. **Recommended Nutrient Intakes for Canadians.** The latest values of recommended levels of dietary nutrients for Canadians are provided.

D. **Nutrient Analysis: Instructions for Keeping Food Records.** This appendix guides students through the process of recording their food intake in sufficient detail to enable further meaningful analysis.

E. **Food Composition Tables.** Nutrient composition of commonly consumed foods in the United States is presented.

F. **Food Composition Tables for Canadians.** This table lists nutrient composition of common Canadian foods with nutrient values different from their United States counterparts. This appendix serves as an adjunct to Appendix E for Canadian students.

G. **Food Sources of Nutrients in Relation to the U.S. RDAs.** This appendix serves as a quick reference for identification of excellent and good food sources of nutrients.

H. **Exchange System Lists.** Lists of foods with comparable amounts of energy-yielding nutrients are presented to assist the student in interpreting many popular diets in the lay literature.

I. **Standards for Triceps Skinfold Measurements.** Standards currently used to interpret skinfold measurements in national surveys and in research studies are provided.

J. **Selected Sources of Reliable Nutrition Information.** This resource lists professional and governmental sources where the interested student can locate sound nutrition information on a variety of topics.

K. **Selected Health and Nutrition Examination Survey III Data.** The major findings on nutrient intakes from the latest Health and Nutrition Examination Survey (1989-1991) conducted by the U.S. Department of Health and Human Services are summarized.

L. **Food Frequency Questionnaire for Calcium Intake Estimation.** A rapid assessment tool for students to estimate daily calcium intake.

ANCILLARY MATERIALS

Instructor's Manual And Test Bank

Prepared by Robin S. Bagby, MEd, RD, of The Pennsylvania State University, this excellent resource contains the following practical features: chapter objectives, chapter outlines; lecture enhancements; critical analysis exercises; lists of current media resources; and self-assessments. A Test Bank of approximately 1000 examination questions includes multiple choice, true/false, matching, and essay questions. Transparency masters highlight key illustrations and charts from the text.

Computerized Test Bank

Qualified adopters of the text receive a computerized test bank package compatible with IBM or Macintosh computers. This advanced-feature test generator allows instructors to add, delete, or edit questions; save and reload tests; and print different versions of each test.

Nutrient Analysis Software

Mosby offers easy-to-use interactive software to allow students to input food intake and physical activities to determine total kcalories consumed and expended in multiple 24-hour periods.

Transparency Acetates

Full-color transparency acetates feature key illustrations from the text with large, easy-to-read labels.

Audiovisual Resources

Qualified adoptees may choose from an excellent selection of videotapes and videodiscs. The *Mosby Multimedia Library: Nutrition II Teaching Videodisc* offers almost 50 animations of important physiologic processes, 280 colorful still images, and several short video clips that will help students apply nutrition concepts.

NUTRI-NEWS

Mosby offers a 16-page semiannual nutrition update with expert opinions on late-breaking or controversial nutrition topics.

ACKNOWLEDGMENTS

The development of *Human Nutrition* was possible because of invaluable assistance from a great many people, several of whom we will inadvertently forget to acknowledge. From the start, we received continual encouragement and support from the capable staff at Mosby, notably Jim Smith, Vicki Malinee, Suzanne Fannin, and especially Terry Eynon, who never wavered in enthusiasm and prodded gently but firmly when appropriate.

We are particularly indebted to the reviewers who provided critical evaluation of the manuscript in a timely fashion and to our colleagues who provided assistance and who shared illustrations, relevant references, and other materials that helped shape the book. Their contributions are contained in each chapter.

Ronette Breifel, Ph.D.
National Center for Health Statistics, U.S. Public Health Service

Danielle Brule, Ph.D.
Health and Welfare Canada

Kim L. Dittus, Ph.D., R.D.
Syracuse University

Jean-Xavier Guinard, Ph.D.
The Pennsylvania State University

K-L. Catherine Jen, Ph.D.
Wayne State University

Michael J. Kelley, Ph.D.
San Diego State University

Kelly Kohls, Ph.D.
Miami University

Roland M. Leach, Jr., Ph.D.
The Pennsylvania State University

Anne Looker, Ph.D.
National Center for Health Statistics, U.S. Public Health Service

Joseph Loomis, Ph.D.
The Pennsylvania State University

Bernadette M. Marriott, Ph.D.
Food and Nutrition Board, National Academy of Sciences

April Mason, Ph.D.
Purdue University

Donald M. Mock, M.D., Ph.D.
University of Arkansas for Medical Sciences and Arkansas Children's Hospital

A. Catherine Ross, Ph.D.
The Pennsylvania State University

John E. Smith, Ph.D.
The Pennsylvania State University

Irene Strycher, Ph.D.
University of Montreal

William A. Verity
Center for Academic Computing
The Pennsylvania State University

Susan Welch, Ph.D.
United States Department of Agriculture

Gorgianna Williams
The Pennsylvania State University

Judith Wolf, Ph.D.
Queens University, Canada

Helen Wright, Ph.D.
The Pennsylvania State University

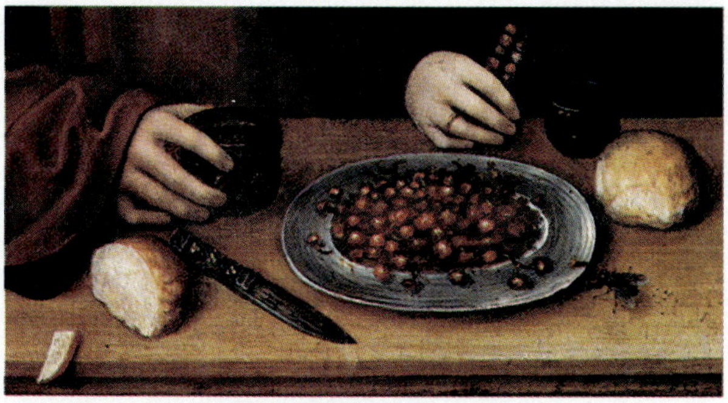

Special acknowledgments are expressed to our families for their continued moral support, encouragement, understanding, and love throughout the entire project. We are also indebted to our students who graciously read and provided their reactions to the content and style presentation.

Helen A. Guthrie

Mary Frances Picciano

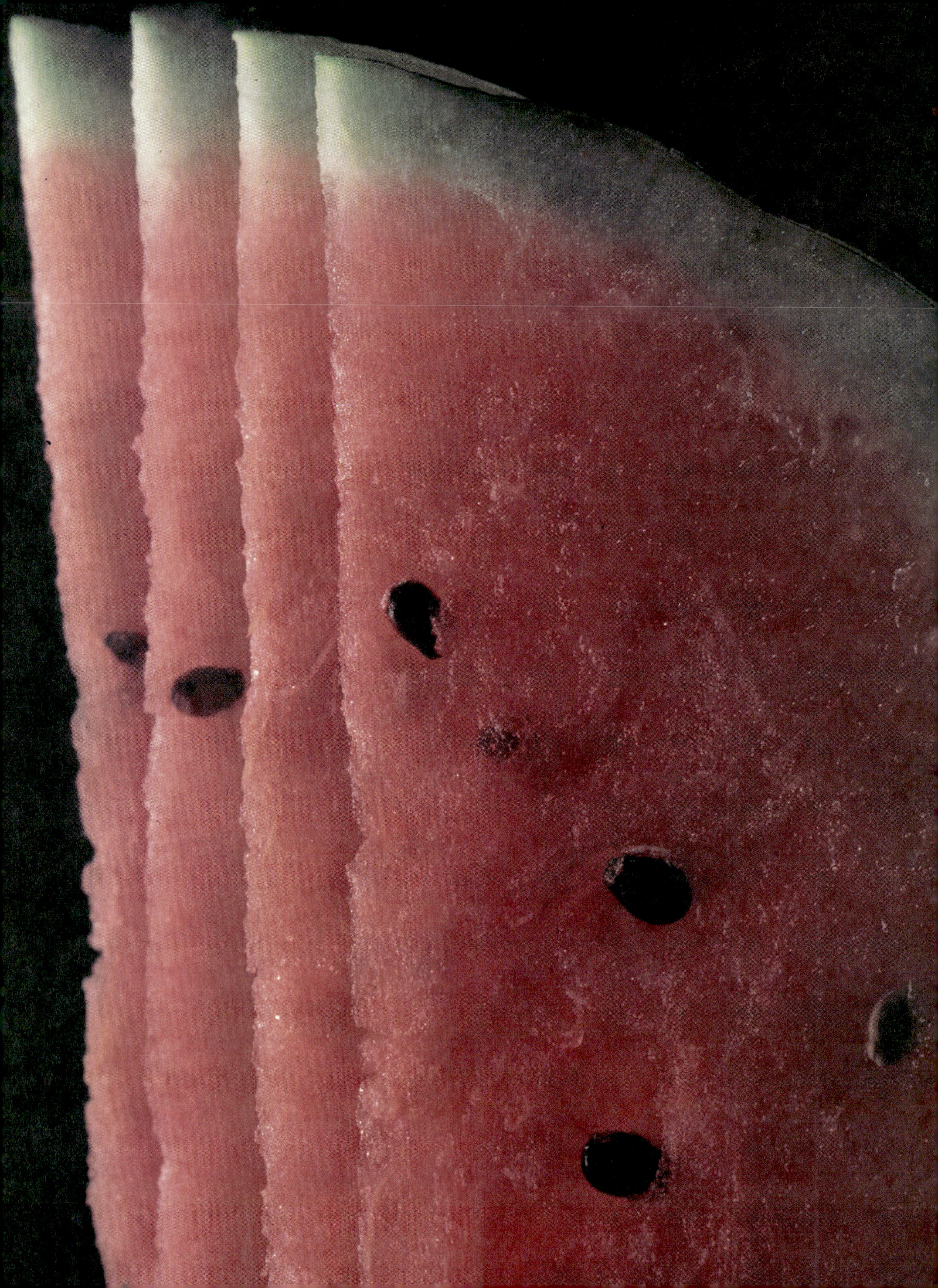

CHAPTER 1

INTRODUCTION TO NUTRITION

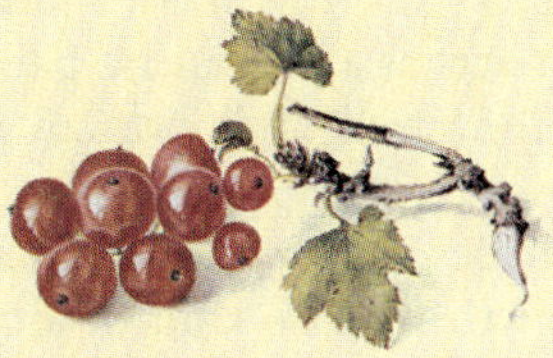

Nutrition has been recognized as a science for at least half a century, but only in the past 25 years has it captured the imagination and interest of the public and policymakers. Today we are surrounded by evidence of great awareness and concern about nutrition: health food stores and magazines flourish; nutrition is discussed at length on television talk shows; the public is turning to nutritionists for counsel and advice; the federal government supports nutrition intervention programs and nutritional research and training; private industry is "selling" nutrition; and career opportunities for nutritionists are expanding. This heightened awareness of nutrition, however, has opened up many opportunities for the promotion of unfounded and unscientific theories. This book is designed to provide the basic nutrition information you need to make informed food choices in the face of an ever-changing food supply promoted with sophisticated marketing techniques.

FOOD AND LIFE

We are made from the chemicals of the earth, which flow through us as we live. We take in food and oxygen, and we give out "wastes" (end products of metabolism) as solids, liquids, and gases. Everything within us and everything we do is sustained by this continual flow of chemicals through our bodies. Apart from oxygen, which we breathe in from the air, all of the chemicals we need are taken in through our mouths as food. This book is about our food, examining what it is composed of, why we need it, and how it allows us to live and grow.

We need food for three main reasons: (1) it acts as a source of energy, which our bodies require to power all activities, just as cars need the energy released from gasoline to make them run, (2) our food provides the chemical raw materials that promote the growth and repair of bodily tissues, and (3) some of the chemicals in food serve to regulate vital processes within the body. The chemicals of food and the energy these chemicals contain are the two central features of our study of the science of nutrition. Appendix A includes a full review of what these chemicals are, what we mean when we talk of the energy they contain, and how they facilitate the processes of life. To begin this introductory chapter of the book, the central principles of chemistry, food, and life are briefly summarized, without going into the details covered in Appendix A.

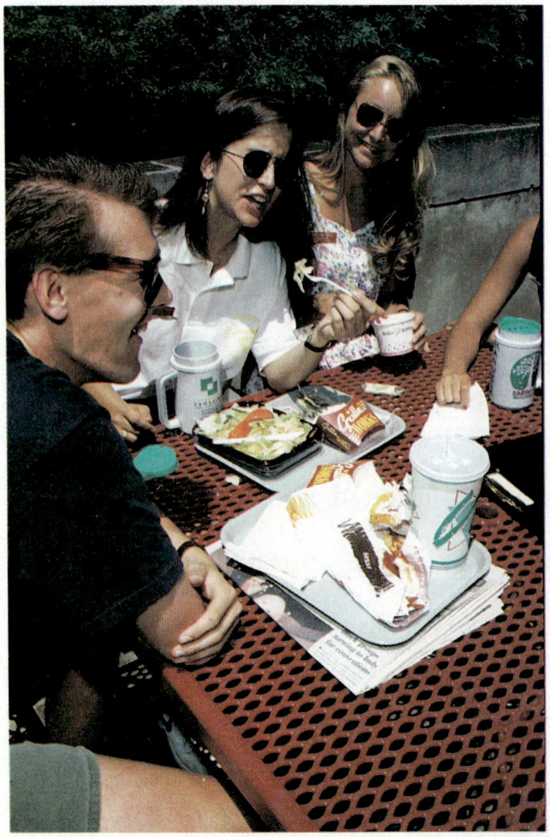

All chemicals are either **elements** or **compounds**. An **element** is a substance composed of only one kind of atom, whereas a **compound** contains two or more kinds of atoms chemically bonded together. Ninety-two different elements naturally occur on Earth, and some of their names are familiar, such as oxygen, calcium, and iron. The names of all the elements, and therefore of all the types of atoms, are listed in the periodic table of the elements (Figure 1-1). The 92 types of atoms listed in the periodic table are the basic building blocks of everything on and in the earth, including human beings. Only some of these atoms, however, are found within the body. Finding out which ones, what compounds they can be part of, and how we get supplies of them is an important part of the study of nutrition.

Most chemicals, including most of the chemicals in the body, are not simple elements containing only one kind of atom. Instead they are chemical "compounds" in which two or more types of atoms are held together by forces known as chemical bonds. **Water** is a chemical compound composed of oxygen atoms bonded to hydrogen atoms. Common table sugar is a chemical compound composed of carbon, hydrogen, and oxygen atoms bonded together. There is an almost limitless variety of chemical compounds on Earth, and many thousands of them are taken into our bodies as food. So although atoms are the basic building blocks of our bodies, many of the atoms we need are taken in as the "locked-up" atoms of compounds rather than the free atoms of individual elements.

The chemicals within food that our bodies can use to help them live and grow are called **nutrients.** Once nutrients are inside of us, they may be built into the material of our bodies directly or immediately used to supply energy. It is more common, however, for them first to be altered in various ways by the chemistry of the body. The cells of the body are able to bring about a wide range of transformations of the nutrients we eat. These transformations shift the atoms about, rearranging them into new compounds more suited to the body's needs.

Some of the nutrients within food are not absolutely essential because the body can make sufficient supplies of them from other chemicals in food. Many nutrients, however, are classified as "essential nutrients" because our bodies either cannot make them at all or cannot make them fast enough to meet our needs. The essential nutrients in the human diet are members of six main categories of chemicals:

- Water
- Carbohydrates
- Lipids
- Proteins
- Minerals
- Vitamins

These nutrients are considered fully in the chapters that follow, but a few words about each are given here.

FIGURE 1-1

The periodic table of the elements, listing the symbols of the 92 naturally occurring elements. Elements found in significant amounts in humans, and therefore required in food, are highlighted in green.

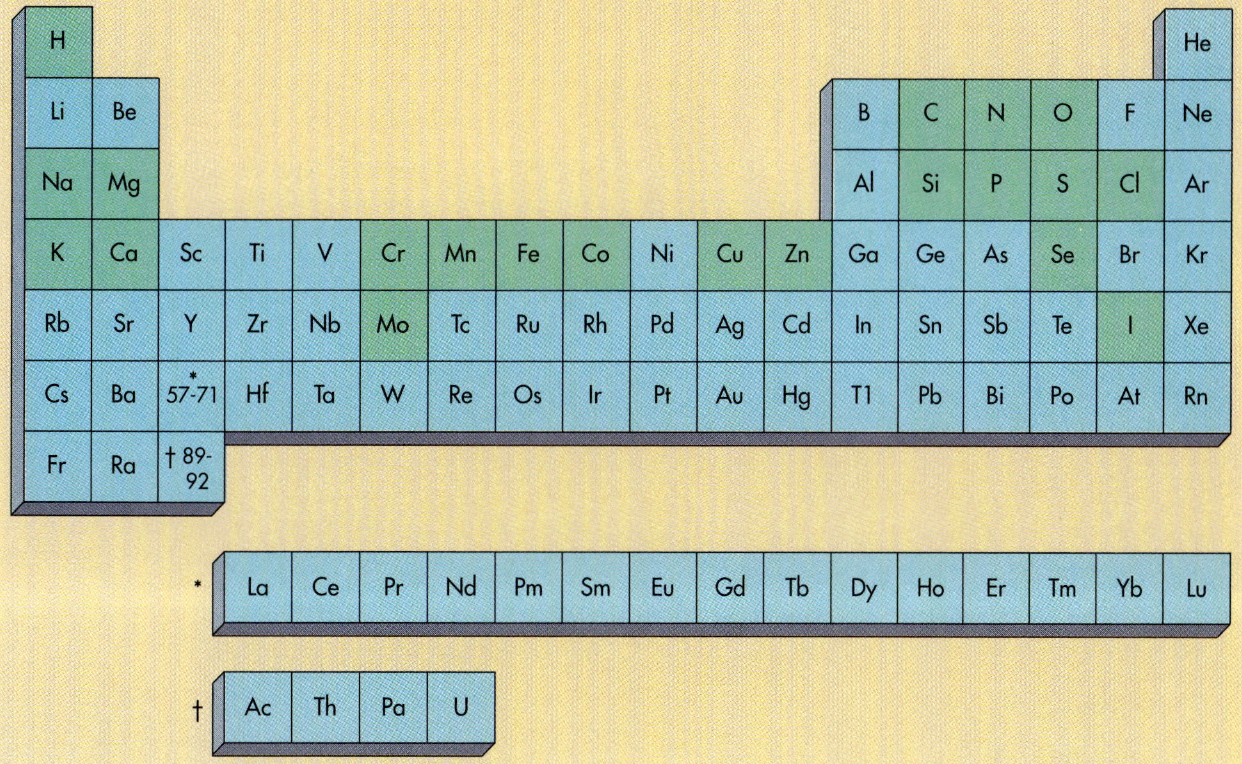

H He
Li Be B C N O F Ne
Na Mg Al Si P S Cl Ar
K Ca Sc Ti V Cr Mn Fe Co Ni Cu Zn Ga Ge As Se Br Kr
Rb Sr Y Zr Nb Mo Tc Ru Rh Pd Ag Cd In Sn Sb Te I Xe
Cs Ba * 57-71 Hf Ta W Re Os Ir Pt Au Hg Tl Pb Bi Po At Rn
Fr Ra † 89-92
* La Ce Pr Nd Pm Sm Eu Gd Tb Dy Ho Er Tm Yb Lu
† Ac Th Pa U

The chemistry of life takes place within the watery medium inside the cells of the body. Without water the cells would dry up and die, and so without water we would quickly die. We could survive without eating food for much longer than we could survive without drinking water. Water is composed of the atoms oxygen and hydrogen; we need these atoms combined into the form of water not as a source of chemical raw materials, but simply to act as the medium in which all the chemistry of life takes place.

Carbohydrates are made of carbon, hydrogen, and oxygen atoms. Sugars and starch are examples of carbohydrates, and they are major sources of energy in our diet.

Lipids include all of the fats and oils we eat. They too are composed largely of carbon, hydrogen, and oxygen atoms. They are rich sources of energy. The "fat" that builds up in the body if the diet is too rich in energy-containing foods is largely composed of lipids. Despite the poor reputation of fatty foods, some of the specific lipids they contain are—in proper amounts—vital parts of a healthful diet. In addition to providing energy, lipids are involved in the growth and maintenance of body tissues and the regulation of body processes in a variety of ways.

Almost all of the body's chemistry is mediated and controlled by chemicals called **proteins**. So one of the main reasons we must eat proteins is to provide the raw materials needed to make the proteins of our own bodies. Proteins are largely composed of carbon, hydrogen, oxygen, nitrogen, and sulfur atoms. Proteins are required for growth and maintenance of our bodies. They are not required as a source of energy but can be used as such, and the levels in excess of needs of proteins normally consumed mean that they are regularly used as sources of energy. Proteins also allow all the interacting chemical processes within the body to be properly regulated.

> Energy-yielding nutrients contain carbon, hydrogen, and oxygen in varying proportions. Protein also contains the minerals nitrogen and sulfur.

As Table 1-1 shows, water, carbohydrates, lipids, and proteins together constitute over 98% of the weight of food. The other two kinds of essential nutrients are minerals and vitamins, which together make up a small part of food. This does not mean that they are any less important. Minerals and vitamins are vital components

TABLE 1-1

Approximate nutrient composition of some representative foods

	WHOLE MILK (%)	BREAD (%)	CARROTS (%)	CHICKEN (%)	BANANAS (%)
Water	87.0	35.8	88.2	69	74
Carbohydrate	5.0	50.4	8.4	0	24
Lipid	3.5	3.2	0.2	8	0.9
Protein	3.7	8.7	1.1	19	0.9
Minerals	0.7	1.1	1.9	1	1
Vitamins	0.1	0.1	0.1	0.1	0.1

TABLE 1-2

List of essential nutrients in each general category of nutrients

CARBOHYDRATE

Glucose

FAT OR LIPID

Linoleic acid
Linolenic acid

PROTEIN

Amino acids
- Leucine
- Isoleucine
- Lysine
- Methionine
- Phenylalanine
- Threonine
- Tryptophan
- Valine
- Histidine

Nonessential amino nitrogen

MINERALS

Macronutrient elements
- Calcium*
- Phosphorus
- Sodium†
- Potassium
- Sulfur
- Chlorine
- Magnesium†

Micronutrient elements
- Iron*
- Selenium
- Zinc†
- Manganese
- Copper
- Cobalt
- Molybdenum
- Iodine‡
- Chromium
- Vanadium
- Tin
- Nickel
- Silicon
- Boron
- Arsenic
- Fluorine

VITAMINS

Fat-soluble
- A (retinol)*
- D (cholecalciferol)‡
- E (tocopherol)
- K

Water-soluble
- Thiamin ‡
- Riboflavin
- Niacin‡
- Biotin
- Folic acid†
- Vitamin B_6 (pyridoxine)*
- Vitamin B_{12} (cobalamin)
- Pantothenic acid
- Vitamin C (ascorbic acid)

WATER

* Most likely to be a problem in the United States (based on Nationwide Food Consumption Survey, 1977-1978).
† Potential problems.
‡ Previous problems; they have now been corrected.

of a healthful diet, and a deficiency in any of them can quickly make the difference between good health and illness.

The essential **minerals** of the diet are all elements (Table 1-2). The **micronutrient minerals** are needed in tiny amounts (less than 50 mg/day). The **macronutrient minerals** are needed in somewhat larger, but still small, amounts (between 350 and 3625 mg/day). These minerals perform a variety of vital functions within the body.

Vitamins—also listed in Table 1-2—are much more complicated substances than minerals, and each is needed to perform some important chemical task required for good health. The vitamins are a chemically

FIGURE 1-2

Relationships among major nutrient groups and main functions of nutrients. Vitamins and minerals are directly involved in supplying energy and in providing growth and maintenance. They are necessary to facilitate the chemical changes involved in these processes.

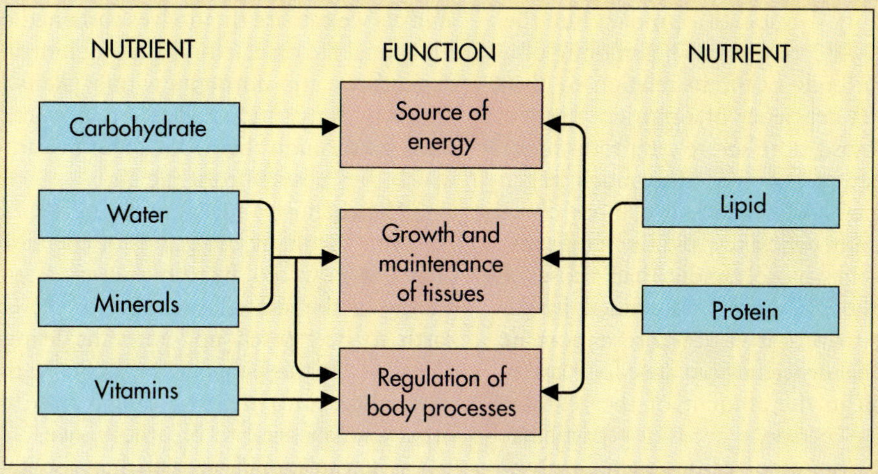

diverse group of compounds, with the only links between them being that they are all organic compounds and are all essential parts of a healthful diet, although required in only small amounts.

Figure 1-2 classifies nutrients according to their main functions, which are the following:

- Acting as a source of energy
- Assisting in the growth and maintenance of tissues
- Helping regulate and facilitate the body's processes

Protein and lipid perform all three functions, certain minerals and water are directly involved in only two, and vitamins and carbohydrate are each directly involved in only one function.

Table 1-2 lists the essential nutrients within each of the main nutrient categories. Some of these nutrients are present in a wide variety of foods, so there is little likelihood of anyone's diet being deficient in them. Others are found in a limited range of foods, so a diet with little variety in certain types of foods—such as fruits, dairy products, and cereals—may well be deficient in one or more essential nutrients. Despite the many opportunities for a diet to be deficient in one or more nutrients, an almost limitless number of different diets (different combinations of foods) can provide adequate nutrition. It is also important to realize that the nutritional needs of different animal species vary considerably. Vitamin C, for example, is a dietary essential for humans and guinea pigs, but not for rats. Throughout this book we concentrate on the nutrients that are essential in the human diet. Nutrients that have been identified as "problem nutrients" in the United States, meaning those we are most likely to suffer a deficiency of or consume an excess of, are identified in Table 1-2.

In the United States amounts of each nutrient estimated to at least meet a person's needs are listed in the **Recommended Dietary Allowances (RDAs)** (see inside cover). The first set of RDAs were established in 1941 and have been revised approximately every 5 years by a committee appointed by the National Academy of Sciences. The RDAs do not consist of single values for each nutrient, but they list a series of values corresponding to the needs of various subgroups of the population that are defined on the basis of gender, age, and whether they are pregnant or lactating women. The RDAs are recommended dietary *intakes,* rather than the amounts our bodies need to absorb and retain. So when the RDAs are set, allowance is made for the efficiency with which the nutrients are absorbed by the body and used within it. The RDAs apply to healthy people only; they do not take into account any increased nutrient needs because of illness or injury. People who are ill or recovering from injury or surgery may need to consume more than the RDA of certain nutrients. The RDAs include a significant margin for error, however, so almost every healthy person consuming the RDA amount of each nutrient is taking in more of each nutrient than the body actually needs. Many other developed countries have their own systems of nutritional recommendations, similar to the RDA system. The World Health Organization (WHO) and the Food and Agricultural Organization (FAO) of the United Nations have also developed practical nutritional standards for use by nations who have not developed their own.

Each of the essential nutrients is needed for a body to live and grow properly, but all are needed in different amounts. The RDA for cobalamin (vitamin B_{12}) for an adult man is about 2 µg (1/14,000,000 oz)/day, but the RDA for protein is 56 g (2 oz)/day. The amount of a nutrient needed by the body bears no relation to that nutrient's importance. A deficiency of a nutrient needed in small amounts may cause more severe symptoms more rapidly than a deficiency of one needed in much larger amounts. Iron deficiency, for instance, is a more common problem than calcium deficiency, and the symptoms of iron deficiency develop more rapidly than those of calcium deficiency, although the recommended intake for calcium is 80 times that for iron. It is also important to know that a nutritional deficiency can arise for reasons other than a reduction in the amount of the relevant nutrient in the diet. A person's needs for particular nutrients may increase for some reason, such as pregnancy, making a previously adequate diet become a deficient one. In addition, the body may begin to absorb a nutrient in decreased amounts or use less of it for various physiological reasons.

*E*ssential nutrients are needed in amounts varying from a few micrograms to 56 grams.

1 ounce		=	28.35 grams
1 kilogram	10^{3}	=	1000 grams
1 gram	10^{0}	=	1000 milligrams
1 milligram	10^{-3}	=	1000 micrograms
1 microgram	10^{-6}	=	1000 nanograms
1 nanogram	10^{-9}	=	1000 picograms
1 picogram	10^{-12}		

One important factor in the development of nutrient deficiencies is how quickly the body's reserves of a nutrient are depleted when the diet is not providing enough. This time can vary from a few days to about 2500 days, depending on the nutrient. Some nutrients are hardly stored at all, whereas others can be stored in large amounts. The site of storage, if there is one, also varies. For example, the liver stores iron, vitamin A, and carbohydrate; the adrenal gland stores vitamin C; and bone stores calcium.

The science of nutrition is based on the twin foundations of chemistry and biology. These foundations are described more fully in Appendix A. Before embarking on an exploration of the detailed chemistry and biology of nutrition, it is worth pausing to consider the few central simplicities that lie at the heart of it:

We are sustained by eating plants and animals. The animals we eat, or perhaps the animals eaten by the animals we eat, are themselves sustained by eating plants. All animal life on Earth, including human life, ultimately depends on the nutrients within plants. Plants are sustained by water and various simple minerals, which they draw up through their roots, and by carbon dioxide gas, which they absorb from the air.

The chemistry that transforms these basic raw materials into the many thousands of chemicals found within plants is powered by the energy of sunlight. So the energy of the sun allows some of the chemicals of the earth to be "raised up" into the living complexity of plant life. As this happens, incidentally, the plants release oxygen gas into the atmosphere, the oxygen we and other animals need to breathe to live.

When an animal eats a plant, it uses the plant's chemicals as the raw materials needed to build and maintain the animal. Also, it combines some of the plant's chemicals with oxygen to provide energy needed to sustain the life of the animal. In doing so the animal releases water and carbon dioxide gas as wastes, in addition to the other chemical wastes it releases in urine and feces. So the waste products of animals are the raw materials needed to sustain plants. This means that animals and plants are locked together in a set of self-sustaining chemical cycles (Figure 1 - 3). Animals eat plants and release chemicals that can be used to build more plants. Plants take up these chemicals and use them to build new plant material that can be eaten by animals. This whole system of cycling, self-sustaining chemistry is powered by the sun's energy, which floods down to Earth and can be captured within the green leaves of plants.

As we delve ever more deeply into the science of nutrition, it is worth keeping in mind the beautiful simplicity of Figure 1 - 3, which illustrates the foundation on which all the details we discuss are overlaid.

NUTRITION DEFINED

The branch of science known as nutrition has been defined in many ways. The simplest definitions emphasize that it is the science of nourishing the body properly. A more detailed definition is as follows:

> Nutrition is the science of food, the nutrients, and other substances within food; their action, interaction, and balance in relation to health and disease; and the processes by which the organism ingests, absorbs, transports, uses, and excretes food substances.

FIGURE 1-3

The cycling of chemicals, powered by energy from the sun, which generates food and sustains life.

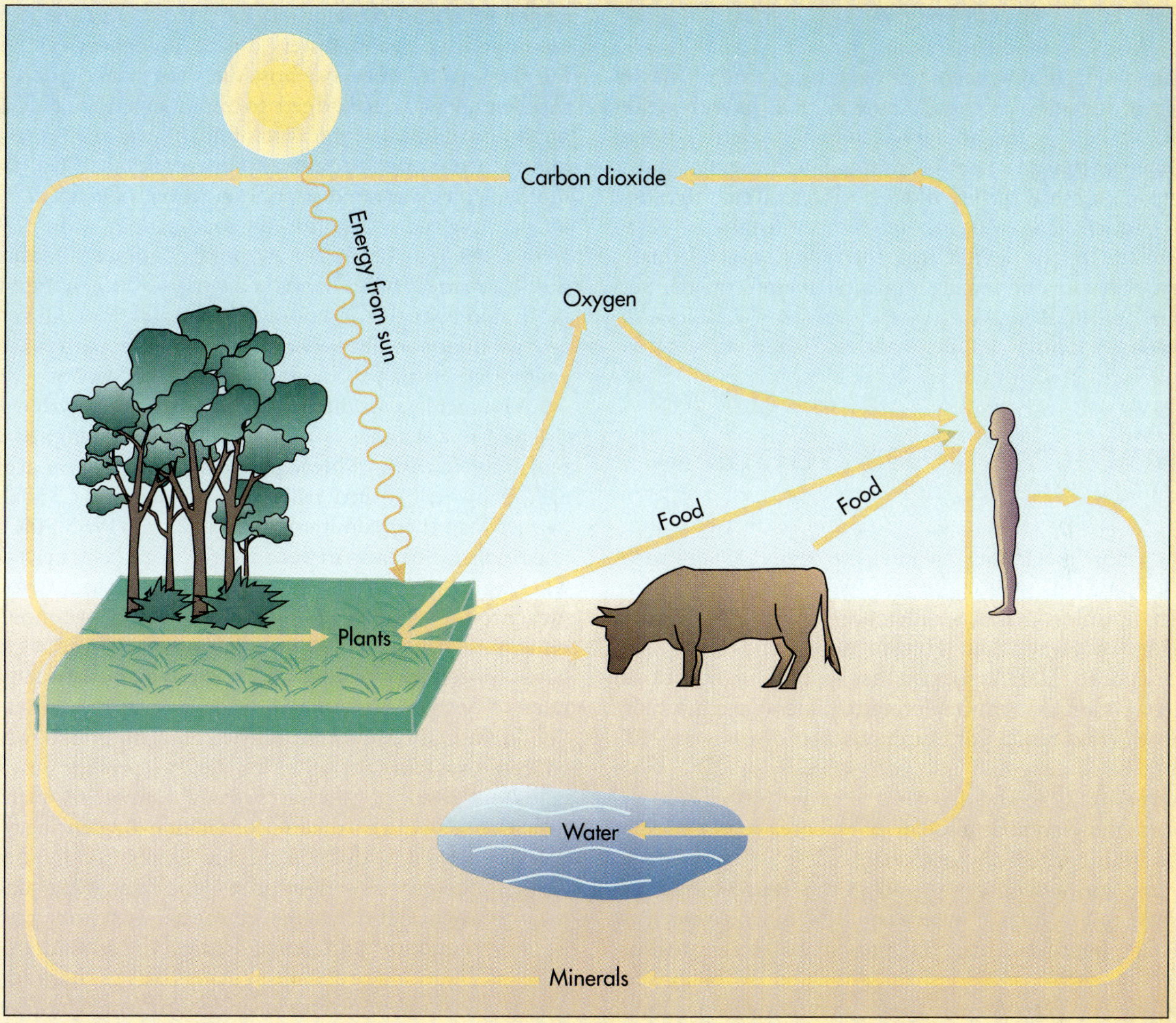

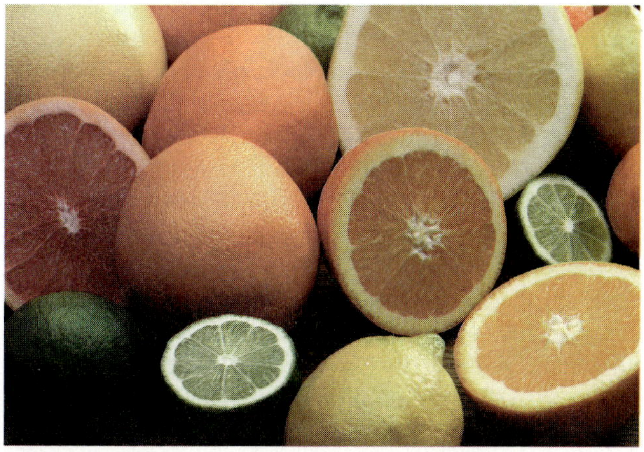

Whatever words are used to define the science of nutrition, there is clear agreement that it is concerned with the way food is produced, with any changes that occur within the food before it is eaten, and with the way the body uses the food until it is used for energy, built into body tissues, or excreted. It includes the study of the digestion, absorption, and transport of nutrients and what happens to the nutrients once they get into the various types of cells in the body. Nutritionists are also becoming increasingly concerned with the factors that determine what food is available to people, what food they choose to eat, and how these factors affect the nutritive quality of a person's diet and his or her state of health or illness. We must remember that people eat food for various reasons, in addition to the basic one of supplying raw materials and energy. We often eat for social or perhaps psychological reasons, for example, even when we are not hungry.

As more is learned about the role of nutrients in maintaining health, there has been rising interest in the role of nutrition in the immune system, its interaction with genetics, and the ways in which nutrition can influence the processes of development, aging, and a person's general quality of life. It is also ironic that one of the challenges facing modern nutritionists is to persuade many people that their diets are adequate, that they do not require nutritional supplements, and that excessive intake of some nutrients can lead to illness.

IMPORTANCE OF GOOD NUTRITION

Before beginning an intensive study of individual nutrients, you might ask, "What evidence is there that nutrition makes a difference?" The U.S. Departments of Health and Human Services (DHHS) and Agriculture (USDA) suggest that appropriate nutritional intervention can reduce morbidity (illness) and mortality (death) that result from cardiovascular diseases by 25%, from respiratory and infectious diseases by 20%, from cancer by 20%, and from diabetes by 50%.[1] Furthermore, the National Academy of Sciences report on diet and health[2] cited cardiovascular diseases, obesity, dental decay, and osteoporosis among the many conditions whose toll of human misery could be much reduced by dietary improvements. The preventable costs attributable to such conditions are estimated at billions of dollars per year. So it appears that knowledge about good nutrition may be one of our most valuable and underused resources in health promotion and disease prevention.

> **Degenerative diseases with some diet-related causes:**
> - Coronary heart disease
> - Atherosclerosis
> - Stroke
> - Some cancers
> - Hypertension
> - Diabetes mellitus
> - Osteoporosis

One of the earliest systematic studies of the relationship between diet and health was performed by Burke and colleagues in the early 1940s.[3] They related the health of newborn infants to the adequacy of the diets consumed by their mothers during pregnancy. Of the infants born to mothers whose diets were rated good or excellent, 94% were judged to be in superior or good physical condition at the time of birth, with the remaining 6% being rated in poor or fair condition. When the mother's diet was rated as poor, however, only 8% of the infants received a superior or good rating, while 92% were judged to be in fair or poor condition. Because people change food habits slowly, even when highly motivated by such conditions as pregnancy, these dietary ratings undoubtedly reflect long-standing patterns of eating, rather than those during pregnancy alone.

The increase in the height of American children in the past few decades is partly attributable to improved nutrition. In 1951 Philadelphia children were, on average, 3 inches (5 cm) taller and 3 pounds (1.35 kg) heavier than their counterparts in 1925. In 1955 30% of male college freshmen were over 6 feet (1.8 m) tall, whereas in 1880 only 5% reached this height.[4] Before giving too much credit to nutrition, however, we should remember that advances in other areas of health care have reduced the incidence of infection and other deterrents to optimal growth at an early age.

In the early days of the science of nutrition the main concern was the alteration of diet to prevent severe deficiency diseases, such as pellagra (caused by niacin deficiency), beriberi (thiamin or vitamin B_1 deficiency), scurvy (vitamin C deficiency), and goiter (iodine deficiency). Anemia caused by iron deficiency is the only major nutrient deficiency that remains a worldwide public health concern,[5] and iodine deficiency[6] and vitamin A deficiency[7] are still problems in many parts of the world. The focus of attention in the developed world has now turned to the role of nutrition in the major causes of death. An increasing body of evidence suggests that diet plays a major role in the maintenance of health and the prevention of disease. Perhaps most convincing is the data relating blood levels of cholesterol and especially the level of low-density lipoprotein cholesterol (risk factors for coronary heart disease) to the saturated fat content of the diet. It now appears clear that the total blood cholesterol level, and specifically the low-density lipoprotein cholesterol level, can be reduced by reducing the level of total fat in the diet to less than 30% of kilocalories and of saturated fat to less than 10% or by raising the content of polyunsaturated fat in the diet up to 10% of kilocalories. Each 1% reduction in the blood cholesterol level is associated with a 2% reduction in coronary heart disease.[8] There is also a growing conviction that adequate, but not excessive, fiber in the diet may reduce the risk of colon cancer.[9] In addition, it has

TABLE 1-3

Summary of specific nutrition objectives in Healthy People 2000

CATEGORY	OBJECTIVES
Health status	1 Reduce heart disease deaths to no more than 100 per 100,000 people.
	2 Reverse the rise in cancer deaths to achieve a rate of no more than 130 per 100,000 people.
	3 Reduce overweight to a prevalence of no more than 20% among people ages 20 years and older and no more than 15% among adolescents ages 12 through 19 years.
	4 Reduce growth retardation among low-income children ages 5 years and younger to less than 10%.
Risk reduction	5 Reduce dietary fat intake to an average of 30% of calories or less and average saturated fat intake to less than 10% of calories among people ages 2 years and older.
	6 Increase complex carbohydrate- and fiber-containing foods in the diets of adults to five or more daily servings for vegetables (including legumes) and fruits and to six or more daily servings for grain products.
	7 Increase the proportion of overweight people ages 12 years and older who have adopted sound dietary practices combined with regular physical activity to attain an appropriate body weight to at least 50%.
	8 Increase calcium intake, so at least 50% of youth ages 12 through 24 and 50% of pregnant and lactating women consume three or more servings daily of foods rich in calcium and at least 50% of people ages 25 years and older consume two or more servings daily.
	9 Decrease salt and sodium intake, so at least 65% of home meal preparers prepare foods without adding salt, at least 80% of people avoid using salt at the table, and at least 40% of adults regularly purchase foods modified or lower in sodium.
	10 Reduce iron deficiency to less than 3% among children ages 1 through 4 years and among women of childbearing age.
	11 Increase to at least 75% the proportion of mothers who breast-feed their babies in the early postpartum period and to at least 50% the proportion who continue breast-feeding until their babies are 5 to 6 months old.
	12 Increase to at least 75% the proportion of parents and caregivers who use feeding practices that prevent baby bottle tooth decay.
	13 Increase to at least 85% the proportion of people ages 18 years and older who use food labels to make nutritious food selections.
Services and protection	14 Achieve useful and informative nutrition labeling for virtually all processed foods and for at least 40% of fresh meats, poultry, fish, fruits, vegetables, baked goods, and ready-to-eat carry-away foods.
	15 Increase the availability of processed food products that are reduced in fat and saturated fat to at least 5000 brand items.
	16 Increase to at least 90% the proportion of restaurants and institutional food service operations that offer identifiable low-fat, low-calorie food choices, consistent with the Dietary Guidelines for Americans.
	17 Increase to at least 90% the proportion of school lunch and breakfast services and child care food services with menus that are consistent with the nutrition principles in the Dietary Guidelines for Americans.
	18 Increase to at least 90% the proportion of school lunch and breakfast services by people ages 65 years and older who have difficulty in preparing their own meals or are otherwise in need of home-delivered meals.
	19 Increase to at least 75% the proportion of the nation's schools that provide nutrition education from preschool through twelfth grade, preferably as part of quality school health education.
	20 Increase to at least 50% the proportion of worksites with 50 or more employees that offer nutrition education and/or weight management programs for employees.
	21 Increase to at least 75% the proportion of primary care providers who provide nutrition assessment and counseling and/or referral to a qualified nutritionist or dietitian.

From U.S. Department of Health and Human Services: *Healthy People 2000: national health promotion and disease prevention objectives,* U.S. Public Health Service Pub No 91-50212, Washington, DC, 1990, U.S. Government Printing Office.

been widely reported that excessive fat intake is a risk factor for obesity and hence diabetes, atherosclerosis, some types of cancer, and possibly gallbladder disease.

Further evidence that health authorities in the United States consider that nutrition really does make a difference is the inclusion of 21 specific nutrition objectives in *Healthy People 2000: National Health Promotion and Disease Prevention Objectives.*[10] This list of key objectives is designed to dramatically cut health care costs, prevent the premature onset of disease and disability, and help all Americans enjoy healthier and more productive lives. The 21 nutrition objectives are shown in Table 1-3.

THE RISE OF INTEREST

The late 1960s saw an upsurge of interest in nutrition in the United States, when a shocked and outraged public began to realize that hunger and malnutrition existed in the midst of plenty. As a result the first White House Conference on Food, Nutrition, and Health was convened in 1969. This conference represented a commitment by the federal government to identify problems of hunger and malnutrition and take steps to alleviate them. A follow-up conference in 1974, to assess what progress had been made, resulted in the initiation of a number of federally supported nutrition activities. These included nutrition programs for elderly persons; a program for women, infants, and children at high risk for malnutrition; standards for nutrient labeling of processed foods; and support for nutrition education in elementary schools. Previously established programs, such as school feeding and food stamps, were expanded.

Dietary Goals for the United States, a statement issued by the Senate Select Committee on Nutrition in Human Needs in 1977 and revised in 1978, gave further evidence of increasing government interest in the nutritional health of the country. In 1981 a joint DHHS and USDA publication, *Dietary Guidelines for Americans,* was issued to help promote health and prevent chronic diseases; this publication was revised in 1985 and 1990.[11] Two National Academy of Sciences (NAS) publications, *Diet, Nutrition and Cancer*[12] and *Diet and Health: Implications for Reducing Chronic Disease Risk,*[2] further highlighted the relationship of nutrition to health problems. Similar governmental initiatives are evident in Canada, Sweden, Finland, New Zealand, and other developed countries, emphasizing the worldwide recognition of the role of nutrition and diet in health maintenance and disease prevention.

Awareness of nutritional issues continues to grow in the United States, but nutritional excesses and imbalances have replaced nutritional deficiencies as the primary concern. We spend ever-increasing amounts on health foods, increasing numbers of people attempt to change their diets in response to nutritional concerns, and there is now a widespread interest in the relationship between nutrition and all aspects of health.

Turning briefly to the global situation, the worldwide distribution of nutritional deficiency diseases is concentrated in tropical countries with a high population density. As might be expected, these countries are also the poorest of the world. The first authorized agency concerned with nutrition within the United Nations was the FAO. In 1944 it was charged with devising ways to improve the nutritional status of the world's population as a pathway to peace. The WHO, another United Nations agency, now allocates some resources to solving problems in nutrition. U.S. groups, such as the U.S. Agency for International Development (USAID), and similar groups in Germany, Canada, and the Netherlands have similar goals. In spite of these efforts, malnutrition and undernutrition—existing alongside a rapidly expanding population, inadequate medical care, and poor sanitation—remain dominant health problems in the modern world.

HISTORICAL BACKGROUND

Nutrition is a relatively new science, achieving recognition as a distinct discipline only in 1934 with the founding of the American Institute of Nutrition. Because it is the science of how food is used by and affects our bodies, nutrition could properly emerge as a science only once the basic chemical and biological principles of life had been uncovered (Appendix A). So the science of nutrition has grown out of the sciences of chemistry and biology and continues to draw on and contribute to many modern branches of chemistry and biology. Biochemistry, microbiology, physiology, cellular and molecular biology, medicine, and food science are just a few of the areas of modern science that overlap in places with the science of nutrition. The rapidly expanding fields of genetic engineering and biotechnology are also offering new tools and challenges to nutritionists.

Most of the organized study of nutrition has occurred in the twentieth century, but general interest in the subject—accompanied by some useful study—goes back much further. The history of nutrition can be divided into four main eras:

- Naturalistic era (400 BC to AD 1750)
- Chemical-analytical era (1750 to 1900)
- Biological era (1900 to 1955)
- Cellular or molecular era (1955 to present)

A few of the most important discoveries of each era are highlighted below to give an overall view of the state of knowledge at each stage. Of course, chemical, analytical, and biological investigations continue to contribute to nutritional knowledge. Although modern nutritional science is founded on a substantial body of well-established information, it is a field of active investigation and much remains unknown or uncertain. Many of the theories of modern nutritionists remain speculative to varying degrees and therefore open to modification as time passes and more is discovered about nutrients and their interaction with the body. The student using this book will learn about a science in progress, rather than a science whose days of speculative excitement and interest are past.

NATURALISTIC ERA (400 BC TO AD 1750)

The naturalistic era was characterized by many vague ideas concerning taboos, magical powers, and medicinal values associated with different foods. Many such ideas were swept aside by discoveries made in later eras, but early men and women did clearly and correctly recognize that food was essential for survival and health. In biblical times, Daniel is reported to have observed that men who ate pulses (vegetables of the pea and bean family) and drank mainly water thrived better than those who ate the king's food and drank a lot of wine. Hippocrates, the father of medicine, considered food as one universal nutrient when he discussed food, health, and disease in 400 BC.

In the early seventeenth century, the Italian physician Sanctorius weighed himself before and after each meal. He reported that his average daily intake was about 8 lb, whereas his excreta (urine and feces) weighed only 3 lb. Because he found no significant change in his weight, there was a daily unexplained disappearance of 5 lb of material. His explanation was that there must be a continual process of weight loss from the body caused by something he called *insensible perspiration:* a loss of water through the skin so slow that it goes unnoticed. During this period such men as Harvey and Spallanzani made key studies of the circulatory and digestive systems that laid important foundations for the development of the science of nutrition. In 1747, at the end of the naturalistic era, the first controlled experiment in nutrition was performed by the British physician, Lind. In attempting to find a cure for scurvy, now known to be caused by vitamin C deficiency, Lind treated 12 sailors suffering from the disease with six different substances, four of which were foods. He found that fruit juice from lemons or limes could cure the scurvy but that oil of vitriol (sulfuric acid), cider, nutmeg, sea water, and vinegar could not. For the first time the rigorous methods of experimental science had entered into the study of nutrition with great success.

CHEMICAL-ANALYTICAL ERA (1750 TO 1900)

The chemical-analytical era was initiated in the eighteenth century by Lavoisier, who became known as the father of nutrition. Lavoisier studied the way in which food provides us with energy. He was the first person to look carefully at the relationship between the oxygen we breathe and the heat our bodies produce. We now know that this heat is produced when oxygen combines with some of the compounds in our food in a process similar to, but much more controlled than, burning.

Early in the nineteenth century, methods were developed to analyze foods to determine the amounts of the elements carbon, hydrogen, and nitrogen they contained. The results of the early analyses led Liebig to suggest that the nutritive value of food was a function of its nitrogen content. He also proposed that an adequate diet must provide what he called *plastic foods* (protein) and *fuel foods* (carbohydrate and fat).

In 1871 the French chemist Dumas tried to produce a synthetic milk. He mixed carbohydrate, fat, and protein in the proportions found in cow's milk, but when the infants fed with this mixture died, Dumas concluded that milk must contain some other unknown nutritive substance. A similar conclusion was reached by Lunin in 1881. He prepared a mixture of purified casein (a protein in milk), milk sugar (a carbohydrate), milk fat, and the minerals found in milk. A group of mice that were fed this mixture died, whereas those that were fed milk thrived. Between 1881 and 1906 various similar experiments in animal nutrition led to one basic conclusion: The addition of "astonishingly" small amounts of natural foods was always necessary to promote growth and maintain health in animals fed experimental diets. So it became obvious that food contained other crucial substances besides water, carbohydrate, fat, protein, and minerals. What these substances were remained a mystery for some time.

BIOLOGICAL ERA (1900 TO 1955)

By 1912 it was well established that there was another essential dietary component, in addition to water, carbohydrate, fat, protein, and minerals. Casimir Funk introduced the term *vitamine* to describe it because it was essential for life (*vita* in Latin) and he believed it to be *amine,* meaning nitrogen-containing. Soon afterwards, two independent studies showed that there were at least two "vitamins." One of the studies demonstrated that some fats—such as butter—contain an essential substance needed to promote growth, whereas other fats—such as lard—do not. This essential fat-soluble substance became known as *vitamin A.* The other study demonstrated that a water-soluble substance in rice bran could prevent beriberi, then a common disease in Asia. This substance was called *vitamin B.*

By 1920 scientists had determined that these substances did not all contain nitrogen, so the final "e" was dropped from the word vitamine. The modified term, *vitamin,* is now a household word.

The concept that such classic deficiency diseases as beriberi, scurvy, rickets, and pellagra were caused by a deficiency of nutrients needed in small amounts stimulated research to identify the chemical nature of these dietary essentials. It soon became clear that several distinct components made up both the fat-soluble vitamin A and the water-soluble vitamin B. By 1940 four fat-soluble and seven water-soluble vitamins had been identified as essential in the human diet, and several others were identified as essential for other species of animals. So differences in the vitamin needs of different species were emerging. Also by 1940 the chemical structure of each vitamin had been established, many of them had been synthesized (made) in the laboratory, and knowledge of their biological functions was accumulating rapidly. Since 1940 only two further essential vitamins, known as *folic acid* and *vitamin B_{12}*, have been identified.

During this same period the mineral requirements for a healthful diet were also under study. Essential minerals, like vitamins, were found to compose a complex mixture. To date, 20 mineral elements have been established as essential in an adequate diet for humans. The status of several others is still uncertain.

CELLULAR OR MOLECULAR ERA (1955 TO PRESENT)

Since 1955 many new techniques have made it possible to study the nutrient needs of individual cells and even of the subcellular components, or organelles, of cells. The electron microscope, for example, allows us to see the contents of cells with astonishing detail. The ultracentrifuge allows the various components of cells to be separated from one another by spinning at high speeds, yielding samples of separated components for individual analysis. These and many other new techniques are allowing a rapid growth in our understanding of the intricacies of cell structure and of the complex and vital roles that nutrients play in the growth, development, and maintenance of healthy cells. Healthy cells are needed to form healthy tissues, which combine to form healthy organs in a healthy body. Good nourishment is required at all levels, with the cellular level being the most fundamental. The failure to form an essential enzyme or other cellular component because of poor nutrition can result in the malfunction or death of cells, which eventually results in specific and obvious physical symptoms and even death.

After 1960 the emphasis of nutrition research turned away from the search for essential dietary components, which is regarded as largely complete. Instead, the research focus turned to such things as the relationships between nutrients, the precise biological roles of nutrients, determination of the optimal amounts of nutrients in the human diet, and the effect of processing on the nutritive quality of food. More recently, efforts have been made to narrow the gap between theoretical knowledge in nutrition and the practical application of that knowledge to actually improve nutrition of the public. Nutritionists have called on the help of educators, communicators, and anthropologists in this task of putting theory into practice.

Remember that although we depend on studies at the molecular level to enhance our understanding of nutrition, foods are the ultimate source of all nourishment. The food we grow, buy, and eat is our only source of many of the nutrients on which cell growth and function depend. Only by understanding why people choose to grow, buy, and eat particular foods are we able to influence food intake in the future.

PRESENT STATUS

A hundred years ago water, carbohydrate, fat, and protein were thought to be the only food components needed for healthy growth and development. Today we know of at least 50 nutrients that must be supplied by our diet, and a vast body of knowledge describes what these are, where they are found, and what happens to them in the body. A deficiency in any one of them, whether it is needed in small or large amounts, can have a serious effect on our health.

Although the last vitamin was discovered over 40 years ago, we are still identifying new essential mineral elements. We also have the challenge of understanding the many complex interactions among the nutrients we require. In some ways an even greater challenge is to translate the knowledge of nutritional needs into meaningful dietary advice for the public. The fact that nutritional deficiency diseases are still occasionally found in wealthy countries, and to a much greater extent in the developing countries, is evidence of our failure to apply all the nutritional information we possess. These diseases, and the problems of overnutrition that occur where people are wealthy enough to overeat, have led nutritionists to seek the help of social scientists in encouraging the behavioral changes that can improve nutrition.

Many new approaches to the study of nutrition are emerging. The realization that people vary in their nutritional needs has stimulated interest in the influence of genetics on these needs. Knowledge of the role of genetics in human development has led to nutritional cures for some metabolic defects. Having discovered which nutrients are required for basic health, nutritionists are beginning to explore the role of nutrition in more subtle and perhaps more complex aspects of life, such as the development of the brain and the behavior and intelligence it sustains, the resistance of the body to infection, and the effects of environmental pollution, drugs, and stress on the body.

Nutrition plays a major role in the onset of what are commonly called the "killer" diseases: cardiovascular disease, hypertension, diabetes, and cancer. Although serious research continues, many premature claims have been made about the effect of specific nutrients on such complex conditions. In fact the modern nutritionist may spend as much time combating misinformation about nutrition as is spent delivering sound nutritional information.

An impression of the growth in nutrition research over recent years can be gained by considering how the number of scientific publications in the field has grown. In 1913 only four papers (articles) on nutrition were published, all by Casimir Funk. By 1993 around 3000 papers on nutrition could be delivered at a single conference. Review articles regularly cite as many as 200 to

500 papers as references, and research papers about vitamin E alone are appearing at the rate of about 700 per year.

The number of investigators who consider nutrition to be their main topic of interest can be deduced from the membership of scientific organizations devoted to nutrition. The American Institute of Nutrition, whose members have made many significant contributions to the field, has more than 3200 members. The Society for Nutrition Education was formed in 1971 to provide a forum for professionals concerned with the application of knowledge in nutrition and has more than 2400 members. The American Dietetic Association has over 65,000 members and is the largest and longest-established professional organization devoted to research in and practice of dietetics—the dietary application of nutritional knowledge.

The money to fund research, training, and education in human nutrition comes from many sources, ranging from national governments to private industry and foundations. Taken together, these provide a growing level of support for the continuing efforts to accumulate nutritional knowledge and disseminate that knowledge to the people who most need to know it.

CONTEMPORARY TOPICS IN NUTRITION

One of the reasons that so many people are interested in nutrition must be that it is one of the few factors influencing health over which we have some direct control. Nutrition scientists, food scientists, physiologists, and many other scientists are busy exploring a wide range of issues concerning nutrients and how they act and interact within our bodies. Some aspects of this work are widely reported in the media, whereas others receive relatively little media attention. A few issues of current concern are summarized here.

IATROGENIC MALNUTRITION

Iatrogenic malnutrition means nutritional problems arising as a result of medical treatment. Although the idea might sound strange at first, the use of drugs and surgery to treat many physical ailments can cause nutritional problems in people who were previously well nourished. For example, the oral contraceptives used by many women can increase the women's requirements for various nutrients. In addition to the effects of such contraceptives on women's immediate nutritional needs, they can also influence their nutritional needs during eventual pregnancies and subsequent lactation. The widespread use of antibiotics provides another example. Antibiotics in the body can interfere with the manufacture (or "synthesis") of some vitamins in the gastrointestinal tract, raising the amounts of these vitamins that must be supplied by the diet. Anticonvulsant drugs, given to control seizures, can considerably increase the amount of folic acid needed in the diet. Bypass surgery to shorten the intestinal tract in obese people can reduce their ability to absorb many nutrients from their food. The practice of providing total parenteral nutrition (TPN), in which patients who have trouble eating or absorbing nutrients are fed entirely through their arteries and veins, has given nutritionists the difficult task of formulating TPN solutions to meet all nutritional needs. These are just a few examples of the sorts of nutritional problems that can be caused by medical intervention. Physicians must be aware of new, unsuspected nutritional complications resulting from the drugs they prescribe or the surgery they perform.

ATHLETIC PERFORMANCE

A relationship between nutrition and physical fitness has been recognized only recently. Athletes are increasingly turning to nutrition to try to gain some competitive advantage. This has generated a new field of nutrition, called *sports nutrition,* concerned with the positive effect of nutrition and eating patterns on athletic performance. Sports nutrition research attempts either to document or to refute much of the anecdotal information underlying the lucrative "sports health" business. Many claims are made on behalf of altered eating patterns and products that might enhance athletic performance. It is important that these claims be investigated by competent research teams that include nutritionists, especially considering the great involvement of young people in athletics.

BEHAVIOR

Interest in the relationship between nutrition and behavior usually falls into one of two distinct areas. First, there is concern that severe malnutrition, especially in the infant, might impair the development of the brain and other parts of the central nervous system. Such impairment might have long-term effects on learning ability, intelligence, and general behavior. Second, there is great interest in the effect on behavior of certain essential nutrients; food additives; normal dietary constituents, such as sucrose; and dietary contaminants such as lead. The possibility that attention deficit disorder (ADD, or hyperactive behavior) in children might sometimes be caused by dietary factors has been under investigation for several decades and is attracting increasing attention. Nutritionists and behaviorists are also investigating the role of diet in the treatment of such problems as autism and Down's syndrome. The effects of simple hunger or chronic anemia on learning and behavior are also under investigation.

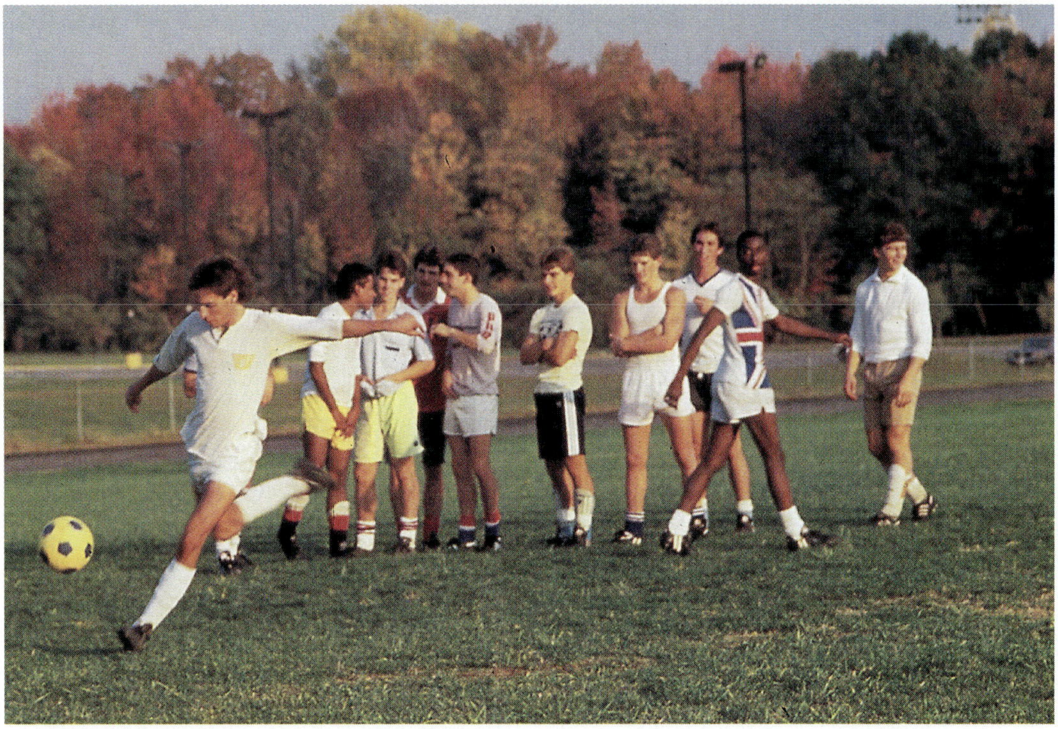

Both professional and amateur athletes are increasingly turning to nutrition to improve their performance.

SPACE EXPLORATION

We live in an era in which some people spend long periods in space, at present in orbiting space flights but perhaps soon on journeys to Mars and beyond. Nutritionists are investigating possible changes in dietary requirements during prolonged travel in space. They are interested in such things as the type of diet required, the form in which food should be supplied, and possible changes in the way the body uses nutrients in the condition of weightlessness. Specific areas of investigation are changes in taste perception, the effects of dehydration and possible loss of appetite, changes in the distribution of blood throughout the body, and changes in dietary energy, calcium, potassium, and protein requirements.[13] The number of us who will have firsthand experience of space flight may be small, but what we learn about the body's use of food in space may well have wider applications on Earth.

SAFETY OF THE FOOD SUPPLY

The Food and Drug Administration (FDA) and the USDA are responsible for ensuring that our food supply is safe and wholesome. There is widespread consumer concern about the use of herbicides and pesticides on crops and antibiotics in animal feed. Such practices help make high-quality food available at reasonable prices, but their safety is under constant evaluation. Another major concern of consumers is the use of a wide range of additives to enhance the keeping qualities, flavor, texture, and palatability of food. Nutritionists and food scientists share these concerns and are constantly assessing the effect of modern agricultural and food preparation techniques on nutrients and their use by the body. Both groups must carefully balance any risks of the modern methods of food preservation and processing against their benefits. Scientists are also becoming increasingly concerned about unintentional or incidental additives, including some naturally occurring toxins and substances that may enter food during processing or arise in it during storage.

HEALTH, ORGANIC, AND NATURAL FOODS

Health, organic, and *natural* are terms applied to various foods that have crept into public perception via advertising, labeling, and popular articles about food and nutrition. Until 1993 in the United States, none of these terms actually had any legal or even generally accepted definition. Their use on food labels and in advertising are now regulated by the FDA and the USDA in the United States and by comparable agencies in most developed countries. These terms are often used loosely and with widely varying interpretations, some of which may be more emotional than scientific. All foods are in fact organic in the biological sense because they are all derived from living matter. Most foods are "natural" in that they are produced in nature, and the vast majority make a positive contribution toward health. When foods do not make a positive contribution to health, it is usually because they are overused rather than because there is

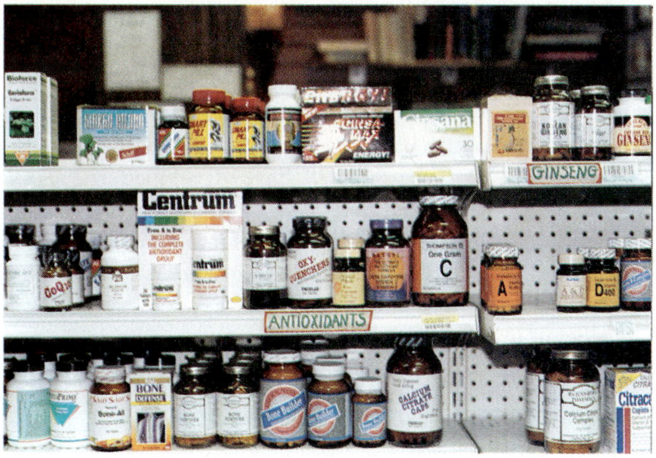

Consumers are presented with a confusing array of nutritional supplements.

anything inherently unhealthful about them. The terms *health food, organic food,* and *natural food* are usually used to imply the absence of something from the food, rather than the presence of something in it. They are used to describe foods produced without the use of inorganic fertilizers, pesticides, or herbicides and produced with minimal processing and without anything being added (such as sugar, preservatives, coloring, or flavoring) or taken away (such as skins on fruits or husks on cereals).

FOOD LABELING

The Nutrition Labeling and Education Act of 1990 initiated a new era in food labeling.[14] In 1993 the FDA and the USDA published 961 pages of final regulations, which became effective in the middle of 1994. These regulations specify what information must be on the nutrition panel, define terms that can be used to describe nutrient content, allow certain health claims about the relationships between nutrients and diseases, standardize serving sizes, require full ingredient listing, and require the total percentage of juice in juice drinks to be shown. It is now possible to read a food label and learn not only what the ingredient and nutrient contents are, but also how they relate to a healthful diet. A visit to the grocery store can easily enhance people's working knowledge of nutrition because they can learn about the nutritional quality of almost all the foods they buy. An example of a typical "Nutrition Facts" panel on a food label is presented in Figure 2-2. The nutrition labeling regulations are discussed in greater detail in Chapter 2.

The FDA has estimated that the new food label will cost FDA-regulated food processors $1.4 billion to $2.3 billion and government $163 million from 1993 to 2013, but that the savings resulting from the benefits to health will well exceed costs.[14] The potential benefits include decreased rates of coronary heart disease, cancer, osteoporosis, obesity, high blood pressure, and allergic reactions to food and decreased risk of deficiencies of such nutrients as iron, calcium, folic acid, and vitamin A, which are currently consumed at less than adequate levels. The USDA estimates that nutrition labeling of meats and poultry for which it has responsibility will cost $218 million to $272 million for the same period.

SUPPLEMENTATION

There are several situations in which nutrient supplements in specified amounts are recommended for certain segments of the population. However, concern about nutrition and its relationship to health has led a great many people to prescribe nutritional supplements—such as vitamin and mineral pills, royal jelly, and pollen—for themselves. The multibillion-dollar food supplement business testifies that many Americans have lost faith in the ability of the everyday food supply to meet their nutritional needs. Many people have also become overconfident in their own ability to diagnose nutritional problems and take appropriate action. In most cases the results are relatively harmless, although a waste of money. In some cases, however, the results are potentially harmful and even fatal. The term *megavitamin*

Dietary supplements include products with the following:

- Proven value in appropriate amounts for at-risk individuals
  - Multinutrients, minerals, or vitamins
  - Individual vitamins and minerals
- Doubtful or limited value
  - Highly fortified cereals
  - Protein powders
  - Herbs
- Unproven value and possible harm
  - Enzymes
  - Glandular material
  - Herbal teas

therapy is used to describe one of the most common and sometimes dangerous practices: dosing oneself with many times more than the actual required amounts of various nutrients. In fact the term is also a misnomer because many of the supplements used contain minerals and nonnutritive substances in addition to vitamins.

IMMUNITY

In the past few years it has become clear that adequate nutrition is important to allow our immune system to protect us against infection and to help us recover as fast as possible when we contract an infectious disease. There is great interest in the search to find out exactly what nutrients are most involved in maintaining a healthy immune system. Until that work is complete, however, the best advice is simply to maintain good general nutrition. The role for nutrition in modifying the course of acquired immunodeficiency syndrome (AIDS) is also attracting much attention.

BIOTECHNOLOGY

Using the well-publicized techniques of genetic engineering, scientists can now transfer genes between organisms almost at will. This has widespread implications for the food industry. Animals are being genetically engineered to help in the production of novel food products, such as eggs with less cholesterol and milk from which calcium can be more easily absorbed. Crop plants are being genetically altered to make them more resistant to pests, higher yielding, longer lasting on supermarket shelves, and perhaps even better tasting. Genetic engineering is being used to alter the animals we eat, generating new breeds of livestock to provide higher yields and leaner cuts of meat. Nutritionists recognize the value of using genetic engineering and other aspects of biotechnology to alter the nutritional value of foods. Public debate about the impact of biotechnology on the food supply is already lively and can be expected to grow. Nutritionists are important participants in this debate.

EDUCATION

Nutrition has long been taught in school during health and home economics classes, but nutritional concepts are increasingly finding their way into classes on science, mathematics, social studies, and reading. Many industries are also emphasizing nutrition during their health promotion and disease prevention programs, partly in recognition of the fact that well-nourished workers are less likely to take sick leave. Nutritional issues are increasingly discussed on television and in newspapers and magazines, as well as in more formal community health programs. Medical schools are increasing the attention they pay to nutrition, and many people are seeking private consultation to learn about the components of an adequate diet.

To assist nutrition and health professionals in communicating fundamental dietary principles and current knowledge of the basic nutritional needs of individuals, the USDA and the DHHS have developed the *Food Guide Pyramid: A Guide to Daily Food Choices* (see Figure 2-4). It reflects the *Dietary Guidelines for Americans* and is an update of the Basic 4, which has been used since the 1950s.[15] The Food Guide Pyramid is discussed in detail in Chapter 2.

CHANGING LIFE-STYLES

Modern life-styles bring with them major changes in eating patterns, as compared with those of previous generations. Nowadays, for example, it is much more common for both parents to be employed outside the home, and there is an increasing number of single-parent homes. These changes have implications for nutrition, many of which may be negative unless appropriate corrective action is taken. Three main concerns are (1) the number of children who are responsible for choosing their own diet without adequate adult supervision, (2) the perceived reliance on food produced by "fast food" or "convenience food" chains, and (3) the number of adults who "eat on the run" or "graze" on food throughout the day. Money spent on meals away from home accounts for over 40% of American food dollars, with the proportion increasing each year. The nutritional effects of these changes, whether good or bad, can be judged only by their influence on the total diet.

DEGENERATIVE DISEASES

One major reason for the growing interest in nutrition over the past 10 years or so has been the possible links between nutrition and the so-called degenerative diseases—cancer, coronary heart disease, hypertension, arthritis, diabetes, and osteoporosis. Several state-of-the-art research papers on these topics have been published and have aroused much public interest. More importantly, these reports have focused the attention of Congress on the need to support investigations into these relationships so that sound nutritional guidance can be given to the public. Dietary modification may benefit people who are genetically susceptible to a particular condition and may also benefit those without any genetic predisposition to the condition. There is a lively debate, however, about how appropriate it is to suggest that everyone change his or her diet if the changes are helpful only to a small proportion of people, but not to the others. For instance, only 20% of the U.S. population is likely to develop hypertension (high blood pressure) because of an excessive intake of sodium or to respond to a reduced sodium intake.

PUBLIC POLICY

The nutritional status of a population is ultimately determined by the availability of an adequate food supply, so it is vital that policymakers are aware of the nutritional implications of their policies. These implications are most obvious in the fields of agricultural subsidy, import-export tariffs, public works, and credit. It is essential that the government develop a national nutrition policy to ensure that everyone has access to a nutritionally adequate diet. Nutritionists who have traditionally avoided becoming involved in politics are increasingly recognizing that they have a responsibility to support programs that are designed to promote a high level of nutritional health.

From this point on, we look in some detail at the nutrients we eat, what happens to them when we eat them, and the consequences for our bodies of a deficient or overabundant supply of them. Most of the information is well established, but because nutrition is a science in progress, some of the information is speculative and perhaps the subject of considerable debate. Failure to include some of the speculative and debatable material deprives students of much of the excitement of the study of nutrition. As we go along, however, guidance about what concepts are based on less firmly established aspects of our knowledge of nutrition is provided.

CAREERS IN NUTRITION

The field of nutrition offers a wide variety of career opportunities, ranging from dietetics to basic research in nutrition. Assuming moderate growth in the U.S. economy, the employment of nutritionists is predicted to increase by 26% between 1992 and 2005.[16] This rate of growth is faster than the average predicted rate for all occupations, so aiming for a career in nutrition could be the basis of a secure future.

DIETITIANS AND NUTRITIONISTS

To become a **dietitian,** a person must complete an undergraduate program that meets the requirements of the American Dietetic Association. He or she must then obtain the necessary experience to qualify for professional registration. After successfully completing a "registration" examination, he or she becomes a **registered dietitian (RD).** The academic requirements consist of a core of courses in basic science, nutrition, and foods, and an introduction to related subjects, such as economics, educational psychology, and management. In addition to being qualified for a variety of positions, an RD has the credentials to justify third-party payments from the many insurance companies that consider nutrition counseling a reimbursable medical expense.

A **nutritionist** is someone who has completed undergraduate or graduate training in nutrition, without necessarily meeting all of the requirements to become an RD. A nutritionist usually has had the same or more advanced training in nutrition than a dietitian but may not have taken the required supporting courses. Unfortunately, there is no restriction on the use of the term *nutritionist,* so many unqualified people call themselves nutritionists.

All dietitians have some experience in counseling people on normal nutrition and therapeutic diets (for conditions such as diabetes or kidney problems). Nutritionists are more likely to have experience in dealing only with the concerns of normal nutrition.

CAREERS IN HOSPITALS AND OTHER INSTITUTIONS

Many of the career opportunities for nutritionists and dietitians are in hospitals and other residential institutions. In these settings the nutritionist or dietitian is concerned with the day-to-day operation of the institution's food service. His or her tasks include planning menus, making food purchase decisions, advising on kitchen layout, and managing some personnel and may also include the individual nutritional counseling of patients or residents.

In hospitals and other institutions there is an increasing division of responsibilities between **clinical nutritionists** and **dietitians** and **administrative dietitians.** Clinical nutritionists and dietitians are responsible for the day-to-day nutritional quality of the meals served and for the nutritional counseling of patients or residents. Administrative dietitians are more concerned with food service and the overall planning and running of those aspects of the institution that are related to nutrition.

THE WIDER SCENE

Until about 20 years ago, career opportunities for nutritionists and dietitians were almost entirely confined to hospitals and other large institutions. Nowadays there are many more opportunities in the world. These additional career options include the following:

- Private nutritional practices, which offer nutritional counseling to the public on a fee-for-service basis
- Physicians' group practices, which are increasingly including nutritionists as part of an integrated health care team
- Small nursing homes and child-care organizations, which often employ nutritionists, at least on a part-time basis
- Voluntary organizations involved in promoting health care

- Summer camps for children, including ones for children with medical or weight problems
- Sports and fitness clubs
- Professional sports teams, such as football teams, which are increasingly employing nutritional consultants
- Health-in-the-worksite programs

ANCILLARY SKILLS

In addition to their knowledge of nutrition, professional nutritionists and dietitians require good communication skills because much of their work involves communicating their knowledge of nutrition to other people. Diplomacy is also often required when counseling people with weight problems or other nutrition-related medical conditions. Many nutritionists and dietitians are also required to manage groups of workers, such as kitchen staff; thus management and general interpersonal skills are also important.

ACADEMIC AND RESEARCH CAREERS

An academic or research career in nutrition usually requires an advanced graduate degree. Obtaining either an undergraduate or an advanced degree can also qualify a person for admission to professional schools of medicine, dentistry, osteopathic medicine, and veterinary medicine. So in addition to leading to an initial qualification in nutrition, the study of nutrition can also open up a variety of other career paths.

ISSUES AND OPINIONS

Nutrition: A New Science?

by William J. Darby, M.D., Ph.D.
Professor Emeritus, Nutrition and Biochemistry
Vanderbilt University, School of Medicine
Nashville, Tennessee

Significant relationships between food and health have been recognized throughout recorded history. Hippocrates (460 to 370 BC) wrote that:

... the art of medicine would not have been invented at all, nor would it have been made a subject of investigation (for there would be no need of it) if when men were indisposed, the same food and other articles of regimen which they eat and drink when in good health were proper for them, and if no other were preferable to these ...

He foreshadowed current concepts in the succinct aphorism:

Growing bodies have the most innate heat; they therefore require more food, for otherwise their bodies are wasted. In old persons the heat is feeble, and therefore they require little fuel, as it were to the flame, for it would be extinguished by much ...

and observed that

Persons who are naturally very fat are apt to die earlier than those who are slender.

Sanctorius (AD 1561 to 1636) of Padua and Venice quantitated his body weight changes, food intake, and weight of excreta over a prolonged period, thus making the first balance studies. The subsequent landmark elucidation of the relationship between the use of oxygen and the production of body heat was initiated during the era of Lavoisier (1743 to 1794).

The effect of fruits and fresh vegetables in curing and preventing scurvy was widely recognized during the 1600s, and the apothecary Moellenbrock crystallized a "salt" from juice of fresh leaves of Cochleoria (scurvy grass) that mistakenly was termed *curative*.

Should nutrition be considered a *new* science?

BY NOW YOU SHOULD KNOW

- At this time at least 50 different nutrients have been identified as essential to human nutrition.
- Essential nutrients are chemicals that must be provided by food.
- Essential minerals and vitamins constitute only 2% of the weight of food.
- Nutrients function in the body to supply energy, promote growth, repair body tissues, and regulate body processes.
- Nutrients fall into six major categories—water, carbohydrate, lipid, protein, minerals, and vitamins.
- Although some nutrients are needed in the body in greater quantities than others, all nutrients are important, working either alone or together to maintain health.
- Recommended Dietary Allowances (RDAs) are the estimates of the needs of healthy people for essential nutrients.
- Plants are the origin of most nutrients in our diet.
- The sun, whose energy is trapped by plants, is the original source of dietary energy.
- Evidence of practical nutrition knowledge dates to biblical times.
- Vitamins were first identified as dietary essentials in 1912.
- Nutrition as a scientific discipline has been recognized only since 1934.
- The United States has selected 21 nutrition objectives to be met by the year 2000.
- Both overnutrition and undernutrition may have an adverse effect on health.
- Interest in nutrition is at an all-time high, ranging from concerns about the relationship between nutrition and degenerative diseases to nutrition for athletes and astronauts.
- This text is designed to provide the fundamentals of nutrition for those planning to pursue a career in a nutrition-related field and for those who wish to acquire sufficient information to help them make informed dietary choices for themselves and their families.

STUDY QUESTIONS

1. Make a time line of the highlights in the development of our knowledge of nutrition.
2. Identify the six major categories of nutrients, and indicate the functions performed by each.
3. Define an essential nutrient.
4. Why and when was the original spelling of "vitamines" changed to "vitamins"?

CRITICAL ANALYSIS

1. Have you or a friend used a nutrition supplement, replacement drink, or energy bar in the last week? List the claims made for the product. Did you use the product to (a) replace part or all of a meal, (b) supplement your normal diet, or (c) replace losses specific to work or athletic training (for example, a sports drink to replace fluid and electrolyte losses after a workout or an energy bar to cover the energy cost of a workout)?
2. The supermarket where you shop sells bananas. A nearby "health" food store also sells produce such as bananas, but the bananas are advertised as "organically grown." State which bananas are organic and why. What is commonly meant by the phrase "organically grown?"

REFERENCES

1. U.S. Department of Health and Human Services: *The surgeon general's report on nutrition and health,* US Public Health Service Pub No 88-50210, Washington, DC, 1988, U.S. Government Printing Office.
2. National Academy of Sciences: *Diet and health: implications for reducing chronic disease risk,* Washington, DC, 1989, National Academy Press.
3. Burke BS, Harding VV, Shart HC: Nutrition studies during pregnancy, *J Pediatr* 23:506, 1943.
4. Roche AF: Secular trends in human growth, maturation, and development, *Monogr Soc Res Child Dev* vol 44, 1979.
5. Hetzel BS, Dunn JT: The iodine deficiency disorders: their nature and prevention, *Ann Rev Nutr* 9:21, 1989.
6. Dallman PK: Iron. In Brown ML, editor: *Present knowledge in nutrition,* ed 6, Washington, DC, 1990, International Life Science Institute, Nutrition Foundation.
7. Sommer A: New imperatives for an old vitamin (A), *J Nutr* 119:96, 1989.
8. Grundy SM and others: Workshop on the impact of dietary cholesterol on plasma lipoproteins and atherogenesis, *Atherosclerosis* 8:95, 1988.
9. Rogers AE, Newberne PM: Dietary effects and nutritional influences on cancer: a review of epidemiological and experimental data, *Lab Invest* 59:729, 1989.
10. U.S. Department of Health and Human Services: *Healthy People 2000: national health promotion and disease prevention objectives,* U.S. Public Health Service Pub No 91-50212, Washington, DC, 1990, U.S. Government Printing Office.
11. U.S. Department of Agriculture and U.S. Department of Health and Human Services: *Dietary guidelines for Americans,* Washington, DC, 1981, 1985, 1990, U.S. Government Printing Office.
12. National Academy of Sciences: *Diet, nutrition and cancer,* Washington, DC, 1992, National Academy Press.
13. Lane HW: Nutrition in space: evidence from the US and the USSR, *Nutr Rev* 50:3, 1992.
14. Mermelstein NH: A new era in food labeling, *Food Tech* 47:81, 1993.
15. Food guide pyramid replaces the basic four circle, *Food Tech* 46:64, 1992.
16. Kornblum TH: Professional demand for dietitians and nutritionists in the year 2005, *J Am Diet Assoc* 94:21, 1994.

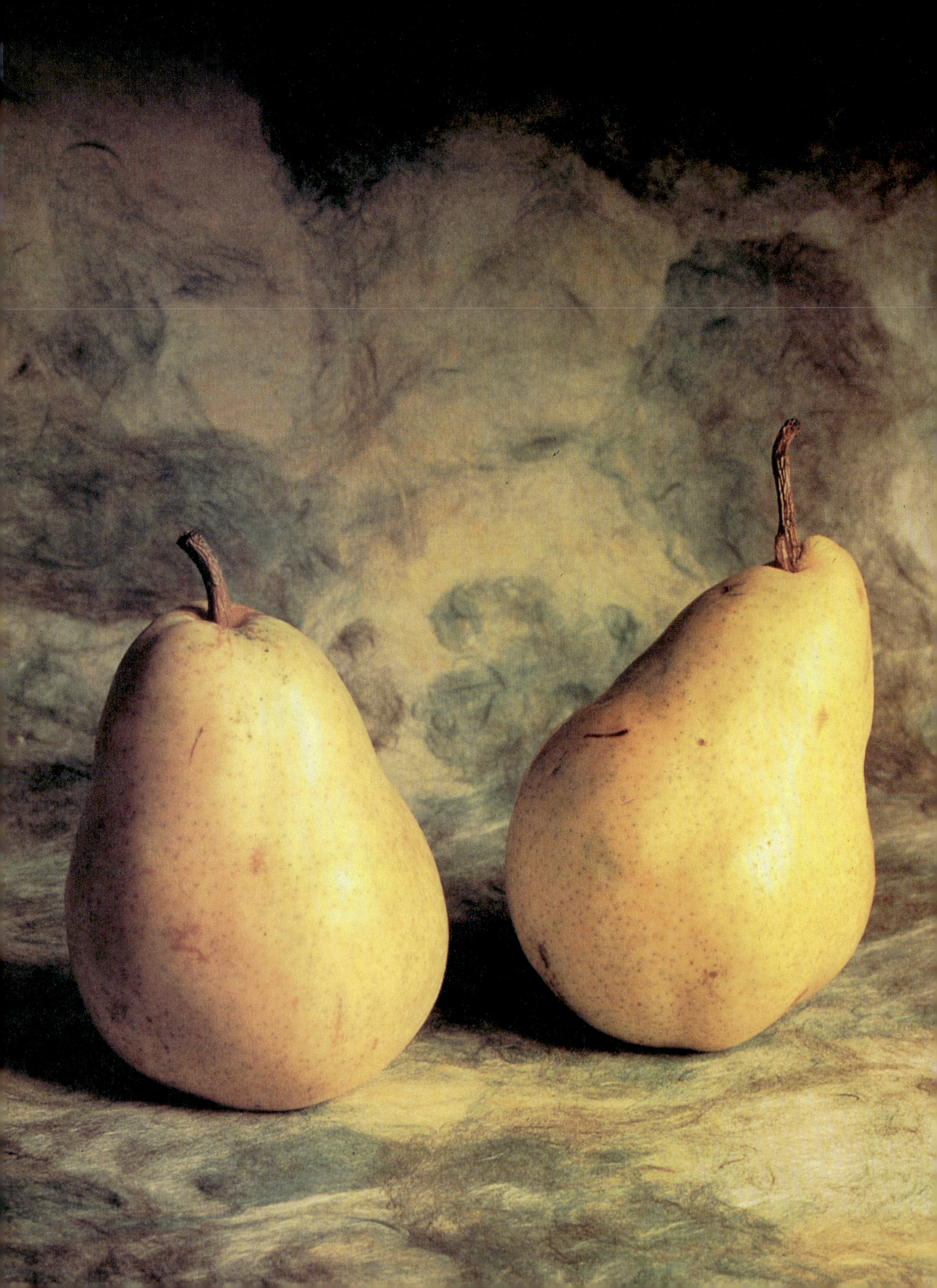

CHAPTER 2

SELECTION OF AN ADEQUATE DIET

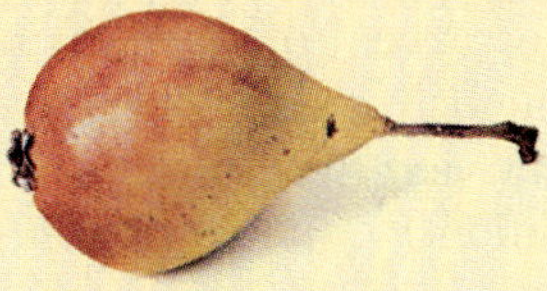

There is considerable public interest in what foods should be eaten to promote optimal health. The practical aspects of nutrition receive wide coverage in all branches of the media: television, radio, newspapers, magazines, and advertising. There has also been a dramatic increase in the number of consumer-oriented subscription newsletters on nutrition and health. The kilocalories and sodium, calcium, cholesterol, fat, and sugar contents in various foods are common topics of everyday conversation.

Five basic questions lie at the heart of most public interest in nutrition:

- How much of each particular nutrient is required to meet the needs for normal growth, development, and the maintenance of health?
- Will consuming some nutrients in amounts greater than those actually required by the body produce additional health benefits?
- Which foods are good sources of specific nutrients?
- How healthful or well-chosen is the typical diet?
- How can the most appropriate diet be most easily selected?

This chapter examines these questions from the nutritionist's point of view, focusing mainly on the dietary standards, food guides, and food surveys of the United States, Canada, and other developed countries.

The wide-ranging information available on the nutrient content of foods provides a base on which to select an adequate diet. In general, the selection can be "food based," with the emphasis on selecting appropriate amounts of food from various food groups, or "nutrient based," focused on the specific intakes of the individual nutrients. Both approaches have a role to play in helping us select an adequate diet, but they can be combined with differing degrees of emphasis. A series of food-based dietary guidelines have been published to help people make appropriate choices as they select the foods in their diet. These guidelines, the most recent of which is the Food Guide Pyramid, are founded on a consensus about the need for various nutrients and their role in health promotion and disease prevention.

DIETARY STANDARDS

The identification of the nutrients essential for human health raised the obvious question of how much of each of them is required. The first large-scale efforts to answer that question were prompted by the threat of war in 1940. This was the result of the recognition that nutritional science could contribute to national security by providing a scientific basis on which to make food choices to promote the health of the population. The U.S. government and public had been appalled by the high proportion of military recruits who were rejected because of health problems related to poor nutrition.

Against this background, 25 scientists met in 1941 as the first Food and Nutrition Board of the National Research Council.[1] Their task was to examine the available information on nutrient needs to decide whether recommendations could be made to the general public about the amount of various nutrients required to maintain health in the majority of the population. They decided there was indeed sufficient information to make useful recommendations. This led to a subcommittee, chaired by Dr. Lydia J. Roberts, at the University of Chicago being charged with establishing dietary standards for evaluating the adequacy of the diet of large population groups, that could provide a rational guide for practical nutrition and the planning of agricultural production. Although they accepted that their first attempt at establishing standards might be based on data that would later need to be modified, they agreed on the need to make the best possible estimates based on the information available at the time. They proposed their first set of standards in the belief and hope that more information would become available to allow the revision of their standards, with a resulting steady improvement in their accuracy.

The deliberations of the subcommittee resulted in the United States' first set of recommended dietary allowances (RDAs), which were published in 1943.[2] RDAs were set for energy and nine specific nutrients. The term *recommended allowances* was chosen, rather than *requirements,* to emphasize that the RDAs were not seen as final figures but would need periodic updating in the light of new information. This was an appropriate decision because the original RDAs have now been revised nine times, with the most recent version released in 1989.[3]

The original RDAs were intended to indicate the quantities of certain nutrients believed to be adequate to meet the known nutritional needs of practically all healthy people in the United States. For each nutrient, specific allowances were set for 17 different categories of person, depending on age, gender, and, for women, whether they were pregnant or lactating. The allowances did not represent mean (average) requirements because these would meet the needs of only about half of the population. Instead, they were set at a level approximately "two standard deviations above the mean requirement." In practice this meant that the allowances should be sufficient to meet the needs of 97.5% of the population (Figure 2-1). The RDAs also included a margin of safety to take into account possible losses of nutrients during cooking and storage and to provide a buffer against increased requirements during illness and other states of nutritional "stress." Other factors considered were the stability of the nutrients, the body's ability to store the nutrients, the range of observed requirements, the availability of the nutrients in the North American diet, any possible hazards associated with excessive intake of any of the nutrients, the difficulties involved in establishing precise requirements, and the scientific validity of the data on which the recommendations were based.

The RDAs were used as target values in the planning of the national food supply and the preparation of meals for large groups of people. If the intake by a group met the RDAs, it could be assumed that practically everyone in the group was consuming amounts of the specified nutrients in excess of actual needs. When the first set of RDAs was announced, it was emphasized that they were not intended for the assessment of the adequacy of individual diets, but only for a population group as a whole. They are now, however, considered to be a useful reference point from which to judge the adequacy of any individual's diet. When RDAs are used to assess the nutrient intake of an individual, it should be remembered that the RDA values exceed the amounts actually required for over 97% of the people in the relevant age and gender group. So a person who consumes less than

FIGURE 2-1

Distribution of actual nutrient requirements with coefficient of variation of 15% around the mean requirement.

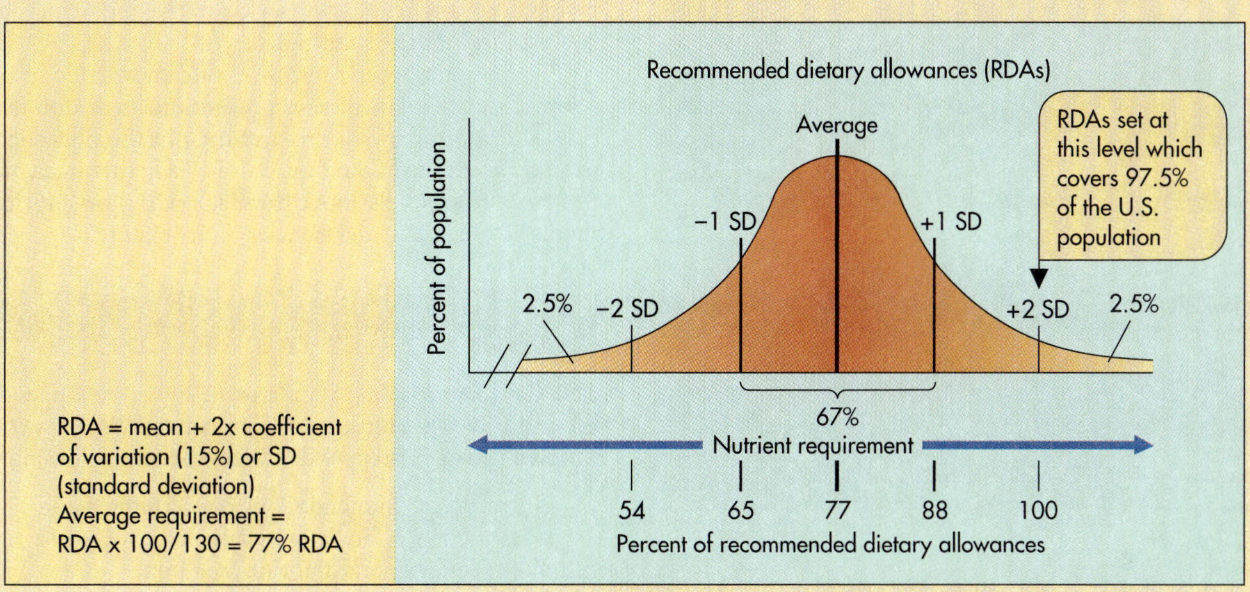

the RDA value of a nutrient is not necessarily deficient in the nutrient. The more the intake falls below the RDA, however, the greater is the risk of suffering from a marginal or deficient intake.[4,5] Biochemical, clinical, or physical evidence is always needed to determine whether a person has a genuine deficiency of any nutrient.

> When recommended dietary allowances (RDAs) are used to assess the nutrient intake of an individual, it should be remembered that the RDA values exceed the amounts actually required for 97.5% of the people in the relevant age and gender group. So a person who consumes less than the RDA value of a nutrient is not necessarily deficient in the nutrient. The more the intake falls below the RDA, however, the greater is the risk of suffering from a marginal or deficient intake.

It is also possible that a small proportion of people have a need for a nutrient that is slightly *greater* than the RDA value. For any one person, however, the likelihood that the RDA fails to meet his or her needs is small, unless a health problem is causing increased need for, increased losses of, or poor absorption of the nutrient concerned.

Now, more than 50 years after publication of the first RDAs, it is still not an easy task to determine the level at which dietary standards should be set. For some nutrients, little information is available, especially to quantify the differing needs of different age and gender groups. For other nutrients, scientists are uncertain about how to interpret the information they have. For others, there is such a wide range of apparent requirements that it is difficult to arrive at meaningful RDAs.

The data on which RDAs are based are obtained from the following sources[6]:

- Surveys of food and therefore nutrient intake by large numbers of apparently healthy individuals
- Surveys that consider both food intake and the biochemical or functional assessment of nutritional status
- Controlled metabolic experiments or nutrient balance studies in limited numbers of individuals
- Relevant nutritional studies on several species of animals
- Epidemiological information about diet and health status within large populations
- Factorial analysis of nutrient needs for growth, the maintenance of body stores, replacement of obligatory losses, and the bioavailability of dietary sources of a nutrient

Improved analytical techniques and increased knowledge about the biological role of most nutrients have been two of the most significant factors behind the periodic changes in RDAs and an increasing confidence in their relevance. The rationale by which the RDAs are set is

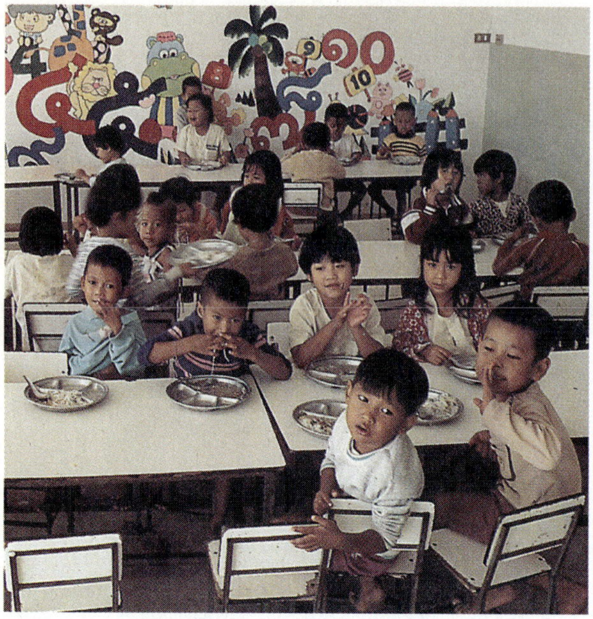

also becoming steadily more consistent across the full range of nutrients considered.

The periodic revision of the original RDAs has been accompanied by an increase in the number of nutrients for which RDAs are set. In 1980, for example, scientists believed they had sufficient information to propose estimated safe and adequate intakes for 12 additional nutrients for a restricted range of age and gender categories.

The current set of RDAs, proposed in 1989,[3] represent the best judgment of the RDA subcommittee on the intakes of nutrients that meet the needs of essentially all healthy people. The allowances are believed to include a sufficient margin of safety to allow for periods of nutritional stress related to physical, emotional, or environmental factors, although they do not meet the additional requirements of people whose reserves are depleted as a result of disease. The subcommittee identified no confirmed benefit from intakes higher than the RDAs. As with the first set of RDAs, the current RDAs are set at a level of two times the coefficient of variation (15%) or two standard deviations (30%) above the mean requirement (Figure 2-1). This means that an intake of 77% ($^{100}/_{130}$) of the RDA provides what is estimated to be the average (mean) requirement for the nutrient.

Although the RDAs may represent neither a minimal nor an optimal level of intake, they have served many useful purposes. They provided a meaningful guide for the planning of diets for large groups of people and are also now widely used for evaluating the adequacy of individual diets. They have provided the rationale for many nutrition intervention programs, such as the school lunch, senior citizen congregate feeding, and Women, Infants, and Children (WIC) programs.[7] They have also provided the scientific basis for formulating regulations governing the composition and labeling of foods and dietary supplements. Although admittedly high for use in conditions of economic stringency or national emergencies, they set desirable and achievable goals under normal conditions.

The continuing expansion of our knowledge of the roles of nutrients in disease prevention, in addition to basic nutrition, may lead to a change in the philosophy behind the RDAs in the future. It is likely that many will be increased to levels above those known to be sufficient simply to prevent deficiencies and maintain general health.[8,9]

CANADIAN DIETARY STANDARDS

The Canadian Dietary Standards (1990) (see Appendix C), also known as Nutrition Recommendations, are set out within a three-part report that comprises the following[10]:

- Nutrition recommendations concerning the intake of energy, fat, saturated fat, alcohol, sodium, caffeine, and fluorine (see box)
- Recommended Nutrient Intakes (RNIs) based on kilocalorie intake for energy, thiamin, riboflavin, niacin, n-3 polyunsaturated fatty acid (PUFA) and n-6 PUFA
- Recommended Nutrient Intakes based on age, gender, and body weight; for protein; vitamins A, D, E, C, and B_{12} and folate; and the minerals calcium, phosphorus, magnesium, iron, iodine, and zinc

These standards are based on a Report of the Committee on Diet and Cardiovascular Disease and the 1983 RNI for Canadians. They are set at levels aimed to maintain health and reduce the risk of chronic disease.

Nutrition Recommendations for Canadians

- The Canadian diet should provide energy consistent with the maintenance of body weight within the recommended range.
- The Canadian diet should include essential nutrients in amounts recommended in this report (Appendix C).
- The Canadian diet should include no more than 30% of energy as fat (33 g/1000 kcal or 39 g/5000 kJ) and no more than 10% as saturated fat (11 g/1000 kcal or 13 g/5000 kJ).
- The Canadian diet should provide 55% of energy as carbohydrate (138 g/1000 kcal or 165 g/5000 kJ) from a variety of sources.
- The sodium content of the Canadian diet should be reduced.
- The Canadian diet should include no more than 5% of total energy as alcohol, or two drinks daily, whichever is less.
- The Canadian diet should contain no more caffeine than the equivalent of four regular cups of coffee per day.
- Community water supplies containing less than 1 mg/L of fluoride should be fluoridated to that level.

TABLE 2-1

Comparison of United States (1989), United Kingdom (1991), Canadian (1990), and FAO/WHO (1957-1989) dietary standards for the adult male and adult female

CLASSIFICATION	Kcal	PROTEIN (g)	CALCIUM (g)	IRON (mg)	VITAMIN A (RE)	THIAMIN (mg)	RIBOFLAVIN (mg)	VITAMIN C (mg)
UNITED STATES								
Female (63 kg, 1.63 m)	2200	50	0.8	15	800	1.1	1.3	60
Male (79 kg, 1.76 m)	2900	63	0.8	10	1000	1.5	1.7	60
UNITED KINGDOM								
Female	1940	45	0.7	14.8	600	0.8	1.1	40
Male	2550	55.5	0.7	8.7	700	1.0	1.3	40
CANADA								
Female (59 kg)	1900	51	0.7	13	800	0.8	1.0	30*
Male (74 kg)	2700	64	0.8	9	1000	1.1	1.4	40*
FAO/WHO								
Female (60 kg)	2200	45	0.4-0.5	18	500	0.9	1.3	30
Male (70 kg)	2700	52.5	0.4-0.5	10	600	1.3	1.8	30

* Nonsmoker; smoker, 50% higher.

BRITISH (UNITED KINGDOM) DIETARY STANDARDS

In 1991 the Committee on Medical Aspects of Food Policy of the U.K. Department of Health released Dietary Reference Values (DRVs) for 41 different dietary components.[11] These were to replace the Recommended Dietary Amounts of Food, Energy, and Nutrients that had served as dietary standards in Britain since 1979. The new report embodies three levels of recommendations:

- Reference Nutrient Intakes (RNIs), which are sufficient to meet the needs of 97% of the population
- Estimated Average Requirements (EARs), which meet the needs of half the population
- Lower Reference Nutrient Intakes (LRNIs), which are adequate for the small proportion of the population with low nutrient needs

The report also makes recommendations for average intakes of fats and carbohydrates.

DIETARY STANDARDS IN OTHER COUNTRIES

Many other countries have established dietary standards for their populations. Any appreciable difference among the standards in different countries is usually a result of the differences in the basis on which the recommendations were established rather than any cultural differences in nutrient requirements.

The Food and Agriculture Organization (FAO) of the United Nations has been given the task of devising standards applicable to all cultures that meet the needs of fully active, healthy individuals.[12] The FAO has worked with the World Health Organization (WHO) to assess the available information. So far, the two organizations have proposed practical allowances for energy (kilocalories), calcium, protein, thiamin, riboflavin, niacin, vitamins A, C, D, and B_{12}, iron, and folate. A comparison of the American, United Kingdom, Canadian, and FAO/WHO standards of selected nutrients for adults is given in Table 2-1.

STANDARDS FOR THE LABELING OF FOOD PRODUCTS

An example of the current label format that is mandatory in the United States is shown in Figure 2-2. Food labels in the United States list the nutrient content of foods as a percentage of a standard amount known as the **Daily Value (DV)** for any particular nutrient. DVs are comprised of two separate sets of standards, Daily Reference Values (DRVs) for macronu-

FIGURE 2-2

An example of the food label format that is currently mandatory in the United States.

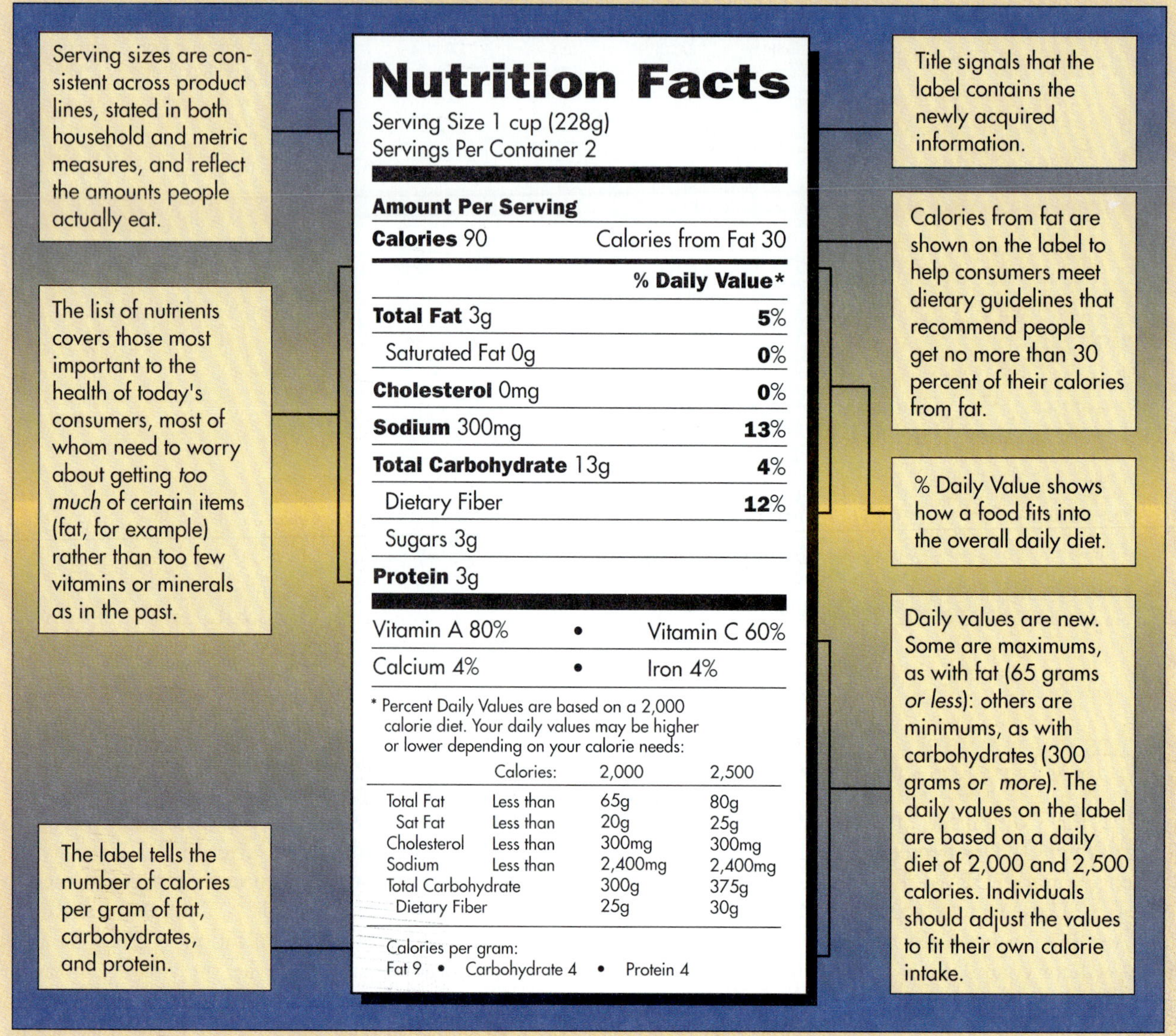
Serving sizes are consistent across product lines, stated in both household and metric measures, and reflect the amounts people actually eat.
The list of nutrients covers those most important to the health of today's consumers, most of whom need to worry about getting *too much* of certain items (fat, for example) rather than too few vitamins or minerals as in the past.
The label tells the number of calories per gram of fat, carbohydrates, and protein.
Nutrition Facts
Serving Size 1 cup (228g)
Servings Per Container 2
Amount Per Serving
Calories 90 Calories from Fat 30
% Daily Value*
Total Fat 3g 5%
Saturated Fat 0g 0%
Cholesterol 0mg 0%
Sodium 300mg 13%
Total Carbohydrate 13g 4%
Dietary Fiber 12%
Sugars 3g
Protein 3g
Vitamin A 80% • Vitamin C 60%
Calcium 4% • Iron 4%
* Percent Daily Values are based on a 2,000 calorie diet. Your daily values may be higher or lower depending on your calorie needs:
Calories: 2,000 2,500
Total Fat Less than 65g 80g
Sat Fat Less than 20g 25g
Cholesterol Less than 300mg 300mg
Sodium Less than 2,400mg 2,400mg
Total Carbohydrate 300g 375g
Dietary Fiber 25g 30g
Calories per gram:
Fat 9 • Carbohydrate 4 • Protein 4
Title signals that the label contains the newly acquired information.
Calories from fat are shown on the label to help consumers meet dietary guidelines that recommend people get no more than 30 percent of their calories from fat.
% Daily Value shows how a food fits into the overall daily diet.
Daily values are new. Some are maximums, as with fat (65 grams *or less*): others are minimums, as with carbohydrates (300 grams *or more*). The daily values on the label are based on a daily diet of 2,000 and 2,500 calories. Individuals should adjust the values to fit their own calorie intake.

trients (carbohydrate, fat, and protein) and electrolytes (sodium and potassium) and Reference Daily Intakes (RDIs) for vitamins, other minerals, and protein for certain groups (Table 2-2). Although frequently (and understandably) confused with the RDAs, the DVs are a distinct set of standards. Whereas the RDAs list separate standards for 17 different age and gender groups (see inside cover), the DVs give only one standard for everyone over the age of 4, apart from pregnant and lactating women. The DVs are thus a simpler set of standards that can reasonably be used on a food label (Figure 2-2).[13,14]

The DV approach is mandated by the Food and Drug Administration (FDA) for the nutrient labeling of all processed foods and drugs. For essential nutrients (proteins, vitamins, and minerals), the DVs, known as *Reference Daily Intakes (RDIs)*, represent the highest RDA (based on the 1968 RDA) for any age or gender group except pregnant and lactating women. The RDI is currently the same as the U.S. RDA value used on food labels before 1994. It is anticipated that RDIs will soon be based on standards such as the most recent RDAs that more accurately reflect current nutritional knowledge. Nutrient content is expressed as a percentage of the RDI for these nutrients.

The way in which the RDI are defined means that the DVs for most essential nutrients correspond to intakes higher than the actual needs for most people, apart from adolescent boys and some adult men. So it is unnecessary for everyone to consume 100% of the DV of each nutrient every day.

The DRVs used as standards for macronutrients and electrolytes include values for total fat, saturated fat, cho-

TABLE 2-2

Daily Values established by the Food and Drug Administration as standards for nutrient labeling purposes

REFERENCE DAILY INTAKES (RDIs)*‡§

NUTRIENT	REFERENCE AMOUNT
Vitamin A‖	5000 International Units (IU)
Vitamin C‖	60 mg
Thiamin	1.5 mg
Riboflavin	1.7 mg
Niacin	20 mg
Calcium‖	1 g
Iron‖	18 mg
Vitamin D	400 IU
Vitamin E	30 IU
Vitamin B_6	2 mg
Folic acid	0.4 mg
Vitamin B_{12}	6 μg
Phosphorus	1 g
Iodine	150 μg
Magnesium	400 mg
Zinc	15 mg
Copper	2 mg
Biotin	0.3 mg
Pantothenic acid	10 mg

DAILY REFERENCE VALUES (DRVs)‡§

NUTRIENT	BASIS FOR CALCULATING DAILY REFERENCE VALUE
Total fat	30% of calories
Saturated fat	10% of calories
Carbohydrate	60% of calories
Dietary fiber	11.5 g of fiber per each 1000 calories
Protein†	10% of calories for adults and children over 4 years

NUTRIENT	2000 CALORIES	2500 CALORIES
Total fat‖	65 g	80 g
Saturated fat‖	20 g	25 g
Cholesterol‖	300 mg	300 mg
Sodium‖	2.4 mg	2.4 mg
Total carbohydrate‖	300 g	375 g
Dietary fiber‖	25 g	30 g
Protein‖	50 g	65 g
Potassium	3.5 mg	3.5 mg

* Based on the National Academy of Sciences' 1968 recommended dietary allowances (same as U.S. RDA used until 1994). Values are highest RDAs except for pregnancy and lactation.

† The DRV for protein does not apply to certain populations. An RDI for protein has been established for these groups: infants under 1 yr, 14 g; children 1-4 yrs, 16 g, pregnant women, 50 g; and nursing mothers, 66 g.

‡ Some Daily Values (DVs) have been rounded to make label reading easier for consumers.

§ DV as used on label includes both Reference Daily Intakes (RDIs) for vitamins and minerals and DRVs for macronutrients and electrolytes.

‖ % DVs must be declared on label. % DV for other nutrients may be provided voluntarily.

The mandatory (**bold**) and voluntary dietary components and order in which they must appear on food labels are the following:

- **Total calories**
- **Calories from fat**
- Calories from saturated fat
- **Total fat**
- **Saturated fat**
- Stearic acid (on meat and poultry products only)
- Polyunsaturated fat
- Monounsaturated fat
- **Cholesterol**
- **Sodium**
- Potassium
- **Total carbohydrate**
- **Dietary fiber**
- Soluble fiber
- Insoluble fiber
- **Sugars**
- Sugar alcohol (for example, the sugar substitutes xylitol, mannitol, and sorbitol)
- Other carbohydrate (the difference between total carbohydrate and the sum of dietary fiber, sugars, and sugar alcohol, if declared)
- **Protein**
- Other essential vitamins and minerals, i.e., calcium
- Vitamins A and C and iron

If a food is fortified or enriched with any of the optional components or if a claim is made about any of them, the pertinent nutrition information then becomes mandatory.

To help consumers focus on nutrients of public health significance, these mandatory and voluntary components are the *only* ones allowed on the nutrition panel. The listing of single amino acids, maltodextrin, calories from polyunsaturated fat, and calories from carbohydrate, for example, may *not* appear on food labels.

FIGURE 2-3

An example of the food label format that is currently mandatory in Canada.

The nutrition label consists of:

- **A Heading**
- **Serving Size**

Nutrient content must be declared per *stated* serving size. Consumers should realize that if they eat more or less than the stated serving size, the nutrient values for fat, iron and other nutrients will change accordingly. Sometimes the serving size for the nutrition label differs from the Food Guide serving size.

- **Values for Energy, Protein, Fat and Carbohydrate**
  The nutrition label may also include:
- **Total fat broken down into Fatty Acids and Cholesterol**
- **Carbohydrate broken down into Sugars, Starch and Dietary Fibre**
- **Sodium and Potassium**

- **Vitamins and Minerals Expressed as a % of Recommended Daily Intake.** The RDI of a vitamin or mineral is a value developed for food labelling only. It is based on the highest Recommended Nutrient Intake (RNI), excluding the needs for pregnancy and breast-feeding.

CEREAL
Source of Fibre
Low in Fat

Ingredients: Whole Wheat, Wheat Bran, Sugar, Salt, Malt,Thiamin, Pyridoxine hydrochloride, Folic Acid, Reduced Iron, BHT.

NUTRITION INFORMATION
per 30 g
Serving Cereal
(175 ml. 3/4 cup)

Energy	Cal	100
	KJ	420
Protein	g	3.0
Fat	g	0.6
Carbohydrate	g	24
Sugars	g	4.4
Starch	g	16.6
Dietary fibre	g	3.0
Sodium	mg	265
Potassium	mg	168

Percentage of Recommended Daily Intake

Thiamin	%	46
Niacin	%	6
Vitamin B_6	%	10
Folacin	%	8
Iron	%	28

lesterol, total carbohydrate, fiber, sodium, potassium, and protein based on either a 2000- or a 2500-kcal diet. For all nutrients with DRVs—except carbohydrate, protein, and fiber—the DV represents the upper limit recommended. For nutrients with RDIs and for carbohydrate, protein, and fiber, the DV reference standard represents a minimal intake goal. Although on a food label, the content of all nutrients is expressed as a percentage of the DV, for those nutrients with DRVs, the actual weights present are also given immediately after the nutrient name.

The label must also indicate the usual amount consumed per serving in household measure, followed by the corresponding metric weight in parentheses and the number of such servings in the package or unit to which the label applies. The comparable Canadian food label format is shown in Figure 2-3.

Accurate labeling of nutrient content can be done only for foods whose composition is relatively stable and can be accurately analyzed. Because of the variability of their nutrient content, fresh foods do not have to carry nutrient labeling. At present, a voluntary program is in place for the labeling of the nutrient content of the 20 most commonly used fruits and the 20 most commonly used vegetables. In these cases, nutrient information is posted in stores in the produce section. If there is insufficient participation in this voluntary program, it

TABLE 2-3

Approved definitions for various nutrient content claims

NUTRIENT	FREE	LOW	REDUCED/LOW	COMMENTS
	Synonyms for "free": "zero," "no," "without," "trivial source of" "negligible sources of," "dietary insignificant source of"	Synonyms for "low": "little" ("few" for calories), "contains a small amount of," "low source of"	Synonyms for "reduced"/"less": "lower" ("fewer" for calories)	For "free," "very low," or "low," must indicate whether food meets a definition without benefit of special processing; e.g., "broccoli, a fat-free food" or "celery, a low-calorie food"
Calories	Less than 5 calories per reference amount and per serving	40 calories or less per reference amount (and per 50 g if reference amount is small)	At least 25% fewer calories per reference amount than an appropriate reference food; uses term "fewer" rather than "less"	"Light" or "lite": if 50% or more of the calories are from fat, fat must be reduced by at least 50% per reference amount. If less than 50% of calories are from fat, fat must be reduced at least 50% of calories or reduced at least ⅓ per reference amount
Total fat	Less than 0.5 g per reference amount and per serving*	3 g or less per reference amount (and per 50 g if reference amount is small)	At least 25% less fat per reference amount than an appropriate reference food	"___% fat free" must meet the requirements for "low fat"
Saturated fat	Less than 0.5 g saturated fat and less than 0.5 g *trans*-fatty acid per reference amount and per serving*	1 g or less per reference amount and 15% or less of calories from saturated fat	At least 25% less saturated fat per reference amount than an appropriate reference food	
Cholesterol	Less than 2 mg per reference amount and per serving*	20 mg or less per reference amount (and per 50 g of food if reference amount is small)	At least 25% less cholesterol per reference amount than an appropriate reference food	Cholesterol claims only allowed when food contains 2 g or less saturated fat per reference amount
Sodium	Less than 5 mg per reference amount and per serving*	140 mg or less per reference amount (and per 50 g if reference amount is small†)	At least 25% less sodium per reference amount than an appropriate reference food	"Light in sodium": if food is reduced by at least 50% per reference amount. "Very low sodium": 35 mg or less per reference amount (and per 50 g if reference amount is small). "Salt free" must meet criterion for "sodium free."
Sugars	"Sugar free": less than 0.5 g sugars per reference amount and per serving*	Not defined; no basis for a recommended intake	At least 25% less sugars per reference amount than an appropriate reference food	

* If an ingredient is present that is understood to contain this nutrient, it must be followed by an asterisk that refers to a footnote stating that it contains a trivial amount of the nutrient.

† "Small reference amount" = reference amount 30 g or less or 2 Tbsp or less.

will become mandatory. Meat, poultry, and eggs, which are under the jurisdiction of the United States Department of Agriculture (USDA), are subject to a set of labeling regulations similar to those for processed foods. Labeling regulations do not apply to single-ingredient products, such as flour, and sugar, which may be labeled voluntarily.

Nutrient labeling can be used by consumers to compare different brands and products and to assess the nutrient content of their diet as a whole. There is, as yet,

TABLE 2-4

Approved terms used on food labels

TERM	DEFINITION
"Lean"	On seafood or game, meat that contains <10 g total fat, 4.5 g or less saturated fat, and <95 mg cholesterol per reference amount and per 100 g
"Extra lean"	On seafood or game meat that contains <5 g total fat, <2 g saturated fat, and <95 mg cholesterol per reference amount and per 100 g
"High," "rich in," or "excellent source of"	Contains 20% or more of the Daily Value (DV) to describe protein, vitamins, minerals, dietary fiber, or potassium per reference amount
"Good source of," "contains," or "provides"	10%-19% of the DV per reference amount
"More," "added"	10% or more of the DV per reference amount
"Light" or "lite"	≥50% less fat per reference amount or ⅓ fewer calories if less than 50% of calories from fat

From Wilkening YL: *Nutr Today* 28(5):13, 1993.

TABLE 2-5

*Health claims approved by the FDA for use on food labels**

APPROVED CLAIM	FOOD REQUIREMENTS	MODEL CLAIM STATEMENTS†
Calcium and osteoporosis	High in calcium Assimilable (bioavailable) Supplements must disintegrate and dissolve Phosphorus content cannot exceed calcium content	Regular exercise and a healthful diet with enough calcium helps teens and young adult white and Asian women maintain good bone health and may reduce their high risk of osteoporosis later in life.
Sodium and hypertension	Low sodium	Diets low in sodium may reduce the risk of high blood pressure, a disease associated with many factors.
Dietary fat and cancer	Low fat Fish and game meats must be "extra lean"	Development of cancer depends on many factors. A diet low in total fat may reduce the risk of some cancers.
Dietary saturated fat and cholesterol and risk of coronary heart disease	Low saturated fat Low cholesterol Low fat Fish and game meats must be "extra lean"	While many factors affect heart disease, diets low in saturated fat and cholesterol may reduce the risk of this disease.

* The term *healthy* (health, healthful, or healthier) may be used only on foods containing no more than 3 g of total fat, no more than 1 g of saturated fat, and no more than 480 mg of sodium per reference serving and at least 10% of the Recommended Daily Intake or Daily Recommended Value of either vitamin A, vitamin C, calcium, iron, protein, or fiber.

† Contains all elements that FDA considers essential to make claim nonmisleading.

From Wilkening YL: *Nutr Today* 28(5): 13, 1993.

TABLE 2-5

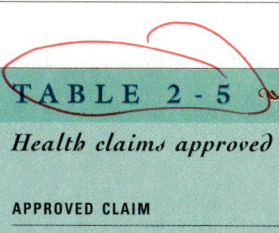

Health claims approved by the FDA for use on food labels (continued)

APPROVED CLAIM	FOOD REQUIREMENTS	MODEL CLAIM STATEMENTS*
Fiber-containing grain products, fruits and vegetables, and cancer	Dietary fiber Low fat Good source of dietary fiber (without fortification)	Low-fat diets rich in fiber-containing grain products, fruits, and vegetables may reduce the risk of some types of cancer, a disease associated with many factors.
Fruits, vegetables, and grain products that contain fiber, particularly soluble fiber, and risk of coronary heart disease	Low saturated fat Low cholesterol Low fat At least 0.6 g of soluble fiber per reference amount (without fortification)	Diets low in saturated fat and cholesterol and rich in fruits, vegetables and grain products that contain some types of dietary fiber, particularly soluble fiber, may reduce the risk of heart disease, a disease associated with many factors.
Fruits and vegetables and cancer	Low fat Good source (without fortification) of at least one of the following: vitamin A, vitamin C, or dietary fiber	Low fat diets rich in fruits and vegetables (foods that are low in fat and may contain dietary fiber, vitamin A, or vitamin C) may reduce the risk of some types of cancer, a disease associated with many factors. Broccoli is high in vitamins A and C, and it is a good source of dietary fiber.
Folate and neural tube defects (NTDs)	Good source of folate	Women who consume adequate amounts of folate throughout their childbearing years may reduce their risk of having a child with NTD. Such birth defects, although uncommon, are serious. Fruits, dark green leafy vegetables, legumes, enriched grain products, fortified cereals, and supplements are good folate sources. Mothers of children with a spinal cord birth defect should consult a physician before becoming pregnant again. Folate intake should be limited to 1000 μg/day.

little information available on how much of the mandatory nutritional information is understood by consumers. It appears, however, that the system of mandatory labeling will be effective only if accompanied by a continuing education campaign.

To help consumers understand claims about nutrient content on food packages and in advertising, the FDA has set approved definitions of the terms *free, low,* and *reduced/low* and has recognized equivalent terms. The limits applying to the use of these terms with reference to calories, total fat, saturated fat, cholesterol, sodium, and sugars are given in Table 2-3. The USDA has also set regulations governing the description of meat and poultry as *lean* or *ultra lean* (Table 2-4). The FDA has evaluated many possible health claims for food labels and approved eight of them (Table 2-5).

FOOD-BASED GUIDANCE

Attempts to translate scientific knowledge of nutrient needs into clear guidelines to help people select an adequate diet date as far back as 1916.[15] The basic guidelines have been revised several times since then, as summarized in Table 2-6, and are considered individually below.

FIVE FOOD GROUPS

In 1916 it was believed that five basic types of nutrients were required for health: protein, carbohydrate, fat, minerals, and organic acids. This led to assurances to the public that if these were all included in the diet, all nutritional needs for energy and materials, including all "unknown" essentials, would be met. To ensure that all of the required nutrients were present in a diet, people were encouraged to make use of five basic food groups in the diet, namely, the following:

- Meat, milk, and other protein-rich foods
- Cereals and other starchy foods
- Vegetables and fruit
- Fatty foods
- Sugars

The emphasis behind this guidance was on the need to obtain sufficient calories and body-building protein.

TWELVE FOOD GROUPS

In 1930 the original five food groups were subdivided to obtain a new list of 12 food groups that should all be represented in a healthful diet, namely, the following:

- Milk
- Lean meat, poultry, and fish

TABLE 2-6

Major food guide systems in the United States from 1916 to 1992

FIVE FOOD GROUPS, 1916*	BASIC SEVEN, 1943*	BASIC FOUR, 1956*	HASSLE-FREE GUIDE, 1979*	FOOD PYRAMID, 1992† (FOOD WHEEL, 1984)
Milk, meat, fish, poultry, eggs, and meat substitutes	Milk and milk products (2) Meat, fish, etc. (2), eggs (4 per week)	Milk and milk products (2) Meat, fish, poultry, eggs (2)	Milk-cheese group (2-4) Meat, poultry, fish, beans, eggs (2)	Milk, cheese, yogurt (2-3) Meat, fish, poultry, eggs (2-3)
Fruits and vegetables	Green and yellow vegetables (1) Citrus fruits and raw cabbage (1) Potatoes, fruit, and other vegetables (2)	Fruits and vegetables (4)	Fruits and vegetables (4)	Fruits (2-4) Vegetables (3-5)
Bread and other cereal foods	Bread, flour, cereal (enriched or whole grain) (3)	Bread, flour, cereal (enriched or whole grain) (4)	Whole grain bread and cereal (4)	Bread, whole grain cereals (6-11)
Butter and wholesome fats	Equivalent of 2 Tbsp butter or fortified margarine			
Simple sugars			Fats, sweets, alcohol (caution)	Fats, sweets, alcohol (moderation)

Recommended number of servings per day in parentheses.
* Foundation diet.
† Total diet.

- Dry mature beans, peas, and nuts
- Eggs
- Flours and cereals
- Leafy green or yellow vegetables
- Potatoes and sweet potatoes
- Tomatoes and citrus fruits
- Other vegetables and fruits
- Butter
- Other fats
- Sugars

Later, as specific minerals and vitamins were identified as essential, the emphasis in food selection shifted away from calories and protein toward the need for foods to provide specific vitamins and minerals. This led to the designation of certain foods as **protective foods** because of their ability to provide significant amounts of vitamins and minerals, in addition to adequate calories and protein.

THE BASIC SEVEN

To support the publication of the first RDAs in 1943, the U.S. Bureau of Home Economics published a food guide that recommended that seven classes of foods be included in the diet in specified amounts. This guide formed the basis of the **Basic Seven** food groups plan, which was promoted in 1943 as part of the National Wartime Nutrition Program of the Department of Agriculture. The basic seven food groups were the following:

- Milk and milk products
- Meat, poultry, fish, eggs, dried beans, peas, and nuts
- Bread, flour, and cereals
- Leafy green or yellow vegetables
- Citrus fruits, tomatoes, cabbage, and salad greens
- Potatoes and other fruits and vegetables
- Butter and fortified margarine

This familiar guide became the basis of practically all public nutrition programs from 1943 until 1956.

THE BASIC FOUR

In 1956 the USDA recommended that the Basic Seven guide be replaced by a simpler guide based on four food groups. The four food groups, soon designated as the **Basic Four,** were the following:

- Milk and milk products
- Meat, fish, poultry, and eggs
- Bread, flour, and cereals
- Fruits and vegetables

This new guide was published in a document entitled *Essentials of an Adequate Diet.*[16] The only differences between the Basic Four guide and the Basic Seven guide were that the Basic Four guide grouped all vegetables and fruits together and did not include the butter and fortified margarine group of the Basic Seven guide. The butter and fortified margarine group was removed because use of foods from the Basic Four groups usually leads to the use of some butter, margarine, or other fats and oils to improve flavor and palatability. Also, the idea that fat consumption might be linked to coronary heart disease was gaining ground. The USDA did not want to encourage the consumption of foods that might later prove to be a cause of degenerative disease (as indeed they have).

The stated purpose of the Basic Four guide was "to translate what is known about nutritional requirements and the composition of foods into a workable plan that will help people select the kinds of foods that will give a nutritionally good diet." Because the choices within the food groups were unlimited, the guide also allowed for considerable diversity, to cater to differing food preferences and eating patterns. At the same time that the Basic Four guidelines were implemented in the United States, Canadians were advised to follow the *Food Guide for Canada,* which was based on a similar four-group plan.

In both cases it was assumed that the foods recommended by the official guidance would form the *foundation* of an adequate diet rather than the entire diet. When foods from the four groups were consumed in the recommended amounts, the diet provided 80% of the RDAs of the eight nutrients for which standards had then been published and a total of 1200 to 1400 kcal of energy. It was assumed that other foods chosen to bring the total kilocalorie content of the diet up to satisfying levels also provided sufficient nutrients to provide adequate nutrition overall. Recent research has confirmed that when the Basic Four guidance is followed, this assumption is valid. It was discouraging to learn, however, that the diets of the 21,000 subjects in the 1977 to 1978 Food Consumption Survey actually adhered to the Basic Four guidelines on only 3% of the 63,000 days for which food intake was analyzed.

Recent Dietary Guidance in the United States

1977	Dietary Goals (Senate Select Committee on Nutrition and Human Needs)
1979	Dietary Goals (revised) Hassle-Free Guide (USDA) Healthy People (Surgeon General)
1980	Toward Healthful Diets (National Academy of Sciences [NAS])
1982	Diet, Nutrition, and Cancer (NAS)
1984	Food Wheel—A Pattern for Daily Food Choices (USDA and American Red Cross)
1985	Nutrition and Your Health: Dietary Guidelines for Americans (USDA and DHHS), (revised)
1988	Surgeon General's Report (DHHS)
1989	Diet and Health (NAS)
1990	Dietary Guidelines for Americans (USDA/DHHS) (revised)
1992	Food Guide Pyramid (USDA)

THE HASSLE-FREE GUIDE

By the late 1970s the Basic Four guidelines were increasingly criticized for not reflecting the developing knowledge of nutrient needs or prevailing patterns of food use. In response to these criticisms the USDA published modified guidance, known as the **Hassle-Free Guide,** in 1979.[17] The detailed advice supporting this guide emphasized the use of whole grain, rather than enriched, cereals and stressed that legumes were reasonable substitutes for more traditional protein-rich foods, such as meat, fish, and milk products. The Hassle-Free Guide also added a fifth food group comprising fats, sweets, and alcohol. This new group was introduced not to encourage its use, but to recognize that the foods within it were widely used and to draw attention to the need to take this use into account in dietary planning. People were encouraged to use foods from this food group sparingly, or not at all. The Hassle-Free Guide was supported by an attractive publication entitled *Food,* which emphasized the need for most people to reduce their intakes of kilocalories, sugar, fat, and sodium but to increase their consumption of fiber.

THE FOOD WHEEL

In 1984 the American Red Cross, in collaboration with the USDA, promoted a food guidance graphic called *The Food Wheel, A Pattern for Daily Food Choices.* This included five major groups of foods, whose consumption was encouraged in the specified amounts, and a sixth group (alcohols, fats, and sweets), to be consumed in moderation, if at all. The Food Wheel was designed to stress the use of fiber-rich foods, in addition to those that provide sufficient vitamins, minerals, and protein. It was also intended to limit the energy obtained from fat to 35% of total kilocalories. It was found that to accomplish these goals using a diet based on the Food Wheel, an adult needed to consume more than 2200 kcal/day. Because this value exceeds the energy needs of some sedentary adults, such people consuming the upper level of recommended servings needed to increase their energy expenditure to avoid gaining weight. The Food

FIGURE 2-4

The Food Guide Pyramid.

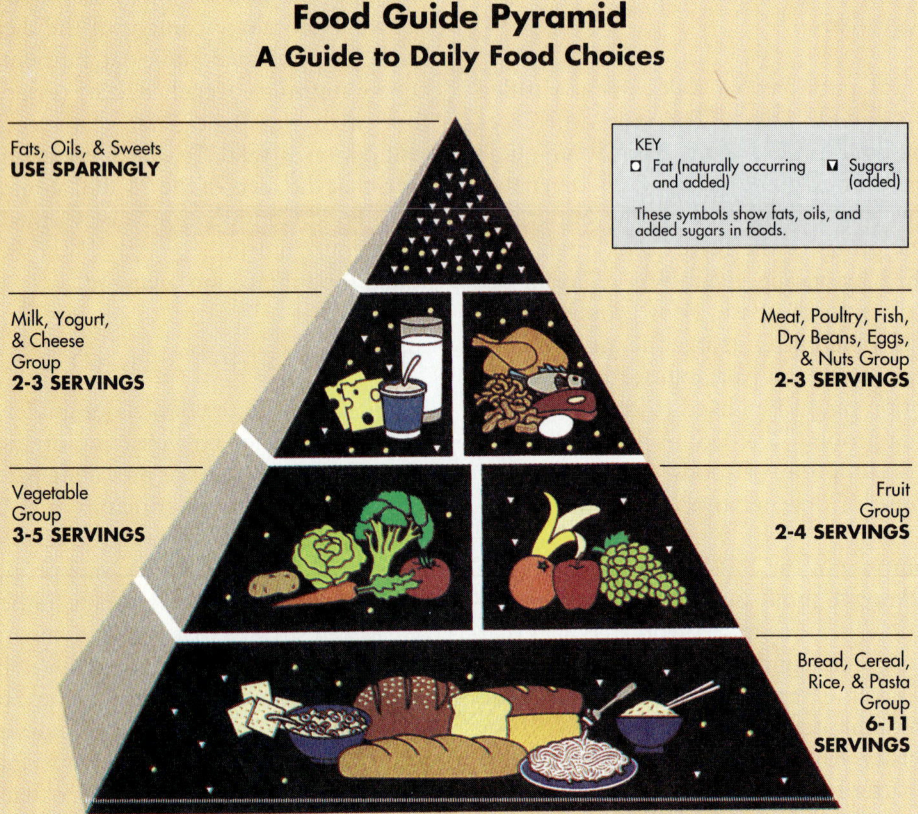

Wheel was never well promoted, and it has now been replaced by the most recent nutritional guidance system, the Food Guide Pyramid.

THE FOOD GUIDE PYRAMID

All previous food guides have now been replaced by the Food Guide Pyramid (Figure 2-4), released by the USDA and the Department of Health and Human Services (DHHS) in 1992.[18] The Food Guide Pyramid organizes foods into five groups and conveys the three essential elements of a healthful diet: *proportionality,* or the appropriate amount of food to choose from each major food group; *variety*—that is, eating a selection of foods from each major group each day; and *moderation* in eating fats, oils, and sweets.

The guidance embodied within the Food Guide Pyramid was based on several years of intensive research to determine the most scientifically sound recommendations and the most appropriate format in which to convey them. Its recommendations are essentially the same as those embodied within the Food Wheel, but they are presented in a different graphic format. The concept that fats and sugars are either contained within or added to many foods represented in the pyramid is conveyed by the small triangles and dots scattered throughout the image of the pyramid.

Choosing the smaller numbers of servings per day results in a diet providing approximately 1600 kcal/day, appropriate for people with the lowest energy requirements. Choosing the larger numbers of servings, on the other hand, provides about 2800 kcal/day, as required by people with the highest energy requirements. Recommendations on the appropriate number of servings from the five food groups at different caloric levels are summarized in Table 2-7.

In developing the Food Guide Pyramid, the USDA and DHHS focused on eight basic goals:

- To promote overall health
- To provide recommendations based on the latest research
- To focus on the total diet rather than specific parts of it

TABLE 2-7

Three diets based on the Food Guide Pyramid providing different total kilocalorie intakes

	PATTERN A	PATTERN B	PATTERN C
Approximate kcal	1600	2200	2800
Bread group (servings)	6	9	11
Vegetable group (servings)	3	4	5
Fruit group (servings)	2	3	4
Milk group (servings)	2-3*	2-3*	2-3*
Meat group (total oz)	5	6	7
Total fat (g)	53	73	93
Total added sugars (tsp)	6	12	18

* Women who are pregnant or breast-feeding, teenagers, and young adults to age 24 need 3 servings.

From Welsh S, Davis C, Shaw A: *Nutr Today* 27(6):12, 1992.

TABLE 2-8

Nutritional goals on which the Food Guide Pyramid is based

NUTRIENT/FOOD COMPONENT	GOALS
NUTRITIONAL ADEQUACY	
Food energy	1300 to 3000 calories
Protein	100% of RDA for gender/age groups over 2 years of age
Vitamins: vitamin A, thiamin, riboflavin, niacin, vitamin B_6, vitamin B_{12}, ascorbic acid, folate, vitamin E	100% of RDA for gender/age groups over 2 years of age
Minerals: calcium, iron, magnesium, phosphorus, zinc, copper	100% of RDA for gender/age groups over 2 years of age
Fiber	Increase consumption
MODERATION	
Fat, total	30% or less of calories
Saturated fatty acids	<10% of calories
Cholesterol	300 mg or less
Sodium	2400 mg or less
Added sugars	To balance calories but not to exceed current consumption

From Welsh S, Davis C, Shaw A: *Nutr Today* 27(6):12, 1992.

- To be of practical use to the target audience
- To meet nutritional goals in a realistic manner
- To allow maximal flexibility in food choices
- To be practical
- To be evolutionary

The specific nutritional goals that should be attainable through use of the Food Guide Pyramid are shown in Table 2-8.

The Food Guide Pyramid has become widely accepted as the graphic embodiment of official nutritional advice in the United States. A slightly different format is used to convey similar information for Canada. This is called **Canada's Food Guide to Healthy Eating** (Figure 2-5).

NUTRIENT-BASED GUIDANCE

In the late 1970s, at about the same time that the USDA released its Hassle-Free Guide, the U.S. Senate Select Committee on Nutrition and Human Needs issued a document entitled *Dietary Goals for the United States.*[19] This document focused on the role of diet in several "killer" diseases—coronary heart disease, hypertension, obesity, diabetes, and cancer—and also on the effect of diet on the incidence of tooth decay. The **dietary goals** were directed toward the distribution of kilocalories obtained from macronutrients, carbohydrate, lipid, and protein and the amount of saturated fat,

FIGURE 2-5

Canada's Food Guide to Healthy Eating.

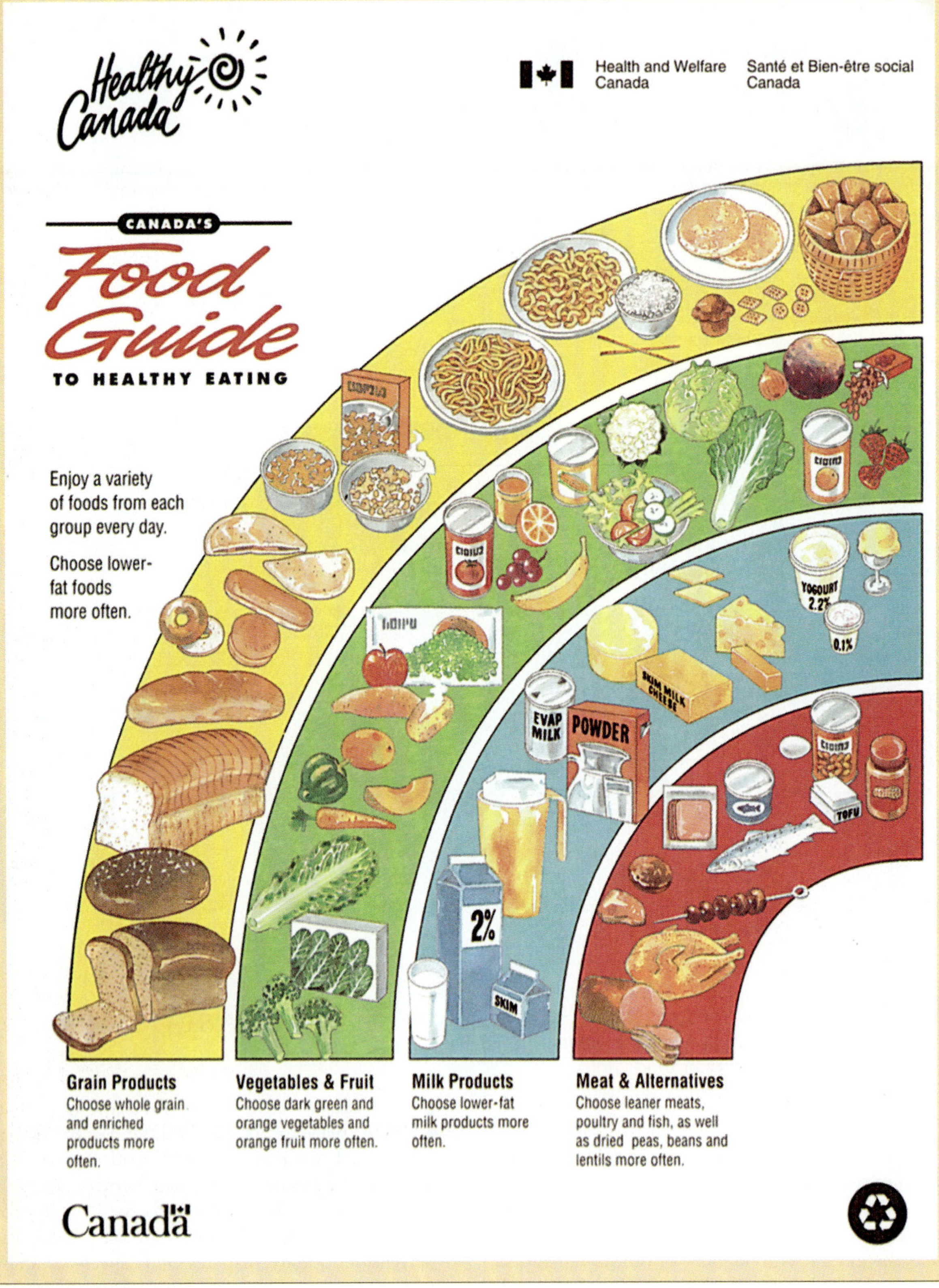
Healthy Canada
Health and Welfare Canada
Santé et Bien-être social Canada
CANADA'S
Food Guide
TO HEALTHY EATING
Enjoy a variety of foods from each group every day.
Choose lower-fat foods more often.
YOGOURT 2.2%
0.1%
SKIM MILK CHEESE
EVAP MILK
POWDER
2%
SKIM
TOFU
Grain Products
Choose whole grain and enriched products more often.
Vegetables & Fruit
Choose dark green and orange vegetables and orange fruit more often.
Milk Products
Choose lower-fat milk products more often.
Meat & Alternatives
Choose leaner meats, poultry and fish, as well as dried peas, beans and lentils more often.
Canada

FIGURE 2-5

Canada's **Food Guide to Healthy Eating** *(continued).*

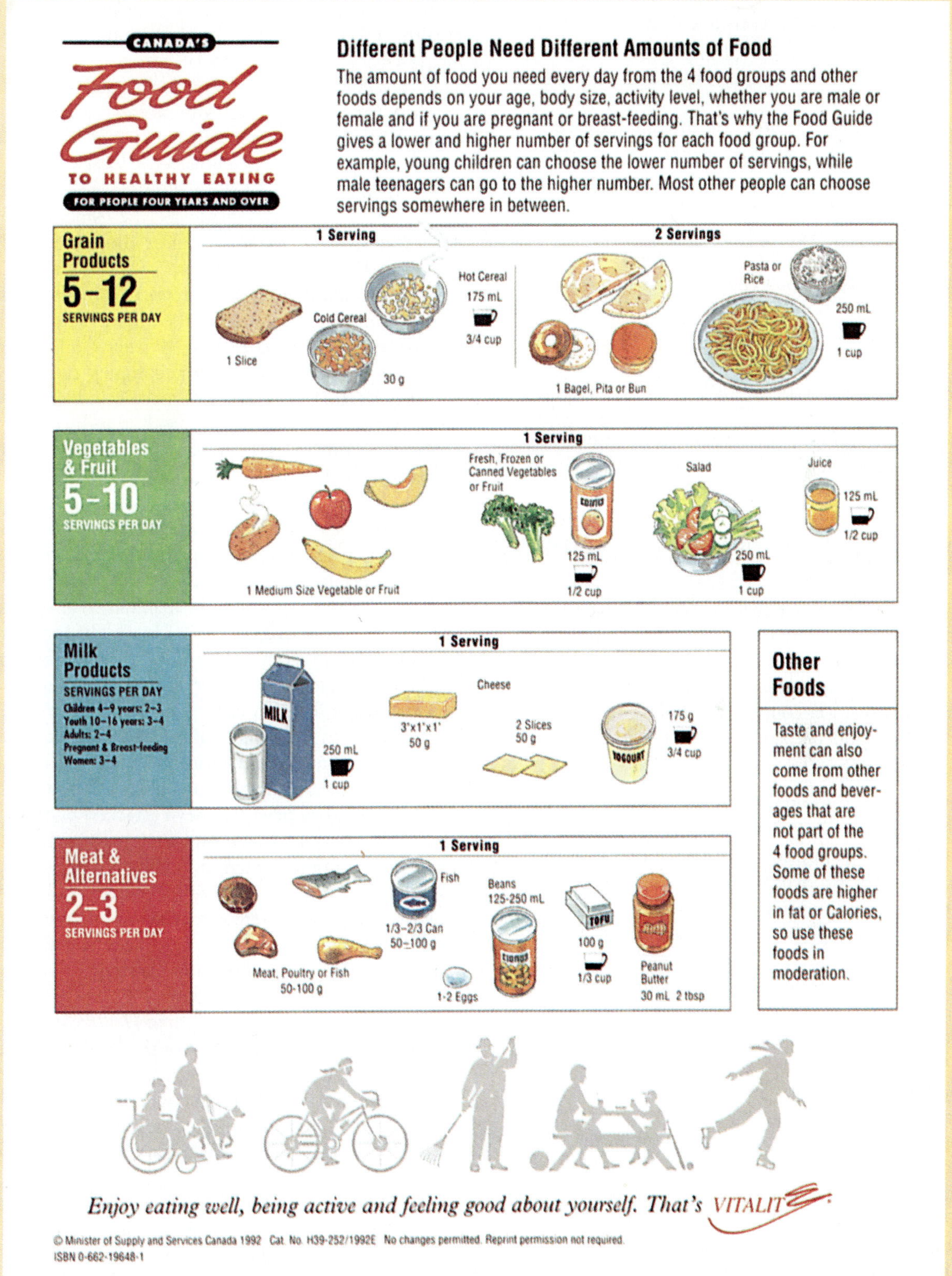
CANADA'S
Food Guide
TO HEALTHY EATING
FOR PEOPLE FOUR YEARS AND OVER
Different People Need Different Amounts of Food
The amount of food you need every day from the 4 food groups and other foods depends on your age, body size, activity level, whether you are male or female and if you are pregnant or breast-feeding. That's why the Food Guide gives a lower and higher number of servings for each food group. For example, young children can choose the lower number of servings, while male teenagers can go to the higher number. Most other people can choose servings somewhere in between.
Grain Products
5–12
SERVINGS PER DAY
1 Serving
1 Slice
Cold Cereal
30 g
Hot Cereal
175 mL
3/4 cup
2 Servings
1 Bagel, Pita or Bun
Pasta or Rice
250 mL
1 cup
Vegetables & Fruit
5–10
SERVINGS PER DAY
1 Serving
1 Medium Size Vegetable or Fruit
Fresh, Frozen or Canned Vegetables or Fruit
125 mL
1/2 cup
Salad
250 mL
1 cup
Juice
125 mL
1/2 cup
Milk Products
SERVINGS PER DAY
Children 4–9 years: 2–3
Youth 10–16 years: 3–4
Adults: 2–4
Pregnant & Breast-feeding Women: 3–4
1 Serving
MILK
250 mL
1 cup
Cheese
3"x1"x1"
50 g
2 Slices
50 g
YOGOURT
175 g
3/4 cup
Meat & Alternatives
2–3
SERVINGS PER DAY
1 Serving
Meat, Poultry or Fish
50-100 g
Fish
1/3–2/3 Can
50–100 g
Beans
125-250 mL
1-2 Eggs
TOFU
100 g
1/3 cup
Peanut Butter
30 mL 2 tbsp
Other Foods
Taste and enjoyment can also come from other foods and beverages that are not part of the 4 food groups. Some of these foods are higher in fat or Calories, so use these foods in moderation.
Enjoy eating well, being active and feeling good about yourself. That's VITALITY.
© Minister of Supply and Services Canada 1992 Cat. No. H39-252/1992E No changes permitted. Reprint permission not required.
ISBN 0-662-19648-1

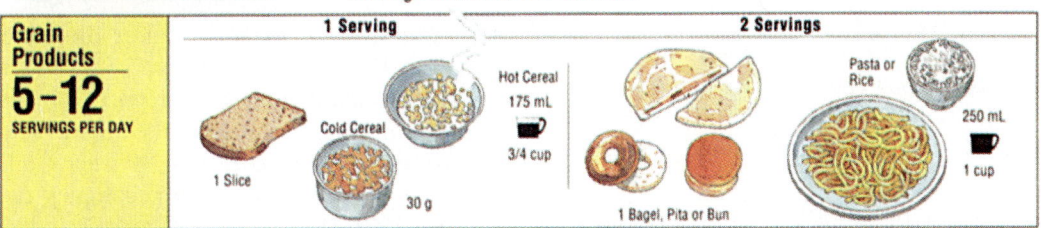

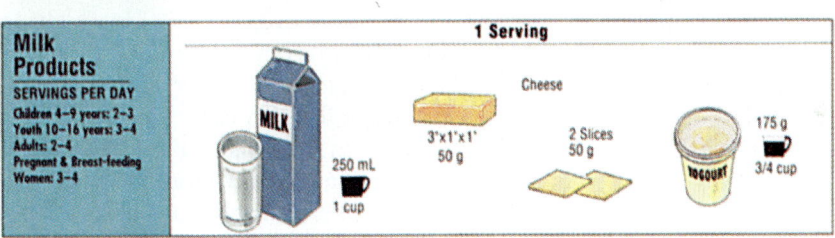

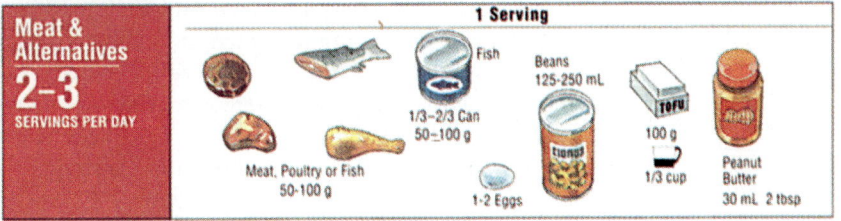

cholesterol, sodium, and sugar in the diet. The original recommendations were slightly modified soon after publication to yield the following list of dietary goals:

- To avoid overweight, consume only as much energy (kilocalories) as is expended; if overweight, decrease energy intake and increase energy expenditure
- To increase the consumption of complex carbohydrates and "naturally occurring" sugars from about 25% to about 48% of energy intake
- To reduce overall fat consumption from approximately 40% to 30% of energy intake
- To reduce saturated fat consumption to account for about 10% of total energy intake and balance that with polyunsaturated and monounsaturated fats, which should account for about 10% of energy intake each
- To reduce cholesterol consumption to about 300 mg/day
- To reduce consumption of refined and processed sugars by about 45% to account for about 10% of total energy intake
- To decrease consumption of salt and foods high in salt content to provide 5 g or less of salt per day

There was considerable debate about whether sufficient scientific evidence existed to justify the quantified recommendations within these dietary goals. Nevertheless, there was general agreement for the general population that it was wise to encourage the following changes in food selection and preparation to attain the previously listed goals:

- Increase consumption of fruits, vegetables, and whole grains
- Decrease consumption of animal fat and choose poultry and fish, which reduces animal fat
- Decrease consumption of foods high in total fat, and partially replace saturated fats with unsaturated fats
- Except for children under 2, substitute low-fat and nonfat milk for whole milk and low-fat dairy products for high-fat dairy products
- Decrease consumption of butterfat, eggs, and other high-cholesterol sources; some consideration should be given to easing the cholesterol-reduction goal for premenopausal women, young children, and elderly persons to obtain the nutritional benefit of eggs in the diet
- Decrease consumption of refined and other processed sugars and foods high in such sugars
- Decrease consumption of salt and foods high in salt content

How the fat, protein, and carbohydrate content of a diet achieving these goals compares with the U.S. diet at the time these goals were set and with the current U.S. diet is shown in Figure 2-6.

At about the same time as the publication of *Dietary Goals for the United States,* a National Institutes of Health (NIH) consensus group recommended similar measures for the reduction of coronary heart disease. They recommended a reduction in total fat intake to account for 30% of total kilocalories, a reduction of saturated fat intake to account for 10% of total kilocalories, and a reduction of cholesterol intake to between 250 and 300 mg/day. Essentially the same recommendations have also been made by the American Heart Association, the National Cancer Institute, and the American Diabetes Association.

Almost simultaneously, a report from the National Academy of Sciences in the United States suggested that 60% of cancers were related to diet.[20] They urged increased consumption of fiber, complex carbohydrate, and **cruciferous vegetables** (broccoli and other members of the cabbage family) and a reduction in fat consumption from the prevailing average of 43% of kilocalorie intake to 35%.

Another panel from the NIH on the health implications of obesity concluded that obesity is closely associated with hypertension, elevated blood cholesterol levels, diabetes, certain cancers, and other medical problems.[21] This panel urged that weight be maintained at levels of no more than 20% above the desirable weight for height.

All of these recommendations have great bearing on the design of nutritional intervention programs in addition to their effects on each individual following them. They have been the subject of intense and often acrimonious debate among nutrition scientists and educators. Although the recommendations have received considerable support, they have also been attacked by those who believe that they are based on inadequate evidence, they could not be implemented in practice, or they may even prove to be counterproductive. There is also concern that they impose a therapeutic dietary regimen on the total population when they may benefit only a small segment of the population with a genetic predisposition for a particular medical problem.

A 1980 report entitled *Toward Healthful Diets* from the Food and Nutrition Board of the National Academy of Sciences simply urged Americans to consume a varied diet in moderation.[22] It maintained that there was inadequate information on the consequences of modifications to macronutrient intake to allow specific recommendations to be made.

The concerns and developing recommendations about the link between nutrition and health have certainly not been confined to the United States. For example, in 1983 the British Health Education Council published a paper entitled *Proposals for Nutritional Guidelines for Health Education.* This suggested an average fat intake accounting for 30% of total kilocalories

FIGURE 2-6

Comparison of current North American diet with the diet proposed in the* Dietary Goals of the United States *document and the North American diet at the time the* Dietary Goals *was published.

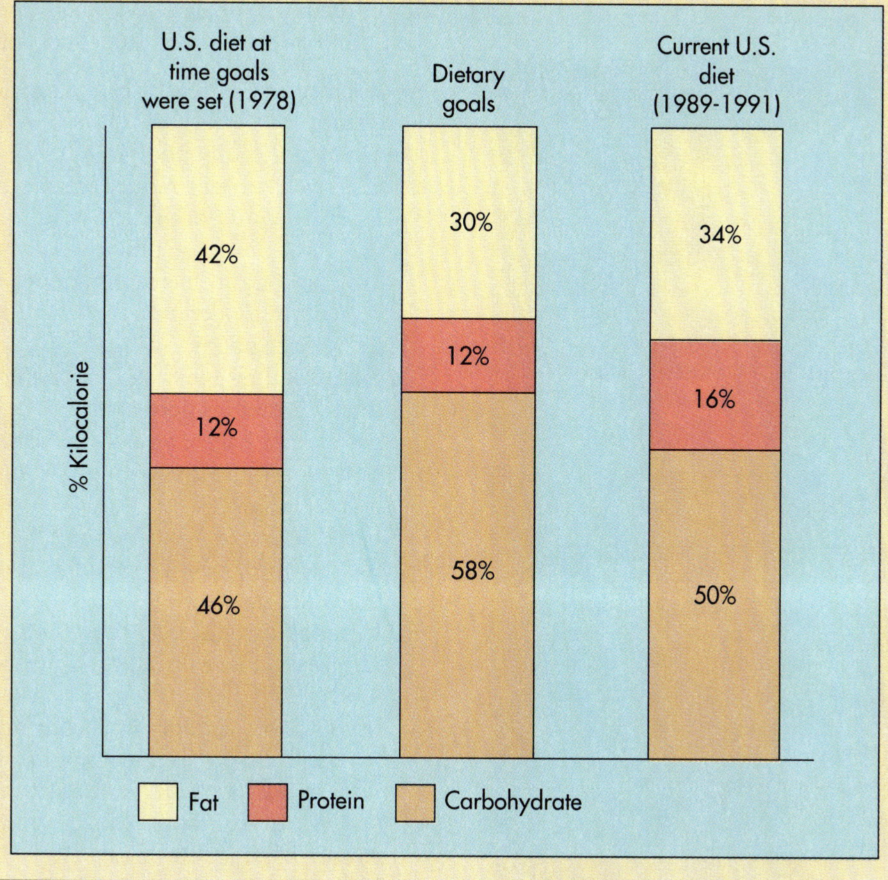

(with saturated fat providing one third of these kilocalories, or 10% overall), a reduction in sugar intake to 44 kg/year, increased intake of fiber to bring it up to 30 g/day, and decreased intake of salt (down to 3 g/day) and alcohol (down to 4% of total kilocalories). No recommendation was made for cholesterol. Like the various U.S. recommendations, this British recommendation stirred up a considerable debate over whether there is sufficient scientifically based knowledge on which to base such advice.

The debate in America surrounding the Dietary Goals, particularly the concern that they were more specific than could be justified, led the DHHS and the USDA to jointly issue a new set of guidelines entitled *Nutrition and Your Health: Dietary Guidelines for Americans,* which recommended certain dietary practices but did not set specific numerical goals for the quantities of nutrients to be consumed. This proved to be a landmark document, representing the first time that the DHHS and USDA had collaborated to provide nutritional guidance. An expert panel of nutritionists appointed to review the guidelines in 1984 produced a slightly modified form of the original guidelines. A further review in 1990 resulted in the current version of the dietary guidelines (Figure 2-7). The recommendations in the latest version are phrased in a slightly more positive manner by encouraging people to "choose" recommended foods or "use in moderation" foods associated with health risks, in place of the strong emphasis on the negative word "avoid," which characterized earlier versions. As can be seen in Figure 2-7, these guidelines continue to focus on macronutrients rather than vitamins and minerals. This reflects the growing concern that overnutrition is a serious health problem.

The Canadian Guidelines for Healthy Eating deliver a similar message, as follows:

- Enjoy a *variety* of foods.
- Emphasize cereals, breads, other grain products, vegetables, and fruits.
- Choose low-fat dairy products, lean meats, and foods prepared with little or no fat.
- Achieve and maintain a healthy body weight by enjoying regular physical activity and healthful eating.
- Limit the intake of salt, alcohol, and caffeine.

FIGURE 2-7

***The recommendations made by the current version of* Nutrition and Your Health: Dietary Guidelines for Americans.**

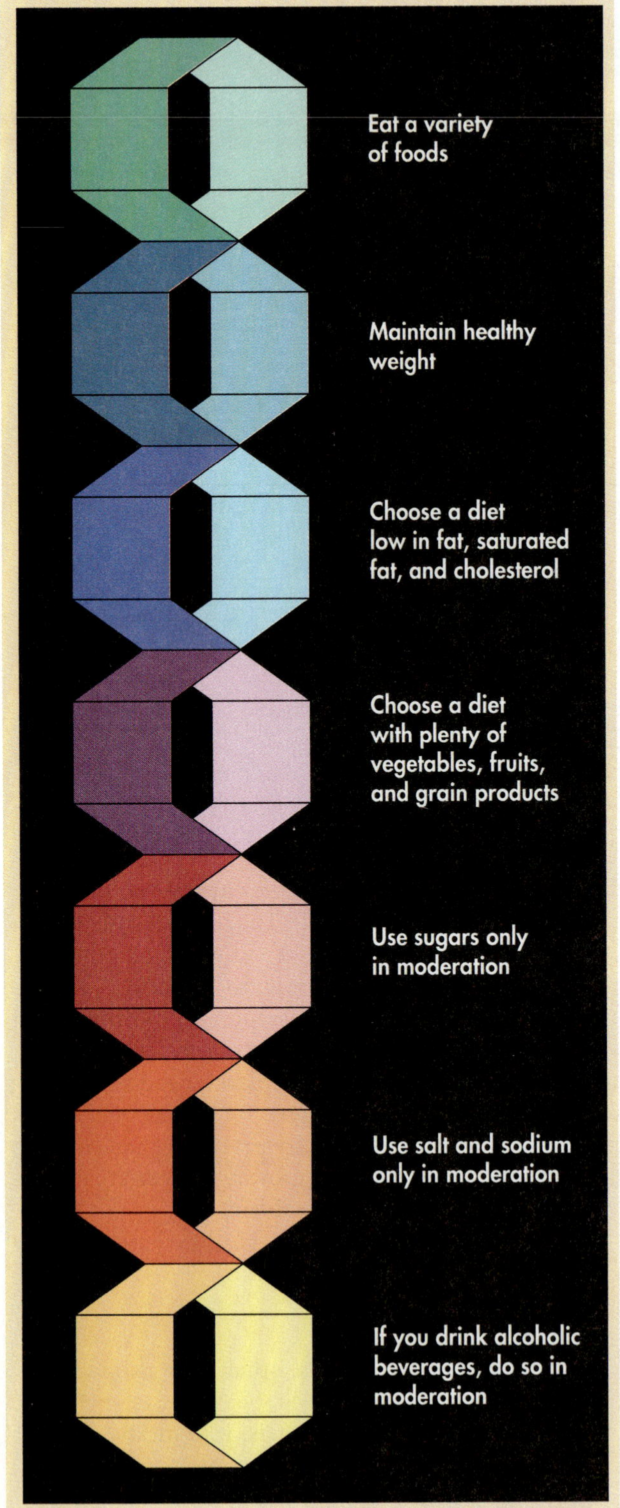
Eat a variety of foods
Maintain healthy weight
Choose a diet low in fat, saturated fat, and cholesterol
Choose a diet with plenty of vegetables, fruits, and grain products
Use sugars only in moderation
Use salt and sodium only in moderation
If you drink alcoholic beverages, do so in moderation

In 1987 the American Dietetic Association believed there were enough unique nutritional requirements for women to justify the development of a set of guidelines specifically designed to improve women's diets and decrease their risk of disease.[24] The association came up with the following set of guidelines for women:

- Eat a variety of foods from all major food groups.
- Maintain healthy body weight. To lose weight effectively, do not reduce intakes to less than 10 kcal/pound of present weight and do not skip meals; increase physical activity (exercise). To gain weight, increase kilocalorie intake and exercise in moderation.
- Exercise regularly.
- Limit total fat intake to less than one third of total kilocalories per day.
- Eat at least half of your daily kilocalories from carbohydrate, with an emphasis on complex carbohydrates.
- Eat a variety of foods rich in fiber.
- Include three or four servings of calcium-rich foods per day.
- Include plenty of iron-rich foods.
- Limit intake of salt- and sodium-containing foods.
- If you drink alcohol, limit your intake to one or two drinks per day (the amount of alcohol in "one drink" is equivalent to 12 oz of beer, 5 oz of wine, or 1½ oz of distilled spirits).
- Avoid smoking.
- If you have questions about the adequacy of your diet, see a registered dietitian.

NUTRITIVE CONTRIBUTION OF FOOD GROUPS

The selection of the food groups used in the various food guides was based primarily on the unique nutritive contributions of the foods within each group (Figure 2-8). The specific nutritive contributions of the four major food groups are considered next.

MILK AND MILK PRODUCTS

The major nutrients provided by milk and milk products are calcium, vitamin D, phosphorus, riboflavin, protein, vitamin B_{12}, zinc, and magnesium (Figure 2-9). It is almost impossible to obtain recommended amounts of calcium from conventional food sources available in developed countries without consuming milk or milk products. Milk is a poor source of iron and vitamin C. It is recommended that adults consume the equivalent of 2 cups of milk per day.

FIGURE 2-8

The major nutritional contribution of major food groups represented in most food guides: Nutrition recommendations for Canadians.

Each food group is essential because it provides its own set of nutrients.

Grain products	Fruits and vegetables	Milk products	Meat, alternatives	The food guide
Protein		Protein	Protein	Protein
		Fat	Fat	Fat
Carbohydrate	Carbohydrate			Carbohydrate
Fiber	Fiber			Fiber
Thiamin	Thiamin		Thiamin	Thiamin
Riboflavin		Riboflavin	Riboflavin	Riboflavin
Niacin			Niacin	Niacin
Folate	Folate		Folate	Folate
		Vitamin B_{12}	Vitamin B_{12}	Vitamin B_{12}
	Vitamin C			Vitamin C
	Vitamin A	Vitamin A		Vitamin A
		Vitamin D		Vitamin D
		Calcium		
Iron	Iron		Iron	Iron
Zinc		Zinc	Zinc	Zinc
Magnesium	Magnesium	Magnesium	Magnesium	Magnesium

Whole milk contains 3.3% fat; low-fat milk, 2% fat; and nonfat milk, less than 0.5% fat. Using low-fat and nonfat milk in place of whole milk provides less energy and reduces fat intake. Chocolate milk provides about 30% more kilocalories than does whole milk but has the same nutritional value as whole milk in other respects. Other flavored milks have the same nutritive value as milk, but they have more kilocalories.

In general, cheese has the same nutritive value as the milk from which it is made, but—depending on the method of processing—some nutrients may be lost in the whey. With cheese (as with milk), the protein, calcium, and riboflavin content increases as the fat content decreases. Cottage cheese, a good source of protein, is a variable source of calcium. The calcium source is good if the curd is first coagulated with the enzyme rennin and poor if acid coagulation is used before rennin is added. Such information is not readily available to the consumer.

Ice cream contains only half as much calcium per kilocalorie as does milk. Its kilocalorie content is increased by the addition of sugar and its high butterfat content. Low-fat and nonfat ice creams have been developed for people who want to reduce their kilocalorie and saturated fat intakes, but they have not proved popular.

Commercially prepared yogurt has often had its fat removed and replaced by nonfat milk, yielding an end product that is somewhat higher in calcium and milk sugar than milk. In yogurt with fruit preparations, up to 50% of the original milk may be replaced by fruit and sugar, thus reducing the content of calcium and other nutrients while increasing the kilocalorie content. Sour cream, cream cheese, and butter do not qualify for inclusion in this food group because of their high fat content and low nutrient density.

The per capita consumption of dairy products has been declining slowly but steadily since 1960, despite increases in the sales of yogurt, low-fat milk, and cheese. The decline has been attributed to concern about obesity and blood cholesterol levels, lack of understanding of the unique nutritive value of milk, competition from other beverages, and the development of dairy substitutes.

FRUITS AND VEGETABLES

Although fruits and vegetables are treated as separate groups in the Food Guide Pyramid, there is sufficient overlap in their nutritional contributions to discuss them together in this section.

The recommendation that the diet should contain three to five servings of vegetables and two to four servings of fruit per day gives no guidance about the most appropriate selection of vegetables and fruits. Foods in this group actually vary widely in their nutrient content. Nutrition education programs should promote the use of at least one daily serving of a fruit or a vegetable high in ascorbic acid and at least one serving of dark green, yellow, or orange vegetable or fruit as a source of vitamin A every other day. It is more realistic to suggest the consumption of the dark green, yellow, or orange vegetables every other day rather than every day

FIGURE 2-9

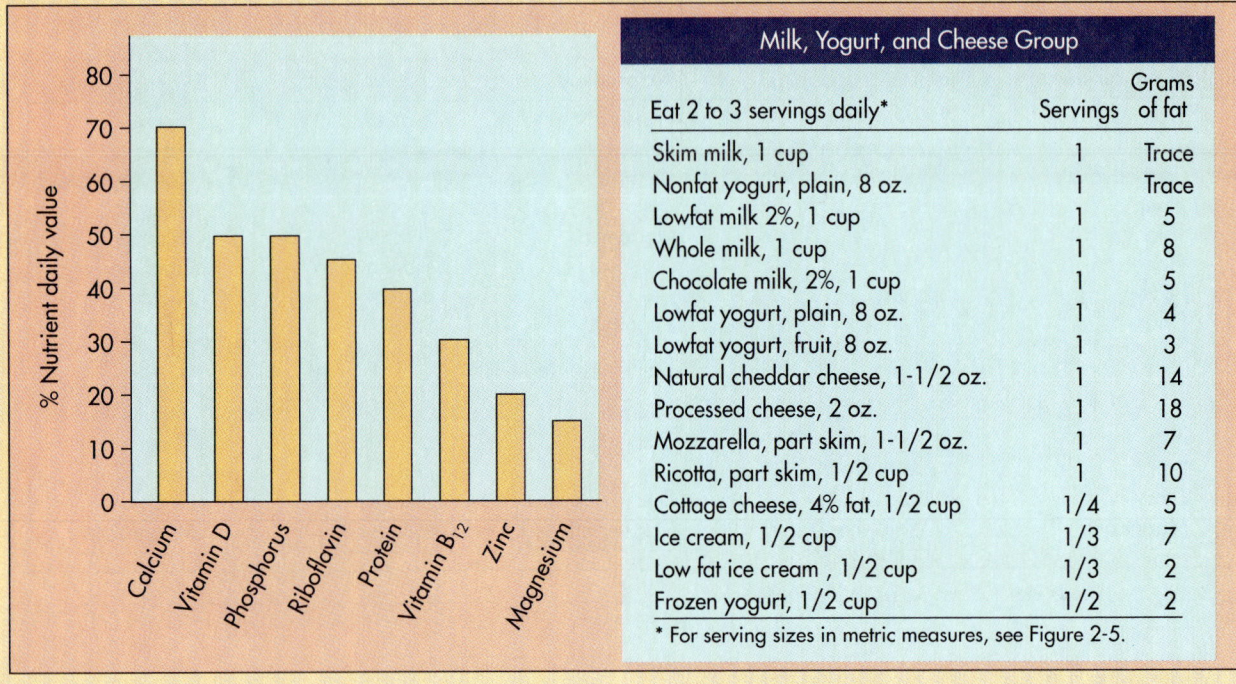

Percentage of RDA typically provided by the major nutrients in milk and milk products. (Based on nutrient analysis of two servings as recommended by USDA for a 2200-kcal diet. Food items were selected from the most frequently mentioned foods from this food group in NFCS, 1987-1988.)

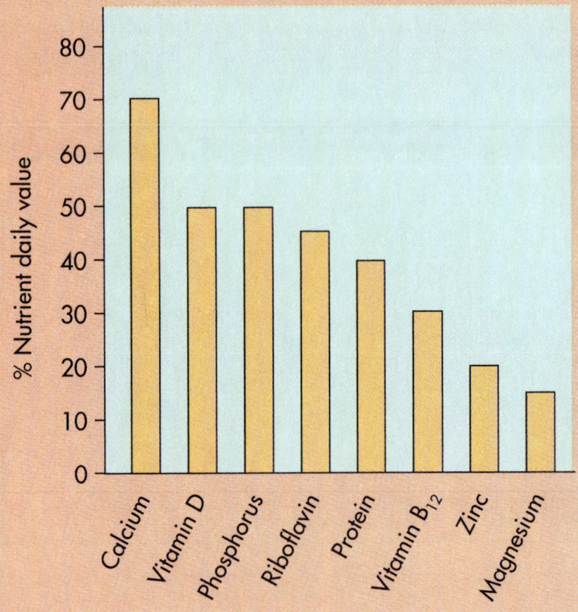

Milk, Yogurt, and Cheese Group

Eat 2 to 3 servings daily*	Servings	Grams of fat
Skim milk, 1 cup	1	Trace
Nonfat yogurt, plain, 8 oz.	1	Trace
Lowfat milk 2%, 1 cup	1	5
Whole milk, 1 cup	1	8
Chocolate milk, 2%, 1 cup	1	5
Lowfat yogurt, plain, 8 oz.	1	4
Lowfat yogurt, fruit, 8 oz.	1	3
Natural cheddar cheese, 1-1/2 oz.	1	14
Processed cheese, 2 oz.	1	18
Mozzarella, part skim, 1-1/2 oz.	1	7
Ricotta, part skim, 1/2 cup	1	10
Cottage cheese, 4% fat, 1/2 cup	1/4	5
Ice cream, 1/2 cup	1/3	7
Low fat ice cream , 1/2 cup	1/3	2
Frozen yogurt, 1/2 cup	1/2	2

* For serving sizes in metric measures, see Figure 2-5.

because they are rarely used on a daily basis. The stability of vitamin A, along with the body's ability to store it and the fact that rich sources of vitamin A usually provide more than 1 day's allowance per serving, also justifies the "every other day" advice. The practice of using butter, margarine, or salad oil to enhance the flavor of vegetables is desirable because fat enhances the absorption of vitamin A.

In general, vegetables and fruits are good sources of vitamins C, A, and B_6 and folate (Figures 2-10 and 2-11). They are also significant sources of dietary fiber.

The recommendation of two to four servings of fruit per day is primarily based on the fact that the most commonly consumed fruits are dependable sources of vitamin C. Because vitamin C is susceptible to oxidation, unstable in alkali, and soluble in water, fruits (and vegetables) need to be stored at low temperatures with limited access to air and sunlight, cooked in small amounts of water, baked or microwaved in relatively large unpeeled pieces, and served as soon as possible if they are to provide the greatest possible amount of vitamin C. In addition to citrus fruits, fruits and vegetables that are rich in vitamin C include strawberries, cantaloupe, cherries, broccoli, asparagus, spinach, and cabbage.

Although a 6-oz serving of fruit juice is considered an average serving in dietary guidance material, in practice servings usually range from 4 to 8 oz. For labeling purposes the FDA defines a serving as 8 oz. Citrus juices are generally rich sources of vitamin C, whereas other fruit juices provide varying amounts of vitamin C. Emphasis should be placed on those juices that provide at least 30 mg of vitamin C in a 4-oz portion, especially if the diet contains no other rich source of vitamin C. Many juices, such as apple and grape juice, that are low in natural vitamin C are now fortified to at least the 30 mg/4-oz level. Fortification with acerola, a tropical fruit rich in vitamin C, has no advantage over fortification with synthetic vitamin C. Current labeling regulations help consumers distinguish between fruit juices that contain only their natural sugars and those to which sugar or artificial coloring and flavoring have been added. There are few nutritional differences between fruit juices and fruit drinks or cocktails with less fruit but added ingredients.

The fruit and vegetable group typically supplies about 15% of the daily requirement of iron as nonheme iron, 25% of folate, 70% of vitamin B_6, and 50% of dietary fiber. The iron content of fruits and vegetables varies between different parts of the plants concerned,

FIGURE 2-10

Percent of RDA typically provided by the major nutrients in vegetables. (Based on nutrition analysis of four servings as recommended by the USDA for a 2200-kcal diet. Food items were selected from the most frequently mentioned foods from this food group in the NFCS, 1987-1988.)

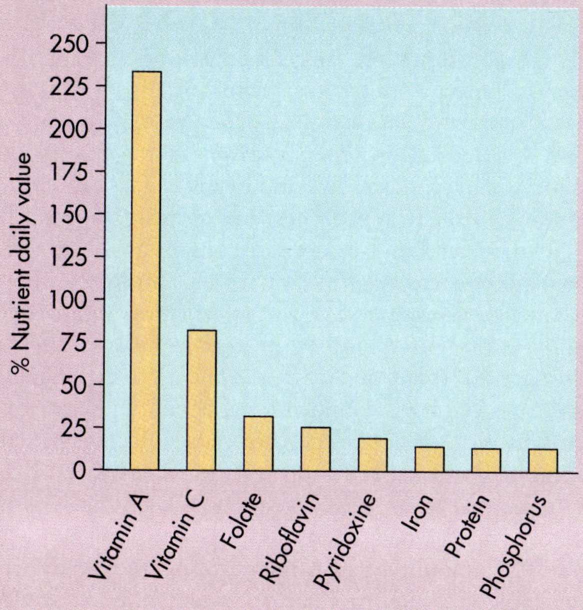

Vegetable Group

Eat 3 to 5 servings daily*	Servings	Grams of fat
Vegetables, cooked, 1/2 cup	1	Trace
Vegetables, leafy, raw, 1 cup	1	Trace
Vegetables, nonleafy, raw, chopped, 1/2 cup	1	Trace
Potatoes, scalloped, 1/2 cup	1	4
Potato salad, 1/2 cup	1	8
French fries, 10	1	8

* For serving sizes in metric measures, see Figure 2-5.

FIGURE 2-11

Percent of RDA prvided by the major nutrients in fruit. (Based on nutrient analysis of samples of three servings as recommended by the USDA for a 2200-kcal diet. Food items were selected from the most frequently mentioned foods from this food group in NFCS, 1987-1988.)

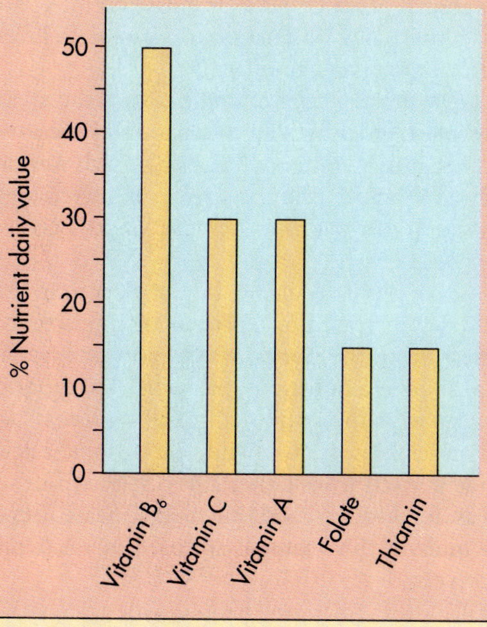

Fruit Group

Eat 2 to 4 servings daily*	Servings	Grams of fat
Whole fruit, medium apple, orange, banana	1	Trace
Fruit, raw or canned, 1/2 cup	1	Trace
Fruit juice, unsweetened, 3/4 cup	1	Trace
Avocado, 1/4, whole	1	9

* For serving sizes in metric measures, see Figure 2-5.

being greater in the leaves and fruits than in stems and roots.

The amount of calcium provided by fruits and vegetables is normally small, when compared with the amounts supplied by the milk and milk products group, but fruits and vegetables become an important source if milk intake is low. The vitamin C in fruits and vegetables offers the additional benefit of facilitating the absorption of iron and calcium from these foods.

The amount of trace minerals in fruits and vegetables depends on the amount in the soil in which the plants were grown. Because the fruits and vegetables on sale in most locations are derived from many different parts of the country and the world, problems caused by low trace mineral levels are unlikely. Such problems were more common when only locally grown produce was consumed.

Fruits and vegetables are generally poor sources of protein, and the protein they contain is of poorer quality than animal protein. Roots and tubers contain 2% protein and 20% carbohydrate, whereas legumes such as fresh peas and beans contain 4% protein and 13% carbohydrate.

The energy content of fruits and vegetables is generally low because of their high proportion of dietary fiber and water and their low fat content. Immature seeds, such as peas and beans, and starchy tubers, such as potatoes, contribute two to eight times as many kilocalories per serving as do celery, carrots, spinach, and cabbage. The kilocalorie content of a vegetable dish may easily be double or triple that of the basic vegetables alone because of such additions as table fats and sauces used during their preparation.

Another important nutritional benefit of fruits and vegetables is the bulk they provide because of their high fiber and water content. This bulk promotes gastrointestinal motility and generally facilitates the passage of food through the gastrointestinal tract, helping to prevent constipation. Recent evidence that diets low in dietary fiber may promote diverticulosis (see Chapter 3) and cancer of the colon is further reason for adequate amounts of fruits and vegetables to be included in the diet.

PROTEIN-RICH FOODS: MEAT, FISH, POULTRY, AND EGGS

The protein-rich foods provide over half of all the protein recommended in the diet, 61% of the vitamin B_{12}, from 33% to 50% of the iron, and 47% of the niacin. The nutritional profile of a typical selection of foods from the protein-rich group is shown in Figure 2-12. An average 3- to 4-oz serving of meat, fish, or poultry provides at least 20 g of protein.

The fat content of meat is variable, ranging from 1% by weight in low-fat processed meat to 40% by weight in prime beef. It depends on the type of animal and its diet, condition at time of slaughter, the cut of meat chosen, the extent to which excess fat is trimmed off, and the method of preparation. In general, the higher the grade of meat, the greater the amount of fat that is marbled throughout the muscle fiber and the higher the kilocalorie value. However, revisions in grading standards have lowered the fat content of higher grades.

Meat alternatives such as eggs, nuts, legumes, and peanut butter contain less protein than does meat per average serving. They are usually consumed in combination with cereal protein, however, so the total protein value of such foods as rice and beans and a peanut butter sandwich usually approaches that of meat and costs less.

Dried peas and beans can contain as much as 35% protein, whereas peanuts contain 15% protein. Although frequently consumed as meat substitutes, legumes contain less protein than does meat per 1000 kcal and their protein is of lower quality than is meat protein. Legumes do, however, have the nutritional benefit of being low in fat and high in fiber. They are most effectively used in combination with cereal protein, as in beans and rice or tofu lasagna or as meat extenders in such meals as chili con carne, in which beans are mixed with meat.

The amount of iron in meat and meat substitutes depends on which product is chosen. The iron content of organ meats (liver, kidney, and so on) is high but that of chicken and fish is low. Pork liver is not only the richest source of iron but also one of the least expensive. It is not a popular dietary item, however, and like all liver, it is high in cholesterol. The heme iron in meat is more efficiently absorbed than is iron from vegetables (23% vs. 8%).

Meat is a major source of zinc and phosphorus. Pork is a good source of thiamin, and vitamin B_{12} is derived only from animal products such as meat and milk. Most meat provides virtually no calcium or vitamin C. Liver is a rich source of iron and riboflavin.

Meat is the most expensive single item in the average diet, so people frequently plan meals around their meat or other protein-rich components. Fish, which was once a relatively low-priced protein source, is increasing in price as its popularity grows because of its perceived health benefits.

The use of meat available in the American food supply has been increased by a process that mechanically removes flesh from the bones of beef and poultry. The resulting product is a nutritious, palatable, and economic form of meat with the same high-quality protein, vitamins, and minerals as meat, in addition to some calcium and fluoride derived from bone. It is often used in such products as frankfurters and luncheon meats. Several million pounds of this material are used in the United States each year.

Typical North American diets provide adequate intakes of protein. There is little reason for promoting the use of additional servings of foods from the protein-rich

FIGURE 2-12

Percentage of RDA typically provided by the major nutrients in protein-rich foods. (Based on nutrient analysis of samples of two to four servings as representing 6 oz of protein as recommended by the USDA for a 2200-kcal diet. Food items were selected from the most frequently mentioned foods from this food group in NFCS, 1987-1988.)

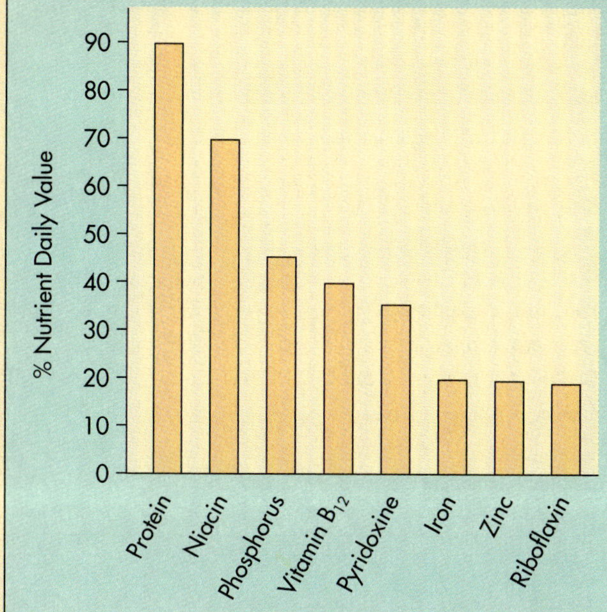

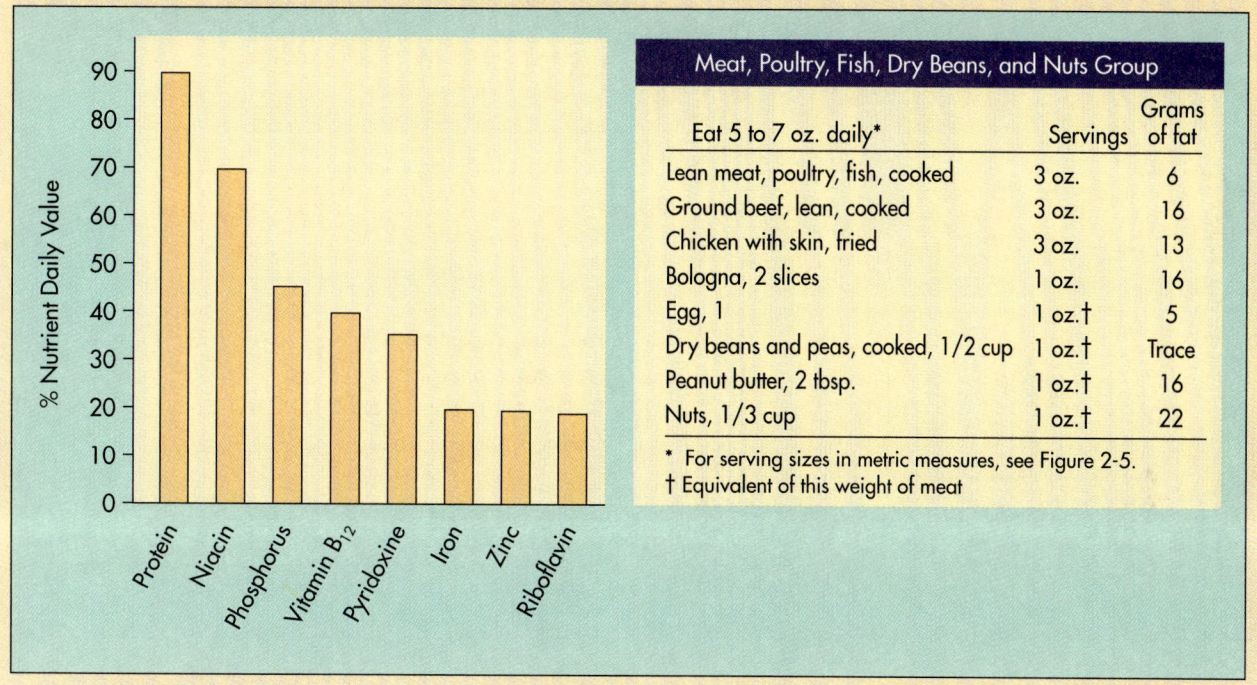

Meat, Poultry, Fish, Dry Beans, and Nuts Group

Eat 5 to 7 oz. daily*	Servings	Grams of fat
Lean meat, poultry, fish, cooked	3 oz.	6
Ground beef, lean, cooked	3 oz.	16
Chicken with skin, fried	3 oz.	13
Bologna, 2 slices	1 oz.	16
Egg, 1	1 oz.†	5
Dry beans and peas, cooked, 1/2 cup	1 oz.†	Trace
Peanut butter, 2 tbsp.	1 oz.†	16
Nuts, 1/3 cup	1 oz.†	22

* For serving sizes in metric measures, see Figure 2-5.
† Equivalent of this weight of meat

group. If meat is excluded from the diet, however, it becomes difficult to obtain sufficient vitamin B_{12} and zinc and iron absorption may become significantly less effective.

Many ecologically minded nutritionists recommend that people should eat foods from "lower on the food chain," using more vegetable protein and less animal products, especially meat. Their recommendations are based on the fact that the energy yield per acre of land is greater when vegetable products are consumed directly, rather than being used to feed animals that are then consumed. Much of the meat we eat, however, is derived from animals that are raised on land that is suitable only for grazing and so would not otherwise contribute to the food supply.

BREAD AND CEREAL PRODUCTS

The Food Guide Pyramid recommends consumption of 6 to 11 servings of cereal products per day, half of which should be whole grain cereals. It does not specifically mention the enriched cereals promoted in earlier guides. This reflects the growing recognition that enriched cereal products are not equivalent to their whole grain counterparts because the fiber, vitamin B_6, magnesium, and trace elements (such as zinc and iron) that are lost in milling are not returned during enrichment.

One of the major justifications for the inclusion of cereal products in the diet is their ability to supply a wide variety of nutrients at low cost. The major nutrient contributions made by members of this food group are shown in Figure 2-13. Foods from this group also make significant contributions to the total protein content of the diet. Although cereals are not themselves effective meat substitutes, they can be combined with other proteins to yield food containing high-quality protein overall. Examples are macaroni with cheese, rice with chicken, egg with toast, and cereal with milk.

The common belief that only such foods as bread, rice, macaroni, and dry or cooked cereal can be used to meet the 6 to 11 servings recommendation is not nutritionally justified. Any product made primarily of flour is included within this group, including waffles, muffins, pancakes, pastries, cakes, and cookies. The use of milk or nonfat milk solids in many baked products increases their calcium and protein content. Unfortunately, the addition of sugar and fat also increases the kilocalories supplied and decreases nutrient density.

The addition of sugar to ready-to-eat cereals has become a highly controversial issue. Opponents of this

FIGURE 2-13

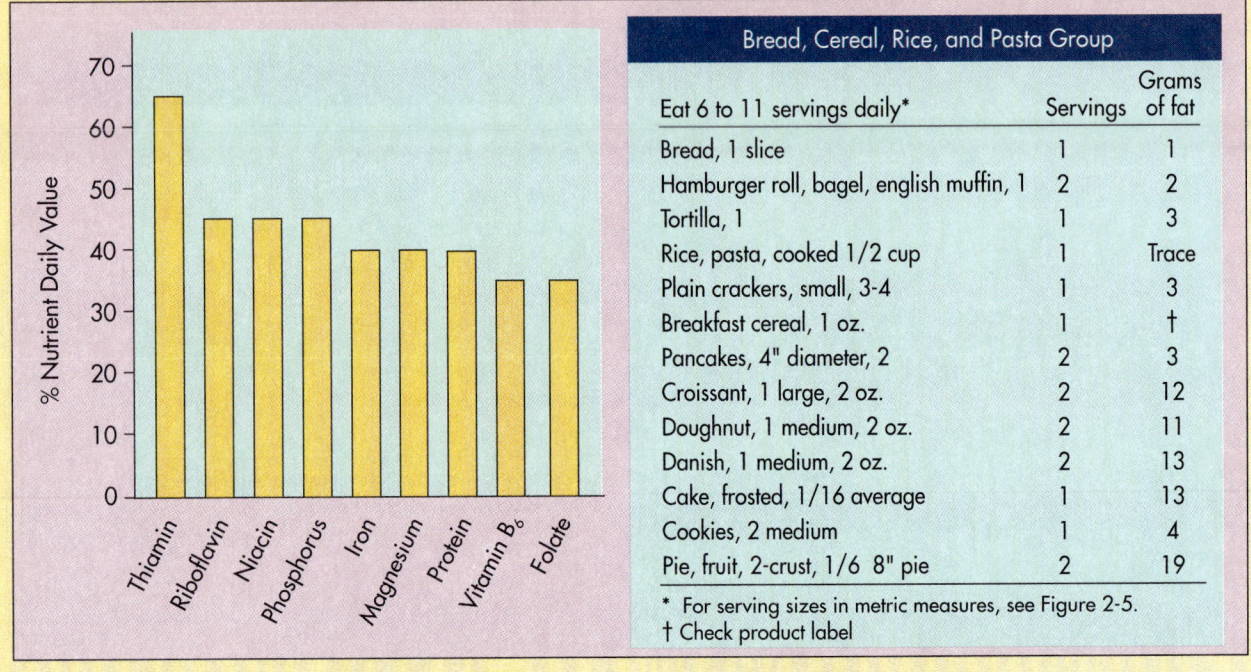

Percentage of RDA typically provided by the major nutrients in cereal products. (Based on nutrient analysis of samples of nine servings as recommended by the USDA for a 2200-kcal diet. Food items were selected from the most frequently mentioned foods in this food group in NFCS, 1987-1988.)

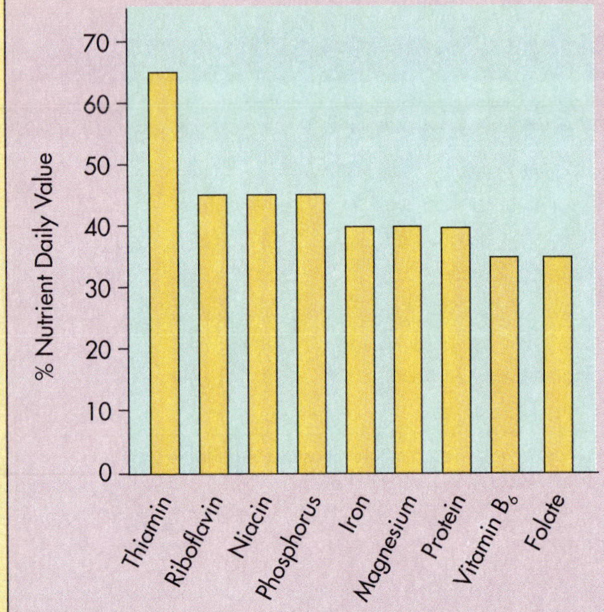

Bread, Cereal, Rice, and Pasta Group

Eat 6 to 11 servings daily*	Servings	Grams of fat
Bread, 1 slice	1	1
Hamburger roll, bagel, english muffin, 1	2	2
Tortilla, 1	1	3
Rice, pasta, cooked 1/2 cup	1	Trace
Plain crackers, small, 3-4	1	3
Breakfast cereal, 1 oz.	1	†
Pancakes, 4" diameter, 2	2	3
Croissant, 1 large, 2 oz.	2	12
Doughnut, 1 medium, 2 oz.	2	11
Danish, 1 medium, 2 oz.	2	13
Cake, frosted, 1/16 average	1	13
Cookies, 2 medium	1	4
Pie, fruit, 2-crust, 1/6 8" pie	2	19

* For serving sizes in metric measures, see Figure 2-5.
† Check product label

practice question the value of including sugar as an integral part of the product, often at excessive levels, especially because people who want sugar can readily add it themselves. Those in favor of the addition of sugar point out that the amount present in the cereal is often less than the amount that people add themselves if none had been added during processing. Cereal with 1 tablespoon of sugar added per 1-oz serving is 50% sugar by weight. Cereal with 1 teaspoon of added sugar per ounce is 16% sugar by weight. Both are widely available. Obviously, any "cereal" that is 50% sugar is also only 50% cereal and so provides a proportionately smaller amount of the nutrients provided by cereal that is 100% cereal.

Converted rice is prepared by parboiling the rice kernels before polishing. During this process the nutrients normally concentrated in the outer husk are driven into the kernel, where they remain when the husk is removed. This produces a refined product that has been enriched with its own original nutrients. Converted rice has been used in India for many years. It should be distinguished from quick-cook rice, which does not retain the nutrients from the husk.

Almost the only people in America who do not obtain the recommended number of servings from the cereal group are some young girls and people on weight-reducing diets, who tend to avoid cereal products unwisely.

FOUNDATIONS OF AN ADEQUATE DIET

Figure 2-14 indicates the percentage of contribution that foods from each food group in the Food Guide Pyramid make to the total intake of various nutrients in the typical North American diet. As it illustrates, an intake close to the RDA of all nutrients can be obtained by consuming each day a 2200-kcal diet that includes the following, as recommended by the USDA:

- Two servings from the milk, yogurt, and cheese group
- Two servings from the meat, poultry, fish, dry beans, eggs, and nuts group (1 serving = 3 oz meat or its equivalent)
- Four servings from the vegetable group
- Three servings from the fruit group
- Nine servings from the bread, cereal, rice, and pasta group

The actual number of servings from each group that is consumed should depend on each person's total energy requirements. Table 2-7 shows how three different diets, each adhering to the recommendations within the Food Guide Pyramid, can lead to intakes of 1600, 2200, or 2800 kcal/day. These examples make it clear that the recommendations of the Food Guide Pyramid

FIGURE 2-14

Complementary contributions of foods from the five food groups of the Food Guide Pyramid to the total content of key nutrients in the typical North American diet.

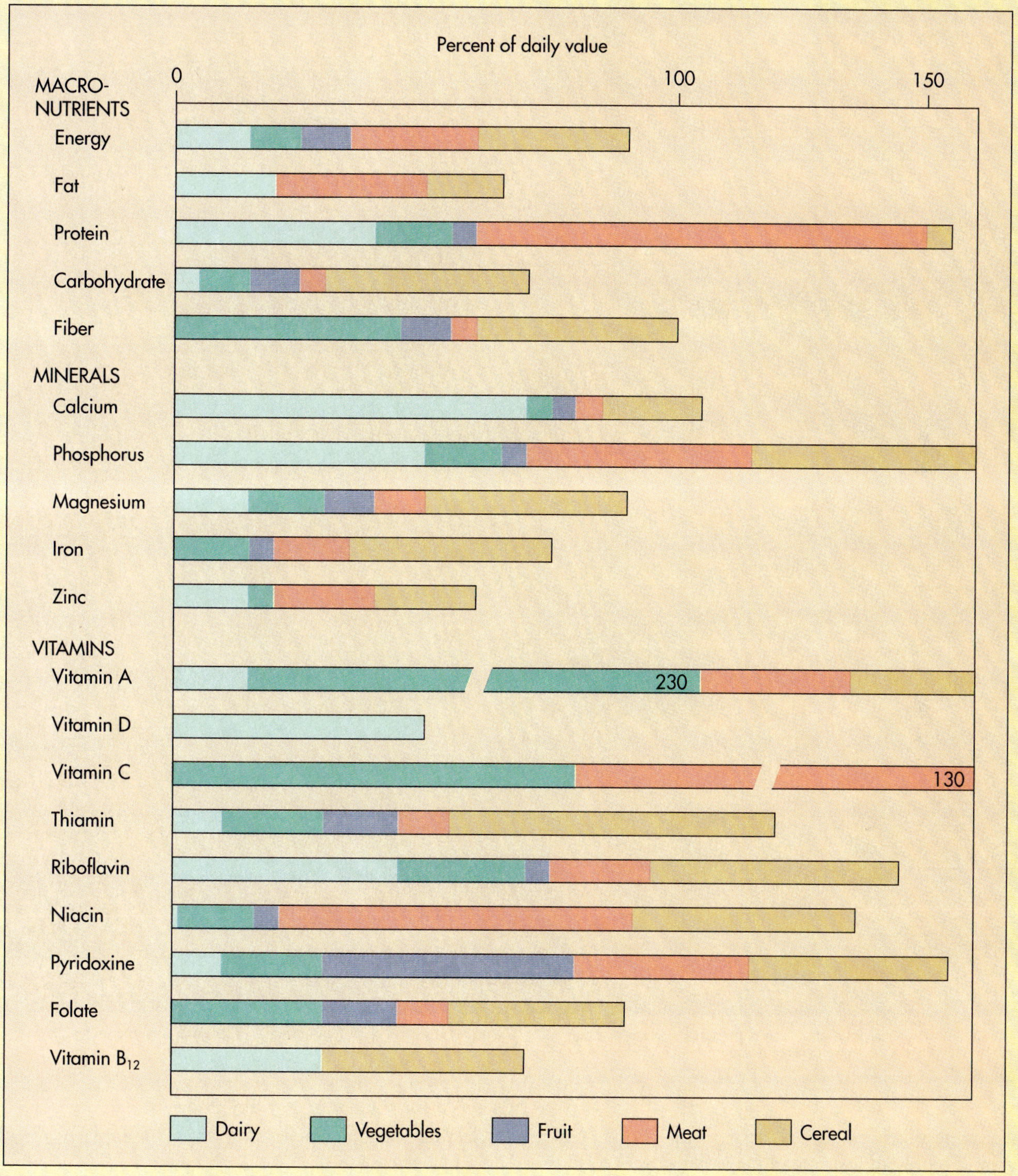

leave plenty of scope for adjusting the total kilocalorie content of the diet to meet individual needs.

The Food Guide Pyramid also allows great variety in the diet. Since the first dietary standards were published, the Food and Nutrition Board has emphasized that the recommended nutritional goals can be met in innumerable different ways using a virtually unlimited number of foods. Following the recommendations within the Food Guide Pyramid definitely does not require a person to eat a limited and unvaried diet. It is also fair to say that

Trade-offs in Food Choices Within Various Food Categories

FOR FRUIT

½ cup frozen sweetened fruit = ½ cup of fresh or frozen unsweetened fruit + 6 tsp sugar
½ cup fruit, canned in heavy syrup = ½ cup unsweetened fruit + 4 tsp sugar
½ cup fruit, canned in light syrup = ½ cup unsweetened fruit + 2 tsp sugar

FOR A STARCHY VEGETABLE

10 French fries = 1 medium boiled potato + 2 tsp fat

FOR MEAT ALTERNATES

½ cup cooked dried beans or peas + 1 tsp fat = 1 oz lean meat, fish, or poultry + 1 slice of bread
2 Tbsp peanut butter = 1 oz lean meat, fish, or poultry + 3 tsp fat
¼ cup seeds = 1 oz lean meat, fish, or poultry + 4 tsp fat
⅓ cup nuts = 1 oz lean meat, fish, or poultry + 5 tsp fat

FOR MEAT, FISH, POULTRY, AND EGGS

2 oz bologna = 1 oz lean meat, fish, or poultry + 3 tsp fat
½ chicken breast, batter fried = ½ breast, roasted + 1 slice white bread + 2 tsp fat

FOR MILK, YOGURT, AND CHEESE

1 cup whole milk = 1 cup skim milk + 2 tsp fat
1 cup 2% milk = 1 cup skim milk + 1 tsp fat
1 cup low-fat (2%) chocolate milk = 1 cup skim milk + 1 tsp fat + 3 tsp sugar
8 oz plain low-fat yogurt = 1 cup skim milk + 1 tsp fat
8 oz low-fat vanilla yogurt = 1 cup skim milk + 1 tsp fat + 4 tsp sugar
8 oz low-fat fruit yogurt = 1 cup skim milk + 1 tsp fat + 7 tsp sugar
1½ oz natural cheese = 1 cup skim milk + 3 tsp fat
2 oz processed American cheese = 1 cup skim milk + 4 tsp fat
Cottage cheese contains less calcium than other cheeses; ½ cup cottage cheese contains only as much calcium as found in ¼ cup of milk, while providing considerably more kilocalories.

FOR DESSERTS AND SNACK FOODS

½ cup ice cream = ⅓ cup skim milk + 2 tsp fat + 3 tsp sugar
½ cup ice milk = ⅓ cup skim milk + 1 tsp fat + 3 tsp sugar
½ cup low-fat frozen yogurt = ⅓ cup skim milk + 4 tsp sugar
1/16 of a white layer cake with chocolate frosting = 1 slice bread + 6 tsp sugar + 3 tsp fat
2 oatmeal cookies = 1 slice bread + 1 tsp sugar + 1 tsp fat
⅙ of 9" apple pie = 2 slices bread + ⅓ medium apple + 6 tsp sugar + 3 tsp fat
18 potato chips = 1 medium boiled potato + 3 tsp fat

FOR FATS

1 tsp mayonnaise = 1 tsp margarine, butter, or oil
2 tsp Italian salad dressing = 1 tsp margarine, butter, or oil
3 tsp cream cheese = 1 tsp margarine, butter, or oil
4 tsp light cream = 1 tsp margarine, butter, or oil
5 tsp sour cream = 1 tsp margarine, butter, or oil

FOR SWEETS

(These trade-offs are based on approximate kilocalorie content.)
1 tsp jam or jelly = 1 tsp sugar, syrup, or molasses
Chocolate bar, 1.05 oz = 5 tsp sugar + 2 tsp fat
12 oz noncarbonated fruit drink, ade, or punch = 12 tsp sugar
12 oz cola = 9 tsp sugar

From USDA Human Nutrition Information Service: *Developing a food guidance system for "Better eating for better health," a nutrition course for adults,* Admin Report No 377, Hyattsville, Md, 1985, U.S. Government Printing Office.

the suggestions embodied within the Food Guide Pyramid represent just one of many patterns of food use that could be devised to provide a nutritionally adequate diet. Following such a plan as the Food Guide Pyramid usually ensures that a person's diet is nutritionally adequate, but the failure to follow that guidance does not necessarily result in a nutritionally deficient diet. The box above outlines alternatives, or trade-offs, in selecting food, which may make compliance with guidelines easier.

It is also relevant to bear in mind that the Food Guide Pyramid is intended to help people in choosing a healthful diet that is compatible with North American tastes, food availability, and culture. Some other cultures have eating patterns that appear to be different from ours, yet still provide an adequate nutrient intake. In most cases, they, too, conform to the recommendations of the Food Guide Pyramid.

TABLES OF FOOD COMPOSITION

To determine whether the amount of a nutrient in any diet is adequate, it is necessary to perform calculations using information on food intake and data from tables listing the nutrient content of different foods. Many tables of food composition, such as that in Appendix E, have been developed to assist in this task. Most are derived from data provided by the USDA and published in a series within the USDA Handbook No. 8, *Composition of Foods—Raw, Processed and Prepared.*

To get useful information from a food composition table, the kind and amount of each food eaten by the person whose diet is being assessed and the way in which the food was prepared must first be known. This requires that an accurate record be kept of all food consumed during some period. This record must include everything added to basic foods, such as table fats (butter, margarine, and so on), mayonnaise, condiments, sweeteners, and all beverages consumed. Many such items are easily overlooked when food intake is recorded. The record must also reflect food actually eaten and not include any food that was served but left uneaten. The record obviously must also include all snack items and all foods eaten at formal mealtimes.

Having recorded the types and amounts of foods consumed as accurately as possible (using actual weights or measures wherever possible, rather than rough estimates), tables of food composition can then be used to calculate an estimate of the amount of any or all of the 17 to 24 nutrients usually listed in such tables that the diet being investigated actually contained. The total amounts of nutrients that were consumed can then be compared with the RDAs for the age, gender, and physiological condition of the person eating the food. This basic system of carefully recording food intake and then calculating nutrient intakes from tables is the least expensive and most widely used method for estimating nutrient intakes.

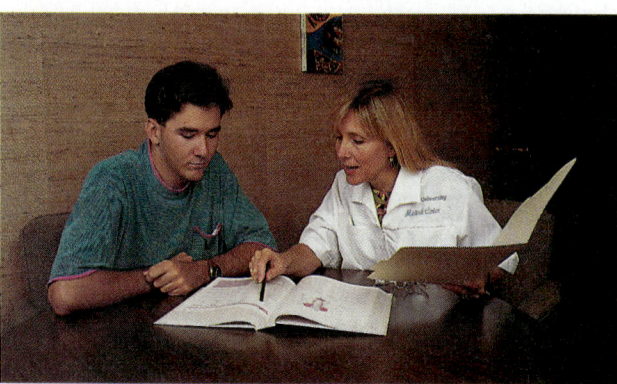

Food tables are an indispensable tool in providing nutrition counseling.

To use food composition tables appropriately, one must understand how they were developed and recognize their limitations. The data within the tables have come from the careful chemical analysis of foods in laboratories of the government, universities, and food industries. The tables list just one figure per nutrient per food, which in reality is an appropriately weighted average of all the relevant analytical results available. Any figure in a table of food composition may not be precisely accurate for a particular sample of the food eaten on a particular day. It is, however, a good estimate of the average amount of nutrient obtained from any food eaten on a regular basis.

These data have been available in the USDA Handbook No. 8, *Composition of Foods—Raw, Processed and Prepared,* originally published in 1916 and revised in 1950 and 1963. A revision involving 21 segments, each devoted to a particular food group, was completed in 1991. These segments provide data on over 60 different nutrients, including vitamins, minerals, and amino acids for over 4000 foods. In addition to providing information on the nutrient content of 1 lb "as purchased" (AP) and of the "edible portion" (EP) of an average serving of a 100-g portion, the tables and many computer programs based on them indicate the number of analyses on which each value was based and the range of values

Available Revised Units of Handbook 8

8-1:	Dairy and egg products
8-2:	Spices and herbs
8-3:	Baby foods
8-4:	Fats and oils
8-5:	Poultry products
8-6:	Soups, sauces, and gravies
8-7:	Sausages and luncheon meats
8-8:	Breakfast cereals
8-9:	Fruits
8-10:	Pork products
8-11:	Vegetables
8-12:	Nuts
8-13:	Beef
8-14:	Beverages
8-15:	Finfish and shellfish
8-16:	Legumes and legume products
8-17:	Lamb, veal, and game products
8-18:	Baked products
8-19:	Snacks and sweets
8-20:	Cereal grains and pasta
8-21:	Fast foods

that has been used to derive the single value listed. Differences in the values given for the same food over time may reflect changes in marketing and processing techniques or improved methods of analysis. For example, the selective breeding of poultry has produced animals with a reduced fat content, the use of dried milk solids in bread has led to an increase in its calcium content, the use of fat substitutes and cooking oil with a higher proportion of unsaturated fatty acids has changed the character of the fat in many food products, and new analytical techniques have provided more accurate information on the iron content of meat.

The USDA has now set up a computerized data bank that can be constantly updated to provide the nutritional information needed by those involved in nutritional evaluation and counseling. Many independent data bases also exist, mainly incorporating the same information. The legal requirement for industries using nutrient labeling to provide analytical data in support of claims on a label has greatly increased the amount of food composition data available and the public's access to it.

The number of analyses used to determine any one value varies widely, depending on the food and nutrient concerned. In some cases, only a few or even just one analytical report was available. In other cases, data were available on several varieties of the same food at different times of the year and from various geographical areas. A wide range of values, for example, was available for the vitamin C content of oranges. The single value appearing in the official table represents a weighted average using marketing information on the extent to which each variety of orange is consumed, the percentage of domestic oranges coming from each geographical area, and the size of the crop in each season. The value in the table may not be accurate for any one specific orange, but it provides an appropriate representative value for oranges consumed in the United States, in general.

In addition to varietal, seasonal, and geographical differences in the nutrient content of foods, other factors that must be considered in some cases are the loss or gain in nutrient content through the various stages of harvesting, handling, commercial processing, packaging, storage, display, home preparation, cooking, and serving. The amount of each nutrient in each food is influenced by such factors in its own unique way. For example, the vitamin A content of sweet potatoes varies with the maturity of the crop at harvest and the conditions in which it is stored, the vitamin A content in butter varies with the seasons of the year, the vitamin C content of oranges varies with the site of production and the time of harvesting, and the amount of vitamin A provided by most plant foods depends on which parts of the plants are consumed.

Niacin values in food composition tables reflect only preformed niacin, not the niacin produced by conversion of the amino acid tryptophan. As a result the niacin values in such tables underestimate the amount of the vitamin available from protein-rich (and therefore tryptophan-rich) foods. Similarly, vitamin C values are for reduced ascorbic acid only and do not include the dehydroascorbic acid in some fruits and vegetables. Thus the vitamin C value of many fruits and vegetables may be underestimated when calculated by the use of tables.

In addition to the food composition tables given in Appendix E or the USDA Handbook No. 8, *Composition of Foods—Raw, Processed and Prepared,* many other similar tables are available that contain comparable and in some cases additional scientifically sound data. The student of nutrition should not be concerned to find small differences between the values listed in different tables. There will always be slight differences in the values obtained by different analytical groups working at different times in different places and perhaps using slightly different techniques. As a general rule, alternative values that differ by no more than 10% can be considered essentially the same. Information on exactly how the data within the tables are obtained can be found in the preface and appendix of each section of the Handbook No. 8, *Composition of Foods—Raw, Processed and Prepared,* which is available from the U.S. Government Printing Office.

In spite of some recognized limitations, as considered previously, the use of food composition tables allows estimates of the nutritive content of diets that prove to be comparable with those obtained (at much greater cost) by direct chemical analysis of an individual's actual diet. The food composition tables are an indispensable tool for everyone who evaluates the nutritional value of food supplies, develops food distribution programs, plans and evaluates food consumption surveys, provides nutritional counseling, and estimates the nutrient content of individual diets. The use of the tables has been greatly facilitated by their availability on computer disks.

Keeping tables of food composition up to date is a continuous task currently being complicated by the arrival of various genetically engineered and other novel foods on the market, because of the impact of biotechnology on food production. Again, however, the speed and power of computer technology greatly assist the USDA in its efforts to make available the accurate food composition data so essential to the work of nutritionists everywhere.

NUTRIENT DENSITY

The information in tables of food composition can be used to assess which of several sources of a nutrient provides the greatest amount of the nutrient relative to kilocalories. Many people who must watch their kilocalorie intake, however, wish to know which sources provide an adequate nutrient intake but a low kilocalorie intake. To provide some guidance to such people, nutritionists have developed the concept of an **index of nutrient quality (INQ)**,[25] which measures the **nutrient density** of a food in terms of its kilocalorie content as follows:

$$\text{INQ} = \frac{\text{\% OF RDA OF A SPECIFIC NUTRIENT PROVIDED BY A FOOD}}{\text{\% OF ENERGY REQUIREMENT PROVIDED BY THE FOOD}}$$

For example, Appendix E tells us that 8 oz of whole milk provides 150 kcal of energy, 291 mg of calcium, and 2 mg of vitamin C. The relevant RDAs for women aged 23 through 50 are 2200 kcal, 800 mg of calcium, and 60 mg of vitamin C. The 8 oz of milk therefore provides 7% of such women's energy needs, 36% of their calcium needs, and 3.3% of their vitamin C needs. The nutrient density (or INQ) of the milk for calcium for such women is therefore $^{36}/_{7}$ = 5, whereas the INQ of the milk for vitamin C is $^{3.3}/_{7}$ = 0.5 (see box).

The higher the INQ value is, the better the food is as a source of the nutrient concerned. Any food that has an INQ of 1 or more for a nutrient is making as great a contribution to the need for that nutrient as it is to the need for energy. This means that if that food is the sole source of energy in the diet, it provides at least the full day's requirement of the nutrient concerned. On the basis of nutrient density, milk is considered a good source of calcium and a fair source of vitamin C.

Calculation of Nutrient Density or Index of Nutrient Quality (INQ)

	Amount Provided in 8 oz Milk (Whole)	RDA* for Women, Age 23-50 yr	Percentage of RDA Provided by 8 oz Milk (Whole)
Calories energy	150 kcal	2200 kcal	$\frac{150}{2200} \times 100 = 7\%$
Calcium	291 mg	800 mg	$\frac{291}{800} \times 100 = 36\%$
Vitamin C	2 mg	60 mg	$\frac{2}{60} \times 100 = 3.3\%$

Nutrient density

$$\text{FOR CALCIUM} = \frac{\text{\% RDA}}{\text{\% ENERGY}} = \frac{36}{7} = 5.0$$

$$\text{FOR VITAMIN C} = \frac{\text{\% RDA}}{\text{\% ENERGY}} = \frac{3.3}{7} = 0.5$$

*RDA used varies with age and gender. Therefore INQ will be different for different people. If calculating the INQ for a population rather than a specific age or gender group, use the RDAs for both nutrient and an appropriate energy value—usually 2200 kcal for women and 3000 kcal for men.

It has been proposed that if a food has an INQ of 1 or more for four nutrients or an INQ of 2 or more for two nutrients, it should be regarded as "nutritious" because it makes a significant contribution to total nutrient intake.[26] Most foods that have been traditionally considered to be nutritionally beneficial are found to meet these quantitative criteria. Foods that do not meet the criteria are foods with a high kilocalorie density, usually because of the addition of sugar, starch, or fat during their preparation. Many foods, however, that do not meet the standard for nutrition, do make significant worthwhile contributions to the total nutritional value of a diet. Thus a food that is not regarded as nutritious in terms of the INQ criteria should not necessarily be regarded as having no nutritional value.

As a general rule, a food is considered as a distinct "source" of a specific nutrient if the INQ value for that nutrient in the food is greater than 1 *and* one serving of the food provides at least 2% of the DV for the nutrient. To qualify as a "good source" or an "excellent source" of the nutrient, the INQ value must be at least 1.5 and the food must provide at least 10% of the DV per serving.[8]

U.S. DIETARY SURVEYS

Most of our information on the adequacy of the American diet comes from two major surveys. One, the **Nationwide Food Consumption Survey (NFCS),** is conducted every 10 years by the USDA. In the 1987-to-1988 NFCS, data were gathered on the food intake of about 8000 individuals over 3 consecutive days. The information obtained was used to assess how closely the nutrient intake by the various age and gender groups corresponded to the appropriate RDAs. The information can also be used to investigate the relationship of nutrition to social factors such as income, education, geographical location, size of a household, and the meal-taking patterns within a household or outside the home. In 1985 the USDA also set up a continuous study of the food intake of women aged 23 through 50 and their children aged 1 through 5. This Continuing Survey of Food Intake of Individuals (CSFII) is performed every year, except for the years in which the regular 10-year survey of households and individuals is being performed.

The second major survey is the **National Health and Nutrition Examination Survey (NHANES),** which is conducted approximately every 5 years on a random sample of the American population by the National Center for Health Statistics (NCHS). It gathers information on the food intake of approximately 20,000 people over a 24-hour period. It also collects data on the health status of the participants and includes analyses of

National Health and Nutrition Examination Survey III

I. DIETARY COMPONENTS

Food energy	Riboflavin
Protein	Niacin
Total fat	Vitamin B_6
Saturated fatty acids	Vitamin B_{12}
Monounsaturated fatty acids	Calcium
	Phosphorus
Polyunsaturated fatty acids	Magnesium
	Iron
Cholesterol	Carotenes
Carbohydrate	Vitamin E
Dietary fiber	Folate
Vitamin A (IU)	Zinc
Vitamin A (RE)	Copper
Vitamin C	Sodium
Thiamin	Potassium

II. HEMATOLOGICAL AND BIOCHEMICAL DATA

Complete blood cell count (WBC, RBC, MCV, MCHC, hematocrit, hemoglobin)
Red blood cell distribution width
Iron and total iron binding capacity (TIBC)
Ferritin
Protoporphyrin
Folate (serum and red blood cell)
Retinol and retinyl ester
Carotenoids (total and individual)
Vitamin E
Vitamin C
25-Hydroxyvitamin D
Calcium (serum and ionized)
Selenium
Cholesterol (total and high-density lipoprotein)
Triglycerides
Apolipoproteins A and B
Lead
Cadmium

III. ANTHROPOMETRIC MEASUREMENTS

Height	Circumference
Standing	Head
Sitting	Mid-thigh
Knee	Calf
Length	Waist
Upper leg	Buttocks
Upper arm	Mid–upper arm
Breadth	Skinfold
Biiliac	Subscapular
Elbow	Suprailiac
Wrist	Mid-thigh
Biacromial	Triceps

blood and urine samples and anthropometric measurements (see box). These data allow possible relationships between dietary habits and specific health problems to be explored. Because of day-to-day variations in people's diets, it is more difficult to assess a person's typical nutrient intake on the basis of such a 1-day survey than on the basis of the longer 3-day period surveyed in the NFCS. From 1985 to 1986 the NCHS also undertook a survey of food intake among the Spanish-speaking population, now referred to as the Hispanic HANES.

NUTRIENT SUPPLEMENTATION—MORE HAZARD THAN HELP?

Forty years ago nutritionists would have found it hard to imagine a time when they would be more concerned about the consequences of the overuse of nutrients than with the problems of nutritional deficiencies. Yet that is the situation facing nutritionists today. The success of their efforts to persuade people of the importance of nutrition has had an unfortunate result: many people have lost confidence in the ability of the normal food supply to provide them with adequate nutrition. Not surprisingly, entrepreneurs have been quick to capitalize on these fears, which have led to the multibillion-dollar business generally referred to as the "health food industry." Annual sales of vitamins alone exceed $4 billion, providing clear evidence of the wide prevalence of what could be called "vitamin mania." It is of great concern that many people decide to take megadoses of vitamins on the basis of their own intuition or skillful advertising, rather than as a result of any scientific consideration of the likely benefits and risks.

Megadoses of vitamins have been available and widely used for a relatively short time, so nutritionists are concerned that we have not yet had time to learn any or all of the possible harmful effects of megavitamin consumption. Harmful effects resulting from megadoses of some vitamins may take years to develop. For example, neurological problems associated with overuse of vitamin B_6 take a long time to appear, and the diarrhea associated with vitamin C overuse was recognized only after many people had consumed large amounts for long periods. Fortunately, megadoses of minerals are less available.

Many users of nutrient supplements turn to them because they fear illness rather than because they are ill. In doing so, they can be exposing themselves to increased health risks rather than protecting their health. Those who do turn to multinutrient mineral/vitamin products because they are already ill may delay seeking the medical guidance that could help them because they have placed their trust in pills instead.

The promotion of megadoses of nutrients for the prevention and cure of a wide range of conditions is frequently based on unreliable anecdotal evidence rather than scientifically sound trials. People who begin to take supplements often embark on several "health-promoting" actions at the same time, making it difficult to distinguish any possible effects of the nutrients from beneficial effects of increased exercise, improved diet, reduced intake of alcohol or use of tobacco, or measures that reduce stress.

Studies have shown that many people taking nutrient supplements are consuming diets that already provide ample amounts of the nutrients concerned but that may provide only marginal amounts of some nutrients that are not present in the supplements being used. This may worsen an existing imbalance in nutrient intake, which can make a person's overall nutritional situation worse rather than better.

The nutrient supplementation industry thrives only in relatively affluent societies, but the poorest members of these societies are often the ones who are enticed into wasting their money on unnecessary supplements. Elderly persons, for example, are targets for door-to-door salespersons who prey on old people's fears that they may become ill and unable to look after themselves. To these persons, any product that promises to maintain their health and independence has tremendous appeal. Similarly, mothers concerned about their children's health are all too willing to accept the assurance of good nutrition that they believe supplements can provide. Many children's supplements are sold as tasty, chewable, candylike pills, which can encourage the child to take more than the prescribed amount. Toxicities resulting from the overuse of vitamin D or iron are just two examples of the potential hazards of self-directed supplementation in both children and adults.

Some substances are promoted as "vitamins" despite there being no evidence to suggest that they play any vitamin-like role in the body. "Vitamin B_{17}," named after a World War II bomber because of the way it was expected to attack a variety of health problems, is an example of such a nonnutrient substance.

Many of the multinutrient supplements being marketed contain an irrational mixture of nutrients. A preparation may contain 10 mg of vitamin B_1, for example, accompanied by labeling stating that this is 10 times the RDA, and also contain 10 mg of vitamin C, which is only one sixth of the RDA. Similarly, a long list of ingredients on a nutritional supplement may mislead customers who choose a product simply on the basis of how many different ingredients it contains. Many of the ingredients may in fact be nonnutrient substances, such as hesperidin or rutin.

Another deceptive practice is the listing of ingredients by the least familiar of their alternative names or in other deceiving ways. Listing all the amino acids within a protein, for example, produces a seemingly impressive array of mysterious-sounding ingredients, yet they are all readily available from any protein-rich food.

The public is also being trained to believe that "natural" vitamins (or sugars, and so on) are desirable, whereas synthetic products are of less benefit or even bad for us. Our cells, however, cannot distinguish between a vitamin derived from a chemistry laboratory and one derived from a natural food.

If people wish to take nutritional supplements, perhaps "just to be sure" they are receiving adequate nutrition, they should be advised to choose a low-level and well-balanced supplement that provides no more than 50% of the RDA of all or most of the vitamins (and perhaps minerals) the body requires. Such products can be hard to find because the higher level supplements tend to sell better to people who always believe that more is better. It is acceptable to divide the pills of a high-level supplement, however, if suitable low-level supplements cannot be found. Everyone should certainly be advised to avoid taking many different pills containing high levels of nutrients.

ISSUES AND OPINIONS

Learning What People Eat

Nutritionists have many reasons for finding out what people are eating. Those who give advice on diet, particularly on dietary modifications, must know what a person is eating to know what aspects of the diet to reinforce and what aspects to try to modify. Nutritionists involved in establishing dietary guidelines for a population must know what the population is eating before they can suggest any desired changes. Nutritionists responsible for setting dietary standards must take into consideration the dietary intakes associated with a high level of health, as well as the level of intake that apparently fails to meet needs. Epidemiologists concerned with identifying which eating habits are associated with health or disease also rely on information about the diet of the population.

How do all of these professionals get the information they need? In general, they **observe** the target audience; they **ask** them what they eat; and they **make inferences** from information on the foods available to specific groups of people. The precision and usefulness of the data obtained influence the confidence with which any judgments on the suitability of diets can be made.

OBSERVATIONS

An investigator who chooses to get information by observing an individual or group must be able to observe the subject in all situations in which the relevant food intake is likely to occur. It is possible to do this unobtrusively by recording eating within a fairly limited living area with the use of hidden cameras. This, however, is an expensive approach that is also seen as an invasion of privacy. Observations may also be done in an institutional setting by recording the food served to the individual and what food is returned uneaten. This relies on the assumption that the person being studied does not have any other source of food or the opportunity to offer the food to someone else. Any attempt to observe an individual by following him or her all day is likely to result in a change in eating behavior and therefore yields unreliable data.

ASKING

Asking what a person eats may be done retrospectively, as in a 24-hour recall, in which the subject has not been warned that he or she will be asked to provide the information at the end of the period. The success of this method is dependent on the person's memory and his or her ability to estimate portion sizes and to describe the food with sufficient accuracy. Few untrained people can supply reliable information based on recall periods longer than 1 day. However, an interviewer who is trained to ask appropriate questions may be able to elicit a more complete response.

Prospective records, prepared after people have been given instruction, are a more common source of information. Respondents are given explicit instructions about the kind of information needed and are encouraged to write down their food intake immediately after each eating occasion. The quality of records usually declines after 4 days unless a subject is highly motivated and interested in the outcome or is providing the information to a health professional to develop an individualized dietary plan. Subjects are often given visual aids to help them visualize and record the amounts of food consumed.

Both prospective and retrospective surveys provide information only on the intake at one point in time, rather than on long-term dietary patterns. To get information on long-term dietary patterns, the investigator often uses a food frequency questionnaire. With this method the subject is given a list of foods or groups of foods and asked to indicate how often, if ever, they are usually consumed in a specified period of time (such as a week, a month, or a year). These lists can be given to subjects to fill out, or the investigator can ask the questions and record the answers (often directly onto a portable computer or a tape recorder for later tabulation).

INFERENCE

Information on the food that is purchased and that is in the home or institution or that is available within a country can be used to estimate the nutritional qualities of the diet available to the specific population groups concerned. The major limitation of this method of assessing what people eat is that it provides no information about how the food was distributed among the members of the group concerned. This makes it difficult to relate the availability of food to any particular health characteristic of members in the group.

INTERPRETATION OF THE INFORMATION

Although information is gathered about what foods are eaten by people, it is the intake of specific nutrients provided by the food that is important to nutritionists. Food composition tables must be used to convert information on food intake into information on nutrient intake. The most common tables provide information on the amounts of between 20 and 40 nutrients or dietary components within several hundred to several thousand different foods. The information is usually related either to common portion sizes or to 100-g portions. The effective use of food composition tables depends on having records in which the foods have been described with sufficient accuracy for them to be matched with the most appropriate items in the food composition tables. For example, it is important to know if the milk consumed was whole milk, 2% milk, or nonfat milk; if peas were fresh, frozen, or canned; and if potatoes were mashed with milk, fried, baked, or scalloped. It is also important that the amounts be recorded in serving sizes that can be related to the amounts in the tables.

The information on the nutrient composition of any one food given in food composition tables represents a *weighted average* that reflects all the relevant analyses available from government, industry, and university sources. For some nutrients the analytical techniques used are well standardized and sensitive to small variations, whereas for others the margin of error is much greater.

The overall nutrient content of the diet and other related values such as the percentage of kilocalories from carbohydrate, fat, and protein and the calcium/phosphorus ratio can be obtained by totaling the content of each nutrient for each food in the diet. The values obtained can then be compared with the appropriate recommended dietary allowances to determine those nutrients that are provided in recommended amounts and to identify those that fall below the standard.

Failure to obtain an intake equal to the recommended level does not mean that a person is deficient in the nutrient concerned because the standard for almost all nutrients is at least 30% above the average requirement for any age and sex group. However, the further the intake falls below the standard, the greater the possibility that the intake is inadequate for that individual. Only when there is some biochemical or physical evidence of a deficiency, however, is there cause for concern.

The methods outlined above are the best available ways to assess dietary intake, despite the limitations in the accuracy of the data (because of such factors as failure to accurately record all food eaten, failure to accurately describe the food and the serving size, and the possibility of errors in selecting the proper items from tables of food composition). These methods have been used widely and successfully to determine the nutrient intake of individuals or groups and to provide indices of health and nutritional status. This information is used in the major nutrition surveys conducted by the U.S. Departments of Agriculture and Health and Human Services as part of the National Nutrition Monitoring System. It is also used by epidemiologists to identify associations, but not prove causes and effects, between food or nutrient intake and various health status variables. Any interpretation of the data, however, should take into account the limitations of the methods of data collection and analysis.

BY NOW YOU SHOULD KNOW

- The RDAs are used as a tool in planning diets for groups and evaluating individual diets.
- Dietary Values (DVs), which include Reference Daily Intakes (RDIs) and Daily Reference Values (DRVs), are used for labeling food products.
- Dietary standards have been set in America and most other developed countries of the world and by the FAO/WHO for developing countries.
- Food guides were developed to allow the public to plan meals based on the inclusion of certain food groups in specified amounts so that they would supply sufficient nutrients to maintain good health.
- The first food guide had five food groups, the second had seven, and the food guide most widely used today—the Food Guide Pyramid—has five food groups.
- The major nutrients in milk and milk products are protein, calcium, and riboflavin.
- The major nutrients in protein-rich foods are protein, vitamin B_{12}, vitamin B_6, zinc, and iron.
- The major nutrients in fruits and vegetables are vitamins C and A.
- The major nutrients in cereal-based foods are vitamin B_1, riboflavin, and iron.
- Information widely available on food groups identifies foods included in the groups, the sizes of "servings," and the number of servings to be eaten per day. Provided the basic rules of selection given in the Food Guide Pyramid are adhered to, the specific foods chosen and methods of preparation used can be adjusted to meet individual tastes.
- The Dietary Goals and Dietary Guidelines were developed to give guidance to help Americans choose foods that promote good health.
- The nutrient density of a food can be determined by calculating the index of nutrient quality of the food.
- Food composition tables can be used to estimate the nutrient intake of individuals or groups.

STUDY QUESTIONS

1. Define RDA, INQ, and nutrient density. What do all of these terms have in common?
2. Why do dietary standards differ among countries?
3. Where do the data in food composition tables and in nutritional computer data banks come from?
4. In what way is the Food Guide Pyramid different from the Basic Four?
5. Name the Dietary Goals for Americans. Explain how they differ from the current pattern of food intake.
6. Name some foods that are considered meat substitutes.

CRITICAL ANALYSIS

1. Here is an exercise that compares your food intake to the goal intakes from the Food Guide Pyramid. Record the number of servings you eat from the following food groups today or tomorrow. For a shorter exercise, you may record intakes from a single meal. If you record intakes from a single meal, ask yourself the following questions: Did I eat approximately ⅓ of the recommended servings for 1 day? If not, did I or will I make up the difference at another meal? Some serving sizes and a record form are provided at the top of p. 59.

Serving sizes

Bread	1 slice, 1 small dinner roll, ½ hamburger bun, bagel, english muffin
Cereal	½ cup of ready-to-eat or hot cereal
Rice	½ cup cooked rice
Pasta	½ cup cooked pasta
Vegetables	½ cup cooked vegetable, 1 cup chopped raw vegetable
Fruits	1 medium apple, orange, pear, banana, ½ cup cut fruit, ¾ cup fruit juice
Dairy	1 cup milk, yogurt, ½ oz cheese
Meat	3 oz lean meat; 2 Tbsp peanut butter or 1 egg equals 1 oz meat

	NUMBER OF SERVINGS				
	BREADS, CEREALS	VEGETABLES	FRUITS	DAIRY	MEATS, MEAT SUBSTITUTES
Breakfast	______	______	______	______	______
Snack	______	______	______	______	______
Lunch	______	______	______	______	______
Snack	______	______	______	______	______
Dinner	______	______	______	______	______
Snack	______	______	______	______	______
Total	______	______	______	______	______
Recommended	6 to 11	3 to 5	2 to 4	2 to 3	2 to 3

How does your diet rate? Although meeting the recommended number of servings for each food group is not a guarantee of an adequate diet, it is likely that your diet is adequate with respect to all known necessary nutrients. An exception to this would be if all of your servings in one food group were from the same food (for example, if you eat three servings per day of fruit, but apples are the only type of fruit you eat). If you fell below the minimum recommended number of servings for any food group, it might be worthwhile to record your intake for 3 or 4 days. The reason is that your intake for any given day is rarely representative of your intake over many days. If your average daily intake over several days still falls below the recommended number of servings for any food group, you might ask yourself if there are any other foods in that group that you like, you would be willing to eat, you can afford to buy, and would be convenient to eat? If you can think of several foods that meet these criteria, try adding a serving of one of those foods each day.

REFERENCES

1. Darby W: Food and Nutrition Board—personal reflections, *Nutr Today* 26(4):30, 1991.

2. National Research Council, Committee in Food and Nutrition: *A yardstick for good nutrition—recommended dietary allowances,* Washington, DC, 1941, National Academy Press.

3. Institute of Medicine, Food and Nutrition Board: *Recommended Dietary Allowances,* ed 10, Washington, DC, 1989, National Academy of Sciences.

4. National Research Council/National Academy of Sciences: *Nutrient adequacy: assessment using food consumption surveys,* Washington, DC, 1985, National Academy Press.

5. U.S. Department of Agriculture and U.S. Department of Health and Human Services: *Nutritional monitoring in the United States—a report from the Joint Nutrition Monitoring Evaluation Committee,* DHHS Pub No 86-1255, Washington, DC, 1986, U.S. Government Printing Office.

6. Guthrie HA: Recommended dietary allowances 1989: changes, consensus and challenges, *Nutr Today* 25(1):43, 1991.

7. Spleth P: Federal food assistance program: a step toward food security for many, *Nutr Today* 29(2):6, 1994.

8. Institute of Medicine, Food and Nutrition Board: *Should the recommended dietary allowances be revised?* Washington, DC, 1994, National Academy Press.

9. Harper AE: Transitions in health status: implications for dietary recommendations, *Am J Clin Nutr* 45:1094, 1987.

10. Health and Welfare Canada: *Nutrition recommendations,* Report of the Scientific Review Committee, Ottawa, Canada, 1990, Supply and Services Canada.

11. Committee on Medical Aspects of Food Policy, Department of Health: *Dietary reference values for food energy and nutrients for the United Kingdom,* Report on Health and Social Subjects No 41, London, 1991, Her Majesty's Stationary Office.

12. FAO/WHO: *Eighth Report of the Joint Expert Committee on Nutrition,* WHO Technical Report Series No 452, Geneva, 1971, World Health Organization.

13. Food and Drug Administration: *Consumer special report: focus on food labeling,* Washington, DC, 1993, The Food and Drug Administration.

14. Wilkening VL: FDA regulations to implement the NLEA, *Nutr Today* 28(5):13, 1993.

15. Haughton B, Gussow JD, Dodds JM: An historical study of the underlying assumptions for United States food guides from 1917 through the Basic Four food group guide, *J Nutr Educ* 19:169, 1987.

16. Page L, Phipard EF: *Essentials of an adequate diet—facts for nutrition programs,* Washington, DC, 1956, USDA Agricultural Research Services.

17. U.S. Department of Agriculture: *Food, the hassle-free guide to a better diet,* Washington, DC, 1979, The U.S. Department of Agriculture.

18. Welsh S, Davis C, Shaw A: Development of the Food Guide Pyramid, *Nutr Today* 27(6):12, 1992.

19. U.S. Senate Select Committee on Nutrition and Human Needs: *Dietary goals for the United States,* ed 2, Washington, DC, 1977, U.S. Government Printing Office.

20. National Academy of Sciences: *Diet, nutrition and cancer,* Washington, DC, 1982, National Academy Press.

21. National Institute of Health: Health implications of obesity, *Ann Intern Med* 103:147, 1994.

22. Food and Nutrition Board, National Research Council: *Toward healthful diets,* Washington, DC, 1980, National Academy of Sciences.

23. U.S. Department of Agriculture and U.S. Department of Health and Human Services: *Nutrition and your health: dietary guidelines for Americans,* ed 3, Home and Garden Bulletin No 232, Washington, DC, 1990, U.S. Government Printing Office.

24. American Dietetic Association: *Recommendation of food choices for women,* Chicago, 1987, The Association.

25. Hansen RG: Why calories count: communicating moderation and a balanced diet, *Food Technol* 45:86, 1991.

26. Guthrie H: Concept of a nutritious food, *J Am Diet Assoc* 71:14, 1977.

ADDITIONAL READINGS

Beaton GH: Human nutrient requirement estimates: derivation, interpretation, and application in evolutionary perspective, *Food Nutr Agriculture* 1:3, 1991.

Beaton GH: Design of nutrition monitoring and surveillance systems: questions to be considered, *J Am Diet Assoc* 51:472, 1990.

Clydesdale FM, Kolasa KM, Ikeda JP: All you want to know about fruit juice, *Nutr Today* 29(2):14, 1994.

Cronin FJ and others: Developing a food guidance system to implement the dietary guidelines, *J Nutr Educ* 19:281, 1987.

FAO/WHO: *Requirements of vitamin A, thiamine, riboflavin and niacin,* FAO Nutrition Meeting Report Series No 41, Rome, 1967, Food and Agriculture Organization.

FAO/WHO: *Requirements of vitamin A, iron, folate, and vitamin* B_{12}, Report of Joint FAO/WHO Expert Consultation, FAO Food Nutrition Series No 23, Rome, 1988, Food and Agriculture Organization.

FAO/WHO and United Nations University: *Energy and protein requirements,* WHO Technical Report Series No 724, Geneva, 1985, World Health Organization.

Harper AE: Nutrition standards for today, *Nutr Today* 26(2):34, 1993.

Hegsted DM: Dietary standards: guidelines for prevention of deficiency or prescription for total health? *J Nutr* 116:482, 1986.

Hepburn FN: The USDA national nutrient data bank, *Am J Clin Nutr* 35:1297, 1982.

International Union of Nutritional Scientists: Recommended dietary intakes around the world, *Nutr Abst Rev Clin Nutr* 53:939, 1983.

Light L, Cronin FJ: Food guidance revisited, *J Nutr Ed* 13:57, 1981.

National Research Council: *Diet and health: implications for reducing chronic disease risk,* Report of Committee on Diet and Health, Washington, DC, 1989, Food and Nutrition Board, National Academy of Sciences.

Report of a WHO Study Group: *Diet, nutrition and the prevention of chronic diseases,* WHO Technical Report Series No 797, Geneva, 1990, World Health Organization.

Rosenberg IH: Behind and beyond the recommended dietary allowances, *Am J Clin Nutr* 41:139, 1985.

Truswell AS: Dietary goals and guidelines, national and international perspectives. In Shils ME, Olson JA, Shike M, editors: *Modern nutrition in health and disease,* ed 8, Philadelphia, 1994, Lea & Febiger.

U.S. Department of Agriculture: *The Food Guide Pyramid,* Home and Garden Bulletin No 252, Washington, DC, 1992, U.S. Government Printing Office.

U.S. Department of Health and Human Services/Public Health Service: *The Surgeon General's Report on Nutrition and Health,* Department of Health and Human Services (Public Health Services), Pub No 88-50210, Superintendent of Documents, Washington, DC, 1988, U.S. Government Printing Office.

Whitehead RG: Dietary allowances: what to recommend, *Acta Paediatr Scand Suppl* 373:25, 1991.

Willett WC: Diet and health: what should we eat? *Science* 264: 532, 1994.

O V E R V I E W

Digestion, Absorption, and Excretion

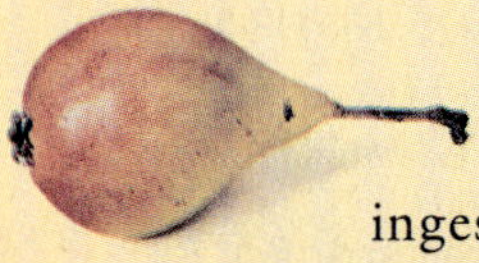

The first step in nourishing the body is the eating, or ingestion, of food. Eating is regulated by hunger and appetite, which are influenced by internal and external stimuli. The internal stimulus to consume food is the sensation of hunger, which accompanies either a drop in blood glucose levels or the contraction of the stomach in the absence of food. When food is eaten and is in the stomach, hunger gives way to feelings of satiety as the blood glucose level rises and physical hunger pangs subside. The external stimuli, or external cues, for eating are complex and varied. For many people the sight or aroma of food triggers the appetite. Others respond to social and environmental cues. People may eat in the following situations:

- In social situations whenever food is available
- At a prescribed time of day or in a prescribed place
- As a defense mechanism against times when food is not available
- As a response to frustration, anxiety, or unhappiness
- As a reward

Some people respond only to internal cues, but for most, eating is triggered by both physiological internal cues and environmental external cues.

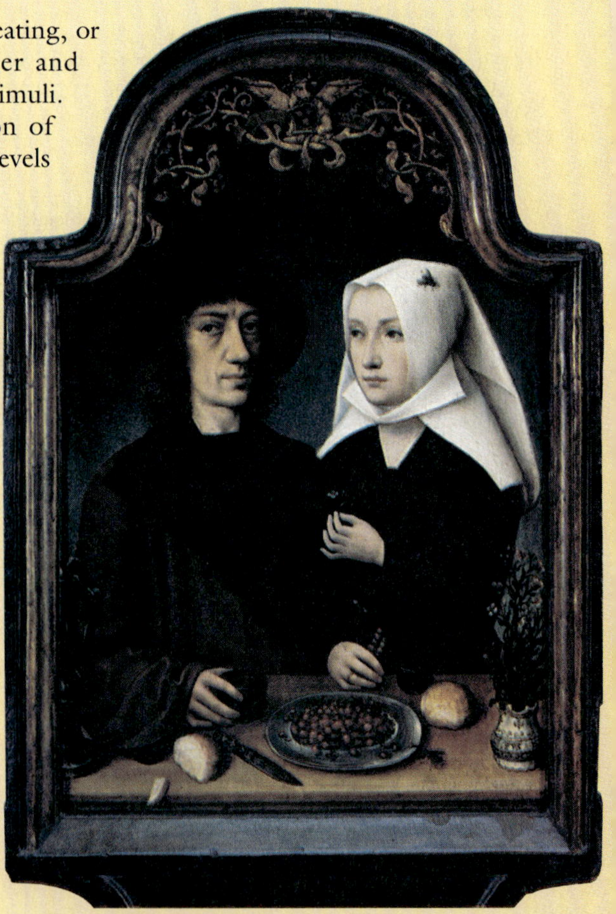

Portrait of the artist and his wife, with cherries. Painted in the late 15th century by Master of Frankfurt.

TABLE OV1-1

Key features of the GI tract

ORGAN	EXOCRINE SECRETIONS	FUNCTIONS
Mouth and pharynx		Used for chewing (mechanical digestion), initiating the swallowing reflex
Salivary glands	Salt and water	Used for moistening food
	Mucus	Lubricates
	Amylase	Used as a polysaccharide-digesting enzyme
Esophagus		Moves bolus of food to stomach by peristaltic waves
	Mucus	Lubricates
Stomach		Stores, mixes, and dissolves food; regulates emptying of homogenized food into small intestine
	HCl	Solubilizes food particles; kills microbes
	Pepsin	Used as a protein-digesting enzyme
	Mucus	Lubricates and protects epithelial surface
Pancreas		Secretes enzymes and bicarbonate:
	Enzymes	Digests carbohydrates, fats, proteins, and nucleic acids
	Bicarbonate	Neutralizes HCl entering small intestine from stomach
Liver		Secretes bile; used for many other nondigestive functions
	Bile salts	Solubilizes water-insoluble fats
	Bicarbonate	Neutralizes HCl entering small intestine from stomach
	Organic waste products and trace metals	Eliminates waste from body
Gallbladder		Stores and concentrates bile between meals; stores bile released by contraction of gallbladder during meal
Small intestine		Digests and absorbs substances; used for mixing and propulsion of contents
	Enzymes (amylase, peptidases, and lipase)	Digests food
	Mucus	Lubricates
Large intestine (colon)		Stores and concentrates undigested matter by absorption of salt and water; used for mixing and propulsion of contents
	Mucus	Lubricates
Rectum		Used for defecation (reflex initiated by distension)

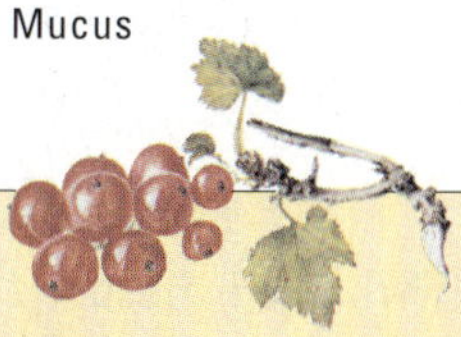

Digestion

Before food can be used by the cells of the body, it must undergo many changes to convert its nutrients to forms that can be absorbed through the intestinal wall. The process of changing the varied and often complex chemicals of food into absorbable chemicals is called **digestion**. The mechanical and chemical changes of digestion occur primarily in the gastrointestinal tract or alimentary canal (Figure Ov1-1). The **gastrointestinal (GI) tract** is essentially a tube about 30 feet (9 m) long that passes through the center of the body from the mouth to the anus. The organs of the GI tract include the oral cavity, pharynx, esophagus, stomach, small intestine, and large intestine. The accessory digestive organs include the teeth, tongue, salivary glands, liver, gallbladder, and pancreas (Table Ov1-1). Food travels through the muscular tube of the GI tract from the time it is swallowed until any undigested residue is excreted in the feces. Until food is absorbed through the walls of the digestive tract and into the blood or lymph, it cannot be used by the cells, and technically is still outside the body. The cells lining the digestive tract control not only the form in which nutrients enter the body, but also, in many cases, the

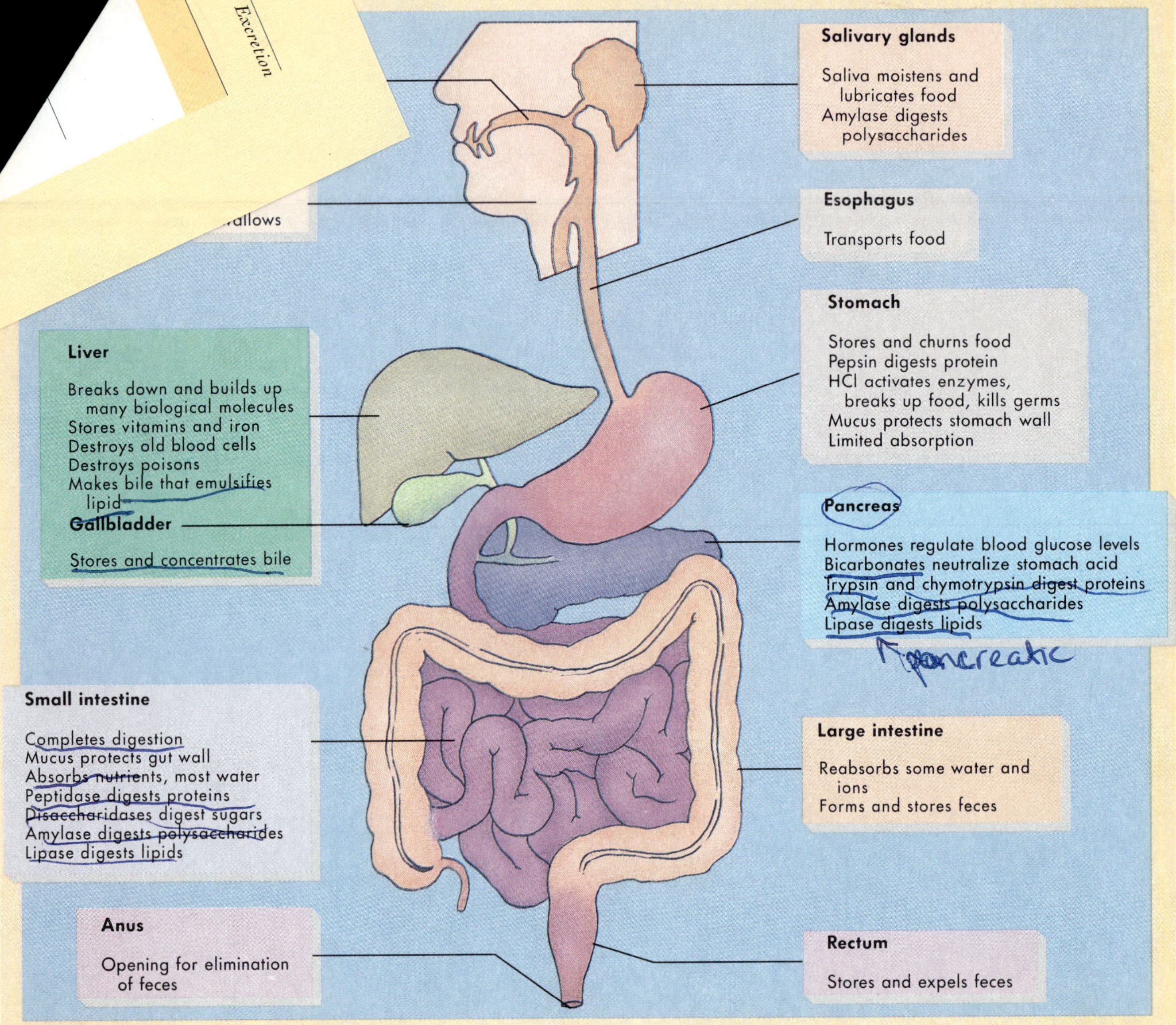

amounts of nutrients that enter. These cells also have the ability to keep substances that are of no value or are potentially dangerous out of the body.

Mouth

The first physiological response to either the anticipation or presence of food is the flow of **saliva** into the mouth. Saliva is a thin, mucuslike fluid secreted by the salivary glands, and it performs three major roles. Its first function is to mix with food, lubricating dry foods and diluting thicker foods. Its second function is to provide the polysaccharide-digesting enzyme α-amylase and the lipid-digesting enzyme lingual lipase. A third function of saliva is to dissolve some molecules in food, allowing them to interact with the chemoreceptors in the mouth to give rise to the sensation of taste. We each secrete approximately 1.5 L of saliva per day. The physical action of chewing (**mastication**) also mechanically divides food into small particles. This serves two purposes: it gives the enzymes that act on food a larger surface area on which to act, and it greatly reduces the distance through which the enzymes must penetrate to reach all of the food particles. Both of these effects speed up the reactions catalyzed by the enzymes.

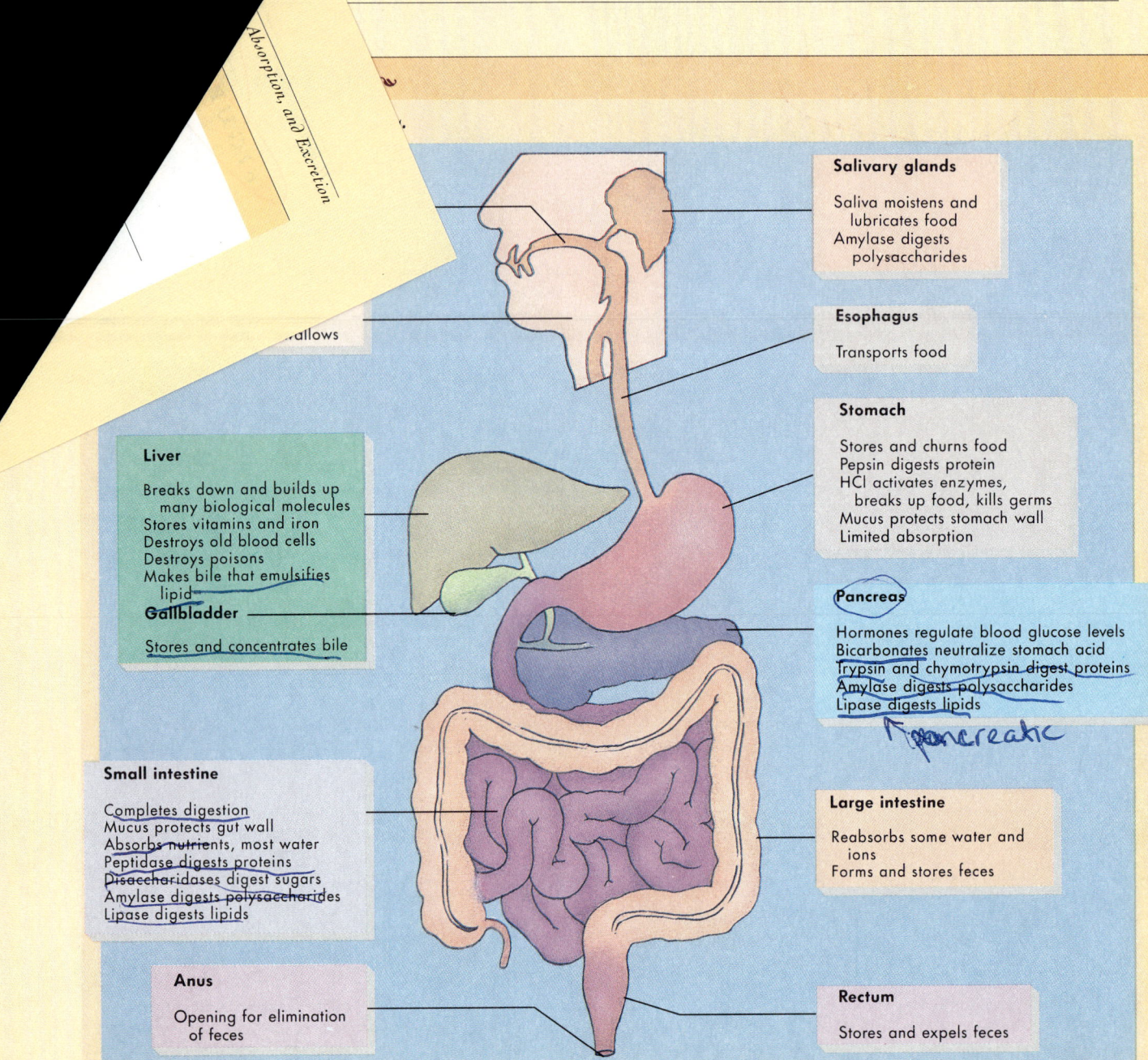

Esophagus

The esophagus is a muscular tube about 10 inches long that connects the mouth to the stomach. Once food has been lubricated with saliva and broken into small pieces by chewing, the tongue can roll it into a small ball (**bolus**) and thrust or toss it to the back of the mouth. From there it can be placed at the top of the esophagus. Simultaneously, a small flap called the *epiglottis* slips over the top of the trachea, or windpipe, which prevents food from entering the respiratory tract and lung. This is how food is directed into the esophagus.

Once the bolus is in the esophagus, it is propelled to the stomach by **peristalsis,** the churning, wavelike action resulting from the contraction and relaxation of the muscles of the GI tract. Peristalsis physically reduces the size of food particles still further and mixes them thoroughly with digestive secretions.

Stomach

Although we often think of the stomach as the major organ or site of digestion, it actually plays a relatively minor role. The stomach, located at the end of the esophagus, consists of three sets of muscles surrounding a cavity that can expand to hold up to 2 quarts of food and fluid. Food arrives in the stomach from the esophagus and mixes with the gastric secretions to form a homogeneous mass called **chyme.** The entry of food into the stomach is controlled by the **cardiac sphincter** muscle that is found where the esophagus joins the stomach. It is called the cardiac sphincter simply because of its close proximity to the heart. The gastric secretions that mix with food in the stomach to form chyme consist of hydrochloric acid (secreted by parietal cells in the gastric **mucosa,** or lining); mucus (secreted by goblet cells); pepsinogen, an inactive form of the enzyme pepsin (secreted from chief cells); the hormone gastrin (secreted by G cells); and intrinsic factor, a protein that is required for the absorption of vitamin B_{12} in the intestine.

The presence of food in the stomach triggers the release of the hormone gastrin, which in turn stimulates the release of hydrochloric acid (HCl) and pepsinogen from the stomach wall. The HCl maintains the pH of the stomach at a strongly acidic level of about 2.0, and this level of acidity performs three main functions. First, it denatures ingested proteins, unfolding the molecules in a way that makes their breakdown during further digestion easier. Second, it causes the pepsinogen molecules to partially digest themselves in a way that converts them into the active enzyme pepsin. The pepsin, which is most active in acidic conditions (optimal pH level of around 2.0), goes on to break down proteins into small peptides and amino acids. Proteins are only partially digested in the stomach, however, whereas carbohydrates and lipids are not digested at all in the stomach. The polysaccharide-digesting enzyme α-amylase, present in saliva, is inactivated by the acidic conditions in the stomach. The complete digestion of food molecules occurs later, once the chyme has entered the small intestine. The wall of the stomach is protected from the strongly acidic environment in the stomach by the secretion of mucus along with the HCl. This mucus forms a protective coat over the lining, or mucosa, of the stomach.

The chyme churns in the stomach for approximately 4 to 6 hours, allowing the digestive secretions and peristalsis to continue to prepare the nutrients in food for their eventual absorption.

Small Intestine

The small intestine is the major organ of digestion. Most of the absorption from the GI tract occurs in the small intestine, whose mucosal surface is highly specialized for this absorptive process. It is 9 to 12 feet in length and is therefore the longest organ in the body. It is called "small" because its diameter (about 1.5 inches) is less than that of the large intestine. The small intestine is divided into three segments: an initial short (8-inch) segment called the **duodenum,** followed by the **jejunum,** and ending in the **ileum,** which is the longest segment.

By the time chyme leaves the stomach and enters the duodenum, it is almost completely liquefied. This liquid then passes slowly, in regulated amounts, through the **pylorus** (a muscular opening that separates the stomach from the small intestine) into the **lumen** (or interior) of the intestinal tract. The enzymes needed to complete the breakdown of complex nutrients into units simple enough to move into and through the intestinal wall are available in the intestine.

TABLE OV1-2

Summary of the sources and activities of the major digestive enzymes

ORGAN	SOURCE	SUBSTRATE	ENZYMES	OPTIMAL pH LEVEL	PRODUCTS
Mouth	Saliva	Starch	Salivary amylase	6.7	Maltose
Stomach	Gastric gland	Protein	Pepsin	1.6-2.4	Shorter polypeptides
Duodenum	Pancreatic juice	Starch	Pancreatic amylase	6.7-7.0	Maltose, maltriose, and oligosaccharides
		Polypeptides	Trypsin, chymotrypsin, carboxypeptidase	8.0	Amino acids, dipeptides, and tripeptides
		Triglyerides	Pancreatic lipase	8.0	Fatty acids and monoglycerides
	Epithelial membranes	Maltose	Maltase	5.0-7.0	Glucose
		Sucrose	Sucrase	5.0-7.0	Glucose and fructose
		Lactose	Lactase	5.8-6.2	Glucose and galactose
		Polypeptides	Aminopeptidase	8.0	Amino acids, dipeptides, and tripeptides

Bile, made in the liver and stored in the gallbladder, is released into the small intestine to aid lipid digestion by breaking fat into small particles. Bile is a solution containing six primary ingredients:

- Bile salts
- Cholesterol
- Lecithin (a phospholipid)
- Bile pigments (end products of the breakdown of hemoglobin)
- Certain minerals such as copper and manganese
- Small amounts of some end products of organic metabolism

The bile salts, cholesterol, and lecithin are manufactured in the liver and are involved in the solubilization of fat before its digestion in the small intestine. The bile pigments, minerals, and end products of organic metabolism are substances that are normally excreted from the body via the anus.

Once the chyme enters the small intestine, two of the gastrointestinal hormones—**secretin** and **cholecystokinin**—are released. These hormones stimulate the pancreas to release its digestive enzymes and stimulate the gallbladder to contract to release its stored bile. The pancreas also releases sodium bicarbonate, an alkali that acts to neutralize the hydrochloric acid in chyme. This, in turn, permits the activation of the digestive enzymes in the lumen of the small intestine, whose optimal pH levels range from 5 to 8. The final stage of digestion, known as *membrane digestion,* takes place in the intestinal wall. This converts nutrients to simple components that can be absorbed into the blood to be transported around the body to nourish the cells. The sites of action, sources, and activities of the major digestive enzymes are summarized in Table Ov1-2. The names and actions of the major gastrointestinal hormones are summarized in Table Ov1-3.

Absorption

Absorption is the process by which the simple nutrient components produced by digestion pass out of the GI tract into the cells lining it and from these cells into the blood or the lymphatic system, which carries the nutrients to the body cells. Most nutrients are absorbed directly into the blood and taken by the **portal vein** to the liver, where further processing occurs within the liver cells. Some nutrients, however, enter the lymphatic system, which is a secondary circulatory system that collects lipids and excess fluids and transports them back to the blood (Figure Ov1-2).

All nutrients eventually pass from the blood into the extracellular fluids between cells. It is from these extracellular fluids that the cells actually obtain supplies of the nutrients they need. The cell membrane, however, acts as a selective barrier that regulates the entrance of nutrients into each cell.

TABLE OV1-3

The gastrointestinal hormones

HORMONE	STIMULI	EFFECTS	ROLE
Gastrin	Amino acids Distension pH >3	↑ Acid secretion ↑ Motility ↑ Pepsinogen secretion	Facilitates gastric digestion
Gastric inhibitory peptide	Glucose Distension Hypertonicity	↑ Motility ↓ Gastric secretion and motility	Limits gastric emptying; prepares the intestine for substrate
Motilin	pH >4.5	↑ Gastric motility ↑ Intestinal motility	Facilitates digestion in intestine
Secretin	Hypertonicity pH <4.5	↑ Pepsinogen secretion ↑ Pancreatic bicarbonate secretion ↓ Gastric motility and secretion	Limits gastric emptying; neutralizes the chyme leaving the stomach
Cholecystokinin	Fats Amino acids	↑ Pancreatic secretion ↑ Intestinal secretion and motility ↓ Gastric secretion and motility ↑ Gallbladder contraction	Limits gastric emptying; promotes digestion in the intestine

Modified from Moffett CL, Moffett DF, Schauf SB: *Human physiology,* ed 2, St Louis, 1993, Mosby.

The small intestine, where the initial absorption of nutrients from the GI tract occurs, is a long coiled tube with an inner structure that greatly increases the surface area through which nutrients can be absorbed. The inner surface, especially in the duodenum and jejunum, has fingerlike projections, or **circular folds,** that extend about halfway around the inner intestinal surface. These folds are 8 to 10 mm in height and increase the intestinal surface area to at least three times what it would be without them. On the surface of these folds and over the rest of the surface of the small intestine are small projections called **villi.** Villi are from 0.5 to 1.5 mm high and are tightly packed at a density of about 20 per 40 mm^2. They further increase the inner surface area of the small intestine to about 15 times what it would be without the villi and circular projections. Each villus is in turn covered with even smaller projections called **microvilli,** which are each 1 mm high and are packed together at a density of 200,000 per mm^2. This further multiplies the inner surface area of the small intestine by 20 times. The combined effect of the circular folds, the villi, and the microvilli is to present a large total surface area through which absorption can occur, which is 300 times the size it would be if the small intestine were simply a smooth-walled tube (Figure Ov1-3). The surface of each villus is made of a one-cell–thick layer of specialized cells. Most of these cells are absorptive cells, although a few produce mucus that lines and protects the inner intestinal wall. Some of the cells produce hormones, whereas others produce chemicals of the immune system that protect against infectious microorganisms and toxins in food.

Enzymes embedded in the microvilli carry out the final stage of digestion necessary for all the nutrients in food to be absorbed into the absorptive cells. The surface (epithelial) cells of the microvilli are the ones that actually perform and control the absorption of nutrients into the blood. They can control the rate of nutrient entry into the blood either by regulating the rate of absorption from the digestive mass in the GI tract or by regulating the rate at which nutrients pass out of the cells and into the blood. Some nutrients are transported rapidly and completely from the GI tract through the absorptive cells and into the blood, whereas others go more slowly and in more variable amounts. The rate at which many minerals and vitamins are absorbed into the cells and passed into the blood depends on the body's need for these nutrients at any particular time. If the body has high stores of these minerals and vitamins, large amounts of many of them remain unabsorbed; however, if supplies are low, the level of absorption is usually high.

FIGURE OVI-2

Relationship between the arteriovenous and lymphatic circulatory systems.

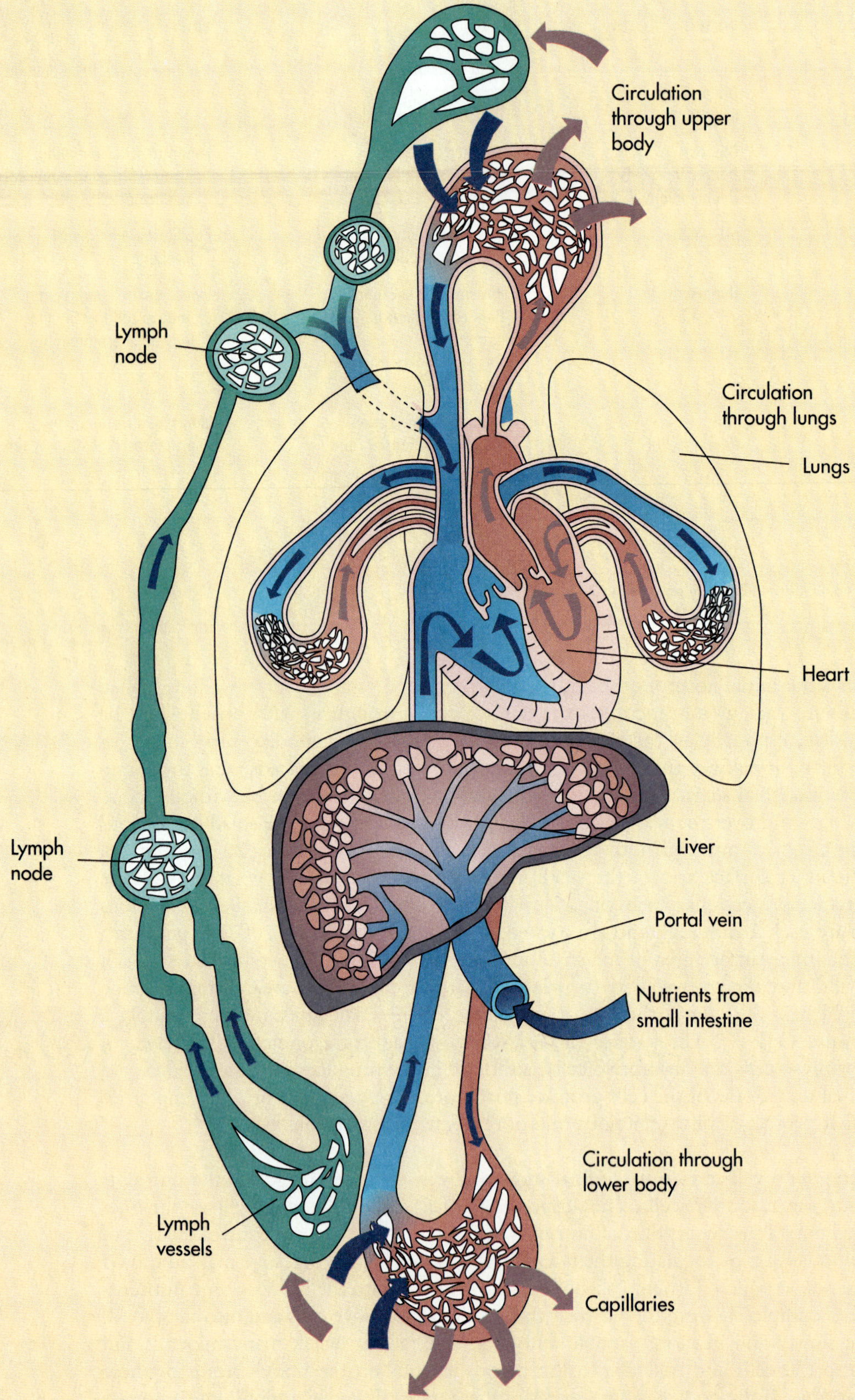

FIGURE Ov1-3

Structure of the intestinal wall.

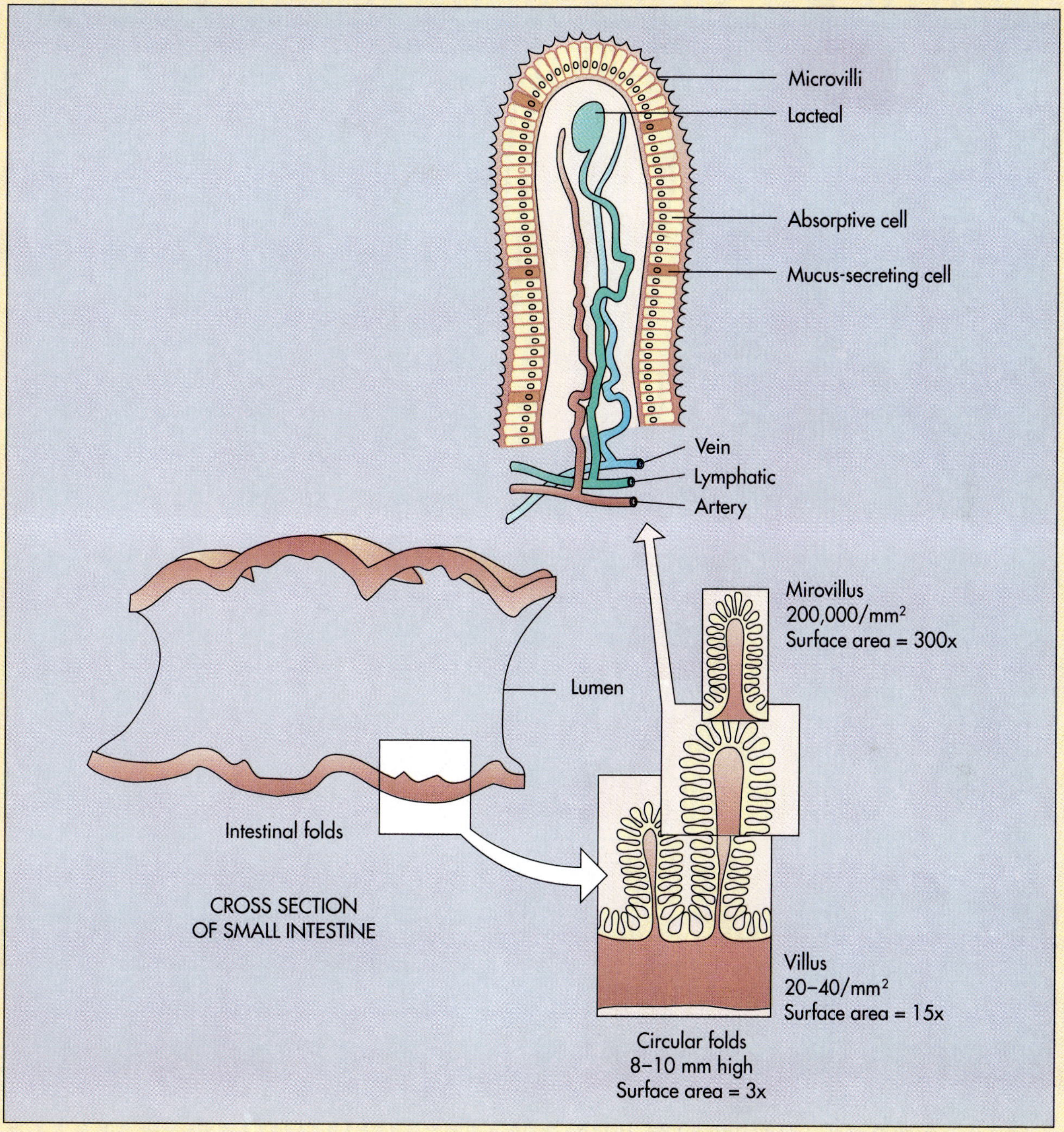

Mechanisms of Absorption

Nutrients are absorbed from the GI tract in several ways: passive diffusion, facilitated diffusion, active transport, and endocytosis (Figure Ov1-4).

Passive diffusion is the free movement of substances that can pass through the cell membrane, a process that automatically causes the substances to move "down their concentration gradient," from the side of the membrane where they are most concentrated to the side where they are less concentrated. This directional diffusion occurs simply because the random motion of particles makes it more likely for them

FIGURE OV1-4

Methods of absorption. Passive diffusion—the net movement of molecules from the region of high concentration to low concentration; facilitated diffusion—the movement of molecules by a carrier protein across the cell membrane from the region of high to low concentration; active transport—the movement of molecules and ions against a concentration gradient that requires the expenditure of cellular energy (i.e., hydrolysis of ATP); and endocytosis—the engulfment of molecules by the cellular membrane folding inward and pinching off within the cell.

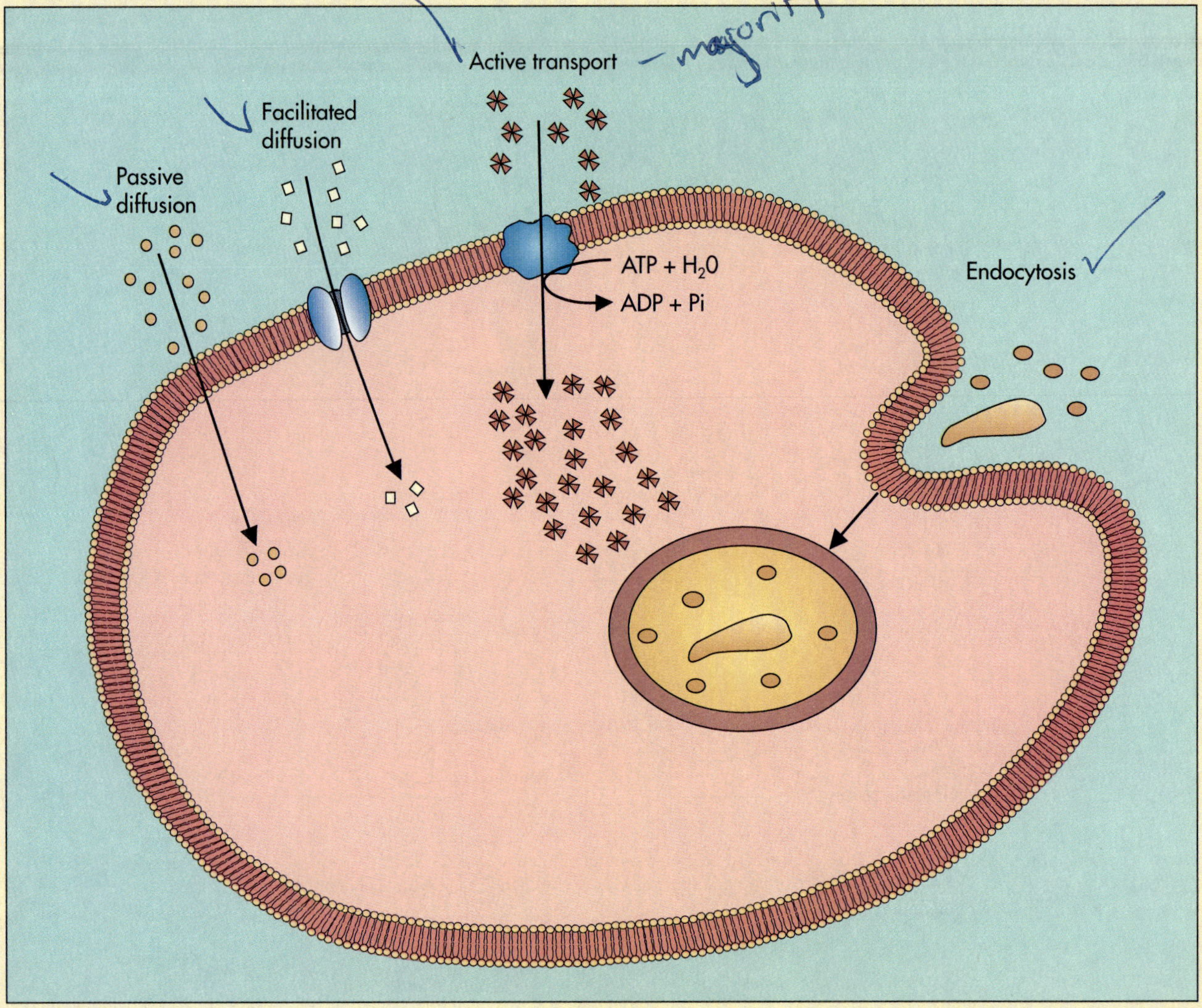

to move from regions of high concentration to regions of low concentration. One special case of passive diffusion is **osmosis,** which is simply the passive diffusion of water across a semipermeable membrane. Passive diffusion can allow nutrients (including water) to move from the GI tract, into the absorptive cells, and then into the blood or lymph, provided their concentration gradients force them to move in that direction. Osmosis is the major mechanism by which water enters the body; but the entry of other nutrients by passive diffusion occurs only when their concentrations in the GI tract are high, and even then, passive diffusion accounts for only a small portion of nutrient absorption.

Most nutrients are absorbed by **carrier-mediated** processes in which a specific carrier protein binds to a nutrient on the outer (intestinal, or mucosal) side of an absorptive cell membrane and transports it into the cell, where it can move across the cell and into the blood or lymph. **Facilitated diffusion** is a carrier-mediated process in which a protein acts as a carrier or shuttle to transport nutrients across the membrane. Because it does not require the expenditure of energy stores to make it happen, it relies on an appropriate concentration gradient to make the nutrients flow out of the GI tract, into the absorptive cells, and into the blood. **Active transport,** on the other hand, involves carriers that can act a bit like "pumps," actively transporting nutrients into the absorptive cell, even if these nutrients are already more concentrated within the cell than in the GI tract. Thus active transport can move nutrients *up* their concentration gradients, in the opposite direction to which they move under the influence of diffusion. This requires the expenditure of energy, however, and all active transport systems are coupled to energy-releasing reactions such as the hydrolysis of adenosine triphosphate (ATP) to adenosine diphosphate (ADP) and inorganic phosphate (P_i). This coupling can be direct or indirect. In direct energy coupling, known as **primary active transport,** the carrier protein binds to and hydrolyzes ATP and directly couples the energy released to the energy-requiring transport process. In **secondary active transport** the energy of ATP is used directly to generate a concentration gradient of particles such as sodium ions by actively transporting them out of the cell. The sodium ions can then bind to some other carrier *along with* some specific nutrient molecule to reenter the cell by moving down the sodium ion concentration gradient. Thus the flow of sodium ions down a previously established concentration gradient can serve to pull associated nutrient molecules along with it.

Carrier-mediated transport systems are used primarily for the absorption of specific nutrients because each carrier can bind to and transport only one specific nutrient or at most a small range of specific nutrients. Carrier-mediated transport systems can also become **saturated** when there are so many of the carried nutrients available that all of the carriers are constantly in use. At this point the rate of transport cannot be increased, regardless of how high the available nutrient concentration becomes.

A mixed "bag" of nutrients can also be taken into cells by a process known as **endocytosis.** In endocytosis a portion of the cell membrane buds inward (invaginates) to form a membrane-bound sac or **vesicle** that pinches off from the membrane and enters the cell. Inside the cell the endocytotic vesicle fuses with a lysosome. A lysosome is a cellular organelle that contains enzymes. Following fusion, the contents of the endocytotic vesicle become exposed to the digestive enzymes of the lysosome. This is a major route by which infectious microorganisms in the GI tract are taken into cells and broken down into materials that are not only harmless, but also can be used as a source of nutrients. The reverse process, known as **exocytosis,** serves as the main route by which secretory products of cells are passed to the exterior. Digestive enzymes, mucus, hormones, and so on can be manufactured within the cell, accumulate in vesicles derived from the internal membranes of the cell, and be released when the membrane of the exocytotic vesicle fuses with the cell membrane.

Once nutrients have passed across the absorptive cells, most are released directly into the blood (via carriers where appropriate) and taken by the portal vein to the liver. From the liver they go either to the cells that need them, to the kidneys to be filtered and either reabsorbed or excreted, or to storage sites such as the liver, kidneys, and bone. Some nutrients, primarily lipids reformed in the absorptive cells and the fat-soluble vitamins, are released to the lacteals, or fat-collecting ducts, of the lymphatic system. The nutrients absorbed into lymph in this way are eventually released into the blood via the thoracic duct on the subclavian vein near the heart.

Excretion

By the time the food mass passes through the **ileocecal valve** at the end of the small intestine to enter the **large intestine,** most nutrients have been absorbed. These include minerals, vitamins, and the products of the digestion of carbohydrate, lipid, and protein. The remaining mass consists mostly of dietary fiber, microorganisms, and water. No further digestion occurs in the large intestine, although the action of microorganisms on material in the large intestine can generate gases as a by-product. As the mass continues through the 10-foot length of the large intestine, water is absorbed into the body, resulting in a progressively more solid mass that eventually reaches the anus as semisolid fecal matter, or **feces.** Dietary fiber within feces does retain some fluid, increasing the bulk of the stools and facilitating their passage through the colon. Lack of fiber in the diet produces dry, hard stools that are passed with difficulty. This results in constipation and sometimes contributes to diverticulitis, an inflammation of abnormal out-pouchings of the intestinal wall of the large intestine.

Feces contain materials derived from food that are excreted from the anus without ever having been absorbed into the cells of the body. Other waste products are the result of the chemical processes of metabolism and are excreted in different ways. The combination of molecules of food with oxygen during catabolism generates carbon dioxide and water as waste products while releasing energy that is stored within ATP. Carbon dioxide, water, and other waste products of cellular metabolism, along with unused nutrients, are released from cells into the extracellular fluid. They enter the capillaries and then the veins of the blood and are eventually excreted from the body, primarily through the lungs and kidneys. Almost all of the carbon dioxide waste and 10% of the excreted water is excreted from the lungs. The kidneys act as efficient and selective filters of the blood. They are able to concentrate the waste products of metabolism and excrete them within urine. They also allow excess nutrients, such as water-soluble vitamins, to leave the body in urine. However, as the blood is filtered through the kidneys, they reabsorb almost all of the glucose and protein present. With some other nutrients, such as sodium, the kidneys reabsorb only the amounts needed to maintain normal blood and tissue levels and excrete any excess in urine. The kidneys are extremely sensitive to the body's needs. They excrete nutrients and metabolites related to nutrients only in amounts appropriate to changing requirements in a way that is partly under the control of various hormones.

Some nutrients are lost from the body through the skin, in perspiration; within **epithelial cells,** which are constantly dying and being shed from the skin; or within hair and nails. Also, the cells lining the intestinal tract are completely replaced every 3 to 4 days, with the old cells and any nutrients they contain being lost in the feces. The feces may also contain nutrients that are part of the various digestive secretions, which are not reabsorbed. Analysis of the kinds and amounts of nutrients lost from the body in these ways can reveal much about the need for various nutrients and the way in which they are changed in the body. It is important to remember that although food must enter through the mouth alone, the products of digestion and metabolism can have several fates, such as being absorbed into the blood or excreted through the lungs (in the breath), the skin (as perspiration, dead skin cells, nail clippings, or lost hair), the kidney (as urine), or the colon (as feces).

The detailed processes of digestion and absorption are more complex than this discussion suggests. The student of nutrition, however, can understand the subject adequately with only the level of information supplied in this overview.

~ BY NOW YOU SHOULD KNOW ~

- The gastrointestinal tract, also known as the digestive tract or alimentary tract, extends from the mouth to the anus.
- Complex nutrients in foods must be reduced to a simpler form by the process of **digestion** before they can be absorbed from the GI tract and transported in the blood for use in individual cells.
- Digestion of food occurs within the lumen and in the walls of the GI tract.
- Specific enzymes, water, and the appropriate acid-base conditions are required for the digestion of various food components.
- The major parts of the digestive tract are the mouth, stomach, small intestine, and large intestine.
- Gastrointestinal hormones regulate the release of enzymes and facilitate their conversion to an active form.
- Absorption of nutrients from the gastrointestinal tract into the blood may occur by passive diffusion, facilitated diffusion, active transport, or endocytosis.

STUDY QUESTIONS

1. Trace the changes that occur in each complex nutrient—carbohydrate, lipid, and protein—from the time it is ingested to when it is either absorbed from the digestive tract or excreted.
2. Describe the lining of the small intestine and how it facilitates absorption.
3. What are the digestive processes occurring in the major parts of the gastrointestinal tract?
4. Describe the roles of the pancreas, gallbladder, and esophagus in the digestive process.
5. List the major digestive enzymes, the substrates on which they act, and the products of their activity.
6. List the gastrointestinal hormones, the conditions that stimulate their release, and the results of their activity.
7. Distinguish the three types of absorption of nutrients: passive diffusion, facilitated diffusion, active transport, and endocytosis.

CRITICAL ANALYSIS

1. While taking a nutrition course, J. W. became interested in weight loss. He began to read journal articles that described studies on the effects of low-calorie diets on short-term weight loss. One of the articles stated that the average daily energy intake of the individuals in the study was 4180 J/day. What was their average energy intake stated in kilocalories?
2. J. W. later went to graduate school where he carried out his research in the area of sports nutrition. He studied the dietary intake of male university rowers and found their average energy intake to be 3000 kcal/day. However, when it was time to submit his findings to a journal for publication, he found that the journal required energy intake to be stated in kilojoules. What was the average daily energy intake of the rowers stated in kilojoules per day?
3. Your friend has recommended that you take a nutrient supplement that contains enzymes. The stated function of the enzymes is to increase energy. Your friend is an excellent athlete who seems to make steady progress in training and always seems to have an abundance of energy. Will this supplement be of benefit to you? What happens to proteins, including enzymes, in the stomach?

ADDITIONAL READINGS

Fox SI: *Human physiology,* ed 2, Dubuque, Ia, 1987, William C Brown.

Ganong WF: *Review of medical physiology,* ed 15, Norwalk, Conn, 1991, Appleton & Lange.

Moffett D, Moffett S, Schauf C: *Human physiology,* ed 2, St Louis, 1993, Mosby.

Thibodeau GA, Patton KT: *Anatomy and physiology,* ed 2, St Louis, 1993, Mosby.

Vander AJ, Sherman JH, Luciano DS: *Human physiology: the mechanisms of body function,* ed 4, New York, 1985, McGraw-Hill.

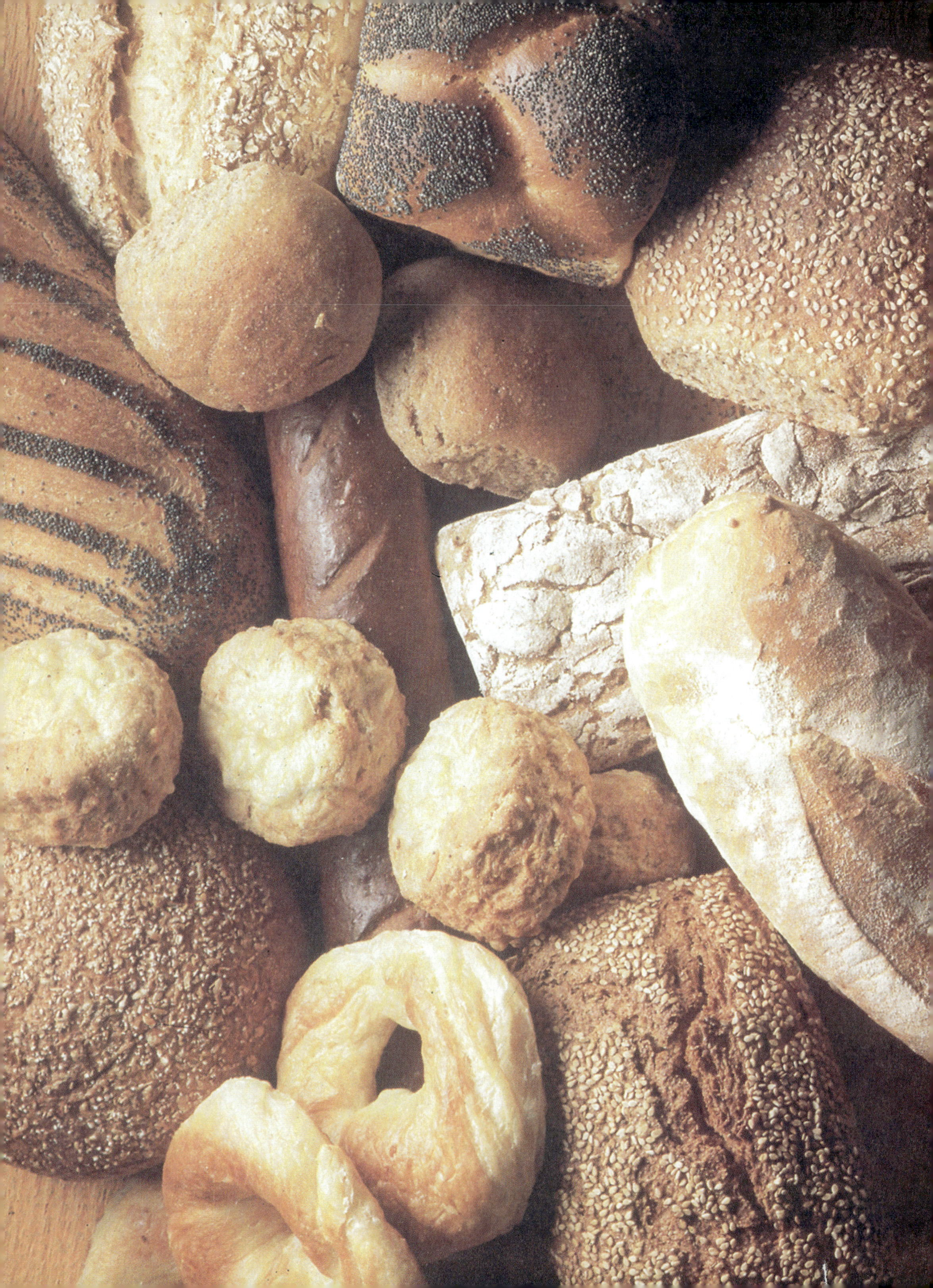

CHAPTER 3

CARBOHYDRATE

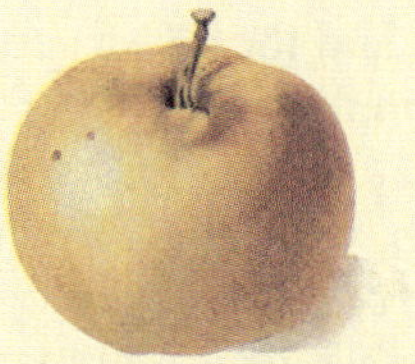

The three major types of dietary carbohydrate are starch, sugar, and fiber. Many people regard starch and sugar as fattening and therefore to be avoided; refined sugar is commonly blamed as a cause of attention deficit disorder (ADD), or hyperactivity, in children; and fiber is known as something to consume to avoid constipation. There is some scientific basis for each of these beliefs, although it is often exaggerated. Carbohydrate is an essential dietary component, but if it is responsible for an energy intake in excess of need, it can cause weight gain. Only a small percentage of children with ADD are actually sensitive to sugar; and although a certain amount of fiber is a good thing, too much can cause problems. Health authorities in most developed countries are encouraging people to increase their intake of carbohydrate but to use sugar in moderation and to include adequate, but not excessive, fiber in their diet. The kind and amount of carbohydrate in the diet play a role in the prevention and/or treatment of tooth decay, diabetes, hypoglycemia, and various other health problems.

Carbohydrate was the first nutrient to be chemically identified, but only recently have dietary recommendations included advice on how much and what type of carbohydrate should be eaten. The term *carbohydrate* has become a part of everyday language. Both singular and plural forms of the word are in common use and mean much the same thing. Nutritionists often talk of the "carbohydrate" in the diet, but dietary carbohydrate consists of a range of different but closely related compounds known collectively as "carbohydrates."

Most people associate the term *carbohydrate* or *carbohydrates* with "starchy," "sugary" food, and they are right to do so because the chemicals in starch and the many types of sugars in nature are indeed all examples of carbohydrates. It is also commonly assumed that foods high in carbohydrates must be "fattening" foods, which is not necessarily the case. Carbohydrates can be considered fattening only when their use is responsible for calorie intakes in excess of energy needs. It is recommended that they account for over 50% of the total caloric intake, and they are an essential part of a healthful diet. To a person with diabetes, carbohydrate is a part of the diet that must be carefully controlled. To a chemist or biochemist, a carbohydrate is simply a compound composed of carbon, hydrogen, and oxygen atoms in certain specific proportions. To a botanist, carbohydrate is the chemical form in which plants store the energy they have captured from the sun. Finally, to a nutritionist, carbohydrate is an essential nutrient that is a major source of energy in the diet and is provided almost entirely by plant-based foods. This chapter explains how these various views of carbohydrate can be reconciled as parts of a wider understanding of the term.

CARBOHYDRATE COMPOUNDS

The term *carbohydrate* covers a large number of different compounds, all composed of carbon, hydrogen, and oxygen atoms. In most carbohydrates the ratio of hydrogen to oxygen is 2:1, meaning there are two hydrogen atoms for every oxygen atom. This is the same ratio in which these atoms occur in water (H_2O), so the ratio of carbon, hydrogen, and oxygen in many carbohydrates can be represented by the general formula $C_x(H_2O)_y$, where x and y represent the numbers found in specific formulas, such as $C_6(H_2O)_6$ or $C_{12}(H_2O)_{11}$. This explains the origin of the term *carbohydrate,* the "carbo" coming from the word *carbon* and the "hydrate" coming from *hydro,* loosely derived from a Greek term meaning "having to do with water." The carbon, hydrogen, and oxygen atoms of carbohydrates are combined in their own special way within carbohydrate molecules: the hydrogen and oxygen atoms of carbohydrates are *not* present in the form of water molecules. The chemical structure of one of the simplest, most common, and most important carbohydrates, **glucose,** is shown in Figure 3-1.

Glucose (blood sugar) is the main form in which carbohydrate is transported in the blood and supplied to the cells of the body. The carbohydrates in our diet, however, comprise a wide range of compounds, each one having its own molecular formula and structure. They include all of the chemicals known as sugars. These sugars are called **simple carbohydrates** because they consist of small molecules with relatively simple chemical structures.

The carbohydrates also include the chemicals known as **starch, glycogen,** and **cellulose.** Starch is the main form in which carbohydrate is stored in many plants, glycogen is the form in which carbohydrate is stored in human beings and other animals, and cellulose is the main component of the indigestible carbohydrate in plants that is called *fiber.* These types of carbohydrates are known as **complex carbohydrates** because they consist of large molecules made when many sugar molecules become linked together into giant chains and more complex three-dimensional networks.

The various types of carbohydrates occur in a wide variety of foods. Starch is found in cereals (both whole grain and refined) and in vegetables. Cellulose, which is one type of **insoluble fiber,** is found in whole grain cereals, fruits, and vegetables. Sugars are found in fruits, vegetables, milk products, and sweeteners.

Apart from water, carbohydrate is the single largest component in the diet. From 45% to 60% of the energy needed by American adults is usually provided by carbohydrate. One gram of carbohydrate provides 4 kcal of energy; thus 300 g (⅔ lb) of carbohydrate provides 1200 kcal. This is 60% of the average American adult's daily energy needs (2000 kcal) and is the proportion that is recommended to be obtained from carbohydrates in the diet. This recommended amount of carbohydrate-derived energy can be provided from just 1½ cups of household or "table" sugar (which is pure carbohydrate), but we normally get most of it in a more palatable form, such as in fruits, vegetables, and cereal products, which also provide many other nutrients.

In some parts of the world, particularly developing countries, many diets contain over a pound of carbohydrate per day, providing 80% or more of daily energy supplies. This is particularly true where locally grown carbohydrate-rich cereals—such as rice, corn, or millet—and root crops—such as cassava or sweet potatoes—provide inexpensive staple foods. At the other extreme are Eskimos, who live where plant life is minimal and animal life is the major source of food. The Eskimos get only about 8% of their energy in the form of carbohydrate. The diets at both of these extremes tend to be much less varied than the diets of people in developed countries.

FIGURE 3-1

Structure of a glucose molecule. A, Linear model. B, Three-dimensional, or space-filling, model. C, Ring structure.

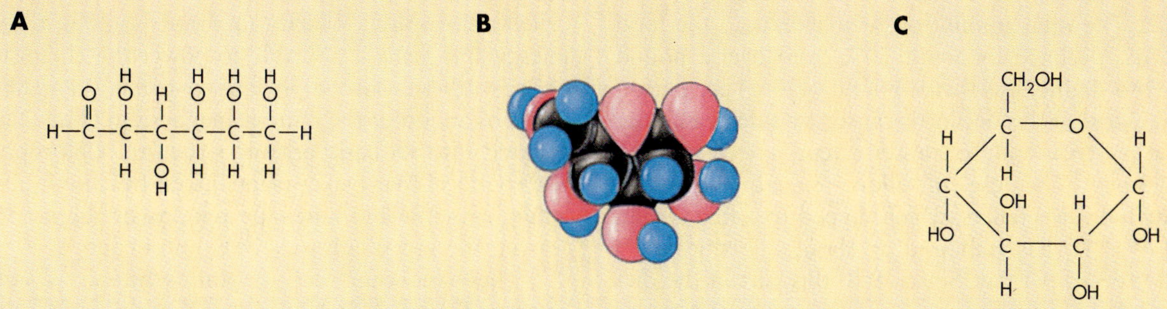

FIGURE 3-2

Use of sugar in the United States with examples of total sugar (% by weight) in some processed foods.

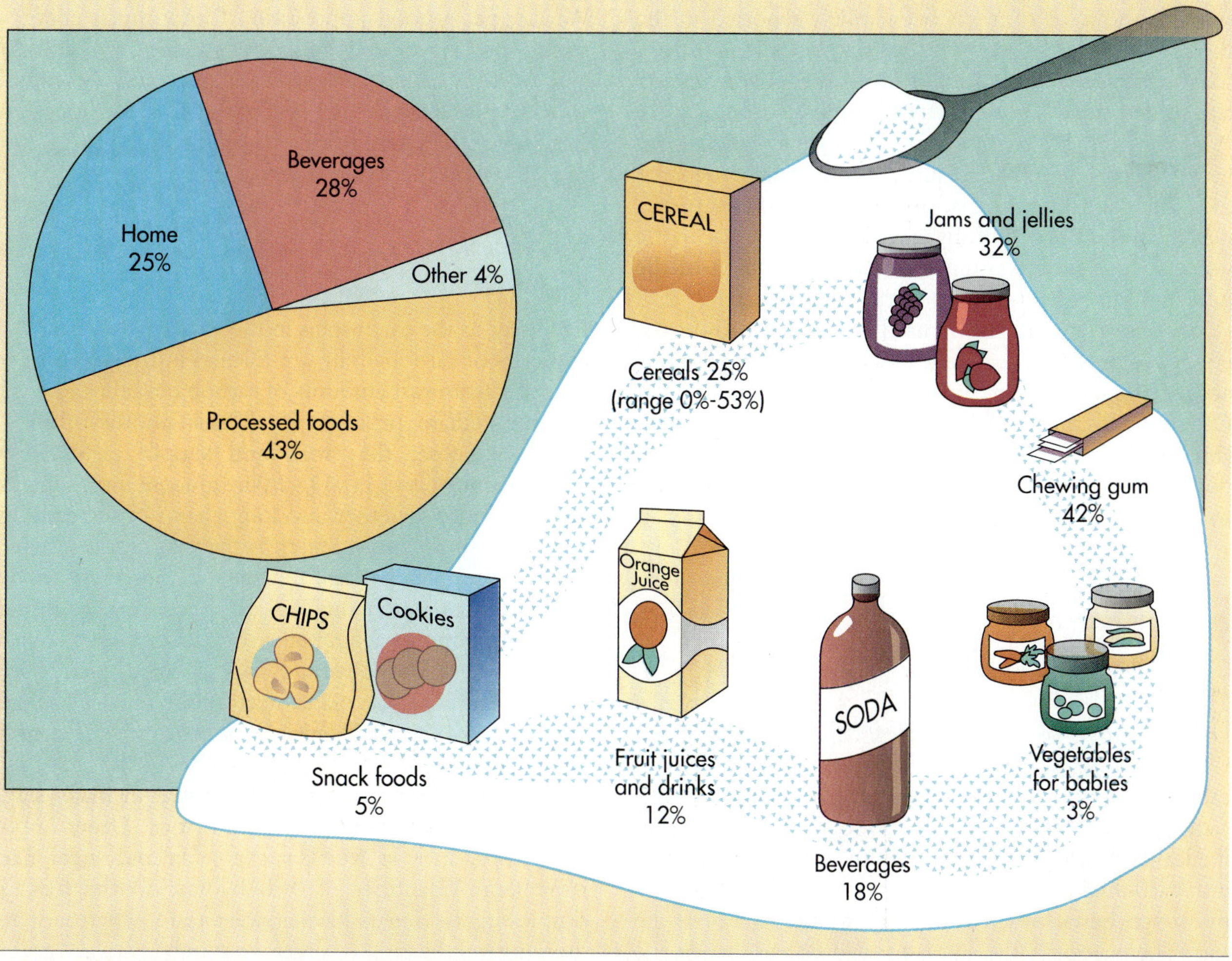

TRENDS IN CARBOHYDRATE CONSUMPTION

Since 1909 there have been some interesting trends in the type of carbohydrate available in the North American diet. The total amount of carbohydrate in the food supply has declined by about 20%, from over a pound (499 g) to slightly less than a pound (425 g) per person per day. Most of this decline is caused by a decreased use of grain products and, to a lesser extent, a decreased use of potatoes. The use of added sugars and other carbohydrate sweeteners, which dipped to a low during World War II, has stabilized at about one third of a pound (163 g) per day. Since 1970 this part of the diet has included increasing amounts of alternative sweeteners to replace common sugar, particularly corn syrups. Corn syrups (including ones high in the sugar known as *fructose*) and other alternative carbohydrate sweeteners (such as dextrose, lactose, and maltose) now account for about one third of all dietary sugar.[1] As a result of these trends, the proportion of total carbohydrate provided by sugar has increased. Added sugars now account for 12% of an average American's daily calorie intake. There has been a clear trend away from grain and vegetable sources of carbohydrates and toward simple carbohydrates, leading to great interest in the possible health implications of this change.[2] Much research has been done on this subject, and a lot of it has been widely reported in the media. The current view of nutritionists is that 60% of total kilocalories should come from carbohydrates and that added sugar should be used in moderation.

Changing life-styles have led to a shift away from home-prepared food and toward commercially prepared food and food eaten out of the home. This has caused a decline in the amount of sugar sold directly for use in the home, which now accounts for only one fourth of the nine million tons of sugar marketed in America each year. Almost all the rest is used by the food industry, either as a preservative or as a sweetener. Beverages alone account for 28% of the sugar used in the United States. Other processed foods account for 43% of the total (Figure 3-2), although the amount of sugar added during processing in each food can vary from around 3% to as much as 42%.

SYNTHESIS OF CARBOHYDRATES

The story of carbohydrates begins in the green leaves of plants. These leaves take in supplies of carbon dioxide gas from the air and are supplied with water from the soil via the plant's roots and stem. Within the leaves the carbon dioxide and water can be converted into carbohydrates and oxygen in the process known as **photosynthesis,** which is powered by the energy of the sun. The energy of the sun is needed because when the atoms involved are in the form of carbohydrate and oxygen, they contain more energy than when in the form of carbon dioxide and water. The extra energy must come from somewhere; so plants contain a chemical called **chlorophyll,** which can absorb some of the sun's energy and make it available to power the chemistry of photosynthesis. Chlorophyll is a green pigment that contains an ion of the mineral magnesium (Mg^{2+}) incorporated into its basic organic structure. Chlorophyll is the chemical that makes plants green because it absorbs sunlight in the red and blue regions of the spectrum, leaving the green light relatively untouched.

The basic chemistry of photosynthesis is summarized in Figure 3-3. Notice that oxygen gas is released into the air and the carbohydrates are stored within the plant. If the process of photosynthesis is *reversed,* with the carbohydrates combining with oxygen to generate carbon dioxide and water, a lot of energy is given out—the energy that went in during the manufacture of the carbohydrate and oxygen. This, indirectly, is what happens when carbohydrates are used as a source of energy in the body during the **oxidation** process known as **respiration,** also summarized in Figure 3-3. Carbohydrates in the body cells are oxidized to generate carbon dioxide, which we breathe out; water; and energy, which our bodies can use in many different ways. We can get a good impression of how much energy is stored within carbohydrates by watching wood burn. The wood is mainly carbohydrate and fiber; it combines with oxygen from the air as it burns, and the hot flames carry away the energy that was originally captured from the sun when the wood was formed.

PRODUCTION OF GLUCOSE AND STARCH

Each day, as the earth spins in the energy of the sun, vast amounts of carbohydrate are formed in the green leaves of plants from vast amounts of carbon dioxide and water. The immediate product of all this photosynthesis is usually glucose, the small and simple carbohydrate whose formula is $C_6H_{12}O_6$. Many glucose molecules can then be linked together into long chains of the carbohydrate known as *starch.* Starch is the main form in which plants store carbohydrate until it is required to provide energy. When starch supplies are used, they are broken down into glucose again before being oxidized to release their energy. Carbohydrates are formed and stored within plants because plants need them, but we can gain the benefit of the plants' photosynthetic efforts by eating the plants.

Large amounts of starch are stored in many staple foods, such as potatoes, wheat, and rice. Other important crops, such as fruits, sugar cane, and sugar beet, store large quantities of carbohydrate in the form of simple sugars. Sugars have a sweet taste, whereas starch does not; so the ratio of sugars to starch in a plant greatly

FIGURE 3-3

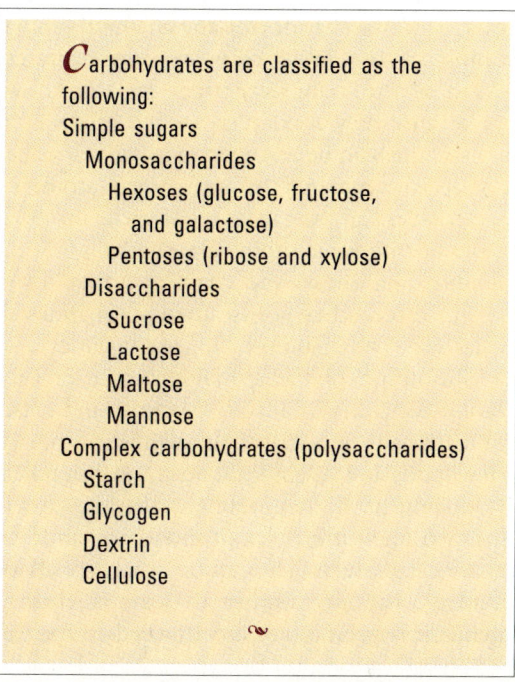

Summary of photosynthesis and respiration.

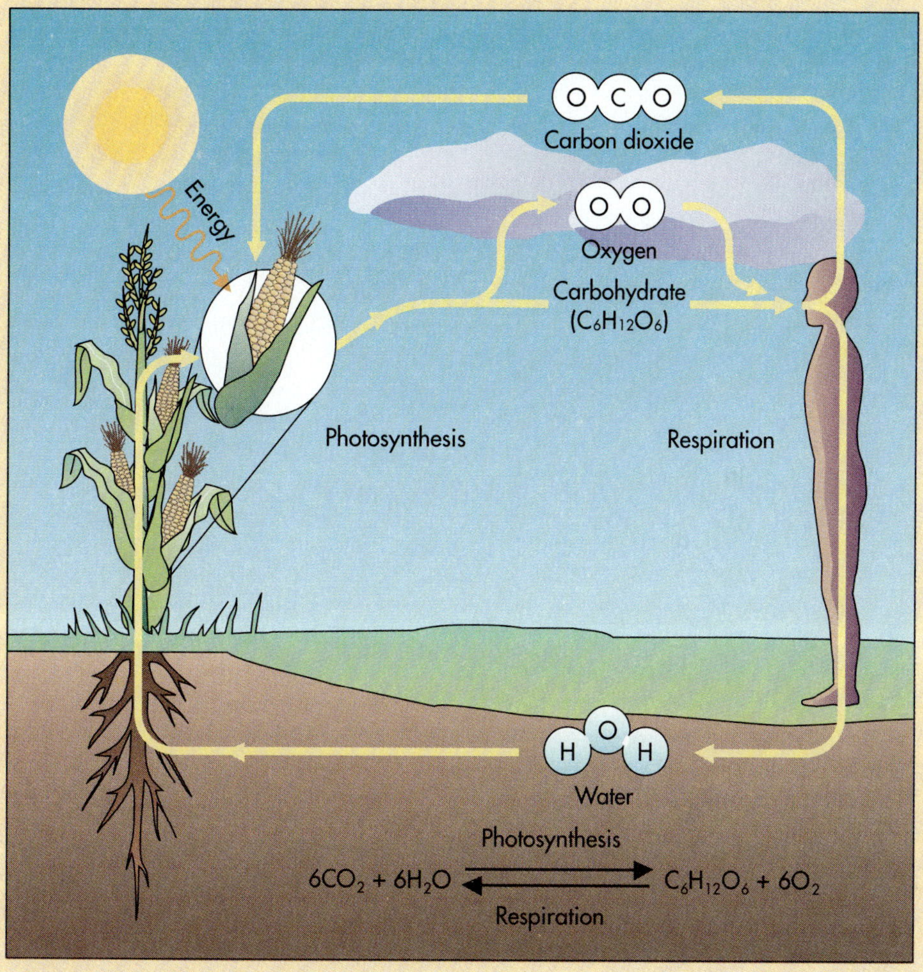

affects its taste. In vegetables such as peas and corn, carbohydrate that is stored initially as sugar is changed to starch as the seed matures. Similarly, the sweetness of carrots declines with age as the sugar in the root is converted into starch. On the other hand, the starch in immature fruits such as bananas, apples, and pears is converted to sugar during the ripening process. This is why the fruits taste better when allowed to ripen. On further ripening, however, the sugar changes to acid or is fermented to alcohol. What we call a "ripe" fruit is simply one that has reached the stage with the sugar content at a level that we find most palatable.

Carbohydrates are classified as the following:

- Simple sugars
  - Monosaccharides
    - Hexoses (glucose, fructose, and galactose)
    - Pentoses (ribose and xylose)
  - Disaccharides
    - Sucrose
    - Lactose
    - Maltose
    - Mannose
- Complex carbohydrates (polysaccharides)
  - Starch
  - Glycogen
  - Dextrin
  - Cellulose

CLASSIFICATION OF CARBOHYDRATES

There are three main categories of carbohydrates: the **monosaccharides,** the **disaccharides,** and the **polysaccharides** (Figure 3-4).

FIGURE 3-4

Summary of monosaccharide, disaccharide, and polysaccharide structure.

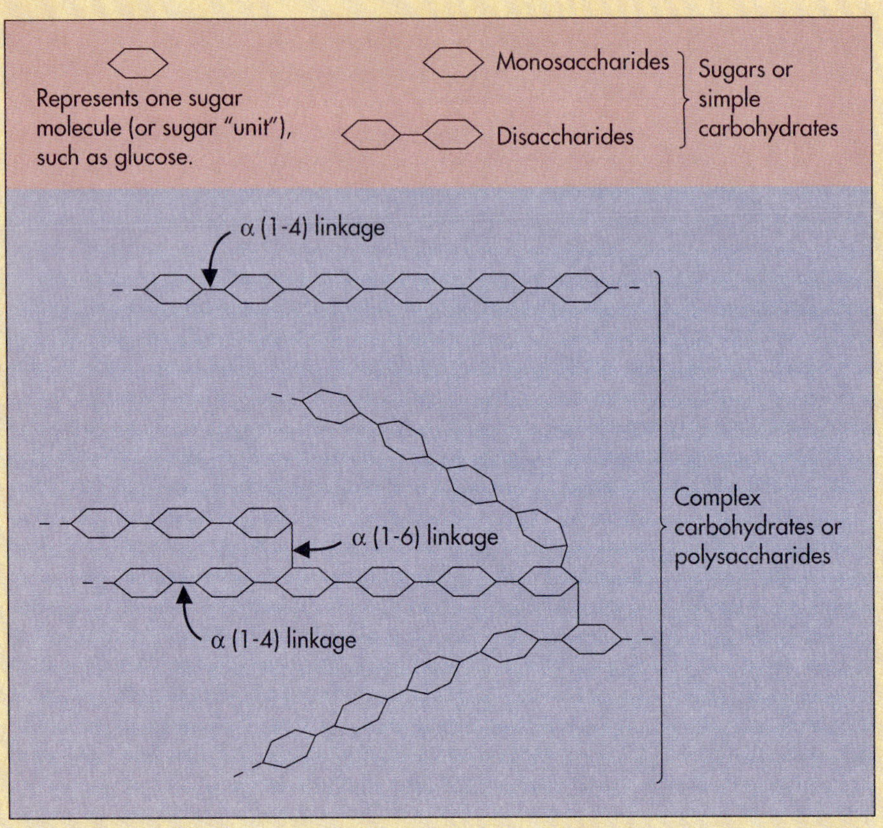

MONOSACCHARIDES

Hexoses

The simplest carbohydrates are the monosaccharides, which means one sugar ("mono" for one, "saccharide" for sugar). Monosaccharides are the chemical units from which most of the more complex carbohydrates are built. Most of the monosaccharides are also known as **hexoses** because they contain six carbon atoms ("hex," meaning six) that can be arranged in a chain or as part of a ring that is completed by an oxygen atom. Many monosaccharides can exist in chain or cyclic forms. Both forms contain the same atoms arranged slightly differently. Figure 3-5 shows the chain and ring forms of glucose and three other hexose monosaccharides: fructose, galactose, and mannose. It also includes a more realistic illustration of the spatial structure of each of these monosaccharides. Glucose, fructose, and galactose are all nutritionally important, but mannose is present in only a few foods and so has little nutritional significance.

By looking at all four monosaccharides in Figure 3-5, the two main principles of monosaccharide structure can be clearly seen. The carbon atoms are all joined or "bonded" to one another to form a chain, and hydrogen and oxygen atoms are attached to the carbon atoms, either as single atoms or within hydroxyl (OH) groups.

All hexoses contain the same number and kind of atoms—6 carbon atoms, 12 hydrogen atoms, and 6 oxygen atoms—so they all have the same molecular formula: $C_6H_{12}O_6$. In each one, however, the atoms are arranged in a different way; so each one has its own chemical structure. The six carbon atoms are always bonded together; thus the differences in structure concern only the way in which the hydrogen and oxygen atoms are bonded to the carbon atoms. The differences in the spatial arrangements of the atoms that can be seen in Figure 3-5 are responsible for the differences in sweetness, solubility, and other properties that distinguish each monosaccharide from all others.

The naturally occurring monosaccharides—found mainly in fruits, vegetables, and milk—make up approximately 10% of dietary carbohydrate. We now take a closer look at the three main monosaccharides: glucose, fructose, and galactose.

Glucose

Glucose (also known as **dextrose, blood sugar,** and **grape sugar**) is found naturally in fruits, vegetables, and

FIGURE 3-5

Chain and ring structures and space-filling models of glucose, fructose, galactose, and mannose.

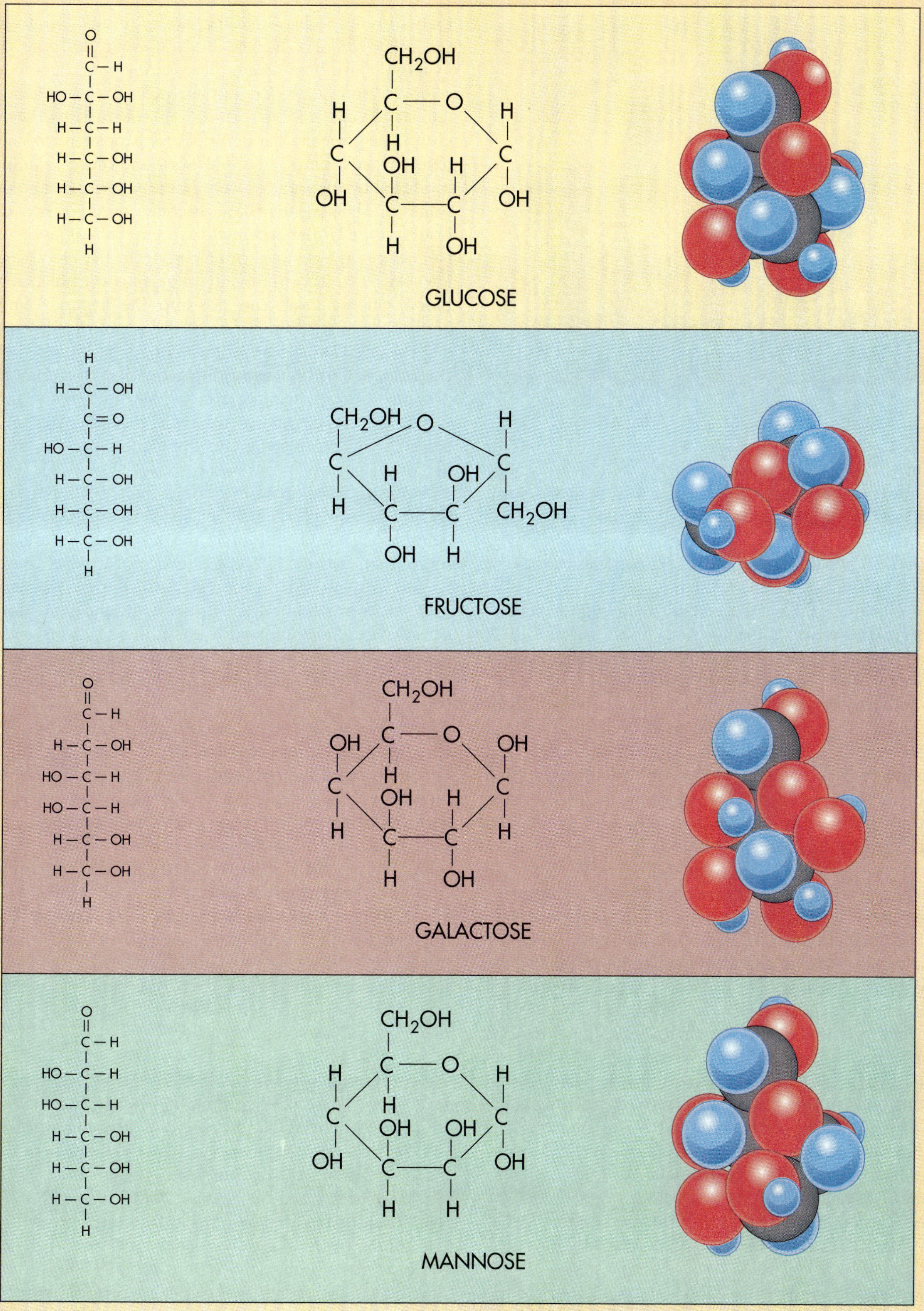

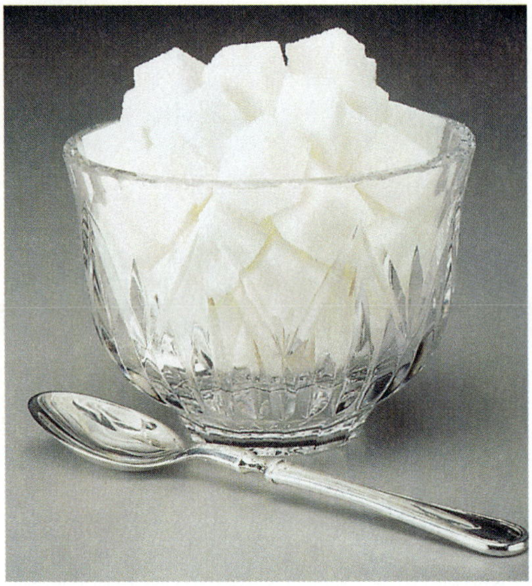

honey. These foods, however, provide us with an average of only 18 g of glucose per day, which is only a small fraction of the glucose used daily in the body. The rest is provided by the breakdown of more complex carbohydrates, by the conversion of other monosaccharides, or by the metabolism of certain amino acids.

Glucose is the main source of energy for the **central nervous system (CNS),** which uses about 140 g (9 Tbsp) of glucose per day. Red blood cells need about 40 g (3 Tbsp) of glucose per day.

Glucose is often referred to as *blood sugar* because it is by far the main form in which carbohydrate is transported within the blood to all the cells, tissues, and organs of the body. Thus most of the carbohydrates that we eat must be converted into glucose before their atoms and energy can be transported in blood and delivered to the cells of the body.

The processes within the body usually serve to maintain a blood glucose concentration of approximately 90 mg of glucose per deciliter of blood. One deciliter (dl) is one tenth of a liter (100 ml). When the required amount of glucose is not being provided by the diet, extra glucose can be generated by the breakdown of carbohydrate stores within the cells of the body or by the chemical conversion of some amino acids into glucose. A blood glucose level of about 90 mg/dl is referred to as the **fasting glucose level** because it is the level that is maintained during fasting. After a meal, when carbohydrates in the diet are being digested and absorbed, the amount of glucose in the blood can rise well above the fasting level. It then falls gradually as glucose is taken into cells and either used as a source of energy or raw materials immediately or converted into complex carbohydrate or fat as storage compounds for future use.

Hyperglycemia If the blood glucose level rises too high, above 200 mg/dl, a condition called **hyperglycemia** (too much glucose in the blood) results. Normally the processes of a healthy body prevent the state of hyperglycemia from arising by ensuring that glucose is removed from the blood and into cells at a suitably fast rate. In people suffering from **diabetes mellitus,** however, hyperglycemia can occur. These people either have deficient supplies of a natural hormone called **insulin,** produced by the pancreas (**type I diabetes mellitus**), or some of their tissues have become unresponsive to insulin (**type II diabetes mellitus**). One role of insulin is to promote the removal of glucose from the blood and into various cells of the body. In persons with diabetes, blood glucose levels can rise into the hyperglycemic zone. One of the first effects of this problem is on the kidneys. The kidneys are where urine is produced, and the kidneys normally reabsorb glucose from the urine to prevent it from being excreted from the body and wasted. In the state of hyperglycemia the kidneys cannot reabsorb the excessive amounts of glucose present; thus glucose begins to appear in the urine.

Testing for glucose in urine is one of the simplest ways to identify people who may be developing diabetes. Another related symptom is the tendency to urinate more frequently. A third consequence of hyperglycemia is thirst caused when more fluid than usual is being excreted from the body as urine. Thus the four most obvious and most immediate symptoms of diabetes are unusually high levels of glucose in the blood, the presence of glucose in urine, frequent urination, and thirst.

Hypoglycemia On the other hand, if the blood glucose level falls much too low, to about 60 mg/dl, a condition called **hypoglycemia** (too little glucose in the blood) results. In addition to feeling hungry, people with hypoglycemia experience weakness, sweating, and light-headedness. Hypoglycemia is not a disease, but a symptom by which various diseases can be diagnosed (just as hyperglycemia is a symptom of diabetes). It is also a danger in persons with diabetes because of the uncertainties that variations in exercise or food intake introduce relative to exogenous (externally supplied) insulin administer to treat the condition. In extreme cases both hypoglycemia and hyperglycemia can cause people to fall into a coma and die.

Reactive hypoglycemia A mild form of hypoglycemia, sometimes called **reactive hypoglycemia,** occurs from time to time in almost everyone. Sometimes this is simply because a person has waited too long between meals. Reactive hypoglycemia occurs when the cells of the body have taken up glucose from the blood faster than it can be replaced by supplies from the liver, where our limited reserves of carbohydrate are stored. It tends to occur several hours after eating and only lasts a short time before correcting itself or being corrected by new supplies from a meal.

Reactive hypoglycemia can also be caused by eating a meal high in carbohydrate, especially simple sugars, which are absorbed from the intestine and converted into blood glucose rapidly. This causes a sudden increase in the blood glucose level, which in turn causes the pancreas to produce and release large amounts of insulin. This insulin serves to prevent hyperglycemia by promoting the rapid uptake of blood glucose into cells. Sometimes, however, the pancreas overreacts and produces large amounts of insulin for longer than is necessary. This causes the blood glucose level to fall low enough to cause symptoms of hypoglycemia. The resulting symptoms usually include a lack of **neuromotor coordination.** This means that the nerves that control muscles and the muscles they control stop working together properly, resulting in uncoordinated movements of the limbs. Because this form of hypoglycemia usually occurs after a meal, it is also known as **postprandial hypoglycemia** ("post," meaning after; "prandium," meaning meal).

Spontaneous hypoglycemia One other form of hypoglycemia, **spontaneous hypoglycemia,** is characterized by chronically low blood glucose levels because the pancreas constantly produces too much insulin. This excessive insulin production occurs whether or not there has been a surge of glucose into the blood to stimulate insulin production. The symptoms are the same as before: weakness, sweating, light-headedness, and loss of neuromotor coordination. These symptoms of hypoglycemia indicate that the brain and nerve cells can use only glucose as a source of energy and are becoming literally starved until they begin to stop working properly. Such symptoms as anxiety, tiredness, weakness, and dizziness are common to both reactive and spontaneous hypoglycemia; thus it is not surprising that many people are misdiagnosed as suffering from spontaneous hypoglycemia when the more easily corrected reactive hypoglycemia is their only problem.

Sorbitol Before leaving the subject of glucose, we should briefly consider **sorbitol.** Sorbitol is a derivative of glucose that is formed when glucose is chemically "reduced" by the addition of one hydrogen atom. Sorbitol occurs naturally in such fruits as apples, pears, and peaches and also in several vegetables. It is absorbed from the intestine and converted in the liver to the monosaccharide fructose before further metabolism. It is not actively absorbed from the gastrointestinal (GI) tract and is absorbed at about one third the rate of glucose absorption. This means that eating food rich in sorbitol allows blood glucose levels to remain above the fasting level for a longer time than does eating food correspondingly rich in glucose. Thus eating sorbitol may delay the onset of hunger. For this reason, sorbitol is an ingredient in some foods designed for use in weight-reducing diets and has been used clinically as a non–insulin-stimulating carbohydrate. Unfortunately, sorbitol also causes flatulence and diarrhea in some people, which considerably reduces its acceptability. Sorbitol is also widely used as a sweetener in chewing gums because it is less likely to promote the formation of dental cavities than is sucrose, the usual sweetening agent.

Fructose

Fructose, another monosaccharide, is also known as **levulose** or **fruit sugar.** It is called fruit sugar because it occurs in many different fruits and berries. It also makes up one third of the sugar in honey. Some years ago it became commercially feasible to convert cornstarch or sucrose (table sugar) into fructose using enzymes. Specific purified enzymes are used to make either pure crystalline fructose or **high-fructose corn syrup** (HFCS). This is sweeter per calorie than normal sugar and was first used commercially in the 1970s. It is now used in a wide variety of processed foods, especially beverages. The extent of its use tends to fluctuate widely, depending on the price of common sugar relative to the price of fructose from corn. The growing popularity of HFCS overall, however, is evident (Figure 3-6). Current use of HFCS is estimated to be 40 lb per person per year.

Insulin is not needed to allow fructose to be transported into cells; so fructose does not cause problems of high blood sugar levels in persons with diabetes. This has led to the idea that diets high in fructose might be a suitable way for those with diabetes to get their supplies of carbohydrate. We have too little experience with the effects of high-fructose diets, however, to be sure that they are safe. There is some evidence that a high fructose intake may increase plasma lipid levels in certain susceptible individuals.

We do know that fructose is less likely to be **cariogenic** (tending to cause tooth decay) than other sugar-based sweeteners. Tooth decay, technically known as **caries,** is produced when bacteria in the mouth act on carbohydrate to produce acid. The level of acid production depends on what carbohydrates are available in the mouth, with fructose resulting in a relatively low level.

It was mentioned earlier that over one third of the sugar in honey is in the form of fructose. Despite what some advertisers suggest, however, there is no proven benefit to be gained from the use of fructose as an "animal sugar" produced by bees. When fructose is sold in crystalline form, it must be considered a processed rather than a natural food product. Honey itself has been advertised as a natural food high in fructose. As far as we know, however, apart from its pleasant flavor there is no reason to promote the use of fructose in preference to other carbohydrates. In fact there may be a drawback in increasing fructose consumption because evidence is growing that it may increase the body's need for the mineral copper.[3]

FIGURE 3-6

Availability of sweeteners for the U.S. population from 1960 to 1990.

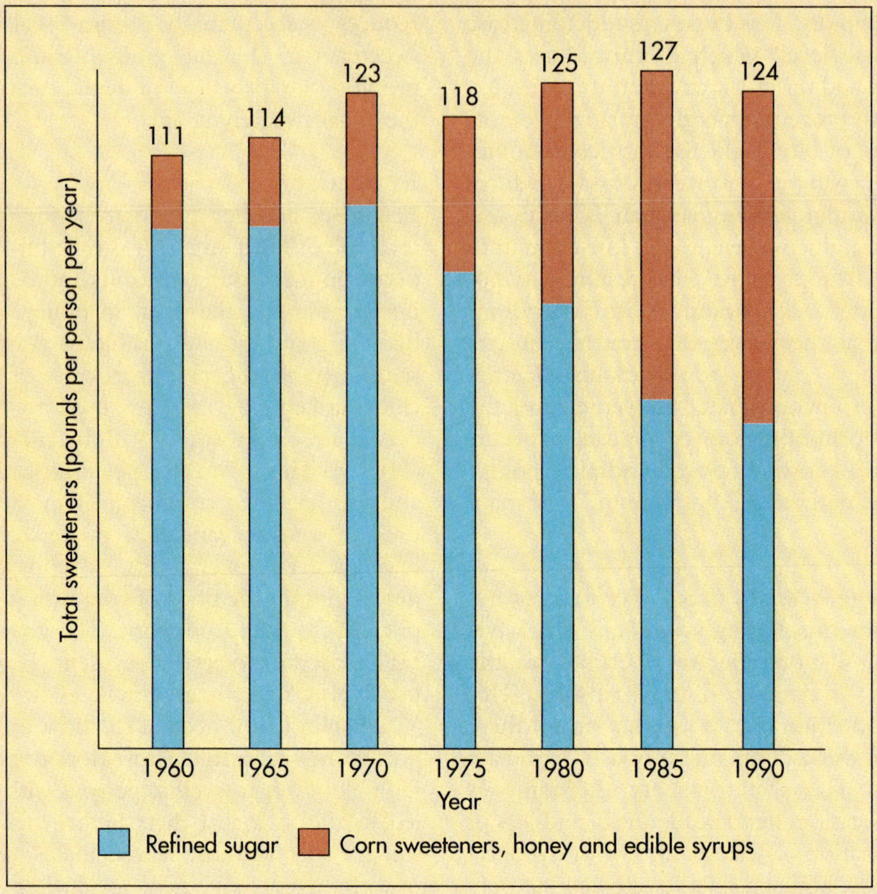

Galactose

Galactose, the third main monosaccharide of nutritional relevance, occurs only as a result of the breakdown during digestion of the disaccharide known as **lactose.** Lactose is the sugar found in milk, and many of us take in significant amounts of it (8 g per cup of milk). Milk, of course, is of animal rather than plant origin, and galactose is the only monosaccharide obtained primarily from animal-based food. Studies using laboratory animals have linked excessive galactose consumption with the development of cataracts. The levels used, however, indicated that this was unlikely to present any problem to humans apart from the few people with a genetic defect of metabolism known as **galactosemia,** which leads to excessive amounts of galactose in the blood.

Pentoses

The hexoses just described are by far the major monosaccharides in food, but food also contains several five-carbon sugars known as **pentoses.** One, called **ribose,** is part of the vitamin riboflavin (vitamin B_2). Ribose is also part of the important chemicals ribonucleic acid (RNA) and in a slightly modified form deoxyribonucleic acid (DNA). RNA acts as the intermediary between the DNA of our genes and the protein molecules whose production is directed by our genes. Ribose can be produced in the body from glucose, which makes its presence in the diet nonessential.

Another pentose sugar called **xylose** is now being produced commercially from the complex polysaccharides cellulose and hemicellulose found in wood, especially birchwood. **Xylitol,** an "alcohol sugar" derived from xylose, is being used as an alternative sweetener in candies and gum because, similar to sorbitol, it does not contribute to tooth decay and does not require insulin for its metabolism. Currently there is no concern about the safety of xylitol at the levels usually consumed.

DISACCHARIDES

Disaccharides are formed when two monosaccharide molecules join together in a chemical reaction that also

FIGURE 3-7

Synthesis and hydrolysis of disaccharides.

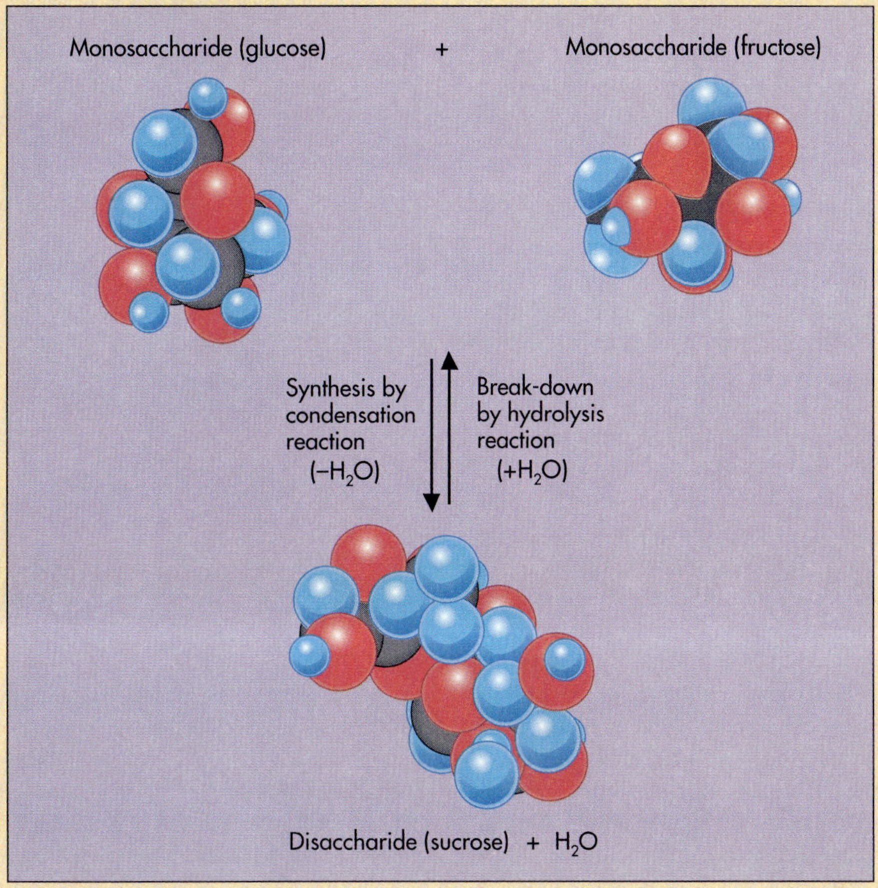

releases one water molecule. So the linkage of monosaccharides into disaccharides is a "condensation" reaction (see Appendix A). It is illustrated diagrammatically in Figure 3-7.

Different disaccharides are produced when different kinds of monosaccharide molecules become joined. Three main disaccharides—known as sucrose, lactose, and maltose—are found in food, each of which contains at least one glucose unit. **Sucrose** is formed when one molecule of glucose combines with a molecule of fructose. **Lactose** is formed when a molecule of glucose combines with a molecule of galactose. **Maltose** is formed when a molecule of glucose combines with another molecule of glucose. Sucrose and maltose are made in plant cells, whereas lactose is the "milk sugar" produced by the mammary glands of mammals. Sucrose, lactose, and maltose have the same molecular formula, namely $C_{12}H_{22}O_{11}$, or put another way $C_{12}(H_2O)_{11}$, but each has its atoms arranged in a distinct way.

Once we have eaten disaccharide sugars, the processes of digestion must reverse the reaction that made them, by adding water to the disaccharide in a way that splits it back into its two original monosaccharides. This is because only monosaccharides are readily absorbed by the intestinal cells and transported to blood. This reversal of the condensation reaction is an hydrolysis reaction.

Sucrose

Sucrose is the most common disaccharide. It is obtained commercially from sugar cane and sugar beets and is mainly purified to produce the familiar white crystals or powder known simply as "sugar." Whether in "granulated" form (composed of readily visible crystals) or fine powdered form, this product is 100% sucrose. Brown sugar, with its more distinctive flavor, is 97% sucrose and is made by partially refining sucrose or by adding some molasses to white refined sugar. Both sugar cane and sugar beets yield far more kilocalories per acre than any other crop, which makes sugar our least expensive source of food energy. Although sugar does not provide any other nutrients, it does much to enhance the palatability of many foods.

On average, each person in the United States consumes 41 g (about ¼ cup) of sucrose per day. The average intake of "total sugar" (sucrose and other sugars, both naturally present in and added to food, but not including lactose) is 80 g per day.[4] There are well-publicized concerns that the amount of sugars in the typical U.S. diet may have adverse effects on health, particularly if the sugars displace foods that provide other essential nutrients besides carbohydrates.

Lactose

Lactose is the disaccharide found only in milk and is composed of glucose combined with galactose. Americans consume an average of 25 g of lactose per day. One effect of dietary lactose is to enhance the intestinal absorption of calcium from foods. It is interesting that milk, our only source of lactose, is also our most dependable source of calcium.

The enzyme **lactase** is produced in the intestinal mucosal cells and is essential for the conversion of dietary lactose into glucose and galactose. In most mammals and in many races of humans, intestinal lactase activity is high at birth, declines to low levels during childhood, and remains low in adulthood. The low levels of lactase in the intestine (**lactase insufficiency**) are associated with intolerance to milk and other milk products containing lactose (**lactose intolerance**). Most Europeans and Americans of European descent retain their intestinal lactase activity. Thus the incidence of lactase insufficiency in people of northern and western European descent is only approximately 15%. The incidence in African-American, Native American, Asian, and Mediterranean populations is 70% to 90%.[5] Lactose intolerance as a result of lactase insufficiency causes undigested lactose, which cannot be absorbed, to accumulate in the GI tract, where it serves as food for microorganisms that thrive there. Some of these microorganisms produce a large amount of gas, resulting in symptoms of flatulence, bloating, and abdominal cramps. Also, because lactose has what is called an *osmotic effect,* which loosely means a tendency to attract water, its presence in the colon leads to retention of water there, with resulting watery stools or diarrhea.

People with lactose intolerance experience a lot of discomfort if they eat large amounts of lactose-containing dairy products. They can eat fermented dairy products, such as cheese, however, because much of the lactose has been converted into lactic acid, which does not cause a problem. They can also eat yogurt that is prepared by fermentation because the fermentative microorganisms convert the original lactose into lactic acid. Yogurt that is manufactured by adding lactic acid, without relying on fermentation, may not be tolerated.

Many people with lactase insufficiency are able to tolerate small amounts of lactose and can consume milk products in moderation. Although they may never begin to produce lactase, they do seem to gradually build up a tolerance to lactose and can consume increasing amounts over time.

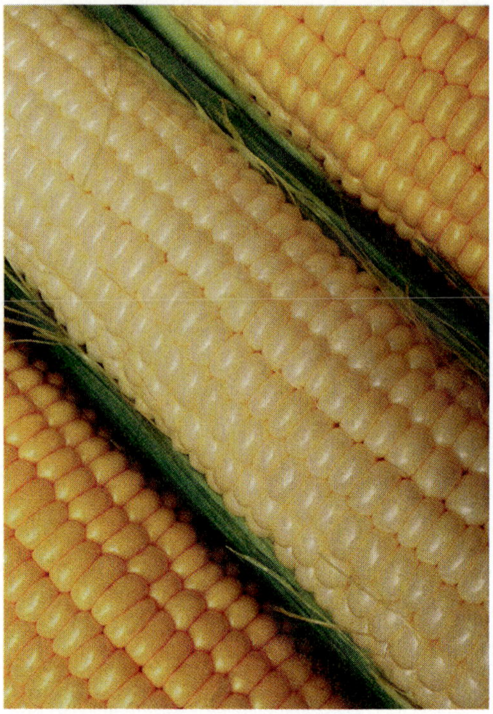

Most infants, including those who become lactase insufficient in later life, do have the appropriate levels of enzymes to thrive solely on milk without any problems. The intolerance to lactose in people with lactase insufficiency develops later, in early childhood. This situation has led many to question the wisdom of providing milk in school feeding programs for population groups in which lactase insufficiency is common. Instead of withholding milk from all children, however, many nutritionists suggest that children who are lactase insufficient should be identified so that milk can be withdrawn from only their diets.

Finally, the availability of the enzyme lactase, purified from yeasts and molds, has made it possible for lactose-intolerant people to drink milk or to eat food made with milk without concern. The enzyme, which is available in tablet or powder form, is taken before or with lactose-containing foods or is mixed with the food before it is consumed. It splits the lactose into glucose and galactose, eliminating the problem and permitting the consumption of milk and milk-containing products, which are valuable sources of dietary calcium and protein.

Maltose

The third nutritionally significant disaccharide is maltose. It is composed of two glucose molecules joined together. It is found only in the germinating seeds of cereals. During the process of germination, starch in the cereal is broken down into maltose molecules. These are then split further into glucose, which serves to nourish the germinating seed. During the fermentation process used to make beer and other malt beverages, the maltose is converted into alcohol by enzymes in brewing yeasts.

The Sweetness of Sugars

All sugars contribute sweetness to food, but the relative sweetening power varies among sugars. In general, the more easily the sugar dissolves in water, the greater its sweetening power. For example, fructose is 75% sweeter than any other sugar. It is soluble in water, difficult to crystallize, and, as a result, expensive. It is useful in syrups and is the type of sugar formed in soft-centered candies. At the other extreme, the least sweet, least soluble sugar is lactose. Lactose is seldom if ever used as a sweetener because it is almost impossible to dissolve in the food to be sweetened.

For a long time, scientists have wondered whether the desire for sweetness in food is something we are born with or a taste we acquire. Recent studies indicate that even in utero (in the womb) and immediately after birth, the fetus and the newborn baby respond favorably to a stimulus from a sweet substance and unfavorably to a bitter substance.[6]

POLYSACCHARIDES

Unlike the monosaccharides and disaccharides, the **polysaccharides,** the third category of carbohydrate, are not sugars. Polysaccharides are known as the **complex carbohydrates** because their molecules are much larger and more complex than those of the monosaccharides or disaccharides. All polysaccharides are made up of many individual sugar molecules, usually glucose, joined together by condensation reactions. This is signified by the name *polysaccharide,* which is made up of "poly" (meaning many) and "saccharide" (meaning sugars). Four types of polysaccharide are nutritionally significant: starch, glycogen, dextrin, and fiber.

Starch

About half of our dietary carbohydrate is composed of the carbohydrates known as **starches.** Although starch molecules can be large (from 2000 to 26,000 glucose units) and look complicated, they are all composed simply of glucose molecules joined together by condensation reactions. If the glucose units in these large molecules are joined into one long chain, the starch is known as an **amylose.** An enormous variety of different amylose molecules can exist, each with a different number of glucose units, but they all have their glucose units linked into a single chain and are all classified as starches. The glucose units in amylose are joined by what are known as **α(1-4) linkages** (Figure 3-4) because they bond together carbon atoms one and four of adjacent molecules, which are in what is called the *α-configuration.* It is also possible for the glucose units to be joined up in a branching pattern. Starches with the branched structure are known as **amylopectins.** They consist of chains of glucose units joined by α(1-4) linkages, with the chains joined to one another in places by an alternative type of linkage known as the **α(1-6) linkage.**

Starches are produced in plants, where they serve as a storage form of carbohydrate. Each plant produces its own characteristic type of starch, depending on the number of glucose units linked together and the pattern of branching, if any. Large numbers of individual starch molecules are found aggregated together into **starch granules.** Granules of potato starch can be distinguished from granules of rice, wheat, cassava, corn, or any other starch by examining the size and shape of the granules under the microscope. Also, the starch from each source has its own characteristic solubility, thickening power, and flavor. Nutritionally, however, there is no difference between starches from different sources. All cooked starches can be broken down in the body into identical glucose molecules for absorption and transport to the body's cells.

Glycogen

Animals, including humans, store some carbohydrate in the form of a polysaccharide known as **glycogen.** Glycogen consists of glucose units linked into a pattern of branching chains by α(1-4) and α(1-6) linkages, much like amylopectin. Glycogen, however, is more highly branched than amylopectin. Glycogen is stored in the liver and muscles. Liver, muscles, milk, and blood are in fact the only parts of animals that contain significant amounts of carbohydrate. Even there, the amounts are not large. The average male human stores a total of only about 500 g of glycogen; one fifth of that is stored in the liver and the remaining four fifths in muscle. The energy stored in the glycogen is sufficient to meet the energy needs of an adult for only about two thirds of a day. The animal muscle or liver that we use as food contains virtually no glycogen because it is converted into lactic acid when the animal is slaughtered.

The capacity of the liver and muscles to store glycogen can be increased by as much as 50% to 100% by a combination of diet control and exercise.[7,8] This procedure is known as **carbohydrate loading** and involves carefully controlled changes in carbohydrate consumption and exercise. For a while it was used routinely by athletes to enhance their performance during endurance activities, such as soccer or long-distance running. These activities demand large amounts of energy over periods of 30 minutes or more of continuous exercise. Increased glycogen supplies could provide some of that energy. Adverse side effects of the carbohydrate loading regimen began to appear, however, and most athletes have abandoned it in favor of regular adherence to a diet high in complex carbohydrates (see Chapter 18).

Dextrin

If the long glucose-containing chains of starch are broken down into shorter chains by removing maltose units (each composed of two glucose units) one after another, a carbohydrate known as **dextrin** results. The partial degradation of starch into dextrin can be accomplished by salivary and pancreatic enzymes during digestion. It is also achieved by the action of dry heat on starch (during the toasting of bread, for example) or during the production of the dry bread known as **zwieback** for infants. Dextrin is slightly soluble in water and is sweeter than the starch from which it comes.

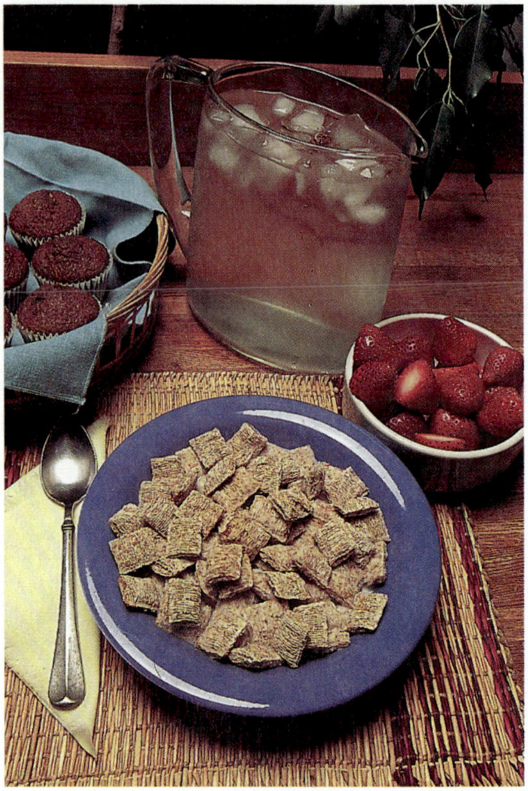

Fiber

Fiber is an indigestible carbohydrate. It is taken in as part of many foods, but most of it simply passes through the digestive tract because we do not possess the enzymes needed to break it down into a form that can be absorbed into the blood. However, some bacteria in the large intestine can degrade some components of fiber, releasing products that can be absorbed into the body and used as an energy source.

Two categories of fiber are found in food: *crude fiber* and *dietary fiber.* The major component of **crude fiber** is the polysaccharide called **cellulose.** Cellulose provides the structural framework for all plant material. In other words, it forms and holds together the shape of a carrot, a bean, a squash, and other plants. Cellulose is the most abundant organic chemical on Earth, being found in fruits, vegetables, and whole grain cereals, as well as in wood and the leaves, stems, and roots of all plant life. Like starch, cellulose is composed of many glucose units, but they are joined together in a different way, by **β(1-4) linkages** rather than the α(1-4) and α(1-6) linkages of starch. This subtle structural difference prevents our digestive enzymes from breaking cellulose down to release its glucose.

Several other carbohydrates and related compounds called **pectins, hemicelluloses,** and **lignins** are found in plant foods and are also resistant to digestion in the human digestive tract. These, together with cellulose, are known collectively as **dietary fiber.** This is a general term that describes any material in food that remains undigested in the intestine. The cellulose that is called *crude fiber* is just a part of dietary fiber as a whole.

Dietary fiber can also be classified into soluble and insoluble fiber. **Soluble fiber** is found in fruits, some legumes, and such grains as oats, rye, and barley. It dissolves in water to form a gel. This gel forms within the digestive tract and serves to slow the rate at which food passes through the small intestine. This in turn increases the rate of absorption of nutrients from the food. Soluble fiber is known to have cholesterol-lowering effects because of its promotion of increased fecal excretion of bile acids, slower cholesterol and lipid absorption, and increased production of short-chain fatty acids by fermentation in the large intestine. The relative importance of these factors in the cholesterol-lowering effect of soluble fiber is unknown.

Insoluble fiber—composed of cellulose, hemicellulose, and lignins—is found in vegetables and wheat bran. It tends to absorb water and increase in bulk, greatly contributing to the volume of stools or feces. This causes insoluble fiber to increase **gastrointestinal motility,** or in other words speed the movement of material through the GI tract, especially the colon.

Balancing fiber intake Most national health authorities recommend that Westerners increase their fiber intake. Only recently, however, have they begun to make quantified recommendations. The advice to increase fiber intake has caused some food processors to add fiber to their foods, largely in the form of bran or wood fiber. However, there is now concern that some people may be consuming too much fiber, which can lead to a condition known as **irritable bowel syndrome.** It is also possible that too much fiber may cause decreased absorption of some mineral elements (magnesium, calcium, zinc, and iron), either by binding to them or by simply speeding the passage of food through the intestinal tract and reducing the opportunity for the mineral elements to be absorbed. At present it is thought that 20 to 30 g of dietary fiber per day maximizes the benefits of fiber while minimizing the possible adverse effects of either excessive or insufficient fiber consumption. This recommended level is considerably more than the current typical intakes of 15 g for men and 10 g for women.[9]

Current intakes of dietary fiber are less than half the recommended levels.

Interest in the role of fiber in the diet has been stimulated by the observation that other cultures with a high consumption of fiber have much lower incidences of both cancer of the colon and diverticulitis. Most attention has focused on fiber itself as the cause of these effects, but it is possible that other components of high-fiber diets are responsible for the protection against cancer.

Cancer of the colon is the second leading cause of death from cancer; it kills 52,000 Americans per year. The link between a lack of dietary fiber and the onset of colon cancer has been attributed to various effects of fiber—namely, changes in the populations of microorganisms in the GI tract, the decreased binding of intestinal bile acids, the increased time for which food residue remains in the colon, decreased stool weight and volume, and decreased frequency of defecation. Scientists postulate that the microorganisms encouraged by a diet low in dietary fiber enhance the formation of cancer-causing substances (**carcinogens**). These microorganisms may also prevent or at least limit the breakdown of carcinogens that are normally destroyed by the microorganisms that thrive when there is more dietary fiber in the diet. The main alternative theory suggests that the beneficial effect of dietary fiber results from its speeding of the passage of feces through the large intestine. The logic behind this idea is that faster passage means less time for any carcinogens present to be in contact with the intestinal wall. Also, the bulk and water of the feces may dilute the carcinogens to a nontoxic level. Other **phytochemicals** (chemicals present in plant foods) such as carotenoids, indoles, and flavonoids might also contribute to the observed protective associations between diets rich in dietary fiber and certain other cancers (of breast, lung, esophagus, stomach, and pancreas).[10]

The condition known as **diverticulosis** affects 30 million Americans per year. It is associated with a weakening of the intestinal wall caused by the pressure from hard stools. The weakened intestinal wall then develops small outpouchings in which fecal material becomes trapped (Figure 3-8). Diverticulitis is an inflammation of the intestinal wall that develops when these outpouchings become irritated or infected. Dietary treatment of diverticulitis involves consuming 20 to 30 g of dietary fiber per day to encourage the formation of softer stools.

FIGURE 3-8

Development of diverticulosis and associated diverticulitis.

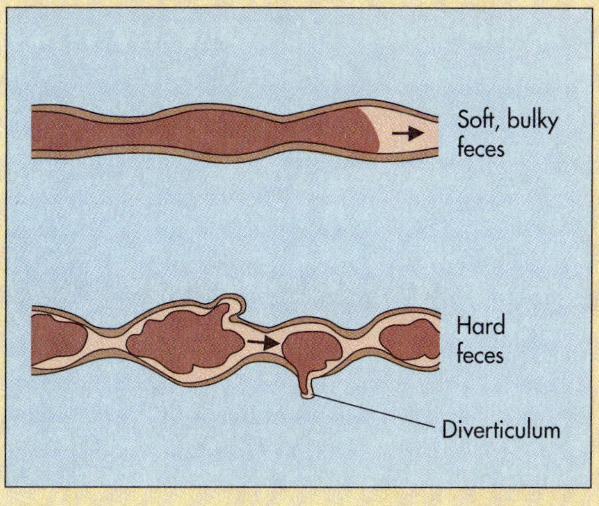

The data on fiber recorded in tables of food consumption have traditionally referred only to crude fiber or cellulose. This is because cellulose resists breakdown by strong acid or alkali in the laboratory; thus it is easy to quantify by analysis. From a nutritional standpoint, however, we are interested in data on dietary fiber, meaning all the fiber that remains undigested in the intestine. In addition to the cellulose of crude fiber, this includes hemicelluloses, pectins, and the noncarbohydrate lignins. Values for dietary fiber (Table 3-1) can be up to 10 times greater than those for crude fiber. It is also important to remember that dietary fiber occurs naturally only in foods of plant origin. It is present in foods of animal origin only if such ingredients as cereals are added during processing.[11]

One of the problems in setting recommended intakes for dietary fiber is the limited data available on the dietary fiber in foods. We know that intakes of 6 to 8 g of crude fiber are usually sufficient to avoid the constipation associated with insufficient dietary fiber. This level of crude fiber intake probably means that around 20 g of dietary fiber are being consumed. U.S. Department of Agriculture (USDA) data indicate that the amount of fiber actually available in the types of foods we eat has declined throughout this century, as has the actual intake by individuals. Current dietary recommendations and the advertising of fiber-rich foods are reversing this trend among the health-conscious sector of the population. As a general guide, experience has shown that a diet providing five daily servings of fruits and vegetables and six daily servings of cereal (at least two of which are whole grain or minimally processed) provide enough fiber.

TABLE 3-1

Carbohydrate content and selected carbohydrate sources of the most frequently used foods in the United States

FOOD	AMOUNT	KCAL	TOTAL CARBOHYDRATE (GRAMS)	DIETARY FIBER (GRAMS)*	SUGAR (GRAMS)†	STARCH (GRAMS)
Whole milk	8 oz	157	4.7	0	4.7	0
2% milk	8 oz	121	5.0	0	5.0	0
Cheddar cheese	1 oz	114	7.2	0	7.2	0
Eggs, fried	1 egg	83	1.2	0	1.2	0
Beef, roast	3 oz	318	0	0	0	0
Hamburger	3 oz	285	0	0	0	0
Chicken	3 oz	242	0	0	0	0
Tuna fish	3 oz	170	0	0	0	0
Peanut butter	2 T	178	5.4	2.1	5.4	0
Bread, white	1 slice	81	15.0	0.8	1.0	13.2
Bread, whole wheat	1 slice	73	13.0	2.4	1.0	9.6
Rice	1 oz	109	24.0	0	1.0	23
Saltine crackers	4 crackers	43	7.0	0	0	7
Corn flakes	1 oz	114	25.0	2.8	1.9	20.3
Shredded wheat	1 biscuit	105	26.0	3.0	0.1	23
Bran flakes	1 oz	90	25.0	8.2	3.4	13.4
All Bran	1 oz	70	22.0	10.0	5.0	7.0
Apple	1 apple	81	21.0	2.6	18.0	0.4
Banana	1 banana	105	26.0	1.4	24.6	0
Orange juice	4 oz	56	15.0	0.5	14.0	0.5
Peach	1 peach	40	10.0	0.6	9.0	0.4
Lettuce	¼ head	8	3.0	1.1	1.9	0
Tomatoes	1 tomato	25	5.3	1.0	4.3	0
Green beans	4 oz	30	10.0	1.8	8.2	0
Green peas	4 oz	110	18.0	5.4	12.6	0
Potato, baked	1 potato	95	21.0	1.4	1.5	18.1
Corn, canned	4 oz	98	19.8	1.3	2.3	14.2

* Includes all fiber not digested by human.

† Naturally occurring monosaccharides and disaccharides.

USDA data, 1984, 1987.

Related Carbohydrates

Mucopolysaccharides and **mucoproteins** are classes of compounds that are chemically related to carbohydrates, do not occur to any significant extent in foods, but are normal constituents of the body. The most common mucopolysaccharides are found in the fluid that lubricates the joints; in the vitreous humor of the eye; in cartilage, skin, bone, and nails; and in the blood as anticoagulants.

Modified starches are starches that have been purposely changed to give them new properties, such as altered texture or improved stability to acid and heat. They are used in many processed foods and are usually regarded as food additives. They typically make up about 4% of a food to which they are added, such as commercially prepared baby foods. Recent survey data indicate that the average consumption of modified starch by infants from commercially prepared baby foods is about 3.6 g/day or 1.8% of the average daily energy intake. This amount is regarded as of little practical significance.[12]

Sugar alcohols such as sorbitol, xylitol, and mannitol are derived from carbohydrates. They are added to some foods largely because of special properties, such as their rate of absorption into the body and their effect on dental health.

DIGESTION AND ABSORPTION OF CARBOHYDRATE

Before carbohydrate can fulfill its role in the body, it must be converted into monosaccharide units that can be absorbed by the intestinal mucosal cells and transported to the blood. The required changes are brought about by the action of certain enzymes found in

TABLE 3-2

Principal carbohydrate digestive enzymes and their products.

SOURCE	ENZYME	PRODUCTS
Salivary glands	Salivary α-amylase	Hydrolyzes α(1-4) linkages, producing α-limited dextrins, maltotriose, and maltose
Pancreas	Pancreatic α-amylase	Hydrolyzes α(1-4) linkages, producing α-limited dextrins, maltotriose, and maltose
Intestinal mucosa	Maltase	Hydrolyzes maltose and maltotriose to glucose
	Lactase	Hydrolyzes lactose to galactose and glucose
	Sucrase*	Hydrolyzes sucrose to glucose and fructose
	α-Limited dextrinase*	Hydrolyzes starch to glucose

* Sucrase and α-limited dextrinase are separate polypeptide chains that are subunits of a single protein.

FIGURE 3-9

Schematic representation of carbohydrate digestion and absorption.

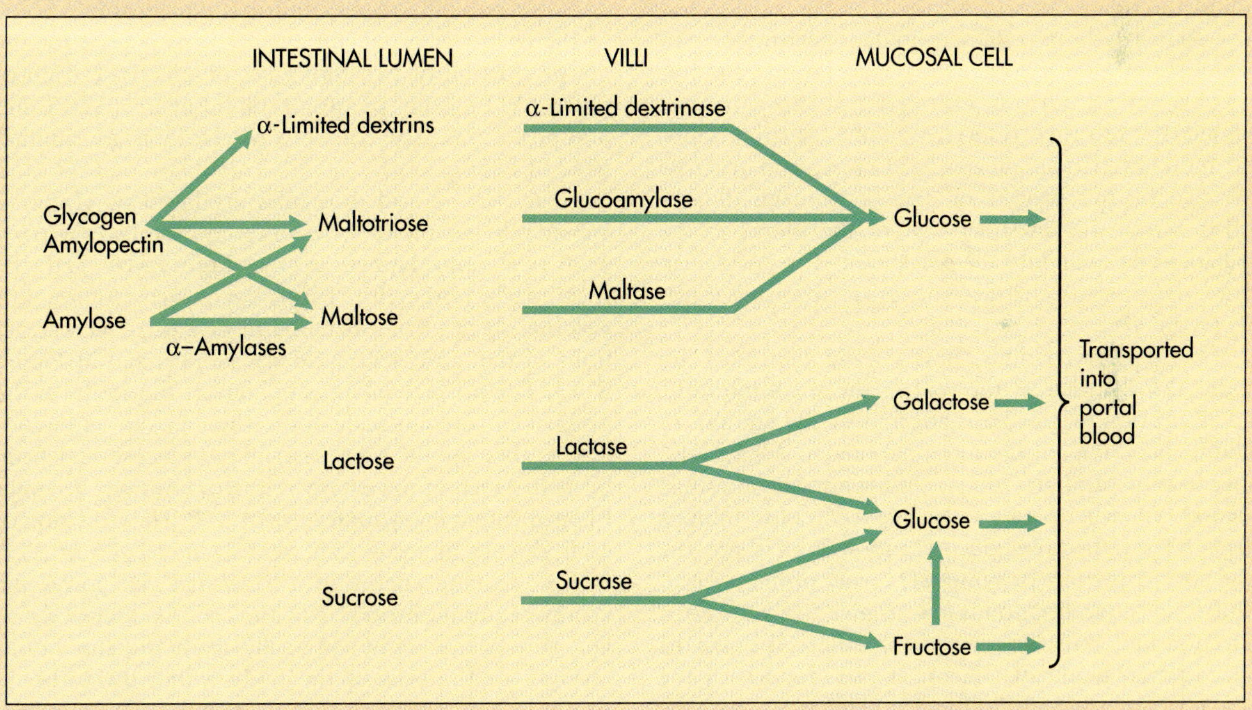

the mouth and the intestine and by the acidity of the stomach contents (Table 3-2 and Figure 3-9).

In the mouth the enzyme known as **α-amylase,** or **ptyalin,** which is present in saliva, partially breaks down starch. It catalyzes the hydrolysis of most α(1-4) linkages but not the final or "terminal" α(1-4) linkages of starch chains, the α(1-4) linkages next to branching points, or the α(1-6) linkages responsible for branching. The eventual end products of α-amylase digestion (salivary and pancreatic) are maltose, maltotriose, and α-limited dextrins (branched polymers containing an average of eight glucose units). In the acid conditions found in the stomach some disaccharides are split into monosaccharides, but the action of α-amylase is inhibited because the optimal pH value of the enzyme is 6.7. In the small intestine the conditions change from acidic to alkaline, and another potent α-amylase released from the pancreas acts to continue the digestion of starch and

FIGURE 3-10

Mechanism of glucose transport across the intestinal mucosal cell.

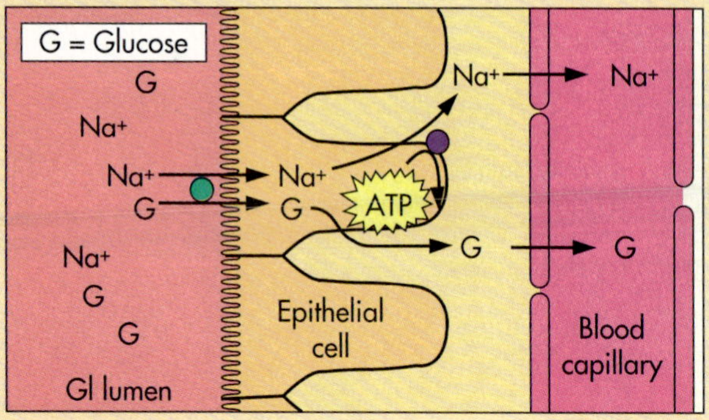

dextrins. Finally the intestinal brush border (the area around the membranes of microvilli in the small intestine) contains the enzymes α-limited dextrinase, glucoamylase, maltase, lactase, and sucrase, which are able to split α-limited dextrins, maltotriose, maltose, lactose, and sucrose into their respective monosaccharide units. The monosaccharides glucose, galactose, and fructose produced by this process of digestion are rapidly absorbed across the intestinal wall to the blood in the capillaries that drain into the portal vein. The portal vein carries the monosaccharides and other absorbed nutrients to the liver.

The monosaccharides (hexoses and pentoses) are rapidly absorbed across the wall of the small intestine. The absorption of glucose is affected by the amount of sodium (Na^+) ions in the intestinal lumen. A high Na^+ concentration facilitates glucose influx into the intestinal mucosal cell, whereas a low Na^+ concentration inhibits influx. This is because glucose and sodium share the same **cotransporter** (or **symport)** carrier protein. Intracellular Na^+ concentration is low relative to the external concentration; thus Na^+ moves into the cell down its concentration gradient. Glucose moves along with the Na^+ and is released inside the cell (Figure 3-10). The glucose transport mechanism also transports galactose. Fructose is transported via a different carrier, and its absorption is independent of Na^+ or the transport of glucose and galactose. Some fructose is converted to glucose in the mucosal cells. Pentoses are absorbed by simple diffusion. Insulin has little effect on intestinal transport of sugars, which is essentially normal in those with diabetes. The maximal rate of glucose absorption from the small intestine is 120 g/hr, or about 4 oz (or ¼ lb)/hr.

When absorbed, monosaccharides reach the liver, and fructose and galactose are converted into glucose, which is then carried in the blood to the rest of the body. These digestive changes and absorption and distribution processes are summarized in Figure 3-11.

ENERGY FROM CARBOHYDRATE

The major function of carbohydrate in the diet is to serve as a source of energy. Digestible carbohydrate is largely converted into glucose, which is released into the blood and delivered to every cell of the body. If the body requires fresh supplies of energy, most of the glucose is used as an energy-releasing fuel immediately. The first steps in this process are known collectively as **glycolysis.** "Lysis" in Greek means "to break," and in glycolysis each glucose molecule, with its six carbon atoms, is broken down into two molecules of **pyruvic acid,** each containing three carbon atoms. This stage of the metabolism of glucose does not require oxygen; thus it is **"anaerobic."** Some of the energy released during glycolysis is used for the net production of two molecules of adenosine triphosphate (ATP) from adenosine diphosphate (ADP) and phosphate ions. The reactions of glycolysis are summarized in Figure 3-12.

The pyruvic acid molecules produced by glycolysis are fed into a complex series of reactions called the *citric acid cycle* (also known as the Krebs cycle and the tricarboxylic acid cycle). This is the oxygen-requiring, or **aerobic,** stage in the metabolism of glucose. The reactions of the citric acid cycle are summarized in Figure 3-13. Their overall effect is to convert the atoms of the original glucose molecule into carbon dioxide and water, just as they would have been if the glucose had been burned. Much of the energy released, however, becomes trapped within many molecules of ATP. The oxidation of each glucose molecule can yield 38 molecules of ATP, each containing energy in a form that can power the energy-requiring processes of the cell. As discussed earlier, this energy came originally from the sun but is brought to the cells of the body within the carbohydrates we eat and the oxygen we breathe. The complete oxidation of glucose, involving both glycolysis and the citric acid cycle, is summarized in Figure 3-14.

When the amount of glucose available exceeds the amount needed to meet the body's immediate energy needs, the glucose molecules can be linked into glycogen by the enzyme **glycogen synthase** and stored in the liver or in muscle. When the capacity of the liver and muscles to store glycogen is saturated and excess glucose is still available, the glucose can be converted into fat. Small quantities of this fat can be stored in most cells, but large quantities can be stored in special fat storage cells known as **adipose cells,** or **adipocytes.** The stores of carbohydrate or fat generated when glucose is available in excess

FIGURE 3-11

Summary of carbohydrate digestion, absorption, and circulation.

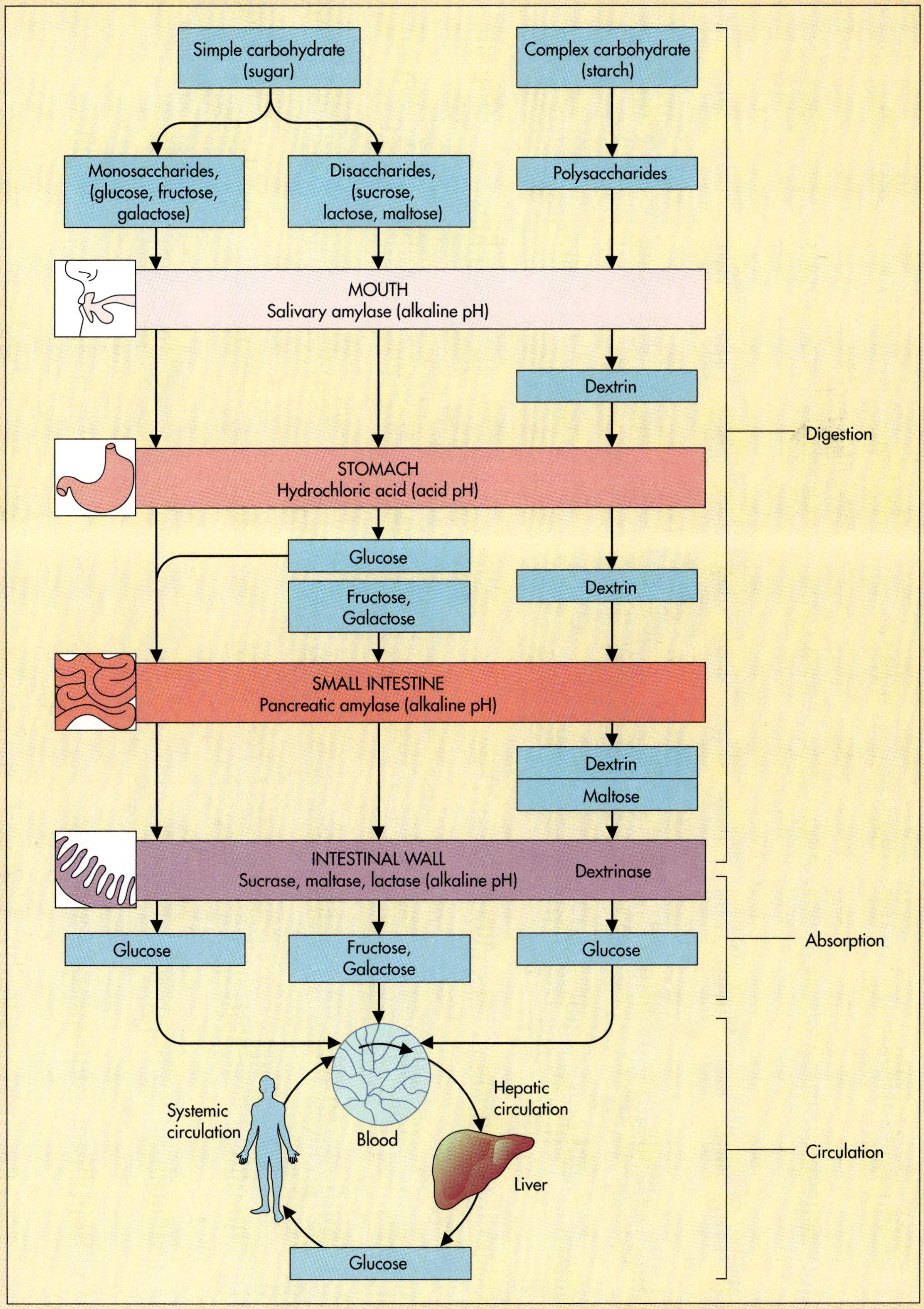

FIGURE 3-12

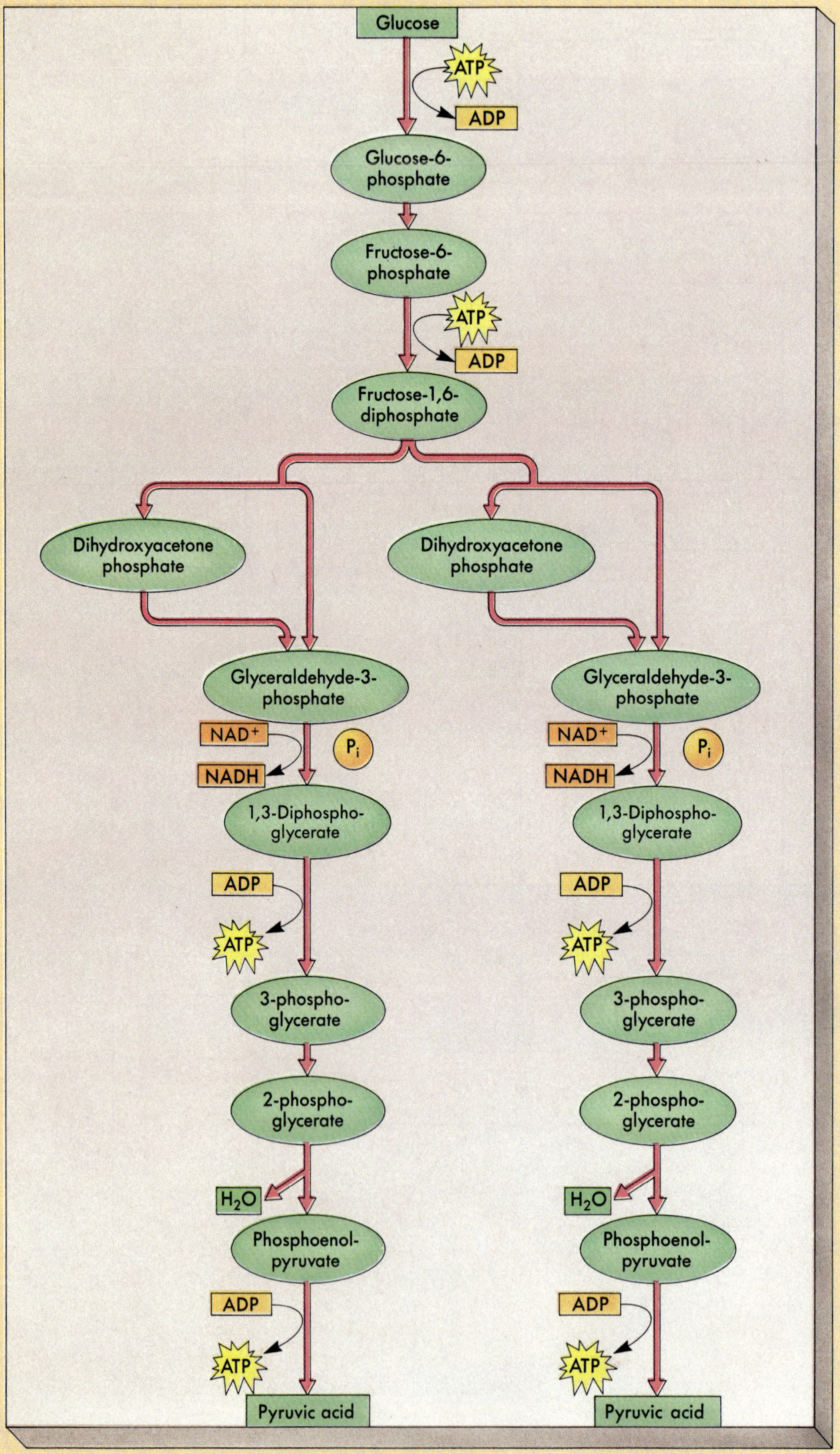
Glucose
ATP
ADP
Glucose-6-phosphate
Fructose-6-phosphate
ATP
ADP
Fructose-1,6-diphosphate
Dihydroxyacetone phosphate
Dihydroxyacetone phosphate
Glyceraldehyde-3-phosphate
Glyceraldehyde-3-phosphate
NAD+
NADH
Pi
NAD+
NADH
Pi
1,3-Diphospho-glycerate
1,3-Diphospho-glycerate
ADP
ATP
ADP
ATP
3-phospho-glycerate
3-phospho-glycerate
2-phospho-glycerate
2-phospho-glycerate
H2O
H2O
Phosphoenol-pyruvate
Phosphoenol-pyruvate
ADP
ATP
ADP
ATP
Pyruvic acid
Pyruvic acid

FIGURE 3-13

Citric acid cycle.

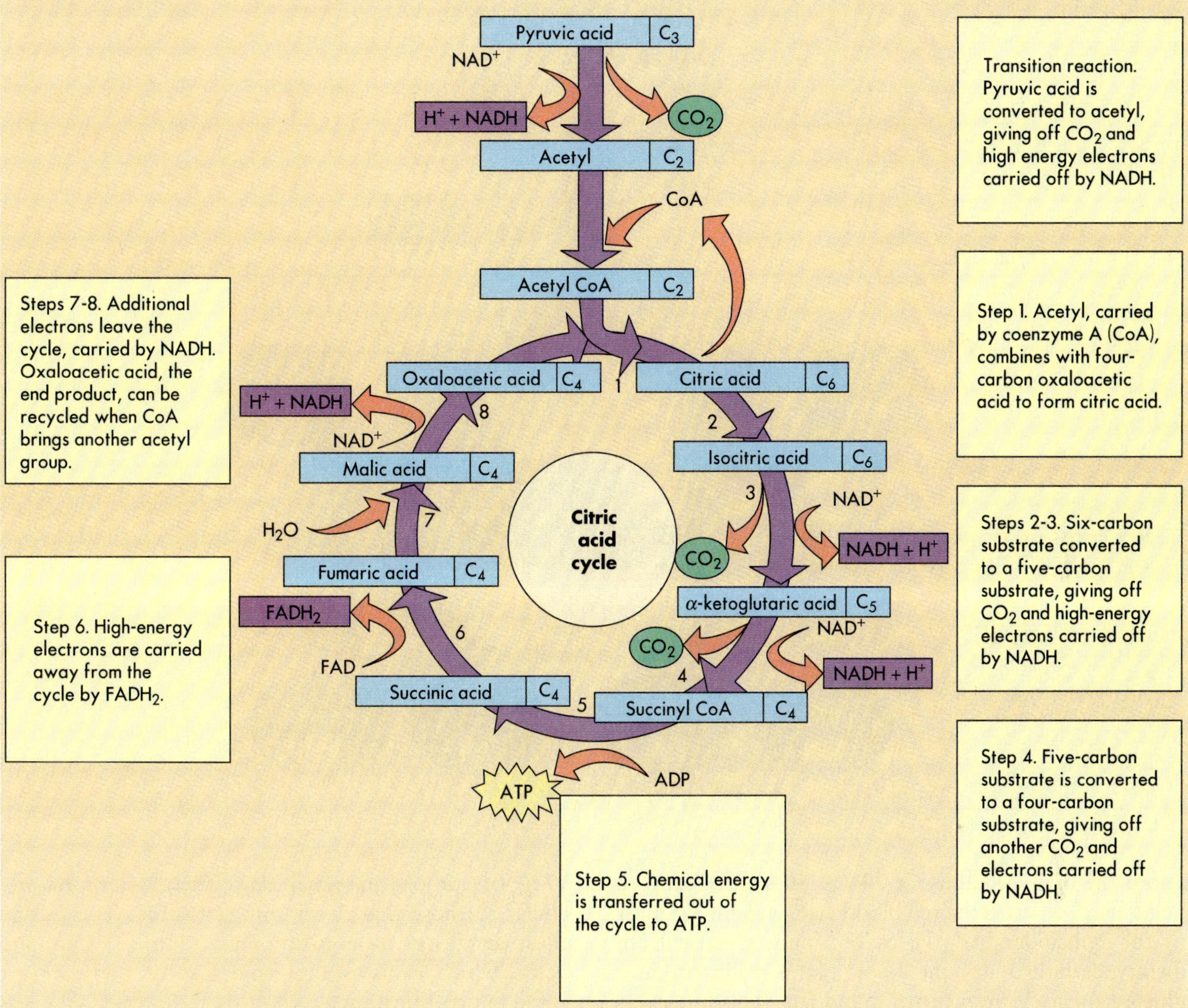
Pyruvic acid | C_3
NAD^+
$H^+ + NADH$
CO_2
Acetyl | C_2
CoA
Acetyl CoA | C_2
Transition reaction. Pyruvic acid is converted to acetyl, giving off CO_2 and high energy electrons carried off by NADH.
Step 1. Acetyl, carried by coenzyme A (CoA), combines with four-carbon oxaloacetic acid to form citric acid.
Steps 7-8. Additional electrons leave the cycle, carried by NADH. Oxaloacetic acid, the end product, can be recycled when CoA brings another acetyl group.
Oxaloacetic acid | C_4
1
Citric acid | C_6
$H^+ + NADH$
8
NAD^+
2
Malic acid | C_4
Isocitric acid | C_6
3
NAD^+
H_2O
7
Citric acid cycle
CO_2
$NADH + H^+$
Steps 2-3. Six-carbon substrate converted to a five-carbon substrate, giving off CO_2 and high-energy electrons carried off by NADH.
Fumaric acid | C_4
$FADH_2$
α-ketoglutaric acid | C_5
NAD^+
Step 6. High-energy electrons are carried away from the cycle by $FADH_2$.
6
CO_2
FAD
4
$NADH + H^+$
Succinic acid | C_4
5
Succinyl CoA | C_4
ATP
ADP
Step 4. Five-carbon substrate is converted to a four-carbon substrate, giving off another CO_2 and electrons carried off by NADH.
Step 5. Chemical energy is transferred out of the cycle to ATP.

can be called on to provide energy when the supplies of glucose from the diet are insufficient to meet the body's energy needs. In a 70-kg man, carbohydrate reserves total about 2000 kcal that are stored in 400 g of muscle glycogen, 100 g of liver glycogen, and 20 g of glucose in circulation. In contrast, 112,000 kcal (about 80% of the body's fuel reserves) are stored in fat, with the remainder of the reserves being in the form of protein. When energy is required to be released from these stores, the glycogen in the liver is broken down into glucose and is used first. When this glycogen is almost all used up, the body switches to using its fat reserves. At this time the blood glucose level falls to the fasting level. This usually stimulates the appetite, causing the individual to eat and to conserve the fat reserves.

It is significant that the anaerobic stage of glucose metabolism, which generates a net gain of only two molecules of ATP, sometimes proceeds when lack of oxygen prevents the aerobic stage from going ahead. During extreme physical exertion such as a 100-m sprint, oxygen is used up so quickly within some muscles that some glucose molecules can complete only the anaerobic stage of their metabolism. The two molecules of ATP generated per glucose molecule can still prove useful. Without their help, the winners of many Olympic sprints would have been losers.

Carbohydrate is not the only nutrient able to provide us with energy, but it is the least expensive source of energy. Glucose is the major source of energy for both nervous tissue and red blood cells. In fasting individuals

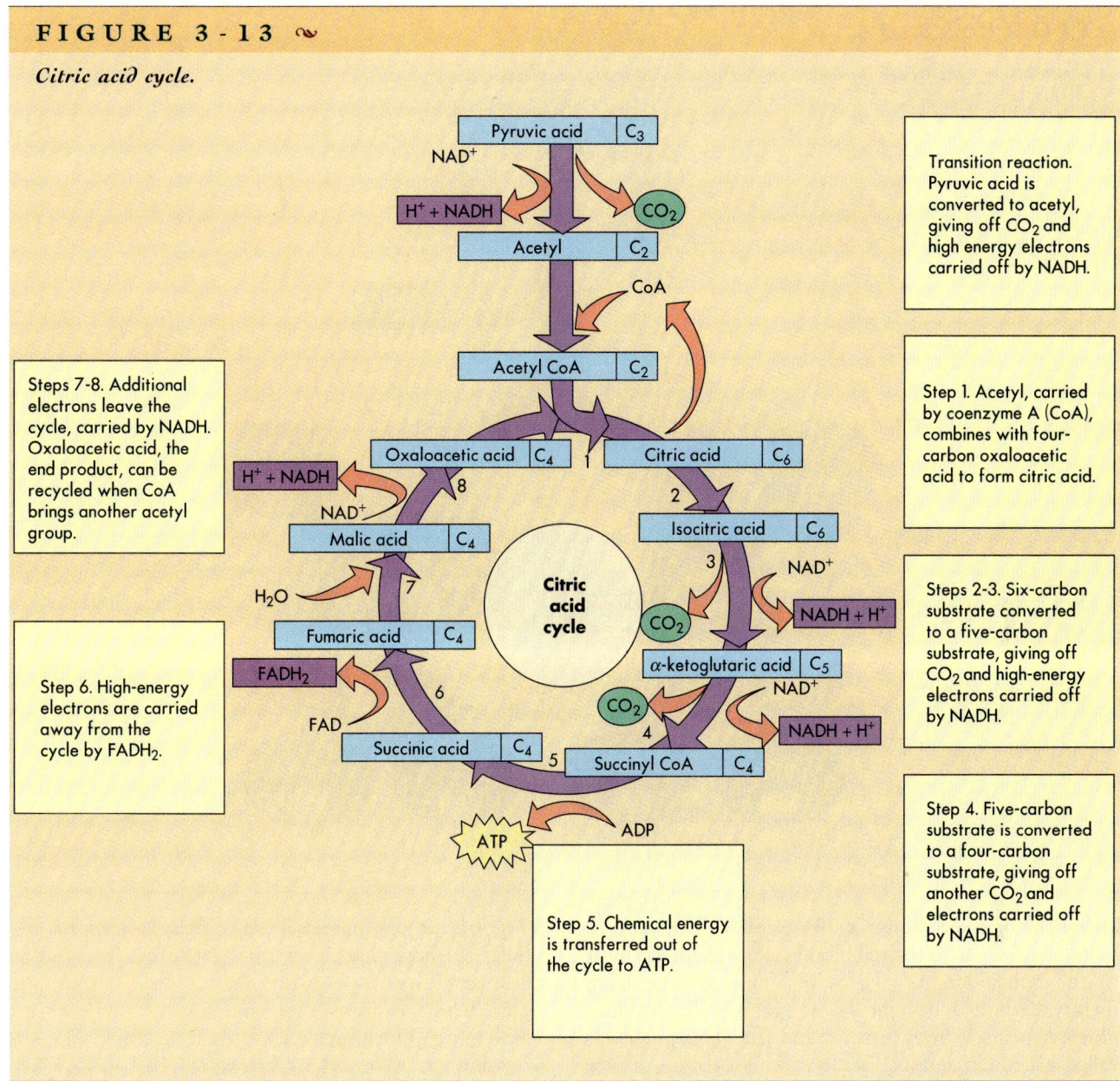

FIGURE 3-14

Catabolism (metabolic breakdown) of glucose during respiration.

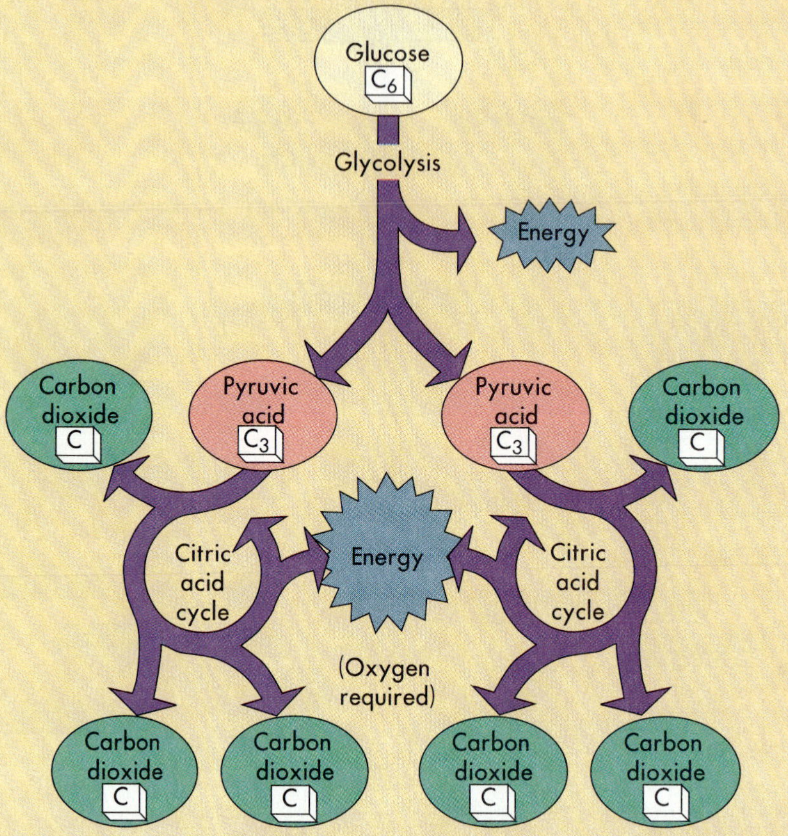

at rest the brain accounts for 70% to 80% of the glucose being used, whereas the red blood cells account for most of the remainder. As well as obtaining glucose from dietary carbohydrate, the body can actually produce glucose for itself from proteins and fats. This process is called **gluconeogenesis,** meaning the formation of new glucose. Thus even the tissues most dependent on glucose supplies, especially the brain tissues, can get along without dietary carbohydrate or the glucose released from glycogen and fat for a short time. Glucose is the most usual source of energy for muscles, but the muscles can also use chemicals called *fatty acids* (see Chapter 4), albeit less efficiently.

REQUIREMENTS FOR CARBOHYDRATE

CARBOHYDRATE AS A DIETARY ESSENTIAL

Although carbohydrate can be replaced as a source of energy by fat or protein, a series of undesirable symptoms appear when the diet consistently provides less than 50 g of carbohydrate per day. These symptoms are similar to those that develop in starvation. There is an unexplained loss of large amounts of both sodium and water, which explains the rapid loss of body weight found in people eating a carbohydrate-free diet. The loss of sodium is followed by a loss of potassium, which usually leads to weakness. At the same time, unless the dietary protein intake is very high, the protein of the body begins to break down. Muscles are largely composed of protein, which leads to muscle wastage, further weakness, and further weight loss. Even more seriously, when carbohydrate is absent, the use of fat to provide energy becomes hindered in the final series of chemical steps normally involved in oxidizing the fat (see Chapter 4). This leads to the accumulation of chemical intermediates of fat oxidation, known as *ketones.* As the ketones build up, they begin to be found as abnormal components of blood and urine. Also, because they change the hydrogen ion balance (or acid-base balance) of tissues, the ketones begin to interfere with the normal functioning of various body processes. People reaching this stage are said to be suffering from **ketosis,** which usually produces symptoms of fatigue and dehydration and a loss of stamina. All these undesirable effects of a carbohydrate-free diet are soon corrected by the return of carbohydrate to the diet—a clear indication that carbohydrate really is a dietary essential.

Intakes of less than 50 g of carbohydrate per day are associated with adverse health effects.

All this information helps us appreciate that low-carbohydrate diets (less than 50 g/day) or starvation diets are a dangerous and unsuccessful way to try to lose weight. Fortunately, because low-carbohydrate diets are unpalatable, people who try them usually soon give up and regain their lost water and weight.

The notion that carbohydrate is not bad for us, but is actually essential, contradicts long-held popular beliefs that have caused many people to try to avoid carbohydrate (or at least talk about trying to avoid it). Many people still regard carbohydrate as somewhat of a dietary villain, but there is now no doubt that it is an essential part of a healthful diet.

TRENDS IN CARBOHYDRATE USE AND RECOMMENDED INTAKES

From 1988-1991 carbohydrate provided 46% to 51% of the kilocalories in a typical American's diet,[13] compared with 56% at the beginning of the century. The proportion of complex carbohydrates in the diet has declined by more than 30% since the early 1900s, with a corresponding increase in the proportion of sugars consumed. These are the main trends in carbohydrate intake, but what levels of intake are actually desirable?

The body can function with much less carbohydrate than usually consumed, but little information is available to establish a minimum dietary standard. The Food and Nutrition Board recommends an intake of 100 g/day simply to prevent ketosis. Because most diets contain at least 200 g of carbohydrate per day, a lack of carbohydrate is unlikely to reach the level where it causes serious problems. Also, because carbohydrate-rich foods are the cheapest source of kilocalories, they tend to be used in amounts that ensure at least a minimum intake, especially among those with low incomes. There is a big difference, however, between eating at least the minimal amount of carbohydrate and eating the optimal amount. The current Dietary Goals of the United States recommend a reversal of the trends in carbohydrate use. They recommend an increase in the consumption of carbohydrate to get the energy provided by carbohydrate back to between 55% and 60% of total kilocalories. They further recommend that added sugar be used in moderation (less than 10% of kilocalories), requiring that more should come from complex carbohydrates and naturally occurring sugars in foods. One gram of carbohydrate provides 4 kcal of energy, regardless of whether it is eaten in the form of polysaccharide, disaccharide, or monosaccharide. Taken together, these facts and guidance mean that in a 2000-kcal diet, an intake of 275 to 300 g of carbohydrate is recommended (providing 1100 to 1200 kcal).

FOOD SOURCES OF CARBOHYDRATE

All the significant sources of carbohydrate in the diet are of plant origin, except for the lactose in milk. Table 3-1 summarizes the carbohydrate content of foods most frequently consumed in the United States and foods generally considered to be good sources of carbohydrate. The figures for total carbohydrate include all the usable starches and sugars, as well as indigestible fiber. As Table 3-3 indicates, many processed foods contain a considerable amount of added sugar, which significantly increases their energy value.

Some foods, such as sugar and cornstarch, contain little or no water and thus are over 80% carbohydrate. Other foods that are known for their carbohydrate content, such as potatoes and boiled rice, have a fairly high water content and are actually less than 20% carbohydrate.

Most of the energy (kilocalories) provided by foods in the cereal, fruit, and vegetable groups listed in Table 3-1 is provided by carbohydrate. However, few of these foods are eaten without the addition of some fat or oil in the form of butter, salad dressing, or a sauce. Such additions to the basic foods can add a considerable number of kilocalories.

Until recently it was thought that the quickly digested simple sugars must be absorbed rapidly and cause an immediate increase in the blood sugar level. On the other hand, it was thought that complex carbohydrates were digested more slowly and caused a slower and steadier rise in blood sugar level. This led to persons with diabetes being advised to avoid foods with simple sugars in favor of complex carbohydrates to prevent undesirable surges in their blood sugar level. The wisdom of this advice has been recently challenged. The values in Table 3-4 show the relative rate at which glucose appears in the blood after the ingestion of various sources of carbohydrate. This rate is known as the **glycemic index** of a food compared with white bread with a glycemic index of 100.

TABLE 3-3

Added sugar in processed foods

PRODUCT (SERVING SIZE)	TOTAL CALORIES IN PRODUCT	TEASPOON SUGAR IN SERVING	CALORIES FROM ADDED SUGAR (%)
Coke (12 oz)	150	9	100
Tonic water (8 oz)	88	5.5	100
Club soda/seltzer water (8 oz)	0	0	0
Jello (½ cup)	83	4.5	87
Vanilla pudding (½ cup)	90	4	71
Cranberry sauce (½ cup)	200	12	96
Catsup (1 T)	16	0.6	61
Yogurt, fruited (8 oz)	260	6.5	40
French dressing (2 T)	134	1.5	18
Instant cocoa powder (1 T)	83	2	38
Instant oatmeal (1 package)	170	4	38
Regular oatmeal (¾ cup)	110	0	0
Cheerios (1¼ cup)	110	0.2-0.3	4
Granola (⅓ cup)	133	1.5	18
Frosted Flakes (¾ cup)	110	2.7	40
Fruit drink (8 oz)	120	7	93
Kool-Aid (8 oz)	96	6	100
Tang (8 oz or 3 rounded tsp)	122	7.6	100

Sugar values taken from resources at the Penn State Nutrition Center.

The glycemic index of a food is the rate at which glucose appears in the blood after the ingestion of a carbohydrate source relative to the rate after ingestion of white bread. The glycemic index for white bread is 100.

The listed values make it obvious that some vegetables, such as potatoes, and some other sources of complex carbohydrate, such as cornflakes and millet, raise blood sugar levels more rapidly than does table sugar (sucrose). Fructose has practically no effect, and many fruits have less effect than previously believed. Another important point is that two forms of the same food, such as mashed and boiled potatoes, do not necessarily have the same effect. Yet another complicating factor being investigated is the effect of consuming foods together, as in eating a meal, rather than one food at a time. Altogether there is convincing evidence that casts doubt on the need for those with diabetes to avoid foods with simple carbohydrates and eat only foods with complex carbohydrates.[14]

Milk, a major source of lactose, is the only animal food that makes a significant and consistent contribution to dietary carbohydrate. Human milk contains 1.5 times as much lactose as cow's milk. Eggs contain a small amount of carbohydrate, and oysters (hardly dietary staples) are the only other animal food with any significant amounts of carbohydrate.

Aside from milk, almost all dietary sources of carbohydrate are of plant origin.

A group of polysaccharide gums related to starch are used widely in food processing. They include **agar** and **carrageenan,** common names on food ingredients labels. Both these gums are derived from algae and are used in fruit fillings, gels, icings, and baked goods to serve as fat stabilizers and gelling agents. **Pectin,** which comes from citrus peel, and **guar gum** from a legume are other gums used as gelling agents.

Methylcellulose is an indigestible synthetic carbohydrate used in low-calorie cookies, mayonnaise, and

TABLE 3-4

Glycemic index of selected foods adjusted to a glycemic index of 100 for white bread*

Milk products		Grains	
Ice cream	69	Cornflakes	121
Yogurt	52	Milled	103
Whole milk	44	Whole wheat bread	100
Sugars		Shredded wheat	97
Maltose	152	Oatmeal	89
Glucose	138	White rice	81
Honey	126	Sweet corn	80
Sucrose (table)	83	Vegetables	
Fructose	26	Potatoes (mashed)	98
Fruits		Potato chips	77
Bananas	84	Baked beans	70
Orange juice	71	Peas	50
Apples	52	Peanuts	15

* The blood glucose response after the feeding of a test dose of the food relative to white bread, which is set at 100.

From Wolever TMS: *World Rev Nutr Diet* 62:120, 1990.

candies to help provide bulk without kilocalories. **Fluffy cellulose** is a newly developed indigestible carbohydrate made from nonwoody plants. It can be used as a noncaloric flour to replace up to 50% of the flour used in baked goods. It does not affect the taste of food but can significantly reduce the kilocalorie content. It absorbs more water than does flour and so produces larger cakes than those made with a similar quantity of flour.

EXCHANGE LISTS

The amount of carbohydrate in different foods varies considerably. Persons with diabetes, who must know the amount of carbohydrate in their diet, are familiar with a system of classifying fruits and vegetables into groups on the basis of their carbohydrate and other energy-yielding nutrient (fat, protein, and alcohol) contents. Various amounts of different foods, all of which contain the same amount of carbohydrate, are arranged in **exchange lists.** Any food on a particular list can be exchanged for any other food on the list, with the same amount of carbohydrate being provided in either case. These lists allow those with diabetes to make appropriate variations in their diet while controlling the amount of carbohydrate, fat, and protein they consume. Exchange lists are also used by people on weight-control diets to help them recognize different foods with approximately the same energy value (see Appendix H).

MILLING OF CEREALS

The cereals corn, wheat, and rice are the major sources of carbohydrate in our diet. From the diagram of a typical cereal grain (Figure 3-15), it is clear that the **endosperm,** or center, makes up the largest portion. The endosperm is composed mainly of starch, which serves as the seed's energy store. There are some other nutrients in the endosperm, but most of the other nutrients of the grain occur in greater amounts in the **bran** layers (mainly in the aleurone and pericarp) and in the **germ.** As a result the contribution of any cereal product to our intake of vitamins and minerals largely depends on the amount of bran that is retained when the cereal is milled. The lower the **extraction** (meaning the higher the proportion of the original grain remaining after milling), the higher the bran and therefore nutrient content of the product. The germ of wheat, or **wheat germ,** which includes the scutellum between the germ and the endosperm, contains large proportions of the thiamin (vitamin B_1) and vitamin E found in the grain. The wheat germ is usually removed during milling because it contains oil, which can quickly become rancid and produce unpleasant flavors. Wheat germ sold on its own is usually marketed in vacuum-packed containers, reducing spoilage but increasing the price.

CARBOHYDRATE EFFECT ON BRAIN FUNCTION AND BEHAVIOR

Recent research has indicated that the kind and amount of carbohydrate in the diet can influence brain function and behavior. This work has been widely publicized in the popular press, especially the possible effects of carbohydrate on overall food intake, mood, and the behavior of children.

Some findings, although largely based on animal studies, have shown that when carbohydrate intake is

FIGURE 3-15

Diagrammatic representation of a cereal grain.

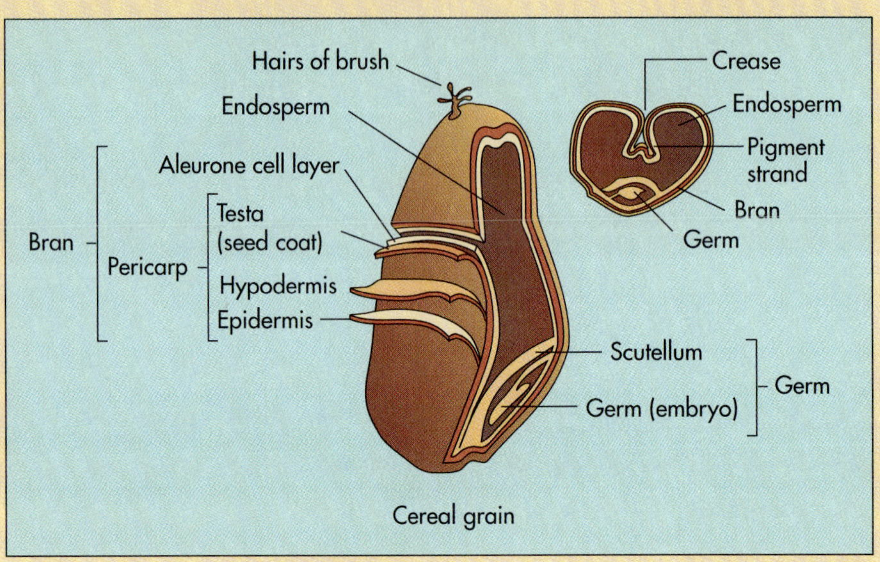

high, comprising 70% to 80% of total kilocalories, the brain produces more of a **neurotransmitter** called **serotonin** than is needed.[15] Neurotransmitters are chemicals that transmit signals between nerve cells, and serotonin is involved in a wide variety of nervous system functions. When produced in excess, serotonin causes a craving for carbohydrate and therefore increased consumption of carbohydrate, which in turn stimulates the production of yet more excess serotonin. This makes a person sleepy and sluggish.[16] This may be the problem with people who have been identified as "carbohydrate cravers." These people may gain weight because of an irresistible urge to eat carbohydrate, and they may have great difficulty adhering to a low-carbohydrate diet.

There is also much interest in how the kinds and amounts of carbohydrates eaten may affect general behavior, particularly in children. Many unconfirmed anecdotal accounts suggest that eating a lot of sugar shortens children's attention span and makes them overactive. Children often eat large quantities of candy or ice cream on special occasions, however, so it may be the occasion rather than the food that causes overstimulation. Controlled studies have failed to show that sugar has an adverse effect on behavior in a significant number of children.[17]

CARBOHYDRATE AND DENTAL HEALTH

Dietary carbohydrate is implicated as a major cause of dental caries, or tooth decay. Before they break through the gums, or "erupt," teeth are nourished by nutrients brought to them in the blood, thus carbohydrate in the mouth has no direct effect on tooth health at this stage. It has an indirect and adverse effect before eruption only when the diet contains simple carbohydrates to the exclusion of foods rich in such nutrients as calcium, vitamin D, and vitamin C. All of these nutrients, together with the use of fluoridated water or other means of fluoride administration, ensure the good health of developing teeth.

Once a tooth has erupted through the gums, it is exposed to the oral environment while retaining only minimal connection to the blood supply. At this stage dietary carbohydrates begin to have a direct effect on tooth health. Research has shown that the following conditions must exist for the formation of dental caries: the presence of fermentable carbohydrate, acid-producing bacteria, and a susceptible tooth. Caries-producing bacteria such as *Streptococcus mutans* metabolize a range of sugars (glucose, fructose, maltose, lactose, and sucrose) to generate acids that demineralize teeth. The unique role of sucrose in promoting dental caries is related to its special ability to be converted by caries-forming bacteria into polysaccharides known as **dextrans,** which stick to the tooth surface to form dental **plaques.**[18] The plaques in turn tend to attract more fermentable carbohydrate. Carbohydrates in solution do not adhere to the tooth surface and cause relatively little harm. Sucrose-rich foods such as caramel and gummy starches, which tend to adhere to the tooth surface, are more cariogenic than those that wash off. The longer that foods high in sugar remain in the mouth, the more likely they are to increase the irritation and progression of tooth decay. Some food sources of complex carbohydrate—such as pasta, which adheres to the tooth surface—are more cariogenic than soft drinks, which have a relatively high sugar content. The sugar in soft drinks is in solution and does not remain in the mouth long enough to cause a problem.

ALTERNATIVE SWEETENERS

The past two decades have seen a continual and steady decline in the use of added sugar and a comparable increase in the use of nonnutritive sweeteners or other sugar substitutes. We currently eat about 43 lb of sugar a year, which accounts for 10% to 12% of our kilocalories. Because the only health consequence of a high intake of sugar in the diet may be its adverse effect on dental health, the use of substitutes seems to reflect our innate desire for sweetness without wanting to consume the energy associated with the use of sugar. The result has been an ongoing search for a "calorie-free" substance of sufficient sweetness to be used in small amounts as a sugar substitute. It must also be proved safe enough to meet the standards of the Food and Drug Administration (FDA) imposed by the Delaney Amendment (see Chapter 19).

Although a great many substances have been proposed and tested as potential sugar substitutes, most interest has focused on four of them: **saccharin, cyclamates, aspartame,** and **acesulfame-K.**[19] Saccharin has been in use since 1879, cyclamates were discovered in 1937, and aspartame and acesulfame-K were discovered in the 1960s. Only saccharin, aspartame, and acesulfame-K are approved for use in the United States, but all are approved for use in Canada. In the United States cyclamates were considered safe at one time but are now banned. The properties of all four alternative sweeteners are listed in Table 3-5.

Saccharin occurs as white crystals or a white crystalline powder and is derived from a by-product of the petroleum industry. It is a relatively stable substance and is 200 to 700 times as sweet as sucrose. It is not metabolized in the body and thus is excreted unchanged in urine. For a time there was concern about the safety of saccharin for human use because some animals fed high doses developed bladder tumors. Subsequently, the FDA proposed a ban on its use. A congressional moratorium on the proposed ban permitted the use of saccharin in beverages and as a tabletop sweetener while its safety was under review. In December 1991 the FDA approved saccharin as an alternative sweetener. Some people find that it has an undesirable metallic aftertaste, which limits its acceptance. Some authorities suggest that it is wise to restrict the use of saccharin by pregnant women and young children until we have more information on its possible effects on the developing fetus or growing child.

Aspartame, which is 180 times as sweet as sucrose, was first approved in 1974 but then banned in 1975, only to be approved again in 1981 after further testing had established its safety. It has been approved for use in beverages and more than 500 different kinds of food product. Aspartame consists of two amino acids, phenylalanine and aspartic acid, that occur in almost all protein-rich foods at appreciably higher levels than could possibly be provided from aspartame-sweetened products. It is unsuitable, however, for the 1 in 15,000 people who have the genetic defect that causes the condition known as **phenylketonuria** (PKU). These people are unable to metabolize amounts of phenylalanine in excess of that required for growth. There were also fears about the possible toxicity of the methanol that is formed when aspartame is metabolized or when aspartame-containing liquids are stored for a long time at high temperatures. These fears should be allayed, however, by the fact that such foods as grape and tomato juice contain up to twice as much naturally occurring methanol as is produced from the aspartame in a 12-oz beverage sweetened with aspartame. Two major disadvantages of aspartame are its instability in acidic conditions and its loss of sweetness during heating. The problem of its loss of sweetness during heating has been addressed by coating aspartame with a vegetable oil, causing the aspartame to be released only in the final stages of baking.

In assessing the safety of food products, the FDA uses a measure known as the level of **acceptable daily intake** (ADI), which is 1/100 of the amount a person could safely consume every day of his or her life. For aspartame the ADI is 50 mg/kg of body weight. This represents the amount of aspartame in 18 cans of sweetened beverage per day for a 60-kg (132-lb) person. Concern about the effect of aspartame on the developing fetus centers on the fact that the fetus concentrates phenylalanine at a level twice that found in maternal blood. Although aspartame has been ruled safe for use in over 500 food products, questions are frequently raised about its safety, accompanied by requests that it be reevaluated by the FDA. Students of nutrition should remain alert to the status of the safety of aspartame, which is sold under the brand name **NutraSweet.**

Acesulfame-K, which in some circumstances appears to have no aftertaste, received FDA approval in 1988, particularly for use in products for patients with diabetes. It was discovered in 1967 and is currently marketed under the brand name **Sunette.** Acesulfame-K is approximately 200 times sweeter than sucrose, and its sweetness does not decrease with increasing temperature. An ADI of 15 mg/kg was awarded by the FDA after review of the safety assessment studies.

Cyclamates, the other widely used nonnutritive sweeteners, were discovered in 1937 but have been banned in the United States since 1969 because it has not been clearly established that they are not carcino-

TABLE 3-5

Properties of alternative sweeteners

SWEETENER	SWEETNESS (SUCROSE = 1)	TASTE CHARACTERISTICS	REGULATORY STATUS	ADI* (mg/kg OF BODY WEIGHT)
Acesulfame-K	130-200	Rapid onset, persistent bitter and metallic tastes at high concentrations	Approved for use in tabletop sweeteners, dry beverage mixes, and chewing gum	15
Aspartame	180	Clean, similar to sucrose, no bitter aftertaste	Approved for use in tabletop sweeteners, dry beverage mixes, chewing gum, beverages, confections, fruit spreads, toppings, and fillings	50
Saccharin	200-700	Slow onset, persistent aftertaste, bitter at high concentrations	Used under congressional moratorium; FDA ban withdrawal in 1991	2.5
Cyclamate	30	Similar to sucrose; however, some bitter and salty attributes	Banned in the United States; food additive petition filed	–

* Acceptable Daily Intake values for aspartame and acesulfame-K are standards established by the FDA, and the value for saccharin is established by the Joint FAO/WHO Expert Committee on Food Additives.

From Giese JH: *Food Tech* 47:113, 1993.

genic. They have, however, been allowed for use as a tabletop sweetener and in drugs in Canada and 40 other countries. Cyclamates are available as calcium cyclamate and sodium cyclamate. Current evaluations conclude that cyclamates are not carcinogenic, but the FDA is awaiting further information on their safety for humans before approving their use.

A great many other sugar substitutes are being researched and tested. Sugars known as **L-sugars**—because they are "left-handed" (in that they rotate a beam of polarized light to the left), in contrast to the naturally occurring **D-sugars** ("right-handed")—have potential as alternative sweeteners. They taste just like the natural D-sugars, but the body cannot use them as a source of energy, they do not initiate tooth decay, they are stable in the presence of heat (and therefore are useful in the preparation of baked products), and they are suitable for people with diabetes. A ruling on their safety is expected from the FDA soon.

Among the other sweeteners currently being developed are the following:

- Other peptide sweeteners similar to aspartame
- The amino acid **tryptophan**
- **Xylitol,** which is derived from cellulose
- **Dihydrochalcones,** many of which come from oranges and grapefruits
- **Thaumatins**
- **Sucralose**

Dihydrochalcones are several hundred times sweeter than sucrose, and their use is approved in Belgium and Argentina, but the FDA has requested additional toxicology tests on them. Thaumatins are sweet proteins obtained from the fruit of the West African plant *Thaumatococcus danielii.* There are at least five thaumatins, and a mixture of two of them is marketed under the brand name **Talin.** Talin has a lingering sweet taste and is 2000 times sweeter than sucrose. **Sucralose** is a white crystalline substance produced by the selective chlorination of the sucrose molecule. It is 600 times sweeter than sucrose, has a sweetness profile similar to that of sucrose, and is very stable. It is predicted to become a preferred alternative sweetener with wide applications. In September of 1991 Canada approved its use in 13 food and beverage categories. It is marketed under the brand name **Splenda** and is currently being reviewed by the FDA for use in the United States.

ALCOHOL

The alcohol within alcoholic beverages is a compound called **ethanol,** which is just one representative of a vast number of compounds known as *alcohols.* Their distinguishing feature is that they have at least one hydroxyl group (OH). Ethanol, whose chemical structure is shown in Figure 3-16, is the only alcohol that may be consumed in significant quantities in the diet. In the discussion that follows, the word *alcohol* should be taken to mean *ethanol.* Ethanol is not a carbohydrate, but it is produced from carbohydrate and therefore is discussed in this chapter. The ethanol in beers, wines, and hard liquors is produced when the microorganisms known as *yeasts* use sugars, such as those present in cereals or grapes, as a source of food. One main waste product of this process is ethanol, but although it is excreted as a waste by the yeast cells, it is to us the most valued ingredient of alcoholic beverages. The process by which sugars are used by yeasts with

FIGURE 3-16

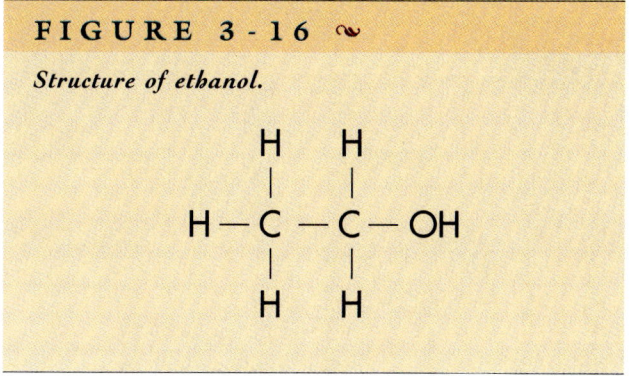

Structure of ethanol.

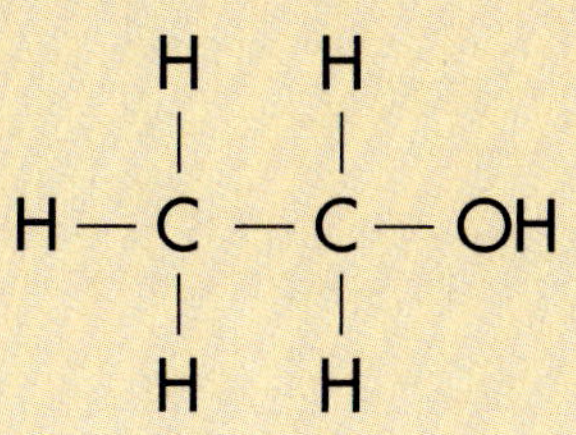

production of ethanol is one example of what are called **fermentations,** which proceed in the absence of oxygen.

It is difficult to get accurate estimates of how much alcohol people consume. Data based on the sale of alcoholic beverages and on surveys of dietary intakes suggest that daily intakes of alcohol range from 0.2 oz to 1 oz of ethanol per person per day.[20] For people who consume alcoholic beverages, it is estimated that alcohol provides from about 5% to 20% of total energy intake, or about 100 to 600 kcal/day. However, 3% of the population over the age of 15 report levels of alcohol consumption that contribute over 1000 kcal daily.

ABSORPTION AND METABOLISM

Ethanol is a small water-soluble molecule that does not require digestion. It is absorbed into the blood quickly throughout the length of the GI tract. As much as 80% of the ethanol consumed is absorbed through the intestinal wall immediately after leaving the stomach. Because alcohol dissolves in water, it immediately disperses throughout the body fluids. Its relative concentration within various tissues is proportional to the water content of these tissues. Thus a large amount of absorbed alcohol is found in the blood, but little is found in fat or bone. Less than 5% of the alcohol taken in is excreted in the breath or in urine. The small amounts that are excreted are important, however, because they are used as the basis of legally accepted tests for the amount of alcohol in the blood. This procedure is acceptable because the level of alcohol in breath and urine, although much smaller than the level in the blood, varies in proportion with the amount in the blood. It is also possible to analyze a blood sample directly, but this is less convenient.

Alcohol is a potent poison. A blood concentration of 0.1% is evidence of intoxication, whereas a concentration of 0.4% is usually fatal. The body is able to convert alcohol into harmless substances. This "detoxification" process begins in the liver, which contains an enzyme called **alcohol dehydrogenase** that is able to convert the alcohol into chemicals that can be used as a source of energy. This makes the energy of alcohol available in safe form for use by muscles. The brain also contains alcohol dehydrogenase, which can prevent the alcohol levels in the brain from rising too high. This is important because the brain is particularly sensitive to alcohol.

Although it is possible for alcohol to be converted into fat and stored, it is usually used immediately as a source of energy in preference to fats or glucose. It therefore spares other energy sources and should indirectly contribute to fat storage and weight gain. Pure alcohol (also known as 200-proof alcohol) provides 7 kcal of energy per gram, or 200 kcal/oz. The energy content of some commonly used alcoholic beverages is given in Table 3-6.

Recent studies in humans suggest that alcohol may cause significant increases in the body's expenditure of energy, possibly because alcohol stimulates the general rate of metabolism. The net result of the use of alcohol as a source of energy is less than expected from its caloric value alone. The difference may be dissipated as heat, produced by the acceleration of metabolism.[21] Thus adding alcohol to a diet already adequate in energy may not necessarily cause a gain in fat storage or weight. Recent epidemiological data support this possibility. A careful analysis of the data from 89,538 women and 48,493 men showed a negative association between alcohol consumption and body mass index (a measure of fatness and leanness based on weight and height) for women and no association for men.[22]

> Recent research suggests that there are health benefits associated with moderate consumption of two or fewer drinks per day. Serious adverse health and social consequences remain a concern with higher levels of alcohol consumption.

Most people are able to metabolize from 45 to 90 mg of alcohol per pound of body weight per hour, or in other units, 100 to 200 mg of alcohol per kilogram of body weight per hour. For a 154-lb (70-kg) man, this is equivalent to the amount of alcohol provided by consuming 800 ml (one fifth) of 100-proof whiskey or 3.5 L (or quarts) of wine per day.

The rate of absorption of alcohol can be modified by other drugs. Contrary to popular belief, however, its rate of metabolism is not affected by physical exercise, vitamin supplementation, thyroid hormone, or caffeine.

TABLE 3-6

Energy, carbohydrate, and alcohol content of alcoholic beverages

BEVERAGE	AMOUNT (OZ)	ALCOHOL (GRAMS)	CARBOHYDRATE (GRAMS)	ENERGY (KCAL)
Beer				
Regular	12	13	14	150
Light	12	10	6	90
Extra light	12	8	3	70
Near	12	2	12	60
Distilled				
Gin, rum, vodka, whiskey	1.5	15	—	105
Brandy, cognac	1.0	11	—	75
Wine				
Red	4	12	1	85
Dry white	4	11	0.5	80
Sweet	4	12	5	103
Sherry	2	9	1.5	75
Port, muscatel	2	7	7	95
Vermouth, sweet	3	12	14	141
Vermouth, dry	3	13	4	105
Manhattan	3	21	2	165
Martini	3	19	1	140
Old-fashioned	3	21	1	180

EFFECT OF ALCOHOL ON NUTRITION

Alcohol can affect nutritional status in various ways. It may depress appetite and therefore food intake; it may displace other foods in the diet and thus lower the intake of nutrients; it may affect the GI tract in a way that impairs the absorption of nutrients; or, through its effects on the liver, it may alter the transport, use, and storage of nutrients. Also, the money spent on alcohol reduces the money available to buy food, which may be a problem in low-income families. Harwood and others[23] estimated that Americans suffer financial losses linked to excessive alcohol intake of more than $80 billion per year.

Some alcoholic drinks actually contribute a small amount of nutrients in addition to acting as an energy source. Only half of the kilocalories of beer come from the alcohol, and it retains some of the nutrients in the malt from which it is made. This allows beer to contribute reasonable amounts of magnesium, phosphorus, and some vitamins to the diet. Wine, which is about 12% alcohol, retains smaller amounts of these nutrients. Hard liquors such as gin, rum, and whiskey, which are made by distilling out the ethanol produced by natural fermentation, contribute nothing of significance to the diet apart from energy.

A body that is suffering from malnutrition is less able to counteract the toxic effects of alcohol than a well-nourished body. This compounds the negative effects of alcohol on a nutritional status that is already poor.

There is increasing evidence that fatty livers and other forms of liver disease are a direct result of excessive alcohol consumption. An otherwise adequate diet does not protect against these problems.

FETAL ALCOHOL SYNDROME

In the past 25 years a condition known as **fetal alcohol syndrome** has been recognized. This syndrome covers a range of problems during the development of a fetus that are caused by the mother's consumption of alcohol. As little as 2 to 3 oz of alcohol (equivalent to 4 to 6 oz of a 100-proof liquor) consumed by the mother each day or indulgence in a single alcohol binge at a critical stage of the pregnancy may be enough to cause the syndrome. A badly affected fetus grows more slowly than normal, has a small head and distorted facial features, and suffers from mental retardation. It is estimated that at least 5000 babies per year are born suffering from one or more of these symptoms of fetal alcohol syndrome. Clearly, all women of childbearing age should be warned of the potential damage their fetus may suffer as a result of alcohol consumption during pregnancy. This issue is discussed further in Chapter 14.

Sugar, Aspartame, and Child Behavior

Refined sugar and artificial sweeteners have been suggested as possible causes of behavioral problems in children. Sucrose and aspartame have received the most attention, being blamed by some people for attention deficit disorder (ADD), or hyperactivity, and other behavior problems such as juvenile delinquency. There have been claims that preschool children are particularly sensitive to sugar, to an extent that may vary with the ratio of sugar to protein and carbohydrate in the food consumed.

It has been suggested that sucrose can cause behavioral problems as a result of a surge in blood glucose levels immediately after consumption, followed by reactive hypoglycemia, or problems resulting from an exaggerated reaction to sucrose. The alleged behavioral problems caused by aspartame have been attributed to its ability to cause high levels of phenylalanine in plasma, which may interfere with the transport of amino acids into the brain and modify mental activity.

Despite many subjective anecdotal accounts of behavioral problems associated with sucrose and aspartame, most controlled studies have failed to detect any consistent effects.* Some of these studies, however, have been criticized for monitoring children for only a short time before and after sucrose or aspartame consumption and for studying the children in unfamiliar laboratory settings.

Despite the lack of supporting evidence, subjective reports of poor child behavior as a result of sucrose or aspartame consumption continue to appear. These reports are of considerable concern to nutritionists and other health professionals because sucrose and aspartame are common components of most children's diets.

The possibility that sucrose or aspartame affects behavior and mental performance in children was evaluated in a recent study.† This involved a group of children who were believed to be sensitive to sugar on the basis of reports from their parents, and a group of "normal" children about whom no such reports had been made. The children were placed on either a high-sucrose diet, a high-aspartame diet, or a normal "placebo" diet. The placebo diet had all the attributes of the high-sucrose or high-aspartame diets, apart from the additional sucrose or aspartame. The study was "double-blind," meaning that neither the children nor the people administering the diets knew which type of diet was being given at which time to which children. All the diets were either essentially free of other dietary components previously alleged to cause ADD (such as artificial colors, artificial flavors, chocolate, and caffeine) or contained extremely low levels of these substances. The children's behavior and mental performance were evaluated weekly for 9 weeks independently by the children's parents, the children's teachers, and the investigators. During the 9 weeks of study, all foods were provided for the subjects and their immediate family. All foods were removed from the home at the end of each week and a new supply delivered. After a period on one diet, the subjects were assigned one of the other diets, but the changeovers between diets were well disguised by sham (dummy) diets. Thirty-nine relevant measures of behavior and mental performance were used to assess the children. Overall the results resoundingly failed to demonstrate significant adverse effects caused by sucrose or aspartame. Not one child produced a detectable adverse reaction, even when the intake of sucrose or aspartame exceeded typical levels.

The overall conclusion of this most recent, carefully designed, and well-controlled study is that neither dietary sucrose nor aspartame affected the children's behavior or mental performance. It remains unclear how many further studies showing no adverse effects of sweet foods on children's behavior are required to put this issue to rest and allow funds to be diverted to finding the real causes of ADD and other behavioral problems in children.

* Gans DA: *Nutr Today* 26:8, 1991.

† Wolraich ML and others: *N Engl J Med* 330:301, 1994.

BY NOW YOU SHOULD KNOW

- Carbohydrates include simple sugars and complex carbohydrates, such as starch and cellulose.
- Carbohydrates are composed of the elements carbon, hydrogen, and oxygen.
- There are three classes of carbohydrates: monosaccharides, disaccharides, and polysaccharides.
- Monosaccharides vary in sweetening power, rate of absorption, and degree of solubility.
- Carbohydrates contribute 45% to 50% of the kilocalories in the typical American diet but up to 80% of the kilocalories in diets in developing countries.
- Sugar occurs naturally in fruits, vegetables, and milk, but much of the sugar consumed is in the form of sucrose added to food.
- Sugar and starch can encourage dental caries.
- Diabetes mellitus is caused by an underproduction of insulin or by certain cells of the body becoming unresponsive to insulin. It is not caused by eating too much sugar.
- Lactose intolerance is caused by lactase insufficiency.
- Refined cereals and refined bread products are low in fiber.
- Fiber is provided in whole grain products, fruits, and vegetables.
- Insoluble fiber enhances gastric motility and reduces the risk of colon cancer. Soluble fiber can help lower blood cholesterol levels.
- The diet should contain at least 100 g of carbohydrate per day, although no RDA has been set.
- Alcohol is formed by the fermentation of naturally occurring sugars.
- Alcohol does not need to be digested and is quickly absorbed into the body and distributed to tissues in amounts dependent on their water content.
- Alcohol abuse can have negative effects on nutrition.
- Dietary guidelines urge Americans to avoid too much sugar, to eat foods with adequate starch and fiber, and if they drink alcoholic beverages to do so in moderation.

STUDY QUESTIONS

1. What is the primary function of carbohydrate in the body?
2. In what form and where is carbohydrate stored in the body?
3. Explain the difference between hypoglycemia and hyperglycemia, and describe the characteristic symptoms of each condition.
4. What symptoms might be produced by adhering to a low-carbohydrate diet for a prolonged period?
5. Outline the changing trends in carbohydrate consumption in the United States since 1900.
6. How does milling alter the nutritive value of cereals? Name three milled cereal products you eat regularly.
7. Explain the relationship between crude fiber and dietary fiber. What foods would you choose to eat to increase your fiber intake? Do the foods you have listed include water-soluble or insoluble dietary fiber? What is the relevance of the distinction between water-soluble and insoluble fiber to blood cholesterol levels?
8. What are the conditions associated with a lack of dietary fiber?
9. What causes lactose intolerance? Give three symptoms that are characteristic of this disorder. What specific foods must be avoided by people with lactose intolerance?
10. Name the specific enzymes involved in the digestion of polysaccharides and disaccharides.
11. What happens to monosaccharides after they are absorbed from the small intestine?
12. How does the fate of sugar consumed when the diet contains excess kilocalories differ from the fate of sugar when the diet is deficient in kilocalories?
13. How is alcohol absorbed and metabolized? Discuss why an alcoholic may suffer from malnutrition.

CRITICAL ANALYSIS

1. A person's daily intake of carbohydrate usually includes both simple and complex carbohydrates. Among the simple carbohydrates, sucrose and lactose (both disaccharides) and fructose (a monosaccharide) are the most commonly consumed. Although many people assume that they consume more than enough carbohydrate daily, this may not be the case. Here is an exercise that compares your carbohydrate intake to the goal intakes from the Food Guide Pyramid. Record the number of servings you eat from the following food groups today or tomorrow (if you have already recorded your diet for a single day or for 3 days, you may use the record for one of those days). For a shorter exercise, you may record intakes from a single meal. If you record intakes from a single meal, ask yourself the following questions: Did I eat approximately ⅓ of the recommended servings? If not, did I or will I make up the difference at another meal? Some serving sizes and a record form are provided below.

	Serving sizes
Bread	1 slice, 1 small dinner roll, ½ hamburger bun, bagel, or english muffin
Cereal	½ cup of ready-to-eat or hot cereal
Rice	½ cup cooked rice
Pasta	½ cup cooked pasta
Vegetables	½ cup cooked vegetable, 1 cup chopped raw vegetable
Fruits	1 medium apple, orange, pear, ½ banana, ½ cup cut fruit, ½ cup fruit juice
Dairy	1 cup milk or yogurt, ½ oz cheese
Meats, meat substitutes	3 oz meat, fish, poultry 1 egg, 2 Tbsp peanut butter

NUMBER OF SERVINGS

	BREADS, CEREALS	VEGETABLES	FRUITS	DAIRY	MEATS, MEAT SUBSTITUTES
Breakfast	______	______	______	______	______
Snack	______	______	______	______	______
Lunch	______	______	______	______	______
Snack	______	______	______	______	______
Dinner	______	______	______	______	______
Snack	______	______	______	______	______
Total	______	______	______	______	______
Recommended	6 to 11	3 to 5	2 to 4	2 to 3	2 to 3

How does your intake of carbohydrates rate? One way to assess your intake is to compare it with the recommended number of servings for each of the carbohydrate-containing food groups. If your intake is below the recommended range for one or more of the food groups and is at the low end of the range for the others, you are probably consuming too little carbohydrate.

Comparing servings eaten with servings recommended is one way to assess your intake, but it is not very precise. You may use the same information to obtain a more quantitative estimate from average amounts of carbohydrate in food groups. These are as follows:

	BREADS, CEREALS	VEGETABLES	FRUITS	DAIRY
Carbohydrate (grams/serving)	15	5	15	12

Multiply the number of servings at each meal for each food group by the grams of carbohydrate per serving to determine grams of carbohydrate from each food group at each meal. The total grams of carbohydrate from each food group for the day can then be calculated. Then add the total grams of carbohydrate from each of the four food groups to obtain an estimate of the total grams of carbohydrate eaten (the fifth group, meats, provides no carbohydrate).

TOTAL CHO GRAMS FROM GRAINS	TOTAL CHO GRAMS FROM FRUITS	TOTAL CHO GRAMS FROM VEGETABLES	TOTAL CHO GRAMS FROM DAIRY PRODUCTS	TOTAL CHO GRAMS FOR 1 DAY
______	______	______	______	______

How does your intake rate according to total grams of carbohydrate? Several recommendations can be used for comparison. For weight loss diets, minimal daily carbohydrate intake should not fall below 150 g/day. This is based on estimated minimum daily needs for glucose. As described in the text, the central nervous system (CNS) and red blood cells use an estimated 180 g of glucose daily, 140 g for the CNS, and 40 g for the blood cells.

A minimal recommendation for athletes is 250 g/day, but a recommendation that better supports training or hard physical labor is 8 g/kg (about 3.6 g/lb) of body weight. Thus for the following example athletes, the calculated recommended intake would be 400 g for a 50-kg (110-lb) athlete, 560 g for a 70-kg (154-lb) athlete, and 800 g for a 100-kg (220-lb) athlete.

Recommendations for carbohydrate are also made on the basis of percent of total caloric intake. Current recommendations by several agencies are for carbohydrate intake to be 55% to 60% of total kilocalories. For a 1500-kcal diet, 60% of kilocalories would be 900 kcal or 225 g of carbohydrate; for a 2000-kcal diet, 60% would be 1200 kcal or 300 g of carbohydrate; for a 3000-kcal diet, 60% would be 1800 kcal or 450 g of carbohydrate.

REFERENCES

1. Black RM: Sucrose in health and nutrition—facts and myths, *Food Tech* 47:130, 1993.
2. Anderson GH: Sugar consumption: are dietary guidelines needed? *J Can Diet Assoc* 50:229, 1989.
3. Reiser S, Hallfrisch J: *Metabolic effect of dietary fructose,* Boca Raton, Fla, 1987, CRC Press.
4. Economic Research Service: Sugar and sweeteners. In *Situation and Outlook Report,* U.S. Department of Agriculture Pub No. SSRV16N4, Washington, DC, 1991, U.S. Government Printing Office.
5. Büller HA, Grand RJ: Lactose intolerance, *Ann Rev Med* 41:141, 1990.
6. Glinsmann WH, Irausquin H, Park YK: Evaluation of health aspects of sugars contained in carbohydrate sweeteners: report of Sugars Task Force, *J Nutr* 116(suppl):S1, 1986.
7. Nilsson LH, Hultman E: Liver glycogen in man: the effect of total starvation or a carbohydrate-poor diet followed by carbohydrate refeeding, *Scand J Clin Lab Invest* 32:325, 1973.
8. Bergstrom J and others: Diet, muscle, glycogen, and physical performance, *Acta Physiol Scand* 71:140, 1967.

9. Wright HS and others: The 1987-1988 Nationwide Food Consumption Survey: an update on the nutrient intake of respondents, *Nutr Today* 26:21, 1990.

10. Klurfeld DM: Dietary fiber-mediated mechanisms in carcinogenesis, *Cancer Res* 52(suppl):S2055, 1992.

11. Marlett J: Content and composition of dietary fiber in 117 frequently consumed foods, *J Am Diet Assoc* 92:175, 1992.

12. Filer LJ: Modified food starch—an update, *J Am Diet Assoc* 88:342, 1988.

13. National Center for Health Statistics: *Energy and macronutrient intakes of persons ages 2 months and older in the United States: 1988-1991,* Advanced Data from Vital and Health Statistics, No 255, Hyattsville, Md, 1994, U.S. Government Printing Office.

14. Loghmani E and others: Glycemic response to sucrose-containing mixed meals in diets of children with insulin-dependent diabetes mellitus, *J Pediatr* 119:531, 1991.

15. Leproham-Greenwood CE, Anderson GH: An overview of mechanisms by which diet affects brain function, *Food Tech* 40:132, 1986.

16. Spring BJ and others: Effects of carbohydrates on mood and behavior, *Nutr Rev* 44(suppl):S51, 1986.

17. Kruese MJP: Carbohydrate intake and children's behavior, *Food Tech* 40:150, 1986.

18. Brown AT: The role of carbohydrates in plaque formation and oral disease, *Nutr Rev* 33:353, 1975.

19. American Dietetic Association: Position statement. Use of nutritive and nonnutritive sweeteners, *J Am Diet Assoc* 93:816, 1993.

20. Dennis BH and others: Nutrient intakes among selected North American populations in the Lipid Research Prevalence Study: composition of energy intake, *Am J Clin Nutr* 41:312, 1985.

21. Suter PM, Scutz Y, Jequier E: The effect of ethanol on fat storage in healthy subjects, *N Engl J Med* 326:983, 1992.

22. Colditz GA and others: Alcohol intake in relation to diet and obesity in women and men, *Am J Clin Nutr* 54:49, 1991.

23. Harwood HJ and others: *Economic costs to society of alcohol and drug abuse and mental illness: 1980,* Research Triangle Park, NC, 1984, Research Triangle Institute.

~ ADDITIONAL READINGS ~

American Diabetes Association: Position statement. Nutrition recommendations and principles for people with diabetes mellitus, *Diabetes Care* 17:519, 1994.

American Dietetics Association: Position statement. Health implications of dietary fiber, *J Am Diet Assoc* 93:1446, 1993.

Anderson GH, editor: *Diet and behavior: multidisciplinary approaches,* London, England, 1990, Springer-Verlag.

Asp NG: Carbohydrates in human nutrition: the importance of food choice, especially in a high-carbohydrate diet, *Am J Clin Nutr* 59(25):679S, 1994.

Beaugeru L and others: Digestion and absorption in the human intestine of three sugar alcohols, *Gastroenterology* 99:717, 1990.

Canty DJ, Chan MM: Effect of consumption of caloric vs. noncaloric sweet drinks on indices of hunger and food consumption in normal adults, *Am J Clin Nutr* 53:1159, 1991.

Coulston AM: Nutrition considerations in the control of diabetes mellitus, *Nutr Today* 29:6, 1994.

Coulston AM and others: Deleterious metabolic effects of high-carbohydrate, sucrose-containing diets in patients with non–insulin-dependent diabetes mellitus, *Am J Med* 82:213, 1987.

Forbes AL, Bowman BA, editors: Health effects of dietary fructose, *Am J Clin Nutr* 58:7215, 1993.

Gans DA: Sucrose and unusual child behavior, *Nutr Today* 26:8, 1991.

Lewis CJ and others: Nutrient intakes and body weight of persons consuming high and moderate levels of added sugar, *J Am Diet Assoc* 92:708, 1992.

London RS: Saccharin and aspartame—are they safe to consume during pregnancy? *J Reprod Med* 33:17, 1988.

Rolls BJ: Effects of intense sweeteners on hunger, food intake, and body weight: a review, *Am J Clin Nutr* 53:872, 1991.

Rolls BJ, Kim S, Federoff IC: Effect of drinks sweetened with sucrose or aspartame on hunger, thirst, and food intake in men, *Physiol Behav* 48:19, 1990.

Stellman SD: Sweetener usage in America: a brief history and current usage patterns. In Williams GM (editor) *Sweeteners: health effects,* Princeton, NJ, 1988, Princeton Scientific Publishing.

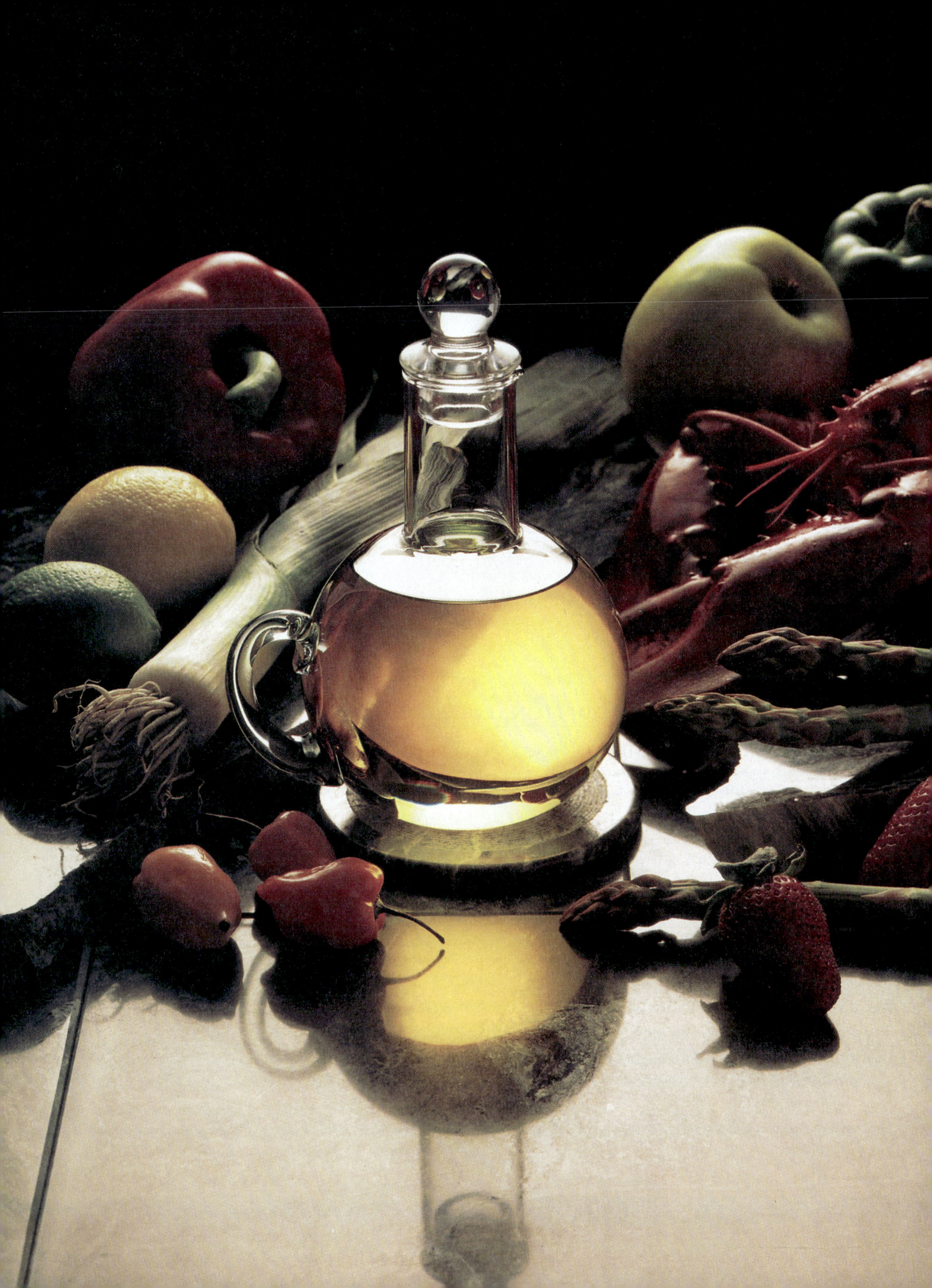

CHAPTER 4

LIPID

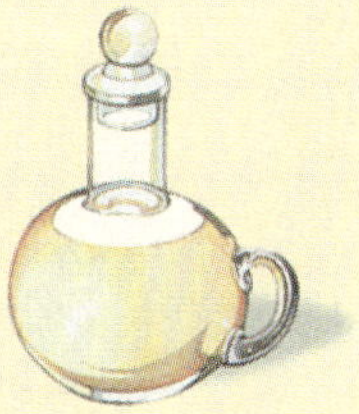

Lipid is the collective name given to a wide variety of water-insoluble chemicals, including all fats and oils in the diet and in the body. Most lipids of nutritional importance are triglycerides, which are formed when three fatty acid molecules combine with glycerol. For a long time, nutritionists believed that lipids in the diet were important only as a concentrated source of energy. They now recognize that at least two fatty acid components of lipid (linoleic acid and linolenic acid) are dietary essentials and that some lipid intake is essential to form and maintain the membranes surrounding and within cells. In nutrition and other health sciences the term *fat* is often used to mean all lipids, including true fats (solid triglycerides) and oils (liquid triglycerides). The type of fat in the diet plays an important role in general health and the onset of several important diseases. The role of dietary fat in health and disease (notably, coronary heart disease, cancer, and obesity) is one of the most active areas of research in modern nutrition. Although still the subject of debate, current dietary guidelines encourage Americans to reduce the total amount of fat in their diets and to substitute monounsaturated and polyunsaturated fat for some of the saturated fat currently consumed.

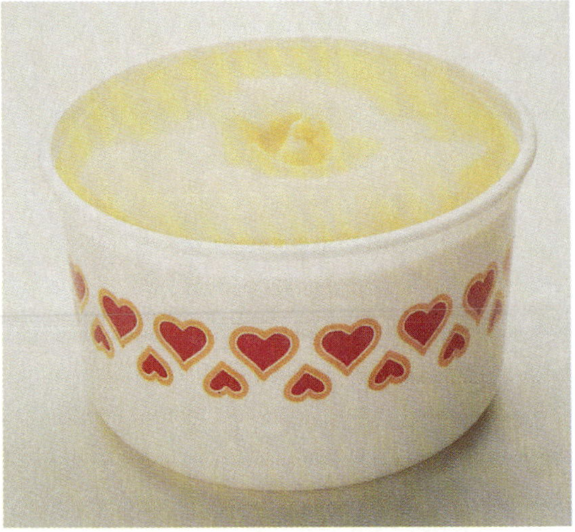

The wide variety of compounds classified as **lipids** (or simply **lipid**) includes all of the substances known as **fats** and **oils.** Most nutritionally important fats and oils are **triglycerides,** as is discussed in this chapter. In chemical terminology, fats are triglycerides that are solids at room temperature, whereas oils are triglycerides that are liquids at room temperature. Both fats and oils, however, with all other lipids are commonly described in nutrition and the health sciences simply as **fat.** This is the sense in which the word *fat* is used throughout this book, except where it is necessary to make the distinction between the solid fats and the liquid oils.

Fat, to most people, means the fats and oils within food and the fat stored within our bodies that becomes particularly noticeable when energy intake exceeds energy requirements over a long period. The middle-aged man working under stress associates fat with the threat of heart disease. To many women, fat represents unwanted deposits under the skin that they believe detract from their appearance. To the biochemist, the lipids that we know of as fat are a diverse range of water-insoluble compounds composed of carbon, hydrogen, and oxygen atoms. To the epidemiologist, fat in the diet and within the body is linked to obesity, heart disease, and cancer. To the nutritionist, fat is an essential part of the diet and a concentrated source of energy.

After water and carbohydrate, fat or lipid is the most plentiful nutrient in the Western food supply. Some sources of fat are easily recognized as visible fats and oils, such as the fat surrounding meat and in butter, margarine, and salad oils. These sources, however, account for less than half the fat in the diet. The rest is "invisible" fat, which includes fat that is interspersed throughout meat fibers, dispersed in finely divided (emulsified) form in egg yolk or homogenized whole milk, and found in whole grain cereals and nuts.

TRIGLYCERIDES

The type of lipids known as **triglycerides** composes the bulk of ingested fat and provides about 95% of the energy derived from dietary fat. Triglycerides, like carbohydrates, are composed of carbon, hydrogen, and oxygen. In triglycerides, and in lipids in general, the ratio of oxygen to carbon and hydrogen is much lower than in carbohydrates. We have already seen that energy is given out when carbon and hydrogen atoms combine with oxygen. Lipids are a more concentrated source of energy than carbohydrate because they begin with less oxygen as a part of their structure and so have a greater capacity to combine with oxygen in energy-yielding oxidation reactions during respiration. When they are oxidized as an energy source, lipids are converted to carbon dioxide gas (CO_2) and water (H_2O), just like carbohydrates.

Many different triglycerides exist, but they all share the same basic structure, formed when a molecule of **glycerol** combines with three molecules of a class of compounds known as **fatty acids** (Figure 4-1). Glycerol is a tri-alcohol compound because it has three hydroxyl (OH) groups, the characteristic group of the alcohols, attached to a simple three-carbon skeleton. Fatty acids have the acidic carboxyl group (COOH) attached to a hydrocarbon chain. A variety of fatty acids are found in food and within the body. These different fatty acids vary in the length of their hydrocarbon chains (**chain length**) and the number of carbon-carbon double bonds within the chain (**degree of unsaturation**).

Triglycerides are also known as **triacylglycerols** because the parts of the triglyceride molecule derived from fatty acids form what are known as **acyl** groups. Triglycerides are also **triesters** because all compounds formed by reaction between a carboxyl group and a hydroxyl group are known as *esters* and are held together by **ester linkages.**

Figure 4-1 reveals that triglycerides are formed from glycerol and fatty acids in a condensation reaction that releases one molecule of water for each acyl group attached (or, in other words, for each ester linkage formed). The reverse process of breaking up a triglyceride into free fatty acids and a glycerol molecule is a hydrolysis reaction.

If all three fatty acids in a triglyceride molecule are identical, which is rare, a **simple triglyceride** is formed. If at least two of the fatty acids differ from one another, a **mixed triglyceride** is formed. Sometimes only two fatty acid groups are attached to the glycerol component, forming a **diglyceride** or **diacylglycerol.** In other cases, only one fatty acid group is present, forming a **monoglyceride** or **monoacylglycerol,** and nothing is attached to the other 2 hydroxyl (–OH) positions on the glycerol molecule. Monoglycerides and diglycerides are

FIGURE 4-1

The basic structural components of glycerol, fatty acids, and triglycerides.

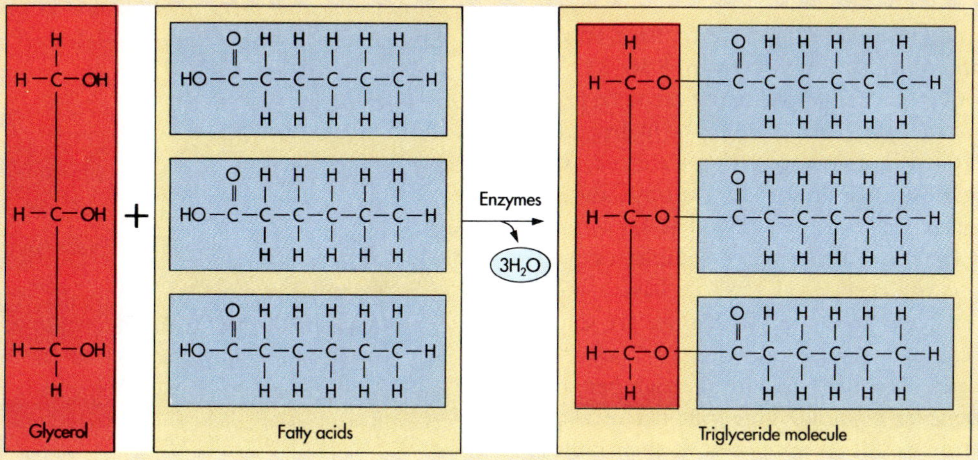

TABLE 4-1

Name, number of carbon atoms and double bonds, and food sources of common fatty acids

NAME	NUMBER OF CARBON ATOMS	NUMBER OF DOUBLE BONDS	FOOD SOURCES
SATURATED			
Short-chain			
Butyric	4		Butter
Caproic	6		Butter
Caprylic	8		Coconut oil
Medium-chain			
Capric*	10		Palm oil
Lauric*	12		Coconut oil
Myristic*	14		Butterfat, nutmeg, coconut oil
Long-chain			
Palmitic	16		Animal fat, vegetable oil
Stearic	18		Animal fat, vegetable oil
Arachidic†	20		Peanut oil, lard
UNSATURATED			
Long-chain			
Palmitoleic	16	1	Butter and seed oils
Oleic	18	1	Most fats and oils
Linoleic	18	2	Seed fats—corn, cottonseed
Linolenic	18	3	Soybean oil
Arachidonic	20	4	Peanut oil, lard
Eicosapentaenoic acid (EPA)†	20	5	Fish oil
Docosahexaenoic acid (DHA)†	22	6	Fish oil

* Sometimes classified as long-chain fatty acids.
† Very long-chain fatty acids.

often listed on food labels because they are used in small amounts as additives in processed foods to achieve the desired texture and consistency.

The fatty acids in foods almost always have an even number of carbon atoms, ranging from 4 to 22. The final carbon atom at the end opposite the carboxyl group is always within a **methyl group:** CH_3. The hydrocarbon chain of a fatty acid is immiscible with water or, more technically, is a **nonpolar** group. In contrast, the carboxyl group mixes well with water and is known as a **polar** group. Glycerol is also a water soluble, or polar, molecule, and so triglycerides as a whole have a mixed affinity for water. Their polar "head" regions are soluble in water, whereas their nonpolar chains, or "tails," are insoluble in water and tend to cluster together away from water whenever possible. This split chemical personality of the triglycerides is important to their biological functions.

One way of classifying fatty acids is by length. Fatty acids with less than 10 carbon atoms are called **short-chain fatty acids,** those with 10 to 14 carbon atoms are called **medium-chain fatty acids,** and those with 16 or more carbon atoms are called **long-chain fatty acids.** The short-chain fatty acids are relatively rare. The medium-chain fatty acids account for 4% to 10% of the fatty acids in food and are more soluble and more readily absorbed than are those with longer chains. The long-chain fatty acids predominate in food. Fatty acids with chains of 20 or more carbon atoms are common in fish and fish oils.

Fatty acids also vary in the number of carbon-carbon double bonds they contain or, in other words, in their degree of "unsaturation." Hydrocarbon chains with carbon-carbon double bonds are said to be unsaturated because they do not have the maximal number of hydrogen atoms attached, whereas those with no double bonds are said to be **saturated** (Figure 4-2). If a fatty acid contains only one double bond, it is a **monounsaturated fatty acid,** whereas if it contains two or more double bonds, it is a **polyunsaturated fatty acid** (**PUFA**). Some very long long-chain fatty acids (20 to 22 carbon atoms), containing five or six double bonds, are classified separately as **highly unsaturated fatty acids** (**HUFAs**). The names, chain lengths, and degree of unsaturation of common dietary fatty acids are shown in Table 4-1.

The degree of unsaturation of the fat within a food was previously expressed as the **P/S ratio,** meaning the ratio of polyunsaturated fatty acids to saturated fatty acids, with the monounsaturated fatty acids being excluded from the calculation. The P/S ratio is not in fact very helpful because the monounsaturated fatty acids often have physiological effects similar to those of the polyunsaturated fatty acids. Use of the P/S ratio is no longer advocated by the nutrition and health professions.

The lipids of different foods contain characteristic amounts of saturated, monounsaturated, and polyunsaturated fatty acids. Of the fatty acids in butter, for example, 55% to 65% are saturated, with the four-carbon short-chain **butyric acid** (so named because it was first isolated from butter) accounting for 6% to 8% of the saturated fatty acids present. Oleic acid, an 18-carbon monounsaturated fatty acid, accounts for 70% to 75% of the fatty acids in olive oil. Linoleic acid, an 18-carbon polyunsaturated fatty acid, accounts for 55% to 60% of the fatty acids in corn oil. There is great interest in the nutritional effect of these differences, especially their possible role in predisposing us to, or protecting us from, various diseases (discussed later in this chapter).

The hydrocarbon chains of fatty acids are often illustrated as perfectly straight structures, as in the linear

FIGURE 4-2

Structural differences between saturated and polyunsaturated fatty acids shown as three-dimensional (space-filling) models and as linear models.

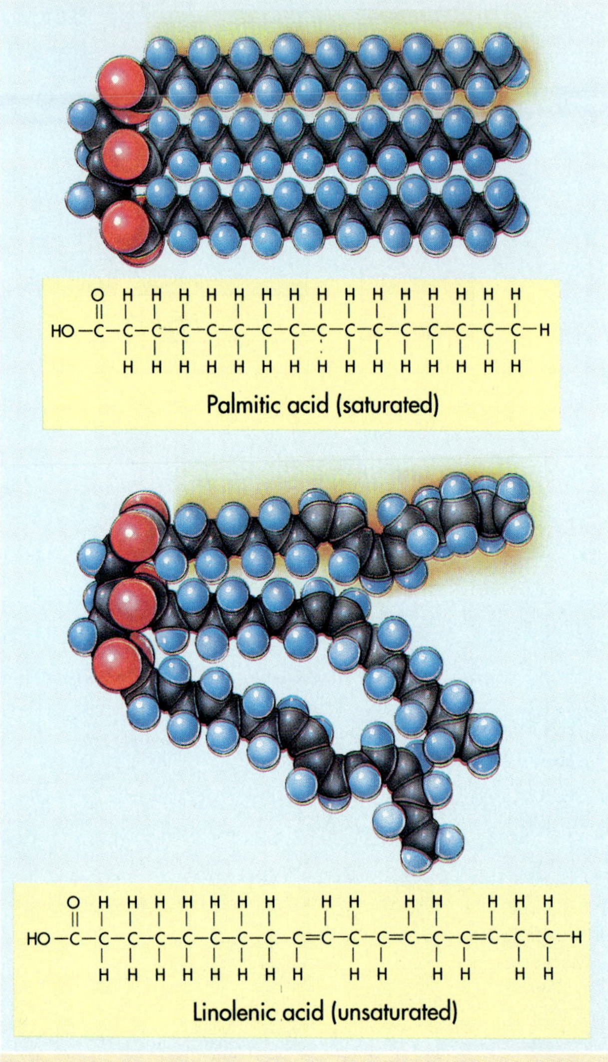

FIGURE 4-3

Space-filling, or three-dimensional models of geometrical implications of* cis *and* trans *configurations within unsaturated fatty acids.* A, *Oleic acid, a* cis *fatty acid.* B, *Elaidic acid, a* trans *fatty acid.

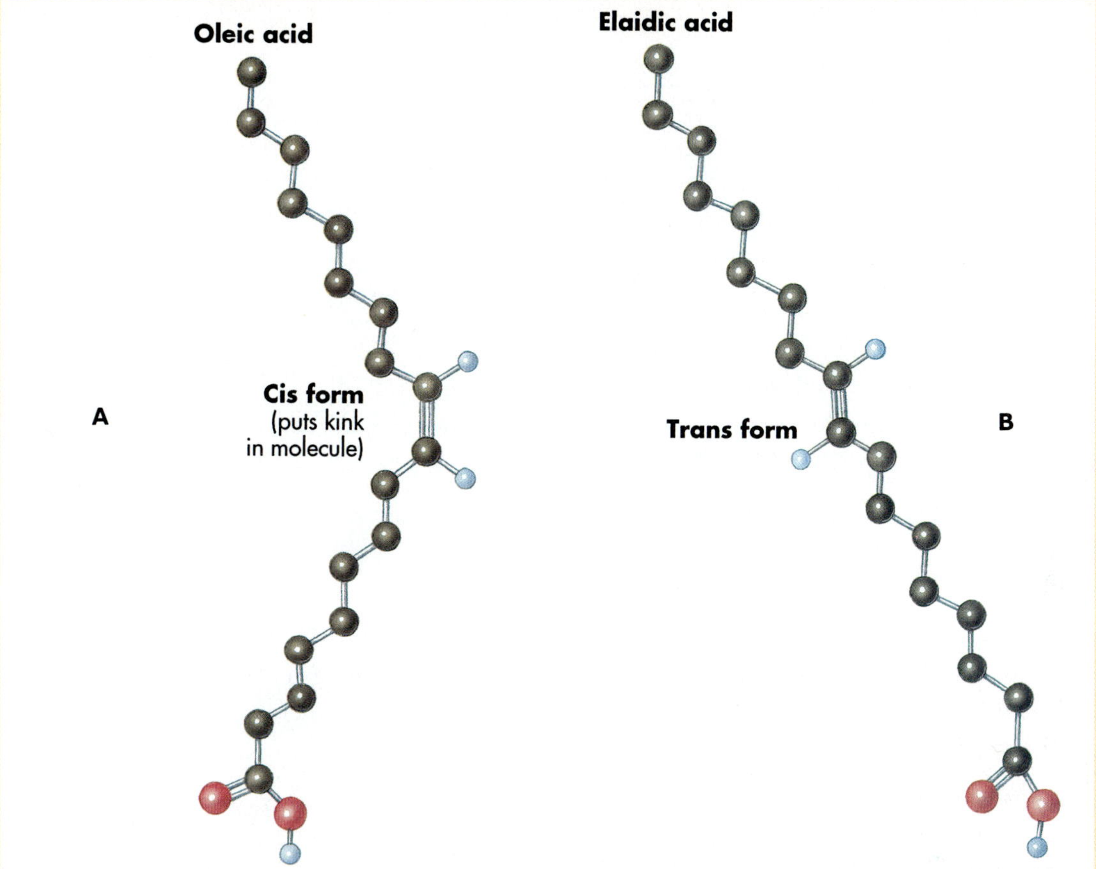

models of Figure 4-2. Such illustrations are not entirely correct because of the difficulty of representing three-dimensional molecules on the two-dimensional surface of a sheet of paper. In reality, the carbon atoms of a saturated hydrocarbon chain are bonded in a zigzag manner, which still forms a long, straight molecule overall (so the inaccuracy in depicting it in a straight line is not very significant). The presence of one or more double bonds, however, introduces significant new possibilities. Each carbon-carbon double bond can be in the **trans** configuration, in which the hydrogen atoms attached to the carbon atoms involved in the bond are on *opposite* sides of the bond, or in the **cis** configuration, in which these hydrogen atoms are on *the same* side of the bond. As the space-filling illustrations in Figures 4-2 and 4-3 indicate, a double bond in the *cis* configuration introduces a kink in the hydrocarbon chain. This kink is a permanent structure because a double bond (unlike a single bond) prevents any rotation of the attached groups relative to one another. Multiple double bonds introduce multiple kinks.

In nature the double bonds of most unsaturated fatty acids are in the *cis* configuration. Therefore they introduce permanent kinks in the hydrocarbon chains of most natural fatty acids. During the manufacture of margarines and shortenings, however, significant amounts of *trans* fatty acids are formed.

Unsaturated fatty acids tend to have lower melting points than do saturated fatty acids with the same length of chain (Table 4-2). This is because natural unsaturated fatty acid molecules, with their *cis* configuration (and their kinked structure), cannot pack together as tightly as the straight-chain saturated fatty acid molecules. This means that it takes less heat energy to disrupt the ordered structure of such unsaturated fatty acids in the solid state and convert them into the less ordered liquid state.

In general, saturated fatty acids containing more that 10 carbon atoms are solids at room temperature. Stearic acid, for example, with 18 carbon atoms does not melt until its temperature rises to 69.5° C. The introduction of just one *cis* double bond forms the 18-carbon unsaturated oleic acid and reduces the melting point by more than 50° C to 13.4° C. Room temperature is usually taken as 25° C, so oleic acid is a liquid at room temperature, whereas stearic acid is a solid. A double

FIGURE 4-4

Numbering and naming of carbon atoms in fatty acids.

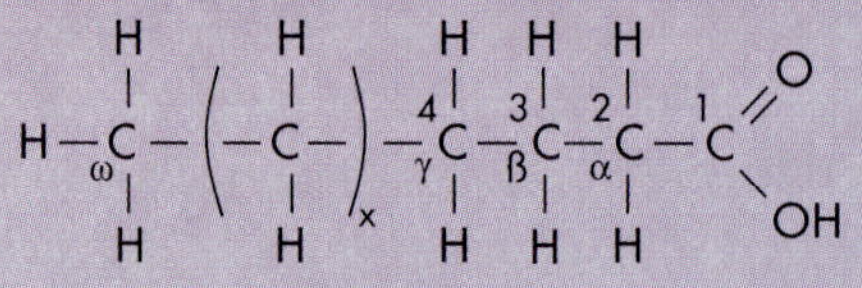

The labels used to identify the carbon atoms of fatty acids

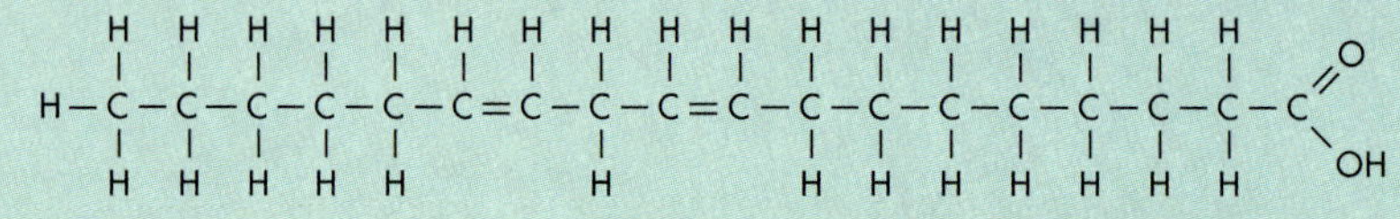

Linoleic acid, a polyunsaturated omega –6 fatty acid, can be variously represented as:

18:2	←	18 carbon atoms, and 2 double bonds
18:2Δ9,Δ12	←	18 carbon atoms, and 2 double bonds between carbons number 9 and 10 and 12 and 13
18:2ω6	←	18 carbon atoms, 2 double bonds and an omega–6 fatty acid
18:2n6	←	18 carbon atoms, 2 double bonds and an omega–6 fatty acid as indicated using *n* in place of ω

TABLE 4-2

The effect of unsaturation on the melting point of a fatty acid

FATTY ACID	NUMERICAL SYMBOL*	MELTING POINT (°C)
Stearic	18:0	69.5
Oleic	18:1 *cis*	13.4
Elaidic	18:1 *trans*	44.5
Linoleic	18:2	–5.0

* The first number refers to the number of carbon atoms, the second to the number of double bonds.

Compiled from a list prepared by Ralph T. Holman, The Hormel Institute, Austin, Minn, by Robert Jensen, Department of Nutritional Sciences, University of Connecticut, Storrs, Conn.

bond in the *trans* configuration, however, forms the 18-carbon elaidic acid, with a melting point only 25° C lower than that of stearic acid. Elaidic acid is a solid at room temperature. The replacement of unsaturated fatty acids in the *cis* configuration by those in the *trans* configuration or by saturated fatty acids (and vice versa) can have important physiological consequences (discussed later in this chapter).

Several systems are used to identify the different carbon atoms in fatty acids and the positions of any double bonds (Figure 4-4). The individual carbon atoms are *numbered* from the carbon atom of the carboxyl group. The position of a double bond can be indicated using the symbol Δ (delta), followed by the lowest-numbered carbon atom involved in the double bond. Thus Δ9 refers to a double bond between carbon atoms number 9 and 10. Carbon atoms 2, 3, and 4 are also known as the α, β, and γ carbon atoms, respectively. An alternative nomenclature system begins at the other end of the fatty acid chain, with the methyl group. The methyl carbon is called the **omega** (ω) carbon. Polyunsaturated fatty acids in which the first double bond occurs between the third and fourth carbon atoms (counting the omega carbon as the first) are called omega-3 (ω-3 or n-3) fatty acids. Those in which the first double bond occurs between the sixth and seventh carbon atoms from the omega end are called omega-6 (ω-6 or n-6) fatty acids, whereas those with the first

TABLE 4-3

Dietary sources, tissue distribution, and metabolic relationships of the common unsaturated fatty acids

FATTY ACID SERIES	MAJOR MEMBERS OF SERIES	TISSUE DISTRIBUTION IN MAMMALS	RICH DIETARY SOURCES
ω-3	α-linolenic acid, 18:3ω3	Minor component of tissues	Some vegetable oil (soy, linseed, rapeseed), leafy vegetables
	Eicosapentaenoic acid, 20:5ω3	Minor component of tissues	Fish, shellfish
	Docosahexaenoic acid, 22:6ω3	Major component of membrane phospholipids in retinal photoreceptors, cerebral gray matter, testes, and sperm	Fish, shellfish
ω-6	Linoleic acid, 18:2ω6	Component of most tissues	Most vegetable oils
	Arachidonic acid, 20:4ω6	Major component of most membrane phospholipids	Meat, liver, brain
	Docosapentaenoic acid, 22:5ω6	Very low in most normal tissues, except testes, rabbit, guinea pig retina, rabbit brain; replaces 22:6ω-3 in n-3 fatty acid deficiency	None
ω-9	Oleic acid, 18:1ω9	Major component of many tissues, including white matter and myelin	Animal and vegetable fats
	Eicosatrienoic acid, 20:3ω9	Accumulates in essential fatty acid deficiency	None

From Neuringer M and others: *Annu Rev Nutr* 8:517, 1988.

double bond between the ninth and tenth carbon atoms from the omega end are omega-9 (ω-9 or n-9) fatty acids. These three families of fatty acids are the only three found in nature; thus all natural unsaturated fatty acids are either ω-3, ω-6, or ω-9. The major members of these families, their tissue distribution, and food sources of them are shown in Table 4-3.

An unsaturated fatty acid with, for example, 18 carbon atoms and three double bonds can be symbolized by 18:3 (or C18:3), and other unsaturated fatty acids can be represented in the same way with the numbers changed appropriately. α-linolenic acid, which is a major fatty acid in the omega-3 series, can be represented as 18:3ω3. The 18:3 part of this designation indicates that it has 18 carbon atoms and three double bonds, as already explained, whereas the ω3 part indicates that the first double bond occurs between the third and fourth carbons when numbered from the omega end of the chain. Using the same system, linoleic acid becomes 18:2ω6 and oleic acid is 18:1ω9.

The other two nutritionally important omega-3 fatty acids, in addition to α-linolenic acid, are eicosapentaenoic acid (EPA), which is 20:5ω3, and docosahexaenoic acid (DHA), which is 22:6ω3. The conversion of α-linolenic acid to EPA and DHA can occur in humans. This transformation occurs slowly, however, because the enzyme catalyzing it also catalyzes conversion of linoleic acid (18:2ω6) to arachidonic acid (20:4ω6); thus the two substrates (α-linolenic and linoleic acids) compete for the same enzyme (see Figure 4-11). The production of arachidonic acid usually wins out, with little EPA and DHA being produced.

The triglycerides within dietary fats contain a mixture of fatty acids with varying chain lengths and varying degrees of saturation. The distribution of the types of fatty acids in fats available in the U.S. food supply is shown in Figure 4-5. Because the glycerol component is common to all triglycerides, the differences between them involve only the type and number of fatty acids and the order in which they are attached to the glycerol core. The characteristics of each type of dietary fat, which may be composed of just one type of triglyceride or a mixture of several different triglycerides, reflect these differences in fatty acid content. A fat containing predominantly fatty acids with one double bond is called a *monounsaturated fat,* even though it almost always contains some saturated and polyunsaturated fatty acids. A fat containing predominantly fatty acids with two or more double bonds is called a *polyunsaturated fat.* The more unsaturated fatty acids there are in a fat, the more likely it is to be a liquid (and so technically an oil) at room temperature. Conversely, the more saturated fatty acids there are in a fat, the more likely it is to be a solid at room temperature. There are exceptions to these general rules,

FIGURE 4-5

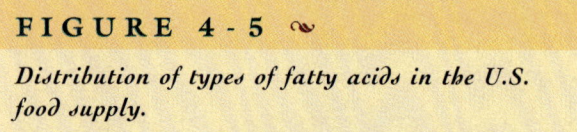

Distribution of types of fatty acids in the U.S. food supply.

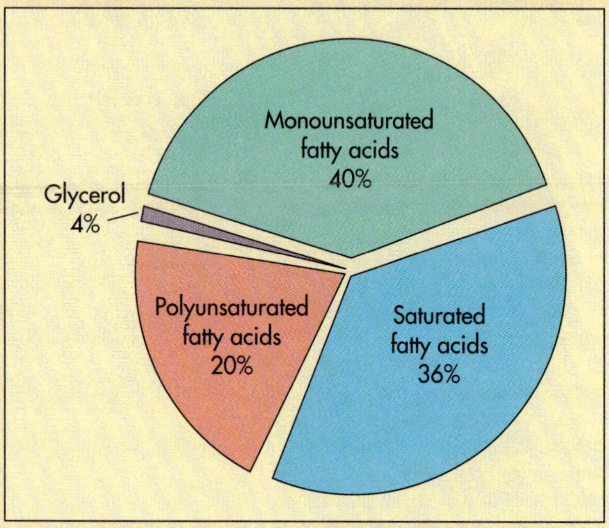

however. Coconut, palm, and palm kernel oils—sometimes called tropical oils—contain 81%, 87%, and 57% saturated fatty acids, respectively; yet they are liquids at room temperature. This is because many of their fatty acids are short-chain fatty acids, which tend to lower the melting point of a fat.

Remember that the nomenclature in this area is a little confused. All triglycerides that are solids at room temperature are fats, whereas all those that are liquid at room temperature are oils; however, oils are usually included as fats when nutritionists talk about the "fat" content of a food. As already stated, the routine use of the word *fat* throughout this book includes the substances that are technically oils and all other lipids.

OTHER DIETARY LIPIDS

In addition to the triglycerides, diglycerides, and monoglycerides, foods also contain smaller amounts of other lipids such as **phospholipids** and **sterols,** the fat-soluble vitamins (A, D, E, and K), some waxes, and other minor lipidic compounds.

PHOSPHOLIPIDS

The average diet provides approximately 1 to 3 g/day of phospholipids, which comprises about 2% of total fat intake. In phospholipids, a phosphate group (PO_4) linked to either a nitrogen-containing or a carbohydrate-like group takes the place of one of the fatty acids of a triglyceride (Figure 4-6). The phosphate and attached groups that replace a fatty acid are more soluble in water than are fatty acids; so the presence of phospholipids serves to increase the ability of lipids to mix with water in a finely divided, **emulsified** form. **Emulsions** are not true solutions, but they consist of tiny particles of substances, such as lipids, suspended throughout water or some other solution. In this emulsified form the "water-loving" polar or **hydrophilic** head groups of lipids and phospholipids tend to interact with water molecules, whereas the "water-hating" nonpolar or **hydrophobic** fatty acid chains cluster together in the center of the emulsified particles, well away from the water molecules.

The best known of the phospholipids are the **lecithins** (known collectively as lecithin), in which a vitamin-like substance called *choline* is the nitrogen-containing group attached to the phosphate. Lecithin serves as a natural emulsifier in eggs and is also present in the cell membranes of the body. Lecithin has become popular as a dietary supplement because of claims that it can prevent the accumulation of fat within artery walls as a result of its properties as an emulsifier. There is no evidence, however, that lecithin should be provided in the diet because it is synthesized from other substances in the liver. In fact, lecithin from many dietary sources is broken down by digestion into glycerol, fatty acids, phosphate, and choline before being absorbed. This makes dietary lecithin supplements useless and unnecessary because they never reach the blood in the form that functions as an emulsifier of fat.

STEROLS

The well-known dietary and body chemical **cholesterol** is one member of another group of lipids known as **sterols.** Their key structural feature is the system of four connected carbon rings, exemplified by the structure of cholesterol (Figure 4-7). Cholesterol is an alcohol lipid because it contains an hydroxyl group. It is present in all animal fats but is not found in vegetable fats. Cholesterol is required for the formation of many essential substances in the body, including steroid hormones (synthesized in the ovaries, testes, and adrenal gland), vitamin D (synthesized in the skin), and bile salts (synthesized in the liver). It is also an integral part of the cell membranes within the body and the **myelin** that forms an insulating sheath around nerve fibers. The myelin sheaths of the body contain around 30 g of cholesterol overall, which is seldom interchanged with cholesterol from other places in the body. The adult body is about 0.2% cholesterol by weight, amounting to about 130 g of cholesterol overall. Cholesterol is not a dietary essential because it can be synthesized in the body, primarily in the liver and in the

FIGURE 4-6

Chemical structure of a phospholipid.

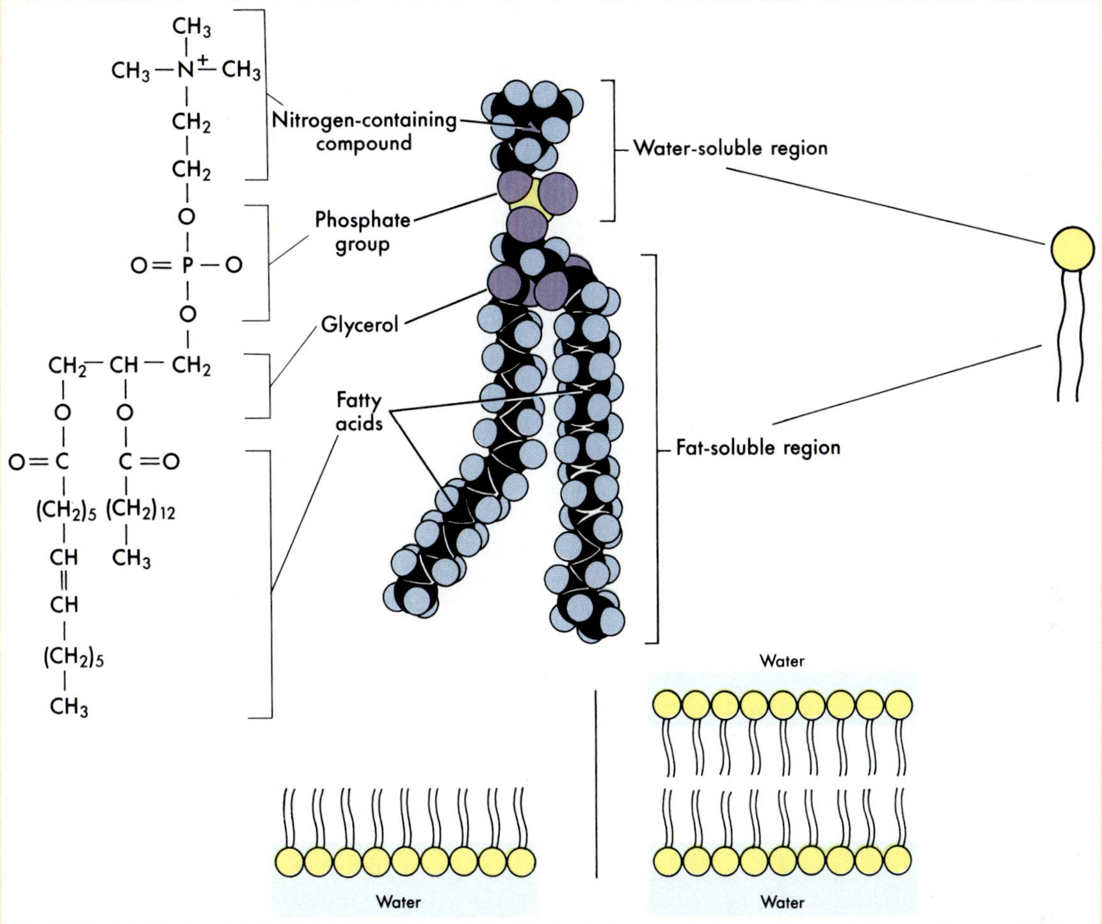

cells lining the small intestine. The amount synthesized depends on the amount required, which in turn depends considerably on the amount available in the diet. Typically, the diet supplies about 300 to 500 mg of cholesterol per day, whereas the body synthesizes between 600 and 1500 mg/day.

Although there has been a steady increase in cholesterol-containing meat in the U.S. food supply, this has been offset by a decline in eggs and the substitution of cholesterol-free vegetable fats in place of many animal fats. As a result, the average amount of cholesterol available from the American food supply—440 mg per person per day—has not changed appreciably in the last 10 years. Data from the most recent national surveys of food consumption patterns of Americans indicate that adult men actually ingest an average of 322-395 mg of cholesterol per day, and adult women ingest an average of 222-249 mg/day.[1,1a]

Phytosterols are a group of sterol lipids found in plants. One of them, sitosterol, apparently competes with cholesterol for absorption, thus causing decreased absorption of cholesterol. Another phytosterol, **ergosterol,** is found in yeast and is a dietary **precursor** of vitamin D (meaning that vitamin D is formed from it).

OTHER FATLIKE SUBSTANCES

Another class of fatlike substances in the diet is some hydrocarbons, which are composed solely of carbon and hydrogen atoms. These are by-products of petroleum refining, and some have such physical characteristics as texture and taste that are similar to true, naturally occurring lipids. Hydrocarbons are not altered by digestive enzymes and cannot be absorbed. Because they do not contribute energy (kilocalories) to the diet, they are sometimes used in place of natural oils to make low-kilocalorie foods, such as salad dressings. Because they have oily characteristics and pass through the digestive tract unchanged, hydrocarbons also act as a digestive "lubricant" or laxative. Unfortunately they also absorb fat-soluble vitamins, which are then excreted along with the undigested hydrocarbons.

FIGURE 4-7

Structure of a cholesterol molecule.

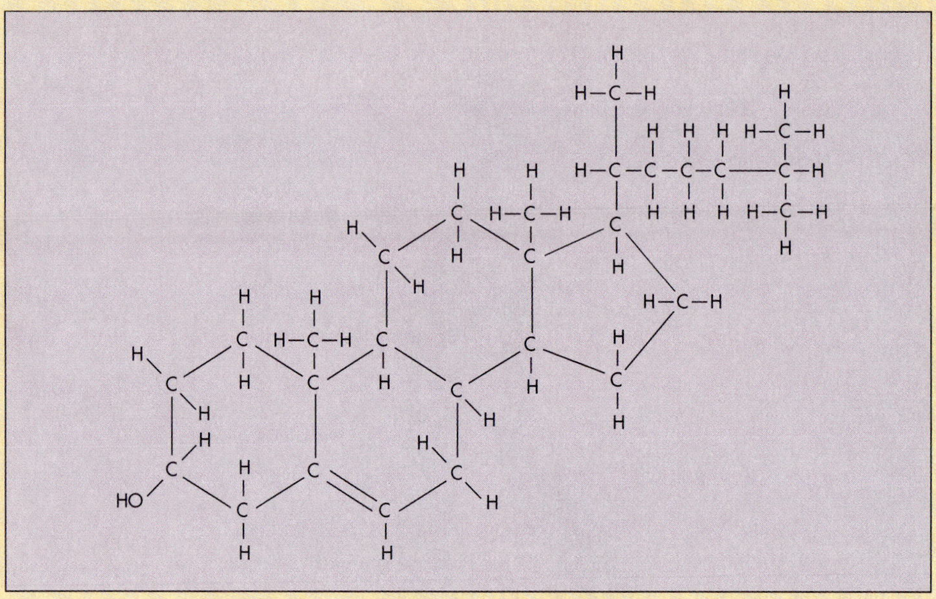

PHYSICAL PROPERTIES OF DIETARY FATS AND THEIR MODIFICATION

Fat is insoluble in water but soluble in solvents such as ether, chloroform, and benzene. Because fats are less dense than water, they rise to the surface of any water-fat mixture, such as salad oil mixed with vinegar.

In such foods as egg yolk the fat is in the form of small particles that are surrounded by a phospholipid-protein complex. This outer layer of phospholipid and protein, which mixes well with water molecules, prevents the particles from clumping together, or *coalescing,* to form visible globules. In other words, the phospholipid and protein coat keeps the fats in the state of an emulsion; such fats are known as **emulsified fats.** Emulsified fats have a much greater surface area than a similar amount of solid or globular fat because they are in the form of many small particles. This allows emulsified fats to be digested much more rapidly than unemulsified fats. Homogenized milk is made from whole milk by mechanically breaking up the large fat globules and allowing them to disperse throughout the milk in an emulsified form that prevents them from coalescing and rising to form a layer of cream. Another example is the oil in mayonnaise, which is mechanically converted to an emulsion that is stabilized by a thin layer of egg protein around each emulsified particle.

Other than in the melting of solid fats, temperatures normally used in cooking do not affect fat. However, heating at temperatures above 400° F (204° C) causes the decomposition of fatty acids and the production of **acrolein** from glycerol. Acrolein is released in the form of pungent fumes that are extremely irritating to the nasal passages and the gastrointestinal (GI) tract. Acrolein is responsible for the coughing attacks that can be caused when fat is burned during the frying of food.

Unsaturated fatty acids slowly alter their structure, or "spoil," more easily than do saturated fatty acids because of the greater chemical reactivity of their double bonds. These react with oxygen from the air in an oxidation process that produces chemicals known as *peroxides,* which cause the rancidity and "off" flavors that can develop in some fats. If unsaturated fats are to be kept for long periods, substances that inhibit the oxidation process, known as **antioxidants,** are often added. Vitamin C or E, butylated hydroxytoluene (BHT), and butylated hydroxyanisole (BHA) are the most common antioxidants. They may be incorporated into the packaging material, rather than mixed throughout the food, but are listed on the label in either case.

Another problem in storing fats is their tendency to absorb other odors and flavors. This is an advantage in distributing flavors throughout food in cooking but a disadvantage when uncovered stored fats pick up unwanted odors and flavors. For example, we want butter to take up the flavor of onion when onions are fried in butter but do not want butter stored in the refrigerator to become tainted with onion flavor and odor.

MODIFICATION OF FATS

Although hydrogen cannot be readily removed from saturated fats to make them unsaturated, it is possible to convert unsaturated fatty acids to saturated ones by the chemical addition of hydrogen. This process is called **hydrogenation** and is used commercially to change less expensive oils such as cottonseed, soybean, and sunflower oils into fats resembling the more expensive, more saturated animal fats. For example, margarine and shortening, which are similar to butter and lard in consistency and texture, are produced by the hydrogenation of vegetable oils. It is possible to control the extent of hydrogenation to retain many of the original unsaturated fatty acids while producing sufficient saturated fatty acids to create the desired texture and spreadability. In most "hydrogenated" fats, only about 30% of the fatty acids have actually been hydrogenated. It is significant, however, that many of the double bonds that escape hydrogenation are converted from the *cis* to the *trans* configuration. *Trans* configuration double bonds, which are relatively rare in nature, can account for as much as 30% to 40% of the double bonds in certain hydrogenated shortenings and frying fats. On the other hand, linoleic acid–rich reduced-fat margarines may contain no *trans* double bonds, only *cis* configuration ones.

The average intake of *trans*-bonded fatty acids in the United States has been estimated to range from about 8 g per person per day[2] to 12 to 15 g per person per day.[3] *Trans*-bonded fatty acids are also found in milk fat (accounting for 2% to 9% of fatty acids) as a result of the action of microorganisms in the rumen of the cow.

Because *trans* fatty acids can function in many of the same ways that *cis* fatty acids do, it has been proposed that food labels should give combined values, without being required to distinguish between them. However, it is only in the last 50 years that hydrogenated fats such as margarine have become dietary staples, and we have given attention to the change of *cis* to *trans* fatty acids only in the last decade. As a result, any possible long-term physiological effects of *trans* fatty acids, especially in young infants, are the subject of intense research.

As well as being affected by the chain length and degree of unsaturation of their fatty acids, the physical properties of triglycerides depend on the distribution of the constituent fatty acids between the three positions of the glycerol molecule. This distribution is not random in natural fats. In vegetable oils, for example, the saturated fatty acids, palmitic acid and stearic acid, are almost exclusively bonded to carbon atoms one and three of glycerol and almost never to carbon atom two (see Figure 4-1 for the numbering of glycerol carbons). The proportion of palmitic and stearic acids at the external positions (that is, carbons one and three) is approximately 1.5 times greater than their overall proportion in the vegetable oil. The specific natural distributions of fatty acids among the three available positions can be converted to a random distribution by the process of **interesterification.** This is used to achieve desirable melting qualities, spreadability, and palatability of margarines. Unlike hydrogenation, interesterification does not change the fatty acid composition of the fats concerned, and no *trans* double bonds are formed. Some of the margarines currently marketed in Europe and Canada contain no *trans* fatty acids, unlike those marketed in the United States. These margarines are manufactured from unhydrogenated sunflower oil, which is made semisolid by mixing with a small amount of saturated fat, followed by interesterification of the fats present.[4]

Each animal tends to produce a fat that is characteristic of its own species. Pork fat, for example, is different from beef or lamb fat. It is possible to modify the nature of the fat laid down by an animal, however, by modifying its diet. This technique has been widely used in the past by animal producers to tailor their products to consumer desires. Today, however, producers are much more likely to use growth hormones that allow them to produce animals with a higher proportion of muscle to fat. This not only yields animals with lower fat content, but also increases the efficiency with which the animals use food energy.

DIGESTION AND ABSORPTION

Fat digestion breaks fats down into substances that can be absorbed by the intestinal mucosal cells. Most dietary fat is in the form of triglycerides, with stearic and palmitic acids being the most common saturated fatty acids within these triglycerides and oleic and linoleic the most common unsaturated fatty acids. The process of emulsification, which breaks ingested fat into small particles, is an essential early step of this digestive process. A series of fat-splitting enzymes called **lipases** then hydrolyzes fatty acids from the glycerol component of triglycerides. About half of the dietary triglycerides are broken down completely to fatty acids and glycerol. The remainder are split into a mixture of monoglycerides, diglycerides, and fatty acids, with monoglycerides predominating over diglycerides.

The digestion of fat is initiated by the lingual lipase enzyme and fat is secreted by **Von Ebner's glands** at the base of the tongue. This enzyme mixes with chewed food and hydrolyzes fatty acids from triglycerides to form diglycerides as the food travels down the esophagus to the stomach. Lingual lipase hydrolyzes short-chain and medium-chain triglycerides more readily than it does long-chain triglycerides. It is resistant to the action of proteolytic enzymes in the stomach and the general

FIGURE 4-8

Summary of the key processes of triglyceride catabolism: action of colipase in allowing pancreatic lipase access to liquid droplets, micelle formation, lipid absorption, and transport of digested lipid to tissue cells and their overall fates there.

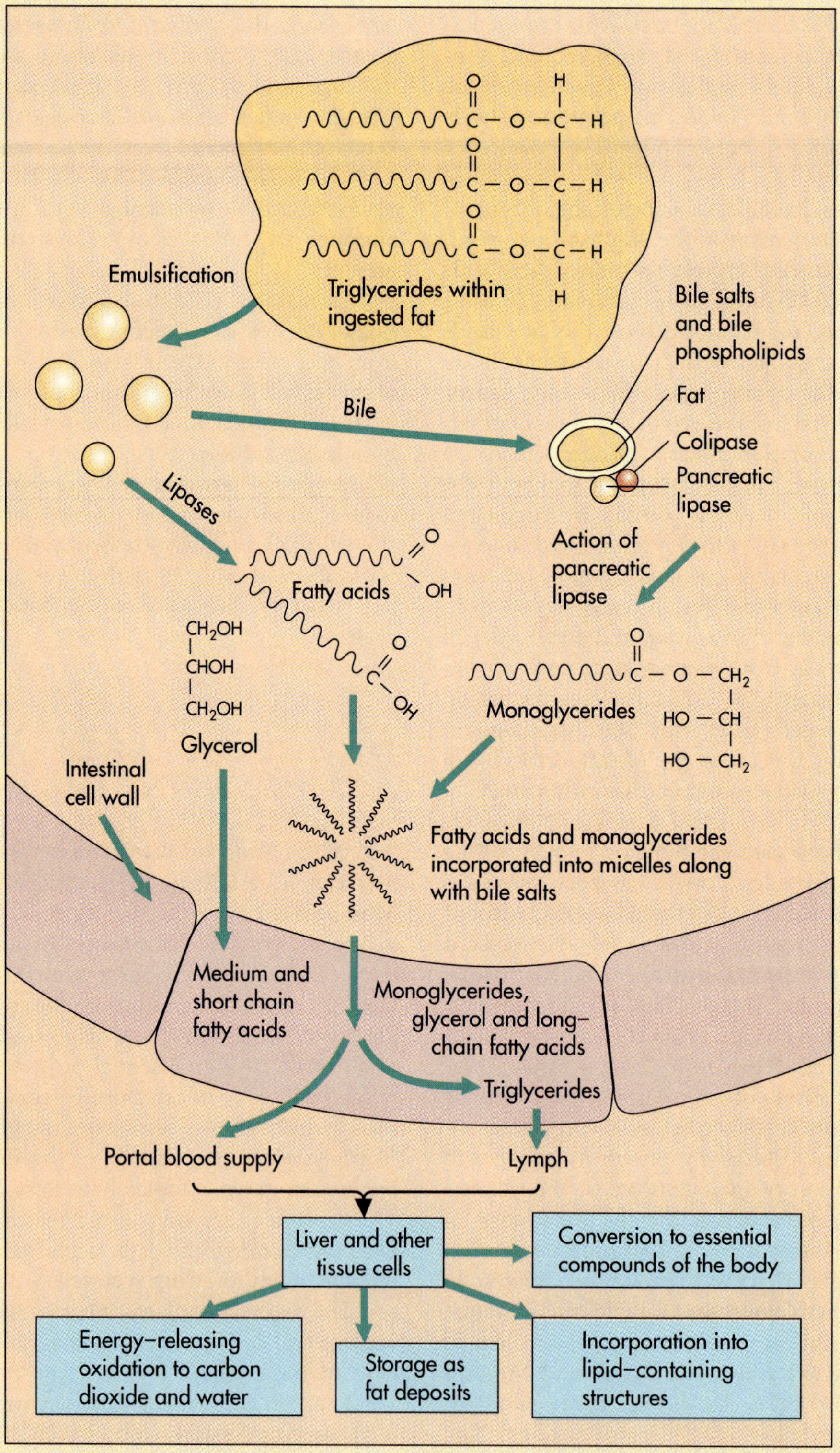

acidity of the stomach's contents and so continues to function after food enters the stomach. After entering the stomach, some of the emulsified fat in the food mass begins to also be digested by the action of the gastric lipase enzyme. Like lingual lipase, gastric lipase is active in an acidic environment and it too hydrolyzes short- and medium-chain triglycerides more quickly than it does long-chain triglycerides.

From the stomach the food mass passes into the small intestine, where the presence of fat stimulates the release of the hormones cholecystokinin and secretin. These hormones, in turn, stimulate the secretion of pancreatic juice from the pancreas and the release of bile, which is synthesized in the liver and stored in and released from the gallbladder. In addition to bile salts and bile pigments, bile contains significant amounts of various phospholipids, including lecithin. As the food mass mixes with bile, the lipid becomes bound within emulsified droplets that are coated in bile salts and bile phospholipids. Pancreatic juice is secreted and it raises the pH value from 5.5 to 6.5, in which pancreatic lipase becomes active. However, pancreatic lipase cannot act until an enzyme, **procolipase** (also secreted by the pancreas), becomes activated to **colipase** by the pancreatic trypsin enzyme. Colipase then combines with pancreatic lipase and the emulsified lipid droplets to permit the lipase to act on the triglycerides within (Figure 4-8). The pancreatic lipase hydrolyzes all lengths of fatty acid chains to yield free fatty acids and monoglycerides.

Bile **micelles** (tiny spherical aggregates of lipids and bile salts) then carry the monoglycerides and free fatty acids across what is called the *unstirred water layer* between the lipid droplets from which they are derived and the membranes of intestinal mucosal cells. This journey is the rate-limiting step in the entire lipid absorption process, meaning that lipid absorption as a whole occurs no faster than the rate of this crucial step. Once absorbed into the intestinal cell, the longer-chain free fatty acids and monoglycerides are combined back into triglycerides, which cannot diffuse in the reverse direction, back into the intestinal lumen. These triglycerides are incorporated into **chylomicrons** (described later in this chapter) and subsequently released inward to the lymph by the process of exocytosis. Medium- and short-chain fatty acids (less than 10 to 12 carbon atoms) are not recombined into triglycerides but move quickly into the blood capillaries that lead to the portal vein and hence to the liver—a faster means of transport than that taken by the long-chain fatty acids.

The rate of absorption of the fatty acids and monoglycerides into the intestinal cells depends on their structures and melting points. In general, long-chain fatty acids with higher melting points are absorbed more slowly than those with lower melting points. *Trans* fatty acids, however, may defy this general rule. On the basis of the melting point, it is predicted that *trans* fatty acids are more slowly absorbed than are their *cis* counterparts. Studies in humans, however, show that both *trans* and *cis* isomers of C18:1 (elaidic and oleic acids, respectively) are well absorbed. This is despite the fact that the melting point of the *trans* fatty acid is about 50° C, which is well above body temperature.[5]

Saturated fatty acids with 18 or more carbon atoms are absorbed relatively slowly in their free form but much more quickly when incorporated within the structure of monoglycerides. Medium-chain fatty acids, derived from medium-chain triglycerides, are absorbed quickly and are also subsequently transported to the liver more quickly than are their longer-chained counterparts, as explained previously.

TRANSPORT AND METABOLISM

Because lipids are insoluble in water, they can be transported in the circulation only if they become associated with specific proteins to form lipoproteins that are miscible with water. Some free fatty acids released from triglycerides (either dietary or derived from stores in adipose tissue) enter the plasma and circulate bound to the plasma albumin protein. Triglycerides and derivatives of cholesterol are transported as parts of much larger **plasma lipoprotein** particles (Figure 4-9). Four classes of plasma lipoproteins are recognized: the **chylomicrons, very low-density lipoproteins (VLDLs), low-density lipoproteins (LDLs),** and **high-density lipoproteins (HDLs).** All four kinds of structure are composed of lipids complexed together with proteins, but they have differing densities determined by the relative amounts of protein and lipid they contain (Table 4-4). Proteins are more dense than lipids, so the more protein a lipoprotein particle contains, the higher is its density and vice versa.

The protein components of lipoproteins are known as **apolipoproteins.** There are four parent classes of apolipoproteins (A, B, C, and E) that are synthesized in the liver and in the intestine. Each class has several related apolipoproteins (such as A-I, A-II, A-IV, B-48, B-100, C-I, C-II, etc.). Several of them are genetically related to one another and share common functions. Apolipoprotein B-48, made in the intestine, and apolipoprotein B-100, made in the liver, become tightly bound within the structure of chylomicrons and VLDLs, respectively, and are essential for their secretion. The other apolipoproteins form much looser associations with lipoprotein particles and can be exchanged between the different kinds of lipoprotein particle. Apolipoproteins play several important roles. They are important determinants of lipoprotein structure, but many of them also act as activators or inhibitors of key enzymes involved in

FIGURE 4-9

Structure of a plasma lipoprotein.

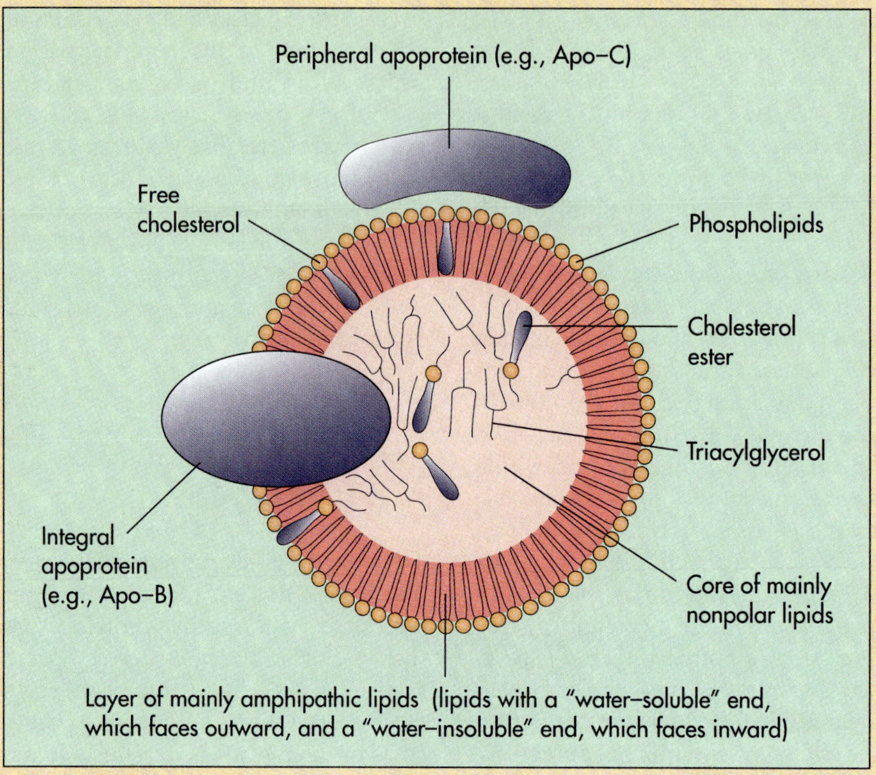

TABLE 4-4

Composition of human serum lipoproteins

			LIPIDS*				APOPROTEIN COMPONENT	
LIPOPROTEIN	DENSITY (g/ml)	PROTEIN*	TRIGLYCERIDE	CHOLESTEROL ESTER	CHOLESTEROL	PHOSPHOLIPIDS	MAJOR	MINOR
Chylomicrons	<0.95	2.0	86	3.0	2.0	7.0	C	A, B, E
Very low-density lipoprotein	0.93-1.0	8-10	55	12.0	7.0	18.0	B, C	E
Low-density lipoprotein	1.02-1.06	22-25	6	42.0	8.0	22.0	B	C, E
High-density lipoprotein Type 2	1.06-1.13	40	5	17.0	5.0	23.0	A	C, D, E
Type 3	1.13-1.21	55	3	13.0	4.5	25.0	A	C, D, E

* Percentage of weight.

lipid metabolism. Several are also involved in the binding of lipoproteins to specific receptors on cell membranes, which allows the lipids to be delivered into the cells concerned. The synthesis of apolipoproteins and their distribution among the different types of lipoprotein seem to be influenced by the quantity and content of a meal. The mechanism by which lipoprotein synthesis is regulated is unclear, but it presumably reflects the body's need to match the profile of lipoproteins available to the amounts and types of lipids needing to be transported.[5a]

Chylomicrons, the lowest-density lipoprotein particles, carry triglycerides whose fatty acids contain more than 10 to 12 carbon atoms, monoglycerides, glycerol, and small amounts of cholesterol and phospholipids. The chylomicrons are released from the intestinal mucosal cells into the lymphatic system and are carried into the general circulation by way of the thoracic duct of the lymphatic system, which leads into the left subclavian vein. Their presence in the blood plasma gives it a characteristic milky appearance for about 1 hour after the consumption of a fat-containing meal. They are quickly broken down in the capillaries of muscle and fat (adipose) tissue, however, and circulate in plasma for only 5 to 10 minutes. The free fatty acids and other lipids released by the breakdown of chylomicrons are taken up by the tissue cells while the glycerol travels on to the liver.

VLDL particles also transport triglycerides but mainly endogenous triglycerides formed in the liver. When both chylomicrons and VLDL particles reach the capillaries of the tissues to which they are delivering lipid, an enzyme called **lipoprotein lipase** plays a key role in breaking them down and releasing their fatty acids and other lipids, such as monoglycerides, for entry into the tissue cells.

HDLs are either secreted from the liver or intestine or formed in plasma from chylomicrons and VLDLs. LDLs are formed from VLDLs. LDL transports cholesterol to the cells of the body, whereas HDL transports cholesterol to the liver. Thus cholesterol can be transported from the liver to other tissues by LDL and from other tissues to the liver by HDL. These two classes of lipoprotein have essentially opposite roles.

Once fatty acids, monoglycerides, and other lipids enter tissue cells, they can be metabolized in one of four different ways:

- They can be used immediately as a source of energy.
- They can be stored as reserve energy supplies within the lipid of the specialized adipose cells of adipose (fat) tissue or, to a lesser extent, within other cells of the body.
- They can become incorporated, as required, into the lipid-containing structures of the cell, particularly its various lipid-based membranes.
- They can be used as raw materials for the synthesis of a variety of essential compounds of the body, including cholesterol.

When fatty acids are used as a source of energy, the net effect is for their atoms to be combined with oxygen to generate carbon dioxide and water. Much of the energy released in this reaction can be trapped within high-energy compounds, especially adenosine triphosphate (ATP), until required by other aspects of cellular metabolism. Like all of the biological oxidations that release energy, the oxidation of fatty acids proceeds via a series of transformations known as a *metabolic pathway.* The metabolic pathway of fatty acid oxidation is known as the **β-oxidation** pathway. This is because it involves removal of two carbon atoms at a time from the fatty acid chain by breaking of the bond between the β and γ atoms of a fatty acid. This process repeatedly cleaves off successive two-carbon units, generating ever-shorter fatty acid molecules until the original fatty acid has been entirely degraded. The two-carbon units become part of **acetyl coenzyme A (acetyl CoA),** which plays a central role in many aspects of metabolism. In fact, the carbon skeletons of fatty acids, carbohydrates, and the amino acids derived from protein digestion all end up as acetyl CoA when these nutrients are being oxidized as a source of energy. The acetyl CoA then enters the series of reactions known as the citric acid cycle (see Chapter 3), eventually leading to the complete oxidation of the carbon and hydrogen atoms derived from fatty acids (or carbohydrates or amino acids) to carbon dioxide and water, with the release of energy as ATP.

The oxidation of fatty acids and carbohydrates are interrelated processes because both eventually generate acetyl CoA that enters the citric acid cycle. (In carbohydrate oxidation, the acetyl CoA is generated from the pyruvic acid, whose formation was discussed in Chapter 3.) Carbohydrates also serve to replenish supplies of the main chemical intermediates of the citric acid cycle. One consequence of this is that fatty acid oxidation cannot proceed properly if an appropriate amount of carbohydrate oxidation is not also taking place. If fatty acid oxidation is hindered because of insufficient accompanying carbohydrate oxidation, some of the fatty acids are instead converted into ketones, leading to the condition known as **ketosis.** The onset of ketosis, when insufficient carbohydrate is in the diet, is one indication that carbohydrate is a dietary essential.

Acetyl CoA is also the precursor of cholesterol, which is of relevance to people following diets intended to reduce blood cholesterol levels. In addition to consuming less cholesterol, these people should reduce the total amount of fat in their diet to prevent the conversion of acetyl CoA derived from excess dietary fat into cholesterol within the body.

ESSENTIAL FATTY ACIDS

The fatty acids linoleic acid, α-linolenic acid, and arachidonic acid have traditionally been regarded as **essential fatty acids (EFAs).** Over 60 years ago experiments suggested that all three of these fatty acids were required to cure **dermatitis** (inflammation of the skin) and to restore growth and fertility in animals that had been fed a very low-fat diet.[6] We now know, however, that arachidonic acid can be formed from linoleic acid; so linoleic acid and α-linolenic acid are now regarded as the two *nutritionally* essential fatty acids able to be converted into other metabolically essential fatty acids (Figure 4-10). Both are required to support growth and reproduction in animals fed fat-free diets, but dermal integrity (good skin condition) requires only linoleic acid. There is still some debate about the essentiality of α-linolenic acid in humans, but the rod and cone cells of the retina and the nerve synapses of the brain do appear to have a specific requirement for the highly unsaturated fatty acids of the omega-3 series, of which α-linolenic acid is the parent molecule.[7]

Both of the nutritionally essential fatty acids serve as precursors of a large group of hormonelike compounds, the eicosanoids, that are discussed later.

> *L*inoleic acid and α-linolenic acid are the nutritionally **essential fatty acids** and are the only lipids that are required components of the human diet.

EFA DEFICIENCY

The characteristic clinical and biochemical features of deficiencies in either the omega-3 or the omega-6 series of fatty acids are presented in Table 4-5. The effects of omega-6 deficiencies, which stem from a deficiency in linoleic acid, have been well characterized in both humans and other animals. The effects of omega-3 deficiencies, stemming basically from a deficiency of α-linolenic acid, are less obvious, have not been so well characterized, and are still the subject of some dispute.

The first study of EFA deficiency in adult humans involved keeping the subjects on an extremely low-fat diet for 6 months and resulted in no dramatic symptoms. Because adults contain more than 2 lb of stored linoleic acid, however, it was suggested that 6 months was not sufficient time for the depletion of these stores that would allow symptoms to appear. The first clear evidence for the nutritional essentiality of linoleic acid was reported by Hansen and colleagues[8] in 1963. These studies involved infants fed one of five proprietary milk formulas that were adequate in all other nutrients but contained varying amounts of linoleic acid. The amounts of linoleic acid varied from 7.3% down to less than 0.1% of total kilocalorie needs. A high proportion of the infants who were fed the formula lowest in linoleic acid for 3 months developed dry, thick, flaking skin and suffered from retarded growth. These clinical problems disappeared, however, when larger amounts of linoleic acid were provided. A level of linoleic acid sufficient to provide 1% to 2% of total kilocalories has proved sufficient to prevent both clinical and biochemical evidence of deficiency in humans. The American Academy of Pediatrics (AAP) and other U.S. and international expert committees recommend that infant milk formula should provide at least 2.7% of total kilocalories in the form of linoleic acid. The suggested intake of omega-6 fatty acids as a whole is between 2% and 6% of total energy intake. It is relevant to note that in human milk, approximately 3.5% to as high as 12% of total kilocalories are provided by linoleic acid and its long-chain polyunsaturated derivatives, depending on the fat composition of the maternal diet.

Although much less thoroughly characterized, a few cases of suspected deficiencies in omega-3 fatty acids have been reported in humans. Holman and colleagues[9] reported a case of peripheral neuropathy and blurred vision in a child receiving total parenteral nutrition devoid of omega-3 fatty acids for 5 months. Bjerve and his coworkers[10] reported linolenic acid deficiency in nine patients fed by gastric tube for 2.5 to 12 years, who had received only 0.025% to 0.09% of their total kilocalories as omega-3 fatty acids. Recent research in rhesus monkeys and preterm (prematurely born) human infants, however, has revealed abnormalities in vision and electroretinograms when the feeding formulas given were low in omega-3 fatty acids.[11] Whatever the true need for omega-3 fatty acids, various studies of the subject have led to the recommendation that from 0.2% to 1% of total kilocalories should be provided by omega-3 fatty acids.[12]

CHOLESTEROL

If the amount of cholesterol in a person's blood exceeds 240 mg/dl, they are said to have **hypercholesterolemia,** which simply means a high level of cholesterol in the blood. Hypercholesterolemia is considered to indicate that a person is at increased risk of coronary heart disease; thus there is a great deal of interest in how the body gains, synthesizes, and metabolizes cholesterol. The study of cholesterol is complicated by the fact that considerable amounts of it are made in the body, supplementing the amounts supplied by animal foods in the

FIGURE 4-10

Metabolic conversion of the omega-6 and omega-3 families of fatty acids.

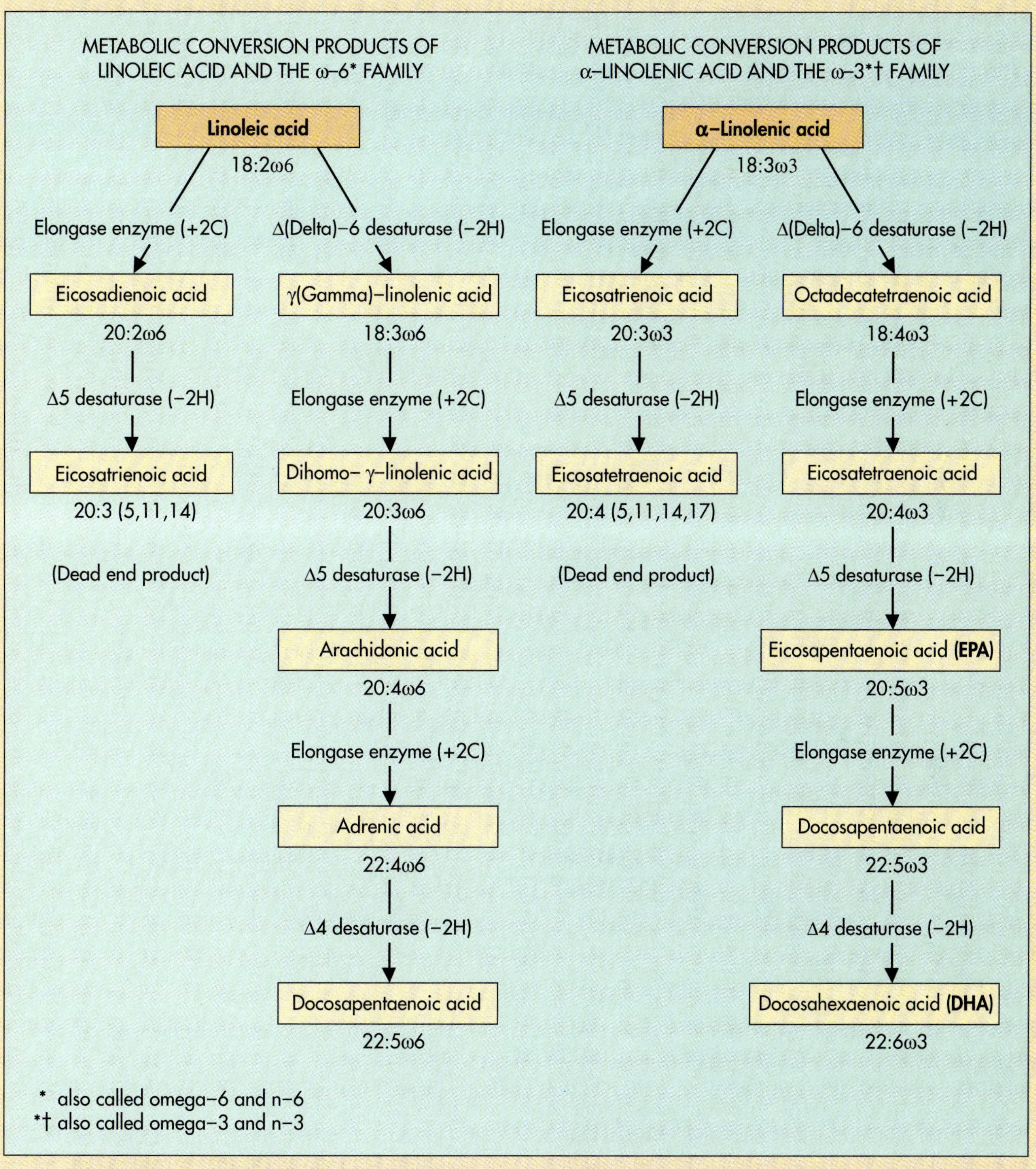

diet. A schematic outline of the metabolism of cholesterol is given in Figure 4-11. Cholesterol from food is absorbed through the intestinal wall and into the lymphatic system, along with reabsorbed cholesterol derived from bile and the breakdown of sloughed intestinal cells. Overall, however, only between 30% and 60% of the cholesterol passing through the intestine is absorbed. Intestinal wall cells regulate the amount absorbed, and once the cholesterol is absorbed, it is incorporated into chylomicrons (which are 7% cholesterol). When the triglycerides within chylomicrons are hydrolyzed in tissue capillaries, the residual particles (chylomicron remnants)—including their cholesterol—are taken up by the liver cells. The liver cells incorporate the cholesterol into VLDL particles,

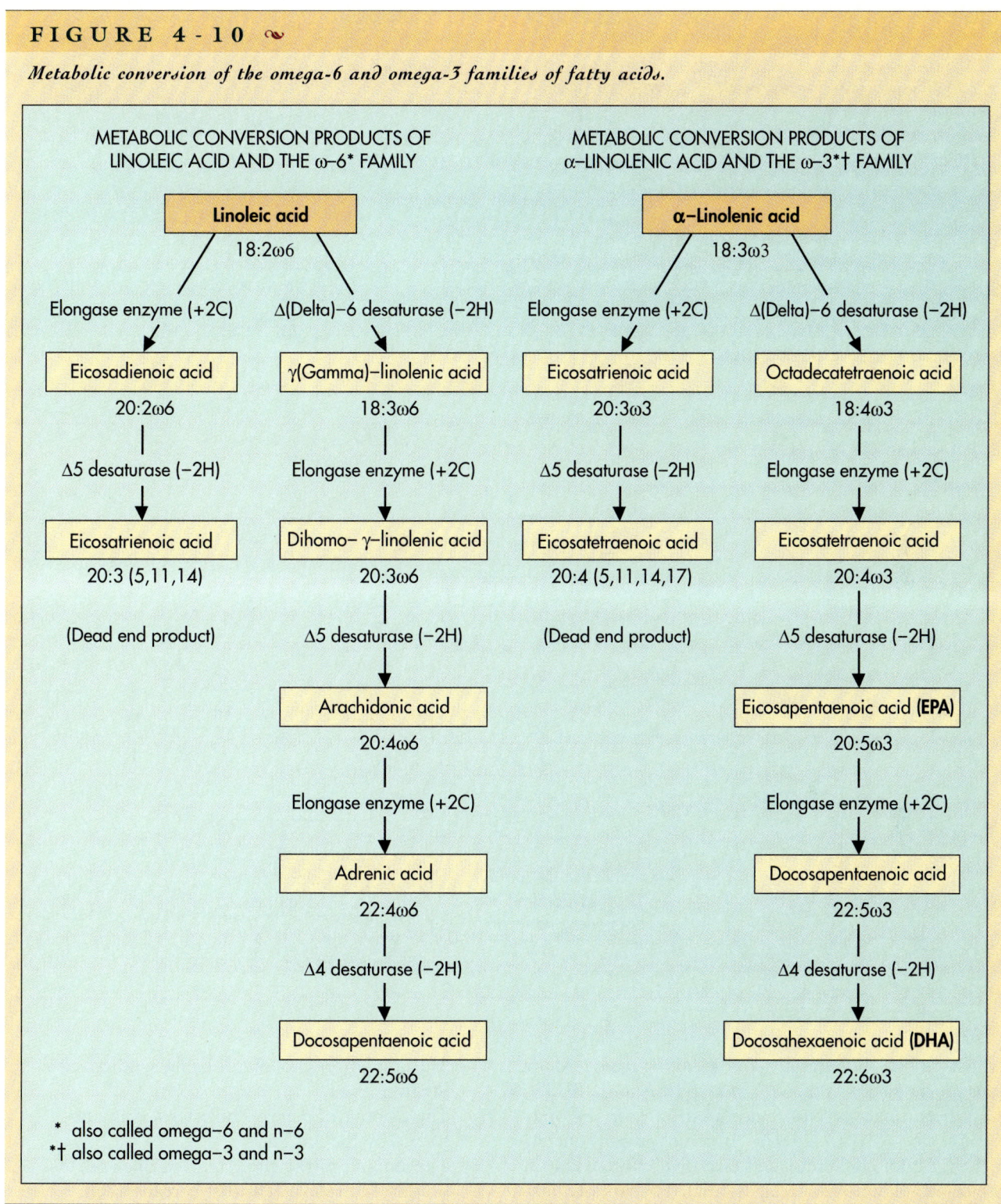

TABLE 4-5

Differing characteristics of ω-3 and ω-6 essential fatty acid deficiencies

	OMEGA-3 (α-LINOLENIC ACID)	OMEGA-6 (LINOLEIC ACID)
Clinical features	Normal skin, growth, reproduction Reduced learning Abnormal electroretinogram Impaired vision Polydipsia	Growth retardation Skin lesions Reproductive failure Fatty liver Polydipsia
Biochemical markers	Decreased 18:3ω-3 and 22:6ω-3 Increased 22:4ω-6 and 22:5ω-7 Increased 20:3ω-9 (only if ω-6 also low)	Decreased 18:2ω-6 and 20:4ω-6 Increased 20:3ω-9 (only if ω-3 also low)

From Conner WE, Neuringer M, Reisbick S: *Nutr Rev* 50:21, 1992.

FIGURE 4-11

Outline of the metabolism of cholesterol.

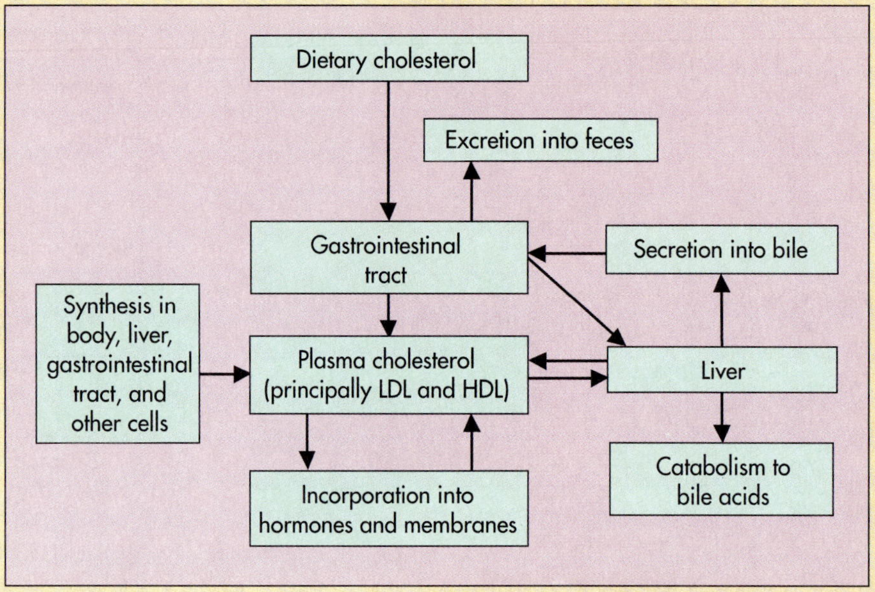

which are 21% cholesterol, before secreting them into the general circulation. When the triglycerides in the VLDL have been removed and transported into various body tissues, the VLDL particles become proportionately richer in both cholesterol and **esterified cholesterol** (in which a cholesterol molecule is bonded by an ester linkage to a fatty acid molecule) and become LDL particles, which are 60% cholesterol. Most of the supplies of cholesterol taken up by body cells reach them in the form of LDL particles. HDL particles, on the other hand (which are around 35% cholesterol), carry smaller amounts of cholesterol away from body cells and back to the liver.

The amount of cholesterol circulating within the various lipoprotein particles depends on four factors:

- The amount of cholesterol being synthesized in the liver
- The amount of dietary cholesterol being absorbed by the intestine
- The amount of the cholesterol in bile and sloughed intestinal cells that is reabsorbed, rather than being excreted in feces
- The amount of cholesterol being removed from the circulation by the various tissues of the body

There is an elaborate interaction among these factors, with the amount of cholesterol synthesized by the body being regulated—within limits—by the amount present within the blood.

TABLE 4-6

Cholesterol and energy (kilocalorie) content of common measures of selected foods

FOOD	AMOUNT	KCAL	CHOLESTEROL (mg)*
Milk (skim, fluid, or reconstituted dry)	1 cup	90	5
Cottage cheese, uncreamed	½ cup	62	5
Yogurt, frozen	½ cup	95	6
Lard	1 T	116	12
Cottage cheese, creamed	½ cup	116	17
Milk, 2%	1 cup	125	18
Cream, light table	2 T	58	20
Cream, half and half	¼ cup	80	24
Ice cream (regular, approximately 10% fat)	½ cup	135	28
Cheese, cheddar	1 oz	114	30
Milk, whole	1 cup	150	33
Butter	1 T	102	31
Oysters	3 oz, cooked	56	42
Tuna	3 oz, cooked	83	55
Chicken, turkey (light meat)	3 oz, cooked	147	72
Lamb, pork, chicken (dark meat)	3 oz, cooked	180	80
Crab	3 oz, cooked	86	85
Shrimp	3 oz, cooked	100	130
Heart, beef	3 oz, cooked	190	230
Egg	1 yolk or 1 egg	80	228
Liver, beef, calf, pork, lamb	3 oz, cooked	195	370
Kidney	3 oz, cooked	180	680
Brains	3 oz, raw	150	More than 1700

* Fruits, vegetables, cereals, and margarines contain no cholesterol.

From Human Nutrition Information Service: *Provisional table on the fatty acid and cholesterol content of selected foods,* Washington, DC, 1984, U.S. Department of Agriculture.

Hypercholesterolemia does not necessarily cause coronary heart disease but does place an individual at increased risk for its development. This seems to be particularly true if the level of LDL cholesterol (that is, cholesterol held within LDL) is high relative to that of HDL cholesterol (LDL/HDL ratios of >4 indicate high risk). Data on the energy and cholesterol content of representative foods are shown in Table 4-6. Note that all these foods come from animal sources.

THE ROLE OF FAT IN THE DIET

SOURCE OF ENERGY

Fat is the most concentrated source of energy in the diet. Each gram of fat, whether animal or vegetable or liquid or solid, releases 9 kcal of energy when completely oxidized to carbon dioxide and water. This is 2.5 times as much energy as is released by an equal amount of carbohydrate or protein. Such fats as butter, sour cream, and salad oil are routinely added to foods such as potatoes and salad greens to enhance their flavor. This can typically cause a two- to threefold increase in the energy content of the food concerned.

Fat is also the main form in which animals, including humans, store excess energy supplies. This means that the amount of fat in an animal we use for food depends on how the animal was fed throughout its life. Virtually all animal foods contain some fat. Even lean steak is 8% fat by weight, which contributes 77% of the total kilocalories provided by the steak. Cheddar cheese is 32% fat by weight, which provides 73% of the total kilocalories provided by the cheese.

Any fat in plant foods is mainly in the form of oil. In cereals, such as corn, or in legumes, such as soybeans, the oil is principally in the germ. Most fruits and vegetables have almost no nutritionally significant quantities of fat. One of the applications of genetic engineering in agriculture is the attempt to modify the kind and amount of fat in certain plants.

SATIETY VALUE

Fat tends to leave the stomach relatively slowly. It can still be released from the stomach for up to 3.5 hours after a meal, with the precise time depending on the size and composition of the meal. This prolonged stay in the stomach helps to delay the onset of hunger pangs and so contributes to a feeling of satiety after a meal. Because of its high kilocalorie value, fat is often reduced or eliminated from diets suggested for weight control. Research has shown, however, that including some fat in a meal (within such foods as low-fat milk, butter, or salad oil) increases the satiety value of low-kilocalorie diets and often makes it easier for people to stick to the diets. This strategy more than compensates for the energy supplied by the fat. Moderate fat-reducing diets are currently considered more successful in weight control than are very low-fat diets.

> Moderate fat-reducing diets are currently considered more successful in weight control than very low-fat diets.

CARRIER OF FAT-SOLUBLE VITAMINS

The dietary essentials include four fat-soluble vitamins: A, D, E, and K. Dietary fat serves as a carrier for these vitamins; thus eliminating fat from the diet leads to reduced intake of them. Also, fat at a level of at least 10% of total energy intake appears to be required for the absorption of vitamin A precursors from nonfat sources such as carrots. Anything that interferes with the absorption or use of fat, such as obstruction of the bile duct, depresses the supply of fat-soluble vitamins to the body.

PALATABILITY

The presence of fat in food, or its addition to food, is responsible for much of the texture and flavor of food. The marbling of fat throughout the lean muscle of a steak contributes greatly to its tenderness and flavor. Conversely, the removal of skin and fat from chicken is considered by many to detract from its flavor. Most uses of fat—in frying, as butter or oil added to vegetables, or as a spread—considerably improve the taste of food. Many of the substances that are responsible for the flavors and aromas of foods are soluble in fat, so the fat tends to carry these flavors and aromas and mix them throughout the food as a whole. It has also been suggested that fat in the diet stimulates the flow of digestive juices. The role of fat in increasing the palatability of the food in most diets is probably best appreciated by those who have tried to adhere to a low-fat diet.

THE ROLE OF FAT IN THE BODY

Fat is an essential constituent of the membranes of every cell in the body, not only the outer membranes of all cells, but also the many internal membranes of the nucleus, endoplasmic reticulum, and the other membrane-bound organelles. In addition to this role as a structural component of cells, fat serves other functions in the body of relevance to nutrition: as an energy reserve, a regulator of body functions, an insulator against heat loss, and a protector against physical shock.

ENERGY RESERVE

Body fat is the primary form in which energy is stored in the body. One pound of stored fat represents 3500 kilocalories of stored energy. Some fat can be stored within most cells, but the body also contains large numbers of specialized fat cells (**adipocytes**) within fat (adipose) tissue, whose main function is the storage of fat. Stored fat can account for up to 90% of the material in an adipocyte (Figure 4-12). The number of adipocytes within the body appears to be genetically determined, but fat cells can increase in size at any time to accommodate increased stores of fat.[13] Adipose cells are found in most parts of the body, but those that increase in size from increased fat content (when energy supplies are in excess) tend to be particularly abundant directly beneath the skin. They form the obvious deposits we associate with "fatness" or obesity.

Within the cells of adipose tissue, fat is stored largely in the form of globules of triglycerides. These may be the result of the resynthesis of triglycerides from glycerol and fatty acids, when dietary supplies of fat are in excess of bodily requirements, or they may be produced by the conversion of excess carbohydrate or protein into fat.

> One pound of stored fat represents 3500 kcal of stored energy.

A considerable amount of body fat (about 18% to 24% of body weight in women and 15% to 18% of body weight in men) is normal and indeed desirable. People

FIGURE 4-12

Structure of an adipose cell.

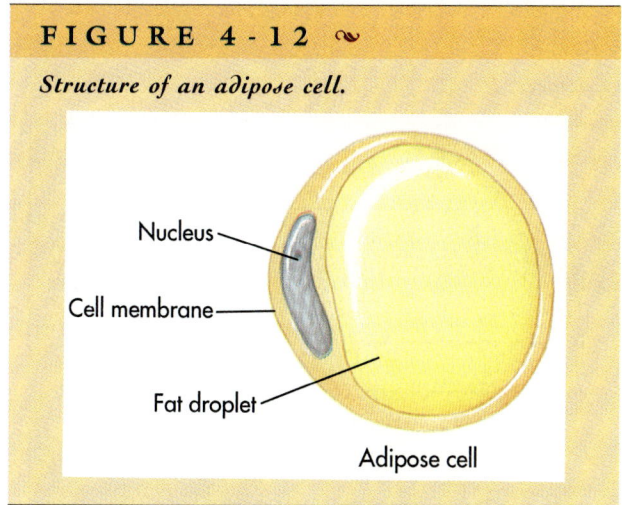

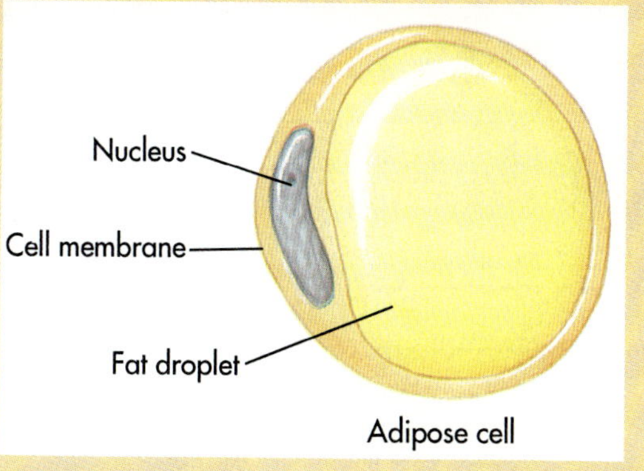

with reserves of fat in excess of these values are considered to be overweight. In extreme cases, when the percentages are very high, they are considered **obese,** a condition associated with many physical, physiological, aesthetic, and psychological disadvantages.

Once reserves of fat have been formed within fat cells, it is not possible for any excess to be removed from the body by excretion. The only way the body's fat reserves can be reduced is by the oxidation of the fat molecules with the accompanying release of energy. This occurs only when the kilocalorie intake of the diet is insufficient to meet the body's energy needs.

Most body fat is what is described as **white fat,** but a small portion—known as **brown fat** because of its generous blood supply—is found in various sites in the upper part of the body. The fat reserves within brown fat can be oxidized at a much faster rate than the fat within white fat. Instead of being used to generate supplies of ATP, however, it seems that most of the energy released by the oxidation of fat within brown fat tissue is simply given out as heat. Also, the fat that is oxidized is constantly replaced by the synthesis of new fat reserves, a process that obviously requires energy. This allows brown fat tissue to serve as a heat-generating system that warms the body as one part of the body's complex system of temperature regulation. Brown fat is also believed to play a role in oxidizing or "burning up" fats when dietary energy intake exceeds the body's needs. Thus the activities of brown fat serve to prevent some of the excess energy from being converted into additional fat reserves.

The oxidation of fat within brown fat tissue to generate heat is an example of **thermogenesis,** the metabolic generation of heat within the body. An increase in the rate of thermogenesis can be initiated either by exposure to cold or by excess dietary energy intake. These two conditions also stimulate the formation of more fat reserves within brown fat tissue so that the body's capacity to produce heat and regulate body weight is increased. These phenomena have been well demonstrated in studies with laboratory animals and are assumed to be a factor in weight control in humans.

Infants have a much higher proportion of brown fat than do adults. There is some evidence that adults contain the same number of brown fat cells as they did when they were children, whereas the number of cells containing white fat increases during growth into adulthood.

REGULATOR OF BODY FUNCTIONS

As an essential component of all cell membranes, fats indirectly help regulate both the flow of materials into and out of cells and changes in cell size and shape, such as those involved in growth.

Specific long-chain omega-6 and omega-3 unsaturated fatty acids also act as the precursors of a range of hormonelike substances, the **eicosanoids,** involved in the regulation of a wide variety of processes in the body. *Eikosi* is the Greek word for 20, and all eicosanoids are based on a skeleton containing 20 carbon atoms. They include the classes of important physiological regulators known as *prostaglandins, prostacyclins, thromboxanes,* and *leukotrienes.*

True hormones are secreted in one location and then transported within blood to other locations, where they bring about specific responses within the cells with which they interact. Eicosanoids, on the other hand, are short-lived substances that act close to their site of synthesis. They have been described as "local hormones," and they perform many functions, including the regulation of blood pressure, the control of important aspects of the reproductive cycle, the stimulation of pain and fever, and the induction of blood clotting.

The most important precursor of eicosanoids in humans is the fatty acid arachidonic acid, which is either obtained directly from animal foods in the diet or synthesized from the linoleic acid found in several vegetable oils. Another group of eicosanoids is synthesized from α-linolenic acid, which is found in such oils as soybean oil and canola oil (also known as *low–erucic acid rapeseed* [or *LEAR*] *oil*); from eicosapentaenoic acid (EPA); or from docosahexaenoic acid (DHA) in fish oils (Figure 4-13).

Prostaglandins, perhaps the best-known eicosanoids, act within the brain, the wall of blood vessels, certain blood cells, and blood platelets. They are involved in promoting conception, inducing labor, effecting spontaneous abortions, regulating the transmission of nervous impulses, and regulating blood pressure. Overproduction of some prostaglandins and other eicosanoids from arachidonic acid may cause excessive clotting of the blood and narrowing of the arteries. The risk of these undesirable consequences can be reduced by EPA and DHA, which are both omega-3 fatty acids found in fish

FIGURE 4-13

Production of eicosanoids from omega-3 and omega-6 fatty acids.

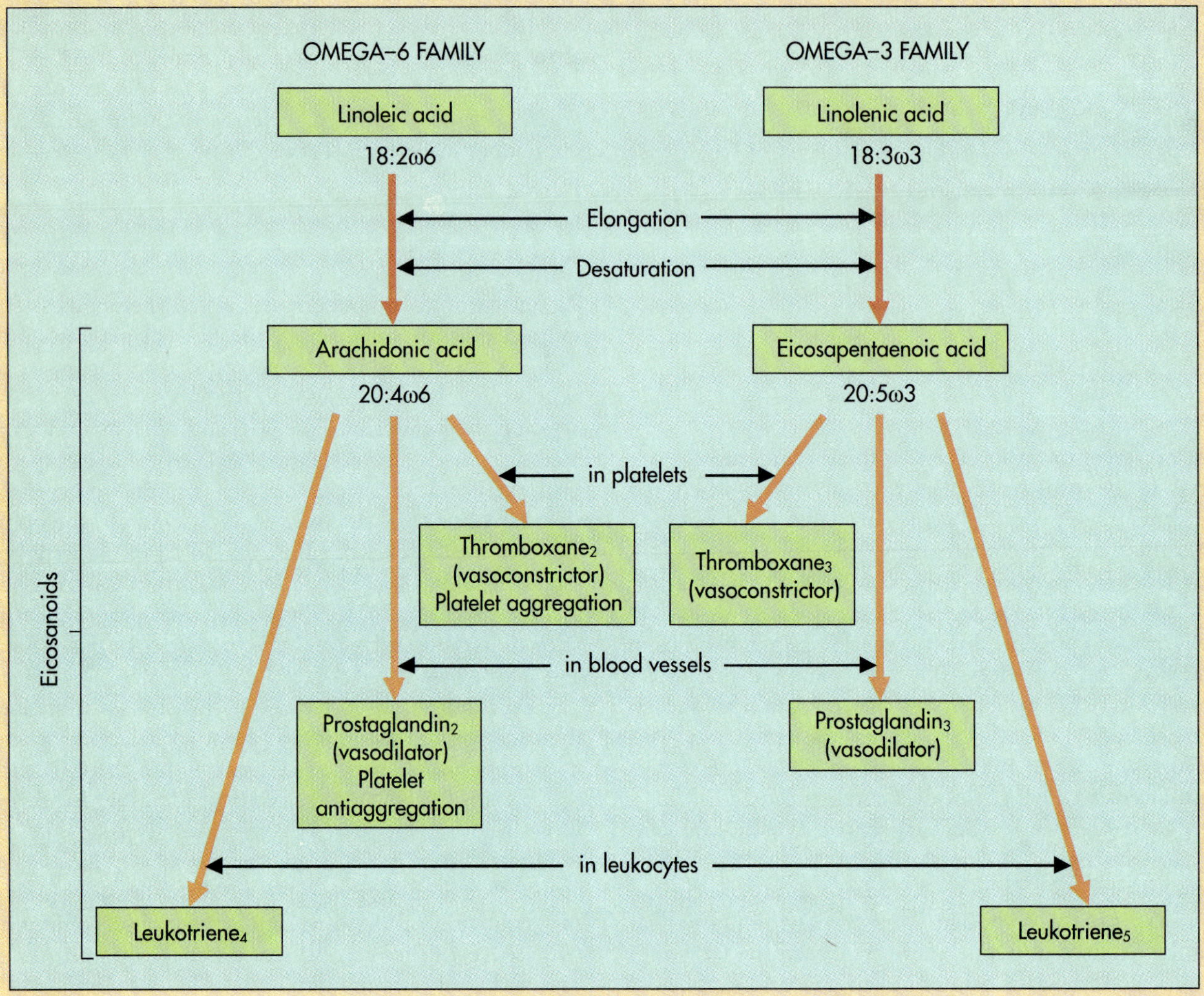

oil. These act to decrease the stickiness of the blood platelets involved in clotting, thus reducing the possibility of a clot that could cause a heart attack.

INSULATOR

Deposits of fat beneath the skin, known as **subcutaneous fat,** serve as an insulating material for the body that is effective at preventing heat loss. A certain minimal layer of fat is desirable, but too thick a layer slows down heat loss too much in hot weather, causing discomfort.

PROTECTOR

Deposits of fat surround certain vital organs, such as the kidneys and heart, serving to hold them in position and protect them from physical shock. These protective deposits are the last to be drawn on for energy supplies when insufficient energy is available in the diet.

FOOD SOURCES OF FAT

The total fat and fatty acid compositions of some commonly used foods are shown in Figure 4-14 and Table 4-7, which also reveal the main kinds of foods that contribute significant amounts of fat to the diet. The polyunsaturated fatty acid linoleic acid, listed separately in Table 4-8, is the predominant essential fatty acid in dietary fats. It is clear from Table 4-8 that coconut, olive, and palm kernel oils contain virtually no EFA, whereas safflower and corn oils contain large amounts. Poultry and game also provide large amounts of EFA. One major source of omega-3 fatty acids is fish, such as salmon, mackerel, and eel. The amount of omega-3 fatty acid in fish and oils is shown in Table 4-8.

It is difficult to present precise data on the fatty acid content of animal fats because of differences caused by variations in each animal's diet. Animals fed on pastures have a fatty acid composition different from that in

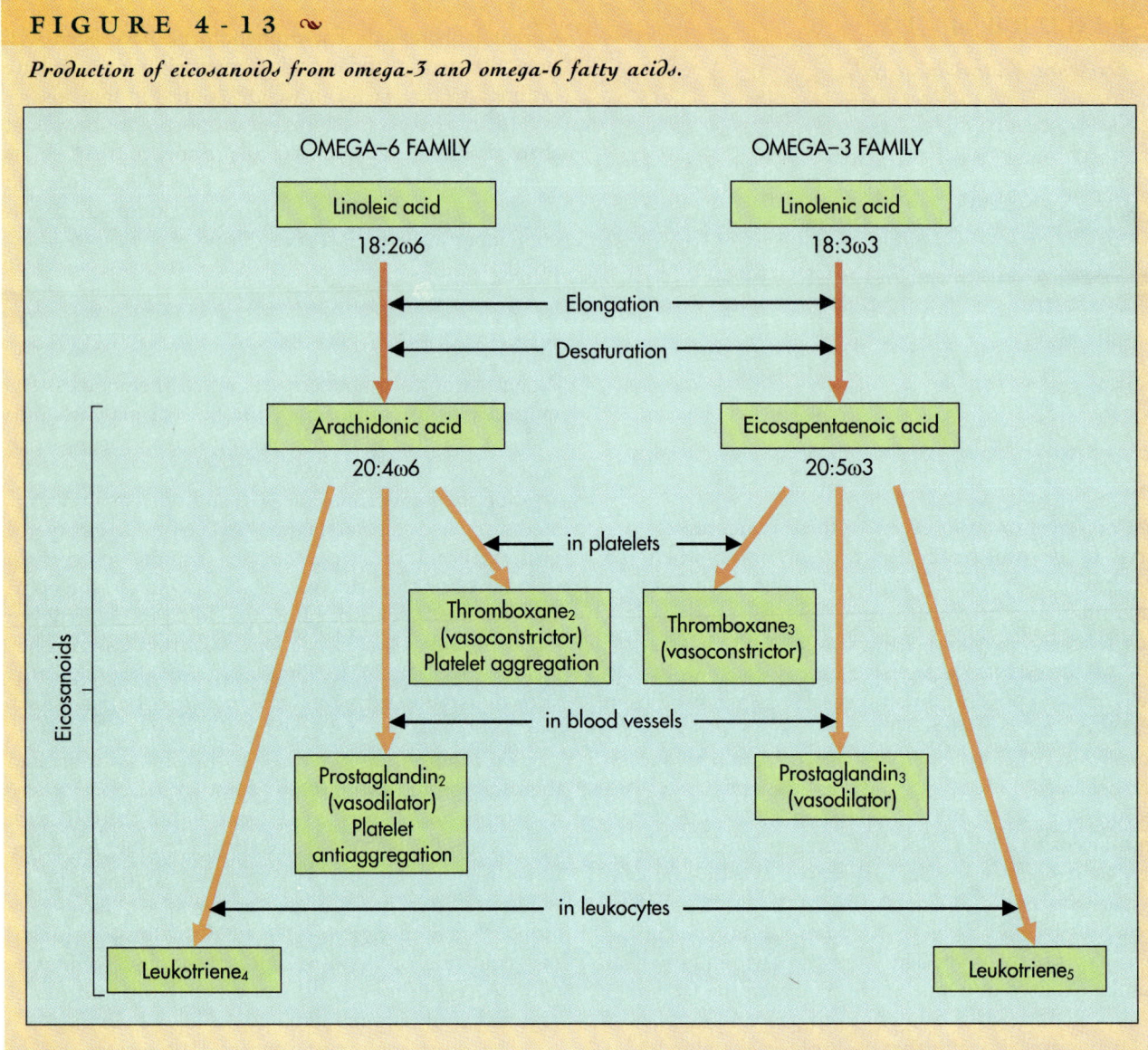

FIGURE 4-14

Profiles of fatty acids in commonly used dietary fats and oils.

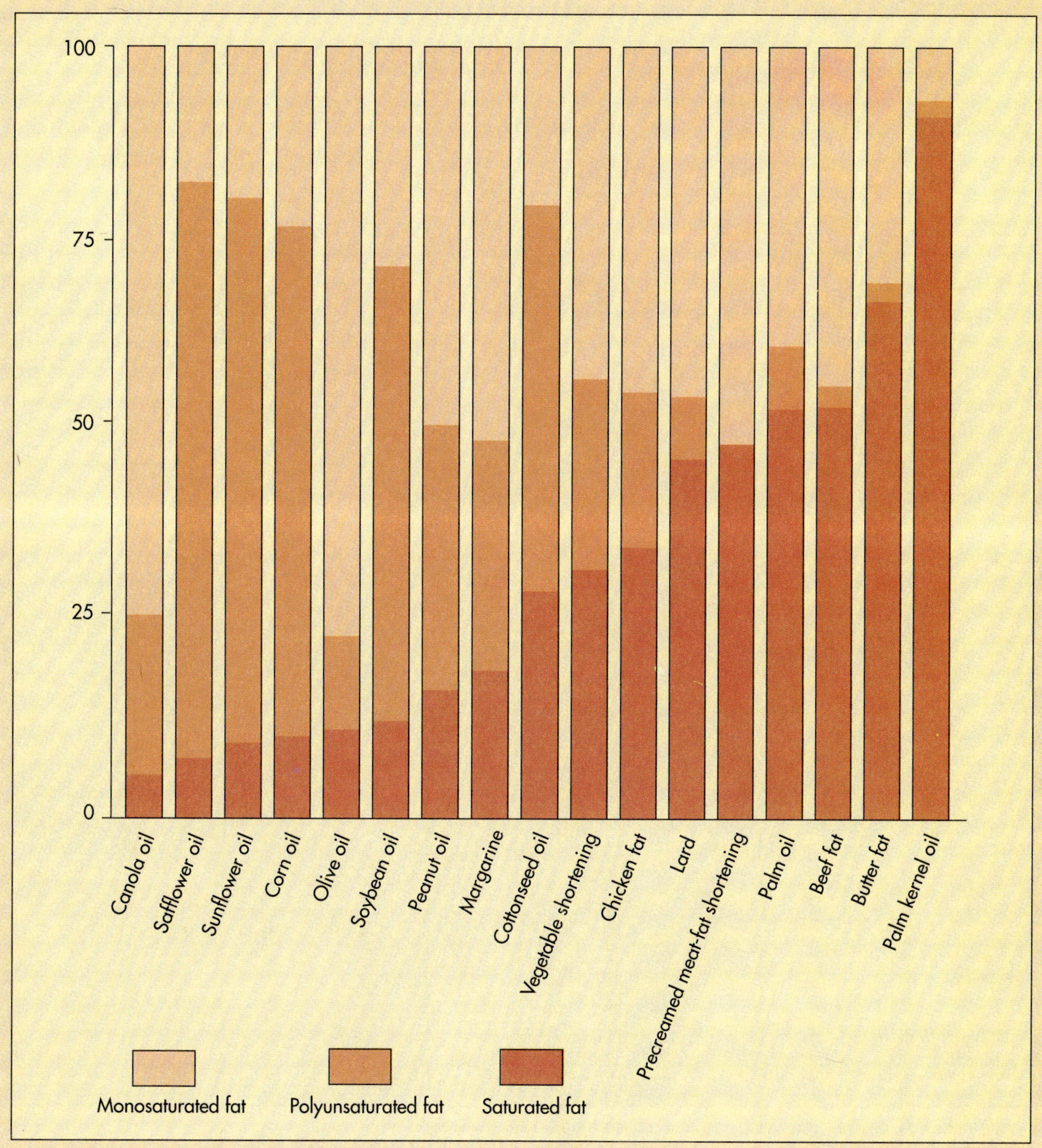

similar animals fed corn and soybean rations. The methods used to process and store food may also affect the fatty acid composition of the food when it is consumed.

Food producers have made many different responses to the public's growing interest in foods with low or no fat content. For example, the number of new low-fat or no-fat foods, which totaled 278 in 1988, more than quadrupled to 1198 in 1991.[14] It is now possible for consumers to select either regular, low-fat, or no-fat versions of such foods as cheese, cookies, mayonnaise, and salad dressings. Generally speaking, however, as the fat content of a food is lowered, so is its palatability as judged by most tastes.

The percentage of kilocalories contributed by fat tends to be relatively high in most foods from animal sources. Whole milk has only 3.2% fat by weight, but this

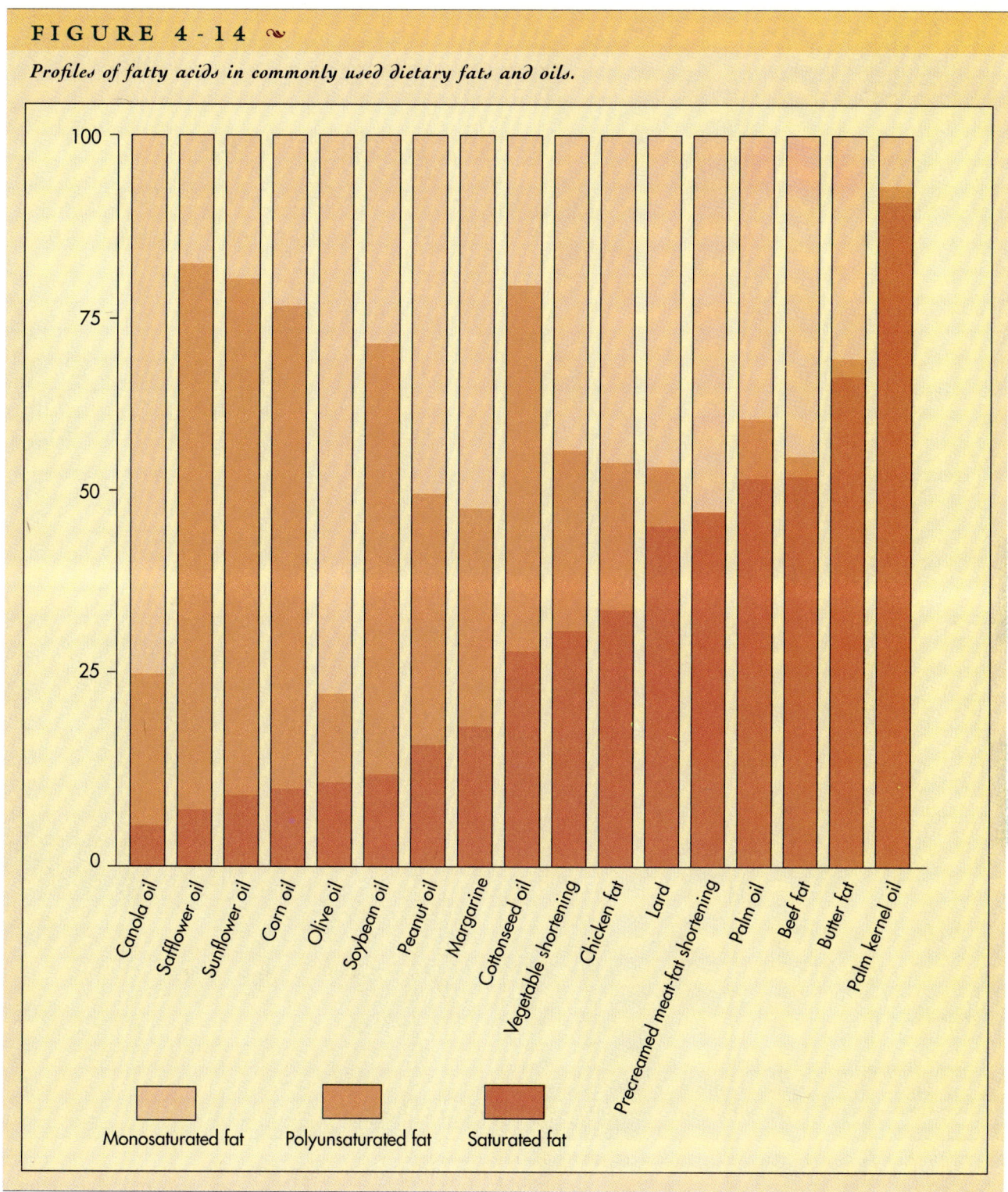

TABLE 4-7

Fat content and major fatty acid composition of selected foods (in decreasing order of linoleic acid content within each group of similar foods)

			FATTY ACIDS*	
			UNSATURATED	
FOOD	TOTAL FAT (%)	SATURATED (%)	MONOUNSATURATED (%)	POLYUNSATURATED (LINOLEIC) (%)
Salad and cooking oils				
Safflower	100	9	12	74
Wheat germ	100	19	15	62
Corn	100	13	24	59
Soybean	100	14	23	58
Cottonseed	100	26	18	52
Sesame	100	14	40	42
Peanut	100	17	46	32
Rapeseed (canola)	100	7	56	33
Palm	100	49	37	9
Olive	100	14	74	8
Coconut	100	87	6	2
Palm kernel	100	81	11	2
Butter	81	51	23	3
Margarine, first ingredient on label				
Safflower oil—tub	80	9	23	44
Corn oil (liquid)—tub	80	14	32	31
Soybean oil—stick	80	17	39	21
Corn oil—stick	80	13	46	18
Lard	100	39	45	11
Animal fats				
Poultry	100	30	37	20
Beef, lamb, pork	100	50	36	3
Fish, raw				
Salmon	9	2	2	4
Mackerel	13	5	3	4
Herring, Pacific	13	4	2	2
Tuna	5	2	1	1
Nuts				
Walnuts, English	64	9	23	63
Peanuts or peanut butter	51	17	46	32
Brazil	67	13	32	17
Pecan	65	4-6	33-48	9-24
Egg yolk	33	10	12	4
Avocado	16	3	7	2

* Total is not expected to equal total fat.

† Polyunsaturated fatty acids: saturated fatty acids (excluding monounsaturated fatty acids).

‡ Polyunsaturated fatty acids plus monounsaturated fatty acids: saturated fatty acids.

From USDA Handbook 8-4: *Composition of fats and oils,* Washington, DC, 1979, U.S. Government Printing Office.

contributes 50% of the milk's kilocalories. Frankfurters are about 30% fat by weight, which accounts for 70% to 80% of their total kilocalories. In cheese, the fat content varies from 1 to 5 g per 4-oz serving of low-fat cheeses—such as cottage, ricotta, and part-skim mozzarella—to 8 g per 1-oz serving of cheddar, Swiss, and Colby, and up to 10 g per 1-oz serving of cream cheese, which is 33% fat (Figure 4-15).

Vegetable foods usually contain less fat than do animal foods. Whole grain cereals contain from 2% to 9% fat, mainly in the germ. The fat content of seeds varies, from 4% in corn to 17% in soybeans. Nuts contain much more fat, with peanuts being 50% fat and pecan nuts 68% fat. The only fruits with any appreciable fat content are avocados, with 16% fat, and ripe olives, with 30% fat.

The contribution of the various food groups to the total fat content of the American food supply is shown in Figure 4-16. The average daily fat consumption found in the U.S. Department of Agriculture (USDA) National

FIGURE 4-15

Fat content of cheeses (grams per ounce).

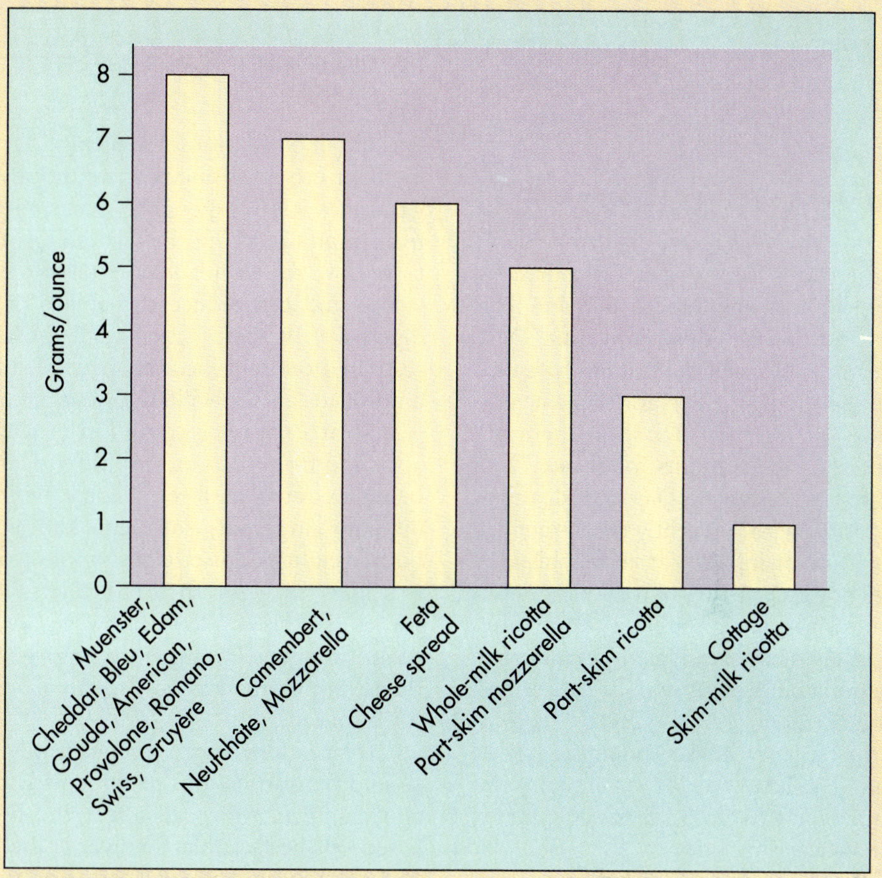

TABLE 4-8

Food sources of omega-3 fatty acids

FOOD	TOTAL LIPID AS OMEGA-3 (%)	
OILS		GRAMS/OZ*
Menhaden	23	6.9
Salmon	22	6.6
Cod liver	20	6.0
Canola	10	3.0
Soybean	7	2.1
Butter fat	2	0.6
Corn	1	0.3
FISH		GRAMS/4 OZ
Cod	42	0.3
Shrimp	38	0.5
Tuna	30	2.3
Pink salmon	29	1
King crab	20	0.6
Mackerel	17	1.8-2.6
Herring	6	1.0-2.0

* 1 oz = 2 tablespoons; 1 oz provides 246 kcal.

FIGURE 4-16

Contribution of various food groups to the fat content of the American diet.

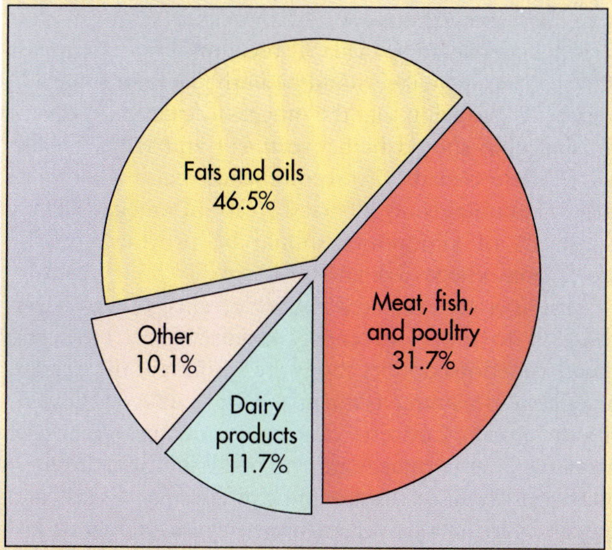

Food Consumption Survey, 1987 - 1988, was 69 to 114 g and in the NHANES III, 1988 - 1991, Health and Nutrition Examination Survey was 57 to 120 g in both cases, varying with age and gender groups.[1,1a] These figures are well below the 168 g available from the food supply, reflecting a relatively large waste of fat during food preparation.

DIETARY REQUIREMENTS

Apart from the need for a dietary source of omega-6 linoleic acid and omega-3 α-linolenic acid, humans do not require fat. A diet providing 1% to 2% of kilocalories from linoleic acid (about 3 to 6 g or 1 tsp) can meet the body's requirements for the omega-6 family of fatty acids. In fact, the average American's intake of omega-6 fatty acids accounts for about 7% of total kilocalories. The Committee on Diet and Health of the Food and Nutrition Board[15] recently recommended that the intake should be maintained at about this level and should certainly not exceed 10% of total kilocalories because of lack of information on the long-term consequences of higher levels of intake. Health and Welfare Canada[16] and the Food and Agricultural Organization/World Health Organization (FAO/WHO)[17] recommend that 3% of total energy intake should be in the form of linoleic acid. The FAO/WHO recommend this should rise to account for 4.5% to 5.7% of total energy intake during pregnancy and lactation.

There is considerable interest in determining how much of the omega-3 fatty acid α-linolenic acid should be consumed. Approximately 1 g/day has been found to be adequate for a 6-year-old girl. Also, the 5:1 ratio of omega-6 to omega-3 fatty acids in human milk is considered to be adequate, although the most appropriate ratio may change with age. The desirable range is certainly believed to be between the ratios of 4:1 and 10:1. The only official body to make a specific recommendation for consumption of the omega-3 fatty acids is Health and Welfare Canada. It recommends that at least 0.5% of energy intake should be in the form of omega-3 fatty acids, agreeing that the omega-6/omega-3 ratio of consumption should be between 4:1 and 10:1. Health and Welfare Canada also recommends that if the diet of an infant contains no 20- or 22-carbon omega-3 fatty-acids, 1% of kilocalories should be provided by the 18-carbon omega-3 α-linolenic acid.

Fat is a concentrated source of energy, which can allow us to meet our energy requirements. However, there are serious doubts about the wisdom of the current practice of obtaining as much as 35% to 40% of kilocalories from fat. Concern centers on the prevalence of excessive energy intake and the possibility that high-fat diets contribute to the risk of cardiovascular disease and cancer. Nutritionists suggest that obtaining 30% or less of total kilocalories from fat is a goal more compatible with good health to provide sufficient essential fatty acids and facilitate the absorption of fat-soluble vitamins.

MODIFICATIONS IN DIETARY FAT INTAKE

Specific modifications of dietary fat may be recommended in several medical conditions. In patients with gallstones who experience recurrent painful episodes from stones blocking the bile duct, surgery is performed to remove the gallbladder. After surgery, bile cannot be stored and can reduce the ability of some patients to digest fat. In these patients, fat intake may need to be restricted or emulsified fats may be substituted for nonemulsified fats to facilitate digestion and absorption.

Steatorrhea is a condition in which fats are poorly absorbed from the gut, resulting in large amounts of fat being excreted in feces. People with steatorrhea have difficulty ingesting sufficient kilocalories to maintain body weight because of the amount of high-energy fats that pass through their GI tracts without being absorbed. In this condition, however, medium- and short-chain fatty acids, which are absorbed more effectively than long-chain fatty acids, can be used as acceptable forms of fat.

It has long been recommended that fat intake should be restricted in patients with hepatitis, cirrhosis, and jaundice, which all affect the liver. This advice is based on the fact that the liver is the major site of fatty acid metabolism and triglyceride synthesis. Its wisdom is now being questioned because people with these conditions often experience malabsorption of fat and resulting steatorrhea, making them prone to deficiencies of the fat-soluble vitamins.

Hyperlipidemia is a term used to describe high blood lipid levels resulting from either high dietary intakes or a range of inherited defects in lipid metabolism. One of the more common inherited forms is **familial combined hyperlipidemia,** a genetically dominant trait that is associated with elevated levels of apolipoprotein B. Individuals with this condition do not always respond to dietary measures designed to lower blood lipid levels and are often treated with blood-lipid–lowering drugs.

TRENDS IN AVAILABILITY AND USE OF DIETARY FAT

Throughout this century, fat has contributed an increasing percentage of total kilocalories available in the U.S. food supply, rising from 32% of available kilocalories in 1909 to 42% in 1988. The current level of about 42% of available kilocalories being in the form of

TABLE 4-9

Average daily fat consumption, 1987-1988

	GRAMS	% KILOCALORIES
Men*	91	38
Women*	61	37
Children	56	35

* Mean intake reported for men and women aged 30 to 39 years.

From Nationwide Food Consumption Survey 1987-1988, U.S. Department of Agriculture, as summarized by Wright HS and others: *Nutr Today* 26(3):21, 1991.

fat contrasts with the recommendation that no more than 30% of kilocalories should come from fat. Fat is a dietary essential that is required in small amounts, and excessive intake is associated with various undesirable health consequences, as considered in more detail later in this chapter.

During this century there has also been a gradual increase in the use of fats from vegetable sources, particularly vegetable oils, largely because of a shift from butter, lard, and cream to vegetable-based margarines, cooking oils, and nondairy creamers. There has also been a slight decrease in the use of animal fats from meat, poultry, eggs, and milk products. Nevertheless, over half the fat available is still derived from animal sources.

In spite of the rise in fat available throughout the century as a whole, the amounts available and actually consumed have fallen a little over the past 10 years. This is largely a result of the shift away from whole milk toward low-fat and nonfat milk and the marketing of leaner and more closely trimmed cuts of meat. It is important to distinguish between fat *availability* and its actual *consumption*. Although about 6 oz (¾ cup) of oil is available per person per day in the U.S. food supply, the average person consumes only 2.5 oz (less than ⅓ cup). This is partly because much of the fats and oils used for frying (especially in the fast-food industry) is never actually consumed. It may also reflect the fact that many people trim most visible fat from foods before consumption, in an attempt to reduce their total fat intake.

In the 1977-1978 Nationwide Food Consumption Survey (NFCS) of more than 25,000 people, over half had diets in which fat contributed more than 40% of total kilocalories. The follow-up 1987-1988 survey (of 8337 people) revealed that the average figure for women had fallen from 42% to 37%, and for men it had fallen from 43% to 38%. In 1987 and 1988 the actual intake of fat averaged from 61 g/day for women and 91 g/day for men (Table 4-9). This compares with average intakes of 72 g for women and 112 g for men in 1977 and 1978. Analyses of national survey data collected in 1988 and 1991 (NHANES III) showed a similar trend with average intakes of total fat for men and women of 95 to 116

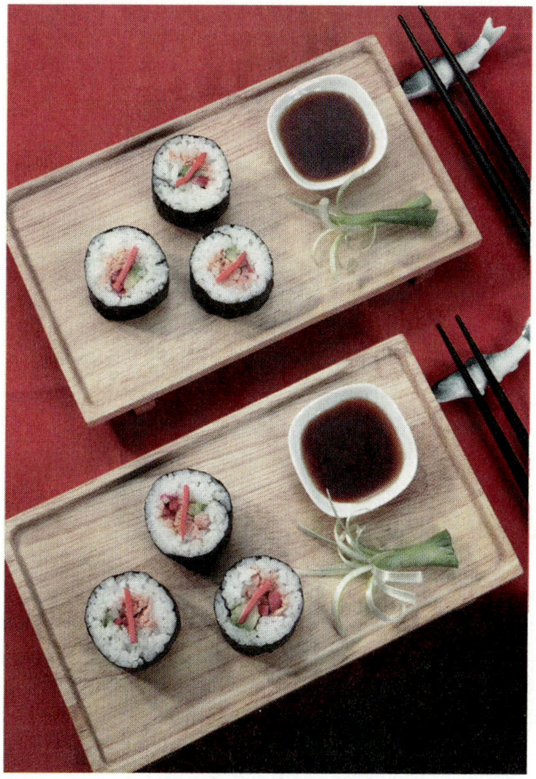

Traditional Japanese food is low in fat.

and 59 to 75 g, respectively. These values correspond to 34% kilocalories from fat. Because the amount of available fat had not declined by an equivalent amount, these figures indicate that the people surveyed (and so presumably the population as a whole) had made a conscious effort to reduce their intake of fat.

The kind and amount of fat in the diet are strongly influenced by social, cultural, geographical, and economic factors, in addition to nutritional concerns. In general, the amount of fat consumed in a country increases in proportion to its wealth, so the total fat intake in the developed world is considerably higher than in the developing world. Within the developed world the Japanese diet is traditionally low in fat, whereas the diet of Italians, who make considerable use of olive oil, is high in fat. In spite of concerns about the health consequences of excessive consumption of animal fat, many Americans still prefer it. They pay a high price for prime-quality meat with fat marbled throughout it, covet desserts with whipping cream, add butter to vegetables and fish, and consider ice cream, sour cream, and whole milk to be dietary staples.

Besides being inappropriate, anyone who has tried knows that it is difficult to eliminate for long all fat from the food we consume: a fat-free diet is unpalatable to most tastes, fails to satisfy our hunger, and may well be deficient in kilocalories. Advice to reduce fat intake was never meant to mean the drastic elimination of dietary fat. Amidst much popular concern about excessive fat consumption, some fat is required to provide us with essential fatty acids and also to act as a carrier of fat-soluble vitamins.

FAT AND DEGENERATIVE DISEASES

A large amount of experimental evidence from epidemiological, clinical, and animal studies suggests that dietary fat is involved in the course of several chronic degenerative diseases, including coronary heart disease, some cancers, and obesity. Based on this evidence, a number of nutrition and health professional organizations and federal agencies have recommended that fat should provide less than 30% of total kilocalories. They also recommend changes in the types of fats consumed, particularly a reduction in the intake of saturated fats. Before summarizing and assessing the evidence implicating dietary lipids as factors in the onset of degenerative diseases, it must be emphasized that the subject is a very active area of research. Nutritional recommendations aimed at preventing and treating these diseases are likely to be modified as we gain a deeper understanding of the complex interrelationships involved in their development and progression and their relationship to diet. Any future modification will simply continue a process of changing recommendations that has occurred in the past.

CORONARY HEART DISEASE

Coronary heart disease (CHD) is the leading cause of death in the United States and other affluent countries of the world. In most instances CHD results from obstruction of coronary blood vessels by **atherosclerosis** or **thrombosis.** Atherosclerosis is characterized by a thickening of artery walls, which causes the arteries to become narrower. These "lesions" (areas affected by disease or injury) eventually accumulate lipid (mostly cholesterol) and become calcified. They are also known as **atherosclerotic plaques.** Thrombosis is the formation of a blood clot caused by the aggregation of blood platelets. The formation of a circulating clot can result in the blockage of a blood vessel, especially at a site where severe narrowing has already occurred because of atherosclerosis. When these events occur in blood vessels leading to the heart, they cause a *heart attack.* If they occur in the vessels leading to the brain, they cause a *stroke.*

CHD is a *process,* not a single event. Its causes are not fully known, but there are distinct relationships between the onset of the disease and high levels of total blood cholesterol and LDL. The arterial wall is permeable to LDL, a situation that promotes atherosclerosis. Conversely, high levels of HDL are associated with a *decreased* risk of coronary heart disease by mechanisms that are not well understood.

TABLE 4-10

Blood cholesterol values as related to relative risk for development of coronary heart disease

	HIGH RISK	MODERATE RISK	LOW RISK
Total cholesterol*	≥240 mg/dl	200-239 mg/dl	<200 mg/dl
High-density lipoprotein cholesterol*	<40 mg/dl	40-49 mg/dl	≥50 mg/dl
Low-density lipoprotein cholesterol*	≥160 mg/dl	130-159 mg/dl	<130 mg/dl
Treatment	Begin a treatment program to reduce levels	Retest, give general diet information	No treatment; reevaluate in 5 years

Sometimes cholesterol and lipoprotein cholesterol are given in measures of mmol/L. To convert mg/dl to mmol/L, multiply mg/dl by 0.026. For example, Cholesterol of 200 mg/dl = 5.2 mmol/L.

In 1908 the first study that linked diet to atherosclerosis was conducted and showed that rabbits fed meat, milk, and eggs developed arterial lesions resembling atherosclerosis in humans. Shortly afterwards, in 1913, cholesterol was identified as the dietary component responsible for hypercholesterolemia and atherosclerosis in rabbits. Because rabbits are herbivorous animals, they do not normally eat cholesterol-containing foods derived from animals. However, it is possible to produce atherosclerotic lesions in a number of omnivorous experimental animals by feeding a diet high in fat and cholesterol. Hypercholesterolemia (high levels of blood cholesterol, currently defined as values greater than or equal to 240 mg/100 ml) is now firmly associated with increased risk for cardiovascular diseases. The relative level of risk associated with various values for blood lipids are presented in Table 4-10.

Increased risk of coronary heart disease is associated with high blood cholesterol and LDL-cholesterol levels. Decreased risk of coronary heart disease is associated with high blood HDL-cholesterol levels.

Early attempts to decrease blood cholesterol levels focused mainly on reducing dietary cholesterol intake from cholesterol-containing foods such as eggs, meat, and liver. Such attempts were not always successful, and it is now known that the liver can itself synthesize up to 2000 mg of cholesterol per day, considerably more than the 400 to 500 mg of cholesterol provided from a typical diet. Synthesis by the liver is stimulated when energy intake is high and reduced when energy intake is low. Despite the ability of the body to synthesize cholesterol for itself, the amount and type of fat in the diet do have an effect on blood cholesterol concentrations. This was shown by the classic studies of Keys and associates[18] and Hegsted and associates.[19] These early studies were mainly concerned with the effect of dietary fats on the total blood cholesterol level (that is, all cholesterol bound within all the different types of lipoproteins), not on the specific lipoproteins carrying cholesterol in plasma. Nonetheless, many of the conclusions remain valid today, especially that dietary saturated fatty acids increase the total blood cholesterol level and dietary polyunsaturated fatty acids decrease it.

In recent years many investigators have reevaluated the effects of dietary fat on total plasma lipoproteins. They have confirmed that saturated fatty acids in the diet raise the total blood cholesterol level. They also show that saturated fatty acids raise the level of LDL, one of the key lipoprotein carriers of cholesterol, and that both of these effects increase the risk of CHD. The mechanisms involved are not completely understood, but the effect of saturated fatty acids appears to involve the receptor on liver cell membranes responsible for binding to LDL before its entry into the cells. The activity of this **LDL receptor**—or in other words, its ability to mediate the entry of LDL—appears to be suppressed by saturated fatty acids. When LDL receptor activity decreases, LDL catabolism decreases and blood levels of LDL increase.

> In general, saturated fats in the diet raise blood cholesterol and LDL-cholesterol levels, but recent clinical studies show that the saturated fatty acid stearic acid actually *lowers* both total blood cholesterol and LDL-cholesterol levels.

Individual saturated fatty acids differ in their ability to change blood LDL-cholesterol levels. Palmitic (16:0), myristic (14:0), and to a lesser degree lauric (12:0) acids increase the LDL-cholesterol level. In contrast, stearic acid (18:0) and medium- to short-chain saturated fatty acids do not. In fact, results of recent clinical studies show that stearic acid actually *lowers* both total blood cholesterol and LDL-cholesterol levels,[20] introducing further complication into what is not a simple story. Variability in responsiveness to dietary saturated fatty acids has been observed in both human and animal studies. The current average intake of saturated fatty acids accounts for approximately 13% to 14% of total energy supplies, which is above the current recommended level of less than 10%.

Monounsaturated fatty acids have either no effect on blood cholesterol levels or a cholesterol-lowering effect. Recent evidence suggests that diets rich in monounsaturated fatty acids can lower total and LDL-cholesterol levels when substituted for saturated fatty acids in the diet. For example, an *inverse* relationship between olive oil (high in oleic acid, 18:1ω9) consumption and blood cholesterol levels has been observed. So consumption of monounsaturated fatty acids may play a preventive role in the battle against CHD. It has also been suggested that monounsaturated fatty acids are a better replacement for saturated fatty acids than polyunsaturated fatty acids because they are less susceptible to oxidation. Oxidized LDL is taken up by macrophages (phagocytic cells of the immune system) and deposited in atherosclerotic plaques. Inhibition of LDL oxidation slows the development of atherosclerosis. The typical American diet contains 14% to 16% of energy as monounsaturated fatty acids, which is more than the current recommended level of 10% or more.

> To minimize risk of coronary heart disease:
> Restrict fat intake to less than 30% of total kilocalories.
> Reduce intake of saturated fats.
> Consume oily fish regularly.
> Make only moderate use of fats high in *trans* fatty acids.

A considerable body of evidence indicates that replacing saturated fatty acids in the diet with polyunsaturated fatty acids, particularly the omega-6 fatty acid linoleic acid (18:2ω6), lowers both total cholesterol and LDL-cholesterol levels. However, very high levels of linoleic acid also lower HDL-cholesterol levels. Evidence linking low levels of HDL cholesterol to CHD is so strong that HDL-cholesterol testing is often endorsed for detection of CHD susceptibility. The HDL-lowering effect of linoleic acid raises concern about its overconsumption. There are also other health-related concerns associated with high levels of polyunsaturated fatty acids, such as cholesterol gallstone formation, promotion of tumor development, and suppression of immunity. Because the long-term health consequences of high polyunsaturated fatty acid consumption are unknown, it is recommended that intake of linoleic acid remain at the current level (7% of energy) and not exceed 10% of energy intake.

In recent years a unique role of the omega-3 polyunsaturated fatty acids in the prevention and treatment of CHD has become evident. α-Linolenic acid (18:3ω3) is the principal polyunsaturated fatty acid in the green tissue of plants, and it also occurs in phytoplankton. In man, animals, and fish, α-linolenic acid is converted to a series of longer-chain polyunsaturated fatty acids, including EPA (20:5ω3) and DHA (22:6ω3). The only concentrated edible sources of these long-chained polyunsaturated derivatives of α-linolenic are oily fish (for example, mackerel and salmon) and the oils derived from them. Early investigations indicated that fish oil lowered LDL-cholesterol and total serum cholesterol levels but not the HDL-cholesterol level. However, it now appears that the total level of cholesterol is reduced only if initial levels are high, and they are lowered because of the lowering of LDL levels alone. Also, fish oils actually increase HDL levels while causing plasma triglyceride levels to decline. The decrease in plasma triglycerides with dietary fish oil intake is apparently caused by a decrease in the capacity of the liver to synthesize triglycerides from diglycerides. Thus the omega-3 polyunsaturated fatty acids have an antiatherogenic effect but do so by mechanisms different from those of the omega-6 polyunsaturated fatty acids.

The omega-3 fatty acids also inhibit thrombosis (they are "antithrombogenic"). Diets high in fish or fish oils containing omega-3 fatty acids reduce platelet aggregation, moderately increase bleeding time, and decrease platelet–vessel wall interactions, all of which reduce the tendency to form clots.

Several investigators suggest that typical American diets contain inadequate amounts of omega-3 fatty acids. Consumption of fish containing omega-3 fatty acids can be used to increase intake, but the use of fish oil supplements is not recommended. The effect of the long-term use of supplemental omega-3 fatty acids is uncertain, and, in view of their potent biological effects, excess consumption is inadvisable, even though no specific problems have yet been identified. The omega-3 fatty acids are potent modulators of the inflammatory and immune responses, and their use may prove to be beneficial in combination with many drug therapies.

There is considerable controversy among investigators about the content and biological effects of *trans* fatty acids in the diet. Estimates of available *trans* fatty acids in the U.S. food supply range from as high as 15.2 g per person per day to as low as 8.1 g per person per day.[2,3] One clinical study compared the effects on cholesterol levels of three diets, one with oleic acid, another with the oleic acid replaced by its *trans*-bonded version, elaidic acid, and the third with the oleic acid replaced by a saturated fatty acid.[21] The saturated fatty acid had its expected cholesterol-raising effect, but the diet containing the *trans* fatty acid also had a cholesterol-raising effect, half as potent as the saturated fatty acid diet. Also, the diet high in *trans* fatty acids increased the LDL-cholesterol level as much as did the diet high in saturated fats and lowered the HDL-cholesterol level appreciably. The results of this study suggest that *trans* fatty acids may have as undesirable an effect on plasma lipoprotein profiles as do saturated fatty acids. Even though the levels of *trans* fatty acid employed in this study were high (three to four times the estimated average intake), the results do suggest that fats high in *trans* fatty acids should not be consumed in excessive amounts. The major sources of such fats are margarines and shortenings prepared by hydrogenation of vegetable oils. Findings from a recent epidemiological study of over 85,000 women also support a positive relationship between *trans* fatty acid intake and the risk of CHD.[22] However, numerous other studies have indicated no adverse health effects of the ingestion of trans fatty acids when the diet provides sufficient essential fatty acids.[23]

The National Cholesterol Education Program Guidelines for the detection, evaluation, and treatment of high blood cholesterol levels are presented in the box above. The American Heart Association Dietary Guidelines aimed at reducing blood cholesterol levels are

National Cholesterol Education Program for Adults

GOAL: Total blood cholesterol level of <200 mg/dl, high-density lipoprotein (HDL)–cholesterol level of > 55 mg/dl, and low-density lipoprotein (LDL)–cholesterol level of <160 mg/dl or <130mg/dl with two or more risk factors

Test LDL-cholesterol level if total blood cholesterol level is >200 mg/dl and individual has two or more of the following risk factors:

- Family history of coronary heart disease
- Smokes cigarettes
- Diabetes
- Obesity
- Hypertension
- Low HDL–cholesterol level
- Male

If LDL-cholesterol level is >130 mg/dl, reduce saturated fat intake to 8% to 10% of total kilocalories, reduce total fat intake to <30% of total kilocalories, and reduce cholesterol intake to <300 mg/day.

If unsuccessful (that is, LDL-cholesterol level is >130 mg/dl), reduce saturated fat intake to <7% of total kilocalories and reduce cholesterol intake to <200 mg/day.

Use drug therapy only on physician's advice.

From U.S. National Cholesterol Education Program: *JAMA* 269:3015, 1993.

American Heart Association Dietary Guidelines for Healthy American Adults

Total fat	<30% calories
Saturated fat	<10% calories
Polyunsaturated fat	≤10% calories
Carbohydrate	≥50% calories
Protein	Remainder of calories
Cholesterol	≤300 mg/day
Sodium	<3 g/day
Ethanol	≤1-2 oz/day
Total calories	Sufficient to maintain recommended body weight

Eat a wide variety of foods

From American Heart Association: *Circulation* 77:721A, 1988.

presented in the box above. To achieve these recommended levels of dietary fat intake, a number of dietary modifications are required. Choice of foods within categories becomes important to reduce total fat intake. Most fat in the Western diet comes from meats, dairy products, snacks, and desserts, so by choosing low-fat alternatives in each of these categories of foods, total fat intake can be reduced. There is controversy surrounding the use of shellfish (for example, shrimp, lobster, and crab) in a blood cholesterol–lowering diet. Shellfish are relatively rich sources of cholesterol, but they are low in fat and kilocalories, so their use in moderation is possible. The method of food preparation can also significantly contribute to dietary fat intake. Recommended methods of cooking include steaming, baking, broiling, grilling, or stir-frying in small amounts of oil low in saturated fat. Deep-fat frying and pan-frying methods should be avoided. Such foods as vegetable salads composed of lettuce, carrots, tomatoes, and cucumbers are low in fat but can become high in total and saturated fat when toppings such as bacon bits, crumbled hard-cooked eggs, cheese, and mayonnaise-based dressings are added. A baked potato is low in fat, but when topped with butter, sour cream, or cheese sauce, the fat content is increased dramatically.

It should be emphasized that some nutrition and health professionals do not wholeheartedly support programs that are aimed at aggressively treating hypercholesterolemia by dietary means.[24] One reason for their lack of support is that only a relatively small reduction in blood lipid levels can be expected to result from dietary measures. The precise value of any reduction varies but is about 10% in many cases, often lower than 10%, and rarely as much as 20%. Another reason is that recent intervention trials demonstrating reduced CHD risk with decreases in blood lipid levels fail to show any differences in overall mortality between control and intervention groups. Also, aggressive intervention programs unnecessarily increase the number of individuals prescribed cholesterol-lowering drugs when dietary measures fail. All of these drugs interfere with cholesterol metabolism in some way. For example, **cholestyramine** binds to cholesterol-containing bile acids and prevents their reabsorption, **clofibrate** decreases VLDL secretion from the liver, and **lovastatin** inhibits 3-hydroxy-3-methylglutaryl CoA reductase, a key enzyme in the biosynthesis of cholesterol. These drugs are expensive and not without side effects. Clofibrate usage has been linked to increased incidences of gastrointestinal cancer and gallbladder disease. A possible side effect of lovostatin is formation of cataracts.

There is also some evidence that reducing blood cholesterol levels may bring risks, as well as benefits. Low plasma cholesterol, or a reduction in plasma cholesterol levels, has recently been linked to increased risk for cancer and elevated rates of depression, suicide, and violent deaths. These linkages may be coincidental, but they underscore the need for further investigations of the relationships among dietary lipids, blood lipoprotein patterns, and mortality from CHD, cancer, and all other causes.

OTHER CHRONIC DEGENERATIVE DISEASES

Controversy surrounds the role of dietary fat in **hypertension** (high blood pressure). The available evidence indicates that a reduction in total fat intake does not lower blood pressure in people with normal or slightly raised blood pressure. However, increasing intake of omega-6 polyunsaturated fatty acids and decreasing total fat intake do appear to cause a reduction of blood pressure in people with true high blood pressure. Reductions in blood pressure and blood viscosity are also associated with increased intakes of omega-3 fatty acids from fish oils. Alterations in eicosanoid production and enhanced excretion of sodium from the kidneys have been implicated as possible mechanisms for this effect.

Fat intake has long been implicated as a factor related positively with the incidence of and mortality caused by **cancers** of the breast, colon, and prostate. Cancer is the second leading cause of death the United States. Studies with experimental animals consistently show that high-fat diets increase the rate of development of cancer at several sites, when compared with low-fat diets. Polyunsaturated fatty acids promote the development of mammary gland tumors more than do saturated fats in experimental animals. Epidemiological studies in humans, however, have yielded more variable results. Studies on the relationship between fat intake and breast cancer range from positive association to no association or negative association, covering all possibilities and so leaving the situation unclear. There is more consistent evidence linking dietary fat to colorectal cancer in humans. There is also cumulative evidence of a relationship between dietary fat intake and prostate cancer in humans. Considerable uncertainty remains to be resolved, however, concerning the links between dietary fat intake and cancer. Many investigators in the field of nutrition and cancer maintain that the data from experimental animals are so strong that the inconclusive evidence from human dietary studies may only reflect multiple sources of error in estimating cancer incidence, mortality, food consumption, and constituent fatty acid intakes. In animal models the effect of dietary fat in carcinogenesis depends on the type of fat and its constituent fatty acids. Although the mechanisms have not been elucidated, high-fat diets enhance carcinogenesis by generating active metabolites that act as promoters, rather than initiators, of tumor development. Omega-3 fatty acid intake, on the other hand, appears to have a tumor inhibitory effect.

It has been suggested that high-fat diets promote obesity by encouraging overeating because satiety is reached at a higher energy intake on high-fat diets than on low-fat, fiber-rich diets. The specific type of dietary fat ingested has also been implicated as a factor in causing human obesity. There is evidence that polyunsaturated fatty acids are oxidized more readily than are saturated fatty acids, indicating that diets high in saturated fatty acids promote fat storage, leading to accumulation of body fat. Not only do high-fat diets have higher energy density than do low-fat diets, they may promote fat storage because deposition of dietary fat in body tissues requires less energy than deposition of fat derived from dietary carbohydrate or protein. Energy is expended to convert dietary protein and carbohydrates to fat. Also, recent evidence suggests that the conversion of dietary carbohydrate to fat may be negligible under certain circumstances.

> *T*he simplest summary of dietary advice about the lipids is to choose a diet low in total fat, saturated fat, and cholesterol.

FAT SUBSTITUTES

Because most people like fat-containing foods but many wish to avoid the kilocalories provided by fat, the food industry has put considerable effort into developing fat substitutes (or "fake fats"), which supply less energy than do real fats. The aim of these efforts is to retain all the normal characteristics of fats such as texture, spreadability, satiety value, and effects on food palatability and avoid the kilocalorie content that usually accompanies them.

The first fat substitutes were made in the 1970s and consisted of starch-based carbohydrate molecules mixed with water to form a bulky fatlike gel. In this form the carbohydrate had a similar feel to fat in the mouth.

In 1991 a starch-based fat substitute called **Stellar** was introduced, which provided only 1 kcal/g, in contrast to the 9 kcal/g supplied by fat. Stellar is made by treating cornstarch with acid, to generate a fine powder that is mixed with water under high pressure. This yields a white and creamy final product, with a smooth, fatlike texture.

The process of mixing carbohydrates with water under high pressure is known as **shearing.** It has also been used to manufacture a pectin-based fat substitute marketed as **Slendid.** Pectin is a carbohydrate obtained from fruits and vegetables, which, when sheared with water and some calcium chloride, yields a very low-kilocalorie, fatlike gel.

Scientists at the USDA have made a similar carbohydrate and water-based gel that they call **Oatrim** because the carbohydrate used is a mixture of oat starch and fiber.

All of these fat substitutes can be used in a wide variety of cold and cooked foods.

A slightly different carbohydrate-based approach is behind a fat substitute known chemically as **sucrose polyester.** This is made by combining the disaccharide sucrose with fatty acids via ester linkages, to produce giant polyester molecules. The commercial name of this product is **Olestra,** and it contains no available kilocalories because the ester linkages hold the sucrose and fatty acid molecules together in a way that cannot be broken down by digestive enzymes. So Olestra behaves in the mouth much like fat but then travels undigested through the GI tract without any of the energy locked up in its structure being made available to the body. One potential drawback is that Olestra reduces the absorption of vitamin E; so vitamin E has been added to Olestra to compensate for this. Olestra also reduces the absorption of cholesterol.

A chemically different approach has been to create protein-based substances with the desired properties of fats. Only one such fat substitute, called **Simplesse,** is available at present. It was introduced in 1990 in a fat-free ice cream.

Food manufacturers are also developing real, although unnatural, fats that contain longer-chain fatty acids than those found in normal food. These products are only partially digestible, and so they provide fewer kilocalories than regular fat while being similar to regular fat in other respects. For example, one such product, called **Caprenin,** contains 5 kcal/g instead of the 9 kcal/g of regular fat. It is currently used in candy bars. Another is SALATRIM, which is a family of structured triacylglycerides produced by the interesterification of short-chain fatty acids (acetic, proprionic, or butyric) and long-chain saturated fatty acids (predominantly stearic).

TABLE 4-11

Information on some fat substitutes currently in use or under review for use in foods in the United States

PRODUCT	COMPOSITION	CHARACTERISTICS	CURRENT USE IN THE UNITED STATES	POTENTIAL USES	FDA STATUS
Simplesse	Whey or egg whites and milk protein	Digestible; 1 to 2 kcal/g; tends to break down at high temperatures	Simple Pleasures frozen dessert	Mayonnaise, salad dressings, yogurt, dips, sour cream, butter, margarine, cheese	FDA affirmed its GRAS standing in 1990
Olestra	Sucrose polyester (sucrose and fatty acids derived therefrom)	Indigestible; 0 kcal/g; withstands high temperatures and can be used for frying	None	Hot and cold foods, deep-fried snack foods, such as potato chips and French fries	Waiting since 1987 for FDA approval as a new food additive
Caprenin	Natural fatty acids	Partially digestible; 5 kcal/g; similar to cocoa butter	Milky Way II candy bar	Candy and confectionery coatings	Manufacturer's request for GRAS standing under review in 1992
Stellar	Water, mixed with a modified food starch made from corn	Digestible; 1 kcal/g; stable in baking but not in deep frying	Commercially prepared salad dressings, Danish pastry, hot dogs, sausages	Puddings, gravies, soups, margarine, dairy products	Meets GRAS standards; no limitations set for its use
Slendid	Pectin—a type of carbohydrate derived from citrus fruit peel—mixed with water and a gelling agent	Digestible; 0 kcal/g; stable for baking but not for deep frying	Cookies, cheese products	Salad dressings, meat products, soups, margarine, sauces, pudding	Meets GRAS standards; no limitations set for its use
Oatrim	Oat bran and flour treated with enzymes	Digestible; 1 kcal/g; stable for baking but not for deep frying	Healthy Choice ground beef product	Frozen desserts, margarine, mayonnaise, cheese, peanut butter, baked goods	Meets GRAS standards; no limitations set for its use

FDA, Food and Drug Administration; *GRAS,* generally regarded as safe.

ISSUES AND OPINIONS

Cardiovascular Disease Kills Women Too

Dr. Penny M. Kris-Etherton
Professor of Nutrition
The Pennsylvania State University

The dangers of cardiovascular disease to men are well publicized, but the threat it poses for women receives less media attention. Despite this relative neglect, cardiovascular disease is the leading cause of death among women in the United States. It causes about 50% of deaths among American women, compared with about 25% caused by cancer. It is also surprising that heart disease kills more American women than American men each year, in a ratio of about 52%:48%. So cardiovascular disease is a considerable danger to women, as well as men.

One reason for the greater prominence given to the risk of cardiovascular disease in men is that men tend to have heart attacks at a younger age than women. Between the ages of 45 and 65, about four times as many men have heart attacks as women. On average, cardiovascular disease tends to arise in women about 11 years later than in men. Beyond the age of 65 the incidence in women steadily rises toward that in men. Although cardiovascular disease occurs later in women than in men on average, many younger women do fall victim to it. One in nine women aged 45 to 64 years has some type of cardiovascular disease.

Another reason for the greater attention given to cardiovascular problems in men is that men are more likely than women to experience acute and dramatic heart attacks. Women are more likely to fall victim to chronic cardiovascular disease, which may worsen gradually until it eventually causes death. The slow worsening of chronic cardiovascular disease can cause years of painful complications and increasing immobility, which ends in a slower and more distressing death than a sudden fatal heart attack. It is obviously important, therefore, to encourage women to take preventive action in their younger years to improve the quality of life in their twilight years.

The major modifiable risk factors for cardiovascular disease are generally the same for women as for men: high blood cholesterol and LDL-cholesterol levels, high blood pressure, and smoking. The major preventive measures involve appropriate nutrition, regular exercise, and giving up smoking. At present, only about 20% of American women are estimated to be consuming diets that offer effective protection against cardiovascular disease. It is clearly important that dietary education programs aimed at preventing cardiovascular disease should be targeted at women, as well as at men.

SALATRIM also delivers approximately 5 kcal/g because short-chain fatty acids provide fewer kilocalories per unit weight than long-chain fatty acids and because stearic acid is poorly absorbed.

As you might expect, these new products are required to undergo extensive tests to establish their safety before they can be used in food. The latest status of these products with the Food and Drug Administration (FDA)—in addition to a summary of their composition, characteristics, and current uses—can be found in Table 4-11.

~ BY NOW YOU SHOULD KNOW ~

- Lipid, or fat, is largely composed of triglycerides but also includes a wide variety of other water-insoluble compounds found in food and in the body.
- Although the term *fat* is used in chemistry to mean triglycerides that are solid at room temperature, and *oil* is used to mean triglycerides that are liquid at room temperature, in nutrition and other health sciences, *fat* is routinely used to mean all lipids.
- Triglycerides are composed of fatty acids bonded by ester linkages to glycerol.
- Fatty acids vary in their chain lengths, number of carbon-carbon double bonds (degree of unsaturation), and the position and configuration (*cis* or *trans*) of any double bonds.
- Saturated fatty acids contain no double bonds, monounsaturated fatty acids contain one double bond, and polyunsaturated fatty acids contain several double bonds.
- Lipids are essential components of the body, and some lipid is required in the diet to provide supplies of the essential fatty acids and also to carry several fat-soluble vitamins.
- Linoleic acid (18:2ω6) and α-linolenic acid (18:3ω3) are the essential fatty acids that must be provided in the diet.
- Almost all animal foods contain lipid, but among plant foods, only nuts, seeds, and avocados are rich sources of lipid.
- Lecithin, a phospholipid, and cholesterol, a sterol, are important examples of nontriglyceride lipids. Both are manufactured by the body, and neither is considered a dietary essential.
- Lipids must be emulsified before their digestive breakdown, and bile released by the gallbladder is an important emulsifying agent.
- Triglyceride lipids are digested by the action of lipase enzymes.
- Because lipids are insoluble in water, absorbed lipids are transported through the circulatory system within lipoprotein particles.
- Fat in the body serves as a source of energy; forms the basic structure of all cell membranes; acts as a precursor of various required body chemicals, including the eicosanoids; and acts as an insulator against heat loss and a protector surrounding the body's organs.
- When oxidized as a source of energy, lipids provide 9 kcal of energy per gram; therefore each pound of stored lipid represents 3500 kcal of stored energy.
- Excessive fat in the diet has been implicated as a cause of several chronic degenerative diseases, particularly coronary heart disease, cancer, hypertension, and obesity. Specific constituent fatty acids are also involved in the initiation and progression of several of these diseases.
- Many vegetable fats such as corn, cottonseed, and soybean oil are liquid at room temperature and are made into solid or semisolid fats by the processes of hydrogenation and interesterification.

STUDY QUESTIONS

1. How have the total consumption and sources of fat in the U.S. diet changed since 1909?
2. What is the relationship between fat consumption and health problems, such as heart disease and cancer?
3. Give examples of food sources of saturated, monounsaturated, and polyunsaturated fatty acids.
4. What food products are produced by the hydrogenation of vegetable oils?
5. What is the significance of the $\omega 3/\omega 6$ ratio?
6. Why are fats a more concentrated source of energy than carbohydrates?
7. Which fatty acids are essential in the diet, and why are they essential?
8. List some important roles of cholesterol in the body.
9. What foods should be avoided in a low-cholesterol diet?
10. Will lowering dietary cholesterol prevent heart disease?
11. What specific dietary recommendations would you make for someone at high risk of developing heart disease?
12. What are some of the important functions of prostaglandins and other eicosanoids?

CRITICAL ANALYSIS

1. How can you reduce the fat in your diet?

There are a number of ways to do this. One way is to reduce the servings of added fat. Examples of added fat are butter or margarine used on bread, potatoes, or pasta; oil used in cooking or salad dressing; and butter, margarine, shortening, or oil used in baking. Many times people find that although they are used to using two pats of butter or margarine on bread, they can use only one pat without sensing a reduction in taste or feeling deprived.

Another strategy is to reduce the fat used in cooking. You have more control over this at home, but most restaurants will honor a request to prepare a meal with reduced fat if they have not already developed new recipes. (You can also choose not to eat at restaurants that continue to serve foods high in fat.) When cooking at home, the amount of fat or oil (fats are solid at room temperature, oils are liquid) used in a recipe can often be reduced with little perceptable effect on the product. A muffin recipe that calls for 3 or 4 Tbsp of oil for 12 muffins can frequently be made with 1½ to 2 Tbsp of oil. Two egg whites can often be substituted for one whole egg (the yolk contains approximately 6 g of fat, whereas the white contains nearly zero). Applesauce, non-fat or low fat yogurt, or purees of prunes, figs, and other fruits have all been used as a substitute for oil or fat in baked goods. Each of these strategies works better with some recipes than with others. However, much of the developmental work has been done and published (and continues to be published) in magazines, newspapers (the food section), and newer cook books.

~ REFERENCES ~

1. Wright HS and others: The 1987-1988 Nationwide Food Consumption Survey: an update on the nutrient intake of respondents, *Nutr Today* 26:21, 1991.

1a. Health and Nutrition Examination Survey: *Energy and macronutrient intakes of persons aged 2 months and older in the United States: 1988-91: advanced data,* No 255, Hyattsville, Md, 1994, Vital and Health Statistics.

2. Hunter JE, Applewhite TH: Isometric fatty acids in the U.S. diet: levels and health perspectives, *Am J Clin Nutr* 44:707, 1986.

3. Enig MG and others: Isomeric trans fatty acids in the U.S. diet, *J Am Coll Nutr* 9:471, 1990.

4. Rozenaal A: Interesterification of oils and fats, *Inform* 3:1232, 1992.

5. Emken EA: Do *trans* acids have adverse health consequences? In Nelson GJ, editor: *Health effects of dietary fatty acids,* Champaign, Ill, 1990, Americal Oil Chemists' Society.

5a. Norum KR: Dietary fat and blood lipids, *Nutr Rev* 50:30, 1992.

6. Sardesai V: Nutritional role of polyunsaturated fatty acids, *J Nutr Biochem* 3:154, 1992.

7. Crawford MA: The role of essential fatty acids in neural development: implication for perinatal nutrition, *Am J Clin Nutr* 57(suppl):S703, 1993.

8. Hansen AE and others: Role of linoleic acid in infant nutrition: clinical and chemical study of 428 infants fed on milk mixtures varying in kind and amount of fat, *Pediatrics* 31:171, 1963.

9. Holman RT, Johnson SB, Hatch TF: A case of human linoleic acid deficiency involving neurological abnormalities, *Am J Clin Nutr* 35:617, 1982.

10. Bjerve KS, Lovold Mostard I, Thorensen I: Alpha-linolenic acid deficiency in patients on long term gastric tube feeding: estimation of linolenic acid and long chain unsaturated n-3 fatty acid requirement in men, *Am J Clin Nutr* 45:66, 1987.

11. Connor WE, Neuringer M, Reisbick S: Essential fatty acids: the importance of n-3 fatty acids in the retina and brain, *Nutr Rev* 50:21, 1992.

12. Neuringer M, Connor WE: N-3 fatty acids in the brain and retina: evidence of their essentiality, *Nutr Rev* 44:285, 1986.

13. Sjöström L: The contribution of fat cells to the determination of body weight, *Psychiatr Clin North Am* 1:493, 1978.

14. Dietary fat and cholesterol, *Prepared Foods,* July 1992.

15. National Research Council: *Diet and health,* Washington, DC, 1989, National Academy Press.

16. Health and Welfare Canada: *Nutrition recommendations,* Ottowa, Canada, 1990, Canadian Government Publishing Center.

17. Food and Agricultural Organization/World Health Organization: *Dietary fats and oils in human nutrition: report of an expert consultation,* Rome, 1977, Food and Agricultural Organization.

18. Keys A, Anderson JT, Grande F: Prediction of serum-cholesterol response of man to changes in fat in the diet, *Lancet* 2:259, 1957.

19. Hegsted DM and others: Quantitative effects of dietary fat on serum cholesterol in man, *Am J Clin Nutr* 17:281, 1965.

20. Kris-Etherton PM, Mustad V, Derr J: Effects of dietary stearic acid on plasma lipids and thrombosis, *Nutr Today* 28:30, 1993.

21. Mensink RP, Katon MB: Effect of dietary *trans* fatty acids on high-density and low-density lipoprotein cholesterol levels in healthy subjects, *N Engl J Med* 323:439, 1990.

22. Willet W and others: Intake of *trans* fatty acids and risk of coronary heart disease among women, *Lancet* 341:581, 1993.

23. Gottenbos JJ: Biological effects of trans fatty acids. In Perkins EG, Visek WJ, editors: *Dietary fats and health,* Champaign, Ill, 1983, American Oil Chemists' Society.

24. Harper AE: Nutrition standards for today—another view, *Nutr Today* 28:29, 1993.

25. Smith RE, Finley JW, Leveille GA: Overview of SALATRIM, a family of low-calorie fats, *J Agri Food Chem* 42:432, 1994.

ADDITIONAL READINGS

Beare-Rogers J, editor: *Dietary fat requirements in health and development,* Champaign, Ill, 1988, American Oil Chemists' Society.

Birch LL and others: Effects of a nonenergy fat substitute on children's energy and macronutrient intake, *Am J Clin Nutr* 58:326, 1993.

Dattilo AM, Kris-Etherton PM: Effects of weight reduction on blood lipids and lipoproteins: a meta-analysis, *Am J Clin Nutr* 56:320, 1992.

Fraser GE: Diet and coronary heart disease: beyond dietary fats and low-density–lipoprotein cholesterol, *Am J Clin Nutr* 59(suppl): 1117S, 1994.

Glore S and others: Soluble fiber and serum lipids: a literature review, *J Am Diet Assoc* 94:425, 1994.

Haskell WL and others: Role of water-soluble dietary fibers in the management of elevated plasma cholesterol in healthy subjects, *Am J Cardiol* 69:433, 1992.

Havel R: Triglyceride-rich lipoproteins and atherosclerosis—new perspectives, *Am J Clin Nutr* 59:795, 1994.

Hunninghake DB and others: The efficacy of intense dietary therapy alone or combined with lovastatin in outpatients with hypercholesterolemia, *N Engl J Med* 328:1213, 1993.

Johnson CL and others: Delining serum total cholesterol levels among U.S. adults: the National Health and Nutrition Examination Survey, *J Am Med Assoc* 269:3002, 1993.

Kromhout D: Dietary fats: long-term implications for health, *Nutr Rev* 50:49, 1992.

Lands WEM: Biosynthesis of prostaglandins, *Annu Rev Nutr* 11:41, 1991.

Liebel RL: Fat as fuel and metabolic signal, *Nutr Rev* 50:12, 1992.

Nelson GL, editor: *Health effects of dietary fatty acids,* Champaign, Ill, 1991, American Oil Chemists' Society.

Nestel PJ: Effects of ω-3 fatty acids on lipid metabolism, *Annu Rev Nutr* 10:149, 1990.

Perkins EG, Visek WJ, editors: *Dietary fats and health,* Champaign, Ill, 1983, American Oil Chemists' Society.

Sardesai VM: Nutritional role of polyunsaturated fatty acids, *J Nutr Biochem* 3:154, 1992.

Simopoulos AP and others: The 1st Congress of the International Society for the Study of Fatty Acids and Lipids (ISSFAL): Fatty Acids and Lipids from Cell Biology to Human Disease, *J Lipid Res* 35:169, 1994.

Smith-Schneider LM, Sigman-Grant MJ, Kris-Etherton PM: Dietary fat reduction strategies, *J Am Diet Assoc* 92:34, 1992.

Spady DK, Wollett LA, Dietschy JM: Regulation of plasma LDL-cholesterol levels by dietary cholesterol and fatty acids, *Annu Rev Nutr* 13:355, 1993.

Ulbricht TLV, Southgate DAT: Coronary heart disease: seven dietary factors, *Lancet* 338:985, 1991.

Vergroesen AJ, Crawford MA, editors: *The role of fats in human nutrition,* London, England, 1989, Academic Press.

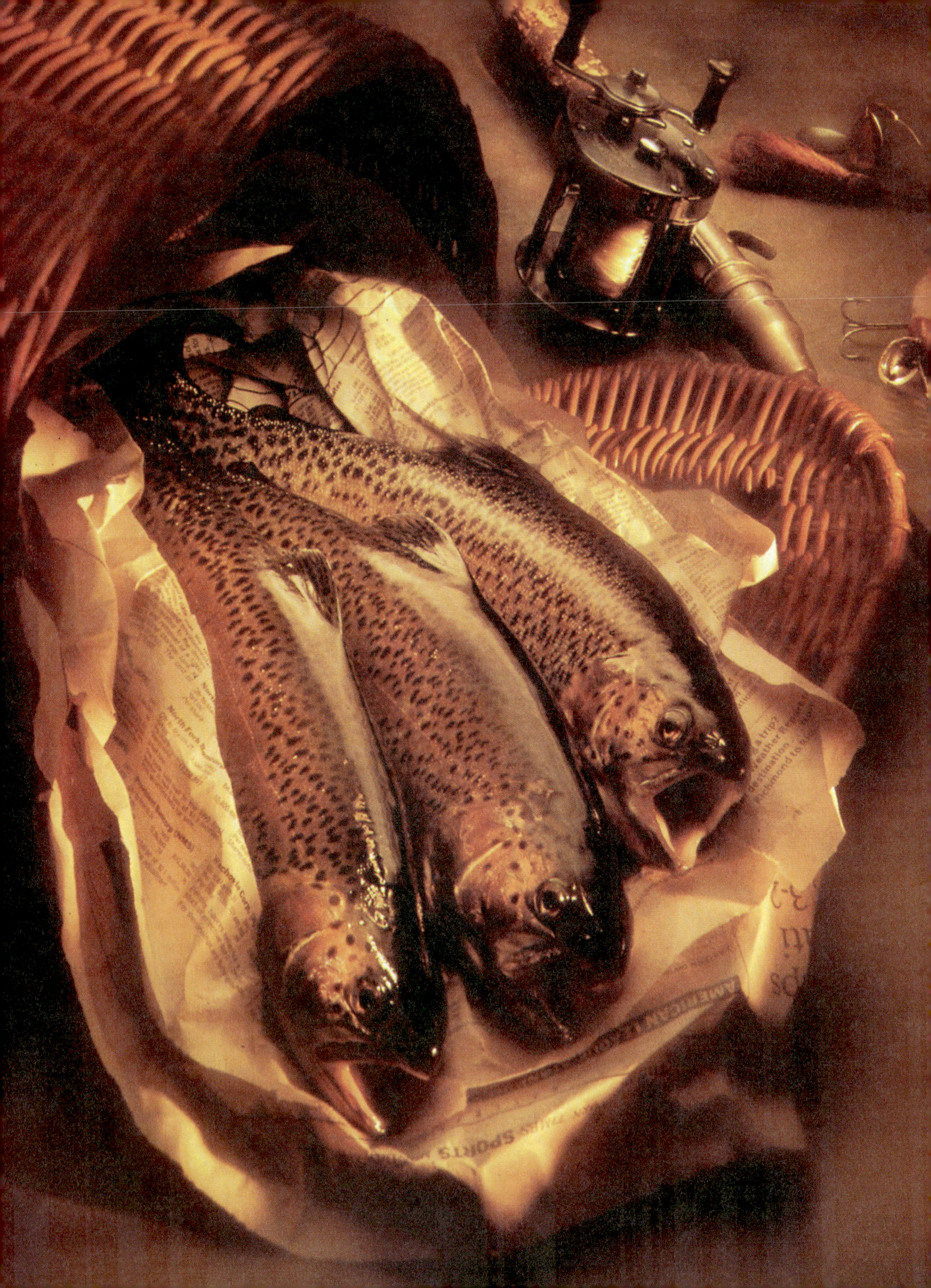

CHAPTER 5

PROTEIN

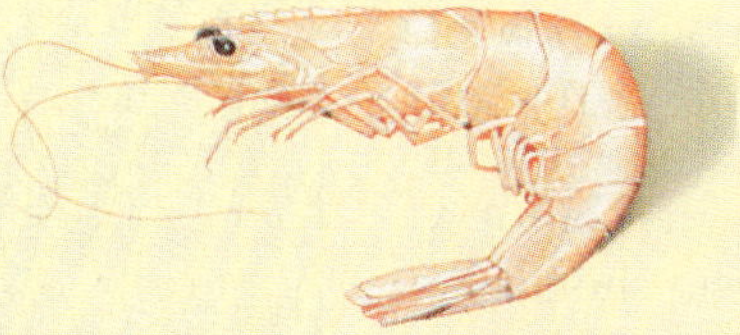

Food contains many different proteins, known collectively as ***protein.*** Protein has been recognized as a dietary essential for well over a century. Proteins perform many different functions in the body. Their main function is to serve as the following: structural components of body tissues (especially in muscles, cartilage, and bone), enzymes, hormones, components of the immune system, transporters of other substances, membrane-bound carriers, and regulators of many biochemical processes. Protein is a source of the amino acids and nitrogen needed for the synthesis of the proteins of the body. Adequate protein intake is particularly important during periods of growth or recovery from disease. The primary role of dietary protein is to supply amino acids for biosynthesis, but it can also be used as a source of energy. Although adequate intake of protein is essential, excessive intake should be avoided.

In contrast to carbohydrate and lipid, which are popularly perceived to have both negative and positive nutritional effects, protein has an almost completely positive image. It helps us to grow, resist infection, and recover from illness or injury. It promotes the development of strong muscles, good skin, shiny hair, and strong nails. It is recognized as an essential and generally beneficial part of a healthful diet. Dietary protein performs all three of the functions of nutrients: It is needed for the growth, maintenance, and repair of body tissue; it regulates key processes within the body; and any excess protein can be used as a source of energy. As a result, many people find it hard to accept the notion that overconsumption of protein can lead to undesirable effects. People who are concerned about the cost or ethics of eating animal protein may favor the use of vegetable sources, but it is rare to hear suggestions that dietary protein should be limited.

The term *protein,* meaning "to take first place," was introduced by the Dutch chemist Mulder in 1838. He defined protein as a nitrogen-containing constituent of food, and he believed it to be of such importance to the functioning of the body that life was impossible without it. He was correct in this belief, but today it is difficult to maintain that protein is more important than other nutrients. All essential nutrients are required for life, but it is true that proteins play a wide range of key roles in almost every aspect of life.

We now know that proteins are by far the most functionally diverse of the various chemicals of life. All enzymes are proteins, and without the catalytic effects of enzymes, none of the chemistry of life would occur. Much of the structural framework of the body within bone, muscle, connective tissue, and skin is composed of proteins. Contractile proteins give muscles the ability to move. Signaling proteins, including many hormones, travel around the body and coordinate the activities of different types of cell. Transport proteins carry key compounds, such as oxygen, from where they are in good supply to where they are in demand. Defensive proteins, such as antibodies, allow the immune system to fight off infectious disease. Proteins act as carriers and receptors within cell membranes, allowing cells to gain supplies of molecules they need and to respond to the environment in an appropriate way. Regulatory proteins can bind to other proteins or genes to control their activities and ensure that the complicated processes of life occur in the right places, at the right times, and at the right speeds.

Every cell of the body contains significant quantities of protein, and protein accounts for one fifth of the total weight of an adult. Around half of that protein is found in muscle, one fifth in bone and cartilage, one tenth in skin, and the rest is distributed throughout the other tissues and fluids of the body (Figure 5-1).

FIGURE 5-1

The distribution of protein in the body.

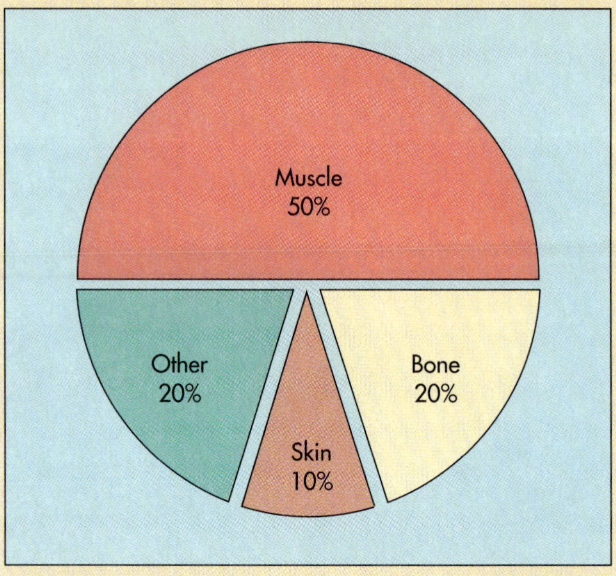

CHEMICAL COMPOSITION OF PROTEIN

All proteins are synthesized from amino acid molecules and 20 different amino acids are used in protein synthesis, although a protein can contain many hundreds of amino acid units (or **residues**) overall. All of the amino acids used in protein synthesis contain carbon, hydrogen, oxygen, and nitrogen atoms, and two of them (cysteine and methionine) also contain a sulfur atom. The fact that all amino acids contain nitrogen is important in the chemical analysis of foods because it distinguishes proteins from carbohydrates and lipids, which contain no nitrogen.

All amino acids contain an amino group (NH_2) a carboxyl group (COOH), and a hydrogen atom (H) attached to a central carbon atom, which is also bonded to the **side chain** or **side group** of the amino acid (Figure 5-2). The side chain is the only part of the structure that varies. It is often represented by the letter *R*. The carboxyl group is acidic and usually exists in its **ionized** form as $-COO^-$, having released a hydrogen ion (H^+). The amino group is basic and usually exists in its ionized form as $-NH_3^+$, having combined with a hydrogen ion. The names, structures, and other details of the amino acids used in protein synthesis are given in Table 5-1. This table also indicates that the side chains of the amino acids fall into eight general chemical categories:

- Aliphatic amino acids, which contain only carbon or hydrogen atoms in their side chain

FIGURE 5-2

General structure of the amino acids within proteins.

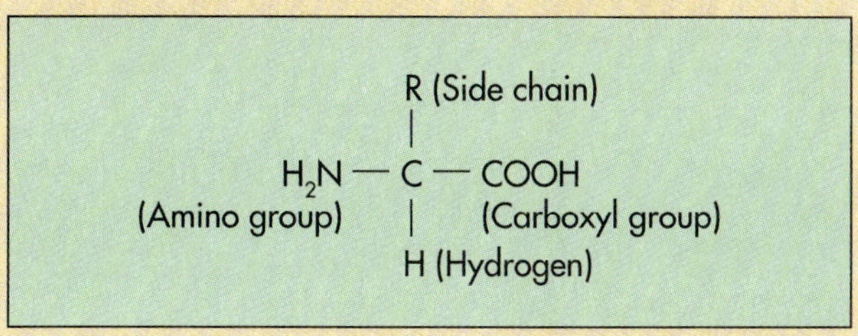

- Hydroxyl-containing amino acids, which contain a hydroxyl group in their side chain
- Sulfur-containing amino acids, which contain a sulfur atom in their side chain
- Aromatic amino acids, which contain an aromatic group (an unsaturated carbon ring system with alternating carbon-carbon double bonds) in their side chain
- Acidic amino acids, which include an acidic carboxyl group in their side chain (these are also known as **diacidic** amino acids because the acidic group in their side chain is in addition to the acidic carboxyl group found in all amino acids)
- Basic amino acids, which include a basic group, such as NH_2, in their side chain (these are also known as **dibasic** amino acids because the basic group in their side chain is in addition to the basic amino group found in all amino acids)
- Amide-containing amino acids, which contain the **amide** ($CONH_2$) group in their side chain
- The imino acid proline, so called because it does not contain a free amino group but it has its nitrogen atoms incorporated into a ring structure (but proline is still commonly referred to as an amino acid)

During the synthesis of proteins, their constituent amino acids are bonded together into long protein chains, as we shall examine in the next main section. During the digestion of the proteins in food, the proteins are broken down into their constituent amino acids again, before being absorbed through the intestinal wall.

NUTRITIONAL CLASSIFICATION OF AMINO ACIDS

From a nutritional point of view, amino acids are classified into two groups: **essential** (indispensable) and **nonessential** (dispensable). Essential amino acids are ones that cannot be synthesized by the body at a rate sufficient to meet the needs for growth and maintenance. It is essential that these amino acids are provided in the diet. Nonessential amino acids are ones that the body can make in adequate amounts from other compounds if necessary. The label *nonessential* does not mean that the body does not need these amino acids—it does. They are "nonessential" only in the sense that they are not essential components of the *diet.* Table 5-1 indicates that 9 of the 20 amino acids are classified as essential components of the diet. Histidine is the most recent addition to the list because it was only recently recognized that adults are unable to synthesize enough histidine to meet their needs over a long period. If sufficient nitrogen is available in the diet, the body can synthesize adequate supplies of the other 11 amino acids. The nitrogen required for this synthesis can come from other nonessential amino acids in food or from an excess of the essential amino acids in the diet. Amino groups can be transferred from these excess dietary amino acids onto the precursors of new amino acids by a process known as **transamination**. Transamination reactions require the participation of vitamin B_6 (see Chapter 12).

> The nine **essential amino acids** are valine, leucine, isoleucine, threonine, methionine, phenylalanine, tryptophan, lysine, and histidine.

In common with many animals, humans can also make use of limited amounts of nitrogen supplied by nonprotein components in the diet, such as urea. The nitrogen needed by the body to synthesize all of the nitrogen-containing substances it needs, including amino acids, is called **indispensable nitrogen**.

PROTEIN SYNTHESIS

To be able to synthesize proteins, a cell or multicellular organism must have access to supplies of nitrogen in an appropriate chemical form. Plants obtain their supplies of nitrogen from the soil, mainly in the form of nitrogen-containing compounds produced by the action of bacteria on decaying organic matter. Air is four fifths nitrogen, and some plants such as the **legumes** (which include peas and beans), can gain access to the nitrogen of the air because of the activities of bacteria that colonize nodules in their roots. These **nitrogen-fixing bacteria** can convert nitrogen (N_2),

TABLE 5-1

Amino acids used in synthesis of proteins

GROUP	NAME	ABBREVIATIONS†	RESIDUE MASS (DALTONS)‡	STRUCTURE (At pH 7)§
ALIPHATIC AMINO ACIDS	Glycine	Gly, G	57	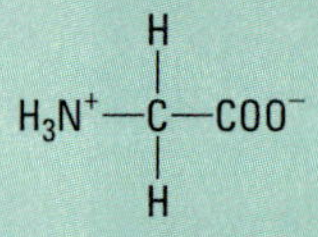
	Alanine	Ala, A	71	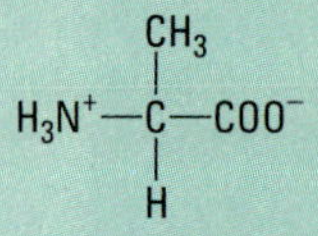
	Valine*	Val, V	99	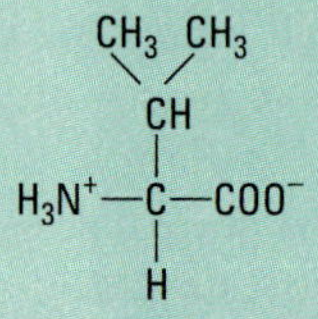
	Leucine*	Leu, L	113	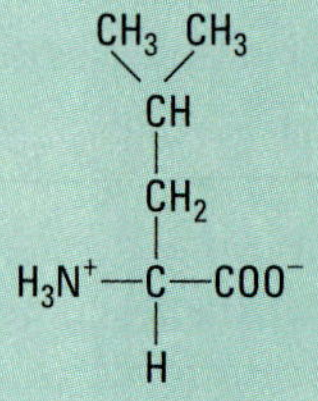
	Isoleucine*	Ile, I	113	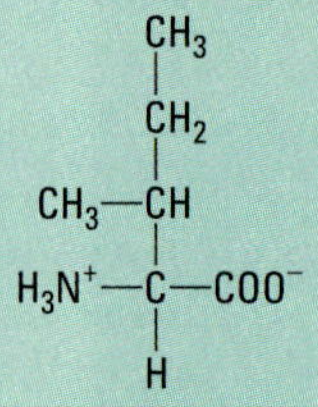
HYDROXYL-CONTAINING AMINO ACIDS	Serine	Ser, S	87	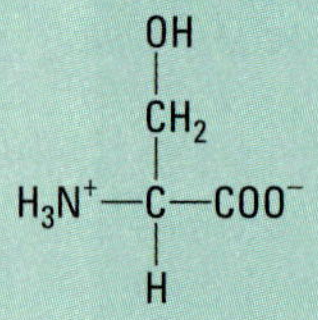
	Threonine*	Thr, T	101	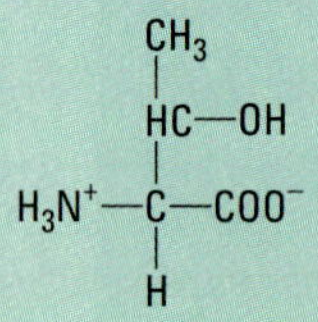

TABLE 5-1

Amino acids used in synthesis of proteins (continued)

GROUP	NAME	ABBREVIATIONS†	RESIDUE MASS (DALTONS)‡	STRUCTURE (At pH 7)§
SULFUR-CONTAINING AMINO ACIDS	Cysteine	Cys, C	103	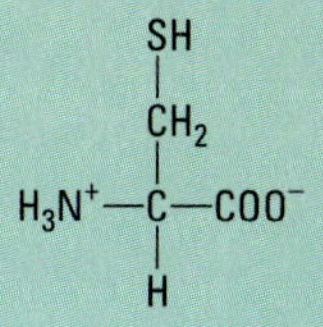
	Methionine*	Met, M	131	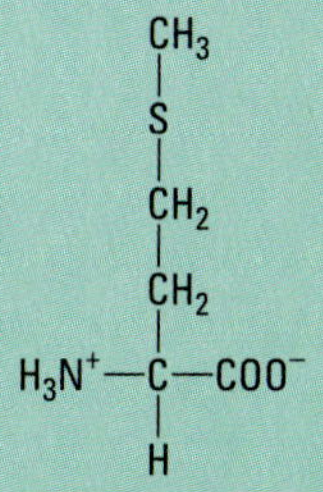
AROMATIC AMINO ACIDS	Phenylalanine*	Phe, F	147	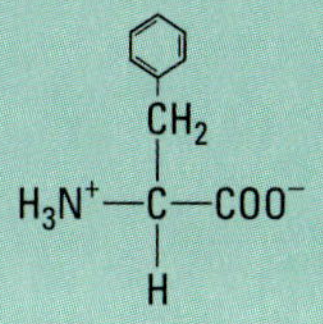
	Tyrosine	Tyr, Y	163	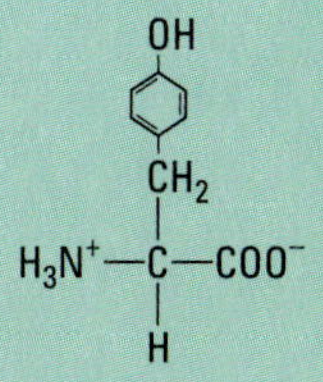
	Tryptophan*	Trp, W	186	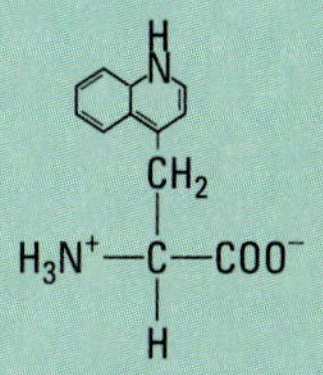
ACIDIC AMINO ACIDS	Aspartic acid	Asp, D	115	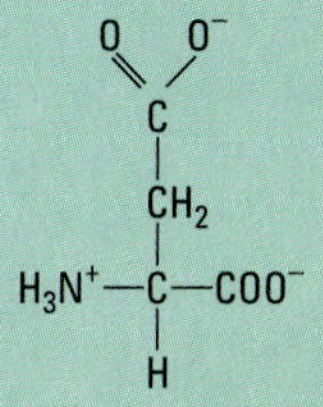
	Glutamic acid	Glu, E	129	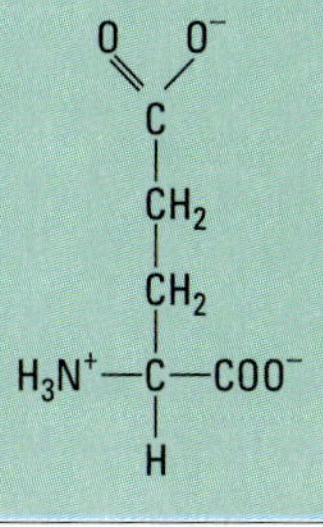

TABLE 5-1

Amino acids used in synthesis of proteins (continued)

GROUP	NAME	ABBREVIATIONS†	RESIDUE MASS (DALTONS)‡	STRUCTURE (At pH 7)§
BASIC AMINO ACIDS	Arginine‖	Arg, R	156	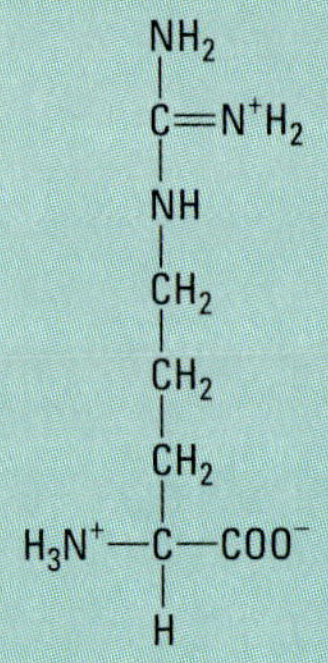
	Lysine*	Lys, K	128	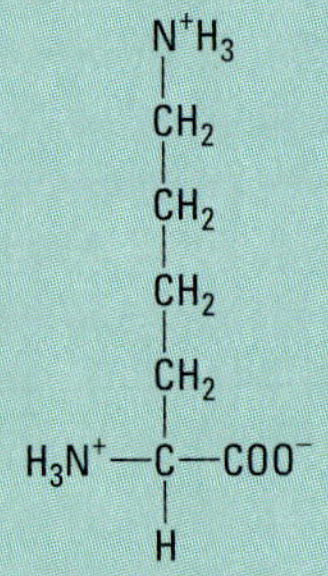
	Histidine*	His, H	137	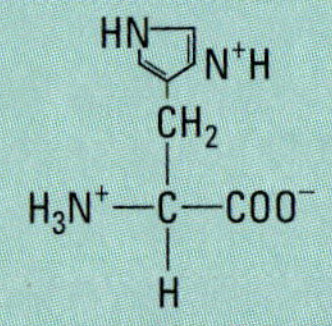
AMIDE-CONTAINING AMINO ACIDS	Asparagine	Asn, N	114	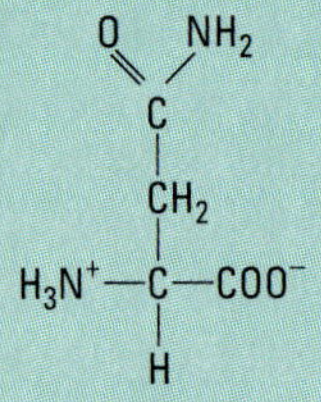
	Glutamine	Gln, G	128	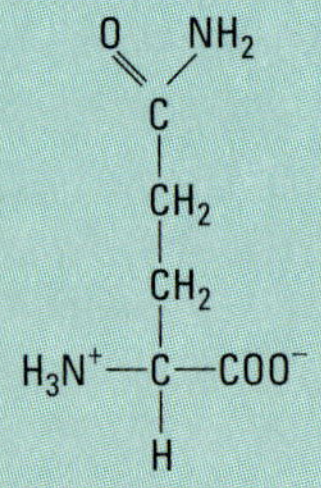
THE IMINO ACID PROLINE (usually called an amino acid)	Proline	Pro, P	97	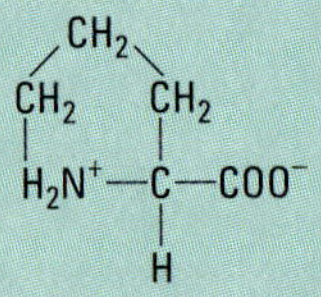

*Nutritionally essential amino acid.

†Alternative three-letter and one-letter standard abbreviations.

‡The mass each amino acid contributes to the overall mass of a protein it is part of. To obtain the mass of the free amino acid, add 18 daltons, for the addition of the atoms of water.

§At pH 7 the basic amino groups have usually gained a hydrogen ion (H^+), while the acidic carboxyl groups have usually lost a hydrogen ion, forming $^-NH3^+$ and COO^- groups.

‖ Arginine is sometimes referred to as semiessential because it may not be synthesized in amounts sufficient for growth.

molecules in the air to ammonia (NH_3), which can then be incorporated into many other organic compounds. The bacteria do this for their own benefit, but the plants with which they live can also draw on the supplies of nitrogen-containing compounds made by the bacteria. The action of lightning on air can also "fix" some nitrogen—or, in other words, incorporate it into compounds that can be used as sources of nitrogen by plants. Where modern agriculture is practiced, these natural sources of usable nitrogen are supplemented by the application of nitrogen-containing fertilizers.

Animals, including humans, obtain most of their nitrogen from the amino acids derived from the plant or animal proteins that they eat. These amino acids can be incorporated directly into new proteins synthesized by the animals, their nitrogen can be transferred to the precursors of other amino acids by the process of transamination, or their nitrogen can be incorporated into the many other important nitrogen-containing chemicals of life.

Like all the other chemicals of life, nitrogen is perpetually *recycled* through living things, back to the soil and atmosphere, and then through living things again. The chemical processes involved in this recycling system are known collectively as the **nitrogen cycle**.

FROM DNA TO PROTEIN

The actual process of protein synthesis within all forms of life requires a good supply of all 20 amino acids used in the process and is controlled by the genes embodied in the structure of deoxyribonucleic acid (DNA). The way in which genes direct the synthesis of specific proteins is complex and is regulated in many different ways, but its key aspects can be summarized simply (Figure 5-3).

DNA exists in the form of a **double helix** composed of two distinct strands of DNA wound around one another (Figure 5-3, *A*). In the center of this structure are chemical groups known as the organic **bases** of DNA, which are strung out along the "backbone" of each strand in specific sequences. The backbone is made of sugar units (deoxyribose) linked by intervening phosphate groups, and is called the **sugar-phosphate backbone** of DNA. Only four different bases are attached to the sugar-phosphate backbone: adenine **(A)**, thymine **(T)**, guanine **(G)**, and cytosine **(C)**. The most vital characteristic of DNA is that these bases can be held together by weak forces of attraction (*not* full covalent bonds) to form **base pairs** that hold the two strands of the double helix together. Adenine can pair only with thymine to form the A-T base pair, whereas guanine can pair only with cytosine to form the G-C base pair. These rules of base pairing are crucial not only to the structure of DNA, but also to the ability of DNA to specify (or "encode") the structure of protein molecules.

One gene is a region of DNA that encodes one particular chain of linked amino acids, which—in the simplest cases—can be one complete functional protein molecule. How this is achieved is examined in outline form.

Because the base pairs of DNA are held together by weak noncovalent forces, they can be broken apart easily, allowing an enzyme called **ribonucleic acid (RNA) polymerase** to enter between the strands of the double helix at the start of a gene. This enzyme catalyzes the manufacture of a strand of RNA that is virtually identical to one of the strands of the DNA (Figure 5-3, *B*). RNA contains additional oxygen atoms to DNA because the sugar in its sugar-phosphate backbone is ribose, rather than deoxyribose. Also, wherever the base thymine (T) appears in DNA, the closely related base uracil **(U)** is found in RNA. Uracil can form an A-U base pair similar to the A-T base pair of DNA.

The manufacture of an RNA copy of a gene is called **transcription.** Transcription is possible, since the rules of base pairing allow a new RNA molecule to be built on the "template" of an existing DNA strand, since the RNA polymerase enzyme links new bases into an RNA molecule only if they can form base pairs with the existing bases of the **complementary** strand of DNA. Complementary strands of DNA or RNA are ones that can bind to one another because their base sequences allow base pairs to form along their length.

The RNA copy of a gene is called **messenger RNA**, or **mRNA**, because once it is formed it leaves the nucleus and takes the chemical "message" stored within a gene out to the cytoplasm, where protein synthesis takes place. One complication is that the mRNA formed by the transcription of a gene usually undergoes various **posttranscriptional modifications** before actually being used in protein synthesis. These modifications do not affect the central principles of what occurs, however, so they are not examined.

DNA and RNA are similar compounds, both known as **nucleic acids.** In the process of transcription the base sequence of one nucleic acid (DNA) is copied into the matching base sequence of another nucleic acid (RNA). To direct the manufacture of a protein, this base sequence must determine the **amino acid sequence** of the protein that the gene encodes. This occurs because each set of three bases in mRNA (known as a **codon**) can direct the incorporation of one specific amino acid into a growing protein chain. This is achieved by a process known as **translation,** which takes place on organelles in the cytoplasm called *ribosomes* (Figure 5-3, *C*).

Ribosomes are complex structures composed of several distinct protein and RNA molecules. They are the sites of protein synthesis, but they cannot catalyze protein synthesis without the assistance of many other enzymes that form temporary associations with the ribosome as protein synthesis occurs. A ribosome becomes

FIGURE 5-3

Summary of the process by which the sequence of the DNA of a gene determines the amino acid sequence of a protein.* A, *The general structure of double-helical DNA.* B, *The process of transcription in which an mRNA copy of the base sequence of a gene is made.* C, *The process of translation in which the base sequence of the RNA molecule determines the order in which tRNA molecules deliver amino acids to the ribosome, where the amino acids are linked in a protein chain.

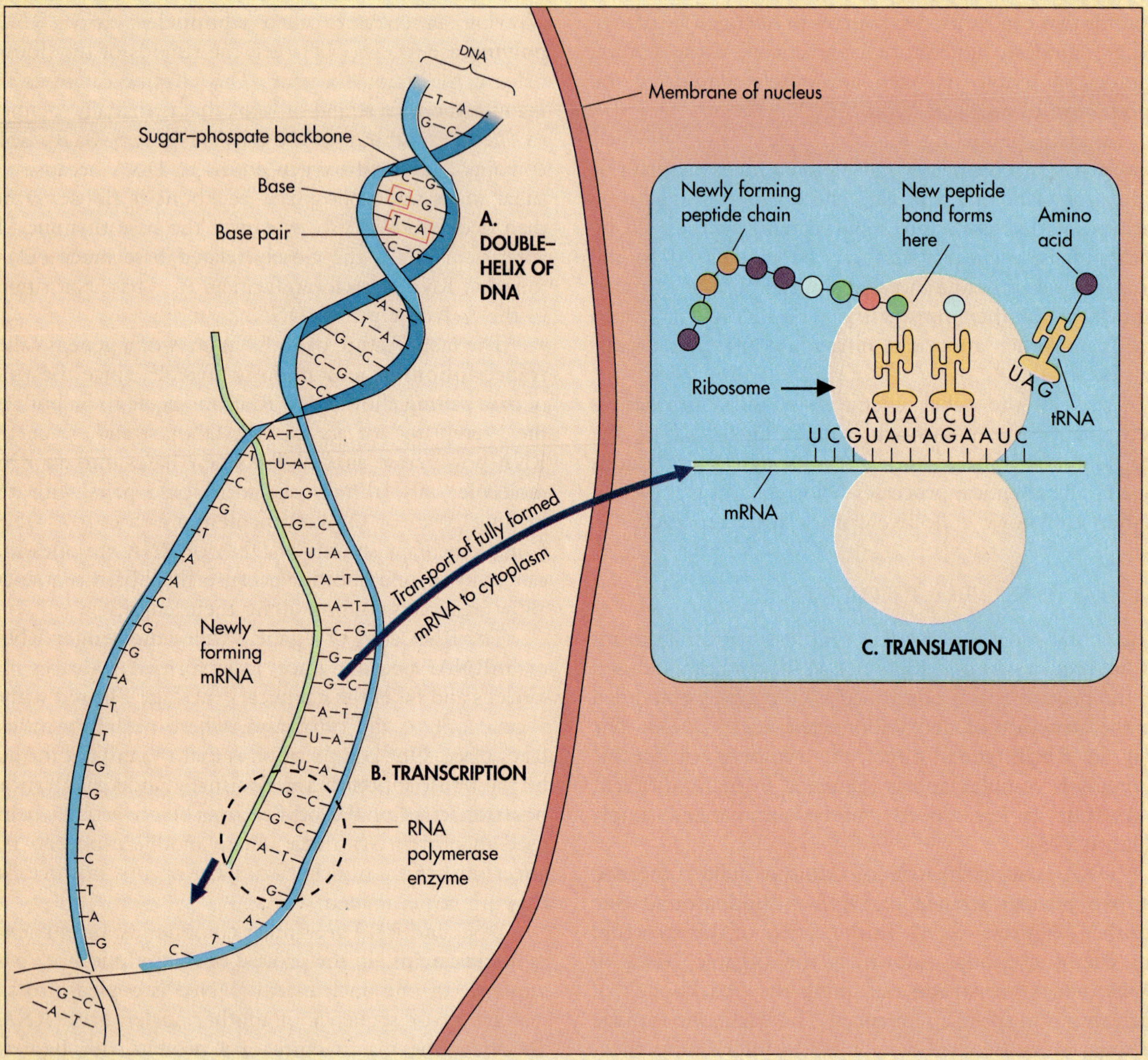

attached at the start of an mRNA molecule and then moves along it. Each time a codon of the mRNA is exposed at a special site on the ribosome, other RNA molecules known as **transfer RNA**, or **tRNA**, molecules can bind to the codon by base pairing. This is possible because each tRNA has a matching set of three bases, an **anticodon**, that is able to form base pairs with one particular codon. Each tRNA molecule is also attached to a specific amino acid molecule, which, when it arrives at the ribosome, is linked up by enzymes into a growing protein chain. So as a ribosome moves along an mRNA molecule, the base sequence of the mRNA determines which tRNA molecules become temporarily bound to the mRNA codons and so determines the order in which amino acids become linked into a protein chain. In this way the base sequence of mRNA, which is a copy of the base sequence of a gene, determines the amino acid sequence of the protein encoded by the gene. This description of transcription and translation conveys only the key essentials of what is in reality a much more complicated process. It does, however, allow us to appreciate the basic features allowing the molecular structure of a gene to determine the corresponding structure of whatever protein it encodes.

During protein synthesis, if any particular amino acid that is needed to form a protein is unavailable and cannot be immediately synthesized within the cell, the synthesis of the protein concerned ceases. This is one main reason why it is vital that the diet provide a plentiful supply of all the essential amino acids.

Each cell of the human body contains around 100,000 genes. Some of these encode functional RNA molecules rather than proteins, and sometimes the proteins encoded by more than one gene must combine to form a functional protein; but at least 30,000 different proteins can be made by human cells where and when appropriate. Genes can be switched "on" and "off" in various ways, usually mediated by the binding of specific proteins. This means that only the genes needed to make a brain cell are active in brain cells, only the genes needed to make a liver cell are active in liver cells, and so on. Genes can also be switched "on" and "off" at different stages in the life cycle of any one type of cell so that the proteins they encode are made only when required and in the quantities required.

THE IMPORTANCE OF PROTEIN STRUCTURE

When amino acids become linked together to form a protein, the individual amino acid "residues" are linked by **peptide bonds,** formed during the condensation reaction between the amino group of one amino acid and the carboxyl group of another. Two amino acid residues joined by a peptide bond form what is called a **dipeptide;** three amino acid residues joined by peptide bonds form a **tripeptide.** Proteins are **polypeptides** because they contain a great many (poly, "many") amino acid residues all joined by peptide bonds. There is no fixed dividing line between the small "peptides" and larger "polypeptides," although a changeover point is customarily set at molecular weights of between 8000 and 10,000 atomic mass units. This molecular weight range corresponds to approximately 175 units of glycine, the smallest amino acid, or about 53 units of tryptophan, one of the largest amino acids. Because all proteins contain many different amino acids, their molecular weights depend on both the type and number of amino acids they contain.

Every polypeptide or protein chain (and every small peptide) has a free amino group at one end (the **amino-terminus**) and a free carboxyl group at the other end (the **carboxy-terminus**). Protein synthesis proceeds from the amino end toward the carboxy end so that the first amino acid to become a part of the protein forms the amino-terminus and the last amino acid to be attached forms the carboxy-terminus (Figure 5-4).

Different proteins are different because they have different amino acid sequences. Although there are only 20 different amino acids available, these can be linked up in an almost infinite variety of ways to form proteins that usually contain several hundred amino acid residues overall. The linear sequence in which amino acids are joined to form any particular protein is known as the **primary structure** of the protein. Once a protein is formed, however, it immediately folds up into the specific three-dimensional configuration that allows it to perform its function (although it may also need to be chemically modified by enzymes, combined with metal ions or coenzymes, or associated with other proteins before it can actually fulfill its role within the cell). This process of protein folding, which is controlled by the amino acid sequence, introduces two new levels of structural organization. Specific regions of a protein chain often fold up into one of a few general patterns of **secondary structures**, such as helices, or sheets (Figure 5-4). Most proteins contain various different secondary structures (a helix, a sheet, then another helix, for example) linked to one another by relatively unstructured regions of the polypeptide chain. Protein folding does not stop with the formation of secondary structures, however, but continues in a way that brings the various secondary structures together into a precisely folded structure overall. This final completely folded structure of the protein in which the different regions of secondary structure are precisely oriented with respect to one another is known as the protein's **tertiary structure**. The folded structure of many proteins is held together in places by the formation of covalent bonds, known as **disulfide bridges**, between sulfur-containing cysteine residues on adjacent regions of the protein.

Many types of protein molecules can also bind to other protein molecules, either identical to themselves or different, to form **multi-subunit** proteins. The way in which the molecular subunits of such a protein are arranged together is called the **quaternary structure** of the protein.

All of the protein folding processes are controlled by the chemical interactions between the amino acids of the primary structure and the way in which these amino acids interact with the water and other molecules in the environment in which the protein is formed. Even when proteins must be chemically modified after they are made, that too is made possible by the folded structure of the original protein, which is in turn determined by the primary structure. So everything about a protein's chemical structure and activity ultimately depends on its primary structure, which is of course encoded by the DNA base sequence of the corresponding gene.

The spatial arrangement of the atoms of a protein (its "shape," in other words) determines what activities it can perform, what reactions it can catalyze if it is an enzyme, what chemicals it can carry into a cell if it is a membrane-bound carrier protein, and so on. This spatial arrangement can be altered by variations in the chemical environment around a protein. Changes in the pH value,

FIGURE 5-4

The four basic levels of protein structure: primary, secondary, tertiary, and quaternary.

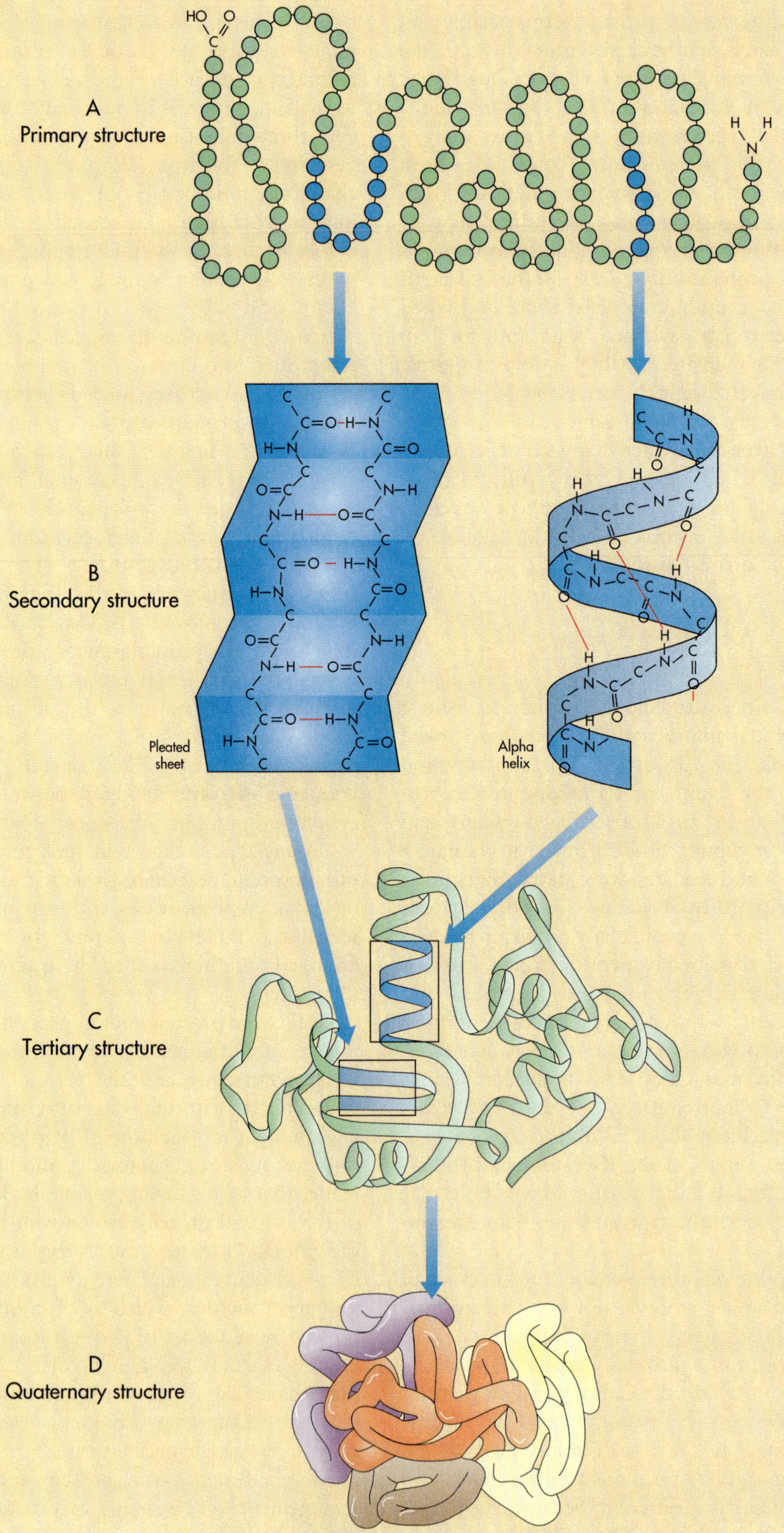

the concentrations of various ions, temperature, or the influence of electromagnetic radiation, such as light and ultraviolet rays, can alter the structure of a protein in ways that alter its ability to perform its usual function. If these influences damage a protein and so prevent it from performing its normal function, the protein is said to be **denatured**. One of the most nutritionally relevant examples of this is the coagulation of egg yolk and egg white on heating. This dramatic change is largely a result of the heat denaturation of the proteins in the egg.

Alterations in the base sequence of a gene (known as **mutations**) can also alter the primary structure and therefore the final tertiary or quaternary structure of a protein. Such changes are believed to provide the novelties required to power the process of **evolution**, but they can also produce the aberrant proteins responsible for genetic disease. In persons with **sickle cell anemia**, for example, the shape of the oxygen-transporting protein of the blood (hemoglobin) is altered because just 1 of its 300 amino acids is changed from glutamic acid to valine. This small change causes a crucial alteration in the shape of the hemoglobin molecule, thereby causing a serious disease.

Our understanding of protein structure and function is still at a comparatively early stage. The first complete primary structure of a small protein (the hormone insulin) was determined in 1953. The first complete three-dimensional structure was determined in 1961, and even today the detailed three-dimensional structure of most proteins remains unknown. In one respect, however, scientists are gaining astonishing and powerful mastery over the process of protein synthesis. The modern techniques of biotechnology, especially the branch known as **genetic engineering** (or **recombinant DNA technology**), allow genes to be moved from species to species and altered at will. Genetic engineering is already being used to synthesize large quantities of proteins that were previously difficult to obtain, usually by inserting the necessary gene into easily grown bacterial cells. Experiments are also being performed using modified genes, which encode modified proteins, whose eventual structures and activities will have been altered by human intervention rather than conventional evolution. These abilities have been exploited mostly in the quest for new medicines but are also being applied to food production. Important crop plants are being genetically manipulated in an attempt to generate better-yielding varieties that are more resistant to diseases and have improved nutritional qualities.

PROTEIN FUNCTION AND ACTIVITY

This section provides further details on some of the activities of proteins that are of particular relevance to the student of nutrition. One key point to remember, which would be tedious to repeat wherever relevant, is that virtually every reaction within the body is catalyzed by a protein enzyme; so the importance of proteins to all aspects of life cannot be overemphasized.

GROWTH AND MAINTENANCE OF TISSUE

Before cells can synthesize new protein, they must have all the nutritionally essential amino acids available simultaneously plus sufficient nitrogen in a suitable form to make any of the nutritionally nonessential amino acids required. Much of the new protein synthesized by cells is used for the **maintenance** of the structures of the cell, in other words, for the continual replacement of existing proteins. This is required because proteins are continually degraded and then resynthesized in a process known as **protein turnover**. The constant breaking down and resynthesis of protein causes about 0.3% to 0.4% of bodily protein to be turned over every day. The turnover of the wall of the intestine alone, which is replaced every 4 to 6 days, requires the synthesis of about 70 g of protein per day. Fortunately the body is efficient at conserving protein, and it reuses most of the amino acids released by the breakdown of proteins for the synthesis of new proteins to replace them. One way in which protein is lost from the body is within the skin, hair, and nails, which are constantly shed from the body's surface. Protein is also lost in the small proportion of the continuously shed intestinal wall cells that are excreted in feces, rather than being broken down for their amino acids to be reabsorbed. Failure to replace any of these losses is reflected in loss of body weight. In addition to the need to replace proteins during turnover, proteins must also be synthesized for the repair of damaged tissue.

New growth, including the buildup of muscles, can occur only when an appropriate mixture of amino acids is available over and above the amount needed for the maintenance and repair of existing tissue. The vital process of cell division is also dependent on proteins. For example, specific proteins form the intracellular scaffolding, or **cytoskeleton**, that is involved in moving the contents of the dividing cell, especially the chromosomes containing the genes, and distributing them properly between the two new cells being formed.

The structural matrix, or framework, within bones and teeth is composed of protein molecules, particularly the protein known as **collagen**. Calcium and phosphorus are deposited within this protein framework, giving bones and teeth their strength and rigidity. Collagen is also the main protein within tendons and ligaments, and it is the intercellular material that binds cells together.

The contractile fibers of muscles are composed of two kinds of protein, **actin** and **myosin**, which slide past one another in a process powered by the hydrolysis of adenosine triphosphate (ATP) to allow muscles to contract.

FORMATION OF ESSENTIAL BODY COMPOUNDS

A wide variety of the compounds needed to keep the body working properly is proteins or amino acids, or they are derived from proteins or amino acids. Enzymes, including those responsible for digestion, are the most obvious examples, but there are many others. Many of the hormones (such as insulin, gastrin, and growth hormone) produced by various glands in the body are proteins or peptides. The oxygen molecules needed to oxidize food molecules during respiration are transported through the blood by the protein hemoglobin, which also gives blood its red color. Almost all of the many substances responsible for the clotting of blood are proteins. The photoreceptors in the eye, which initiate the nervous signals responsible for the sense of vision when they absorb light, are proteins. Epinephrine (adrenaline), a hormone secreted by the adrenal gland, is derived from the amino acid tyrosine. The amino acid tryptophan serves as the precursor for the vitamin niacin and also for serotonin, a vital neurotransmitter that is involved in transmitting nerve signals from one nerve cell to another.

The list of proteins and compounds derived from proteins that are vital to the functioning and regulation of the body is virtually endless. Specific attention is drawn to only a few of the better-known examples. If the diet is deficient in protein, the synthesis of the most vital of these body compounds seems to take priority over the synthesis of less important proteins such as those in skin and hair. Thus a deterioration in the condition of skin and hair is one of the earliest signs of protein deficiency.

TRANSPORT OF NUTRIENTS

Proteins play an essential role in the transport of nutrients from the intestine across the intestinal wall to the blood, from the blood to the tissues of the body, and across the membranes of the cells of the tissues. Most of the many substances involved in nutrient transport are proteins. These transport and membrane-bound carrier proteins are usually specific to one nutrient. Retinol-binding protein, for example, binds to and transports only retinol (one form of vitamin A). Some proteins, however, can carry several different nutrients such as the metallothionein protein, which transports both copper and zinc ions. In such cases the various transported substances may have to compete for a limited supply of the carrier protein. Other proteins can transport many different members of a wide group of related substances, such as the lipoproteins, which can transport many different lipid molecules. If a deficiency of such transport and membrane-bound carrier proteins occurs because of a general lack of protein in the diet, the absorption or transport of some vital nutrients is reduced, which may make the original deficiency worse.

REGULATION OF WATER BALANCE

Fluid in the body is distributed between two types of compartments: the **intracellular** compartments (within each cell) and the **extracellular** compartment (outside of the cells). The extracellular compartment is itself divided into the **intercellular** (between the cells) and the **intravascular** (within the blood vessels) compartments. These compartments are separated from one another by cell membranes, and the distribution of fluid between them must be kept in balance. This balance is achieved by a complex network of control systems involving both dissolved proteins and dissolved ions (**electrolytes**), primarily sodium (Na^+) and potassium (K^+) ions. Protein molecules in the blood that are too large to pass out of the blood into the intercellular space exert an **oncotic pressure,** drawing water from the intercellular space back into the blood. This is essentially just a form of osmosis in which water diffuses into the blood because of the higher concentration of proteins (and other large molecules) within the blood. A **hydrostatic pressure,** pushing fluid in the opposite direction out of the blood and into the intercellular space, is also always present because of the pumping action of the heart. The net direction of fluid flow depends on the relative values of these opposing pressures (Figure 5-5). When the level of protein in the blood is low, the hydrostatic pressure dominates and pushes fluid out of the blood. This causes an accumulation of fluid within the tissues, making them soft and spongy with a bloated appearance. This condition, known as **edema,** is recognized as an early sign of protein deficiency, although it can also be caused by several other factors.

MAINTENANCE OF APPROPRIATE pH

Proteins in the blood serve as **buffers,** which are compounds that resist changes in pH values, and therefore tend to maintain pH values, even if small amounts of acids or alkalis are added to them. Buffers achieve their effects because they can combine with, and so "mop up," *both* hydrogen ions and hydroxide ions if the concentration of either of these determinants of the pH value should rise. This buffering action is an extremely important aspect of protein function because much of the biology of the body is sensitive to changes in pH value, operating properly only within a relatively narrow pH value range. The buffering action of proteins in the blood ensures that there is normally no significant change in the pH value of blood despite the continual transport of many different substances, including both alkalis and bases, through blood.

FIGURE 5-5

The role of protein in maintaining fluid balance between capillaries and intercellular spaces.

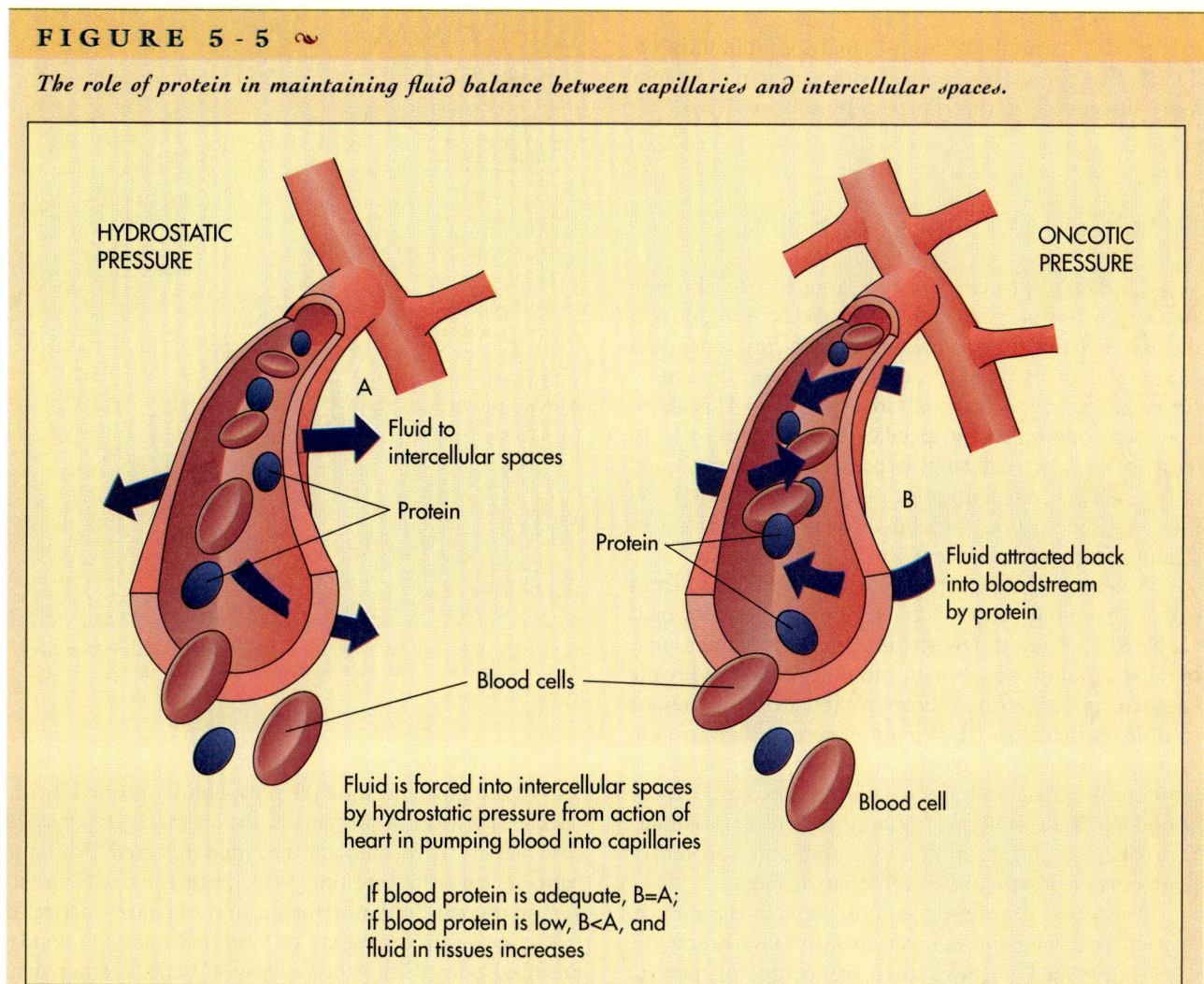

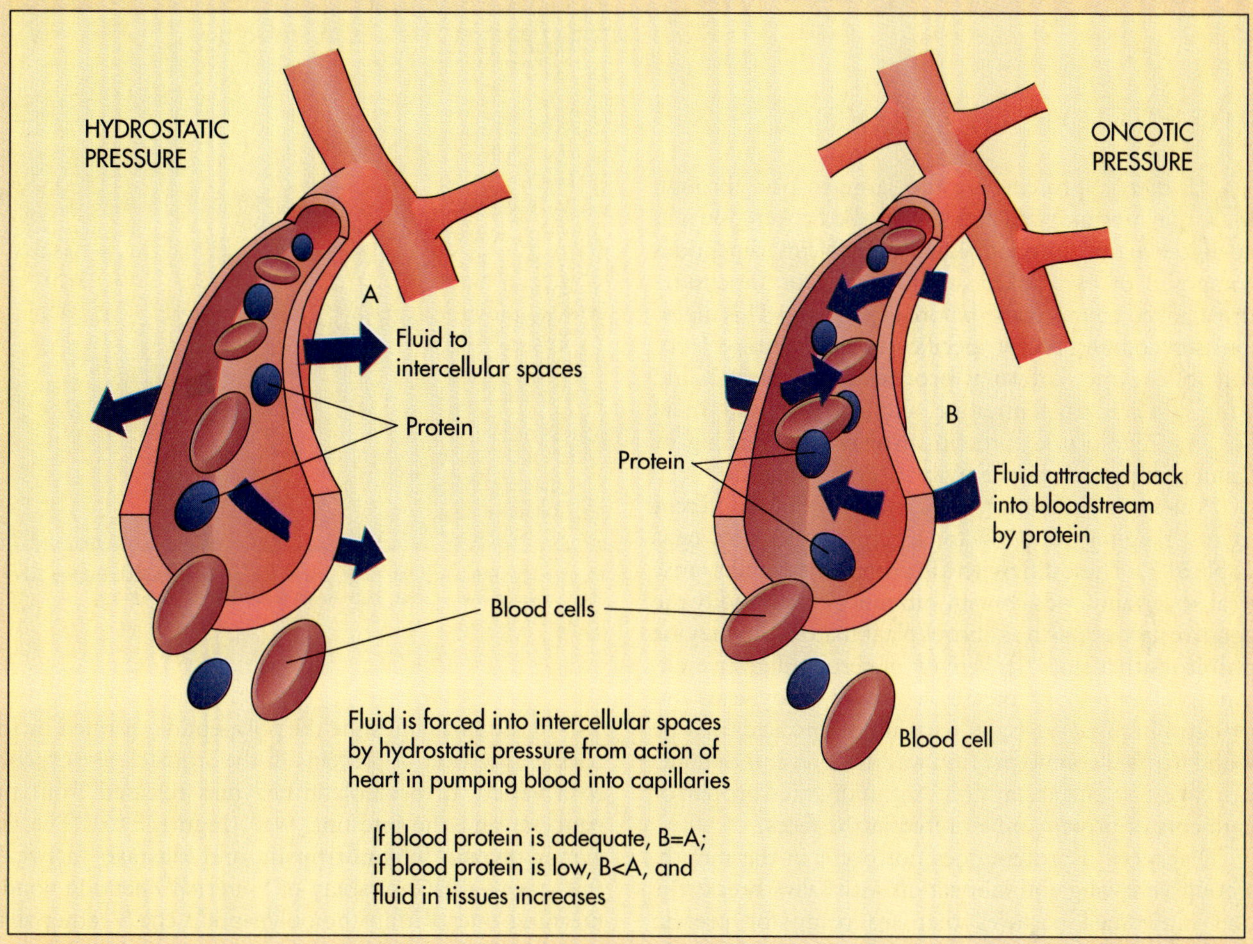
HYDROSTATIC PRESSURE
A
Fluid to intercellular spaces
Protein
Blood cells
Fluid is forced into intercellular spaces by hydrostatic pressure from action of heart in pumping blood into capillaries
If blood protein is adequate, B=A; if blood protein is low, B<A, and fluid in tissues increases
ONCOTIC PRESSURE
B
Protein
Fluid attracted back into bloodstream by protein
Blood cell

> *Proteins in the blood serve as **buffers,** which are chemicals able to resist changes in the pH value.*

DEFENSE AND DETOXIFICATION

The body's ability to fight off infection depends on its immune system, most noticeably the ability of the immune system to produce a diverse array of defensive proteins known as **antibodies**. Each antibody is able to bind to specific parts of infectious organisms or other foreign chemicals known collectively as **antigens**. Once bound to an antigen, an antibody assists in the elimination of the antigen in a variety of ways. Because a specific antibody is required for each specific antigen, the body can produce an astonishing diversity of antibodies, which requires a considerable amount of protein synthesis. Complicated control systems ensure that the level of most antibodies is normally low, but whichever antibodies are needed to meet a specific threat are quickly manufactured in large amounts in response to the arrival of the threat. This means that a healthy immune system depends on a good supply of the amino acids needed to synthesize new antibodies. Malnourished young children, particularly in developing countries, are known to have a lowered resistance to infection, which leaves them unable to fight off many infections. This lowered resistance to infection is attributed to an inability to produce adequate supplies of antibodies and other defensive proteins, which can in turn be attributed to a protein deficiency in their diets.

The health of the body is also threatened by various toxic compounds that are found within foods, including completely natural foods, and in the environment at large. These toxins are normally **detoxified** by enzymes found mainly in the liver, which convert them into harmless substances. If protein synthesis is restricted because of a nutritional deficiency, the ability of the body to detoxify harmful chemicals can be significantly reduced. This also makes a person with a protein deficiency more susceptible to the effects of poisons or drugs.

DIGESTION OF PROTEINS

All dietary proteins are too large to pass through the intestinal wall and so must be broken down in the digestive tract into individual amino acids, dipeptides (composed of two linked amino acids), or tripeptides (three linked amino acids) before absorption. This digestion is accomplished by specific protein-splitting (proteolytic) enzymes known as **proteases**, which are found in the stomach, small intestine, and intestinal wall. In all cases the digestion of protein involves the breaking or cleaning of peptide bonds by hydrolysis reactions.

Proteins in different foods are digestible to different extents, ranging from 78% for legumes to 97% for eggs (Table 5-2). These differences in protein digestibility arise because certain foods contain substances that modify the digestive process, such as fibrous plant material or **enzyme inhibitors** that slow the activity of certain digestive enzymes. Inhibitors of proteases are found in soybeans and raw eggs. In some foods, proteins and amino acids may be bound to other compounds in a way that prevents or limits their digestion and absorption. Any undigested protein or fragments of protein are excreted in the feces.

Digestion of protein does not occur in the mouth, although chewing and lubrication with saliva breaks the food into small particles that are ready for protein digestion to begin in the stomach. In the stomach, **pepsin** enzymes (a class of proteases) cleave some of the peptide bonds within proteins. A **gelatinase** enzyme that liquefies **gelatin** (a mixture of animal proteins) is also present in the stomach.

Pepsins and many other enzymes involved in protein digestion are secreted in the form of **proenzymes**, which are inactive enzyme precursors that become activated within the gastrointestinal (GI) tract. The precursors of pepsins are called **pepsinogens** and become active on exposure to the acid environment in the stomach. The lining of the human stomach contains several related pepsinogens.

Pepsins hydrolyze peptide bonds, linking one of the aromatic amino acids (phenylalanine, tryptophan, or tyrosine) to any other amino acid. The products of pepsin digestion are largely polypeptides, like the original protein, but are significantly smaller than the polypeptide chain of the original protein. The size and number of fragments produced from the digestion of any particular protein depends on the location of the aromatic amino acids within that protein. The optimal range of the pH value of pepsins is 1.6 to 3.2, so they quickly stop working when the acidic contents of the stomach are mixed with the alkaline pancreatic juice in the duodenum and jejunum of the small intestine.

TABLE 5-2

*Values for the digestibility of protein in humans**

PROTEIN SOURCE	TRUE DIGESTIBILITY (%)
Egg	97 ± 3
Milk, cheese	95 ± 3
Meat, fish	94 ± 3
Maize	85 ± 6
Rice, polished	88 ± 4
Wheat, whole	86 ± 5
Wheat, refined	96 ± 4
Oatmeal	86 ± 7
Peanut butter	95†
Soyflour	86 ± 7
Beans	78†
Mixed U.S. diet	96†‡

* -x ± SD.
† Standard deviation not available.
‡ Calculated value.

Modified from FAO/WHO/UNU: *Energy and protein requirements,* Technical Rep Series 724, Geneva, Switzerland, 1985, World Health Organization.

In the small intestine the polypeptides formed by the partial digestion of proteins in the stomach are exposed to a variety of proteolytic enzymes released from the pancreas and the intestinal wall (Figure 5-6). The enzymes **trypsin**, **chymotrypsin**, and **elastase**—active at this stage—cleave a variety of "internal" peptide bonds, meaning ones within the polypeptide chain rather than at either end of it. Such enzymes are called **endopeptidases**. In contrast, the **carboxypeptidase** enzymes released from the pancreas and the **aminopeptidases** of the intestinal wall are **exopeptidases**, meaning that they hydrolyze the *final* peptide bonds of a polypeptide or peptide chain. Carboxypeptidases hydrolyze the bond at the carboxy-terminus of a chain, whereas aminopeptidases hydrolyze the bond at the amino-terminus. Exopeptidases can work their way along a protein chain, cleaving off one amino acid at a time.

Endopeptidases break specific internal peptide bonds of a polypeptide chain. **Exopeptidases** break the final peptide bonds of a polypeptide chain. **Carboxypeptidases** are exopeptidases that act at the carboxy-terminus of a polypeptide. **Aminopeptidases** are exopeptidases that act at the amino-terminus of a polypeptide.

FIGURE 5-6

Activation of the pancreatic proteases in the lumen of the duodenum.

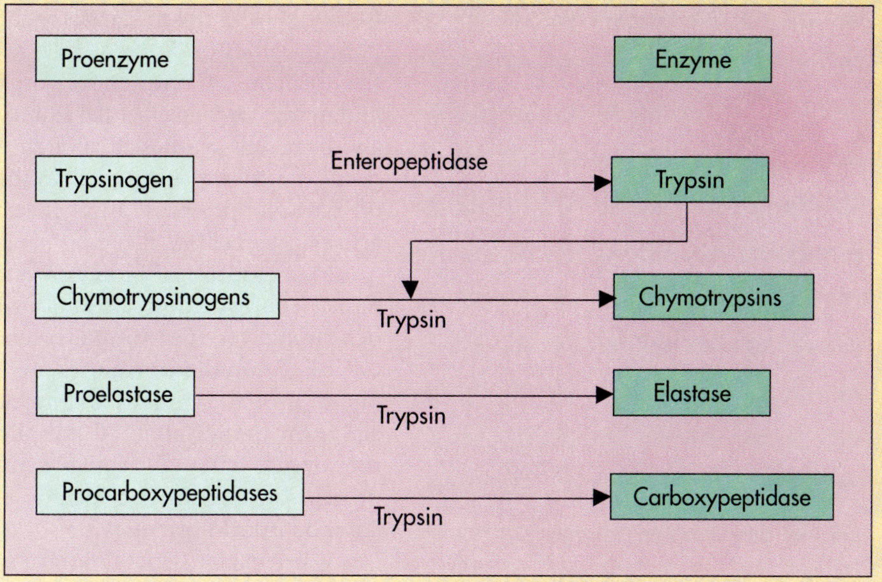

Some free amino acids are released in the lumen of the intestine, whereas others are released at the intestinal wall cell surface by the **aminopeptidase** and **dipeptidase** enzymes found there. Aminopeptidase enzymes hydrolyze peptides from the amino-terminus, whereas dipeptidases cleave dipeptides into their individual amino acids.

The body produces all of the digestive enzymes it needs; so there is no point in buying them in pills.

ABSORPTION OF PROTEINS

Some dipeptides and tripeptides are transported into the cells of the intestinal wall and then are hydrolyzed to amino acids by peptidase enzymes within the cells. Most ingested protein, however, is digested down to individual amino acids that are then absorbed into the intestinal cells. The necessary transport across the cell membranes is achieved by various different carrier proteins. Some of these, including a carrier of aliphatic amino acids and a carrier of phenylalanine and methionine, transport amino acids, along with sodium ions (Na^+), in a manner similar to the cotransport of glucose and Na^+ (see Chapter 3). Other Na^+-independent carriers include one for basic amino acids and an alternative aliphatic amino acid carrier. A different system of carriers transports dipeptides and tripeptides into the intestinal cells. From the intestinal cells the amino acids pass into the blood capillaries that lead to the portal vein, which takes them to the liver. The level of amino acids in the blood of the hepatic portal vein rises quickly after the ingestion and digestion of protein. Once the amino acids reach the liver, some are synthesized into **plasma proteins**, which are proteins found in the plasma of blood. The remainder are transported via the blood to the individual cells of the body, where they are used to synthesize the specific proteins that the body needs.

A considerable proportion of the new proteins synthesized by the body are secreted back into the GI tract as the enzymes and other proteins involved in digestion are lost into the GI tract as a result of the shedding of intestinal mucosal cells. This is shown in Table 5-3, although the values given are only rough estimates.

METABOLISM OF PROTEINS

Early ideas about protein and amino acid metabolism maintained that body proteins were relatively static, changing only slowly, if at all. When radioactive isotopes became available, allowing the fate of individual atoms to be monitored, it was soon learned that body proteins are constantly being "turned over," or degraded and resynthesized. Monitoring the fate of nitrogen atoms revealed a constant interchange of nitrogen between different tissues and between newly absorbed

TABLE 5-3

Daily protein exchange in the digestion of food by a 70-kg man compared with his turnover of body proteins

COMPONENT	AMOUNT OF PROTEIN (g/DAY)
Protein secreted into gastrointestinal tract	
Saliva	3
Gastric juice	5
Bile	1
Pancreatic juice	8
Mucosal shedding	50
Balance sheet of protein entering and leaving gastrointestinal (GI) tract	
Average daily intake	90
Total secreted into GI tract	67
Fecal output	10
Amount absorbed (157-10)	147
Total body protein turnover	210-280

From Fauconneau G, Michel MC: The role of the gastrointestinal tract in the regulation of protein metabolism. In Munro HN, editor: *Mammalian protein metabolism,* vol 4, New York, 1970, Academic Press; and Millward DJ and others: *Nutr Res Rev* 2:109, 1989.

amino acids and body proteins. There is no major storage site for the accumulation of proteins, although the liver increases in size when extra protein is available and some tissue proteins such as plasma albumin act as small, **labile** (easily degraded) protein reserves. If the body suffers a deficiency of either protein as a whole or of specific amino acids, these limited supplies of "storage" protein are quickly broken down and used.

The amount of protein in the body of adults normally changes very little, but the rate of protein turnover does vary significantly from tissue to tissue. Some proteins such as those in the intestinal tract, pancreas, and liver turn over rapidly, whereas collagen and muscle proteins turn over more slowly. The overall rate of protein turnover in the adult male is estimated at 3 to 4 g/kg of body weight per day. This amounts to a total of 245 g/day or 8.75 oz/day for a 70-kg man.

The main processes of protein and amino acid metabolism in the human body are summarized in Figure 5-7. Although these look complex at first sight, they can be largely subdivided into three main categories of reaction that amino acids undergo after absorption:

- Protein synthesis
- Synthesis of small nitrogen-containing molecules
- Degradative reactions in which nitrogen atoms become incorporated into urea while the amino acid carbon skeletons are converted to carbon dioxide or deposited in body tissues in the form of carbohydrate or fat

The flow of amino acids through these alternative routes is closely interrelated so that an increase in flow in one route is balanced by decreased flow in others. Although the body consists of many different cells and tissues, its network of protein metabolism is best regarded as an integrated whole in which materials flow to and from tissues as circumstances require. The varying metabolic activities of different cells and tissues cooperate to the benefit of the entire organism. For example, glutamine is not an essential amino acid because intestinal and liver cells synthesize enough glutamine to meet the needs of other tissues as well as their own. The synthesis of tyrosine provides another example, being largely achieved by cells of the liver, pancreas, and kidney.

Many aspects of protein metabolism are under hormonal control whose effects can be dramatic or subtle depending on the hormones and target tissues concerned. **Anabolic hormones** are ones that increase the rate of protein synthesis and include insulin, androgens, and growth hormone. **Catabolic hormones** decrease the overall rate of protein synthesis by accelerating protein breakdown and include thyroid hormones and adrenocortical hormones.

When dietary energy intake is adequate, the amino acids derived from dietary proteins are immediately used for whatever protein synthesis is required for growth and maintenance of body tissues. Amino acids in excess of immediate needs undergo **deamination** in which they lose their amino groups. These are ultimately incorporated by the liver into urea, which is subsequently excreted by the kidneys. The remaining nitrogen-free portions of the amino acids enter the same metabolic pathways as carbohydrates and lipids to be used as a source of energy or to be incorporated into storage carbohydrates or fat. When the amino acids are used as a source of energy, the fate of their carbon and hydrogen atoms is the same overall as that of the carbon and hydrogen of carbohydrate or fat: They are oxidized in respiration to generate carbon dioxide and water, releasing energy that can be trapped within ATP.

More than half of the amino acids are **glucogenic** amino acids, meaning that after deamination they can be used for the formation of glucose. The remaining amino acids can, after deamination, be broken down into two-carbon fragments that can eventually form the "acetyl" part of the key intermediate of metabolism, acetyl CoA. Like lipids, these amino acids can be converted into ketones, which can be used as a source of energy in the brain. They are therefore known as **ketogenic** amino acids. Any excess ketones produced in this way can be excreted in urine. Some amino acids are both glucogenic and ketogenic. The fate of glucogenic and ketogenic amino acids is considered more fully in Chapter 6.

In general, amino acids are deaminated and used as an energy source when the following situations occur:

- Insufficient fat and carbohydrate are available to meet immediate energy needs.
- Amounts of essential amino acids are insufficient to synthesize required proteins.

FIGURE 5-7

Summary of the main pathways of protein and amino acid metabolism.

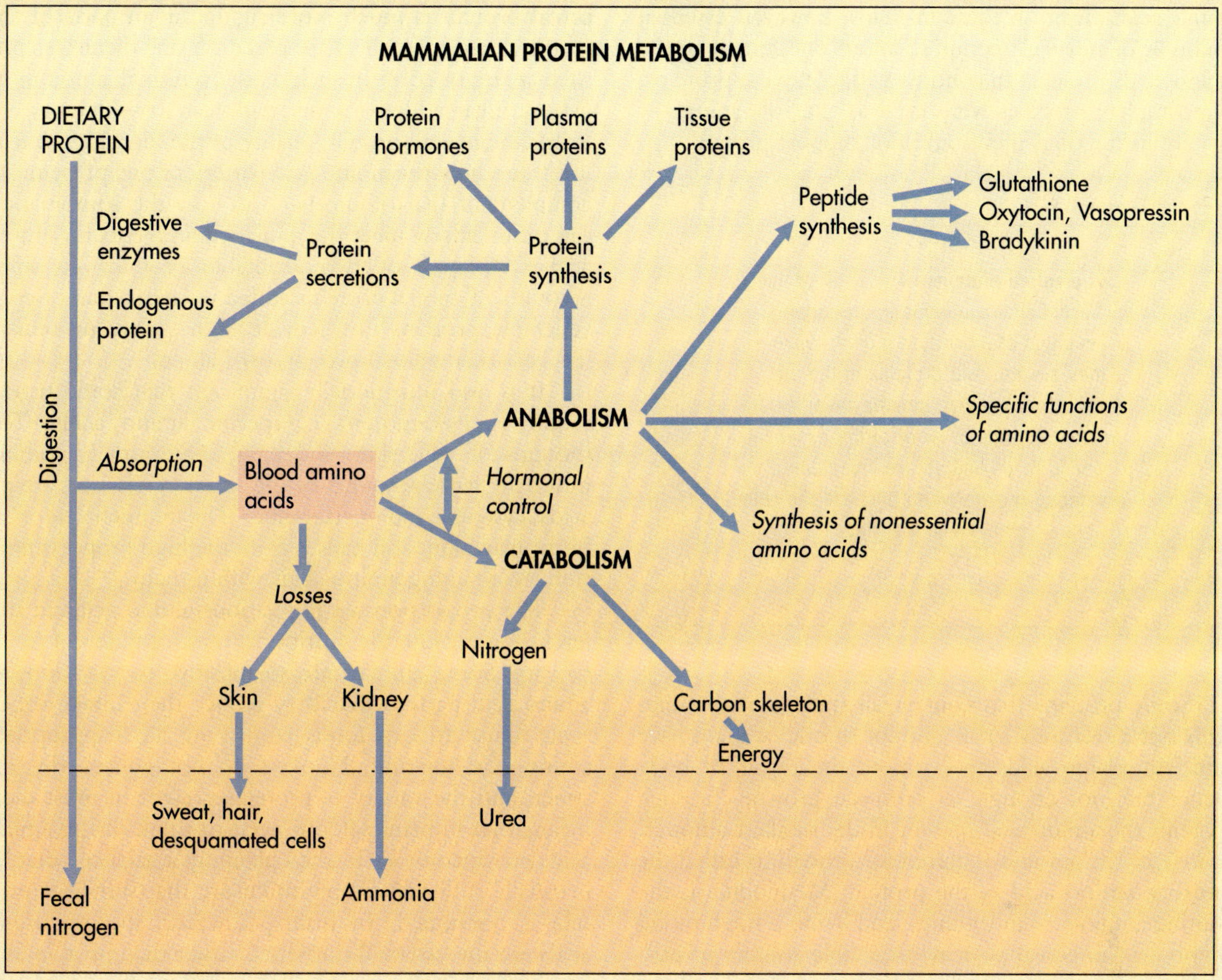

- The diet provides more amino acids than are needed for growth or maintenance and the synthesis of essential body compounds.

PROTEIN QUALITY

The **quality** of a dietary protein is determined by the kind of amino acids it contains and the proportions in which they are present. Good-quality proteins contain all of the essential amino acids in proportions capable of promoting growth when they are the only proteins in the diet. Such proteins are known as **complete proteins** and proteins of **high biological value**. Essential amino acids normally compose about one third of the amino acids in such proteins.

All animal proteins, except gelatin (which has limited amounts of tryptophan and lysine), are complete proteins. This means that if animal foods are used as the sole source of protein in sufficient amounts to meet our total protein needs, they usually provide enough of all the essential amino acids. Any excess amount of the essential amino acids can be used to synthesize nonessential amino acids, if necessary. The essential amino acid content of a protein is known as the protein's amino acid **pattern** or amino acid **profile**.

The **amino acid pattern** of a protein is the relative proportions in which the essential amino acids are present in the protein.

Poor-quality proteins, described as **incomplete proteins** or **proteins of low biological value**, are those that lack or have limited amounts of one or more essential amino acids. Even in these proteins, however, essential amino acids normally compose about one fourth of the amino acids present. In contrast with complete proteins, if incomplete proteins were used as the sole source of protein in the diet, they could not support growth.

> **Complete proteins** contain all of the essential amino acids in proportions capable of promoting growth when they are the sole proteins in the diet. **Incomplete proteins** lack or have limited amounts of one or more of the essential amino acids and so are incapable of promoting growth when they are the sole proteins in the diet.

Some proteins that contain all the essential amino acids but a relatively small amount of one of them have sufficient amino acids to promote the repair of body tissues but not enough to promote growth. In such proteins the amino acid present in the smallest amount, relative to the amount required for growth, is called the **limiting amino acid** of the protein. Methionine is the limiting amino acid in legumes, and lysine is the limiting amino acid in cereal protein. Vegetable sources of proteins such as soybeans and nuts contain some of all the essential amino acids, but they do not have enough of one or more of them to be effective in meeting the needs for growth.

An understanding of the concept of limiting amino acids helps us understand why it is important to have a combination of different vegetable proteins throughout the day, rather than only one. By combining two proteins that are limiting in different amino acids, it is possible to simulate a complete protein. In this way, vegetarian diets can be as adequate in protein as diets containing both animal and vegetable proteins. For example, wheat has ample methionine but lacks lysine, and soybeans have ample lysine but are limited in methionine, so a combination of wheat and soybeans provides a mixture of amino acids capable of promoting growth. Also, adding a small amount of milk, which contains all of the essential amino acids, to a wheat cereal provides enough lysine to greatly enhance the ability of the wheat protein to promote growth. We practice this type of protein combination (or **complementation**) constantly when we eat combined foods, such as cereal with milk, macaroni with cheese, beans with rice, peanut butter on bread, or an egg sandwich.

The use of small amounts of animal protein with cereal protein is much more significant in parts of the world where most diets are based on one dietary staple, such as rice or corn. In such diets, even small amounts of fish or meat added to the staple can considerably enhance the overall protein quality of the diet. Figure 5-8 illustrates how the amino acid pattern of one protein can complement that of another and how the combination can more closely meet the adult requirements for amino acids. Mixtures of two vegetable proteins or small amounts of animal proteins added to larger quantities of vegetable proteins can provide high-quality protein at less cost than animal protein used alone.

It is also nutritionally significant that some tissues require large amounts of specific amino acids. The proteins of hair, skin, and nails, for example, contain unusually large amounts of the sulfur-containing amino acids cysteine and methionine. The pungent odor of burnt hair, skin, and nails is from the high proportion of sulfur-containing amino acids within them.

The proportions of the various amino acids in different foods cause the nutritional value of different foods to vary. Some animals are so sensitive to variations in amino acid pattern that they reduce their intake of, or even refuse to eat, foods containing an inappropriate amino acid mixture. Humans do not possess this instinct, and the variety of proteins present in most diets means that humans seldom need to think of the amino acids provided by each when planning a balanced diet. It is usually sufficient simply to ensure that sufficient protein is consumed. In reality, however, specific amino acids are the essential nutrients, rather than protein as a whole. It is the amount and proportion of amino acids present in the diet that ultimately determine the nutritional adequacy of the protein we consume.

EVALUATION OF PROTEIN QUALITY

Several biological and chemical measures are used to measure protein quality.[2] The most commonly used are the **biological value (BV), net protein utilization (NPU), protein efficiency ratio (PER),** and **amino acid score.**

$$\text{Biological value (BV)} = \frac{\text{Nitrogen retained}}{\text{Nitrogen absorbed}} \times 100$$

$$\text{Net protein use (NPU)} = \frac{\text{Nitrogen retained}}{\text{nitrogen intake}} \times 100$$

$$\text{Protein efficiency ratio (PER)} = \frac{\text{Weight gain in grams}}{\text{Protein intake in grams}}$$

$$\text{Chemical score} = \frac{\text{Actual milligrams of amino acid per gram of protein}}{\text{required milligrams or amino acid per gram of protein}}$$

FIGURE 5-8

Mutual complementation of low-quality protein A (such as wheat protein) lacking in lysine and low-quality protein B (such as bean protein) lacking in methionine. The two low-quality proteins complement each other to provide a good-quality protein overall.

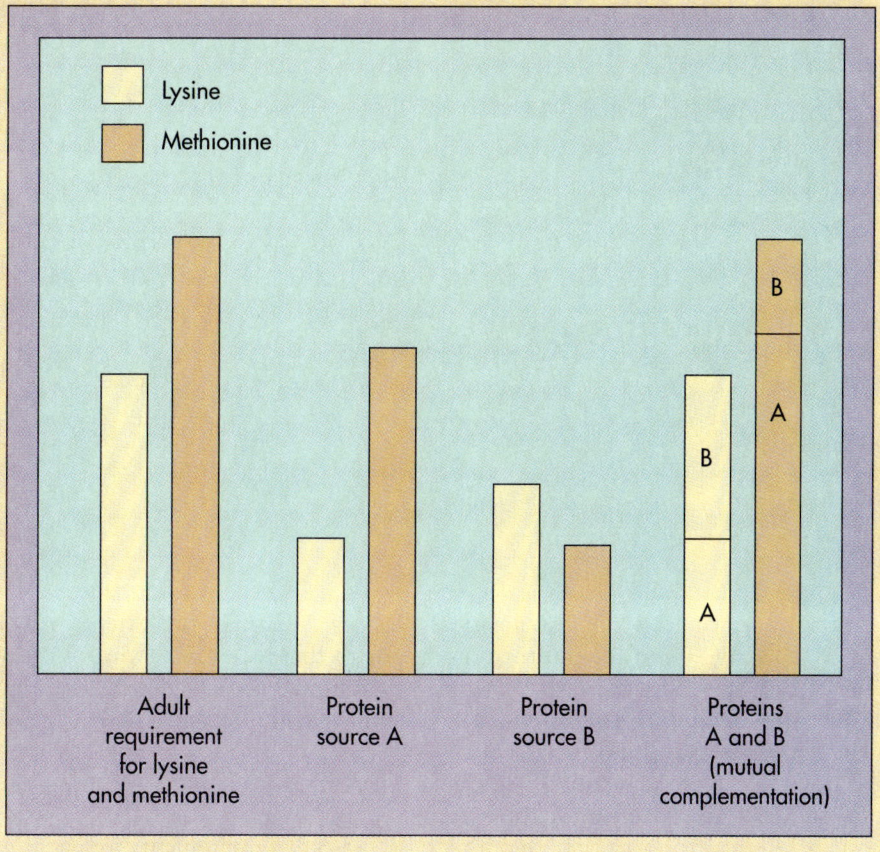

Biological Value

The BV of a protein is measured as the percentage of *absorbed* nitrogen that is retained (that is, not excreted) for use in growth or maintenance. This indicator is based on the assumption that more nitrogen is retained when the essential amino acids are present in sufficient amounts to meet the needs for growth. Determination of the BV of a protein involves controlled animal feeding studies, which makes it a costly and time-consuming procedure. A food or diet with a BV of 70 or more (meaning that 70% of the absorbed nitrogen is retained) is considered capable of supporting growth, assuming that the diet provides sufficient energy.

Net Protein Utilization

NPU is the percentage of *ingested* nitrogen that is retained. Because it does not take into account differences in the digestibility of proteins, it gives a poorly digested but good-quality protein a false low value.

Protein Efficiency Ratio

The PER is the simplest measure of protein quality, but it has some limitations. It is the ratio of the weight gain in grams to the grams of protein ingested in young rats. Casein, a high-quality protein in milk, has a PER of 2.5 and is the standard used for nutrient labeling purposes. The PER is based on the unproved assumption that weight gain in a growing animal is proportional to the gain in body protein.

Amino Acid Score

The amino acid score (or **chemical score**) method of assessing protein quality is based on measurements of the actual amounts of individual amino acids in a food or in the diet as a whole. The amino acid score is usually expressed as the ratio of milligrams of an amino acid per gram of protein in a food to the milligrams of the amino acid required per gram of protein for the age and gender group whose diet is being evaluated. This calculation yields a score for each essential amino acid, but the score

TABLE 5-4

Pattern of amino acid requirements at various ages, compared with the pattern of amino acids in beef, wheat, and the U.S. food supply (milligrams of amino acid per gram of protein)

	INFANT	PRESCHOOL (2-5 YR)	CHILD (10-12 YR)	ADULT	U.S. FOOD SUPPLY	BEEF	WHEAT
Histidine	26	20	18	16	30	34	19
Isoleucine	46	30	29	13	49	48	37
Leucine	93	70	46	19	87	81	61
Lysine	66	62	46	16	68	89	25
Methionine and cysteine	42	26	23	17	35	40	36
Phenylalanine and tyrosine	72	66	23	19	90	80	74
Threonine	43	36	29	9	42	46	31
Tryptophan	17	12	9	5	12	11	11
Valine	55	37	26	13	55	50	43
Total							
With histidine	460	359	244	127	468	479	337
Without histidine	434	339	226	111	438	445	318

From FAO/WHO/UNU, *Energy and protein requirements,* Tech Rep Series No 724, Geneva, Switzerland, 1985, World Health Organization. Values (mg/g of nitrogen [N]) can be calculated from these using the following formula: N – Protein × 6.25.
U.S. food supply is calculated from FAO Food Balance Sheets (FAO, 1980) using a simplified diet structure.
Beef and Wheat: Amino acid content of foods and biological data on proteins (FAO, 1970).

for the food or protein as a whole is the *lowest* ratio found (the limiting amino acid). From the information given in Table 5-4, it can be seen that for a 10- to 12-year-old child, the score for wheat (in which lysine is the limiting amino acid) is 0.54 (that is, 25/46). In contrast, it exceeds 1.0 (25/16 = 1.56) for an adult. Scores greater than or equal to 1 indicate that an amount of the lowest scoring amino acid equal to or greater than the required amount is supplied. Therefore wheat protein could meet the needs of an adult but is not adequate for a growing child. The scores may also be quoted as percentages, with 1.0 becoming 100%, 0.54 becoming 54%, and so on.

The fact that there are so many different ways of assessing protein quality indicates that it is a complex task. Although the chemical score is the easiest to calculate, even if the analytical data required is available, there is unfortunately little evidence that animals—including humans—use protein as predicted by the score.

FACTORS AFFECTING PROTEIN USE

The amino acids generated from the breakdown of dietary protein and existing body protein (during turnover) can be used for the synthesis of new proteins or of nonprotein, nitrogen-containing compounds or deaminated and used as energy supplies. Five main factors determine the extent to which amino acids are put to these uses in varying situations[3]: (1) amino acid pattern, (2) energy adequacy, (3) immobility, (4) injury, and (5) emotional stress.

AMINO ACID PATTERN

A person's requirements for each individual amino acid varies with age and physiological state (stage of growth, pregnancy, lactation, and so on). So the value of a specific food in sustaining protein synthesis for growth or maintenance varies, depending on how close its amino acid pattern matches a person's requirements at any particular time. A food may have an amino acid pattern that meets the needs of one group of people (such as adults) while being inadequate to support the needs of another group (such as growing boys who are synthesizing considerable protein-rich tissues).

ENERGY ADEQUACY

The suitability of the protein content of a diet cannot be evaluated without considering the adequacy of the total energy intake, meaning the total amount of energy available from all the food consumed. Not only does the protein eaten have the potential to be used as an energy source, but also energy is required for the synthesis of protein and for these reasons the rate of protein turnover is sensitive to the energy content of the diet. When kilocalorie intake falls below a certain critical level, amino acids are deaminated and used as a source of energy. This happens in individuals on low-energy diets, even if the protein content of the diet is increased.

IMMOBILITY

The ability to synthesize protein is greatly reduced in people who are immobile. Older people who are bedridden lose protein mass, even when dietary protein and caloric intake seem adequate. Astronauts have experienced a similar problem, losing protein as a result of both weightlessness and relative immobility during space flight.[4]

INJURY

Physical injury causes an increase in the rate of nitrogen loss in urine, presumably correlated with protein loss. Infection, fever, and surgical trauma can also result in significant nitrogen loss and increased use of energy sources. This loss occurs at a time when a person's need for protein and energy is itself increased because of the additional demand for protein synthesis to replace and repair damaged tissues.

EMOTIONAL STRESS

Emotional stresses such as fear, anxiety, and anger increase the secretion of epinephrine (adrenaline) from the adrenal gland. This in turn causes a series of changes that results in increased nitrogen loss via the urine. Students lose additional nitrogen when under the stress of examinations and in other anxiety-producing situations. Severe pain, the reversal of biological rhythms during night-shift work, and air travel across time zones are also capable of increasing nitrogen loss.

PROTEIN REQUIREMENTS

The need for protein and amino acids is estimated in three different ways for infants, children, and adults. For young infants growing at a satisfactory rate, the amount of protein and the pattern of amino acids in human milk are considered appropriate for optimal growth. Therefore recommendations for infants are based on the total protein content and amino acid pattern of the average daily intake of human milk. This amounts to 750 ml of milk per day during the first 6 months and 600 ml during the second 6 months. For children the **factorial method** is used. This involves an estimate of all the unavoidable nitrogen losses through urine, feces, and skin, plus an allowance for growth. In adults, **nitrogen balance** measured at various levels of protein intake has supplied most of the information on which estimates of protein needs are based.

NITROGEN BALANCE

Because all proteins contain around 16% nitrogen by weight, a simple chemical analysis for nitrogen can be used as a means of calculating how much protein the nitrogen has come from or could be converted into. Nitrogen values are converted to protein values simply by multiplying by 6.25 (which is 100/16).

> In **positive nitrogen balance,** nitrogen intake exceeds nitrogen loss. In **negative nitrogen balance,** nitrogen loss exceeds nitrogen intake. In **nitrogen equilibrium,** nitrogen intake exactly matches nitrogen loss.

Nitrogen balance is a measure of the relationship between the amount of nitrogen taken into the body and the amount excreted in urine or feces or from the surface of the skin. When nitrogen intake exceeds nitrogen loss, a person is in **positive nitrogen balance**. When nitrogen loss exceeds nitrogen intake, a person is in **negative nitrogen balance**. If nitrogen intake exactly matches nitrogen loss, a person is in **nitrogen equilibrium** (Figure 5-9).

All nitrogen intake comes from food, and nitrogen losses occur for various reasons. Losses through the urine include nitrogen released from the breakdown of body proteins because of protein turnover. Such nitrogen, derived from inside the body, is termed **endogenous** nitrogen. Some urinary nitrogen, however, is derived from dietary or **exogenous** nitrogen, which is taken in within proteins that are in excess of the requirements for growth and maintenance; these proteins are deaminated, and their nitrogen is passed to the urine. Exogenous nitrogen also appears in the urine when energy intake is so low that some of the absorbed amino acids are immediately deaminated to be used as a source of energy, with the nitrogen again being lost in urine. Fecal losses include endogenous nitrogen derived from proteins secreted during digestion and within sloughed intestinal cells and exogenous nitrogen within dietary protein that is not digested. Other losses of nitrogen from the body include nitrogen in skin cells shed from the surface of the skin, lost hair, nail clippings, saliva, and perspiration. Obligatory nitrogen losses in young adults fed diets con-

FIGURE 5-9

Diagrammatic representation of nitrogen balance.

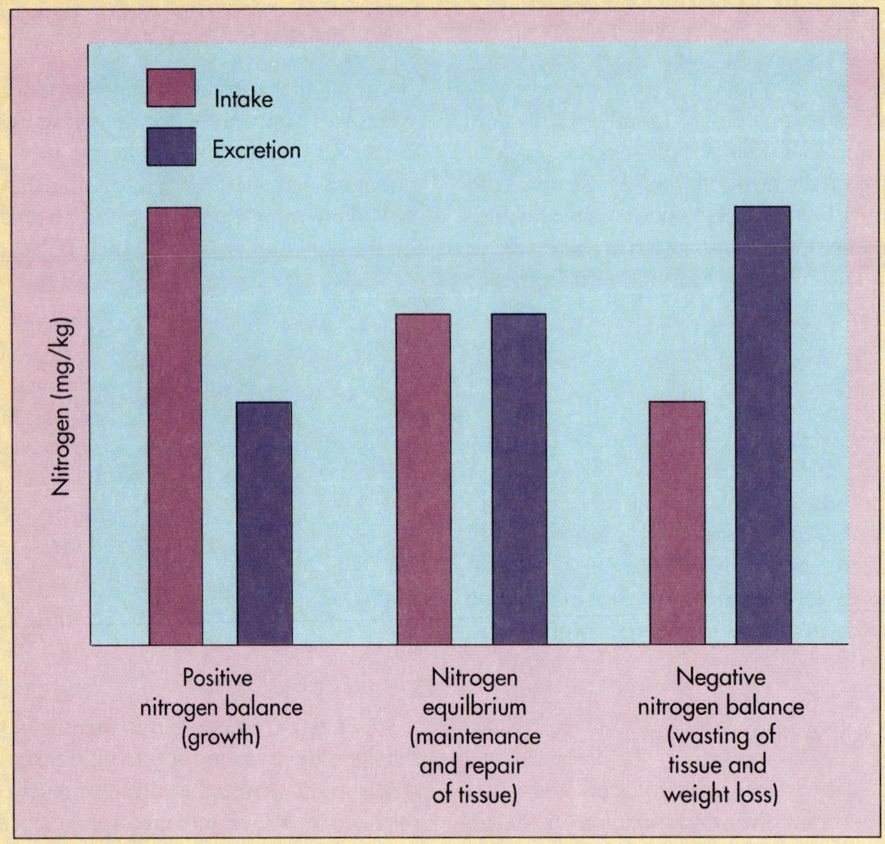

taining no protein average 53 mg/kg of body weight per day. This represents about 23 g of protein (about 4/5 of an ounce) lost by a 70-kg man per day.

The state of nitrogen equilibrium, in which nitrogen intake equals nitrogen losses, occurs in adults who are receiving as much dietary protein as they need, or more. In this state the intake of protein is sufficient to replace net loss of protein, but no growth is occurring.

The state of positive nitrogen balance, in which nitrogen intake exceeds nitrogen losses, indicates that growth is occurring. The excess nitrogen retained within the body must be converted into additional protein during growth. A positive balance should occur throughout infancy, childhood, and adolescence and during pregnancy. It also occurs during recovery from an illness in which protein has been lost. A positive nitrogen balance, known as **adult growth**, is sometimes seen in adults for no obvious reason.

The state of negative nitrogen balance, in which nitrogen losses exceed nitrogen intake, occurs when the proteins of the body are being broken down at a faster rate than they are being replaced. Prolonged negative nitrogen balance shows up as a loss of weight. This occurs most often when there is a severe energy deficiency in the diet, especially when the protein intake is also low. People who are immobile, under emotional stress, or have suffered an injury are especially prone to a loss of body protein that reflects in a negative nitrogen balance.

Nitrogen balance studies give information on changes in body protein mass but provide no indication of a shift of body proteins from one tissue to another. For example, levels of plasma albumin protein may drop, even though a person is in nitrogen equilibrium, if a person's labile protein pool has been depleted to meet the needs of other tissues.

The need for protein has always been considered to be just below the lowest level of intake that results in nitrogen equilibrium and just above the highest level of intake that results in negative nitrogen balance. The nitrogen equilibrium point can be carefully determined by a series of nitrogen balance studies in which the amount of dietary protein is reduced step by step until a negative balance occurs. The intake is then increased in another series of experiments, each of which usually takes 1 to 3 weeks, until positive balance is restored. The real required intake lies between these two levels of intake. This conforms to the definition proposed by the Food and Agriculture Organization/World Health Organization/United Nations University (FAO/WHO/UNU) Committee on Protein and Energy Requirements.[5] The FAO/WHO/UNU definition states that the "requirement for protein is the intake needed to prevent loss of body protein and to allow for adequate deposition or production of protein during growth, pregnancy, or lactation."

Based on both long-term and short-term nitrogen balance studies, the protein requirement for adults appears to be 0.75 g of a high-quality protein per kilogram of body weight per day. This figure provides a 25% margin of safety, representing two standard deviations above the mean of 0.63 g/kg/day. It is assumed that this intake meets the needs of all healthy adults. However, because the total amounts of protein in most diets include some low-quality protein, it is important to increase intake sufficiently above the recommended figure to allow for this.

The quality of protein in a diet depends on the pattern of amino acids in the diet compared with the pattern of amino acid requirements.[6] Because the pattern of requirements varies depending on age and physiological state, the quality of any given diet also varies depending on who is consuming it. Also, the typical pattern of amino acids in the diet varies among different countries. The typical amino acid pattern of diets in the United States was computed using the data reported in the Nationwide Food Consumption Study (NFCS). After making further correction to allow for the fact that protein is about 92% digestible (85% digestible in a vegetarian diet), it is possible to arrive at a final figure representing the need for protein in the diet. Table 5-5 shows the recommended protein intakes of U.S. citizens calculated using the approach recommended by the FAO/WHO/UNU Committee on Protein and Energy Requirements. Average body weights and food protein quality scores appropriate to the United States are shown. Recommended dietary allowances (RDAs) for protein are given as daily grams per kilogram values and also as total grams per day values. Table 5-6 shows the comparable calculations made for Canadian citizens based on usual protein intake of Canadians.[7] The levels of dietary protein recommended by Health and Welfare Canada are slightly higher than those recommended for U.S. citizens.

There is now evidence that protein requirements should be set slightly higher to allow for the fact that even when high-quality protein is being consumed, some is used as a source of energy.[8] So not all of the amino acids absorbed are available for the synthesis of protein and other vital nitrogen-containing compounds in the body.

Although we have traditionally assessed the adequacy of the diet in terms of protein and continue to do so, many nutritionists believe that essential amino acid requirements should be focused on rather than protein requirements. This is a much more complex task because we would have to deal with nine requirements rather than just one. However, the information to estimate amino acid requirements is available. It has been obtained in the same way that estimates of protein requirements were, by eliminating one amino acid from the diet until negative nitrogen balance occurs and then adding progressively larger amounts of the amino acid until nitrogen equilibrium (in most adults) or positive nitrogen balance (if growth is occurring) is restored. Estimates of amino acid requirements for people living in the United States, based on the recommendations of the FAO/WHO/UNU, are presented in Table 5-4. This table makes it clear that amino acid requirements vary with age. Experience has shown that in addition to the need for essential amino acids, there is a need for nitrogen for the synthesis of nonessential amino acids. It is also evident that the amino acids that are likely to be limiting in the diet are lysine, cysteine and methionine (the two sulfur-containing amino acids), threonine, and tryptophan. However, few diets consumed in the United States are low in essential amino acids.

Throughout growth the proportion of the total protein intake needed for growth decreases, whereas that needed for body maintenance increases (Figure 5-10).

FIGURE 5-10

Protein needs for growth and maintenance of the body throughout the life cycle.

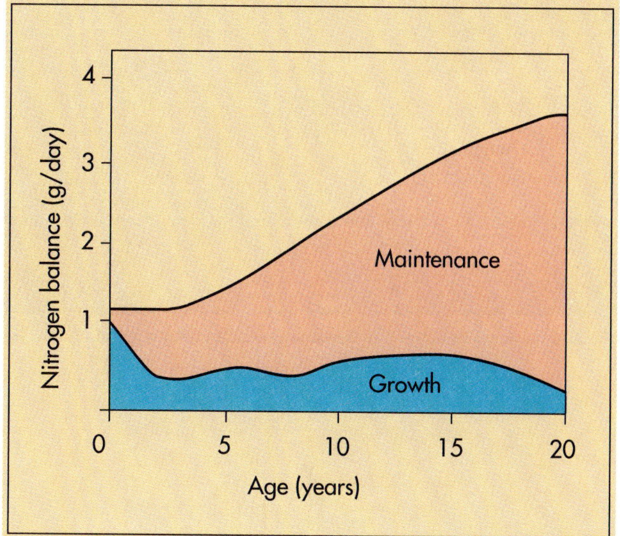

TABLE 5-5

Derivation of the recommended allowances of U.S. dietary protein

AGE (YEARS)	WEIGHT (kg)	SAFE ALLOWANCE OF REFERENCE PROTEIN g/kg	SAFE ALLOWANCE OF REFERENCE PROTEIN g/DAY	SCORE*	ESTIMATED NPU†	RECOMMENDED ALLOWANCE g/kg	RECOMMENDED ALLOWANCE g/DAY
INFANT‡							
0.5	6.0	2.20	13.2	1.00	0.90	2.0	13
0.5-1	9.0	1.56		0.78	0.70	1.64	14
CHILDREN							
1-3	13	1.14	13.0	0.82	0.74	1.2	16
4-6	20	1.03		0.99	0.90	1.1	24
7-10	28	1.00	28.0	1.00	0.90	1.0	28
MALES							
11-14	45	0.98	45.0	1.00	0.90	1.0	45
15-18	66	0.86	53.0	1.00	0.90	0.83	59
19-24	72	0.75	55.0	1.00	0.90	0.83	58
25-50	79	0.75	59.0	1.00	0.90	0.83	63
51+	77	0.75	58.0	1.00	0.90	0.83	63
FEMALES							
11-14	46	0.94	42.0	1.00	0.90	0.83	46
15-18	55	0.81	47.0	1.00	0.90	0.83	44
19-24	58	0.75	44.0	1.00	0.90	0.83	48
25-50	63	0.75	47.0	1.00	0.90	0.83	46
51+	65	0.75	49.0	1.00	0.90	0.83	50
PREGNANCY							
First trimester			+ 1.3	0.70	0.63		+2
Second trimester			+ 6.1	0.70	0.63		+10
Third trimester			+10.7	0.70	0.63		+17
LACTATION							
First 6 months			+14.7	0.70	0.63		+22
Second 6 months			+11.8	0.70	0.63		+13

* Amino acid score based on comparison of intake pattern for various ages in United States to requirement.

† Net protein utilization (NPU) = Amino acid score × Coefficient of digestion of 0.9.

‡ Breast milk consumption assumed.

From National Academy of Sciences: *Recommended dietary allowances,* ed 10, 1989, Washington, DC, National Academy Press.

TABLE 5-6

Derivation of the recommended intake of Canadian dietary protein

AGE	MAINTENANCE (mg/kg/DAY)	GROWTH (mg/kg/DAY)	AVERAGE NITROGEN REQUIREMENT (mg/kg/DAY)	+2SD (mg/kg/DAY)	CV%*	RECOMMENDED INTAKE OF EGG OR MILK PROTEIN (g/kg/DAY)	STATE LEVEL OF DIETARY PROTEIN: QUALITY ADJUSTMENT	STATE LEVEL OF DIETARY PROTEIN: (g/kg/DAY)
MONTHS								
0-2	100	147	247	334	19.7	2.15	1.0	2.15†
3-5	100	64	164	212	14.6	1.32	1.1	1.46†
5-8	100	48	148	188	13.4	1.17	1.2	1.41
9-11	100	39	139	174	12.7	1.09	1.26	1.37
YEARS								
1	100	24	124	153	11.8	0.96	1.26	1.21
2-3	100	19	119	147	11.7	0.92	1.26	1.16
4-6	100	13	113	139	11.7	0.87	1.22	1.06
7-9	100	11	111	137	11.7	0.86	1.20	1.03
10-12 M	100	11	111	137	11.7	0.86	1.18	1.01
F	100	12	112	138	11.7	0.86	1.18	1.01
13-15 M	100	12	112	138	11.7	0.86	1.14	0.98
F	100	8	108	133	11.8	0.83	1.14	0.95
16-18 M	100	7	107	132	11.9	0.83	1.12	0.93
F	100	1	101	126	12.4	0.79	1.12	0.86
19+	100	0	100	125	12.5	0.78	1.10	0.86

* Coefficient of variation (CV) for maintenance taken as 12.5%; CV for growth taken as 32%.

$$CV_{TOTAL} = \frac{\sqrt{(\text{Maintenance} \times \text{CV Maintenance})^2 + (\text{Growth} \times \text{CV Growth})^2}}{\text{Maintenance} + \text{Growth}}$$

† Safe level of protein intake in infants up to 4 months of age is based on the assumption that human breast milk is providing the sole source of protein. If other protein sources are being consumed, the safe level of intake must be calculated correcting for the essential amino acid profile and digestibility of the protein sources in question.

FOOD SOURCES OF PROTEIN

The protein content of the most frequently used foods within the major food groups is shown in Table 5-7, and the relative amounts of protein per serving of some foods are shown in Figure 5-11. In assessing the amount of protein in a food, one must keep in mind that foods containing all the essential amino acids are more useful than those with low or limiting amounts of one or more essential amino acids. Thus as a general rule proteins from animal sources are better suited to the amino acid requirements of humans than are proteins from vegetable sources. Within each group, however, different proteins have a wide range of biological value. Most Western diets provide ample protein, and even when the use of animal protein is limited, the quantity and quality of protein intake is of little concern. In the absence of liver or kidney diseases, the human body can metabolize much more protein than the recommended intake without any risk of harm.

Because protein-rich foods are usually the most expensive items in the diet, it is useful to compare the relative costs of equal amounts of protein from various food sources. This is especially helpful if someone is trying to plan nutritionally adequate meals on a limited food budget.

The relatively high cost of protein may explain why meals are described in terms of the major protein component (ham dinner, chicken casserole, cheese fondue, and so on). It may also explain why meals have a tendency to be planned around a protein item, rather than starting the planning with a less expensive salad or dessert item.

In assessing the adequacy of protein in a diet, one must look at the protein sources. Although a knowledgeable person can plan a diet with protein of high biological value using vegetable foods alone, it is usually recommended that about one third of protein should be of animal origin. As can be seen in Figure 5-12, about three fourths of the protein in the American diet is of

TABLE 5-7

Protein in average servings and per 100 kcal of foods most frequently used foods within the major food groups and other recommended sources

FOOD	AMOUNT	KCAL	PER SERVING (GRAMS)	PER 100 KCAL	INQ*
EGGS, MEAT, POULTRY, FISH, NUTS					
Egg, fried	1 large	95	6	6	2.6
Beef, roast	3 oz	315	19	6	2.8
Hamburger	3 oz	230	21	9	4.0
Chicken	3 oz	140	27	19	8.5
Tuna	3 oz	65	24	14	6.4
Peanut butter	2 T	190	10	5	2.2
Bacon	3 slices	110	6	5	2.2
Pork†	3 oz	295	23	7.7	2.5
CEREAL PRODUCTS					
Beans, kidney†	½ cup	115	7.5	6.5	2.0
Cornflakes	1 cup	110	2	2	0.6
Shredded wheat	1 biscuit	100	3	3	0.9
Saltines (10 g)	4 crackers	50	1	2	0.6
Rice	1 oz dry (½ cup cooked)	109	2	2	0.6
White bread	1 slice	65	2	3	0.9
Whole wheat bread	1 slice	70	3	4	1.2
DAIRY PRODUCTS					
Whole milk	8 oz	150	8.0	5	2.2
2% fat milk	8 oz	120	8.0	7	3.0
Cheddar cheese	1 oz	115	7.0	6	2.6
FRUITS					
Apple	1 medium	80	0.3	0.4	0.1
Banana	1 medium	105	1.1	1.0	0.3
Orange juice, frozen	4 oz	55	0.8	1.4	0.4
Peach	1 medium	35	0.6	1.7	0.5
VEGETABLES					
Corn, canned	4 oz (½ cup)	82	2.5	3	1.1
Green beans	4 oz (½ cup)	22	1	5	1.5
Green peas	4 oz (½ cup)	62	4	6	1.8
Lettuce	¼ head	20	1	5	1.5
Tomatoes	1 medium	25	1	4	0.8
Potato, baked	1 medium	130	3	2	0.7

* Index of nutrient quality (INQ) = RDA (%) for protein (45 g animal protein or 65 g vegetable protein)/energy requirement (%) (2000 kcal).

† Other recommended sources.

FIGURE 5-11

Relative amounts of protein in average servings of various foods.

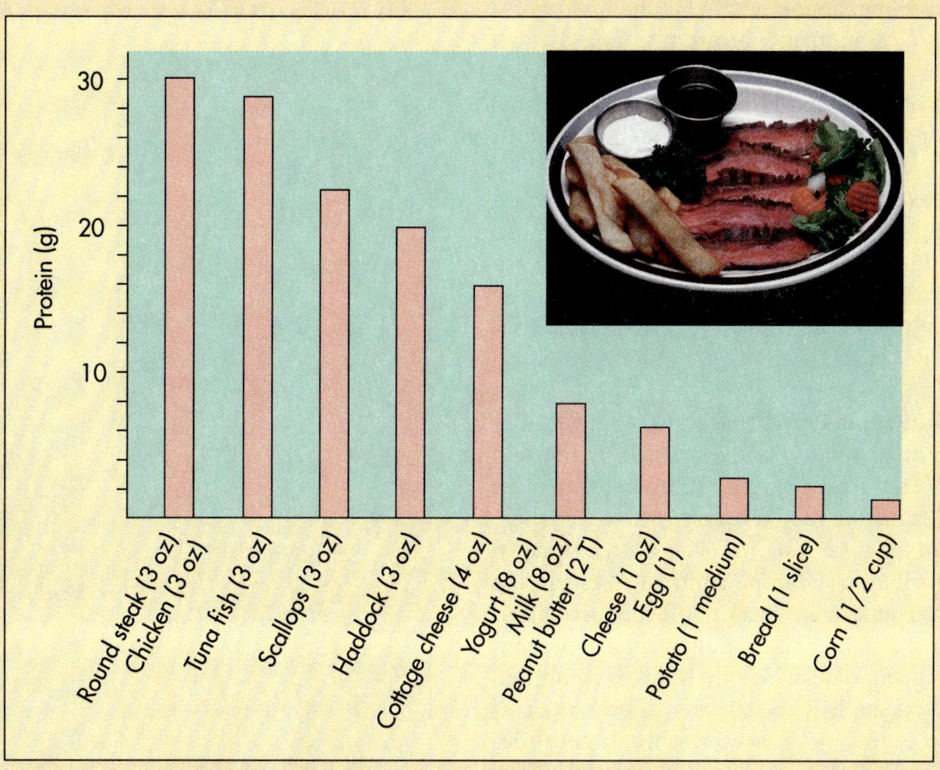

FIGURE 5-12

The contribution of various food groups to the protein available in the U.S. food supply in 1988.

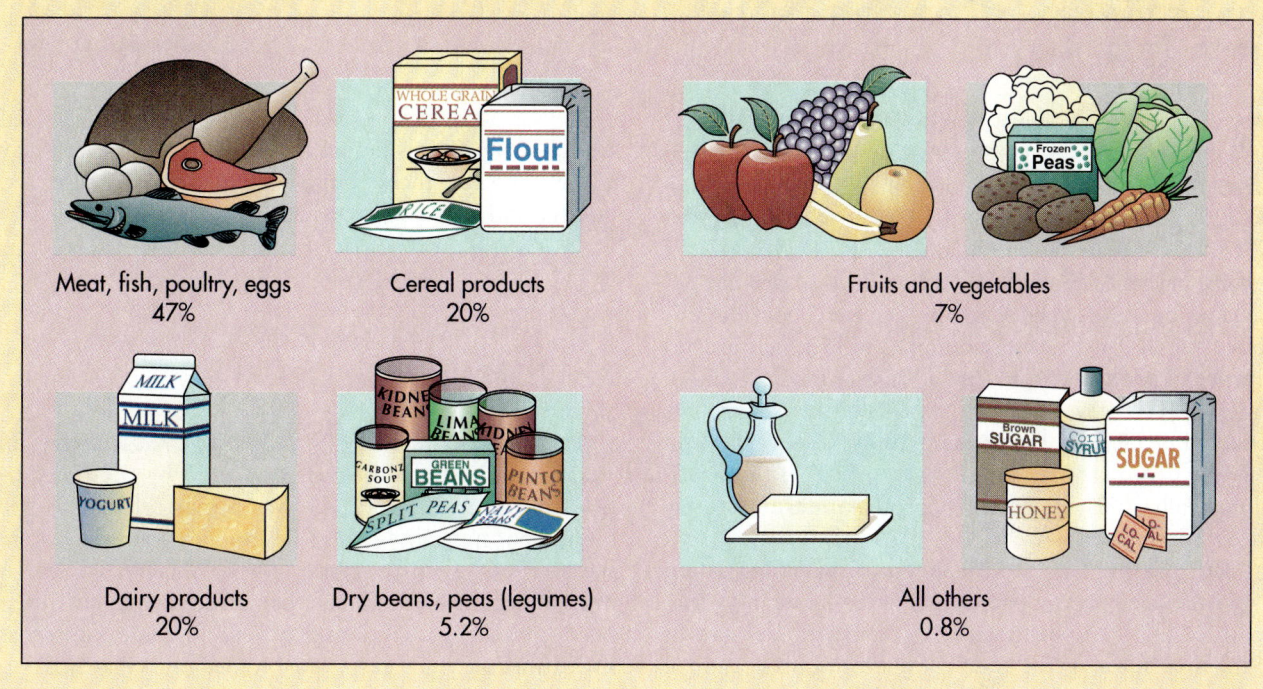

animal origin. Whatever foods are consumed, they should be distributed in such a way that daily meals contain all the essential amino acids. The increasing use of dried milk solids in many bread products, which belong to the cereal group, gives these bread products a protein content of enhanced biological value. Similarly, flour products made with eggs or milk contain good-quality protein.

Such seeds as pumpkin, sunflower, and sesame are often promoted as rich protein sources. They do indeed have a high percentage of protein but are not a practical source of large quantities of protein because they are also high in fat and relatively expensive. Also, some people find that seed fiber causes intestinal irritation.

The efforts of some entrepreneurs to promote the addition of limiting amino acids, especially lysine and methionine, to cereals and legumes to enhance protein quality are not justified in the Western world where there is no dietary problem as a result of poor protein quality. Also, if supplementation with one amino acid creates an amino acid imbalance, the quality of the protein is decreased rather than improved. Amino acid supplementation may be appropriate when the diet is composed primarily of a cereal staple with little animal protein. This supplementation is feasible, however, only in countries where dietary staples are processed in relatively few centers so that the addition of nutrients can be monitored and controlled.

FIGURE 5-13

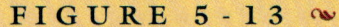

Sources of protein in the U.S. food supply in 1988 and at the start of the twentieth century.

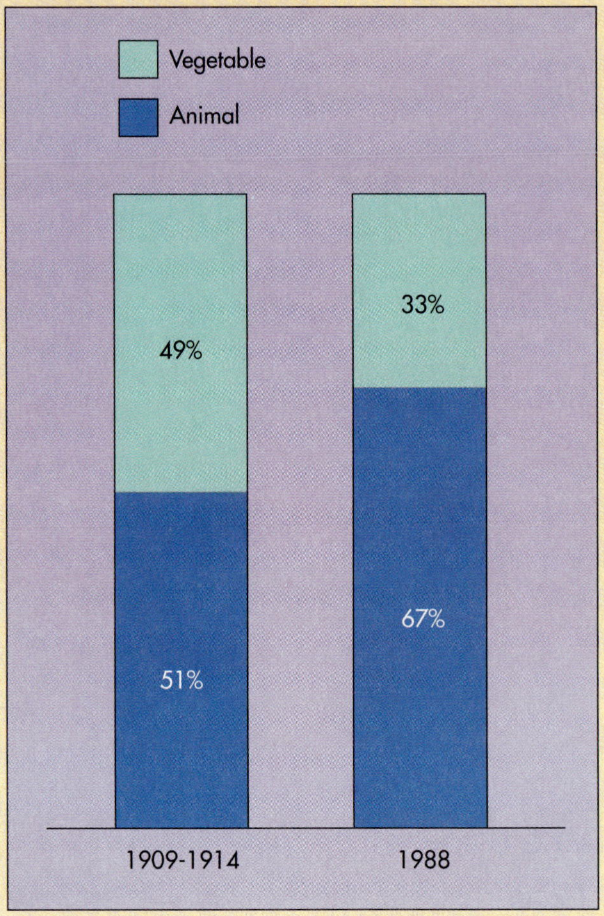

ADEQUACY OF PROTEIN IN THE U.S. DIET

The analysis of data from both the NHANES III and the NFCS 1987-1988 surveys showed that there was no deficiency of protein in the more than 50,000 people studied in the United States. In the NHANES III survey, mean intakes of 74 to 110 g of protein per day for males and 58 to 70 g of protein per day for females, depending on age, were considerably above the RDAs. Serum albumin levels, which are indicative of protein status, were all above standard values. In the NFCS 1987-1988 survey, 88% of the participants reported protein intakes meeting 100% of the RDA, and only 2% had diets providing less than 80% of the RDA. Almost all of those with low protein intake had low kilocalorie intakes as well.[9]

In 1988 the U.S. food supply provided about 105 g of protein per person per day.[10] This is similar to that provided in 1909, which was 99 g per person per day. In 1988 two thirds of the total protein came from animal sources, whereas at the beginning of the century animal and vegetable sources contributed roughly equal amounts of protein (Figure 5-13). This change is largely a result of the increased consumption of cheese and poultry and decreased consumption of grain products.

PROTEIN-ENERGY MALNUTRITION

During the late 1940s and early 1950s interest in protein nutrition was stimulated by the observation that protein deficiency was a major factor in the high infant mortality rate of developing countries where starch roots, such as cassava, were dietary staples. A protein deficiency condition that affected young children between the ages of 2 and 5 years became known as **kwashiorkor**. This term was coined by Ghanaians to describe an illness that struck the firstborn child when a second child was born. The literal translation of *kwash-*

iorkor is "first-second." Once it was recognized that the condition developed within 3 to 4 months after the older child was abruptly weaned from the breast, which was its only source of good-quality protein, the condition was identified as a protein deficiency. Children suffering from kwashiorkor fail to gain weight and may in fact lose weight and become apathetic, listless, and withdrawn. Most important, these children become increasingly susceptible to infection. Such conditions as fever and measles, which are only temporarily disruptive in the lives of well-fed children, are severely debilitating and often fatal for a child with kwashiorkor.

It was soon recognized that kwashiorkor is closely related to another condition called **marasmus**, whose name comes from the Greek word for "wasting." Marasmus is caused by a chronic lack of energy in the diet. When energy intake is insufficient, protein is diverted from its role in growth and maintenance to be used as a source of energy, thus causing a protein deficiency.

Kwashiorkor and marasmus are examples of what is now termed **protein-energy malnutrition (PEM)** as a result of our increasing knowledge of the complex interrelationship between protein deficiency and energy deficiency.[11] Deficits of either protein or energy, or both, are major problems that affect as many as half the children in Third World countries.[12]

Regardless of whether the primary deficit is in energy, protein, or protein quality, the main clinical symptoms associated with PEM are as follows:

- Failure to grow in height and in weight
- Behavioral changes ranging from the irritability of kwashiorkor to the apathy of marasmus
- Edema, which is the accumulation of fluid in the tissues that causes them to be soft and spongy (especially in the lower abdomen, arms, and legs)
- Skin changes, including changes in color, lack of color, drying, peeling, and the eventual formation of ulcers that heal slowly (if at all) and allow a point of entry for infectious microorganisms
- Changes in the hair, which becomes dry and sparse and either loses its pigmentation (which gives it its normal color) or takes on a characteristic red color
- Vomiting, diarrhea, and loss of appetite, all of which result in severe dehydration and loss of sodium and potassium
- Enlargement of the liver
- Anemia
- Increased susceptibility to infection and fever, which follow a much more devastating course than normal

FIGURE 5-14

Children suffering from kwashiorkor (left) and marasmus (right) as a result of inadequate energy intake.

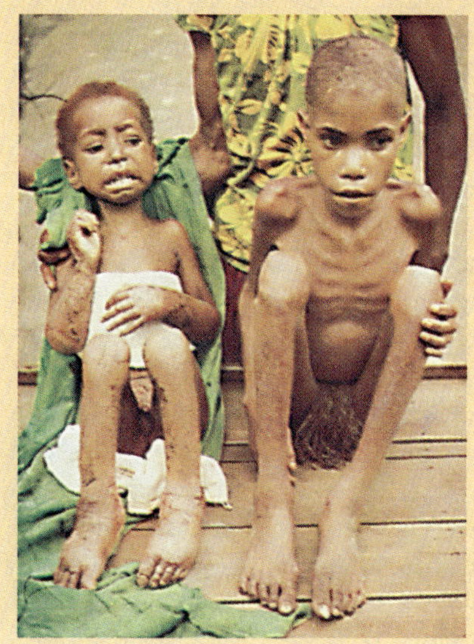

The effect of this severe malnutrition is evident in the photograph of a child with kwashiorkor (Figure 5-14, *left*). This can be contrasted with the effect of marasmus, an energy deficit, illustrated in Figure 5-14, *right*. Children affected by PEM but who survive to age 5, when they can compete more effectively for food and can forage for themselves, do reasonably well thereafter. However, they are seldom able to make up the growth deficit of their earlier years. The causes of severe undernutrition and malnutrition in developing countries are many and varied and are discussed in more detail by Torun and Chew.[14]

VEGETARIANISM

Vegetarianism, or the reliance on foods of vegetable origin for nourishment, has been practiced throughout history by a wide variety of people for different reasons, particularly focused on religion, health concerns, and ethical qualms about the welfare and killing of animals.

In the latter half of this century many people have become vegetarians because they are concerned about our ability to feed the world's population if we continue to eat animals that themselves eat other animals or forage on potential crops for food. These people choose vegetarianism for a combination of ecological, political, economical, and ethical reasons.

Although many people call themselves vegetarians (several million in the United States alone), only a small number are actually true vegetarians—or **vegans**—in the sense that they eat no animal-based foods. Vegans avoid milk, cheese, butter, eggs, and all other products derived from animal sources, even though animals are not killed to produce them. An even more restrictive diet is that of the **fruitarians,** who do not eat animals, animal-based products, vegetables, or cereals, leaving them with a diet of only dried fruit, nuts, and perhaps honey.

Much more common than vegans are the **ovolactovegetarians.** They do not eat any food obtained by slaughtering animals but have no objection to consuming products derived from animals without slaughter, such as eggs, *ovo*, and milk, *lacto* (in Latin).

Ovolactopollovegetarians eat poultry in addition to eggs and milk, whereas **pescovegetarians** consider fish an acceptable food (and perhaps also eggs, milk, cheese, and so on) but not any land animals.

Macrobiotic diets are vegetarian diets based on a balance of foods with opposing "**yin**" (weak) and "**yang**" (strong) characteristics. Macrobiotic diets consist mostly of whole grains and vegetables but include the use of special teas, herbs, seaweed, and fermented soybean products. Most adherents to this diet participate in a series of rituals and eat at least one meal per day in a communal setting. An extreme form is the **Zen macrobiotic diet,** which requires its adherents to proceed in 7 to 10 steps to reduce the variety of foods in the diet until only brown (whole grain) rice is consumed or a balance of "strong" and "weak" food is achieved. Many followers of this diet believe that it can cure any disease because it is supposed to rid the body of toxins. Although such a diet is deficient in vitamins, calcium, and high-quality protein, the lack of vitamin C is the first deficiency to become apparent. Scurvy (vitamin C deficiency) has been reported among those who follow this diet, especially pregnant women and young children. The restricted fluid intake designed to "spare" the kidneys presents an additional hazard because this diet is high in sodium, which increases thirst and the need for fluid. The use of seaweed, with its high salt content, to alleviate thirst only makes the problem worse.

The NFCS respondents were asked whether they were vegetarians. Of the 2% to 3% who indicated that they were, 90% reported eating animal-based foods over a 3-day period. This suggests that the use of the term *vegetarian* is loosely interpreted by the lay person.

What, if any, are the nutritional consequences of eating a vegetarian diet, rather than the omnivorous (animal and vegetable) diet consumed by most Westerners? The answer depends on what degree of vegetarianism is adhered to and also on the age of the vegetarian.

The true vegetarian (vegan) diet probably poses the greatest risks to young, growing children and pregnant women. It is possible to design a strictly vegetarian diet for a young child that meets the needs for all nutrients apart from calcium and vitamin B_{12}. Such a diet is so bulky, however, that it is unlikely that enough food is consumed to meet the energy needs of a young child. As was discussed earlier, if the diet does not provide adequate energy, some of the protein that normally is used for growth is diverted for use as an energy source. This is even more of a problem when the quality of the protein is marginal. Thus we find that many young vegetarian children are at about only the fifth percentile in weight and height for their age and gender; so almost all of the children in their age and gender group are taller and heavier.

Part of the growth retardation in vegetarian children may reflect the low calcium content of their diet and the fact that calcium is poorly absorbed from vegetable foods. The poor absorption of calcium is a particular problem with such vegetables as spinach, which contain significant amounts of **oxalic acid**, an organic acid that binds to calcium. **Phytic acid**, found in the outer husk of grain and therefore present in whole grain cereals, also binds to calcium and other minerals and so reduces their absorption into the body. Because calcium is essential for bone growth, it is easy to understand why there might be decreased stature among vegetarian children.

The role of vitamin D in bone growth cannot be overlooked either. Studies in Boston have found cases of rickets, a vitamin D–deficiency disease, among vegetarian children who are not allowed to drink milk. Vitamin D can be synthesized within the body on exposure to the ultraviolet rays of the sun, but in a northern city, such as Boston, where exposure to the sun is limited, milk may be the only significant source of vitamin D.

In a vegetarian diet, zinc—which is obtained principally from animal foods—is present in inadequate amounts, as is vitamin B_{12}, which comes only from animal foods.[13] It is possible that a breast-fed child may build up a substantial store of vitamin B_{12} during the nursing period to last through the first few postweaning years.

A lack of vitamin B_{12} could be a partial explanation for the "anemia" observed in certain people after relatively short periods on a meatless diet. Another factor contributing to anemia is the bulk or fiber content of a vegetarian diet, which tends to bind iron and other trace minerals and greatly reduce the amount absorbed. Also, fiber stimulates the passage of food through the GI tract, further reducing the absorption of trace minerals and other nutrients. The total amount of iron in the vegetarian diet, which almost certainly falls below the 15 mg/day recommended for adult women, and the absence of meat, which normally enhances iron absorption, increase the possibility that a vegetarian diet will contribute to anemia.

Why then do vegetarians believe that there are nutritional benefits that justify their diet? For children the disadvantages clearly seem to outweigh any advantages. For adults, concern over the relationship between cholesterol and heart disease is one common motivation for avoiding animal products. Cholesterol does not occur in plant foods, and the adult body is capable of synthesizing sufficient cholesterol, which—despite its bad reputation—is a vital component of body chemistry. In addition to being devoid of cholesterol, a vegetarian diet is usually low in fat, with the only fat coming from whole grain cereals, nuts, vegetable oils, and the occasional use of avocados. Vegetable oils and margarines, however, can contribute a large amount of fatty acids if used liberally to increase the palatability of vegetarian meals. These fatty acids, however, are primarily unsaturated, except for those in hydrogenated oils within margarines and in the rarely used coconut oil and palm oil. It is now recommended that polyunsaturated fatty acids should not account for more than 10% of total energy intake. This is based on evidence that health problems may be associated with a high polyunsaturated fatty acid intake because of the tendency of unsaturated fatty acids to become oxidized to substances whose safety has not been established. This offers a possible explanation for the reported increase in colon cancer among people with low serum cholesterol levels.

For adults the advantages of a strict vegetarian diet are that it is low in energy, fat, and cholesterol and that it contains adequate fiber. These advantages must be weighed against the disadvantages of decreased zinc content, poor availability of trace minerals and calcium, and the virtually complete lack of vitamin B_{12}. Most people who call themselves vegetarians are not vegans, however, because they eat amounts of such foods as eggs, milk, and cheese that vary greatly from person to person. The variability of such diets makes it impossible to generalize about their advantages and disadvantages overall.

ISSUES AND OPINIONS

Protein Needs of the Athlete

The protein needs of athletes during training, competition, and recovery after competition have been the subject of many scientific investigations over the past decade. The results indicate that the protein needs of athletes are somewhat higher than those of typical, moderately active people. The increased need for protein can be easily met by diets containing "everyday" foods without the use of specific protein or amino acid supplements.

Normal, healthy people who are not athletes require about 0.8 g of protein per kilogram of body weight. Bodybuilders who train to increase muscle mass and strength need about 1.12 times the normal amount. Endurance athletes—such as long-distance runners and cyclists, who train to develop skeletal and cardiac muscle—need 1.67 times the normal amount. The high-energy intake of athletes almost guarantees that they consume the required amount of additional protein. For a typical 80-kg athlete on a 3000-kcal diet with 55% of the energy coming from carbohydrate, 30% from fat, and 15% from protein, total protein intake is approximately 112 g. The estimated daily protein requirement of an 80-kg bodybuilder is 72 g (1.12 × 0.8 g/kg = 0.9 g/kg), and of an 80-kg long-distance runner is 104 g (1.67 × 0.8 g/kg = 1.3 g/kg). So a typical mixed diet normally provides more than enough protein, even for the endurance athlete.

Amino acid supplements and purified liquid and powdered protein supplements are among the most popular ergogenic (work-enhancing) aids currently being promoted for endurance athletes and bodybuilders. It is claimed that the supplements can build muscle, stimulate fat loss, and speed muscle repair. So these supplements are promoted as legal, ethical, and healthful alternatives to banned anabolic steroids.

The amino acid supplements currently promoted to athletes contain either single amino acids or a combination of different amino acids. They fall into two groups: those which supposedly stimulate growth hormone release (arginine and ornithine) and the branch-chained amino acids (BCAAs) (leucine, valine, and isoleucine), which are supposedly the preferred energy source for muscle during endurance exercise.

It is true that arginine and ornithine stimulate growth hormone production but only when infused in amounts well above normal physiological levels (30 g or more of arginine, for example). Also, both endurance and resistance exercises alone increase serum growth hormone levels to an extent only slightly less than that achieved by infusion of large doses of arginine. So athletes are unlikely to benefit from gram doses of oral arginine, when infusion of 30 to 60 times as much produces only a modest effect over and above the effect of exercise alone.

There is strong evidence that protein synthesis in muscle is decreased by endurance exercise but not necessarily by resistance exercise. This decrease in protein synthesis is accompanied by increased oxidation of BCAAs to provide energy. Greater amino acid oxidation occurs when glycogen stores are depleted and in people who have not trained. The amino acid oxidation stops during the recovery phase. However, because athletes are likely to consume more BCAAs than they need simply by eating a typical diet, the use of specific BCAA supplements is unnecessary and has not been proved to enhance performance.

The amino acid tryptophan is promoted to athletes as a natural tranquilizer to be taken before competition. The logic behind this is that tryptophan is a precursor of the neurotransmitter and neuromodulator serotonin. A tryptophan supplement offers no more value, however, than consuming a food source rich in tryptophan, such as a glass of milk or a piece of lean meat.

Contrary to popular belief, eating extra protein does not build muscle, stimulate the production of growth hormone, or provide a superior fuel for exercising muscle. There is simply no evidence that a well-nourished athlete needs to consume expensive protein or amino acid supplements of no proven benefit. In Canada the sale of all single or combination amino acid supplements (except tryptophan) is banned. Such products are available in the United States because a 1975 court ruling stopped the Food and Drug Administration (FDA) from regulating these supplements (except for pregnant and lactating women and children under 12 years of age).

From Napeer K: *Priorities* 4:36, 1992; and Hauston ME: *Nutr Today* 27:36, 1992.

BY NOW YOU SHOULD KNOW

- Protein is essential for the growth and maintenance of all body tissues and for the manufacture of all enzymes and many hormones.
- Dietary protein and new proteins synthesized by the body are composed of varying amounts of 20 different amino acids.
- Amino acids, and therefore proteins, contain nitrogen atoms, unlike carbohydrates and lipids.
- The R group, or side chain, makes each amino acid unique.
- There are nine amino acids that are essential in the diet because they cannot be synthesized by the body.
- There are 11 amino acids that are not essential in the diet because they can be synthesized in the body, provided that sufficient nitrogen and energy are available.
- Protein needs are determined by nitrogen balance studies, which involve measuring the intake of dietary nitrogen in relation to the excretion of nitrogen in urine and feces and in other unavoidable ways.
- Proteins are synthesized in the body under the direction of the base sequence of the genes that are composed of deoxyribonucleic acid (DNA) and are found in the cell nucleus.
- Protein synthesis occurs on the ribosomes, where the base sequence of a messenger ribonucleic acid (RNA) copy of a gene determines the sequence in which amino acids are incorporated into a growing protein chain.
- Proteins perform a wide variety of vital functions involved in the growth and maintenance of tissues, the formation of essential body compounds, the regulation of water balance, the transport of nutrients, the maintenance of pH values, defense against infection, and detoxification of toxic compounds.
- Protein digestion begins in the acidic environment of the stomach.
- Amino acids are absorbed in the small intestine.
- If energy intake is sufficient, absorbed amino acids are used for protein synthesis. If energy intake is insufficient to meet energy needs or if absorbed amino acids are in excess of needs, the absorbed amino acids are deaminated. The nitrogen atoms are excreted as urea within urine, whereas the carbon and hydrogen atoms are oxidized to release energy or stored as carbohydrate or fat.
- The amount of dietary protein recommended for adults to maintain body tissue is 0.83 g/kg of body weight per day.
- Additional protein is needed for growth during childhood, adolescence, and pregnancy and for milk production during breast-feeding.
- Dietary proteins are of differing "quality," depending on the pattern of amino acids they contain.
- Good sources of dietary protein are meat, fish, poultry, eggs, cereals, legumes, seeds, and nuts.
- There is no evidence of protein deficiency in the North American diet.
- Kwashiorkor and marasmus are protein-energy deficiency diseases that occur most often in young children in developing countries.

STUDY QUESTIONS

1. How is the chemical composition of protein different from that of carbohydrate or fat? How does this difference affect the biological function of protein?
2. How is nitrogen cycled from plants to animals?
3. Why are some amino acids considered essential in the diet? Why is it necessary to consider the amino acid pattern of the protein in food when determining protein requirements?
4. Under what conditions is protein broken down and used for energy?
5. How does animal protein differ from vegetable protein?
6. What is meant by protein complementation?
7. What is meant by nitrogen balance? Describe the situations that alter nitrogen balance.
8. Trace the digestion and absorption of a protein-rich meal.
9. How is protein quality evaluated?
10. Differentiate between kwashiorkor, marasmus, and protein-energy malnutrition.
11. Suggest some possible solutions that may decrease the incidence of protein-energy malnutrition in developing countries.

CRITICAL ANALYSIS

How does your intake of protein compare to your RDA? A quick way to check would be to estimate your intake for one third of a day and compare it to ⅓ of your RDA. Recall lunch today or dinner last night. Count the number of servings you ate from the following food groups. Multiply the number of servings by the grams of protein per serving to get grams of protein from each food group. Add these numbers to get the total grams of protein consumed.

	NO. OF SERVINGS	GRAMS OF PROTEIN PER SERVING	GRAMS OF PROTEIN FROM THIS GROUP
Grains	________	× 3 =	________
Vegetables	________	× 3 =	________
Meats/ substitutes	________	× 3 =	________
Dairy	________	× 3 =	________
		Total grams of protein =	________

Calculate your RDA for protein based on 0.8 grams of protein per kg of body weight (divide body weight in pounds by 2.2 to get kilograms).
______ (body weight in lbs) = ______ kg
______ kg × 0.8 = ______ grams of protein recommended per day (your RDA)
Divide your RDA by 3 and compare it to the total grams of protein you calculated from the meal above.

(⅓ of your RDA vs grams of protein for ⅓ hours)

Did your protein intake at dinner equal ⅓ or more of your RDA? Many people consume their largest meal and, therefore, most of their protein at dinner. If this is your dietary pattern and you received less than ⅓ of your RDA from dinner, it might be worthwhile to complete a 3 day food intake record and analyze it to get a much better estimate of your protein intake. The current exercise is quick and easy, but it is not able to accurately tell you when your intake is too low. Most healthy adults in the United States exceed their RDA for protein.

REFERENCES

1. Munro HN, editor: *Mammalian protein metabolism,* vol 4, New York, 1970, Academic Press.

2. *Nutritional evaluation of protein foods,* Washington, DC, 1978, National Academy of Sciences.

3. Millward DJ, Rivers JPW: The nutritional role of indispensable amino acids and the metabolic basis for their requirements, *Eur J Clin Nutr* 42:367, 1988.

4. Leonard JI, Leach CS, Rambaut PC: Quantification of tissue loss during prolonged space flight, *Am J Clin Nutr* 38:667, 1983.

5. FAO/WHO/UNU: *Energy and protein requirements,* Tech Rep Series #724, Geneva, Switzerland, 1985, World Health Organization.

6. Reeds PJ: Amino acid needs and protein scoring patterns, *Proc Nutr Soc* 49:489, 1990.

7. Health and Welfare Canada: *Nutritional recommendations,* Ottawa, Canada, 1990, Canadian Government Publishing Center.

8. Young VR, Bier DM, Pellet PL: A theoretical basis for increasing current estimates of the amino acid requirements in adult men with experimental support, *Am J Clin Nutr* 50:80, 1989.

9. Wright HS and others: The 1987-1988 Nationwide Food Consumption Survey: an update on the nutrient intake of respondents, *Nutr Today* 26:21, 1991.

10. Raper NR, Zizza C, Rourke J: *Nutrient content of U.S. food supply, 1909-1988,* USDA Home Economics Research Report Washington, DC, 1992 U.S. Government Printing Office.

11. Latham MC: Protein-energy malnutrition. In Brown ML, editor: *Present knowledge In nutrition,* ed 6, Washington, DC, 1990, International Life Sciences Institute.

12. Grant J: *The state of the world's children,* New York, 1985, United Nations International Children's Fund.

13. Herbert V: Vitamin B_{12}: plant sources, requirements, and assay, *Am J Clin Nutr* 48:852, 1988.

14. Torun B, Chew F: Protein energy malnutrition. In Shils ME, Olson JA, Shike M, editors: *Modern nutrition in health and disease,* ed 8, Philadelphia, 1994, Lea & Febiger.

ADDITIONAL READINGS

Allen LH: The nutrition CRSP: what is marginal malnutrition and does it affect human functions? *Nutr Rev* 51:255, 1993.

American Dietetic Association: Position of American Dietetic Association: vegetarianism diets, *J Am Diet Assoc* 93:1317, 1993.

Beaton GH, Calloway DH, Murphy SP: Estimated protein intakes of toddlers: predicted prevalence of inadequate intakes in village populations in Egypt, Kenya, and Mexico, *Am J Clin Nutr* 55:902, 1992.

Beaton GH, Chery A: Protein requirements of infants: a recrimination of concepts and approaches, *Am J Clin Nutr* 48:1403, 1988.

Christensen HN: Amino acid nutrition: a two-step absorption process, *Nutr Rev* 51:95, 1993.

Dwyer JT: Nutritional consequences of vegetarianism, *Annu Rev Nutr* 11:61, 1991.

Olson, R, editor: *Protein-calorie malnutrition,* New York, 1975, Academic Press.

Schrimshaw NS: On the occasion of the 1991 world food prize, *Nutr Today,* 28(3):35, 1994.

Young VR, Pellett PL: Protein intake and requirements with reference to diet and health, *Am J Clin Nutr* 45:1323, 1987.

Young VR, Pellett PL: Mechanisms and nutritional significance of metabolic responses to altered intakes of protein and amino acids, with reference to nutritional adaptation in humans, *Am J Clin Nutr* 51:270, 1990.

Young VR, Pellett PL: Plant proteins in relation to human protein and amino acid nutrition, *Am J Clin Nutr* 59(suppl):1203S, 1994.

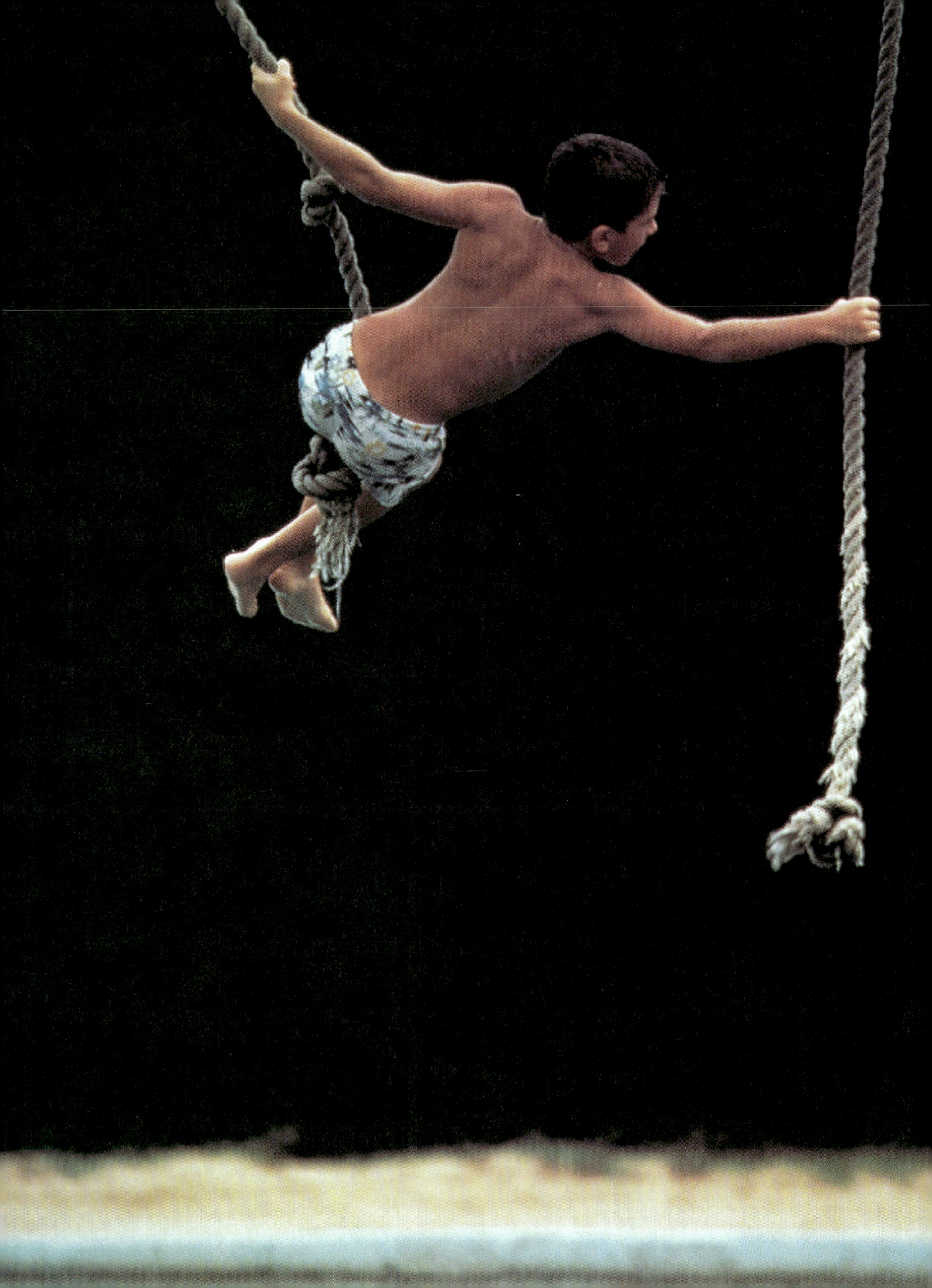

CHAPTER 6

ENERGY BALANCE

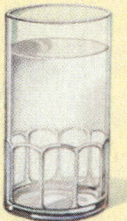

The relationship between the energy content of food and body weight has long been the aspect of nutrition of most concern to the public. There seem to be more "instant experts" on this subject than on any other in nutrition. Scientists are working to understand the different ways in which people use energy and why there are differences in the energy requirements of apparently similar people. Meanwhile, however, the public is being bombarded with advice and help from many sources aimed at solving their problems related to energy balance. The sedentary life-styles that have resulted from the growing mechanization of technologically advanced societies have decreased total energy requirements. This has led to concern that reduced intakes of energy may result in deficient intakes of some vital nutrients. There is a growing view that moderate exercise programs should be encouraged to increase energy needs to levels that correspond more closely to our desire for food and permit increased intake of nutrients.

Energy is a rather subtle property of physical systems that is defined as "the ability to do work." Physicists say "work" is done when a **force** is applied through some distance. This means that the energy of a system is a property of the system that is able to "make changes happen" through the application of forces. There are two basic forms of energy: **kinetic energy** and **potential energy**. Kinetic energy is the energy things possess because they are moving, whereas potential energy is the energy systems contain because of the *positions* of their parts. The student of nutrition is primarily interested in the energy contained within the chemicals of food, which can be released from food to become embodied within the chemicals of the body or used to heat the body or allow it to move. So consideration of energy in nutrition is focused on *chemical* energy and the kinetic energy of motion.

All chemicals contain some **internal energy** resulting from the movement of their electrons (kinetic energy) and the way in which their negatively charged electrons and positively charged nuclei are arranged relative to one another (potential energy). Chemicals also contain some additional kinetic energy, known as **heat energy,** resulting from the *overall* motion of the atoms, molecules, or ions they contain. So when nutritionists talk about the energy contained in food, the energy released from food, the energy required to make certain chemicals of the body, and so on, they are referring to the internal energy contained within chemicals and the heat energy that can be released from or taken up by compounds as chemical reactions proceed (see Appendix A).

What has been said so far should make it clear that energy is a precisely defined property of chemicals and other physical systems. It is also, however, a term used in everyday language. To most people, energy means pep and vitality. People talk of feeling "full of energy" or of "not having the energy" to undertake some strenuous or tiresome activity. Energy is usually measured in units called kilocalories, or calories (1 kilocalorie = 1000 calories). *Calories* is another term used in everyday language. People talk of food being high in calories or low-calorie, and so on, and often use the terms *calories* and *energy* interchangeably. There is a distinction between energy and calories because energy is a specific fundamental physical property, whereas the calorie is a unit used for the measurement of energy. To say that energy and calories mean the same thing is like saying distance means the same as miles, or money means the same as dollars—it is not strictly correct but causes no real confusion in practice. Thus the loose usage of the terms *energy* and *calories* in everyday language can be readily traced back to the precisely defined physical property known as energy, which is usually measured in kilocalories or calories.

People have different attitudes about the energy (or kilocalories) in food, depending on their circumstances. To nutritionists, the energy content of food is one of its most vital properties that is required to build and maintain a healthy body, although certainly undesirable in excess. Athletes value "high-calorie" foods for their ability to supply the energy required to win, and young mothers know that their children need calories to grow and be active. However, to many people who fear or are troubled by weight gain, calories are the worst of food villains to be avoided as much as possible.

The carbohydrate, lipid, protein, and alcohol in the diet, discussed in the preceding three chapters, are the components of the diet responsible for its energy content. Water, vitamins, and minerals provide no energy, although they are essential for other reasons. The energy of carbohydrates, lipids, proteins, and alcohol is made available to the body when these chemicals are oxidized in the energy-releasing reactions of respiration. Overall, these reactions achieve the same chemical transformation as burning; so we need only watch foods burn to realize how much energy they contain within them. This basic chemical link between respiration and burning (more technically, combustion) also justifies everyday talk of "burning up" food or "burning off" excess fat by exercising.

The four energy-containing components of a food (carbohydrate, lipid, protein, and alcohol) together account for widely varying proportions of the chemicals present in foods overall. Only 4% of the weight of lettuce, for example, is made up of these energy-providing nutrients, whereas sugar, salad oil, and dry gelatin are composed entirely of energy-providing substances. The proportion of a food that does not provide energy is composed of varying amounts of water, minerals, vitamins, and fiber. Fiber is largely cellulose, which is a carbohydrate, but one that cannot be digested by humans. It is important to remember that not all of the carbohydrate within a food is in a form that can be used as a source of energy by humans.

In the typical diet consumed in North America, carbohydrate provides 43% to 58% of dietary energy supplies, protein provides 12%, and fat provides 30% to 45% (Figure 6-1). Since the turn of the century the amount of fat has increased from 122 to 168 g/person/day. The amount of carbohydrate decreased from 493 g/person/day around the turn of the century to 382 g/person/day in 1970 but then increased again to reach 425 g/person/day by 1988. The availability of protein throughout the century has remained essentially constant, at around 99 to 105 g/person/day.[1]

The sources of energy within diets vary among individuals as well as among different ethnic and socioeconomic groups. In countries in which cereal is a dietary staple, for example, carbohydrate makes a large contribution to total energy intake. In countries in which many dairy products are available, protein ac-

FIGURE 6-1

Percentages of energy (kilocalories) contributed by carbohydrate, fat, and protein in the typical North American diet.

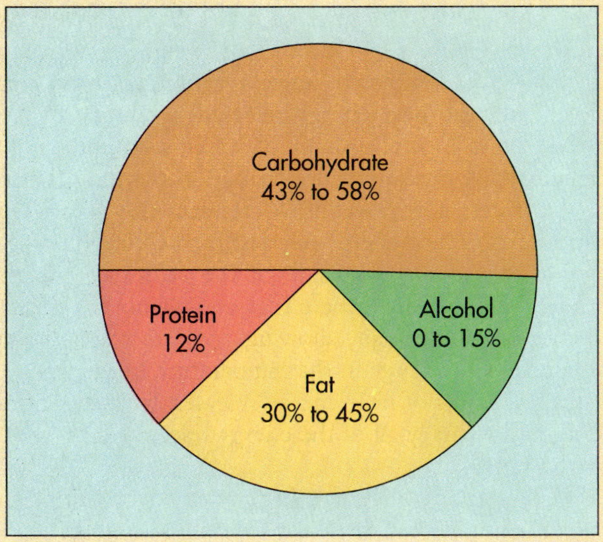

counts for a larger proportion of energy supplies. In Italy, where extensive use is made of oils, more energy is provided by fats than in many other countries. In the United States the amount of money available for the purchase of food has generally increased over the years, resulting in an increased use of animal foods, an increased proportion of kilocalories being provided by protein, and a decreased consumption of complex carbohydrates. More recently, however, concern about the ability of the world food supply to meet the needs of an ever-increasing population has led many North Americans to reduce their intake of animal protein and replace it with cereal grains. People concerned about the relationship between fat intake and health problems, such as heart disease and cancer, are also reducing their intake of fat and increasing their intake of carbohydrate.

MEASURING ENERGY

The energy value of food, meaning the amount of energy that can be obtained from food for use by the body, is expressed in kilocalories (kcal). All forms of energy are interconvertible, but 1 kcal of energy is usually defined in terms of the amount of *heat energy* to which it corresponds. One kilocalorie is defined as the amount of heat energy required to raise the temperature of 1 kg of water 1° C at normal atmospheric pressure. The kilocalorie is also known as the *Calorie*, with a capital *C*, whereas the calorie (lower case *c*) is one thousandth of a kilocalorie (or Calorie), or 0.001 kcal.

In many discussions of nutrition the terms *kilocalorie, Calorie,* and *calorie* are used interchangeably, with the assumption that their definitions are well enough known that no distinction need be made. When quoting specific energy values, however, it is obviously important to know exactly what unit is being used. In this book, as in all nutrition books, we use the kilocalorie as the standard specified unit of energy. All the values quoted in kilocalories are identical to values in Calories (because 1 kilocalorie equals 1 Calorie) but must be divided by 1000 to convert them into calories.

The amount of heat energy required to raise the temperature of 1 kg of water 1° C at normal atmospheric pressure is 1 kilocalorie (kcal):

1 kcal = 1000 calories
1 kcal = 1 Calorie
1 Calorie = 1000 calories
1 calorie = 0.001 kcal
1 kcal = 4.18 kJ
1 calorie = 4.18 joules

There is a growing trend in all countries except the United States to use the kilojoule (kJ) as the standard unit of energy, instead of the kilocalorie. The kilojoule (which equals 1000 joules) is normally defined in terms of the amount of "work" the energy could do, which depends on what physical force it could exert over a given distance. One kilojoule is defined as the energy required to push against a force of 1 Newton (N) for a distance of 1 meter (m). Although the kilojoule is defined in terms of physical work and the kilocalorie in terms of heat, it is important to realize that they are simply alternative units for exactly the same thing, namely energy. Physical work and changing temperatures are just two different effects of the transfer of energy from place to place. One kilocalorie is equal to 4.18 kJ; so 1 calorie equals 4.18 J. Where the kilojoule has been adopted in place of the kilocalorie, all the kilocalorie values simply need to be multiplied by 4.18 to convert them to kilojoule values. Thus a 2000-kcal/day diet is equivalent to a 8360-kJ/day diet. Some food scientists have suggested that a larger unit of energy be used, the megajoule (mJ), as our standard unit. A megajoule equals 1000 kJ, or 1 million J. If this suggestion is ever adopted, all of our energy values will look much smaller, with a 2000-kcal/day diet becoming an 8.36-mJ/day diet. It is the absolute amount of *energy* provided by the diet or used by the body that is the important thing, however, not the particular unit in which we choose to measure it.

It will undoubtedly be some time before the term *calorie,* as used in popular literature, becomes replaced by the more correct *kilocalorie,* or even *Calorie.* It will probably take even longer before the concept of the kilojoule receives popular acceptance in the United States. It is important, however, for the student of nutrition to be aware of the various alternative ways of measuring and quoting energy values because they all appear in various places within the literature of nutrition.

A general appreciation of the amount of energy available from foods can be gained by noting that 2 Tbsp of sugar releases 100 kcal of energy when fully oxidized to carbon dioxide and water (either via respiration or by burning in air). If it were all released in the form of heat energy, this would be sufficient to raise the temperature of slightly more than 4 cups of water from 0° C (its freezing temperature) to 100° C (its boiling temperature). The same amount of energy would be released from the oxidation of 1 Tbsp of fat or 4.5 cups of shredded cabbage. In humans as much as 80% of the energy provided by our food is released immediately in the form of heat, with the rest being used to drive the energy-requiring biochemical processes that sustain the body and allow us to move. Apart from the actual amount of chemical energy stored within the chemicals of the body, *all* the energy of our food is eventually released as heat, and even the chemicals of the body eventually give up their energy as heat after death, when the body decomposes or is cremated. This is an important point of biochemical energetics: Each individual living thing is a temporary high-energy structure that is sustained by the continual *flow* of energy through it.

DIRECT CALORIMETRY

Much of our information about how much energy can be released from foods is obtained by a technique called **direct calorimetry,** which means the direct measurement of heat. This is based on the fact that the chemical changes that occur when carbohydrate or fat is oxidized during respiration in the body are identical *overall* to the chemical changes when these chemicals are burned in air. Thus the maximal energy that can be released by these foods in the body can be calculated by measuring how much heat energy they release when they burn. For protein, the situation is slightly different. When protein burns in air, its nitrogen is combined with oxygen, releasing energy. This does not happen to dietary nitrogen in the body. Nevertheless, once an appropriate correction has been made, as discussed below, calorimetry data can also yield information about the energy available to the body from protein. Thus the burning of a certain amount of food under controlled conditions can tell us how much energy the body could obtain from that food.

The instrument used to perform direct calorimetry measurements is the **bomb calorimeter,** which is a highly insulated boxlike container about 1 cubic foot in size. The essential features of a bomb calorimeter are shown in Figure 6-4. A precisely weighed sample of dried food is completely burned within a central container, and the heat energy released is completely absorbed by a known amount of water surrounding the container. By measuring the change in the temperature of the water, it is possible to calculate the number of kilocalories of heat energy released by the burning of the sample. Because the outside of the calorimeter is extremely well insulated, there is essentially no loss of heat to the surrounding air, allowing accurate results to be obtained. The change in the temperature of the water is entirely a result of heat energy released by the burning food, and virtually all of the energy released is absorbed by the water.

The amount of heat energy released by burning a known amount of a particular food in a bomb calorimeter is known as the food's **heat of combustion,** usually measured in kilocalories per gram. When samples of pure carbohydrate, fat, or protein are analyzed in this way, the heat of combustion values differ among the three types of nutrient but are always the same for samples of any one nutrient taken from different sources. Standard values have been obtained by burning representative samples of each nutrient, such as table sugar for carbohydrate, corn oil for fat, and egg albumin for protein. The generally accepted heat of combustion value obtained for carbohydrate is 4.1 kcal/g, for fat is 9.45 kcal/g, and for protein is 5.65 kcal/g. The value for alcohol is 6.93 kcal/g.

For carbohydrate, fat, and alcohol, the heat of combustion values obtained by calorimetry accurately reflect the *maximal* amount of energy that absorbed molecules of these foods can release within the body. This is because when these nutrients burn, their atoms are oxidized to only carbon dioxide and water, a process that also occurs in the body. As has been previously mentioned, however, nitrogen atoms in dietary protein are not oxidized in the body to release energy, but they are when protein is burned in a calorimeter. The oxidation of nitrogen atoms in a calorimeter (Figure 6-2) accounts for 1.3 kcal per gram of the energy released. This means that the maximal amount of energy available to the body from dietary protein is actually 4.35 kcal/g, which is 1.3 kcal lower than the heat of combustion value.

The process of digestion does not proceed with 100% efficiency, and so the entire amount of any ingested nutrient does not eventually become available to the body's cells. This means that when the amount of energy that is really available to the body from a given amount of food is calculated, the efficiency with which it

FIGURE 6-2

Cross-section of a bomb calorimeter. Food is completely burned in the inner section, the heat produced is absorbed by the known volume of water in the surrounding section, and the change in the temperature of the water is measured and used to calculate the amount of heat energy produced.

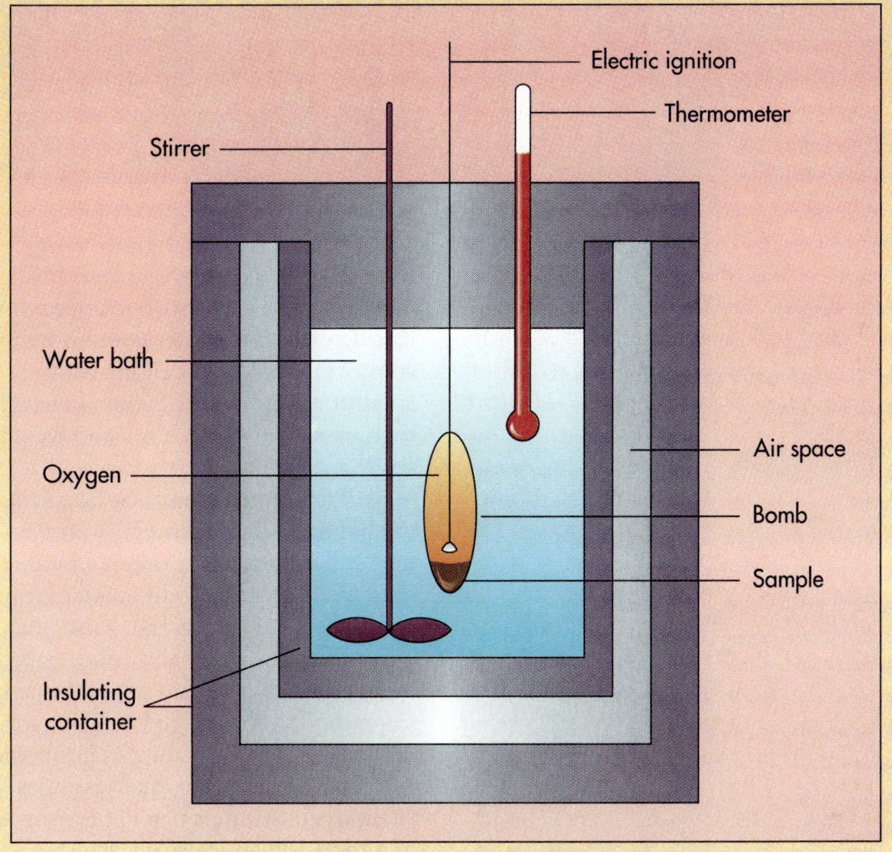

is digested must be taken into account. This varies for different nutrients and is also influenced by the food in which a nutrient is present. For example, the protein of egg, meat, or milk is more readily digested (or **bioavailable**) than protein from such plant sources as wheat, rice, and vegetables. A representative average figure, called the **coefficient of digestibility,** is used to express the proportion of an ingested nutrient that ultimately becomes available to the body's cells. For carbohydrate, the coefficient of digestibility is 0.98 (indicating that 98% of ingested carbohydrate becomes available). For fat, the coefficient of digestibility is 0.95 (95% becomes available), and for protein it is 0.92 (92% becomes available).

The important value from the point of view of human nutrition is the amount of energy actually *available* to the body from a given amount of nutrient. This is known as the **physiological fuel value** of the nutrient. It is calculated from the heat of combustion and coefficient of digestibility values for carbohydrate, fat, and alcohol, with an additional correction for the nonavailability of energy from the oxidation of nitrogen being made for protein (Table 6-1 and Figure 6-3). The slightly rounded off values of 4 kcal per gram of carbohydrate, 9 kcal per gram of fat, 4 kcal per gram of protein, and 7 kcal per gram of alcohol are widely used in nutrition and dietetics to plan and evaluate the energy content of diets.

The **physiological fuel value** of a food component is the maximal amount of energy that can be released to the body by the oxidation of the component concerned. The physiological fuel values of the four energy-releasing components of food are as follows:

- Carbohydrate: 4 kcal/g
- Fat: 9 kcal/g
- Protein: 4 kcal/g
- Alcohol: 7 kcal/g

TABLE 6-1

Calculation of the physiological fuel value of nutrients (kcal/g)

	CARBOHYDRATE	FAT	PROTEIN	ALCOHOL
Heat of combustion	4.15	9.45	5.65	6.93
Energy from combustion of nitrogen unavailable to the body	—	—	1.30	—
Net heat of combustion	4.15	9.45	4.35	6.93
Coefficient of digestibility	0.98	0.95	0.92	1.00
Physiological fuel value (kcal)	4.0	9.0	4.0	7
Physiological fuel value (kJ)	17.0	38.0	17	30

FIGURE 6-3

Amounts of energy (kilocalories) available per gram of the energy-yielding nutrients.

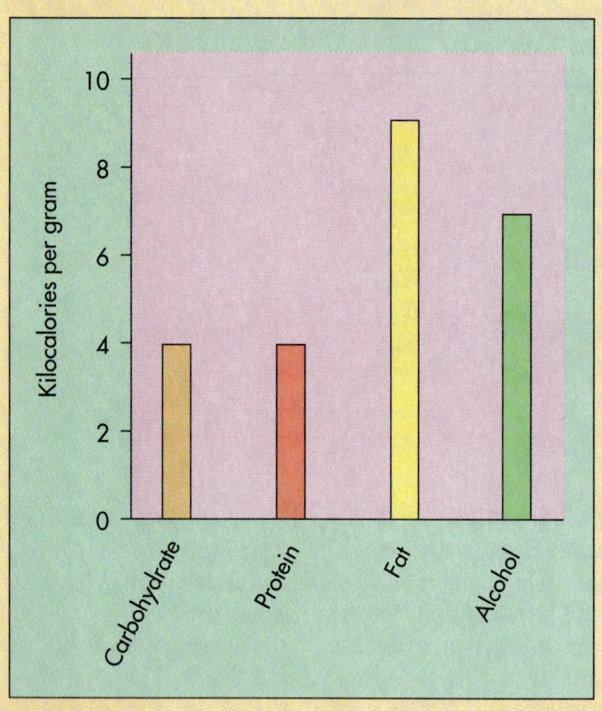

ENERGY VALUE OF FOODS

The amount of energy available from any particular food can be calculated by multiplying the physiological fuel values of the energy-yielding components of food by the amounts of each component present in any food. The amounts present can be determined by chemical analysis. The amount of fat in a food is determined directly by extracting the fat into suitable solvents. The amount of protein in a food is estimated by analytical determination of the amount of nitrogen present and then calculation of protein content from the knowledge that protein is on average 16% nitrogen by weight. To determine the carbohydrate content of a food, one must first determine its water content by drying the food and comparing its dry weight with its wet weight. The amount of crude fiber is then determined by boiling the food in acid and then alkali and weighing the crude fiber (mainly cellulose) that survives this treatment. The carbohydrate content can then be calculated by subtracting the amount of fat, protein, water, and crude fiber from the total weight of the original food. The figure obtained for carbohydrate content includes some dietary fiber that is not crude fiber in the sense that it does not resist breakdown by acid and alkali (see Chapter 3). This means that values for available carbohydrate may be somewhat overestimated and so are less accurate than the fat and protein values. The method of determining carbohydrate content also assumes that minerals and vitamins constitute a negligible proportion of the weight of a food, which is usually the case.

The results of analysis, as outlined previously, reveal what is called the **proximate composition** (proximate means approximate) of a food in terms of the percentages of carbohydrate, fat, protein, fiber, and water present in a typical sample of the food. Only the carbohydrate, fat, and protein, of course, are a source of energy. Table 6-2 shows how the proximate composition of a food can be used to calculate the energy value of the food by simply multiplying the amount of each energy-yielding component in 100 g of the food by the physiological fuel values of each component and then adding the results together. This yields a total energy value for the food in the form of kilocalories per 100 g, a figure that can then, by appropriate multiplication, reveal the energy value of any weighed amount of the food.

By calculating the total amounts of carbohydrate, fat, and protein in a person's diet, one can determine both the total kilocalorie content of the diet and the number of kilocalories provided by each nutrient group. This, in turn, allows us to calculate the percentage of total kilocalories provided by each nutrient group, as demonstrated in the box on p. 193. The boxed calculation also demonstrates that it is only necessary to know

TABLE 6-2

Calculation of the energy value of 100 g (3/4 cup) of ice cream from proximate analysis (percentage composition)

NUTRIENT	PERCENTAGE IN FOOD*	AMOUNT IN 100 g (GRAMS) A	ENERGY VALUE/GRAM (KCAL) B	ENERGY VALUE OF 100 g (KCAL) A × B
Carbohydrate	24	24	4	96
Fat	10	10	9	90
Protein	4	4	4	16
TOTAL ENERGY				202

* Remaining 62% is made up of water, which does not provide energy.

Calculation of Percentage of Total Calories Contributed by One Nutrient Group

PROBLEM

Given the information that a diet provides 2000 kcal and contains 200 g of carbohydrate and 100 g of fat, calculate the amount of protein and the percentage of calories from carbohydrate, protein, and fat in the diet.

SOLUTION

Carbohydrate provides 200 × 4 = 800 kcal.
Fat provides 100 × 9 = 900 kcal.
Because protein is the only other component in food to provide calories, the remaining kilocalories were provided by protein.
2000 − (800 + 900) = 300 kcal
Because 4 kcal are provided by each gram of protein, 300 kcal would be provided by 300/4 = 75 g protein.
The determination of the precentage of calories from a nutrient involves the following equation:

$$\frac{\text{Kcal from a nutrient}}{\text{Total kcal}} \times 100$$

The percentage of kilocalories from carbohydrate is 800/2000 × 100 = 40%.
The percentage of kilocalories from fat is 900/2000 × 100 = 45%.
The percentage of kilocalories from protein is 300/2000 × 100 = 15%.

the values for any three of the four relevant variables (carbohydrate content, fat content, protein content, and total energy value) in a diet to calculate the percentage of kilocalories provided by each of the three main energy-yielding nutrient groups. The value of the unknown variable is easily calculated from knowledge of the other three. If alcohol were present in the diet, of course, then it also must be taken into account.

VARIATION IN ENERGY VALUE

Different foods vary in their energy content because of the differing amounts of carbohydrate, fat, protein, and alcohol they contain. The differing energy values of foods can be expressed in terms of their differing values of kilocalories per 100 g, which relate energy content to the *weight* of a food. The differences can also be expressed, however, using the **energy density** or **caloric density** of a food, which relates its energy content to the *volume* of the food and can be quoted in kcal/dl or kcal/ml.

Foods with a high percentage of fat or a low water content are concentrated sources of energy because small amounts of such foods yield a relatively large number of kilocalories. They are often erroneously identified as "fattening" foods. Although it is easier to consume excess kilocalories by eating foods high in fat or low in water content, the foods themselves—such as cheese, butter, and peanut butter—should not simply be condemned as fattening. In suitable amounts they can be acceptable parts of weight-maintaining and even weight-reducing diets. Only diets as a whole can be described as fattening and then only if the energy provided by the diet exceeds the energy needs of the particular person consuming it.

Some idea of the variability of the energy content of common foods can be gained from Table 6-3, which shows the amounts of various foods required to provide 100 kcal and the size and energy values of average servings. It is clear that consuming foods near the bottom of the table—such as butter, mayonnaise, and salad oil—can readily increase our kilocalorie intake by a significant amount, even when used in small amounts. Such food items, with their concentrated kilocalories, are often used to enhance the palatability of such foods as bread and lettuce that are relatively low in both fat and kilocalories. Such foods as apples and carrots, at the top of Table 6-3, provide much fewer kilocalories per serving than those at the bottom but can provide satisfaction

TABLE 6-3

Size and caloric value of an average serving of various foods and the amount of each food needed to provide 100 kcal

FOOD	AVERAGE SERVING	KCAL/SERVING	AMOUNT TO PROVIDE 100 KCAL
Lettuce	⅛ head	10	1¼ heads
Cabbage	½ cup	10	5 cups, shredded
Asparagus	4 spears	15	25 spears
Carrots	1 medium	30	3½ medium
Sugar	1 Tbsp	50	2 Tbsp
Bread	1 slice	70	1½ slices
Apple	1 medium	80	1¼ apples (7 cm in diameter)
Egg	1 large	80	1¼ large
Potato	1 medium	85	1⅓ medium
Nonfat milk	1 cup	90	1+ cup
Pear	1 medium	100	1
Dates	4	100	4
Butter	1 Tbsp	100	1 Tbsp
Mayonnaise	1 Tbsp	100	1 Tbsp
Banana	1 medium	105	1 small
Salad oil	1 Tbsp	120	⅚ Tbsp
Whole milk	1 cup	150	⅔ cup
Chicken breast	1	160	1.7 oz
Pork chop	1	305	0.9 oz.

From *Nutritive value of foods,* Home and Garden Bulletin No. 72, Agriculture Research Service, Washington DC, 1985, U.S. Department of Agriculture.

TABLE 6-4

The energy value provided by an average serving of apple or potato eaten alone or cooked in various ways, or combined with other foods during food preparation

FOOD	KCAL	FOOD	KCAL
Apple	80	Potato (1 medium)	
Applesauce	195	Boiled	120
Baked apple	225	Baked with skin	150
Apple pie	330	French fried (10 strips)	160
Apple crisp	350	Mashed with 1 tsp butter	170
Apple pie à la mode	440	Baked (served with 1 pat butter)	195
		Creamed	210

From *Nutritive value of foods,* Home and Garden Bulletin No. 72, Agriculture Research Service, Washington DC, 1985, U.S. Department of Agriculture.

because of their bulk in the stomach and the fact that they require considerable chewing.

What is done to a food during its preparation, meaning what is added to it and how it is cooked, can significantly change the eventual kilocalorie content from that of the original main food. Examples of such effects of food preparation are shown in Table 6-4.

The relationship between the weight of some foods and their energy content is revealed in Table 6-5, showing the energy content per 100 g of a variety of foods. As can be expected, foods low in fat and high in water and fiber content have the lowest values of kilocalories per 100 g (shown at the top of Table 6-5), whereas those high in fat and low in water and fiber content have the highest values of kilocalories per 100 g (shown at the bottom of Table 6-5). The relative amounts of energy available from the various food groups in the U.S. food supply are shown in Table 6-6.

EXCHANGE LISTS

People with the metabolic disease diabetes are often advised to regulate carbohydrate, fat, and protein intake in addition to their total energy intake. To assist them in this task, the American Diabetes Association and the American Dietetic Association have developed exchange lists so that people with diabetes do not constantly need to calculate their intake of energy and the various

TABLE 6-5

Caloric value and measure of 100-g (3.5-oz) portions of various foods

FOOD	SERVING SIZE	CALORIC VALUE/100 g
Lettuce	½ head	14
Asparagus	6 spears	20
Cabbage	1½ cups, shredded	24
Carrots	1½	42
Nonfat milk or buttermilk	⅖ cup	36
Milk 3.7% fat	⅖ cup	66
Peas	⅝ cup	68
Potato	1 small	90
Lamb	1 serving	197
Chicken	1 serving	208
Pork	1 serving	236
Bread	4 slices	250
Dates	10	274
Sugar	½ cup	400
Butter	7 Tbsp	716
Mayonnaise	7 Tbsp	718
Salad oil	7 Tbsp	884

From Adams C: *Nutritive value of American foods.* USDA Handbook No. 456, Washington, DC, 1975, U.S. Department of Agriculture, updated with values from Handbook Nos. 8-1 to 8-16, 1976-87.

TABLE 6-6

Contribution of various food groups to the energy content of the U.S. food supply

SUPPLY	PERCENTAGE
Meat, fish, poultry, and eggs	20.2
Cereal products	21.1
Fats and oils	19.3
Sugar	17.7
Dairy products	9.6
Vegetables	4.8
Fruits	3.2
Legumes and nuts	3.0
Other	1.1

From Raper NR, Zizza C, Rourke J: *Nutrient content of the U.S. food supply, 1909-1988,* USDA Home Economics Research Rep No 50 Washington, DC, 1992, U.S. Department of Agriculture.

nutrients. The concept of exchange lists was introduced in Chapter 3. The exchange list system is also useful to people who are not diabetic and are on other therapeutic diets in helping them recognize foods of similar energy and carbohydrate, fat, and protein contents that can be used interchangeably in their diets. The exchange lists divide foods into six categories: (1) starch and bread, (2) meat, (3) vegetable, (4) fruit, (5) milk, and (6) fat. Within each group the lists indicate various kinds and amounts of foods that have similar energy, carbohydrate, fat, and protein content. Such exchange lists can be

TABLE 6-7

Proximate analysis of diabetic food exchange groups

EXCHANGE	CARBOHYDRATE (GRAMS)	PROTEIN (GRAMS)	LIPID (GRAMS)	ENERGY (KCAL)
Nonfat milk	12	8	0	80
Vegetables	5	2	0	25
Fruit	15	0	0	60
Bread	15	3	0	80
Lean meat	0	7	3	55
Fat	0	0	5	45

With permission of the American Diabetes Association and the American Dietetics of Association, 1986.

found in Appendix H. Table 6-7 lists the approximate values for the carbohydrate, fat, protein, and kilocalorie content of the foods in each group.

THE BODY'S NEED FOR ENERGY

The human body's total energy needs can be subdivided into three separate categories of need, each of which can be estimated separately and varies, depending on the person's circumstances and behavior. The three categories of energy requirement are the following:

- The energy required to maintain **basal metabolism:** the basic essential metabolic processes required to keep the body alive and healthy and, where applicable, growing at an appropriate rate
- The energy required to power physical **activity,** meaning all of the muscle movements in addition to those such as involuntary breathing and heart beat required simply to keep us alive
- The energy that is necessarily released as a result of the **thermic effect of food,** which is a process of increased energy expenditure and therefore heat release that inevitably occurs between 1 to 3 hours after a meal because of the stimulating effect that the nutrients of food have on metabolism in general

The value of these three categories of energy requirement depends, among other things, on a person's size (a larger person always requires more energy than a smaller person, all other factors being equal) and age (energy needs are generally higher in younger people).

In general, a person's total daily requirement for energy is the average amount of energy needed to balance the amount expended each day in the three ways listed. This amount of energy maintains body weight in adults, sustains adequate development of the fetus in pregnant females, allows sufficient milk production in lactating females, and supports appropriate growth in children. If there is a consistent pattern of imbalance between energy requirements and energy intake over a long period, the person concerned either gains weight, if intake is in excess of requirements, or loses weight, if intake is less than requirements. In most people these losses and gains in weight are largely a result of changes in the amount of fat stored by the body. If energy expenditure is increased beyond energy intake because of increased physical activity, however, a loss of body fat may be accompanied by an increase in muscle mass.

BASAL METABOLISM

The energy needed to power basal metabolism is the amount required to sustain the basic essential metabolic processes involved in keeping the body alive and healthy and, where applicable, growing at an appropriate rate. The basal metabolic energy need includes the energy needed to maintain required nervous activity; ventilate the lungs; keep the heart pumping to circulate the blood; maintain minimal levels of protein synthesis, hormone production, glandular secretion, nutrient uptake, and waste excretion; and generally keep the internal environment of the body, including all its cells, in a functioning biochemical condition. In essence, it is the energy needed to keep the body alive and ready for more vigorous action. It includes a certain amount of energy needed to maintain what is called **muscle tonus,** or **muscle tone.** No matter how motionless and relaxed a person is, his or her muscles are still maintained in a slightly contracted state. Without this muscle tone, the body would become a loose, floppy mass. The energy required to sustain basal metabolism is also known as the **basal metabolic rate (BMR).**

> Total energy need = need resulting from basal metabolism + need resulting from activity + need resulting from thermic effect of food

Measurement of Basal Metabolism

Basal metabolism, or the basal metabolic rate or basal metabolic energy need, is measured under defined conditions. It is measured while the subjects are reclining in bed, immediately after awakening, in a state of physical and emotional relaxation. They should not have participated in any formal exercise in the 24 hours immediately before the measurement and should have fasted for the 12 hours immediately before the measurement. The actual measurement can be done by a process of **direct calorimetry,** which requires the heat produced by the person's body to be measured directly. However, it is usually measured by **indirect calorimetry,** which measures how much oxygen the person consumes and how much carbon dioxide the person expires. These values are then used to calculate how much energy is being released by the oxidation of the energy-yielding nutrients in the body.

Direct calorimetric methods are based on the assumption that all of the energy being used to maintain the body ultimately is released in the form of heat.[2] Some comes out as heat immediately on its release from food. Some becomes temporarily trapped within adenosine triphosphate (ATP), is used to power various body processes, and is then released as heat, but it all ends up as heat eventually. The direct calorimetric methods require the subjects to be in a **human calorimeter** or **respiration chamber,** which is a small insulated room that operates on the same basic principles as the bomb calorimeter. The heat given off by the subject causes a change in the temperature of a heat reservoir, such as water, surrounding the chamber, allowing the amount of energy released to be easily calculated. In addition to total energy released, the amounts of oxygen used and carbon dioxide released by the subjects are often measured. This allows the calculation of a value known as the **respiratory quotient (RQ),** which is the ratio of carbon dioxide produced to oxygen consumed (that is, CO_2 produced divided by O_2 consumed). Determining the RQ value makes it possible to determine whether carbohydrate, fat, or protein is being used to provide the energy released or to estimate what mixture of these nutrients is used. If carbohydrate is being used as the sole source of fuel, the RQ value is 1.0. If only fat is being used, the RQ value is 0.7, whereas if only protein is used—which almost never happens in practice—the RQ value is around 0.8 (the precise value depends on the particular amino acid mixture involved). Under normal conditions in normal subjects, both carbohydrate and fat are being used as fuels, yielding an RQ that is usually 0.82.

The cost of operating a respiration calorimeter is high, so only a few are available and they are used only under carefully controlled experimental conditions. The room calorimeter at the Human Nutrition Research Center in Beltsville, Maryland, for example, is a 9- × 10- × 8-ft chamber where United States Department of Agriculture scientists measure the energy expenditure of volunteers on awakening after an overnight stay (Figure 6-4). It is also used to measure the total energy expenditure of volunteers over a 24-hour period, when they are engaged in a variety of activities such as eating, exercising, and sleeping. Such measurements yield not only BMR values, but also some other measures of energy expenditure that are discussed below.

FIGURE 6-4

A room calorimeter at U.S. Department of Agriculture Human Nutrition Center in Beltsville, Md.

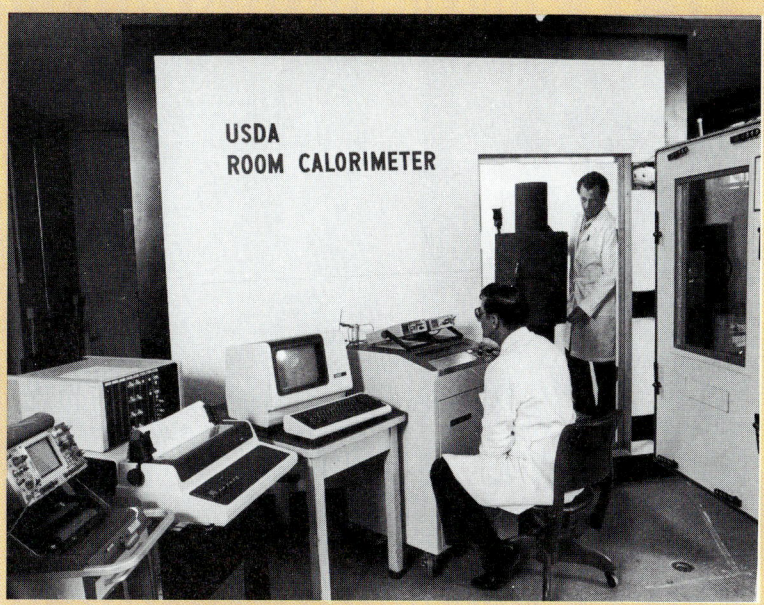

FIGURE 6-5

A metabolic chamber.

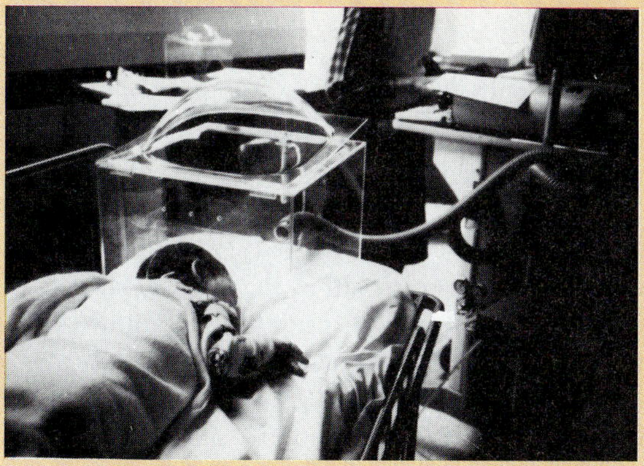

A modified version of the respiration chamber is the **metabolic chamber** in which the heat given off by the subject is measured using thermocouples and heat-exchange disks attached to the skin. Figure 6-5 illustrates one type of metabolic chamber in use. Similar to the respiration chamber the metabolic chamber can be used to determine BMRs and also energy expenditure during various activities, provided that they can be performed in the relatively limited space available.

Indirect calorimetry, in which oxygen consumption, rather than heat release, is measured, is a much simpler and less costly method of determining rates of energy expenditure. For many years the **Benedict-Roth respiration apparatus** was the standard machine used for indirect calorimetry. This is a closed-circuit system in which the subject receives oxygen only from a measured source of oxygen-rich air and exhales into a container in which the waste carbon dioxide and water are removed while the remaining oxygen and nitrogen are recirculated. The amount of oxygen in the air mixture is measured before and after each standard 6-minute test, allowing the amount of oxygen consumed to be determined. The use of 1 L of oxygen under normal conditions of temperature and pressure corresponds to the release of 4.82 kcal of energy when the RQ is 0.82 under basal conditions. Thus the kilocalories released during the consumption of any volume of oxygen can be readily calculated under these conditions.

Another and an equally effective way to determine oxygen use is **open-circuit indirect calorimetry.** In this method, normal room air is breathed in and the exhaled carbon dioxide generated from it is collected and measured. Knowing the amount of carbon dioxide produced in a given time allows calculation of the amount of oxygen consumed to generate that carbon dioxide, and thus the amount of energy released can be calculated as above. The open-circuit indirect method is even less expensive than either direct calorimetry or closed-circuit indirect calorimetry. It also reduces the possibility of errors as a result of stimulation of metabolism caused by the use of oxygen-rich air in the closed-circuit method. Typical instruments used in open-circuit calorimetry are shown in Figure 6-6. These can be used to determine either BMRs or energy expenditure during various activities.

FIGURE 6-6

Respiration meter being used to measure energy expenditure during mild exercise.

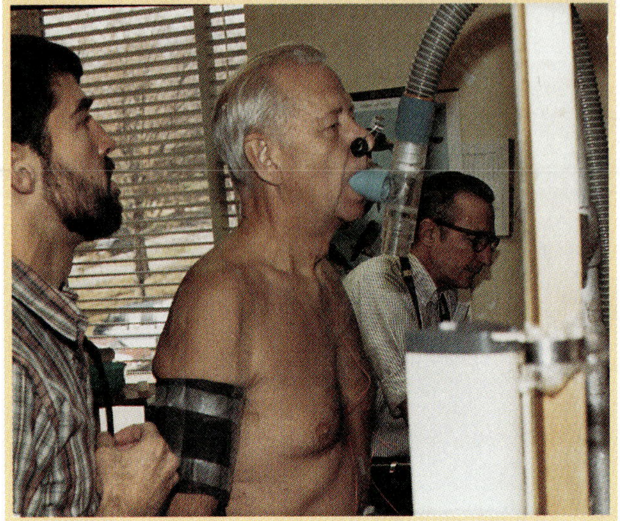

TABLE 6-8

Comparison of methods of estimating basal metabolic needs

METHOD	SUBJECT X*	SUBJECT Y*
A. Body weight 1 kcal/kg/hr	1680	2400
B. Harris-Benedict equation (for males)† 66.5 + [13.5 × wt (kg)] + (5.0 × ht (cm)] − [6.75 × age]	1564	1969
C. Metabolic body size 70 × wt in kg$^{3/4}$	1694	2212
D. FAO/WHO/UNU equation (for males)‡ 11.6 × wt (kg) + 879	1691	2039

* X and Y are both 50-year-old men and are 5′10″ (178 cm) tall. X weighs 154 lb (70 kg), and Y weighs 220 lb (100 kg).

† For females: Resting energy expenditure (REE) = 655.1 + [9.56 × wt (kg)] + [1.85 × ht (cm)] − [4.68 × age (yr)].

‡ For females: 8.7 × w (kg) + 829 (see Table 6-9).

The true BMR of a subject is his or her energy expenditure under the conditions described earlier, when the subject is resting immediately after awakening. A slightly different measurement is the **sleeping metabolic rate (SMR),** measured when the subject is asleep. A third, slightly different measurement is the **resting metabolic rate (RMR),** in which the subject is permitted to walk about (be ambulatory) immediately before the measurement. The RMR value is slightly higher than the BMR value, which in turn is slightly higher than the SMR value. It is not uncommon to find the terms *basal metabolic rate, sleeping metabolic rate,* and *resting metabolic rate* being used as if they mean exactly the same thing. There is a difference between them, however, and their values for any one person can differ across a range of about 10%.

Data from many measurements of BMR have provided enough information for us to predict BMRs from measurements of body weight, height, and other simply measured factors. Four formulas are available for the estimation of basal metabolic energy needs (Table 6-8). The first and simplest method (method A) is most appropriate for people of average body build and hence average body composition. It predicts a basal energy need on the basis of 1 kcal/kg/hr for men and 0.9 kcal/kg/hr for women. When this method is applied to someone whose body build is either more fat or more muscular than average, it becomes increasingly inaccurate with increasing deviation from average build. This is apparently because the simple measurement of body weight does not accurately reflect significant differences in body composition that influence basal energy needs.

A more precise formula developed in 1909 by Harris and Benedict (method B) is still considered one of the best predictors of basal energy needs. This method uses two formulas, one for males over 10 years of age and one for females of all ages. The formula uses measured body weight, height, and age in combination with four constant values to calculate the basal metabolic energy need.

Method C uses a value known as **metabolic body size.** This is defined as the body weight in kilograms raised to the power of three-fourths. Basal metabolic need is predicted to be 70 times the metabolic body size value. Values for basal metabolic energy needs obtained in this way seem to be remarkably applicable for different body builds and can be applied to almost all animals.

After an extensive evaluation of energy requirements, an expert committee of the FAO/WHO/UNU developed a set of equations (method D) based on 11,000 technically acceptable basal metabolism measurements of subjects of all ages and both genders. The committee found that within each age-group the most useful indicator of BMR was body weight. Calculations of predicted BMR based on the FAO/WHO/UNU equations applied to six age-groups of both genders (Table 6-9).[3]

The final two columns of Table 6-8 show the BMRs calculated by these four methods for two men aged 50 years of differing height and weight. The data indicate that the values obtained by the different methods can vary by as much as 22%, a considerable degree of disagreement.

TABLE 6-9

FAO/WHO/UNU equations for predicting basal metabolic rate from body weight in kilograms (W)*

AGE RANGE (YEARS)	KCAL/DAY	AGE RANGE (YEARS)	KCAL/DAY
MALES		FEMALES	
0-3	60.9 W − 54	0-3	61.0 W − 51
3-10	22.7 W + 495	3-10	22.5 W + 499
10-18	17.5 W + 651	10-18	12.2 W + 746
18-30	15.3 W + 679	18-30	14.7 W + 496
30-60	11.6 W + 879	30-60	8.7 W + 829
>60	13.5 W + 487	>60	10.5 W + 596

* Used for resting energy expenditure in developing recommended dietary allowances (National Research Council/Institute of Medicine: *Recommended dietary allowances*, ed 10, Washington, DC, 1989, National Academy of Sciences).

From Report of a Joint FAO/WHO/UNU Expert Consultation: *Energy and protein requirements.* Technical Rep Series 724, Geneva, Switzerland, 1985, World Health Organization.

Factors Affecting Basal Energy Needs

Body composition All body tissues are metabolically active, being constantly maintained, and their components degraded and resynthesized, with an accompanying requirement for energy. These processes occur at different rates in different tissues, however. Muscle, the brain, and various glands and organs such as the liver are relatively active metabolically, consuming large amounts of oxygen per unit of weight and producing more heat than do less active tissues. Various other tissues, such as bone tissue and adipose tissue, are relatively inactive metabolically and so require less oxygen per unit weight to maintain their basal metabolism and release less heat in the process. Total basal energy requirements per unit of body weight are higher when muscle tissue accounts for a higher proportion of total weight and lower when fat or bone account for a higher proportion of total weight.

Body condition A person in good physical condition has usually developed a greater proportion of muscle tissue than someone in poor condition caused by a lack of exercise. Suppose two men are the same age, height, and weight, but one is a construction worker, whose job involves much physical activity, and the other is an accountant, which is an essentially sedentary occupation. More of the weight of the accountant is from fat tissue than muscle, compared with the proportions of these tissues in the construction worker. Thus the accountant has the lower BMR.

Gender There are well-documented differences in body composition that are generally found between men and women of the same age, height, and weight. Women characteristically develop more adipose tissue and less muscle tissue than men. Between the ages of 20 to 25 years, fat accounts for about 10 kg of the weight of a typical 70-kg man and about 15 to 20 kg of the weight of a typical 63-kg woman. So young adult males contain about 14% fat by weight, whereas young adult females contain about 23% to 32% fat by weight. The BMRs for women are correspondingly about 10% to 12% lower than those for men of the same age, height, and weight.

Hormonal secretions Hormones are synthesized by various glands of the endocrine system and secreted into the blood to be carried to specific target tissues where they serve to control and integrate a wide variety of body processes. The hormonal secretions of the adrenal and thyroid glands have more influence on basal energy needs than does any other single factor. The secretions from both glands have a stimulating effect on metabolic rate.

The hormone epinephrine (also known as adrenaline), which is secreted by the adrenal gland, is produced in response to intense emotional stimuli such as anger or fear. This results in an intense but relatively short-lived stimulation of metabolism, which then returns to its normal state within 2 or 3 hours.

The iodine-containing hormone thyroxin, which is secreted by the thyroid gland, is a powerful stimulator of metabolism. Any marked deviation from predicted basal energy needs is usually attributed to oversecretion or undersecretion of thyroxin from the thyroid gland (although other causes are possible). Deviations in basal metabolism of more than 20% from normal predicted levels almost always indicate some problem in thyroid functioning. A condition known as **hypothyroidism,** in which the BMR may be depressed by as much as 30%, results from undersecretion of thyroxin. Because the energy required to power basal metabolism may be 30% less than normal, people with hypothyroidism have unusually low total energy needs and so tend to gain weight easily. The condition can be treated by the careful use of thyroxin pills, which are available only under medical supervision. **Hyperthyroidism** (also known as **exophthalmic goiter**), on the other hand, is a condition in which basal metabolism is elevated by as much as 50% to 75% above normal because of oversecretion of thyroxin. People with hyperthyroidism have high energy requirements and have trouble gaining and maintaining weight. Hyperthyroidism is a more difficult condition to correct. Drugs are available that can interfere with the uptake of iodine, which is needed to produce thyroxin, but it is difficult to control their effects. Alternative approaches to the treatment of hyperthyroidism are **athyroidectomy,** which is the removal of all or part of the thyroid gland, or a limitation in iodine intake to reduce the amount available for the synthesis of thyroxin.

TABLE 6-10

Metabolic rates (MRs) of organs and tissues in adults and newborn infants

ORGAN	ADULT WEIGHT (kg)	ADULT MR/DAY KCAL (kJ)	ADULT % OF WHOLE BODY MR	NEONATE WEIGHT (kg)	NEONATE MR/DAY KCAL (kJ)	NEONATE % OF WHOLE BODY MR
Liver	1.6	482(2017)	27	0.14	42(176)	20
Brain	1.4	338(1414)	19	0.35	84(352)	44
Heart	0.32	122(510)	7	0.02	8(33)	4
Kidney	0.29	187(782)	10	0.024	15(63)	7
Muscle	30.00	324(1356)	18	0.8	9(38)	5
Miscellaneous (by difference)			19			20
TOTAL	70.00	1800(7530)		3.5	197(824)	

From FAO/WHO/UNU: *Energy and protein requirements,* Technical Rep Series 724, Geneva, Switzerland, 1985, World Health Organization.

Sleep Measurements of BMR are made when the subject is awake but physically and emotionally relaxed. During sleep, both muscular and emotional relaxation are even greater, causing a further drop in energy needs. In some people, however, these losses may be compensated for by increased needs caused by involuntary tossing and turning during sleep.

Age The BMR changes with age. This is largely because of changes in the proportion of different tissues with different degrees of metabolic activity. Table 6-10 indicates the metabolic rates of individual organs and tissues in adults and newborn infants (neonates). It also illustrates that infants have a relatively high proportion of the most metabolically active tissues, as compared with adults. This results in infants having high metabolic rates compared with adults. In general, the BMR is high at birth, increases until the subject is 2 years of age, and then gradually declines throughout life, apart from a brief rise during puberty. One of the major factors underlying the decline in BMR with age is the steady decline in lean body mass (the mass of all tissues of the body, except adipose tissue). At age 85, for example, the lean body mass declines to about 75% of that in the same person as a young adult aged 20 to 25. For a man who is 5 feet 10 inches in height, the BMR is about 25 kcal/kg/day between the ages of 18 and 30 and gradually declines to 20 kcal/kg/day between the ages of 30 and 60.

Pregnancy During the sixth to ninth months of pregnancy, basal metabolism increases to 20% above normal. This is caused either by the high metabolic activity of the fetus and placenta or by an increase in the metabolic activity in maternal tissues or by some combination of these factors.

Undernutrition and overnutrition After long periods when energy intake is less than requirements (prolonged caloric undernutrition), the BMR may fall to at least 20% to 30% below normal predicted levels. This phenomenon, known as **privo conservation,** apparently reflects the body's adaptive efforts to conserve energy in response to an energy deficiency and may explain the ability of people with chronic undernutrition to maintain their body weight on caloric intakes below predicted requirements. Privo conservation was first demonstrated by the classic studies of Keys and associates[4] at the University of Minnesota, performed on conscientious objectors during World War II. Men who had previously been normally nourished were found to be able to achieve energy balance on half their usual energy intake after 6 months. This was accomplished by a large decrease in body weight (including the loss of some lean tissue), a reduction in physical activity, and the metabolic adaptation revealed by the reduction in BMR. Privo conservation explains why some people on diets designed to bring about weight reduction hit "plateaus" in weight loss and maintain their weight on what are theoretically insufficient kilocalorie intakes.

Conversely, the concept of a long-term effect on energy use, called **luxus consumption,** has been introduced to explain why some people on diets containing *excess* kilocalories do not gain weight as predicted. The luxus consumption theory maintains that when kilocalorie intake is greater than needs, some people's bodies adapt by using more kilocalories and thus avoid the deposition of as much fat as would otherwise be formed. The use of the kilocalories may involve "futile" or unproductive metabolic activity that allows the energy to be wasted as heat. Such a phenomenon certainly helps explain why some people appear to be able to eat well beyond reasonable needs without any increase in body weight.

The phenomena of privo conservation and luxus consumption are presumably natural adaptations, acquired through the course of evolution, that allow the body to compensate for periods of overconsumption or underconsumption of kilocalories in a way that maintains weight. If so, they are genetically inherited, at least in

TABLE 6-11

Factors affecting basal metabolism

FACTORS THAT INCREASE BASAL METABOLISM	FACTORS THAT DECREASE BASAL METABOLISM
Increase in muscle mass	Increase in body fat
Good physical condition	Poor physical condition
Being a male	Being a female
Hyperthyroidism	Hypothyroidism
Pregnancy	Sleep
Puberty	Aging
Extremes of environmental temperature	Undernutrition
Smoking	

part, although environmental factors may influence how effectively they operate.

Body temperature Because all chemical reactions speed up with increasing temperature, it is not surprising to find that BMR increases with increasing body temperature. A rise of 1° F in body temperature leads on average to an increase of 7% in BMR, although increases as high as 15% have been observed. An average increase of 13% in BMR is found for each rise of 1° C in body temperature. These figures make it obvious that a person with fever has an increased need for energy.

Environmental temperature BMR is also affected by the environmental temperature of subjects, which usually means the air temperature around them. The lowest metabolic rates are obtained at an environmental temperature of 78° F (26° C), with higher metabolic rates being reported at temperatures both above and below that figure. A sudden decrease in environmental temperature, if not compensated for by additional clothing, causes shivering and a temporary process of heat production (thermogenesis) with a resulting increase in BMR. This adaptive response of the body to lowered environmental temperature is called **cold-induced thermogenesis** and serves to generate heat, which can prevent the body's temperature from falling too much, despite the fall in environmental temperature.

Smoking Research indicates that habitual smokers who then stop smoking have a tendency to gain weight. This may be caused by the fact that the nicotine taken in when smoking tends to increase the BMR by approximately 10%. This explanation dispels a widely held belief that the effect is a result of a suppression of normal appetite by nicotine.

In summary, many different factors affect basal energy needs, including body composition and condition, gender, hormonal secretions, sleep, age, pregnancy, undernutrition, body temperature, environmental temperature, and smoking. The effects of various factors on BMR are summarized in Table 6-11. For most people, however, a fairly accurate prediction of basal energy needs can be made on the basis of their body weight. For many people, especially those who are sedentary or engaged in only moderate activity, basal energy needs account for 50% to 70% of their total energy requirements.

ENERGY NEEDS FOR ACTIVITY

The second category of energy requirement that must be taken into account when estimating total energy needs is the amount of energy needed to power physical activity. The energy requirements for activity include the energy required by all of the muscular movements involved in the activity, plus a small amount of energy because of the increased heart rate and breathing during strenuous activity. For many activities the energy requirement depends on body size and how strenuous the activity actually is.

The energy requirements for various activities, often called the energy "costs" of the activities, have been determined by a series of tests based on measurements of oxygen consumption. This information has been used to compile tables that list the average energy cost of a wide range of activities in terms of kilocalories per kilogram of body weight per hour (Table 6-12). To estimate the energy cost of an activity that is not listed, the value for an activity that is listed and that involves similar muscles and a similar degree of exertion can be used. The values in Table 6-12 are fairly accurate for such activities as walking and running, in which moving the whole body accounts for about 75% of the energy costs. For such activities as knitting or piano playing, however, which involve moving only a small proportion of the body mass and for which energy costs are not proportional to body size, Table 6-12 probably overestimates the costs for larger individuals.

Alternative tables provide information on total energy expenditure when a person participates in an activity for a certain length of time, regardless of body size (Table 6-13). These tables are more accurate for activities in which the energy costs are not directly proportional to body size. Such tables underestimate the energy required by a large person for activities that involve moving the whole body, such as running or playing tennis. Whatever type of table is used, the overall accuracy of calculations based on it depends not only on the accuracy of information in the tables, but also on the accuracy of the record that is kept of the kinds of activities participated in and the time spent on each.

It is important to appreciate the limitations of such tables as Tables 6-12 and 6-13. Although the energy costs shown do represent the best average estimates available, they do not reflect many individual differences between people, including the differing efficiencies with which people perform the various activities. We also

TABLE 6-12

Energy cost of activities exclusive of basal metabolism and influence of food

ACTIVITY	Kcal/kg/hr	ACTIVITY	Kcal/kg/hr
Bicycling (century run)	7.6	Piano playing (Liszt's "Tarantella")	2.0
Bicycling (moderate speed)	2.5	Reading aloud	0.4
Bookbinding	0.8	Rowing in race	16.0
Boxing	11.4	Running	7.0
Carpentry (heavy)	2.3	Sawing wood	5.7
Cello playing	1.3	Sewing, hand	0.4
Crocheting	0.4	Sewing, foot-driven machine	0.6
Dancing, foxtrot	3.8	Sewing, motor-driven machine	0.4
Dancing, waltz	3.0	Shoemaking	1.0
Dishwashing	1.0	Singing in a loud voice	0.8
Dressing and undressing	0.7	Sitting quietly	0.4
Driving automobile	0.9	Skating	3.5
Eating	0.4	Standing at attention	0.6
Fencing	7.3	Standing relaxed	0.5
Horseback riding, walk	1.4	Stone masonry	4.7
Horseback riding, trot	4.3	Sweeping with broom, bare floor	1.4
Horseback riding, gallop	6.7	Sweeping with carpet sweeper	1.6
Ironing (5-lb iron)	1.0	Sweeping with vacuum sweeper	2.7
Knitting sweater	0.7	Swimming (2 mph)	7.9
Laundry, light	1.3	Tailoring	0.9
Lying still, awake	0.1	Typewriting rapidly	1.0
Organ playing (30% to 40% of energy hand work)	1.5	Violin playing	0.6
		Walking (3 mph)	2.0
Painting furniture	1.5	Walking rapidly (4 mph)	3.4
Paring potatoes	0.6	Walking at high speed (5.3 mph)	9.3
Playing Ping-Pong	4.4	Walking downstairs	*
Piano playing (Mendelssohn's songs)	0.8	Walking upstairs	†
		Washing floors	1.2
Piano playing (Beethoven's "Apassionata")	1.4	Writing	0.4

* Allow 0.012 kcal/kg for an ordinary staircase with 15 steps without regard to time.

† Allow 0.036 kcal/kg for an ordinary staircase with 15 steps without regard to time.

From Taylor CM, G McLeod: *Rose's laboratory handbook for dietetics,* ed 5, New York, 1949, Macmillan.
To estimate energy costs of activities not listed here, choose one that involves a comparable amount of muscular activity.

know that while a 198-lb (90-kg) man requires more energy to walk a mile than a 132-lb (60-kg) man does, the increase is not 50% more, as is predicted from the tables. The energy costs listed in the tables are based on few observations; so they should not be considered as precise measurements that apply to the activity every time it is performed and whoever performs it. Rather, they are representative results, averaging what has been found to be the case in a few individuals. It is also relevant whether a person engages in a particular activity continuously or intermittently, over the time he or she carried out the activity. For example, someone who reports that he or she was swimming for an hour may really have been in motion for the full hour or may have spent much of the time resting. Such factors as these have been found to account for the differences in energy expenditure in obese and nonobese people who report spending the same time on the same or similar activities.

Many people are dismayed to learn how few kilocalories are actually required for some activities that they consider rather strenuous. The energy cost of walking at 3 miles per hour, for example, is only 2 kcal/kg/hr more than the cost of simply being awake while lying down. Thus a 132-lb (60-kg) woman uses only an additional 120 kcal during a 1-hour walk at that speed. Even skating for 1 hour requires only an additional 210 kcal for this person and bicycling only an extra 150 kcal. In spite of these seemingly low figures, a 30-minute walk every day for a year would require the energy stored in 6 to 7 pounds of body fat. Many people, especially students, are even more disappointed to learn that intense mental activity requires almost no more energy than does daydreaming. Any extra energy costs may well be a result of increased muscular tension associated with mental stress, rather than with the nervous activity in the brain itself.

TABLE 6-13

Energy expenditure in specified activities, including basal metabolic rate and the thermic effect of food

	Kcal/MIN	kJ/MIN
MAN (65 kg, OR 143 lb)		
In bed asleep or resting	1.1	4.52
Sitting quietly	1.4	5.82
Standing quietly	1.7	7.32
Walking 3 miles/hr (4.9 km/hr)	3.7	15.5
Walking 3 miles/hr (4.9 km/hr) with a 10-kg load	4.0	16.7
Office work (sedentary)	1.8	7.5
Domestic work		
Cooking	2.1	8.8
Light cleaning	3.1	13.0
Moderate cleaning (such as polishing and window cleaning)	4.3	18.0
Industry		
Garage work (repairs)	4.1	17.2
Carpentry	4.0	16.7
Electrical and machine tool industry	3.6	15.1
Laboratory work	2.3	9.6
Construction work	6.0	25.1
Bricklaying	3.8	15.9
Driving tractor	2.4	10.0
Feeding animals	4.1	17.2
Planting	4.7	19.7
Sawing—hand saw	8.6	36.0
power saw	4.8	20.1
Shoveling	6.5	27.2
Recreation		
Sedentary	2.5	10.5
Light (playing pool, bowling, golf, sailing)	2.5-5.0	10.5-21.0
Moderate (such as dancing, horseback riding, swimming, and tennis)	5.0-7.5	21.0-31.5
Heavy (such as athletics, football, and rowing)	7.5+	31.5
WOMAN (55 kg, OR 110 lb)		
In bed asleep or resting	0.9	3.7
Sitting quietly	1.2	4.8
Standing quietly	1.4	5.7
Walking 3 miles/hour (4.9 km/hr)	3.0	12.6
Walking 3 miles/hour (4.9 km/hr) with 10-kg load	3.4	14.2
Office work (sedentary)	1.6	6.7
Domestic work		
Cooking	1.7	7.1
Light cleaning	2.5	10.5
Moderate cleaning (such as polishing and window cleaning)	3.5	14.6
Light industry		
Bakery work	2.3	9.6
Laundry work	3.2	13.4
Machine tool industry	2.5	10.5
Recreation		
Sedentary	2.0	8.3
Light (playing pool, bowling, golf, sailing)	2.0-4.0	8.3-16.7
Moderate (such as canoeing, dancing, horseback riding, swimming, and tennis)	4.0-6.0	16.7-25.1
Heavy (such as athletics, football, rowing)	6.0+	25+

From Durnin JVGA, Passmore R: *Energy, work, and leisure,* London, 1967, as reported in FAO/WHO: *Energy and protein requirements,* Technical Rep No 522, Geneva, Switzerland, 1973, World Health Organization.

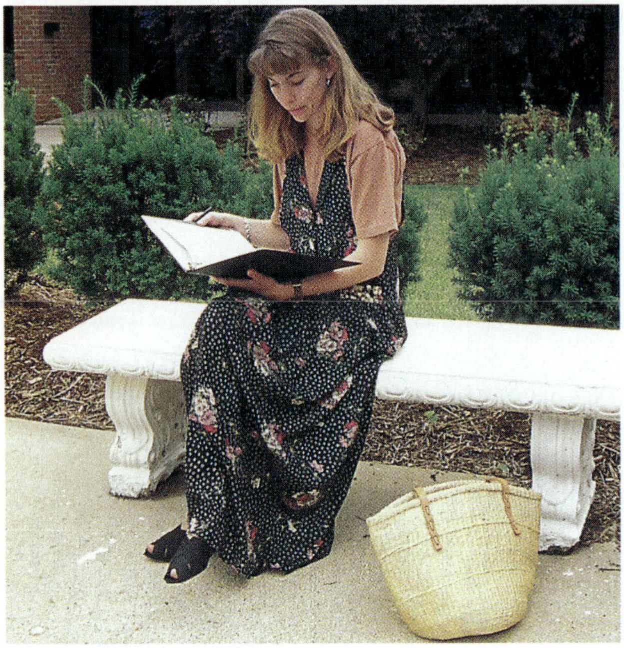

Studying often requires intense concentration, yet this "mental energy" burns no more calories than watching television or daydreaming!

THERMIC EFFECT OF FOOD

The third category of energy requirement to be taken into account when estimating total energy needs is the energy needed to provide the thermic effect of food. It is well known that a food intake that is sufficient to meet the combined needs of basal metabolism and activity is inadequate to meet total needs and leads to weight loss if not supplemented by additional kilocalorie intake. This is because of the thermic effect of food, which is the stimulation of metabolism and therefore increased heat production that occurs from 1 to 3 hours after a meal as a result of the processing of food in the stomach and intestine and of nutrients in the blood and body cells. The energy corresponding to the thermic effect of food includes the energy costs of the absorption, metabolism, and storage of nutrients within the body. The magnitude of the thermic effect of food overall is about 10% of needs for basal metabolism and activity. So the final step in calculating total energy needs is to add 10% on top of the total for basal metabolism and activity.

The thermic effect of food has been subdivided into two components: **obligatory thermogenesis** and **facultative thermogenesis.** The obligatory component is the unavoidable energy cost associated with absorption and transport of nutrients and the synthesis of protein, fat, and carbohydrate required for the renewal of body tissues and the storage of energy. Facultative thermogenesis is thought to be partially mediated by "futile" heat-releasing metabolic cycles and the activity of the nervous system. The magnitude of the facultative thermic effect of food depends on several factors, including the kilocalorie content of the meal itself, how well nourished a person is, and what diet they have been following (that is, whether the energy comes primarily from fat, carbohydrate, or protein or the usual distribution of these).

There is evidence to suggest that the magnitude of the thermic effect of food as a whole is genetically determined. In studies with identical twins, large variations in the thermic effect were noted between different pairs of twins, but *within* pairs the response was remarkably consistent.

Although the thermic response to food is a small portion of the total daily energy expenditure, variations in it are thought to be important in the regulation of human energy balance. In some people the expected effects of an increased energy intake may be offset by an increase in the thermic effect of food. In other people this does not appear to happen to any significant extent.

The thermic effect of food was originally called the **specific dynamic effect of food** because it was believed that the stimulation of heat production varied with the composition of the diet and was greatest when a high proportion of the kilocalories were provided by protein.

ESTIMATION OF TOTAL ENERGY NEEDS

As previously discussed, a person's total energy needs comprise the energy required to maintain basal metabolism, the energy required for activity, and the energy required for the thermic effect of food. Over the years many methods have been developed to measure total energy expenditure. The most accurate methods are the same ones that are used to determine BMR, but the subjects participate in activities and eat, rather than just rest, after fasting. These methods are direct calorimetry, in which the heat released by the body is measured directly, and indirect calorimetry, involving **respiratory gas exchange** (the measurement of oxygen gas consumed or carbon dioxide gas exhaled). With both of these classic methods the total energy expenditure, or energy use, of confined subjects is measured while they perform a range of activities over several hours or days. The major disadvantage of both methods is that the subjects cannot perform all of their habitual activities because of their confinement in a small chamber or the need for them to wear a cumbersome apparatus. To overcome the disadvantage and because the energy needed for activity is the most variable component in total energy needs, various "field" methods have been developed to measure total energy expenditure under free-living conditions. These field methods include **factorial methods, energy intake and energy balance**

methods, heart rate monitoring, and the newly developed **doubly-labeled water technique.**

FACTORIAL METHODS

A factorial method of measuring total energy expenditure involves calculation of each of the three categories of energy need: basal metabolic need, activity need, and the thermic effect of food. The basal metabolic need (BMR) is calculated from the equations in Table 6-8 and below. The energy required for activity is derived from published values such as those in Tables 6-12 and 6-13, combined with a record of activities performed over a day or a number of days. The thermic effect of food is taken to be 10% of the combined value for basal needs and activity, as discussed earlier. The types of calculations involved in the factorial method are as follows:

1. **Calculate basal metabolism using one of the following methods:**
   Method A (kcal/kg/hr method), in which BMR for males = body weight (kg) × 1.0 × 24, and BMR for females = body weight (kg) × 0.9 × 24

   Method B (Harris-Benedict formula), in which BMR for males = 66.4 + [13.7 × weight (kg)] + [5.0 × height (cm)] – (6.8 × age), and BMR for females = 655.0 + [9.6 × weight (kg)] + [1.8 × height (cm)] – [4.7 × age]

   Method C (metabolic body size method), in which BMR = 70 × $[\text{weight (kg)}]^{3/4}$

   Method D (FAO/WHO/UNU equations): see text on p. 198 and Table 6–8

> **M**etabolic body size = weight in kilograms raised to the power of ¾ (i.e., $kg^{3/4}$). To calculate your metabolic body size, follow these steps:
> - Calculate your weight in kilograms (i.e., your weight in pounds divided by 2.2).
> - "Cube" your weight in kilograms (i.e., weight [kg] × weight [kg] × weight [kg]).
> - Find the square root of the answer from the above line.
> - Again, find the square root of the answer from the above line, and the result is your metabolic body size.
>
> For example, for a 70-kg man, metabolic body size is as follows:
> - 70 × 70 × 70 = 343,000
> - Square root of 343,000 = 585.662
> - Square root of 585.662 = 24.2
> - Metabolic body size = 24.

2. **Calculate activity costs based on a record of all activity over a 24-hour period:**

ENERGY COST

ACTIVITY	TIME (hr) (A)	Kcal/kg/hr (B)	Kcal/kg (A) × (B)
Dressing	1.5	0.7	1.05
Sitting	6.0	0.4	2.4
Skating	0.5	3.5	1.7
Walking (3 mph)	2.0	2.0	4.0
Standing	1.0	0.5	0.5
Typing	4.0	1.0	4.0
Sleeping	8.0	—	—
Playing piano	0.5	2.0	1.0
Eating	0.5	0.4	0.2
TOTAL	24		14.85

Energy cost for activity = Body weight (kg) × 14.85 for this example

3. **Calculate thermic effect of food,** which equals 10% of basal energy cost (calculated in step 1, above) + activity energy cost (calculated in step 2, above), that is, 0.1 × (basal needs + activity needs)
4. **Calculate total energy expenditure,** by adding the basal energy needs (calculated in step 1, above) + activity energy needs (calculated in step 2, above) + thermic effect of food (calculated in step 3, above).

For people who want a quick answer, although almost certainly a less accurate one, without having to record their activities over a period, there is a "rule of thumb" method that does give a relatively good prediction of total energy expenditure for people of relatively normal body weight. It is as follows:

ENERGY NEED = BODY WEIGHT (LB) × 12 (FOR A SEDENTARY WOMAN)
× 14 (SEDENTARY MAN)
× 15 (MODERATELY ACTIVE WOMAN)
× 17 (MODERATELY ACTIVE MAN)
× 18 (ACTIVE WOMAN)
× 20 (ACTIVE MAN)

To give an accurate answer, of course, a person must be able to choose which level of activity is most appropriate for him or her.

A factorial method was used by the FAO/WHO/UNU Expert Committee to estimate total energy requirements. The same method was adopted by the Food and Nutrition Board of the U.S. National Academy of Sciences to establish Recommended Daily Energy Allowances for U.S. citizens. The FAO/WHO/UNU calculations used a new quantity, the **resting energy expenditure (REE).** The REE is basically a combination of basal energy needs, plus the thermic effect of food, plus a small amount of energy needed to perform the most basic sedentary activities, such as

TABLE 6-14

Factors for estimating total daily energy allowances at various levels of physical activity

LEVEL OF ACTIVITY	ACTIVITY FACTOR (× REE)	ENERGY EXPENDITURE (Kcal/kg/DAY)
VERY LIGHT		
Men	1.3	31
Women	1.3	30
LIGHT		
Men	1.6	38
Women	1.5	35
MODERATE		
Men	1.7	41
Women	1.6	37
HEAVY		
Men	2.1	50
Women	1.9	44
EXCEPTIONAL		
Men	2.4	58
Women	2.2	51

From FAO/WHO/UNU: *Energy and protein* requirements, Technical Rep Series 724, Geneva, Switzerland, 1985, World Health Organization.

sitting quietly. In this system the equation for total energy needs is simplified to the following:

TOTAL ENERGY NEEDS = REE + NEEDS FOR ACTIVITY

The total energy expenditure associated with various activities can be represented as *a multiple* of the REE value (that is, REE × some factor). Tables have also been drawn up that allow us to calculate a person's total energy requirements by matching his or her typical level of activity with various levels that have been found to match specific multiples of REE (Table 6-14). Patterns of activity typical of U.S. citizens fall into the "light" category (indicating total average energy requirements of 1.5 to 1.6 × REE) or "moderate" category (1.6 to 1.7 × REE). These patterns of activity formed the basis of the recommended energy intakes for U.S. citizens made by the Food and Nutrition Board.

A factorial method of estimating total energy need can be fairly accurate when the observations of activity are performed under controlled laboratory conditions. When applied "in the field" (that is, when the subjects are going about their normal lives), however, there are likely to be significant errors in the reporting of time spent on each activity and how strenuously the activities were pursued. Errors may also be caused by the fact that modern activity charts reflecting modern lifestyles and activities are not available.

ENERGY INTAKE AND ENERGY BALANCE METHOD

The energy intake and energy balance method of estimating total energy needs is based on comparison of total energy intake over several days with the amount of energy required for any observed change in body composition.[5] Essentially, total kilocalorie intake over a number of days is measured, any change in body composition is measured, sufficient kilocalories are subtracted or added to account for the change in body composition (subtracting if weight is gained, adding if weight is lost), and then the remaining figure is divided by the number of days of the trial. The accuracy of this procedure obviously depends on the accuracy of the food intake record and the accuracy of measurements of change in body composition. The methods for measuring changes in body composition are discussed fully in Chapter 7. They involve careful and sophisticated measurements made before and after the trial. Errors in these measurements can introduce significant errors to the final estimate of total energy expenditure. For example, an error of plus or minus 2% in measuring the body composition of a 70-kg man introduces an error of approximately 12,600 kcal, corresponding to an error of 900 kcal/day in a 14-day trial. Nevertheless, this method can yield relatively accurate predictions of total energy needs when it is performed under strictly controlled conditions. It has been shown to be less accurate, and therefore of only limited use, under free-living conditions. This is primarily because of people's underestimation of the amount of food they consumed or their failure to keep accurate records.

HEART RATE MONITORING METHOD

Estimating total energy needs by constantly monitoring the heart rate is based on the strong positive correlation that exists between heart rate and oxygen consumption and therefore energy release from food or energy stores.[6] The relationship between heart rate and oxygen consumption can be explained by the fact that the oxygen needed to release energy from food is transported through the blood; increased oxygen consumption requires increased blood flow powered by an increase in heart rate. In principle, continuous monitoring of heart rate offers an excellent way to estimate total energy needs in a free-living subject connected to an appropriately small, portable apparatus. Before undertaking such free-living studies, however, the relationship between an individual's heart rate and level of oxygen consumption must be determined in laboratory trials. During such trials heart rate and oxygen consumption are both directly monitored while the subject undertakes a series of increasingly strenuous activities, from sitting, to walking on a treadmill, to running on a treadmill or stepping on and off a block, for example. The activities are designed to produce heart rates ranging from the resting rate to more than 160 beats per minute. A mathematical equation describing the relationship between heart rate and oxygen consumption can then be derived that is unique to the individual subject concerned by comparing the heart rate and oxygen consumption data obtained. This equation allows an approximate level of oxygen consumption to be predicted for any heart rate across the entire range.[6] A trial of free-living subjects spanning 24 hours or longer can then be conducted, with heart rate being continuously monitored through a transmitter worn around the chest and a watchlike receiver on the wrist. At the end of the trial the continuous record of heart rate is used in conjunction with the previously determined equation to determine approximate energy consumption rates and hence total daily energy expenditure and therefore need.

DOUBLY-LABELED WATER TECHNIQUE

The doubly-labeled water technique was developed by Lifson[7] to measure carbon dioxide production by animals. It is based on the fact that hydrogen atoms of body water leave the body via the usual routes of water loss—within urine, sweat, and saliva and as evaporated water (such as that in exhalations)— while the oxygen atoms of body water leave the body by these same routes but also as carbon dioxide gas. Oxygen atoms can be transferred from body water into carbon dioxide gas because of the action of an enzyme called *carbonic anhydrase*. Knowledge of this fact allowed Lifson to predict that carbon dioxide gas production could be indirectly measured by "labeling" some of the water in the body with the two stable isotopes, ^{2}H (deuterium) and ^{18}O. These isotopes are uncommon forms of hydrogen and oxygen atoms, with different masses (the superscript numbers) from the most common isotopes, which are ^{1}H and ^{16}O. The presence of these isotopes is readily detectable; so labeling a small proportion of body water molecules with them allows the respective fates of hydrogen and oxygen atoms in the water to be monitored. This indirectly allows carbon dioxide production to be measured, as was first demonstrated in experiments with mice. Although it appeared that the technique was also successful in humans, it was not economically feasible until technological improvements reduced the cost of the instruments, called *mass spectrometers,* used to measure the abundance of the two isotopes in fluid samples. The validity of the method in humans was first established by Schoeller and Van Santen[8] in 1982. Four subjects were given "loading" doses of the two isotopes incorporated into water, and the different rates at which the oxygen and hydrogen labels were eliminated were determined by analysis of urine. This allowed calculation of the levels of carbon dioxide production over 14 days, and the results obtained in this way were validated by comparison with a controlled energy intake and energy balance measurement. Only a 2.1% difference between the results from the doubly-labeled water technique and energy intake and energy balance methods was found.

The doubly-labeled water technique can yield a reliable average measure of a person's energy needs over approximately 1 to 3 weeks. The subjects must provide periodic urine samples but do not need to record their food intake or the activities they perform or wear any apparatus. The results obtained by this method have been summarized by Schoeller and Field.[9] The reliability of this method has been repeatedly confirmed in humans, including pregnant women, infants, children, and the elderly. Unfortunately, it is a relatively expensive method, largely because of the high cost of the mass spectrometers and the ^{18}O isotope and the technical skill required to measure the isotope abundances in urine. Overall, however, the doubly-labeled water technique is the best available method of assessing the energy costs of activity.

Almost all of the available estimates of energy needs are for moderately active and healthy individuals living in comfortable environmental temperatures. Estimates should be adjusted upward for people living in cold temperatures and for those who are appreciably larger than the average man (69 kg) or average woman (59 kg). Estimates should be revised downward for people over 50 years old and for those smaller than the average man or woman.

The best personal estimate of energy need is obtained simply by determining the level of energy intake that maintains body weight at the desired level. A person who is neither gaining nor losing weight over a long period and whose weight is close to the recommended level has clearly achieved the correct balance between intake and need. Those who are overweight or underweight should obviously adjust their intake downward or upward as appropriate.

ENERGY NEEDS OF SPECIAL GROUPS

Pregnant Women

The additional energy needs during pregnancy correspond to the energy needed by the developing fetus in addition to that needed for the growth of the placenta and the formation of other additional tissues in the mother. These energy needs are calculated to total approximately 80,000 kcal over the 9 months of pregnancy, based on a pregnant woman's gaining 12.5 kg in weight and giving birth to a 3.3-kg infant. This estimate was used to derive a recommended additional energy allowance for pregnant women of 300 kcal/day during the second and third trimesters of pregnancy.

TABLE 6-15

Mean heights and weights and estimated daily energy allowances

	WEIGHT		HEIGHT				ESTIMATED ENERGY ALLOWANCE (WITH RANGE)		
	kg	lb	cm	in	RESTING ENERGY EXPENDITURE (Kcal/DAY)	MEAN ACTIVITY FACTOR	Kcal/DAY	Kcal/kg	MJ/DAY
INFANTS (MO)									
0-2.9	4.5	10	55	22	—	—	500 (400-700)	110	2.1
3-5.9	6.6	15	64	25	—	—	650 (500-850)	100	2.7
6-8.9	7.9	17	69	27	—	—	750 (600-1000)	95	3.1
9-11.9	9.0	20	73	29	—	—	900 (700-1200)	100	3.8
CHILDREN (YR)									
1-1.9	11	24	82	32	600	2.0	1200 (900-1600)	105	4.8
2-3.9	14	31	96	38	700	2.0	1400 (1100-1900)	100	5.9
4-5.9	18	40	109	43	830	2.0	1700 (1300-2300)	92	7.1
6-7.9	22	49	121	48	930	2.0	1800 (1400-2400)	83	7.5
8-9.9	28	62	132	52	1050	1.8	1900 (1400-2500)	69	7.9
MALES (YR)									
10-11.9	36	79	143	56	1200	1.8	2200 (1700-2900)	61	9.2
12-16.9	57	126	169	67	1580	1.7	2700 (2000-3600)	47	11.3
17-24.9	70	155	177	70	1750	1.6	2800 (2400-3200)	40	11.7
25-49.9	69	152	176	69	1620	1.6	2600 (2200-3100)	38	10.9
50-69.9	68	149	173	68	1440	1.6	2300 (1900-2700)	34	9.6
>70	66	146	171	67	1310	1.5	2000 (1600-2400)	30	8.4
FEMALES (YR)									
10-13.9	42	96	155	62	1300	1.7	2200 (1700-2900)	50	9.2
14-16.9	56	123	162	64	1410	1.6	2200 (1700-3000)	41	9.6
17-24.9	58	128	163	64	1420	1.6	2300 (1900-2700)	39	9.6
25-49.9	59	130	163	64	1350	1.6	2200 (1800-2600)	37	9.2
50-69.9	59	130	160	63	1220	1.6	2000 (1600-2400)	34	8.4
<70	59	130	158	62	1140	1.5	1700 (1300-2100)	30	7.1
Pregnancy	1st trimester							+ 300	+ 1.3
	2nd trimester							+ 300	+ 1.3
	3rd trimester							+ 300	+ 1.3
Lactation	1st 6 months							+ 400	+ 1.7
	2nd 6 months							+ 600	+ 2.5

From FAO/WHO/UNU: *Energy and protein requirements,* Technical Rep Series 724, Geneva, Switzerland, 1985, World Health Organization.

Breast-Feeding Women

The additional energy requirements during lactation are proportional to the quantity of milk produced. It is assumed that average milk production is 750 ml/day during the first 6 months of lactation and 600 ml/day during the second 6 months. The average energy content of human milk is 70 kcal/100 ml, and the efficiency of milk production is estimated to be 80%. Thus the additional energy requirements during lactation are about 650 kcal/day during the first 6 months of lactation and 525 kcal/day during the second 6 months of lactation. Of these amounts, up to 150 kcal/day can be provided during the first 6 months of lactation by the extra fat accumulated during pregnancy. This leaves a net requirement to be met by additional energy intake of around 500 kcal/day during the first 6 months.

Infants

An infant's energy requirement at birth is approximately 115 kcal/kg/day. This declines to about 95 kcal/kg/day by the time the baby is 6 months old and then rises again to 100 kcal/kg/day during the first year to meet the demands of the high growth rate at this time. The recommended daily energy allowances for infants are average values of 108 kcal/kg/day during the first 6 months of life and 98 kcal/kg/day during the second 6 months. From the age of 2 years onward the energy required per kilogram of body weight continues to decline, apart from a brief rise during puberty. Most estimates of the energy needs of infants and children have come from studies of reported intakes of infants and children who were growing at satisfactory rates. A child whose growth consistently follows one developmental line on the standard growth curves, regardless of where in the standard range that line falls (see Chapter 15), is assumed to be getting adequate kilocalories. As soon as energy intake becomes either inadequate or excessive, growth deviates from the normal pattern and so leaves the growth curve that was previously being followed.

Children and Adolescents

For children 10 years old and over, estimated energy needs equal REE × 1.7 for girls and REE × 1.8 for boys. The needs for growth account for less than 3% of the total of basal needs plus activity needs. Children's total energy needs per kilogram of body weight gradually decrease to the adult levels of REE × 1.5 for young women and REE × 1.6 for young men, attained at an age of about 17 years. A wide variation in activity needs throughout childhood, however, makes it difficult to estimate the total energy needs of individual children. The most sensitive measure of the adequacy or inadequacy of energy intake is the pattern of an individual's growth. Children who show a tendency toward obesity should be encouraged to increase their activity and practice moderation in total energy intake until their weight returns to expected levels. They should seldom be encouraged to actually lose weight, but rather to stabilize it until they "grow into it."

Table 6-15 lists the estimated energy needs for all ages and both genders. The figures are based on the formula prepared by the FAO/WHO/UNU and are applied to people of average weights and heights in the United States. It should be stressed that the recommended energy intakes are *average* requirements for people engaged in light activity at a comfortable environmental temperature, so, unlike the recommended intakes of specific nutrients, the recommended energy intakes may be insufficient for many people, especially those engaged in strenuous physical activity. The important notion that there is a wide variation in individuals' energy requirements, largely because of differences in their levels of activity, is reinforced by presentation of a *range* of acceptable intakes for each gender and age category (Table 6-15). The table makes it obvious that energy requirements per unit of body weight decrease with age. For children and adolescents the energy allowances are sufficiently high to permit appropriate growth, assuming that the level of activity corresponds to that deemed to be typical in the United States.

The Nationwide Food Consumption Study (1987-1988) showed an average energy intake of 84% of the recommended dietary allowances (RDAs). Energy intakes reported in NHANES III (1988-1991) are similarly below recommended levels. This may be explained by a failure to report food intake accurately, lower than anticipated energy expenditure, or unrealistically high recommended intakes. If food intakes were in fact accurately reported, these results raise the obvious question of why there is a high incidence of obesity in a population that eats less than nutritional advice suggests. Almost all studies comparing actual with reported intakes identify underreporting as much more common than overreporting of actual intakes.

TABLE 6-16

Canadian Dietary Standards for average energy requirements

	Kcal/kg BODY WEIGHT	
AGE (YR)	MEN	WOMEN
13-15	57	46
16-18	51	40
19-24	42	36
25-49	36	32
50-74	31	29
75+	29	23

The recommended energy intakes for Canadians are presented in Table 6-16.[10] These are based on energy intake studies of large numbers of Canadians. The Canadian standards are close to the United States standards, although they were derived in a different way. The Canadian standards are based on the results of surveys of large samples of the population in which the energy intakes were evaluated.

THE RELEASE OF ENERGY FROM FOOD

The previous three chapters have been focused on carbohydrate, lipid, and protein, which are the three main energy-yielding components in food (the only other one being alcohol, also considered in Chapter 3). This chapter has discussed how much energy these substances can release to the body, how we measure the body's energy needs, and what these needs actually are in a variety of situations. It has been said that, in general, carbohydrate, lipid, protein, and alcohol release energy when they are oxidized to form carbon dioxide and water. This oxidation process, however, occurs via a series of many chemical reactions that allow much of the energy to be trapped within ATP. We now investigate in more detail how the process of energy capture actually takes place and some of the biochemical consequences of overnutrition and undernutrition. The basic chemical principles involved are summarized in Appendix A.

Before their use as energy-releasing fuels, carbohydrates are digested to glucose, the triglycerides that comprise most dietary lipids are digested to fatty acids and glycerol, and proteins are digested to amino acids. Thus glucose, fatty acids, glycerol, and amino acids are the four main chemicals whose oxidation must be considered to understand how energy is released from food.

METABOLISM OF GLUCOSE

The overall chemical reaction involved in the oxidation of glucose is as follows:

$$C_6H_{12}O_6 + 6O_2 \rightarrow 6CO_2 + 6H_2O + 38\ ATP$$

This indicates that one molecule of glucose ($C_6H_{12}O_6$) reacts indirectly with six molecules of oxygen to generate six molecules of carbon dioxide and six molecules of water. The energy released during this net oxidation process can be used to manufacture up to 38 molecules of ATP from adenosine diphosphate (ADP) and inorganic phosphate. The conversion of glucose to carbon dioxide and water, which proceeds in one step when glucose is burned, is achieved within cells by the combined effect of three multistep processes:

- **Glycolysis**
- **The citric acid cycle**
- **Oxidative phosphorylation** (powered by the transfer of electrons down the **electron transport chain**)

The key chemical steps involved (although certainly not all of them) are outlined in Figure 6-7.

In the process known as glycolysis, the six-carbon glucose molecule is converted into two molecules of the three-carbon compound pyruvic acid (also known as pyruvate). This transformation is achieved by 10 individual chemical steps, each one catalyzed by a specific enzyme. Energy is given out during the conversion of glucose into pyruvic acid, some of which serves to power the net formation of two molecules of ATP.

The conversion of glucose to pyruvic acid also involves the removal of four hydrogen atoms. These hydrogen atoms are removed during reaction with the niacin-containing coenzyme NAD^+ (**nicotinamide adenine dinucleotide**), although one of them ends up in the form of a hydrogen ion (H^+), rather than being directly bound to the coenzyme. NAD^+ is involved in many hydrogen-transfer reactions in the body, being interconverted between its "oxidized form" (NAD^+) and its hydrogen-carrying "reduced" form ($NADH + H^+$), as appropriate. Niacin is a vitamin because it is needed for the formation of this essential coenzyme.

Although glycolysis takes the atoms derived from glucose through the first steps that lead to their eventual complete oxidation, no combination with oxygen is actually involved in glycolysis. This means that oxygen is not required for glycolysis to proceed, a situation described by saying that glycolysis is an **anaerobic** process (one not requiring the presence of oxygen). This is important to athletes such as sprinters because during strenuous activity the rate at which the complete oxidation of glucose can proceed is limited by the rate at which oxygen can be breathed in and transported to muscle cells. The rate of glycolysis is not limited by oxygen availability. So glycolysis can supply some extra ATP from the *partial* breakdown of glucose in addition to the amount that is available from the complete oxidation of glucose. The amounts of ATP concerned are small, compared with the amounts released by the complete oxidation of glucose, but without their help many winners of sprint races would certainly have been losers.

The reactions of glycolysis occur in the cytoplasm of the cell, but subsequent events in the oxidation of glucose take place in the membrane-bound organelles within the cell known as *mitochondria*. These subsequent events compose the **aerobic** phase of glucose metabolism because they require the presence of oxygen obtained from the air. The necessary chemical transformations begin when pyruvic acid is transported into mitochondria, where it reacts with a coenzyme known as **Coenzyme A** (CoA) to form acetyl CoA. This reaction also releases one carbon dioxide molecule per pyruvic acid reacted, and so it leaves only two carbon atoms of the original three in pyruvic acid attached to the CoA. As the name acetyl CoA implies, these two carbon atoms are bound in the form of an **acetyl** group (see Figure 6-8). The conversion of pyruvic acid to acetyl CoA also involves two more hydrogen atoms being passed onto NAD^+, one coming from pyruvic acid and one from CoA itself.

As was stated in Chapter 4, carbohydrates, fatty acids, and amino acids are *all* converted into acetyl CoA when these nutrients are oxidized as a source of energy. So acetyl CoA is obviously a central chemical involved in the release of energy from food. One component of CoA that is needed to form acetyl CoA is the vitamin known as *pantothenic acid*.

Acetyl CoA enters the series of reactions known as the *citric acid cycle,* which is also known as the *Krebs cycle* (after Hans Krebs, who discovered it), and the *tricarboxylic acid (TCA) cycle.* In the first step of this cycle the acetyl CoA reacts with the four-carbon compound oxaloacetic acid to release the CoA and generate the citric acid that gives the citric acid cycle one of its names. A series of eight individual reactions then proceeds to regenerate the oxaloacetic acid needed to react with another molecule of acetyl CoA. This series of reactions is called a "cycle" because it regenerates the original oxaloacetic acid. During the course of each "turn" of the cycle the carbon atoms derived from the two-carbon acetate unit (donated by acetyl CoA) are converted into carbon dioxide. The hydrogen atoms of the acetate unit become transferred to the NAD^+ coenzyme or a different riboflavin-containing coenzyme known as **flavin adenine dinucleotide (FAD).** FAD performs a role similar to that of NAD^+, picking up hydrogen atoms to be converted into its "reduced" form, $FADH_2$. Riboflavin is a vitamin because it is needed for the formation of this essential coenzyme. The flow of the atoms derived

FIGURE 6-7

Summary of the key biochemical steps in the oxidative metabolism of glucose, fatty acids, glycerol, and amino acids.

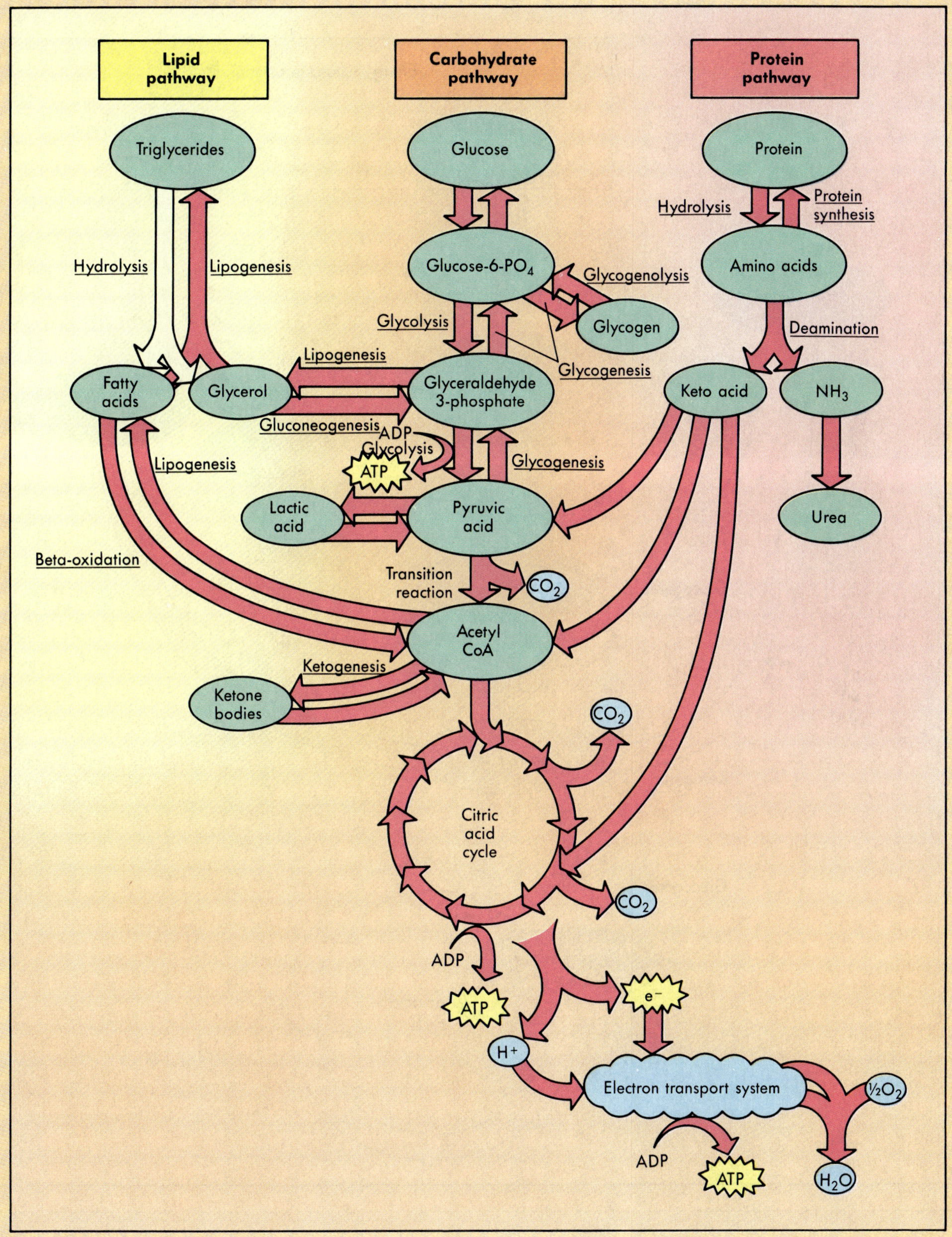

FIGURE 6-8

Pathways by which glucose, amino acids, fatty acids, and glycerol can be converted into storage compounds during overnutrition.

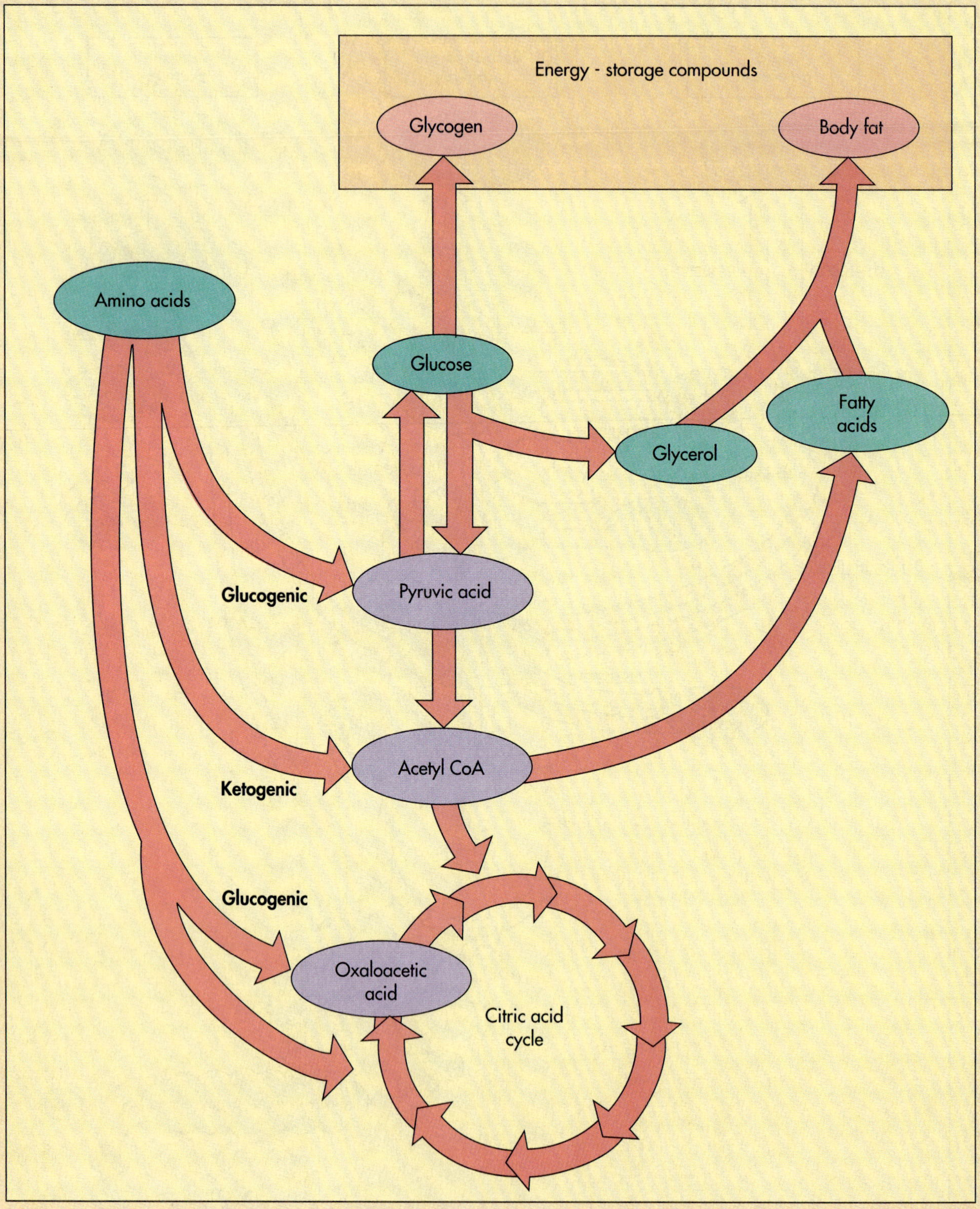

originally from glucose through glycolysis and then the citric acid cycle converts all of the carbon atoms into the form of carbon dioxide, as required by the overall equation for the oxidation of glucose.

During each turn of the citric acid cycle, sufficient energy is given out to form one molecule of ATP from ADP and P_i. Most of the energy-generating steps of oxidative metabolism, however, are still to come. They come in the final of the three stages identified previously, known as *oxidative phosphorylation*. The overall effect of oxidative phosphorylation is for the hydrogen atoms carried in the form of NADH + H^+ and $FADH_2$ to be combined with oxygen to generate water. This overall effect is achieved in an indirect way, however, composed of many individual small steps. Electrons from the hydrogen atoms carried by NADH and $FADH_2$ are transferred to a series of proteins and other compounds embedded in the innermost of the two membranes possessed by mitochondria. These electron-carrying proteins and other compounds form what is known as the **electron-transport chain,** or **respiratory chain.** The electrons being transported down this chain eventually reunite with hydrogen ions and oxygen atoms to form water. The operation of the electron transport chain, however, allows a considerable amount of energy to be trapped within the structure of ATP that is formed from ADP and P_i. This process is known as oxidative phosphorylation because it is a chemically *oxidative* process, with the hydrogen that goes in at the start eventually combining with oxygen to form water and the energy thereby released powering the *phosphorylation* of ADP to form ATP. The details of how this happens are complex and still the subject of much research and debate. As we have seen, however, the essential chemical principle involved is simple: a chemical process that releases a lot of energy is achieved by a series of small coupled steps, which allows much of the energy to be stored within the high-energy structure of ATP, rather than being immediately dissipated as heat. This statement summarizes the basic chemical principle that lies at the heart of not only oxidative phosphorylation, but also the entire oxidation of glucose to carbon dioxide and water via glycolysis, the citric acid cycle, and oxidative phosphorylation.

METABOLISM OF FATTY ACIDS AND GLYCEROL

Of the lipid in the diet, 95% is in the form of triglycerides, which are split into fatty acids and glycerol before entering the oxidative pathways that allow them to serve as a source of energy. Glycerol can enter the pathway of glycolysis at one of the intermediate steps between glucose and pyruvic acid. Thus glycerol derived from dietary fat is converted into pyruvic acid and is then used as a source of energy in exactly the same way as the pyruvic acid derived from carbohydrate.

As was discussed in Chapter 4, fatty acids are degraded by the **β-oxidation** pathway, during which successive two-carbon units are cleaved from the fatty acid molecule to become the acetyl units of acetyl CoA. This acetyl CoA enters the citric acid cycle, allowing its energy to be released in exactly the same way as already outlined for the metabolism of glucose. The oxidation of one molecule of a short-chain, six-carbon fatty acid generates a maximum of 44 molecules of ATP in contrast to the maximum of 38 ATP molecules generated by the oxidation of a molecule of glucose. A six-carbon fatty acid was chosen in the above comparison because glucose also contains six carbon atoms. Most fatty acid molecules are considerably longer, and so yield several times as many ATP molecules as does a molecule of glucose.

METABOLISM OF AMINO ACIDS

When the energy intake of the diet is adequate, the amino acids derived from dietary protein are used for the synthesis of proteins in the body in preference to being used as an energy source. If excess amino acids are available in the diet, however, they can be oxidatively degraded as a source of energy (see Chapter 5).

The first step in the use of amino acids as an energy source is the process of deamination in which their nitrogen-containing amino groups are removed. The remaining nitrogen-free portions of the amino acids enter the same metabolic pathways as carbohydrates and lipids, but they do so at various places, depending on which amino acid is concerned (and some can enter at more than one place). The details of where the deaminated products of the various amino acids can enter the common degradative pathways are shown in Figure 6-7. In general, some are converted into pyruvic acid, some into various intermediates of the citric acid cycle, and some into the acetyl groups that can become incorporated into acetyl CoA.

It should now be clear that the metabolic pathways summarized in Figure 6-8 represent the heart of energy-yielding metabolism into which atoms destined for oxidation flow from carbohydrates, fats, and proteins. Alcohol, the only other dietary energy source, also fits into this scheme. It is converted into acetate units, which can then become incorporated into acetyl CoA. Thus there is a pleasing unity about the biochemical events that allow the energy stored within food to be transferred into ATP for use by the cells and tissues of the body as required.

METABOLIC EFFECTS OF OVERNUTRITION AND UNDERNUTRITION

When kilocalorie intake does not exactly balance kilocalorie expenditure, significant alterations in metabolism occur. When food intake provides more kilocalories than the body requires, the metabolism of all three of the energy-yielding nutrients is altered, (Figure 6-8). Glucose derived from excess dietary carbohydrate is converted into the storage carbohydrate glycogen in the liver and muscle. The capacity of the body to store glycogen is relatively limited, however. Excess glucose can also flow down the normal pathway of glycolysis, some of it being converted all the way to pyruvic acid and then acetyl CoA, and some can be diverted into the form of glycerol, one of the components needed to build storage triglycerides in adipose tissue. The other components needed to form storage triglycerides are fatty acids. These can be synthesized from the acetyl units of acetyl CoA in a process that, overall, reverses the breakdown of fatty acids to acetyl CoA, which occurs when they are being used as a source of energy. Thus glucose derived from excess dietary carbohydrate can be converted into the storage triglycerides of adipose tissue. Fatty acids and glycerol derived from excess dietary fats can be converted back into triglycerides and stored in adipose tissue. Some dietary triglycerides are only degraded to monoglycerides and fatty acids by digestion, a process that can also be reversed to generate new triglyceride stores in adipose tissue.

Excess amino acids that can be converted into pyruvic acid or intermediates of the citric acid cycle are known as *glucogenic amino acids* (see Chapter 5). This means that these amino acids can be used for the synthesis of glucose and therefore glycogen. In the case of those amino acids which are converted into intermediates of the citric acid cycle, their conversion into glucose depends on the fact that oxaloacetate can be converted into a derivative of pyruvic acid. The reactions of **gluconeogenesis** then reverse the net effect of glycolysis to form glucose. The glucogenic amino acids, however, can also be diverted into the formation of storage triglycerides because this can happen to glucose itself. The remaining amino acids, known as the *ketogenic* ones, can be converted into acetyl CoA and from there into storage triglycerides. Thus by a variety of metabolic routes excess protein in the diet can be converted into fat stores. In the process the nitrogen atoms are removed from the amino acids by deamination and either used for the synthesis of other nitrogen-containing components of the body or excreted as urea in the urine.

When energy intake is insufficient to meet immediate energy needs, all of the glucose, fatty acids, glycerol, and amino acids derived from digested food can be used immediately as a source of energy, but the body must also draw on supplies from elsewhere. There are three alternative sources: carbohydrate stored as glycogen in the liver and muscles, fat stored within adipose tissue, and body protein. The carbohydrate glycogen reserves are used first, being broken down into glucose, which is then metabolized as normal. Fat reserves are called on next, with the triglycerides that form the bulk of these reserves being split into fatty acids and glycerol, which are then metabolized to yield energy in the way considered already. While fat reserves are being broken down, there is a steady loss in body weight that is proportional to the amount of fat used. The protein of the body is degraded to amino acids for use as an energy source only as a last resort.

One complicating factor during undernutrition is introduced by the fact that the brain needs a continual supply of glucose as an energy source. The carbohydrate present in the diet is often sufficient to meet the brain's need for glucose, even when the total kilocalories in the diet do not meet all of the body's energy needs. If the diet is low in carbohydrate (less than about 100 g/day), however, once the glycogen stores have been depleted, metabolism changes to provide an alternative source of glucose for the brain. This glucose can be formed from glucogenic amino acids derived from the diet from the breakdown of body protein or by the conversion of glycerol from triglycerides into pyruvic acid and then glucose. Glycerol, however, represents only 5% of a triglyceride molecule, and so when glycerol is being used in this way to generate glucose, the acetyl CoA derived from the breakdown of fatty acids can begin to accumulate. This causes the acetyl CoA to be diverted from its normal oxidative pathway of metabolism into the formation of ketones (see Chapters 3 to 5). After a period of adaptation some of these ketones can be used as an alternative energy source by the brain, reducing—but not completely eliminating—its need for glucose. However, an excess of ketones changes the pH value of the blood, affects the functioning of some enzymes, and depresses hunger. Excess ketones must be excreted, which requires a large volume of fluid. Thus people following low-carbohydrate diets and who must metabolize fat to provide fuel for the brain experience extreme weight loss, which is partially a result of loss of water, rather than loss of fat tissue. All of these changes are essentially caused by a deficiency of carbohydrate in the diet and can be quickly reversed by an increase in carbohydrate intake.

The use of glucogenic amino acids to produce the glucose needed by the brain can lead to the breakdown of body protein to supply the amino acids. This also results in loss of some of the large amounts of water stored in body protein and also produces mineral loss, particularly of potassium. Thus a rapid loss of weight and muscle weakness results. Also, the ketogenic amino acids that are necessarily also released during protein breakdown contribute to the formation of ketones and the associated problems already discussed.

In summary, when the diet is deficient in kilocalories, the body draws on its carbohydrate fuel reserves first, followed by its much larger fat stores. When carbohydrate intake is too low to meet the brain's need for glucose, the use of fat and glucogenic amino acids to generate glucose leads to loss of body water and rapid weight loss. When carbohydrate intakes are sufficient to meet the needs of the brain, weight loss results from the continuing mobilization of stored fat as a fuel supply and so varies in proportion to the amount of fat consumed.

THE ROLE OF VITAMINS AND MINERALS

The metabolic pathways involved in the release of energy from food can operate properly only if adequate supplies of certain vitamins and minerals are available in the diet. The key roles played by three vitamins have been already mentioned: Niacin is required to form the coenzyme NAD^+, riboflavin is required to form the coenzyme FAD, and pantothenic acid is required to form coenzyme A. These are only three of the most prominent examples. A variety of other vitamins and also various minerals are required for normal functioning of the processes of digestion, absorption, and the release of energy or formation of energy stores from food (Table 6-17). The precise roles of these vitamins and minerals is discussed fully in the vitamins and minerals overviews and in Chapters 9 to 13.

TABLE 6-17

Vitamins and minerals required to facilitate the processes of digestion, absorption, and the metabolism involved in energy release and storage

PROCESS	VITAMIN	MINERAL
Digestion		Chloride
		Zinc*
Absorption		Sodium
Anabolism		
Glycogenesis	Riboflavin	Magnesium
	Niacin	Manganese
	Pyridoxine	Cobalt
Catabolism		
Glycolysis	Niacin	Potassium
	Lipoic acid	Magnesium
	Thiamin	
	Pantothenic acid	
Citric acid cycle	Pantothenic acid	Manganese
	Niacin	Iron
	Lipoic acid	Magnesium
	Thiamin	
	Riboflavin	
Electron transport	Niacin	Iron*
	Riboflavin	Copper

* Functions as an essential part of the enzyme.

ISSUES AND OPINIONS

Does Early Overfeeding Increase Fat Cell Number and Destine Us to Obesity in Adulthood?

The effect of feeding in infancy on the amount of body fat during adulthood has attracted a great deal of interest over the years. The earliest studies into this issue were performed mainly on small animals. They indicated that overnutrition or overfeeding of the young animals led to the development of more fat cells (adipocytes), undernutrition produced fewer adipocytes, and these effects persisted into adulthood. These findings led to the hypothesis that infancy was a critical period in determining fat cell number. It was also believed that overeating in infancy caused considerable increases in adipocyte numbers, and that overeating in childhood resulted only in increased size of adipocytes. In other words, it became widely believed that overfeeding in infancy led to irreversible lifelong consequences resulting from the increase in adipocyte numbers.

In all species studied, adipocyte size changes more readily than does adipocyte number, and obese people have larger adipocytes than people of normal weight. A normal adipocyte contains about 0.5 µg of lipid, whereas the adipocytes of extremely obese people can contain more than 2 µg of lipid. Massively obese individuals must store more than four times the amount of lipid stored by people of normal weight, which requires increases in adipocyte number as well as size.

In a study of male and female infants examined at 1, 3, 6, 9, 12, and 18 months, it was found that the average increase in body fat from 0.7 kg at 1 month of age to 2.5 kg at 12 months of age was a result of an increase in fat cell weight from 0.15 to 0.5 µg, whereas fat cell number was stable at 6×10^{10}. A further increase in body fat to 3 kg at 18 months of age was entirely caused by an increase in fat cell number. Data on people aged 22 years indicate that accumulation of body fat from age 1 to 22 is caused by an increase in the number of adipocytes, and the average adipocyte weight does not increase between these ages.

Epidemiological studies tracking body fatness in specific individuals from infancy to adulthood have generally found that no more than 15% of the infants classified as "heavy" were also classified as "obese" or "overweight" as adults. Studies designed to identify early indicators of adult overweight problems indicate that the rate of weight gain in infancy is a poor indicator and so are the type of milk fed (human milk or formula) and the age at which solid foods were fed in addition to milk. So, in general, long-held beliefs that formula-fed infants, who grow more rapidly than human milk–fed infants and are introduced to solid foods early in life (supposedly supplementing energy intake), develop more adipocytes and become overweight adults are not supported by the most recent evidence.

From Häger and others: *Metabolism* 26:607, 1977; and Rolland-Cachera M-F and others: *Ann Hum Biol* 14:219, 1987.

BY NOW YOU SHOULD KNOW

- The energy content of the diet is provided by carbohydrate, lipid, protein, and alcohol.
- The energy available from food is measured in kilocalories (kcal) or kilojoules (kJ).
- Energy needs are divided into three main groups: those for basal, or resting metabolism; those for activity; and those for the thermic effect of food.
- The energy content of food can be determined directly in a bomb calorimeter or indirectly by multiplying the physiological fuel values of carbohydrate (4 kcal/g), lipid (9 kcal/g), and protein (4 kcal/g) by the amount of each of these energy-yielding nutrients in any food found in tables of food composition.
- Energy requirements for basal resting metabolism can be (1) determined by direct calorimetry, (2) obtained indirectly from measurement of oxygen consumption or carbon dioxide generation, or (3) calculated from metabolic body size or the Harris-Benedict equation that incorporates height and weight measurements.
- Energy expenditure during activity varies with the duration of the activity, the intensity of the activity, and the amount of weight being moved.
- Energy needs for activities are calculated from tables listing the energy costs of different activities and records of activity patterns.
- Energy intake beyond the body's needs is stored as body fat. When intake is insufficient to meet needs, body fat is metabolized to yield 3500 kcal/lb.
- Carbohydrates and fatty acids are all converted to acetyl CoA when these nutrients are used as a source of energy.
- The release of energy from carbohydrates, fatty acids, and amino acids involves many chemical steps within the cells of the body, and much of the released energy is trapped within the high-energy molecule ATP.
- The three processes that liberate energy from carbohydrates, fatty acids, and amino acids are glycolysis, the citric acid cycle, and oxidative phosphorylation.
- Minerals and vitamins serve as catalysts for many of the metabolic reactions within the cell.

STUDY QUESTIONS

1. Explain the distinction between the calorie, Calorie, kilocalorie, and kilojoule.
2. Explain why the heat of combustion for protein is 5.65 kcal/g but the net energy available from the oxidation of protein in the body is 4.35 kcal/g.
3. How are the physiological fuel values of carbohydrate, lipid, and protein determined?
4. What are the three components of energy expenditure?
5. Explain the relationship between direct and indirect calorimetry.
6. Name the factors involved in determining basal metabolism and how they affect basal metabolism.
7. Explain the difference between basal metabolic rate (BMR) and resting energy expenditure (REE).
8. Explain how the fate of a teaspoon of sugar consumed when total kilocalorie intake is in excess of requirements differs from its fate when total kilocalorie intake exactly matches requirements.
9. How could the use of the Exchange System help people plan their food intake?
10. Compare the energy needs of certain special groups of people to the needs of normal healthy adults.

CRITICAL ANALYSIS

1. How much energy do you need each day to maintain your body weight? The measurement of energy expenditure with different equipment normally yields only an estimate—precise measurements are extremely difficult to make. In practice, dietitians, athletic trainers, and others usually use methods of calculations that have been previously verified by measurements with instruments. Here is one way to estimate your daily energy expenditure and, therefore, the number of kilocalories you need to consumer daily to maintain your body weight.

- First calculate your basal metabolic rate (BMR):
  ______________(lbs) ÷ 2.2 = ______________ kg
  Your body weight — Your body weight
- ______________ kg × ________ kcal/kg/hour =
  Your body weight — Energy factor 1.0 (males) 0.9 (females) kcal/hour
  ________ kcal/hour × 24 hours = ________ kcal/24 hours
- Then multiply your BMR by the factor that most accurately estimates your daily activity level. The factors, along with corresponding descriptions of daily activities, are listed in Table 6-14.
  ________ kcal/24 hours × ________ Activity factor

REFERENCES

1. Raper NR, Zizza C, Rourke J: *Nutrient content of U.S. food supply, 1909-1988,* Home Economics Research Rep No 50, Washington, DC, 1992, U.S. Department of Agriculture.
2. Webb P: *Human calorimeter,* Westport, Conn, 1985, Praeger Publishers.
3. FAO/WHO/UNU: *Energy and protein requirements,* Technical Rep Series 724, Geneva, Switzerland, 1985, World Health Organization.
4. Keys A and others: *The biology of human starvation,* vol 1, Minneapolis, 1950, University of Minnesota Press.
5. Acheson KJ and others: The measurement of food and energy intake in man: an evaluation of some techniques, *Am J Clin Nutr* 33:1147, 1980.
6. Bradfield RB: A technique for determination of usual daily energy expenditure in the field, *Am J Clin Nutr* 24:1148, 1971.
7. Lifson N: Theory of use of the turnover rates of body water for measuring energy and material balance, *J Theoret Biol* 12:46, 1966.
8. Schoeller DA, Van Santen E: Measurement of energy expenditure in humans by doubly-labeled water method, *J Appl Physiol* 53:955, 1982.
9. Schoeller DA, Field CR: Human energy metabolism: what we have learned from the doubly-labeled water method? *Annu Rev Nutr* 11:355, 1991.
10. Health and Welfare Canada: *Nutrition recommendations,* Ottawa, Canada, 1990, Canadian Government Publishing Center.
11. Häger A and others: Body fat and tissue cellularity in infants: a longitudinal study, *Metabolism* 26:607, 1977.
12. Sjostrom L: The contribution of fat cell to the determination of body weight, *Psychiatr Clin North Am* 1:493, 1978.
13. Kramer MS and others: Determinants of weight and adiposity in the first year of life, *J Pediatr* 106:10, 1985.

ADDITIONAL READINGS

Alpert S: Growth, thermogenesis, and hyperphagia, *Am J Clin Nutr* 52:784, 1990.

Campbell WW and others: Increased energy requirements and changes in body composition with resistance training in older adults, *Am J Clin Nutr* 60:167, 1994.

Carlson MG and others: Fuel and energy metabolism in fasting humans, *Am J Clin Nutr* 60:29, 1994.

Durnin JVGA: Indirect calorimetry in man: a critique of practical problems, *Proc Nutr Soc* 37:5, 1978.

Durnin JVGA, Passmore R: *Energy, work and leisure,* London, 1967, Heinemann Educational Books.

Edholm OG: Energy expenditure and food intake. In Apfelbaum M, editor: *Energy balance in man,* Paris, 1973, Masson.

Hellerstedt WL, Jeffery RW, Murray DM: The association between alcohol intake and adiposity in the general population, *Am J Epidemiol* 132:594, 1990.

Kendall A and others: Weight loss on a low fat diet: consequence of the imprecision of the control of food intake in humans, *Am J Clin Nutr* 53:1124, 1991.

Keys A, Taylor HL, Grande F: Basal metabolism and age of adult men, *Metabolism* 22:5979, 1987.

Schofield WN: Predicting basal metabolic rate: new standards and review of previous work, *Hum Nutr: Clin Nutr* 39C(suppl 1):5, 1985.

Segal KR and others: Thermic effects of food and exercise in lean and obese men of similar lean body mass, *Am J Physiol* 252:E110, 1987.

Thörne A: Diet-induced thermogenesis: an experimental study in healthy and obese individuals, *Acta Chir Scand Suppl* 558:6, 1990.

Vaughan L, Zurlo F, Ravussin E: Aging and energy expenditure, *Am J Clin Nutr* 53:821, 1991.

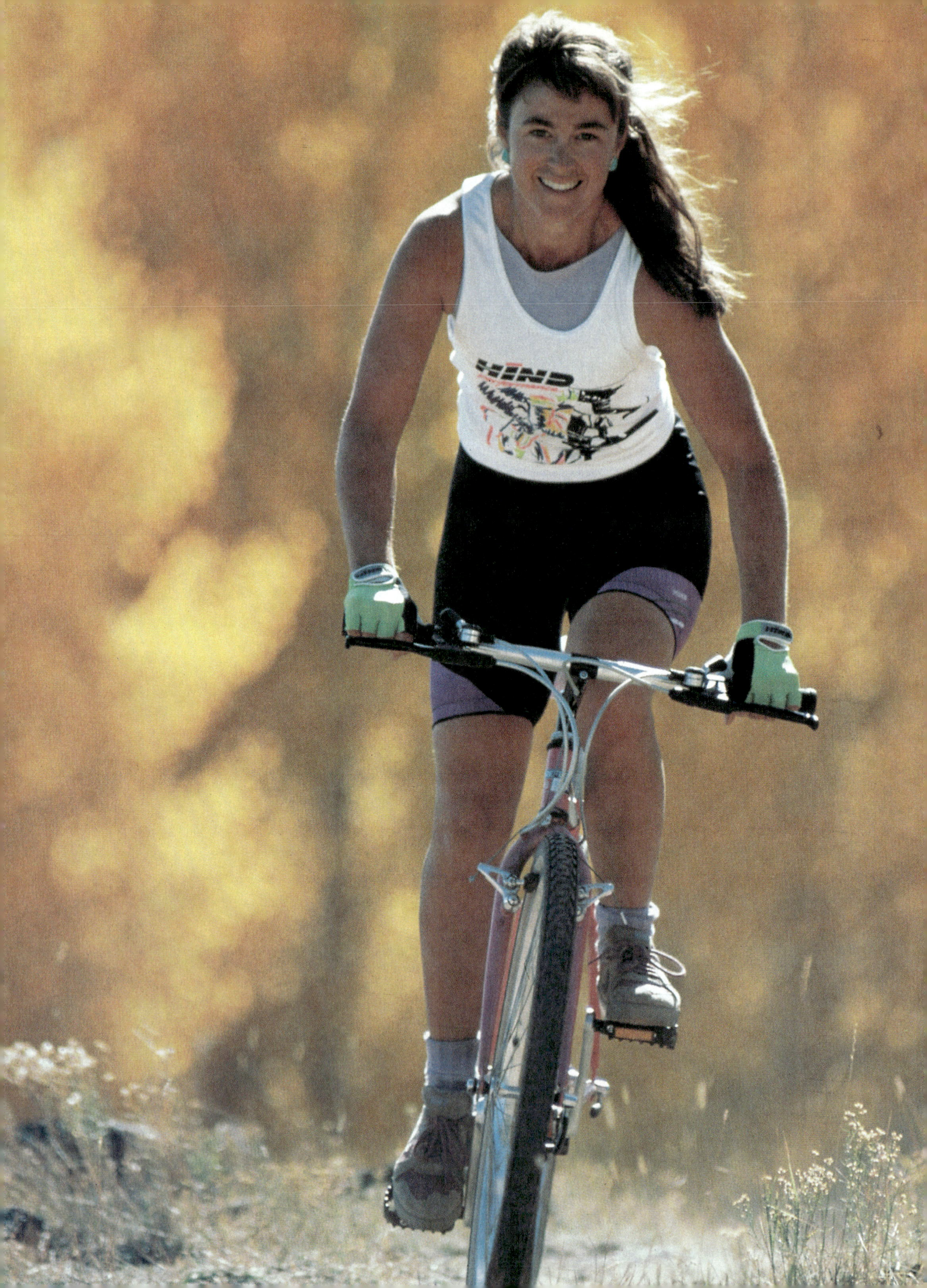
HIND

CHAPTER 7

WEIGHT CONTROL

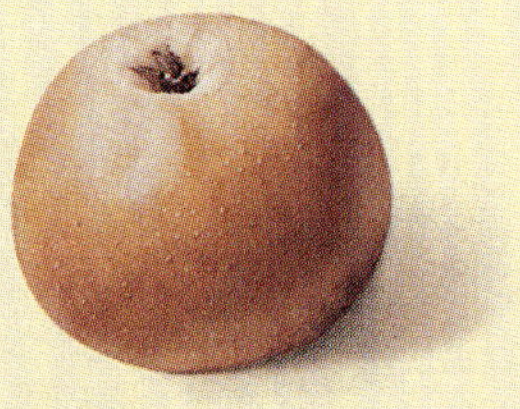

Both obesity and its precursor, overweight, are considered major health problems in the United States. They affect more than 30 million American adults (26%) and from 10% to 40% of the population in various age groups. Obesity and overweight have serious health consequences, and they present a challenge to nutritionists who are trying to understand their causes and advise people affected by them. In these efforts nutritionists are increasingly working with psychologists, exercise physiologists, and other specialists, reflecting the multifaceted nature of the field. Although weight control is a major problem for many people, most people achieve reasonable weight control with little effort or thought. This reflects the amazing sensitivity and subtlety of the body's physiological, behavioral, and psychological control system because small discrepancies between energy intake and expenditure can result in large changes in weight over time. Weight control is an aspect of nutrition about which many people are profoundly concerned, for reasons of personal appearance and esteem, as well as health. Many people wage a constant battle to gain control over their weight, punctuated by many lapses and disappointments. Unfortunately, the widespread public interest in weight control is characterized by much misinformation. Entrepreneurs regularly capitalize on any approach that can be made to sound plausible, regardless of whether there is any evidence of its effectiveness. Undernutrition is also a problem of weight control, although it is not as prevalent and does not arouse as much public concern. Undernutrition can be associated with health problems as severe as those linked to overweight and obesity, and it too demands attention from nutritionists as they develop methods of prevention and treatment.

Weight control is a term used to describe efforts to maintain or attain a body weight within the limits associated with optimal health. The branch of medicine concerned with weight control is known as **bariatrics.** Over the past 50 years weight control has become a national preoccupation in the affluent, developed countries. It is one of the most common topics of everyday conversation and features prominently on television, in newspapers and magazines, and in a steady stream of books devoted to diets, exercise regimens, and health. Grocery stores offer a growing range of products designed to assist in weight control. Most physicians' offices display posters and leaflets encouraging us to gain control over our weight and offering guidance on how to do so. Diet centers, health clubs, and exercise spas grow increasingly popular. Many of these indications of our preoccupation with weight control are the result of ambitious business people catering to, and possibly creating, the market for a vast array of products, including energy-controlled foods, books, magazines, diet pills, exercise devices, psychological aids, specialized clothing, and much more. Many of these weight-control "aids" promise an easy solution to a problem that, for many people, has no easy solution. In general, they are more likely to bring success to the seller than to the buyer. This modern preoccupation with weight control in such countries as the United States and Canada is largely concerned with the desire of people who believe they are overweight to lose weight. It should not blind us to the fact that people in many countries have problems in obtaining enough food to maintain desirable weight and that excesses and deficits in body weight are viewed differently under different cultural and social conditions. Through the centuries some cultures have given higher status to those with excess body weight, whereas other cultures and subcultures have valued slimness.

It is estimated that about 12.5 million adults in the United States are obese. This figure is obtained using the common definition of obesity as body weight of more than 120% of the desirable weight for a person's height (Table 7-1).

There is currently some confusion about the most appropriate weight standard with the two currently

TABLE 7-1

Comparison of body weight standards proposed in dietary guidelines for Americans: A, 1985; B, 1990

A. DESIRABLE BODY WEIGHT RANGES*			B. SUGGESTED WEIGHTS FOR ADULTS		
	WEIGHT WITHOUT CLOTHES			WEIGHT IN POUNDS WITHOUT CLOTHES	
HEIGHT WITHOUT SHOES	MEN (lbs)	WOMEN (lbs)	HEIGHT WITHOUT SHOES	19 TO 34 YEARS	35 YEARS AND OVER
4′10″		92-121			
4′11″		95-124			
5′0″		98-127	5′0″	97-128†	108-138
5′1″	105-134	101-130	5′1″	101-132	111-143
5′2″	108-137	104-134	5′2″	104-137	115-148
5′3″	111-141	107-138	5′3″	107-141	119-152
5′4″	114-145	110-142	5′4″	111-146	122-157
5′5″	117-149	114-146	5′5″	114-150	126-162
5′6″	121-154	118-150	5′6″	118-155	130-167
5′7″	125-159	122-154	5′7″	121-160	134-172
5′8″	129-163	126-159	5′8″	125-164	138-178
5′9″	133-167	130-164	5′9″	129-169	142-183
5′10″	137-172	134-169	5′10″	132-174	146-188
5′11″	141-177		5′11″	136-179	151-194
6′0″	145-182		6′0″	140-184	155-199
6′1″	149-187		6′1″	144-189	159-205
6′2″	153-192		6′2″	148-195	164-210
6′3″	157-197		6′3″	152-200	168-216
			6′4″	156-205	173-222
			6′5″	160-211	177-228
			6′6″	164-216	182-234

* Note: For women 18 to 25 years, subtract 1 lb for each year under 25.

† The higher weights in the ranges generally apply to men, who tend to have more muscle and bone; the lower weights more often apply to women, who have less muscle and bone.

From Metropolitan Life Insurance Company: *Stat Bull NY Metropol Life Ins Co* 40:1, 1959; National Research Council: *Diet and health,* Washington, DC, 1989, National Academy Press; U.S. Department of Agriculture and U.S. Department of Health and Human Services: *Nutrition and your health: dietary guidelines for Americans,* Washington, DC, 1985 and 1990, U.S. Government Printing Office.

proposed standards that are identified in Table 7-1. Standard A, the 1985 *Desirable Body Weight Ranges,* is based on the 1959 Metropolitan relative weights associated with the lowest morbidity and mortality. It has recently been validated with data from the *Framingham Heart Study* and the *Nurse's Health Study,* both of which indicate that even a small increase in adiposity is associated with an increased risk of obesity-related diseases such as coronary heart disease, hypertension, and non-insulin–dependent diabetes mellitus. Standard B is the unisex standard endorsed in the 1990 Dietary Guidelines for Americans developed by the U.S. Department of Agriculture and the U.S. Department of Health and Human Services. Standard B provides a more liberal range of acceptable weights for people as they age. The basis for these recommendations is unclear, but the recommenda-

TABLE 7-2

Relationship among height in inches, weight in pounds, and body mass index

HEIGHT (in)	BODY MASS INDEX (kg/m^2) 19	20	21	22	23	24	25	26	27	28	29	30	35	40
	BODY WEIGHT (lb)*													
58	91	96	100	105	110	115	119	124	129	134	138	143	167	191
59	94	99	104	109	114	119	124	128	133	138	143	148	173	198
60	97	102	107	112	118	123	128	133	138	143	148	153	179	204
61	100	106	111	116	122	127	132	137	143	148	153	158	185	211
62	104	109	115	120	126	131	136	142	147	153	158	164	191	218
63	107	113	118	124	130	135	141	146	152	158	163	169	197	225
64	110	116	122	128	134	140	145	151	157	163	169	174	204	232
65	114	120	126	132	138	144	150	156	162	168	174	180	210	240
66	118	124	130	136	142	148	155	161	167	173	179	186	216	247
67	121	127	134	140	146	153	159	166	172	178	185	191	223	255
68	125	131	138	144	151	158	164	171	177	184	190	197	230	262
69	128	135	142	149	155	162	169	176	182	189	196	203	236	270
70	132	139	146	153	160	167	174	181	188	195	202	207	243	278
71	136	143	150	157	165	172	179	186	193	200	208	215	250	286
72	140	147	154	162	169	177	184	191	199	206	213	221	258	294
73	144	151	159	166	174	182	189	197	204	212	219	227	265	302
74	148	155	163	171	179	186	194	202	210	218	225	233	272	311
75	152	160	168	176	184	192	200	208	216	224	232	240	279	319
76	156	164	172	180	189	197	205	213	221	230	238	246	287	328

* Each entry gives the body weight in pounds (lb) for a person of a given height and body mass index. Pounds have been rounded off. To use the table, find the appropriate height in the left-hand column. Move across the row to a given weight. The number at the top of the column is the body mass index for the height and weight.

From Bray GA, Gray DS: *West J Med* 149:429, 1988.

tions may be based on age-specific analyses of life insurance data that failed to account for the effect of smoking or the relation between body weight and mortality (Figure 7-9). An alternative, but broadly similar, definition says that obesity begins when a value known as the **body mass index,** or BMI (Table 7-2), exceeds 31.1 for men or 32.3 for women.

Another 21.5 million people are overweight, although not obese, with overweight defined as body weight of more than 110% but less than 120% of the desirable weight for a person's height. People who are overweight, of course, may eventually become obese unless they take measures to stop or reverse the weight gain trend that made them overweight.

Of equal concern are the many others who actually have a reasonably acceptable weight for their height but erroneously think that they are overweight. It seems that most people are either "on a diet" now, have been on a diet recently, or think they should be on a diet. We are all on a diet of some sort, of course because our diet is simply what we eat; however, to be "on a diet" has become the general term for following a specifically modified diet aimed at achieving weight control. It is estimated that 47.7 million Americans went on a diet aimed at achieving weight loss in 1992. About 50% of females and 25% of males in America are trying to lose weight at any given time. Among adolescents, 62% of girls and 28% of boys reported dieting in the past year. Some of these people do need to take steps to control their weight, but many people who go on "diets" do not need to.[1]

Most adults achieve reasonably successful weight control with little or no conscious effort. This is an impressive feat, considering that most people consume about ¾ million kcal/year, and a daily excess or deficiency of just 10 kcal/day (0.5% of the needs of a sedentary woman) should produce a net gain or loss of just under 1 pound (0.45 kg) over a year. An excess or deficiency of 100 kcal/day (which is the energy in 1 tablespoon of butter or one large apple) results in a change of 11 pounds (5 kg/year). The cumulative effects of even such small deviations from energy requirements can become significant over periods of 10 years and longer. As fat accumulates, there may be some automatic adjustment in the body's use of energy, but initially the theoretical equivalent of 1 pound of fat gained or lost per 3500 kcal is found to hold true. There is a limit to the amount of weight that can be lost without severe wasting of the body, but there is no apparent upper limit to the amount of weight that can be gained. The health hazards of weight gain increase in proportion to the amount of weight gained above a certain critical point, usually set at the level of 40% overweight.

Health professionals are as concerned about underweight individuals as they are about overweight individuals, but considerably more research is done on the health problems of obesity than on those of undernutrition.

CLASSIFICATION AND EVALUATION OF OVERWEIGHT AND OBESITY

It is generally accepted that weight gain and obesity occur only when energy intake exceeds energy expenditure consistently over time. Because this is a simple principle, obesity was originally described as **simple obesity.** It is now recognized, however, that obesity is a complex condition with a variety of causes, including factors associated with physiology, psychology, a person's environment, and his or her exposure to disease. The treatment of obesity takes many forms, reflecting the variety of causes and the varying responses of different individuals to treatment.

DEFINITIONS

Obesity is defined in general terms as an excessive amount of fat (adipose tissue) in the body. As stated earlier, obesity is also commonly defined as corresponding to body weights of greater than 120% of desirable weight, with the milder state of overweight corresponding to between 110% and 120% of desirable weight. There is considerable debate about the actual amount of body fat that should delineate the boundary between overweight and obesity. Sophisticated and expensive techniques are required to accurately measure the amount of body fat; so they are not routinely used in assessing people for obesity. A somewhat more sophisticated assessment of obesity than those already mentioned involves deriving a value known as the *BMI* (*or Quetelet index*), which is simply a person's weight in kilograms divided by height in meters squared. Table 7-2 presents the weight for various heights, corresponding to specific body mass indexes. The National Center for Health Statistics has developed a statistical definition for the terms *overweight* and *severe overweight* (usually synonomous with obesity) as follows:

- **Overweight** corresponds to a BMI of greater than the eighty-fifth percentile values of the BMI distributions for adults aged 20 to 29 years: 27.8 for men and 27.3 for women.
- **Severe overweight** (obesity) corresponds to a BMI of greater than or equal to the ninety-fifth percentile values of the BMI distributions for adults aged 20 to 29 years: 31.1 for men and 32.3 for women.

People between 20 and 29 years old were used as the reference group in determining the statistical range of BMI across the population. This age range was selected because it corresponds to the decade after normal growth has ceased and during which most excess weight results from the accumulation of adipose tissue.

Approximately one fourth of U.S. adults aged 20 to 74 years are overweight (34 million), and approximately 9% are obese (12.5 million). BMI values of greater than 28 correspond to being approximately 20% above the body weight that is often described as "desirable," "ideal," or "healthy" because of their association with

To determine your body mass index (BMI):

1. Divide your weight in pounds by 2.2, to convert it into kilograms.
2. Multiply your height in inches by 2.54 and divide the result by 100, to convert your height to meters; then multiply your height in meters by itself (that is, square it).
3. Divide your weight in kilograms (result of step 1) by the square of your height in meters (result of step 2). The result is your BMI.

$$\text{BMI} = \frac{\text{Body weight (kg)}}{\text{Height (m)} \times \text{Height (m)}}$$

Obesity is variously defined as the following:

- An excessive amount of fat (adipose tissue) in the body
- Body weights of greater than 120% of desirable weight
- Body mass index of greater than 31.1 for men and greater than 32.3 for women

TABLE 7-3

Recommended body mass indexes for adults

CLASSIFICATION	GENDER	AGE-GROUP (YEARS)	RECOMMENDED BMI (kg/m²)
U.S. Departments of Agriculture and Health and Human Services (USDA/DHHS)	Both	19-34	19-25
		≥ 35	21-27
National Academy of Sciences (NAS)	Both	19-24	19-24
		25-34	20-25
		35-44	21-26
		45-54	22-27
		55-64	23-28
		≥ 65	24-29
National Center for Health Statistics (NCHS)	Male	20-74	20.7-27.8
	Female	20-74	19.1-27.3
World Health Organization (WHO)	Both	Adults	20-25
Ministry of National Health and Welfare Canada (Canadian)	Both	20-65	20-27

From Sichieri R, Everhart JE, Hubbard VS: *Int J Obes* 16:303, 1992.

TABLE 7-4

Proposed classification of obesity according to body mass index and the associated level of medical risk

	BODY MASS INDEX (kg/m²)				
	20-25	25-30	30-35	35-40	>40
Class*	0	I	II	III	IV
Grade†	0	I	2	2	3
Risk	Very low	Low	Moderate	High	Very high
Fat cell number‡	Normal	Normal	Normal or ↑	↑	↑

* American Heart Association classification.

† European system of grading.

‡ Increased or normal.

From Bray GA: *Am J Clin Nutr* 55:488S, 1992.

the lowest mortality rates. A number of agencies have published recommended BMI levels based on several population studies of the relationship between body weight and mortality rates (Table 7-3).

ASSESSMENT OF RISK

It has been clearly demonstrated that obesity is associated with various health risks. It is associated with an increased prevalence of high blood pressure and blood lipid abnormalities that are recognized to increase the risk of developing cardiovascular disease. It is also associated with an increased prevalence of gallbladder disease, diabetes, and cancer. Obesity increases overall mortality rates among obese persons, relative to those found in nonobese people of the same age and gender.

Bray[2] proposed a system for classifying the general level of health risk associated with five different BMI ranges (Table 7-4). As can be seen from Table 7-4, four of the BMI ranges correspond to four classes of obesity: Class I (BMI of 25 to 30), Class II (BMI of 30 to 35), Class III (BMI of 35 to 40), and Class IV (BMI of greater than 40). The American Heart Association proposed the use of Classes 0 to IV for BMIs ranging between 20 and 40, whereas the European system designates the categories as Grades 0 to 3, with Classes II and III combined into Grade 2. The use of these categories of obesity eliminates the need to use such imprecise and sometimes offensive terms as *severe obesity, morbid obesity, extreme obesity, gross obesity,* and *massive obesity.* Bray also developed a "risk assessment algorithm" (an algorithm is simply a set of rules used to perform some task), allowing us to gain a rough idea of the risks associated with the five BMI classes when the presence of any of four complicating factors is taken into account (Figure 7-1). The complicating factors move a person into the next higher category of risk, compared with the one they would be in if the complicating factors were absent. The complicating factors are being under

FIGURE 7-1

Bray's risk classification algorithm, relating relative health risk to body mass index and taking into account the presence of complicating factors (being male or under age 40 at onset of obesity, having a high waist-to-hip ratio, or suffering from other medical complications.

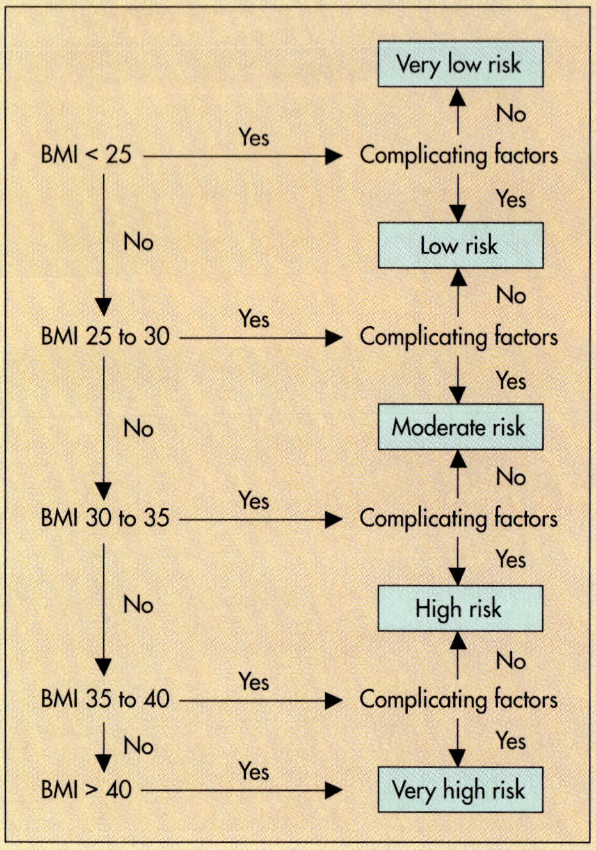

40 years old at the onset of obesity, being male, having an unfavorable regional fat distribution (i.e., high waist/hip ratio), or having other medical complications. The health risks associated with any given level of obesity seem to be significantly greater if a person first becomes obese when younger than 40, when compared with people whose obesity develops later in life.

From puberty onward, women tend to have a greater proportion of body fat than do men and tend to gain more fat during adult life. Nevertheless, women are at less risk of weight-related health problems than are men with a similar percentage of body fat. It has been shown, for example, that for a woman and a man to have the same level of impairment in glucose tolerance or rise in blood pressure, the woman needs to accumulate 20 more kilograms of fat than does the man. This difference in risk between the genders may be explained partly by differences in fat distribution, which is the third complicating factor.

It has been known for a long time that people differ in the way in which fat is distributed within their bodies. The differences between the genders are most obvious: men have more abdominal fat, whereas women tend to have greater amounts around their hips in what is termed the *gluteal region*. These differences can be expressed in terms of a **waist-to-hip ratio (WHR),** also known as the abdominal-gluteal ratio or the android-gynoid ratio (android for man, gynoid for woman). An unusually high WHR (greater than 0.95 for males and greater than 0.8 for females) is regarded as a complicating factor when using the risk classification algorithm. In the last decade the relationship between fat distribution and health risk has become increasingly apparent. Abdominal, central, or upper body obesity is associated with a greater risk of cardiovascular disease and diabetes than is obesity in the gluteal, femoral, peripheral, or lower body regions. These two types of fat distribution have become known as the apple-shaped or android (characteristically male) and pear-shaped or gynoid (characteristically female) distributions.

FAT CELL SIZE AND NUMBER

It is possible to estimate the number and size of fat cells in a person's body by examining a sample of adipose tissue obtained by needle biopsy in which a needle is used to extract a small amount of subcutaneous fat. The total number of fat cells in the body can be estimated by dividing the total weight of body fat by the average weight of a fat cell. Between the ages of 1 month and 1 year, increases in body fat result from an increase in fat cell *size*. From age 1 to age 22 years, further increases in total body fat result from increases in fat cell *number.* In adults who become overweight or obese from an excess of up to 30 kg of body fat, the increased weight of fat is largely accounted for by increased fat cell weight and therefore size. This form of obesity is known as **hypertrophic obesity,** which essentially means it is caused by an additional *growth* of individual fat cells. More severe obesity is usually associated with an increase in fat cell number, a situation known as **hyperplastic obesity.**[3] Hyperplastic obesity is presumed to exist in anyone whose BMI exceeds 35, corresponding to a weight of more than 75% above desirable weight.

THE PREVALENCE OF OVERWEIGHT AND OBESITY

The U.S. National Center for Health Statistics estimates that 26% of the adult population (24% of men and 27% of women) are either overweight or obese, but it recognizes that there is considerable variation among different regions of the country. For example, the prevalence of overweight

FIGURE 7-2

Prevalence of overweight in the United States according to gender and age.

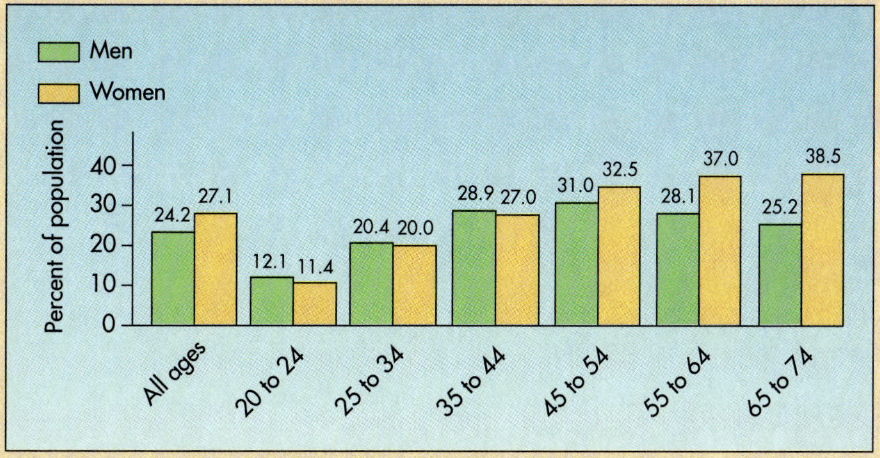

or obesity in Wisconsin and Indiana is estimated at 25.7%, whereas in Arizona, at 15.1%, presumably because of differences in eating patterns and exercise practices.[4]

A national health objective for the nation for the year 2000 is to reduce the prevalence of overweight and obesity to no more than 20% of the adult population. However, data from NHANES III (1988-1991) indicate that prevalence of overweight and obesity actually increased in the United States to 34%.

The incidence of overweight increases throughout adulthood and peaks for men at age 45 but continues to increase for women at least up until age 74 (Figure 7-2). The decline in obesity in males over 45 years of age may be caused by the higher mortality rate among obese middle-aged men.

Of those Americans who are obese, about 0.9% are Class I obese, 90% are Class II obese, 9% are Class III obese, and only 0.1% are Class IV obese (Figure 7-3). The incidence of obesity is considerably higher for African-American and Hispanic populations and for people whose income is below the poverty line. Approximately one third of overweight and obese African-American and Hispanic women also have incomes below the poverty line.

At 1 year of age, infants are now on average 50% heavier than they were a generation ago. The incidence of obesity in children is reported to be increasing in the United States. Estimates suggest that 27% of 6- to 11-year-olds and 22% of 12- to 18-year-olds are overweight or obese.[5] Some studies have suggested that this increase is correlated with the increase in the time children spend in sedentary activities, such as watching television. The relative risk of an obese child becoming an obese adult increases with the age of the onset of obesity. Individuals who first become obese during adolescence are more likely to be obese as adults than those whose obesity first arose earlier in childhood.

FIGURE 7-3

Cumulative percentage of body weight.

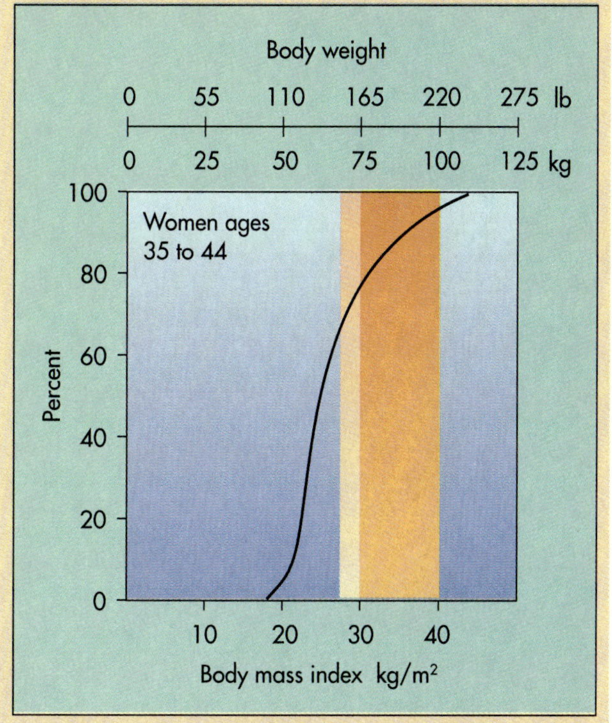

The reported weight gain among women increases with each successive birth by about 2 lbs above that normally gained with age.

TABLE 7-5

Summary of direct methods of body composition measurement

METHOD AND PROCEDURES	LIMITATIONS	RELATIVE COST	EASE OF USE	ACCURACY	REGIONAL FAT*
TOTAL BODY WATER (TBW)					
Tracer dose of water—labeled with ^{3}H, ^{2}H, or ^{18}O—is given orally or intravenously and then equilibrated. Concentration of isotope measured in serum, urine, saliva, or breath (for ^{18}O). TBW calculated from dilution observed.	Involves radiation to the subject if ^{3}H is used. Water content of fat-free tissue is increased during obesity, pregnancy, and wasting disease, leading to an underestimate of fat.	$$	Moderate	High	No
UNDERWATER WEIGHING					
Subject is weighed in air and then when totally submerged in water. Body volume calculated from the apparent loss of weight in water. Body density calculated from body mass and body volume measurements. Correction factors for water temperature, volume of air trapped in gastrointestinal tract. Preferable to measure residual lung volume.	Requires high degree of cooperation from subject. Not suitable for young children and elderly and sick patients.	$$	Moderate	High	No
TOTAL BODY POTASSIUM (TBK)					
TBK measured by counting radiation from naturally occurring ^{40}K in a whole body counter. Fat-free mass (FFM) derived from assumption that average potassium concentration of FFM is constant.	Required equipment is expensive. Obese and elderly subjects have lower potassium concentrations, leading to overestimates of total body fat.	$$$	Difficult	High	No
TOTAL BODY ELECTRICAL CONDUCTIVITY (TOBEC)					
Subject lies supine in a solenoid coil through which a 5 MHz current is passed. The latter induces a current in the subject, which creates a secondary magnetic field. The conductivity value of the subject is obtained by subtracting the background value when the coil is empty. Conductivity value is proportional to body electrolyte content and hence reflects amount of fat-free tissue.	Edema, dehydration, and electrolyte balance will alter conductivity and interfere with reading. Extent to which variation in body shape and size affects readings not yet known. Variations in bone mass may affect readings.	$$$	Moderate	Moderate	No

*Regional fat refers to the localized distribution of fat in the body (i.e., abdomen, hips, etc.).

TABLE 7-5

Summary of direct methods of body composition measurement (continued)

METHOD AND PROCEDURES	LIMITATIONS	RELATIVE COST	EASE OF USE	ACCURACY	REGIONAL FAT*
BIOELECTRICAL IMPEDANCE (BEI)					
The impedance to a weak electrical current passed between the right ankle and right wrist of subject in supine position is measured. Impedance is proportional to the square of the length of the conductor—a function of the height of the subject—divided by the volume.	Edema and dehydration will alter the resistance measurements and invalidate the method. Sensitivity of BEI to detect changes in body composition during nutrition intervention or physical training unknown.	$$	Easy	Moderate	No
NEUTRON ACTIVATION ANALYSIS					
Radioactive isotopes of N, P, Na, Cl, and Ca are created by irradiating the subject. The radioactivity of the element is measured using a whole body counter.	Subjects exposed to radioactivity. Elements are not uniformly activated, and thus sensitivity varies.	$$$$	Difficult	High	No
COMPUTED TOMOGRAPHY (CT)					
Method measures attenuation of x-rays as they pass through tissues, the degree of attenuation being related to differences in physical density of the tissues. Image reconstructed from matrix of picture elements (pixels), which vary in their shading.	Exposure to ionizing radiation limits use of CT for whole body scans, multiple scans in same person, and scans of pregnant women or children. Equipment is not readily available. The CT does not provide information on chemical composition of the structures.	$$$$	Difficult	High	Yes
ULTRASOUND					
High-frequency sound waves from an ultrasound meter pass through adipose tissue to adipose-muscle tissue interface. At interface, some sound waves reflected back as echoes, which are translated into depth readings via a transducer.	Validity of technique for subjects with wide range of body fatness unknown. Technique does not provide same degree of structure resolution possible with computerized tomography.	$$$	Moderate	Moderate	Yes

$$*, Moderate cost; *$$$*, high cost; *$$$$, very high cost.

* Regional fat refers to the localized distribution of fat in the body (i.e., abdomen, hips, etc.).

From Gibson R: *Principles of nutritional assessment,* New York, 1990, Oxford University Press, and Bray GA: *Am J Clin Nutr* 55:488S, 1992.

DIAGNOSIS OF OBESITY BY BODY COMPOSITION MEASUREMENTS

Because obesity is defined in general terms as an excessive amount of fat in the body, its proper diagnosis depends on methods of measuring body composition. Direct methods are expensive, require considerable technical skill, and are often uncomfortable for the subject. As a result the most commonly used methods of measuring body composition are indirect ones, primarily based on measurements of height, weight, the circumference of parts of the body, and skinfold thickness.

Direct Methods of Measuring Body Composition

Table 7-5 summarizes and assesses the various direct methods used to measure body composition and fat distribution.[6] The methods with the lowest cost are usually the least accurate.

The direct methods currently in use consider the body to be composed of either two main compartments—body fat and fat free tissue—or four main compartments—fat, water, protein, and minerals. The proportion of total body mass in each of the chosen compartments is then measured.

The densities of body fat, water, protein, and minerals at 37° C (normal body temperature) are as follows:

- Fat—900 kg/m^3
- Water—993 kg/m^3
- Protein—1304 kg/m^3
- Minerals—3000 kg/m^3

Knowledge of these values allows interconversion between estimates of mass and volume for each component. If the fat-free mass is being considered as one compartment, its density obviously depends on the relative proportions of water, protein, and minerals present. In most healthy people these proportions are fairly constant, at around 73% water, 20% protein, and 7% minerals. These proportions give the fat-free mass an average density of approximately 1100 kg/m^3 at 37° C.

Table 7-6 summarizes the distribution of body fat between its various main locations in a "reference" man of 70 kg and a reference woman of 56.8 kg. The body fat content is its most variable component, however, so there can be wide variations from these reference figures in real people. Fat within the body is found in two main locations, one containing large quantities of the essential fatty acids and the other serving as a general fat-storage site. The essential fatty acids are found concentrated in bone marrow, the central nervous system, mammary glands, and other organs of the body, where they are required for the normal biochemical and physiological operation of the body. Fat in these sites accounts for about 9% of the body weight of the reference woman and 3% of the body weight of the reference man. General fat stores are concentrated in the subcutaneous fat directly beneath the skin, in fat surrounding the major organs (rather than inside them), and in intramuscular and intermuscular fat deposits. This general storage fat accounts for a fairly constant 12% of total body weight in males and 15% of total body weight in females. Subcutaneous fat, which forms the most obviously visible deposits of fat, accounts for one third of the total body fat in the reference man and woman.

TABLE 7-6

Distribution of body fat in reference man and woman

FAT LOCATION	REFERENCE MAN (kg)	REFERENCE WOMAN (kg)
Essential fat (lipids of the bone marrow, central nervous system, mammary glands, and other organs)	2.1	4.9
Storage fat (depot)	8.2	10.4
Subcutaneous	3.1	5.1
Intermuscular	3.3	3.5
Intramuscular	0.8	0.6
Fat of thoracic and abdominal cavity	1.0	1.2
Total fat	10.3	15.3
Body weight	70.0	56.8
Percentage of fat	(14.7)	(26.9)

From Gibson R: *Principles of nutritional assessment,* New York, 1990, Oxford University Press.

A limited number of studies of body composition have been performed on humans after death. Most of these were done between the 1940s and 1960s on adults who had died from some illness, raising doubts about the validity of applying the results to healthy people. Results of direct analysis of six adults are shown in Table 7-7.[7] These show a fairly constant composition for the fat-free tissues, contrasting with widely varying amounts of fat (from 4% to 28% of total body weight). The vast majority of studies of body composition, however, are performed on living subjects using the methods summarized in Table 7-5. These methods are considered individually.

Underwater weighing This is the most commonly used method for the direct determination of total body fat. The subject is weighed in air first, to determine body weight. He or she is then submerged in water and instructed to expel as much air as possible from the lungs; the subject's weight in water is then recorded (Figure 7-4). With a principle of physics known as *Archimedes' principle,* the volume of the body in liters can be calculated from the difference between its weight (in kilograms) in air and its weight in water. This allows the density of the body (D) to be calculated by dividing its

TABLE 7-7

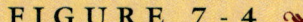

The contribution of water and protein to the fat-free weights of six adult cadavers

GENDER	AGE (YR)	WATER (g/kg)	PROTEIN (g/kg)	REMAINDER (g/kg)	DENSITY (kg/m³)	POTASSIUM (mmol/kg)
Male	25	728	195	77	1120	71.5
Male	35	775	165	60	1083	—
Female	42	733	192	75	1103	73.0
Male	46	674	234	92	1131	66.5
Male	48	730	206	64	1099	—
Male	60	704	238	58	1104	66.6
Mean		724	205	71	1106	69.4
SD		34	28	3	17	3.3

From Garrow JS: *Nutr Abstr Rev* 53:697, 1983.

FIGURE 7-4

Underwater weighing to determine body fat content.

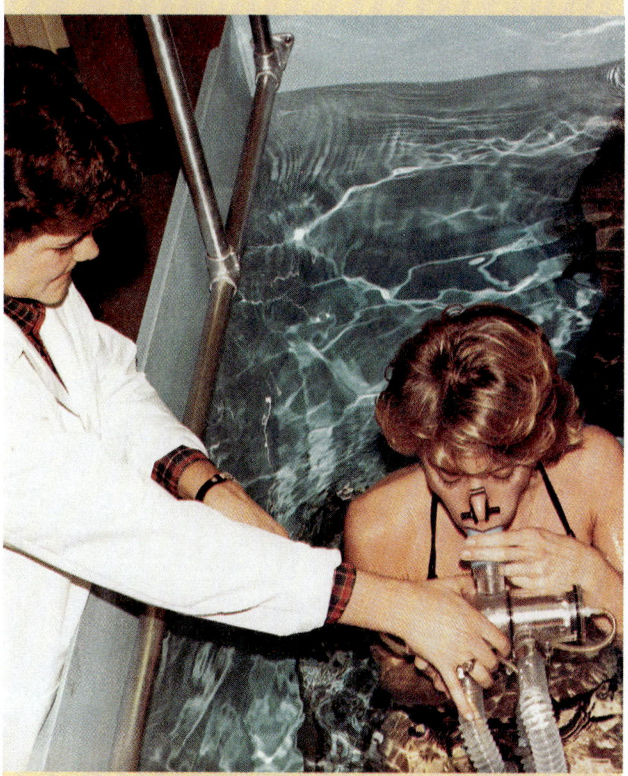

weight in air by its calculated volume. Three slightly different equations have been derived by different groups of researchers to allow the percentage of body fat to be determined from the body density value obtained in this way. The most commonly used equation is as follows[8]:

$$\text{FAT (\%)} = \left(\frac{4.95}{D} - 4.95\right) \times 100$$

The weight of total body fat is then easily derived from the figure for the percentage of fat as follows:

$$\text{TOTAL BODY FAT (kg)} = \frac{\text{BODY WEIGHT (kg)} \times \text{BODY FAT (\%)}}{100}$$

The fat-free weight can then be derived by subtracting the value for toal body fat from that for the total body weight.

Determining total body water by isotope dilution The human body is approximately 73% water by weight, but virtually all of this water is in the fat-free mass. This allows the fat-free mass of the body to be determined by measuring the amount of water in the body (total body water) and performing the following calculation:

$$\text{FAT-FREE MASS (kg)} = \frac{\text{TOTAL BODY WATER (kg)}}{0.73}$$

Knowing the fat-free mass allows the weight of body fat to be calculated by subtraction:

$$\text{BODY FAT (kg)} = \text{BODY WEIGHT (kg)} - \text{FAT-FREE MASS (kg)}$$

The percentage of body fat can then be calculated as follows:

$$\text{BODY FAT (\%)} = \frac{\text{TOTAL BODY FAT (kg)} \times 100}{\text{BODY WEIGHT (kg)}}$$

The total body water value needed to perform these calculations can be determined using what is known as an isotope dilution method. Subjects fast overnight, restrict their fluid intake, and empty their bladder in the morning immediately before the test. They then either drink or are injected with a sample of water that has a known amount of some readily detectable isotope of hydrogen or oxygen incorporated within some of the water molecules. The stable ^{18}O isotope of oxygen, the stable ^{2}H isotope of hydrogen (known as deuterium), or the radioactive ^{3}H isotope of hydrogen (known as tritium) can be used. The isotope "label" is allowed to become evenly distributed (to "equilibrate") throughout the body water over several hours, during which no further water intake is permitted. After equilibration, a sample of urine, saliva, or blood is collected and the amount of isotope contained within it is determined by mass spectrometry (for the stable isotopes) or measurement of radioactivity (for tritium). The collected sample contains a lower concentration of the administered isotope than the original dose of isotope taken in because the isotope has been diluted by mixing with all the water of the body. The extent of this dilution obviously depends on how much water the body contains. Thus the total water content of the subject can be calculated.

Determining total body potassium The mineral element potassium is present in the body almost entirely in the form of potassium ions (K^{+}) within the cells of muscles and the major organs. This potassium contains a virtually constant proportion (68.1 mEq/kg) of the radioactive ^{40}K isotope of potassium.[9] This radioactive isotope has a long half-life, about 1.3 billion years, and as it decays it emits gamma rays with a specific and readily detectable energy. Measuring the level of gamma radiation released by this naturally present radioactive isotope allows total body potassium to be determined. This figure can then be used to calculate the total fat-free mass of the body, on the assumption that the potassium content of a given amount of the fat-free mass is constant.

Determining total body nitrogen Protein is 16% nitrogen by weight; therefore determining the total nitrogen content of the body can be used to calculate the total amount of protein in the body. A procedure known as **neutron activation** can be used to measure total body nitrogen in the living body. The subject lies on a flat bed and is bombarded with a low-dose beam of the subatomic particles called *neutrons,* which can be produced in a variety of ways. Within the body, some of the neutrons are captured by a proportion of the body's nitrogen atoms. This can convert the most abundant nitrogen isotope—^{14}N—into an energetically excited ^{15}N isotope. These excited ^{15}N atoms immediately lose energy by emitting gamma rays of a specific and readily detectable energy, and these gamma rays are detected. The total amount of nitrogen in the body can be calculated from the number of gamma rays emitted.

Total body electrical conductivity The fat and fat-free components of the body have different electrical properties, including different electrical conductivities. These form the basis of the total body electrical conductivity (TOBEC) technique in which the subject is moved through an electromagnetic field, and differences in the electrical conductivity of the body are monitored (Figure 7-5). The results allow estimation of the fat-free mass and total body fat, and the method is simple, quick, and safe. One major drawback is that the TOBEC instrument is expensive. Also, experimental results to validate the technique for different age and gender groups are still rather limited.

FIGURE 7-5

Total body electrical conductivity (TOBEC) apparatus.

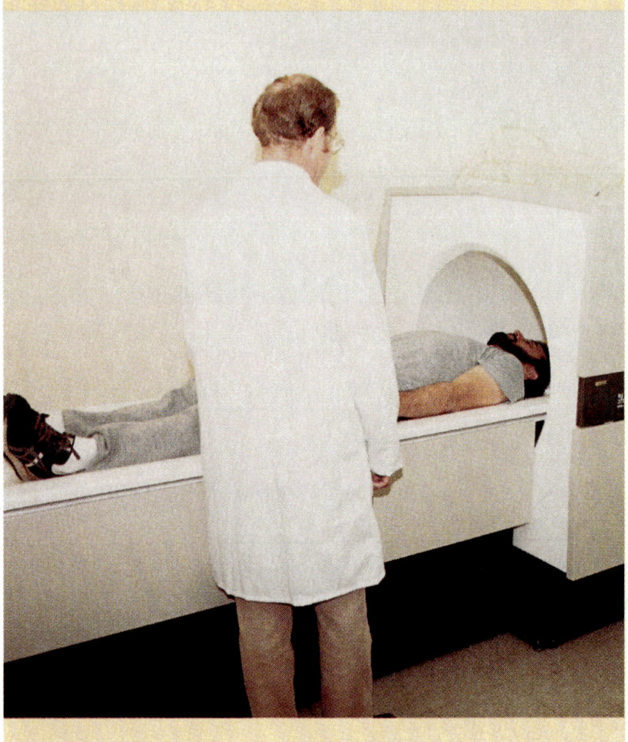

FIGURE 7-6

Bioelectrical impedance measurement in progress.

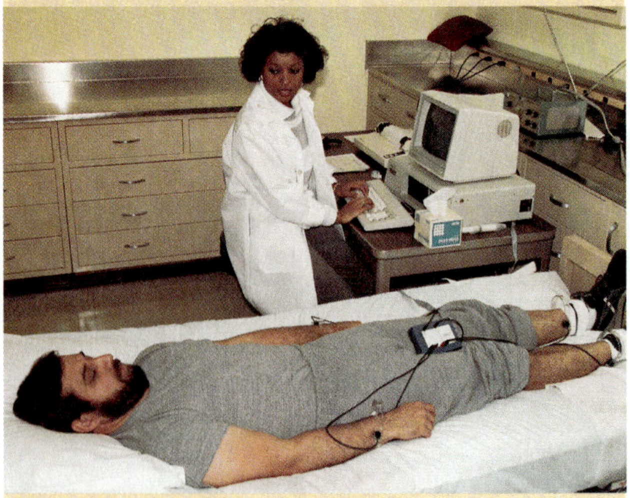

FIGURE 7-7

Measuring skinfold thickness with calipers at A, triceps, and B, subscapular region.

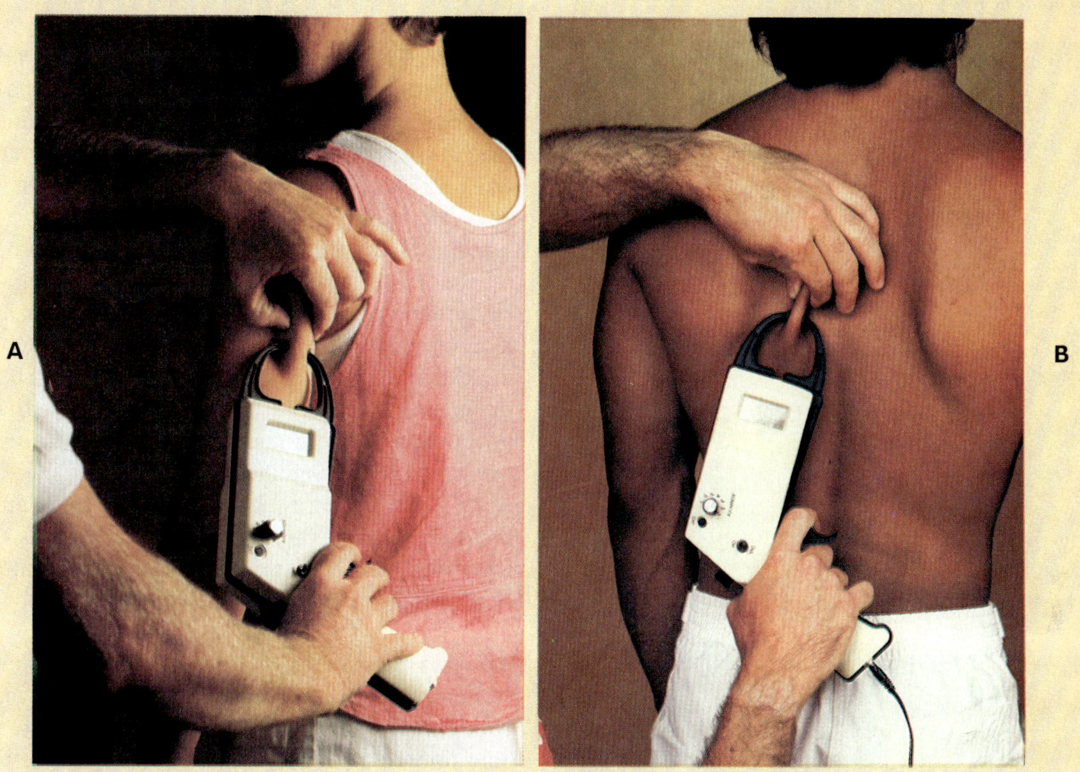

Bioelectrical impedance Bioelectrical impedance is another technique based on the different electrical properties of fat and the fat-free mass. It measures the electrical property known as impedance, using a weak current of electricity passed through the body between electrodes on the wrist and ankle (Figure 7-6). The impedance values are influenced by the amount of water in the body, and because only the fat-free mass contains water, it is possible to derive a relationship between the results obtained and the amount of fat present. Again, the validity of this method has not been as firmly established as that of some alternative methods.

Ultrasound High-frequency sound waves emitted from an "ultrasound" source can be used to measure the thickness of both subcutaneous fat and muscle tissue. This method is based on the reflection of sound waves from the boundary between subcutaneous fat and muscle, with the reflected waves being detected. Comparison with results obtained by various other direct and indirect techniques suggests that ultrasound methods give reasonably accurate results and may be superior to skinfold caliper methods for measuring subcutaneous fat in obese subjects.

Computed tomography Computed tomography (CT) scanning has become a familiar technique of noninvasive internal investigation of the body. It is a complex procedure based on the extent to which x rays pass through regions of the body with differing densities. Sophisticated computer manipulation of the results is used to build up a visual image of the anatomy of the scanned area. This method has been used to measure the volume of various tissues and organs, allowing the total volumes of fat and fat-free tissue to be determined. Its use of ionizing radiation, however, makes it unsuitable for use on pregnant women or children or for multiple scans of the same subject. It is also expensive.

Indirect Methods of Measuring Body Composition

Although a wide variety of direct methods of measuring body composition exist, most routine estimations of body composition still rely on well-established indirect methods based on measuring skinfold thickness, height, and weight. These have the advantages of being relatively quick, noninvasive, cheap, and easily performed by a skillful worker with a minimal amount of equipment.

Skinfold thickness measurement The technique of skinfold thickness measurement involves using a **caliper** to pinch out and measure the thickness of a double fold of fat plus skin on various parts of the body (Figure 7-7). The results allow estimation of the subcutaneous

FIGURE 7-8

Sites and types of anthropometric measurements used to assess body composition.

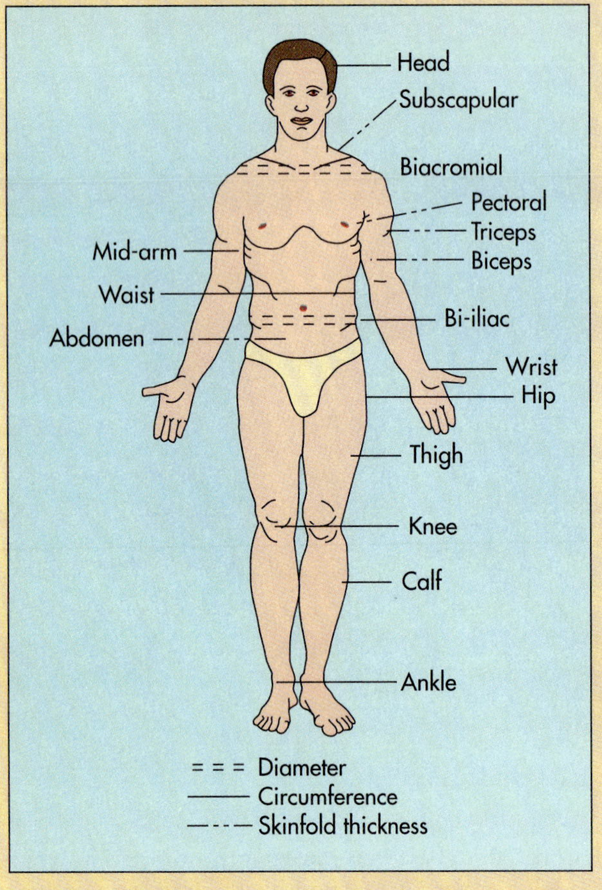

fat content of the body, although their accuracy depends on the skill of the technician in the correct use of the caliper. Skinfold measurements are most frequently made over the triceps muscle on the outside back of the arm, over the biceps muscle on the front of the arm, or in the subscapular region beneath the shoulder blades. An average of several measurements is usually compared with values in standard tables, such as that in Appendix I, to determine the extent to which the subject is overweight or obese. The results can also be incorporated into equations used to predict the percentage of body fat within the subject. Some equations require measurements from as many as 10 different sites (Figure 7-8), but these are not practical for routine assessment. The single most frequently used site is the triceps skinfold because subjects willingly permit this measurement. Many are less enthusiastic about the use of other sites that require undressing.

There is no general agreement about what single skinfold site or combination of sites gives the most accurate results for the assessment of total body fat. In general, however, some combination of measurements is more accurate than a single measurement.

Waist-hip circumference ratio The relative distribution of fat among different locations can be evaluated by calculating the WHR, already mentioned. This is the ratio of the circumference of the body around the waist to the circumference around the hips. The waist circumference is measured by tape, encircling the body horizontally at the visible waist or at the narrowest part of the torso when viewed from the front. The hip circumference is measured in a similar way, but at the level of maximal circumference in the hip region, including the buttocks. A WHR of greater than 0.80 in women or greater than 0.95 in men indicates that a high proportion of abdominal fat is likely to be present and is associated with a significant health risk.[10] Health professionals are currently being advised to include WHR measurements in their evaluation of patients to identify those for whom aggressive weight-reduction treatment is advisable.

Weight and height measurements Skinfold measurements are difficult to make on infants and young children, and appropriate standard values are not available for some groups of people. Because of these difficulties, the routine assessment of body fat levels still relies almost totally on the interpretation of simple measurements of weight and height. The standards used for the interpretation of measurements on infants and children are based on data from several large studies performed by the National Center for Health Statistics. These data have been used to prepare growth curves, indicating normal healthy ranges of weight and height during infancy and childhood (see Chapters 15 and 16). Using these growth curves makes it easy to detect a trend toward undernutrition or overnutrition in an individual before it becomes a serious problem.

For adults the standards are based on data from the 1979 Body Build and Blood Pressure Study, which in turn was based on data obtained by insurance companies showing the weight-for-height values associated with the lowest mortality. People with body weights in excess of 110% of the midpoint of the standard for their weight, height, gender, and age are considered overweight. Those with weights in excess of 120% of the appropriate standard are considered obese (see inside back cover). The applicability of these tables has been questioned, particularly for elderly persons. Several investigators have pointed out that the tables are flawed because they do not take into account the effects of cigarette smoking.[11] Smokers tend to weigh less than do nonsmokers of the same gender, age, and height but suffer a higher death rate because of smoking-related diseases. This tends to cause a smoking-related increase in mortality among lighter people and so shifts the optimal weight toward a higher level. Because the effects of smoking accumulate over many decades, this bias in the tables is greatest for older people and least for the young. A number of studies of U.S. citizens indicate that weights below the average are correlated with greatest longevity, provided that the low weights are not caused by or associated with an illness. Despite these reservations, the 1983 Metropolitan Life Insurance desirable weight ranges are below the average weights revealed from National Center for Health Statistics data. The samples used to gather these data (National Health and Nutrition Examination Survey [NHANES] I and II surveys, 1971 - 1974 and 1976 - 1980) were representative of noninstitutionalized U.S. civilians aged 25 to 74 years.

As an alternative to tables, a quick guide to standard desirable weight for any given height can be obtained.

> A quick guide to standard desirable weight for any given height can be obtained from the following calculations:
>
> *For men:* 105 lbs plus 6 lbs for every inch over 60 inches, *or* 105 lbs minus 6 lbs for every inch under 60 inches
>
> *For women:* 100 lbs plus 5 lbs for every inch over 60 inches, *or* 100 lbs minus 5 lbs for every inch under 60 inches

These standards can be increased by 10% for people with large frames and decreased by 10% for people with small frames.

Another simple test is to place a ruler on the chest and abdomen while the subject is lying down. If the ruler slants upward toward the feet, a weight problem is indicated.

When obesity is severe, merely looking in the mirror is sufficient to indicate its presence; however, when it is marginal, such subjective measures are of little value.

Other standards based on weight and height measurements have been developed for specific uses. These include the BMI, already discussed, and the **ponderal index.** The ponderel index is the ratio of height (in meters) to the cube root of the weight (in kilograms). The BMI is the ratio of weight in kilograms to the square of height in meters. Many investigators consider the BMI to be the most useful standard. Obesity is indicated by a BMI of greater than 30 kg/m^2 and is associated with a significantly increased health risk (Tables 7-3 and 7-4 and Figures 7-1 and 7-9). The BMI is also useful as an indicator of obesity in children over 6 years of age; however, it offers no advantage over standard weight-for-length measurements in infants under 6 months of age. Infant obesity has been defined by Fomon[12] as a weight-for-length value above the ninety-fifth percentile, whereas infant overweight is defined as a weight-for-length value between the ninetieth and ninety-fifth percentiles. In the United States infants are more likely to be overweight than underweight; so the reference data on infant weight-for-height values are probably biased in favor of high values.

DISADVANTAGES OF OBESITY

Before people can be motivated to try to reverse or prevent obesity, they must be convinced that the disadvantages of obesity are sufficiently great to justify the self-discipline required. Weight reduction requires willpower, family support, and perseverance over a long period and often involves disappointing setbacks, periodic plateaus, or slight gains in weight. There are in fact many disadvantages associated with obesity—physical, psychological, economic, and social—in addition to the well-recognized health risks.

HEALTH HAZARDS

Many studies have demonstrated that obesity is clearly associated with increased prevalence of cardiovascular disease, including hypertension (high blood pressure), and also diabetes mellitus and gallbladder disease. Obese males, regardless of their smoking habits, also have a higher mortality rate from cancer of the colon, rectum, and prostate than do nonobese males. Similarly, mortality rates from cancer of the breast, uterus, ovaries, gallbladder, cervix, and endometrium are higher in obese females than in nonobese females. Women who are obese when they become pregnant are at greater risk of obstetrical problems because of their increased risk of hypertension, diabetes, pulmonary complications, and postpartum (after birth) infections. Restriction in weight gain during pregnancy may cause problems, however, and is not recommended. While outlining the various risks of obesity, however, it should be pointed out that overweight or obese people are at *less* risk of suffering from osteoporosis, tuberculosis, and other respiratory diseases than the nonobese population.[13]

Although the health problems associated with obesity have been known for a long time, there is still considerable uncertainty about the stage at which weight gain begins to become a significant health hazard. The relationship is complicated by the effects of smoking and of diseases, but as the BMI rises between 25 and 30, the mortality rate clearly rises (Figure 7-9).

FIGURE 7-9

Relationship between body mass index (BMI) and mortality rate. The lowest mortality rates are associated with BMIs between 19 and 27 kg/m².

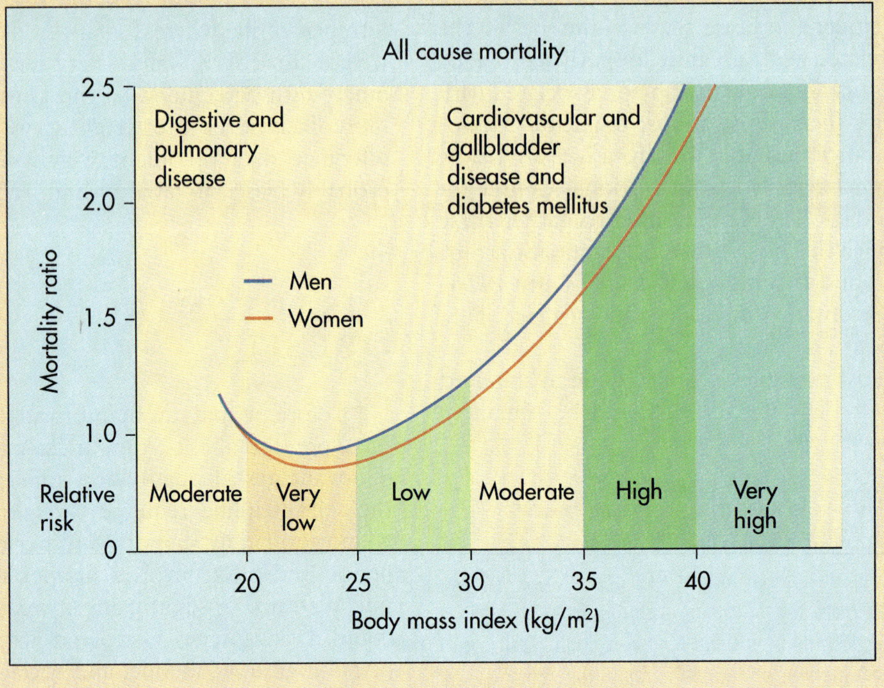

PSYCHOSOCIAL DISADVANTAGES

The social and psychological costs of obesity can be high.[14] Obese people are constantly exposed to advertisements, newspaper and magazine articles, television programs, and movies that in both obvious and subtle ways promote the ideal of slimness. Many also have to contend with pressure from relatives, friends, and doctors forever exhorting them to lose weight. Obese individuals in the United States and other industrialized countries are victims of prejudice and discrimination. There is evidence that obese applicants are less likely to be accepted into prestigious colleges than nonobese applicants with equivalent qualifications. In a 1974 study of executive incomes (when incomes were lower than those of today), only 9% of those earning $25,000 to $50,000 per year were 10 pounds or more overweight, in contrast to 39% of those earning $10,000 to $20,000. Although many factors must influence such statistics, they are taken as evidence of discrimination in the workplace. Airlines, the police, and armed forces do not hire significantly obese people and often discharge employees if they fail to maintain an "appropriate" weight. When obese women marry, their socioeconomic status is twice as likely to fall as it is to rise. Children as young as 6 years old commonly describe obese people as lazy, stupid, ugly, and "cheats."

Because of the many pressures and prejudices obese people face, it is commonly believed that they must suffer higher-than-average levels of depression and other psychological disturbances and lower-than-average levels of general self-esteem. Research using standard personality and psychopathology inventories, however, does not support this widely held belief. In general, recent population studies have shown no significant differences in the psychological status of obese and nonobese adults and children. Where emotional disturbances have been noted in obese people, it has usually been in those seeking surgical treatment to achieve weight loss. Most such studies have lacked proper comparison with "control" groups of obese people not seeking surgical treatment for weight loss. The need for such controls is critical because a certain level of psychological disturbance can be expected in any sample of people seeking surgical treatment.

The fact that obese individuals generally show no increased level of psychological disturbance is surprising, given the intense psychological assault to which they are exposed. Although suffering no greater level of psychological disturbance than the general population overall, however, obese and overweight people do suffer from a variety of psychological problems specific to obesity. These problems must take the place of other problems more common in the general population, and they include binge eating and disparagement of body image, among other disorders.

Binge eating is characterized by the following:

- Eating within a specific amount of time (any 2-hour period, for example) an amount of food that is well in excess of an amount most people eat in a similar amount of time
- A feeling that what is being eaten and how much is being eaten during the binge-eating episode is out of the control of the person doing the eating

Disparagement of body image is defined as the belief that one's body is grotesque and loathsome and that others view it with hostility and contempt. This disturbance is most common among child-onset obese individuals (that is, those who become obese in childhood). It appears to develop in adolescence and represents an internalization of criticism received from parents and peers. It then persists, even if the criticism ceases. Other psychosocial problems experienced by overweight and obese individuals, which are not measured by standard personality and psychopathology inventories, include the following:

- Lack of confidence resulting from the inability to maintain weight loss
- A sense of isolation resulting from the inability of family and friends to understand the frustration caused by a weight problem or the humiliation that arises from the inability to fit into standard sized clothing, seating, and so on.

It is surprising that obese people often only fully recognize the extent of their suffering in retrospect, once they have achieved successful weight reduction. This aspect of obesity is summarized succinctly by the conclusion of the 1985 National Institutes of Health Consensus Conference on the Health Consequences of Obesity as follows: "Obesity creates an enormous psychological burden. . . . In terms of suffering, this burden may be the greatest adverse effect of obesity."[15]

ECONOMIC DISADVANTAGES

In addition to being denied access to many jobs and to encountering discrimination when seeking promotion, obese people suffer a variety of other economic disadvantages. Those who are severely obese may need to buy more expensive clothes from specialized stores. Some also need to purchase special furniture, customized automobiles, and wider first-class seats on airlines and pay increased insurance rates because of the increased health risks. Many also spend a lot of money on expensive "weight-reducing aids." These are only the most obvious of many additional costs that contribute to a generally higher cost of living for obese individuals. Obesity also presents an economic cost to society because of the health care and welfare costs of coping with the diseases associated with obesity, the costs of time lost from work because of illness, and so on. In the United States these costs were estimated in 1986 at $39.3 billion, or 5% of the total cost of illness.[16]

CAUSES OF OBESITY

The underlying cause of all obesity is the long-term persistence of a state of **positive energy balance.** In other words, obesity is caused by the prolonged intake of kilocalories in excess of kilocalorie expenditure. This simple statement does not explain *why* some people consistently consume excess kilocalories or why they have so much trouble in maintaining a desirable body weight when many other people do so automatically.

GENETICS

Recent studies from a number of research centers have shown that a considerable proportion of human obesity, accounting for perhaps as much as 50% to 79% of cases, has a genetic component, meaning that genetics plays some significant role as a cause of the obesity. Genetic factors, which involve the inheritance of genes received from our parents, may *predispose* a person to obesity in the sense that they make it more likely for offspring to become obese. They rarely, if ever, *condemn* a person to obesity because whether a genetically predisposed person actually becomes obese depends on the physical, social, and psychological environment to which he or she is exposed. Thus the development of obesity involves a complex interaction between the genetic factors within a susceptible individual and an environment that fosters obesity. Two major obesity-promoting environmental factors are modern sedentary life-styles and the availability of palatable diets high in fat and sugar.

A role for genetics in obesity is often suggested by examining members of one family with similar body builds. A carefully conducted and controlled study of monozygotic ("identical") and dizygotic ("nonidentical") twins reared either together or apart in Sweden focused attention on the genetic contribution to body weight and size.[17] Monozygotic twins share the same genetic makeup and were found to share significant similarities in BMIs, regardless of whether they were reared together or apart. On the other hand, the BMIs of dizygotic twins, who have differing genetic makeups, did not share such significant similarities. Overall, these

FIGURE 7-10

Physical characteristics of individuals with endomorphic features (tendency to obesity) and ectomorphic features (tendency to thinness).

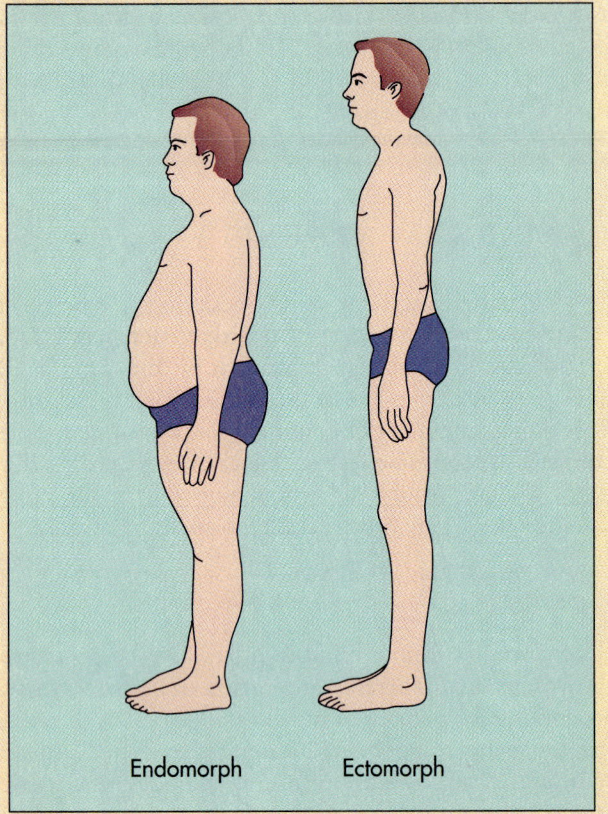

studies suggest a strong genetic component in the development of obesity.

Obese people usually have predominantly **endomorphic** features, which contribute to a short, stocky stature (Figure 7-10). The tendency toward endomorphic, as opposed to **ectomorphic,** body type is presumed to be strongly influenced by genetics. It is less evident what impact genetics has on the different ways in which peoples' bodies use food and the amount of satisfaction they get from food. There is strong evidence suggesting that many obese people, or those who gain weight easily, do not eat more food than those who are not obese and maintain desirable weight with ease. The distinction between these two types of people seems to be that food is used more efficiently in the bodies of those who are obese or who readily gain weight and that these people tend to store fat more quickly and mobilize body fat as an energy source much less effectively. This does not mean that people who inherit a predisposition to obesity are certain to become obese, but it does mean that to avoid obesity, they must engage in a constant and difficult struggle against the accumulation of fat. Such people are more likely to produce additional fat cells (experience hyperplasia) or have larger fat cells (experience hypertrophy) than other people.

Many people with a genetic predisposition to obesity have raised levels of the enzyme lipoprotein lipase. As discussed in Chapter 4, this enzyme plays a key role in breaking down lipoproteins in the blood to release their fatty acids and other lipids for entry into tissue cells. Thus raised levels of lipoprotein lipase increase the efficiency with which tissue cells take up lipids for incorporation into fat stores. Such people also show a marked taste preference for fat-containing foods and dislike sweet-tasting solutions.

Infants born to obese mothers can have a lower energy expenditure than infants born to lean mothers by the time they are 3 months old. Infants who become overweight by the age of 1 year also have lower energy expenditure levels than those who do not become overweight. It has also been shown that many overweight adults have a lower energy expenditure, both basal and total, than predicted on the basis of their height, weight, and activity level. These observations and others provide evidence that a person's rate of energy expenditure is under strong genetic control and so is inherited through the generations.

SEDENTARY LIFE-STYLES

Obesity has become a serious and widespread health problem principally in technologically advanced societies: those characterized by modern economies, sophisticated technological systems, affluence, food surpluses, and social stratification. Numerous studies of traditional societies undergoing the process of economic modernization have found accompanying rapid increases in the prevalence of obesity. There is considerable evidence that the sedentary life-style of many people in modern affluent societies may be a key factor in this trend toward obesity.

There is also, as mentioned previously, much evidence that the weight gain that leads to obesity is caused by a low energy expenditure, rather than obvious overeating. Although the energy expenditure of many activities seems small, the figures involved can mount up over longer periods so that seemingly minor reductions in activity can cause significant weight gain in the long term. For example, 1 hour of playing tennis uses approximately an additional 350 kcal of energy per hour, whereas walking 3 miles uses about an extra 140 kcal. If a 154-pound man played tennis for just 15 minutes every day of the year, this would use up the energy within 9 pounds (4 kg) of body fat. Walking just half a mile every day accounts for 2½ pounds of body fat. These figures demonstrate that *giving up* such activities, or similarly strenuous ones, can soon lead to consider-

TABLE 7-8

Activity equivalents of specific amounts of various foods

		ACTIVITY				
FOOD	KCAL*	WALKING† (MIN)	RIDING A BICYCLE‡ (MIN)	SWIMMING§ (MIN)	RUNNING‖ (MIN)	RECLINING¶ (MIN)
Apple (large) or banana (medium)	101	19	12	9	5	78
Bacon (2 strips)	96	18	12	9	5	74
Beer (1 glass)	114	22	14	10	6	88
Bread and butter	78	115	10	7	4	60
Cake (1/12, 2-layer)	356	68	43	32	18	274
Carbonated beverage (1 glass)	106	20	13	9	5	82
Cereal, dry (½ cup) with milk and sugar	200	38	24	18	10	154
Cheese, cheddar (1 oz)	111	21	14	10	6	85
Chicken, fried (½ breast)	232	45	28	21	12	178
Cookie, chocolate chip	51	10	6	5	3	39
Doughnut	151	29	18	13	8	116
Egg, fried	110	121	13	10	6	85
Ham (2 slices)	167	32	20	15	9	128
Ice cream (⅔ cup)	193	37	24	17	10	148
Malted milk shake	502	97	61	45	26	386
Mayonnaise (1 Tbsp)	92	18	11	8	5	71
Milk, whole (1 cup)	150	32	20	15	9	128
Orange juice (1 glass)	120	23	15	11	6	92
Pie, apple (⅙)	377	73	46	34	19	290
Pizza, cheese (⅛)	180	35	22	16	9	138
Pork chop, loin	314	60	38	28	16	242
Potato chips (1 serving)	108	21	13	10	6	83
Sandwiches						
Club	590	113	72	53	30	454
Hamburger	350	67	43	31	18	269
Tuna fish salad	278	53	34	25	14	214
Sherbet (⅔ cup)	177	34	22	16	9	136
Spaghetti (1 + cup)	396	76	48	35	20	305
Steak, T-bone	235	45	29	21	12	181

* To convert kilocalories to kilojoules, multiply by 4.2; to convert kilocalories to joules, multiply by 4200.
† Energy cost of walking for a 70-kg individual equals 5.2 kcal/min at 3.5 mph.
‡ Energy cost of riding a bicycle equals 8.2 kcal/min.
§ Energy cost of swimming equals 11.2 kcal/min.
‖ Energy cost of running equals 19.4 kcal/min.
¶ Energy cost of reclining equals 1.3 kcal/min.

From Konishi F: *J Am Diet Assoc* 46:186, 1965.

able weight gain over several years if no compensating adjustment of food intake is made. Almost all effective weight control programs involve additional exercise, as well as diet, to raise daily energy needs from the low levels associated with sedentary life-styles. Table 7-8 gives some examples of the **activity equivalents** of various foods, meaning the amount of activity needed to use up the energy supplied by the food.

INTAKE OF ENERGY-YIELDING NUTRIENTS

In some forms of obesity it appears that obesity develops regardless of the type of diet available. In other cases the onset of obesity appears to be strongly influenced by the composition of the diet, particularly the relative proportions of the various energy-yielding nutrients.

The relative proportions of the main energy-yielding nutrients (carbohydrate, fat, and protein) in a typical diet are shown on the left of Figure 7-11. On the right the figure quantifies these daily intakes as a percentage of the body's stores of the nutrients. It can be seen that a typical daily diet supplies an amount of carbohydrate equal to the total amount stored in the body but amounts of fat and protein that represent only a small proportion of the total amounts stored in the body. When allowance is made for normal dietary variation, it can be said that daily carbohydrate intake normally corresponds to between 50% and 100% of the amount held in glycogen stores, whereas fat and protein intakes

FIGURE 7-11

Relationship of nutrient intake to nutrient stores.

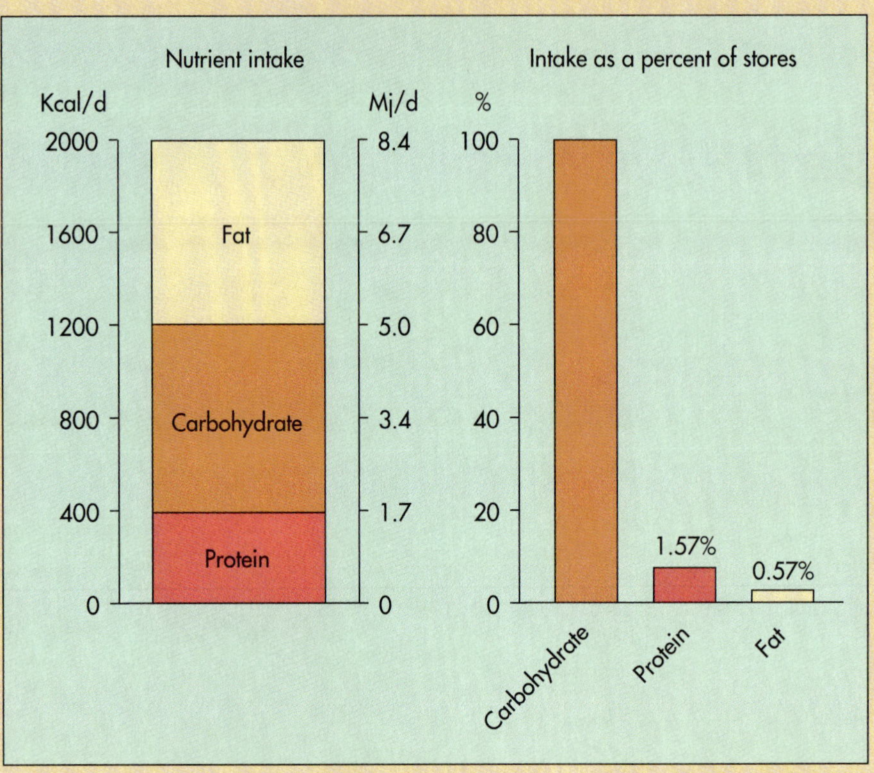

correspond to between 0.5% and 2% of the amount present in storage form. The amounts of carbohydrate and protein held in storage form are tightly regulated. When an excess of these nutrients is ingested, it is either oxidized as an immediate source of energy or converted to storage fat. This conversion of carbohydrate or protein to fat is itself an energetically expensive process in the sense that it consumes significant quantities of adenosine triphosphate (ATP). It appears to occur only when energy intake is excessive. Fat is processed differently from the other energy-yielding nutrients in that excess intake is not oxidized or converted to other substances but is stored as fat. The main stimulus for the oxidation of fat is not the intake of fat in the diet but either an energy deficit in the body in general or energy requirements resulting from increased muscular activity. This reflects the key role of storage fat as the body's main energy storage material.

To achieve **net energy balance,** the net level of oxidation of each of the energy-yielding nutrients must correspond to the average amount of the nutrient present in the diet. Thus a high-fat diet requires greater oxidation of fat than does a low-fat diet, if net energy nutrient balance is to be maintained. Recent evidence indicates that there are major differences among individuals in their ability to increase the rate of fat oxidation after beginning a high-fat diet. These differences appear to be largely genetically determined, and a person with a slow response to increased fat intake obviously is more likely to gain weight on a high-fat diet than is one with a fast response.

Several human feeding trials have found that fat intake is higher in obese subjects, when compared with lean subjects. Also, subjects were found to gain weight and have a higher kilocalorie intake when allowed to eat to satiety a high-fat diet, compared with a low-fat diet of similar palatability. Palatability, which means "pleasing to the palate or taste," is also believed to be a major environmental factor contributing to obesity. It is determined by both the flavor (including taste, aroma, and texture) of food and the effects of the food after ingestion that give rise to a feeling of satiety. There is evidence from animal experiments to indicate that the palatability of foods in a diet contributes to overeating and obesity. In essence, if it tastes good, more of it is likely to be eaten. For example, it is possible to produce overeating and obesity in rats by feeding a "cafeteria-style" diet (composed of supermarket foods, such as chocolate, cookies, and bread), while feeding the animals a less palatable high-fat or high-sugar diet does not produce overeating and obesity to the same extent. The effectiveness of the cafeteria-style diet in promoting overeating and obesity is believed to be caused by the high palatability of the food *combined* with the fact that it is high in fat or sugar, or both.

HUNGER AND SATIETY

Some people become obese because a genetic predisposition to obesity is combined with unlimited access to palatable foods high in fat or sugar content, with a sedentary life-style as an additional contributory factor in many cases. As reported in many studies, obesity in the United States and other developed countries is certainly becoming more prevalent, yet the fact remains that most people maintain a relatively stable and acceptable body weight. This implies that in most people, food intake and energy balance are tightly regulated. This regulation is believed to be achieved by an automatic system allowing the intake of food to be stimulated by *hunger* but inhibited at an appropriate point by the sensation of *satiety*. Recent research indicates that the integration of internal and external stimuli to achieve this regulation depends on a complex network of chemical and physiological effects.

Early investigations suggested that food intake is regulated by two centers in the brain: the **lateral hypothalamic feeding center** and the **medial hypothalamic satiety center** (both parts of the hypothalamus). This conclusion was drawn from studies in animals, showing that destruction of the feeding center abolished voluntary feeding behavior, whereas destruction of the satiety center led to overfeeding and obesity. Thus the feeding center appeared to be required to stimulate appropriate feeding, whereas the satiety center was apparently required to bring a halt to feeding once an appropriate amount of food was consumed. It was later learned that the prolonged period of reduced or zero food intake after destruction of the lateral hypothalamic region was actually caused by destruction of a region of brain tissue that controls *many* voluntary activities, not just feeding. Later studies also showed that the obesity caused by destruction in the medial hypothalamic region seemed to be caused in part by "hyperinsulinism" (high insulin production). This directs energy-yielding nutrients into the lipid storage pathways, rather than allowing them to be used to meet prevailing energy needs.

These early ideas about the systems that regulate food intake have been replaced by more recent ones, but the brain remains central to current theories. These treat the brain as a central "controller" of the "controlled system," which incorporates the body's processes for food intake, storage, and oxidation (Figure 7-12). As

FIGURE 7-12

Summary of the "controller/controlled system" approach to the modeling of the control of food intake.

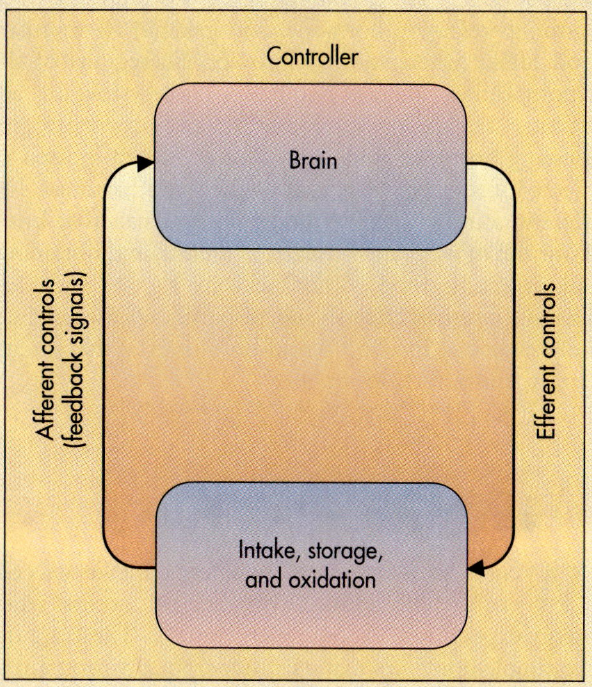

the controller, the brain receives signals (afferent controls) from the controlled system, reflecting the state of that system (levels of food intake, oxidation, storage, current energy needs, and so on), and the brain sends out signals (efferent controls) that regulate the intake of food and its metabolic fate. A detailed discussion of these control systems is beyond the scope of this text, but the essential features are summarized. Those interested in the details should consult the review article on the topic by Bray.[18]

As already stated, the brain is believed to act as the central controller of food intake, serving to integrate chemical and nervous signals from many different sources (the afferent controls) and, in response, produce the efferent control signals that regulate the level of food intake and adjust the balance between food oxidation and storage as appropriate. The afferent controls include sensory signals (such as the sight and smell of food), gastrointestinal signals (such as gastric distention and hunger), cholecystokinin release from the gastrointestinal tract, and nutrients released from the digestion of food. Both cholecystokinin and nutrients, such as glucose and fatty acids (and products formed from them), are known to act as signals that initiate a feeling of satiety. A number of specific neurotransmitters are known to be involved in the integration and control of hunger and satiety, including gamma-aminobutyric acid, norepinephrine (noradrenaline), serotonin, and histamine. Several neuropeptides (regulatory peptides able to affect the nervous system) are also known to be involved: neuropeptide Y, β-endorphin, dynorphin, growth hormone–releasing hormone, and gallanin all stimulate food intake when injected into specific regions of the hypothalamus; whereas bombesin, cholecystokinin, anorectin, calcitonin, neurotensin, and corticotropin-releasing hormone inhibit food intake when infused or injected into specific regions of the hypothalamus. The efferent controls include the nervous signals that bring about the movements involved in identifying, obtaining, and ingesting food; other nervous signals with less obvious internal effects; and also the release of hormones, such as insulin, steroid hormones of the adrenal glands, and growth hormone.

WEIGHT REDUCTION

Weight gain occurs when energy intake exceeds energy expenditure. Weight loss occurs when energy expenditure exceeds energy intake. These are the two simple principles that must underpin any program of weight control. Energy intake depends on the amount of energy-yielding nutrients (carbohydrate, fat, protein, and alcohol) consumed. Energy expenditure equals the basal metabolic rate, plus energy used by the thermic effect of food, plus energy required for activity. Weight loss can be brought about by lowering energy intake or increasing energy expenditure by increasing one's level of activity, or both. Most successful weight loss programs employ a *combination* of strict intake control and increased activity.

If energy intake and expenditure are not equally balanced, a deficit or excess of 3500 kcal normally causes a loss or gain of 1 pound of body fat. So, to result in weight loss, a person's food intake and activity level must cause energy expenditure to be 3500 kcal greater than energy intake for every pound of weight loss. These figures assume that stored body fat is the source of the energy needed to make up for the deficit, which is the case in people who are overweight or obese. If muscle or other fat-free mass is being broken down to supply energy, however, then a deficit of only 580 kcal results in a loss of 1 pound of weight. This reflects the lower energy content of fat-free tissue, which is 70% water. Loss of fat-free tissue produces the fast weight loss seen in starvation or severe malnutrition. Muscle loss is undesirable and in fact dangerous if there is appreciable loss, especially because it can affect the vital muscles of the heart. Weight reduction programs for overweight or obese persons are designed to cause weight loss that is due to fat loss, while maintaining muscle mass at its preexisting level.

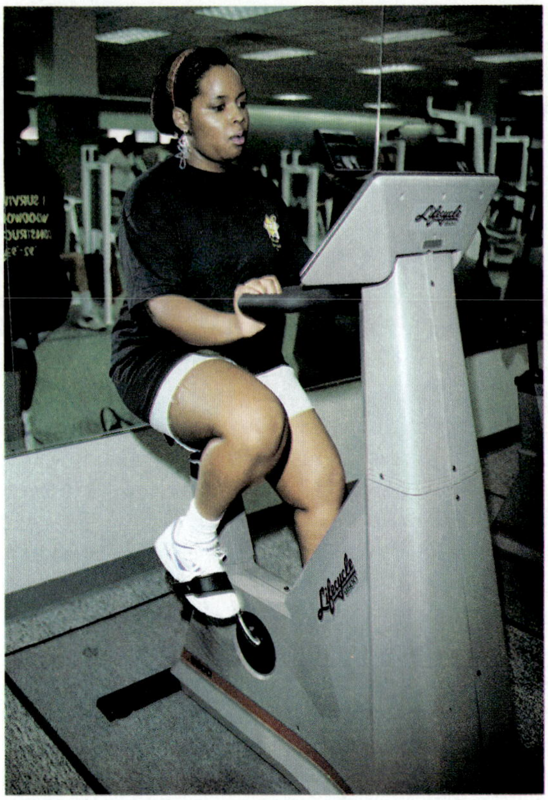

Most successful weight loss plans combine increased physical activity with decreased food intake.

- Weight gain occurs when energy intake exceeds energy expenditure. Weight loss occurs when energy expenditure exceeds energy intake.
- One pound of fat stores 3500 kcal of available energy; so consuming 3500 kcal in excess of expenditure produces a weight gain of 1 pound, whereas consuming 3500 kcal less than expenditure produces a weight loss of 1 pound.

In general, weight that is lost quickly (more than 1 to 2 pounds per week) is more rapidly regained and more likely to be regained than is weight lost more gradually. Gradual but persistent weight loss is the key to successful weight reduction. Despite this, Americans spend over $30 billion every year on commercial weight reduction products and programs, many of which promise fast results indeed. This figure does not include the substantial sums spent on weight-reducing surgery but does include an estimated $5 billion to $6 billion wasted on entirely fraudulent products. The $30 billion is spent on such things as special foods, exercise devices, appetite suppressants, formula diets, health clubs and spas, camps for children, and a wide variety of counseling services. Sadly, the single most obvious factor that all of these products have in common is their failure to produce the desired effect: only 5% of people trying to lose weight are found to maintain any weight loss for more than 3 years.

> Gradual but persistent weight loss is the key to successful weight reduction.

Contrary to the claims made by many advertisements, there have been no breakthroughs in weight control and there are no easy solutions. On the contrary, science is providing an increasingly convincing body of evidence to explain why it is extremely difficult for many people to achieve and maintain their desired body weight. In general, approaches that combine decreased energy intake with increased energy expenditure are the most likely to succeed. That general statement summarizes a wide variety of individual approaches. Only the most common of these are discussed.

> Be wary of any diet, device, or pill that promises quick and easy weight loss. There is no easy route to weight loss; it is a slow process that requires persistence. It has been found that success is most likely if the individual is:
> - Young
> - Single
> - In the higher levels of socioeconomic status
> - Making a first attempt
> - Less than 60% in excess of desirable weight
> - Emotionally well adjusted

CRITERIA FOR SUCCESSFUL DIETS

At any one time, headlines can be found in several magazines proclaiming new weight reduction diets that promise instant and continuing success. Almost all of these, however, are reruns of diets that have been promoted repeatedly over the years.

Any diet that meets the following seven criteria is probably nutritionally adequate and leads to steady weight loss at a reasonable rate with a good possibility of long-term success:

> Criteria for assessing weight-reducing diets include the following:
> - Must be deficient in kilocalories
> - Must have adequate amounts of nutrients, although being deficient in total kilocalories
> - Must have sufficient fat or bulk to provide satiety
> - Must be able to be adapted from family meals and food available when eating out
> - Must be reasonable in cost
> - Must be a diet that can be adhered to for a sufficient time to lose weight
> - Must retrain the individual into a new and sustainable eating pattern

- The diet must be deficient in kilocalories, meaning that it supplies fewer kilocalories per day than are required by the individual following the diet. This can be determined only by comparing the kilocalorie content of the diet with a reasonable estimate of the person's needs. A diet that is deficient in kilocalories for one person is not necessarily so for another. A daily deficit of 500 kcal, amounting to a deficit of 3500 kcal per week, should result in the loss of 1 pound of body fat per week. The body has a temporary tendency to replace this lost fat with water, causing obvious discouragement to people following a diet. If the diet is continued for long enough, however (sometimes as long as 4 to 5 weeks is required), the total predicted loss will eventually occur, sometimes all at once.
- The diet should be adequate in all nutrients, although deficient in total kilocalories. This is difficult to check precisely, but a reasonable indication can be gained by checking that the diet includes at least two servings per day from each of the following food groups: milk and dairy products; fruit and vegetables; cereal products; and meat, fish, poultry, and eggs (and eggs with any additional food coming from fruits, veg-

etables, or cereal products). As the total kilocalorie content of a diet drops, it does become increasingly difficult to choose a nutritionally adequate diet. Even with a total kilocalorie content as low as 1400 kcal, however, it is possible—with a careful choice of foods—to achieve a diet that meets the recommended dietary allowances (RDAs) for all nutrients. If energy intake is restricted to less than 1000 kcal/day, the diet should be supplemented with protective amounts of minerals and vitamins (but not more than 100% of the RDA).
- The diet should have a high satiety value. Diets containing some fat and relatively high levels of protein delay the onset of hunger pangs longer than do diets with the same total kilocalorie content (known as **isocaloric** diets) but composed primarily of carbohydrate. It is easier to adhere to a diet of high satiety value than to one with foods that leave the stomach rapidly or have little bulk.
- The diet should be one that can be adapted readily from family meals and food obtained in public eating places. Any diet that sets dieters apart from the people with whom they eat or that imposes extra work on whoever prepares the food is less likely to be followed than a diet that allows people to eat inconspicuously alongside family and friends in all social situations.
- The diet must be reasonable in cost. If it makes use of seasonal foods and everyday staple items, it is more acceptable and more likely to be adhered to than a diet that requires special purchases of expensive, out-of-season, and unfamiliar foods.
- The diet should be one that can be adhered to for a sufficient time to permit the desired weight loss. It is recommended that, except in extreme obesity, the rate of weight loss should not exceed 1 to 1½ pounds (0.5 to 0.7 kg)/week. This means that a person wishing to lose 20 pounds (9 kg), for example, should try to accomplish the loss over a period of at least 15 weeks. Crash diets that limit dieters to a restricted range of foods, such as cottage cheese and peaches or steak, egg, and tomatoes, are nutritionally inadequate and also so monotonous that their psychological appeal lasts for only a short time. It is almost impossible for a person to remain on such a limited selection of foods long enough to achieve the desired weight loss.
- Most important of all, if dieters are to achieve long-term success, the diet chosen should represent a sufficient departure from their former eating patterns. To achieve success, dieters need to be retrained into a new set of eating patterns that they can expect to adhere to, with slight modifications, as a maintenance diet for a lifetime. The various liquid formula diets available ultimately fail largely because, even if temporary success is dramatic, they do not lead to any permanent weight loss. This can be attributed partly to the fact that they do not substitute a new socially acceptable and satisfying pattern of eating for the old one that led to weight gain.

It is obvious that a diet that meets the criteria previously outlined leads to success only if it is followed long enough to achieve the desired weight loss and establish a new pattern of eating.

An analysis of some of the most popular weight loss programs is presented in Table 7-9 and of popular diet books in Table 7-10. Those diets that meet all seven criteria are rated as "reasonable," those that meet only a few of the criteria are rated as "questionable," and those that are deemed unsafe for general nutritional health, or are fraudulent, are rated "unreasonable." As new weight loss programs and diet books appear, the dieter should assess their merits using these seven criteria.

It is important to warn prospective dieters about the characteristics of some diets that are almost certainly doomed to failure. The following key points allow the identification of such diets:

- There is no single food that facilitates weight loss by "burning fat," stimulating metabolism, or causing fat to "melt away." Any diet composed of a single food certainly causes weight loss but is usually only followed for a short period. Unfortunately, it almost certainly also results in a deficiency of one or more essential nutrients, with potentially negative health consequences.
- A diet accompanied by the promise that "you can eat as much as you want" is almost certainly composed of foods so unpalatable nobody would want to eat large amounts of them or so few foods that monotony would limit their use.
- Total fasting is appropriate only for the most severely obese people. In such people, it should be undertaken only under strict medical supervision. Protein-sparing modified fasts designed to prevent loss of lean body mass or nutritional deficiencies are much more acceptable for such people but also require constant monitoring to prevent adverse health effects.
- Very-low-calorie diets (VLCDs) of less than 500 kcal/day do not establish sustainable new eating patterns and are deficient in nutrients, unless specific supplements are included. They may also lead to ketosis, a condition in which ketones produced by fat metabolism appear in the blood and urine. As discussed in previous chapters, ketosis is associated with various undesir-

TABLE 7-9

Analyses of some popular weight loss programs

DIET	ENTRY CRITERIA	COST	MEDICAL SUPERVISION?	NUTRITION EDUCATION, BEHAVIOR MODIFICATION, EXERCISE INCLUDED?	DESCRIPTION, COMMENTS
<600-800 kcal/day					
Reasonable:					
Health Management Resources (HMR)	20% above ideal body weight or 40 lb overweight for VLCD diet	$115/week for medically supervised program, $90/week for moderate program	Yes	Yes	Medically supervised VLCD (520 to 800 kcal) program and moderate program with less intensive supervision (800 to 1,000 kcal) available. Three phases: Weight loss Refeeding Maintenance Use of liquid formula diet or HMR frozen entrees (150 to 230 kcal)
Medifast	20% above ideal body weight	$62.50 to $75/week	Yes	Prescribed but not necessarily provided by a multidisciplinary team of professionals	Four-phase program: Medical evaluation Weight reduction (450-kcal liquid diet for women; 480-kcal liquid diet for men) Realimentation Maintenance
Optifast	30% above ideal body weight; 20% if medically at risk or 60 lb overweight	$100/week	Yes	Yes	Four-phase program: Modified fast (420- to 800-kcal liquid diet) Refeeding Stabilization Maintenance (optional)
Unreasonable:					
Total fasting	Not appropriate for anyone	—	No	No	Not advised because of high loss of lean body mass, vitamin and mineral deficiencies, and other complications
800-1200 kcal/day					
Reasonable:					
Diet Center	Physician approval needed for individuals more than 40% or 60 lb overweight or who have preexisting health problems	$50/week for reducing phase; less for other phases	? (Nurse travels to different sites)	Prescribed but not necessarily provided by a multidisciplinary team of professionals	Four-phase program: Conditioning (unlimited kcal) Reducing (minimum of 1000 kcal) Stabilizing Maintenance Individual differences in caloric needs are taken into consideration for all phases. Vitamin/mineral supplement taken daily. 1000 mg of vitamin C is recommended daily, which seems excessive

TABLE 7-9

Analyses of some popular weight loss programs (continued)

DIET	ENTRY CRITERIA	COST	MEDICAL SUPERVISION?	NUTRITION EDUCATION, BEHAVIOR MODIFICATION, EXERCISE INCLUDED?	DESCRIPTION, COMMENTS
Diet Workshop	Physician approval needed for individuals with preexisting health problems	Registration fee of $14, $9/week	No	Prescribed but not provided by a multidisciplinary team of professionals	Based on system of food "units" Reducing phase (900 to 1000 kcal) Increased gradually to 1200 kcal until goal weight is achieved Maintenance (kcal according to individual needs) Vitamin/mineral supplement recommended
Jenny Craig Weight Loss Centers	Physician approval needed for individuals with preexisting medical conditions	$185 for membership; $60 to $70/week for food	No	Prescribed but not provided by a multidisciplinary team of professionals	Two phases: Reducing (about 1000 kcal for women; 1200 to 1400 kcal for men) Maintenance (kcal according to individual needs) Complete reliance on packaged foods initially
Nutri/System	Physician approval needed for individuals more than 100 lb overweight or who have preexisting medical problems	Variable according to location and goal weight; $60 to $69/week for food	No	Prescribed but not provided by a multidisciplinary team of professionals	Two phases: Weight loss (minimum of 1000 kcal for women; 1200 kcal for men) Maintenance (kcal according to individual needs) Complete reliance on packaged foods until maintenance phase; low-fat (14%) high-carbohydrate (61%) diet; special diet modifications for medical conditions
Weight Watchers	More than 10 lb overweight	$12 to $20 registration fee, $7 to $9/week	No	Prescribed but not provided by a multidisciplinary team of professionals	Based on system of food exchanges Weight loss (1040 to 1450 kcal for women; 1440 to 1910 kcal for men) Maintenance (kcal according to individual needs)
Not recommended					
Slim Fast/Ultra Slim Fast	Physician approval recommended for individuals who are pregnant, nursing, under 18 years old, have health problems, or want to lose more than 30 lb or more than 15% of their body weight	$8 to $12/week	No	Limited	Over-the-counter meal replacement is mixed with low-fat milk (Slim Fast) or water (Ultra Slim Fast). Slim Fast is 190 kcal/serving, Ultra Slim Fast is 220 kcal/serving. Two phases: Weight loss (2 to 3 formulas, 1 fruit, 1 meal of 410 kcal; 1100 to 1200 kcal/day) Maintenance (1 to 2 formulas, 2 meals; 3 fruits; 6 oz milk; 1450 to 1520 kcal/day) Frozen entrees (230 to 400 kcal) also available. This diet can be dangerous if instructions are not followed properly.

From Dwyer JT, Lu D: Popular diets for weight loss from nutritionally hazardous to healthful. In Stunkard AJ, Wadden TA (editors): *Obesity: theory and therapy,* ed 2, New York, 1993, Raven Press.

TABLE 7-10

Analyses of some popular diet books

DIET	MEETS FOOD GROUP GOALS?	NUTRITION EDUCATION, BEHAVIOR MODIFICATION, EXERCISE INCLUDED?	DESCRIPTION, COMMENTS
800-1200 kcal/day			
Questionable:			
Hilton Head Over-35 Diet by Peter Miller. New York: Warner Books, 1989	No—low in milk and fruit/vegetable groups during low-calorie phase	Yes—but limited behavior modification	Three phases: Low calorie (rotates between 900 kcal/day on weekdays and 1200 kcal/day on weekends) Reentry (about halfway between low-calorie and maintenance phases) Maintenance (kcal equal to resting metabolic rate plus activity factor) Varying energy intakes in weight loss has not been proved to prevent drops in resting metabolic rate (RMR)
The New Pritikin Program by Robert Pritikin. New York: Simon and Schuster, 1990	Yes—heavy emphasis on fruit/vegetable and bread/cereal groups	Yes	Energy intakes of 1000 kcal/day for women, 1200 kcal/day for men on "maximum weight loss" plan. Does not take individual needs for weight loss into account. Low-fat (10%), high-carbohydrate (75% to 80%) diet that is also low in sodium and high in fiber. May be difficult to follow such a low-fat diet
Unreasonable:			
Dr. Berger's Immune Power Diet by Stewart Berger. New York: New American Library, 1985	No—low in milk and bread/cereal groups	Limited	Diet to improve immune system but includes weight loss as an added benefit based on unsupported claims that certain foods affect immune system and levels of energy, creativity, mood, and emotion Three phases: Elimination (about 1050 kcal/day) Reintroduction (about 1400 kcal/day) Maintenance (about 1650 kcal/day) Individual differences in caloric needs for weight loss are not considered; recommends megadoses of supplements, which can be dangerous
Rotation Diet by Martin Katahn. New York: Bantam Books, 1987	No—low in milk and bread/cereal groups for most phases	Yes	Energy intakes of 600 to 1500 kcal/day rotated over 4 weeks; maintenance level is 1800 kcal/day. Individual differences in caloric needs for weight loss are not considered. Varying energy intakes in weight loss has not been proved to prevent drops in RMR
> 1200 kcal/day			
Reasonable:			
Fat Attack Plan by Annete Natow and Jo-Ann Hestin. New York: Pocket Books, 1990	May be low in meat or bread/cereal group, depending on what dieter chooses	Yes	Teaches dieter to count grams of fat in foods Three phases: "Super start" (about 1350 kcal/day) "Getting ahead"—15 g fat (about 1400 kcal/day) "In control"—45 g of fat for women (about 1700 kcal/day), 60 g of fat for men (about 1300 kcal/day) May be difficult to follow such a low-fat diet

TABLE 7-10

Analyses of some popular diet books (continued)

DIET	MEETS FOOD GROUP GOALS?	NUTRITION EDUCATION, BEHAVIOR MODIFICATION, EXERCISE INCLUDED?	DESCRIPTION, COMMENTS
Fit or Fat Target Diet by Covert Bailey. Boston: Houghton and Mifflin, 1984	Yes	Limited—more guidance may be needed for weight loss; focus is on long-term weight management	Emphasis on healthful balanced diet rather than weight loss. Recommended minimum calorie level to promote weight loss is 1000 to 1400 kcal/day for women, 1400 to 1800 kcal/day for men. Diet is based on basic four food groups, with emphasis on low-fat, low-sugar, and high-fiber foods (about 1500 kcal/day)
Set Point Diet by Gilbert Leveille. New York: Ballantine Books, 1985	Yes	Yes	1200 to 2400 kcal/day food plans. Maintenance adds 300 kcal/day. More research is needed regarding the set-point theory of body weight being confined to narrow range, and whether diet can lower one's set-point weight
T-Factor Diet by Martin Katahn. New York: WW Norton, 1989	Yes	Yes	Two diets provided: T-factor diet is relatively low in calories and involves counting fat grams (20 to 40 g fat for women or about 1200 kcal/day, 30 to 60 g fat or about 1800 kcal/day for men). "Quick Melt Diet" restricts women to 1000 to 1300 kcal/day and men to 1500 to 1800 kcal/day. Does not take individual caloric differences for weight control into account. May be difficult to follow such low-fat diet. Based on thermogenesis studies suggesting that dietary fat is more efficiently converted into body fat than carbohydrates.
Callaway Diet by Wayne Callaway. New York: Bantam Books, 1990	No—low in milk group	Yes—but limited advice on maintenance	1400- to 2000- kcal/day menus. Geared toward dieters who are "starvers" (periodically fast or near fast with VLCD), "stuffers" (compulsive eaters), or "skippers" (skip meals)
Unreasonable:			
Fit For Life by Harvey and Marilyn Diamond. New York: Warner Books, 1985	No—low in milk, meat, and bread/cereal groups; very high in fruit/vegetable groups	Yes—but little emphasis on behavior modification and weight maintenance	Based on unsupported claims that fat deposits are caused by improper food combinations. Diet is high in fat (41%) and lacks variety. Individual differences in caloric needs for weight control are not considered, and high bulk may make it difficult to consume adequate calories

From Dwyer JT, Lu D: Popular diets for weight loss from nutritionally hazardous to healthful. In Stunkard AJ, Wadden TA, editors: *Obesity: theory and therapy,* ed 2, New York, 1993, Raven Press.

Guidelines for Evaluating Commercial Weight Loss Promotions

AVOID COMMERICAL WEIGHT LOSS OR CONTROL PROGRAMS THAT DO THE FOLLOWING:

1. Promise or imply dramatic, rapid weight loss (that is, substantially more than 1% of total body weight per week).
2. Promote diets that are extremely low in calories (that is, below 800 calories/day; 1200 calories/day diets are preferred) unless under the supervision of competent medical experts.
3. Attempt to make clients dependent on special products rather than teaching how to make good choices from the conventional food supply (this does not condemn the marketing of low-calorie convenience foods which may be chosen by consumers).
4. Do not encourage permanent, realistic life-style changes including regular exercise and the behavior aspects of eating wherein food may be used as a coping device (that is, programs should focus on changing the *causes* of overweight rather than simply the *effects,* which is the overweight itself).
5. Misrepresent salespeople as "counselors" supposedly qualified to give guidance in nutrition or general health. Even if adequately trained, such "counselors" are still objectionable because of the obvious conflict of interest that exists when providers profit directly from products they recommend and sell.
6. Require large sums of money at the start or require that clients sign contracts for expensive, long-term programs. Such practices too often have been abused as salespeople focus attention on signing up new people rather than delivering continuing, satisfactory service to consumers. Programs should be on a pay-as-you-go basis.
7. Fail to inform clients about the risks associated with weight loss in general or the specific program being promoted.
8. Promote unproven or spurious weight loss aids such as human chorionic gonadotrophin hormone (HCG), starch blockers, diuretics, sauna belts, body wraps, passive exercise, ear stapling, acupuncture, Electric Muscle Stimulating (EMS) devices, spirulina, amino acid supplements (for example, arginine and ornithine), glucomannan, and so forth.
9. Claim that "cellulite" exists in the body.
10. Claim that use of an appetite suppressant or methylcellulose (a "bulking agent") enables a person to lose body fat without restricting accustomed caloric intake.
11. Claim that a weight control product contains a unique ingredient or component unless it is unavailable in other weight control products.

Courtesy National Center Against Health Frauds, Loma Linda, Calif.

able effects on metabolism. VLCDs can also cause problems with water balance and disturbances in cardiac function (the working of the heart). If VLCDs are to be followed, it is important that they contain about 50% protein of good quality to guard against the loss of muscle tissue. In the mid-1970s deaths were reported as being caused by use of some liquid protein supplements—sold in drug stores or door to door—that contained poor-quality protein and were deficient in vitamins and minerals.

WEIGHT CYCLING (YO-YO DIETING)

One common problem associated with dieting is the so-called yo-yo phenomenon in which a large and rapidly achieved loss of weight is followed by an at least equally large and rapid gain in weight as soon as the dieter relaxes control. Such swings or cycles of weight loss and gain can keep repeating themselves over long periods. As discussed in Chapter 6, many people who achieve considerable weight loss experience a reduction in energy requirements. This allows the lost weight to be regained in a much shorter time than it was lost and means that it takes longer to lose the same amount of weight again on a second attempt. Weight cycling is also associated with an undesirable loss of lean body mass when weight is being lost, which is replaced by fat as the weight is gained. The reason for this effect is unknown. Recent studies have provided evidence that weight cycling may increase the risk of heart disease and premature death in both men and women.[19] Further studies currently underway will hopefully reveal the relative health risks of weight cycling and stable obesity.

BEHAVIOR MODIFICATION

Behavior modification is an approach to dieting that was introduced in the early 1970s. It starts with an analysis of the conditions under which an obese or overweight person eats, including both emotional state and physical location. This requires a careful record to be kept over at least 1 week. On the basis of this record, modification of behavior is suggested to avoid or minimize those combinations of circumstances which lead to inappropriate eating. The dieter is set specific reasonable goals for modifying behavior and food intake, accompanied by a schedule of "reinforcements" designed to aid in the achievement of the goals. These reinforcements can be positive rewards for success, although in some cases it is more appropriate for them to be negative consequences of failure. The success of the method relies on accurately identifying aspects of behavior that contribute to overeating, and then, most important, on *sensitizing* the subjects to these aspects of their behavior, meaning that they become aware of the behavior patterns that cause problems and accept the need to avoid them. Examples of behavioral changes that may be recommended are eating more slowly, putting the fork down between bites, trying to avoid eating alone, eating only at specified times or places, resisting opening the refrigerator between meals, and reducing the amount and frequency of use of foods that are often eaten in excess.

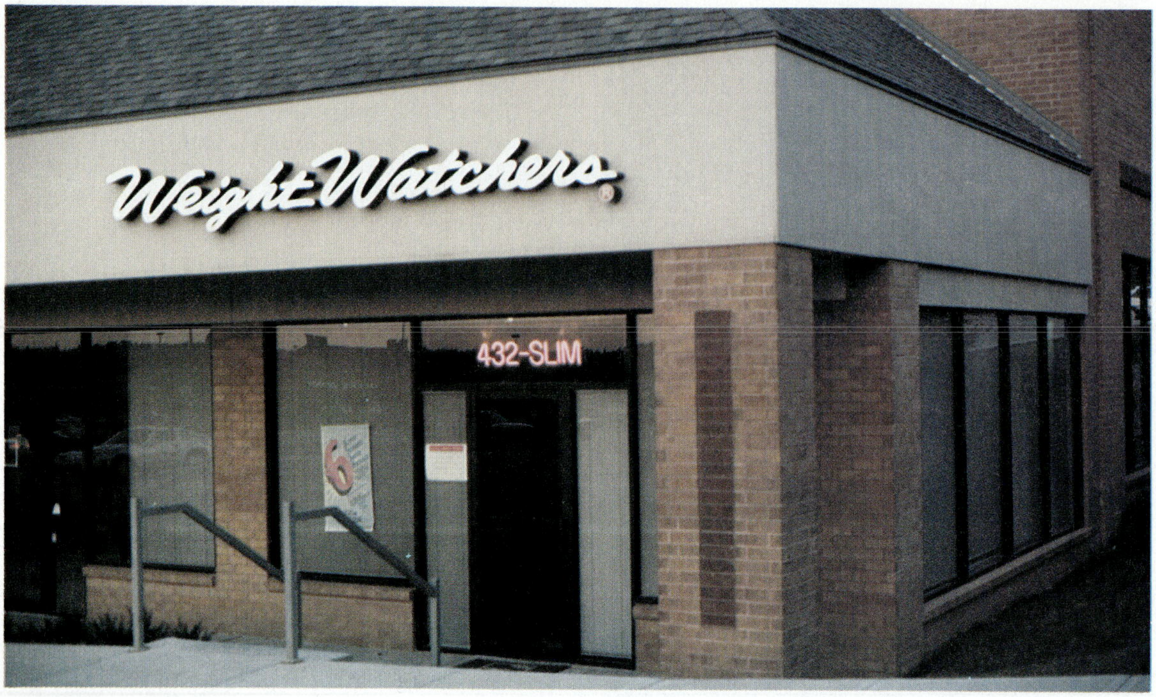

CONSERVATIVE TREATMENTS

As a result of experience with behavior modification, an approach to dieting designated as "conservative" has been developed. This is an individualized dietary approach, incorporating behavior modification where appropriate but recommending for everyone a target weight loss of 1% of total body weight per week using a diet that provides approximately 50% (never less than 40%) of maintenance energy needs. Meeting these targets minimizes the loss of lean body mass. Because this approach results in a slow and steady weight loss, it enhances the possibility of achieving and maintaining significant weight loss over a long period. Conservative treatments involve seven elements overall:

- Self-monitoring or record keeping of behavior
- Control of the stimuli that initiate eating
- Development of techniques to control eating
- Reinforcement of prescribed behaviors
- Alteration of attitude to promote the expectation of success
- Nutrition education
- Increased physical activity

SELF-HELP GROUPS

Such groups as TOPS (Taking Off Pounds Sensibly), Overeaters Anonymous, and Weight Watchers have provided the group support that has helped many people to achieve the weight control that they had been unable to achieve on their own.

TOPS participants are provided with encouragement: those who succeed each week are applauded, whereas those who do not are helped to recognize where they have a problem. TOPS offers little dietary advice or guidance.

Overeaters Anonymous is based on the same principle as Alcoholics Anonymous. Although the support system itself is beneficial, participants are encouraged to seek medical advice on nutrition. The nutritional quality of the program then depends on what advice, if any, is obtained.

In Weight Watchers, group support is reinforced by a prescribed diet that nevertheless permits members to make choices within categories to suit their own preferences. This group also makes available portion-controlled, low-calorie entrees and other menu items that can be used as a basis for a diet and as an aid in learning new eating habits.

For children and some adult groups, summer camps and spas providing a program of activity and a controlled eating environment can help establish a new life-style conducive to weight control.

ACTIVITY

Increasing energy expenditure can achieve the same weight loss as an equivalent decrease in energy intake. As concern has grown that very-low-kilocalorie diets may provide insufficient nutrients for health, increasing emphasis has been placed on recommending increased energy expenditure as a route to weight loss. The required increases in energy expenditure can be produced by formal exercise or by changes in daily routine, such as walking short journeys instead of using transport and climbing stairs instead of using elevators. One well-established benefit of regular exercise is a gradual increase in lean body mass and muscle tone. Recent research has also shown that short bouts of vigorous exercise may result in increased resting metabolic energy expenditure and may stimulate the thermic effect of food eaten around the same time as the exercise. Thus exercise can result in a greater weight loss than is predicted from the amount of energy used during the exercise alone.

The effectiveness and feasibility of achieving weight loss by increasing activity have been alternately underrated and overrated through the years. The 3500 kcal of energy stored within each pound of fat is sufficient to meet the additional energy needs of many hours of vigorous activity. This tends to discourage many people from considering exercise as a means of losing weight. Such people do not fully recognize that weight loss is a long-term process, involving a lifetime commitment, and that seemingly small changes in daily energy expenditure can amount to large total changes over months or years. Most 132-pound women consider walking 90 miles to be an unreasonable way to lose 1 pound in weight. Walking just one fourth of a mile every day for a year, however, would achieve the same effect. The importance of establishing a life-style that involves consistent mild exercise cannot be overemphasized. It is a particularly effective way of avoiding the gradual gain in weight that often accompanies the steady decline in energy needs as we grow older. Increased activity also brings the additional benefit of an enhanced feeling of vitality. Exercise does have an effect on appetite, however, with strenuous exercise usually causing a temporary reduction in appetite, which is then replaced by an enhanced appetite, which if satisfied can lead to increased food intake that counterbalances some of the benefits of the exercise. Care must be taken to moderate the effects of any increased appetite caused by increased activity.

Efforts to cope with impending obesity in schoolchildren have been successful when the approach taken has been to increase activity and reduce intake to allow the children to "grow into" their existing weight, rather than attempting to bring about any reduction in weight.

It is relatively easy to calculate the additional energy cost of any activity from Table 6-14. Such tables as Table 7-7, indicating how many kilocalories are expended by various activities during 10 minutes, and Table 7-8, indicating how long it is necessary to participate in various activities to use up the energy within various foods, are also useful.

The importance of combining dieting with increased activity is now well recognized by most health clubs and spas and is stressed in many worksite health programs. Many worksite programs now also provide nutritional information in cafeterias and offer a host of education opportunities to ensure that employees have a good understanding of the combined effect of diet and exercise on body weight, fitness, productivity, and attendance at work.

SURGICAL APPROACHES

Approximately 30 different surgical methods have been described for the treatment of obesity. They fall into two broad categories:

- Physical or mechanical procedures that remove fat tissue or restrict food intake
- Procedures that reduce the absorption of nutrients into the body

The surgical removal of excess fat is known as **lipectomy** and mainly involves removal of fat from the abdominal area. **Liposuction** is an alternative technique involving the suctioning off of subcutaneous fat, usually during cosmetic surgery. Both of these methods were introduced relatively recently but are considered of questionable value and involve significant risk. The major risks are wound infections and respiratory complications, which in severe cases can cause death.

Jejunoileal bypass is a surgical procedure in which the beginning of the jejunum is connected directly to the terminal portion of the ileum. This reduces the length of the absorptive surface of the intestine by as much as 20 feet. It is intended to reduce the proportion of energy-yielding nutrients in the diet that are actually absorbed into the body. It can lead to substantial weight loss, but serious metabolic, biochemical, and physical side effects mean that it should be used for only the most extreme cases of obesity. **Gastric banding** (in which a plastic collar is placed around the stomach) and **gastroplasty** (the surgical reduction of the stomach size) can be used to close off most of the stomach, leaving a volume large enough to hold only a small amount of food. This can produce considerable weight loss and involves fewer complications than does a jejunoileal bypass. Unfortunately, both gastric banding and jejunoileal bypass can lead to serious vitamin and mineral deficiencies if the patients do not consume appropriate supplements. So people who have undergone these procedures may need to submit to lifelong surveillance and supplementation to ensure that serious deficiencies do not develop.

Many of the beneficial effects of surgical procedures to restrict food intake and absorption can be obtained by inserting a small balloon into the stomach and inflating it. This has the great advantage of being readily reversible, although that advantage also leaves the patient at risk of regaining lost weight once the balloon is removed.

Jaw wiring holds a person's jaws together and so limits him or her to a liquid diet. It is mainly used to bring about some initial weight loss before other surgical procedures. It can also be used over a period of 6 to 10 months as a drastic measure, but it is of questionable value, even in the most extreme cases of obesity.

DIET AIDS

Diet aids fall into two main categories: those that are reported to suppress the appetite and those that stimulate metabolism and so increase energy expenditure. A third category of "useless" diet aids might well be added because many products available are of no help in dieting, despite being part of the multibillion dollar diet aid market.

The most common **appetite suppressants** are the monosaccharide glucose and the disaccharide sucrose. Several diet aids are merely candy to which vitamins and minerals have been added, allowing claims that they are "balanced" products. If taken half an hour before mealtime, these suppressants do introduce a feeling of satiety from the glucose either within them or released from them on digestion. The same effect, however, could be obtained less expensively by eating half a teaspoon of sugar or three jelly beans or by drinking half a cup of fruit juice.

The difficulties of dietary control and its widespread failure have led to the use of a variety of drugs to provide assistance. In general, however, these have had little or no success. The most common drugs used are listed and assessed below:

- **Tranquilizers** are intended to reduce anxiety-caused nibbling.
- **Phenylethylamines** depress the appetite but have serious side effects.
- **Bulking agents,** such as methylcellulose, give a feeling of fullness but cause flatulence.
- **Adrenaline** and **thyroxin** increase metabolic rate but *must* be used only under medical supervision.
- **Growth hormone releasers** are largely proteins containing high levels of the amino acid arginine. They are taken at night to stimulate the secretion of growth hormone, which increases metabolic rate. They are promoted for use by older people, whose natural level of growth hormone secretion is low. The amino acids arginine and ornithine are also promoted for their ability to stimulate the production of growth hormone but are of no proven benefit.
- **Amphetamines** (i.e., Benzedrine and Dexedrine) are available only by prescription. They dull the appetite but are addictive and have adverse effects on the heart and nervous system.
- **Human chorionic gonadotrophin (HCG),** a hormone purified from the urine of pregnant women, is given by injection but is neither safe nor effective for promotion of weight loss. Despite claims to the contrary, it does not reduce hunger or "melt" fat.
- **Phenylpropanolamine (PPA)** is the active ingredient in many cold remedies. It is considered a safe and effective appetite suppressant by the FDA but should not be taken by people with high blood pressure, diabetes, or thyroid or kidney problems. Almost all weight control products based on PPA guarantee results *if* the subjects follow the accompanying instructions, which invariably include restricting energy intake and increasing energy expenditure in ways that lead to weight loss in any case.
- **Phentermine** is an appetite suppressant that has been used successfully in patients with moderate hypertension and diabetes. Side effects include insomnia, nervousness, irritability, and headache.
- **Fenfluramine** is an appetite suppressant that, in contrast to most others, does not stimulate the central nervous system. It does, however, have side effects, including drowsiness, lethargy, and depression. Combinations of fenfluramine and phentermine seem to cancel out each other's side effects and provide enhanced appetite suppression. To maintain weight loss with this combination, however, the drugs must be continued for the rest of the individual's life.
- **Starch blockers,** now deemed to be illegal drugs, were at one time promoted as agents able to block the digestive breakdown of starch and thus reduce the number of kilocalories available for absorption.
- **Dehydroepiandrosterone (DHEA)** is a breakdown product of a sex hormone normally excreted in urine. It reduces fatty acid use but is unproven as a weight reduction aid and is not approved by the FDA.
- **Cholecystokinin (CCK)** is a polypeptide hormone normally secreted in the small intestine in response to the presence of fat. It stimulates the pancreas and gallbladder to increase their secretion of digestive enzymes. As a dietary drug it has not been proven to meet the claim that it can cause sudden and dramatic weight loss. There is some evidence that as it normally functions in the body, CCK may act on the brain to depress the appetite. Because it is a protein, any CCK taken orally is digested to peptides and amino acids and thus never reaches the brain as CCK.

Other products on the market that are designed to promote weight loss are low-calorie foods (with less than 40 kcal per serving); reduced-calorie foods (with less than 75% of the calories of the foods they replace); diuretics, which bring about temporary and sometimes dangerous weight loss by causing the loss of body water; bulk-producing substances, which swell in the stomach to produce a feeling of satiety; and premeasured foods, such as frozen entrees, that help eliminate errors in judgment when estimating serving sizes. Some of these products are useless and harmful, some are useless but harmless, and fortunately some are useful and harmless.

The most widely used of these products are low-calorie and reduced-calorie foods, which include foods sweetened with noncaloric sweeteners such as aspartame and saccharin and foods containing modified fats with reduced calories or fat substitutes and high quantities of fiber or artificial bulking agents. These can all prove useful in the battle to restrict kilocalorie intake. Some other specific products that the student of nutrition should know about are the following:

- **Spirulina,** a protein powder produced from algae, is sold as an appetite suppressant on account of its high content of the amino acid phenylalanine.
- **Glucomannan** comes from a Japanese root called *konjac* and is sold as an "Oriental weight loss secret" but does nothing more than create a sense of fullness.
- **Pectin** is a natural polysaccharide with the ability to attract and hold water. Pectin is widely used as a gelling agent in preserves but has surfaced as a supposed weight control agent because of the belief that it attracts water and forms bulk in the stomach in a way that suppresses appetite.
- **Benzocaine** is a local anesthetic used in many diet gums and candies to numb the surface of the tongue and so destroy or diminish the sense of taste and so reduce food intake.
- **Aerosol sprays** of many popular food flavors sprayed on the tongue are promoted as a way to satisfy the desire for frequent tasty morsels ("the munchies") while avoiding the kilocalories.

In addition to being encouraged to buy many special foods often of questionable benefit, many people have been duped into buying expensive but worthless devices. These include eyeglasses that reflect an image supposed to dampen the desire to eat; electrical muscle stimulators, which pose a risk of electrical shock and burns if misused; wraps and garments that, along with special creams, supposedly "burn" off fat; and belts and sweatsuits that induce sweating and hence temporary weight loss as a result of water loss. No doubt creative entrepreneurs will continue to invent new devices for those with weight problems. The most effective route to weight loss is straightforward and inexpensive: reduce your intake of kilocalories and increase your level of activity as part of a sustainable modified life-style. Sadly, the route is found by many to be easier to describe than to follow.

> Weight loss is best achieved through a reduced intake of kilocalories, combined with an increased level of activity, as part of a sustainable modified life-style. It involves no great secret and no need for additional expense.

PREVENTION OF OVERWEIGHT AND OBESITY

From a public health point of view, the most appropriate solution to the problem of overweight and obesity is to foster its prevention. As our knowledge of the epidemiology of obesity increases, it should be possible to identify the groups to be targeted with preventive education and guidance and the points of access to them. The best preventive approaches combine dietary and exercise components but exploit our knowledge of the responsiveness of various groups to different approaches.

Because there is clearly a strong genetic component to obesity, pediatricians are centrally placed to alert parents to the problem before it actually arises in children. They can encourage the parents to promote eating and activity patterns that combine caloric restriction with raised energy expenditure. School authorities with access to school growth records are also well placed to identify students at risk and guide them into appropriate preventive programs.

Obstetricians and gynecologists have the opportunity to sensitize their patients to the risk of inappropriate weight gain both during pregnancy and at menopause. Physicians dealing with middle-aged men who are working under stress also have an excellent opportunity to provide them with nutritional guidance to help prevent the weight gain that brings increased risk of cardiovascular disease and other degenerative diseases.

Because weight control problems stem as much from low energy expenditure as from high energy intake, nutritionists and exercise physiologists should work together in planning and delivering weight control programs.

UNDERWEIGHT

People who are underweight, generally regarded as being more than 15% below desirable weight for height, are not subjected to the same social pressures as overweight or obese people but nevertheless do have a weight control problem. Being underweight can cause health problems that are just as severe as those associated with overweight and obesity. It is true that underweight persons are at lower risk for hypertension, diabetes, and cardiovascular disease. However, they are much more susceptible to respiratory problems, ranging from the common cold to tuberculosis; they may have difficulty maintaining a comfortable body temperature; and they may suffer from reduced fertility, immune suppression, and a variety of problems associated with insufficient intake of essential nutrients. People who suffer from undernutrition tend to have their problem ignored by most of the population, perhaps partly because there is less of a market for weight gain aids and gimmicks than for those designed to bring about weight loss.

> **Underweight** is defined as less than 85% of desirable weight for height.

Two eating disorders associated with weight loss that have received a lot of attention and publicity are anorexia nervosa (AN) and bulimia nervosa (BN). Because these are most commonly (although not exclusively) found in adolescents, they are discussed in Chapter 15.

TREATMENT

The treatment of underweight people involves creating a positive energy balance by increasing kilocalorie intake. The use of smaller but more frequent meals can in some cases help to increase total kilocalorie intake. Meals can also be enriched with calorie-dense foods such as butter, cheese, nuts, dried fruits, sugar, and cream, although these are best used at the end of the meal because they cause a feeling of satiety that is undesirable early in the meal. Many commercial food products designed for use by postoperative patients can also be used to help underweight people gain weight. Because many foods with a high-kilocalorie content are also the ones associated with increased risk of cardiovascular disease, underweight people should be cautioned about the danger of consuming excessive quantities of saturated fats and should be encouraged to have their cholesterol level checked periodically. When weight is being gained, it is important that it is gained gradually and that the diet producing the weight gain is nutritionally balanced and high in kilocalories.

Because exercise increases kilocalorie expenditure and is advised as an aid to losing weight, some people might assume that exercise should be discouraged in those trying to gain weight. This is completely wrong. It is as important for those trying to gain weight to take regular exercise as it is for those trying to lose weight. Exercise in underweight people with a high kilocalorie intake ensures that lean body mass is built up and not just fat. So the general message about exercise is that regular moderate exercise should be encouraged in people of all weights, accompanied by increased kilocalorie intake for underweight persons but decreased kilocalorie intake for overweight or obese persons.

ISSUES AND OPINIONS

Anorexia Nervosa and Bulimia—The Price of Our Desire to be Thin

The eating disorders anorexia nervosa (AN) and bulimia nervosa (BN) are serious conditions with complex causes.

Anorexia nervosa is characterized by the relentless pursuit of a thinner body. This is achieved by dieting, often combined with induced vomiting, laxative abuse, and obsessive exercising. The resulting weight loss often leads to extreme emaciation and sometimes causes death. The drive for thinness is accompanied by a general dissatisfaction with the body and a distortion in the perception of body shape. People with AN generally perceive their bodies or parts of their bodies to be much larger than they actually are. The clinical criteria used to diagnose AN include an obsessive drive for thinness, distorted perception of body shape, weight loss to 85% of expected weight, failure to attain expected weight, and (in females) a period of amenorrhea during the time of weight loss.

Bulimia nervosa is characterized by less complex concerns about body weight and shape, resulting in a drive for thinness or a phobic fear of fatness. The most obvious symptom of BN is "binging": the consumption of large amounts of food in short periods, accompanied by a sense of "losing control" over what is eaten. The foods consumed during binges are usually those forbidden to individuals by their diet. The binging episodes are usually followed by purging via vomiting, the use of laxatives or diuretics, and a period of strict dieting or vigorous exercise. People with BN may be of normal weight, overweight, obese, or underweight. They may also suffer from AN.

AN occurs in approximately 1% of women aged 15 to 40, whereas BN occurs in about 2% to 3% of those in the same age group. Both disorders also occur in men but less often than in women. There is perhaps 1 male with AN for every 20 females and 1 male with BN for every 10 females. Why women should be so much more prone to AN and BN is unknown, but it is widely acknowledged that males tend to be less concerned about their weight and less likely to diet than females. Nearly half the women with BN have a history of AN, whereas about half of female AN patients also suffer from BN.

The clinically obvious cases of AN and BN are only part of the story of these conditions. About 5% of women are estimated to suffer from a subclinical case of either condition. These people exhibit the behaviors and psychological disturbances of the illnesses but at levels slightly below those required for a formal diagnosis.

AN and BN are typically thought to occur in the 18- to 25-year-old age group, but they often first arise during the earlier teenage years. A significant proportion of patients, however, have their first episode of AN or BN well into adulthood. Both AN and BN have traditionally been regarded as disorders of the upper and middle social classes, but in the past 15 years, cases have been widely distributed among all social classes.

Many people with AN or BN do not seek medical help until years after the illnesses first begin. Both illnesses tend to follow a chronic course, gradually worsening until they cause serious health problems or even death. Studies following the long-term fates of people with AN and BN suggest that 15% die for reasons related to AN or BN over a period of 30 years. The deaths associated with AN are often linked to the long-term damage done to the body by years of near starvation. Most of the deaths in BN patients are related to metabolic disturbances linked to their purging episodes. People with either condition often tend to withdraw from social life and experience difficulties in coping at work. They are all at increased risk for depression and suicide.

Research performed over the past 15 years has considerably improved our knowledge about AN and BN. It suggests that both disorders are becoming more common and represent a significant health risk among specific subgroups of the population. Those at greatest risk include athletes, dancers, models, and all other people who are unusually concerned about their weight and shape. Fortunately, increasingly effective strategies for treating AN and BN are also being developed. However, both conditions are likely to remain serious medical problems associated with the widespread desire to be thin.

BY NOW YOU SHOULD KNOW

- Approximately one fourth of the North American population is either overweight or obese.
- The incidence of overweight and obesity peaks for men at age 45 but continues to increase until age 74 for women.
- The most commonly used methods for assessing the amount of body fat are indirect measures based on height, weight, circumference of parts of the body, and skinfold thickness.
- Because overweight leads to obesity, it increases the risk of degenerative diseases, such as coronary heart disease, hypertension, adult-onset diabetes, cancer, and gallbladder disease.
- The development of obesity involves a complex interaction of genetic factors within a susceptible individual and an environment that fosters obesity.
- The regulation of food intake and weight control is not clearly understood, but many theories are now being studied.
- A gain of 1 lb in body fat results from an excess of 3500 dietary kcal, and a loss of 1 lb of body fat requires a deficit of 3500 dietary kcal.
- The ultimate goal in weight loss is to adjust energy expenditure or energy intake so that intake is less than expenditure until desired body weight is reached.
- There are specific criteria for assessing weight-reducing diets.
- People who are considered underweight are less than 85% of their desirable weight for their height.

STUDY QUESTIONS

1. Differentiate between overweight and obesity.
2. Compare direct and indirect methods of diagnosing obesity.
3. List the disadvantages of being obese.
4. List the health hazards of obesity.
5. Differentiate between endomorphic and ectomorphic body types.
6. Differentiate between hyperplastic and hypertrophic obesity.
7. Your friend tells you he has gained 3 pounds in the past 2 weeks. How many extra kilocalories must he have eaten to gain this much weight?
8. If an individual drank 2 beers (240 kcal) every day in addition to the kilocalories necessary to maintain body weight, how much weight would he or she gain in 1 year?

~ CRITICAL ANALYSIS ~

1. How much do you need to eat less, exercise more, or both, to lose a specific amount of weight? The answer to this question seems to be worth a great deal, but as you understand by now, losing weight is not simply a matter of calculating amount of food and exercise. It is however, necessary to start there. Below is how you would begin the process, with attention to an issue that is rarely raised.

   One pound of body fat is considered to contain approximately 3500 kcal of stored fat (1 lb of adipose tissue weighs 454 g. Of adipose tissue, 90% is normally stored fat; so 0.9 × 454 g = 409 g. Because fat contains 9 kcal/g, 9 kcal/g × 409 g = 3681 kcal. (This is rounded down to 3500 kcal for ease in calculations.)

   To lose 1 lb/week, it is necessary to expend 3500 kcal more than you take in; thus you must expend 3500 kcal/7 days, which equals 500 kcal/day more than you take in. To lose 2 lb/week, you must double the daily caloric deficit; so you must expend 1000 kcal/day more.

   How much of this daily caloric deficit should be from exercise (or an increase in exercise) and how much from a decrease in food intake? Although calculations cannot necessarily tell you precisely how to go about this, they can help you decide. How long must you engage in the following activities to expend 500 calories?

ACTIVITY	APPROXIMATE kcal/MIN	MINUTES REQUIRED TO EXPEND 500 kcal
Walking 3 mph	4.2	$\frac{500\text{ kcal}}{4.2\text{ kcal/min}}$ = ________ min
Running 7.5 mph	14.1	$\frac{500\text{ kcal}}{14.1\text{ kcal/min}}$ = ________ min
Bicycling 15 mph	16.5	$\frac{500\text{ kcal}}{16.5\text{ kcal/min}}$ = ________ min
Swimming 50 yd/min	5.4	$\frac{500\text{ kcal}}{5.4\text{ kcal/min}}$ = ________ min
Aerobics	9.4	$\frac{500\text{ kcal}}{9.5\text{ kcal/min}}$ = ________ min

   If someone is relatively sedentary to begin with, how likely is he or she to increase their activity by this amount daily and carry through with this activity every day of the week for the next 3 months, 6 months, 9 months, or more?

   Aerobic exercise derives between 50% and 70% of energy from fat (less in the untrained individual and more in the trained athlete). Therefore it is possible that the expenditure of 500 kcal used only 250 to 300 kcal from fat, for a loss of about 30 (1 oz) of fat. This brings out the importance of program of activity and diet that can be sustained over a long period, hopefully, a lifetime.

2. Can you safely cut 500 to 1000 kcal from your diet daily? This depends. With an initial daily intake of 3000 to 4000 kcal, perhaps your diet can be reduced by that much. However, if you fill out a 3-day food record that indicates a daily intake of 1500 to 2000 kcal/day, a reduction of 500 to 1000 kcal/day becomes harder to accomplish and could result in a diet that is very low in energy and nutrients. Diets in the range of 500 to 1000 kcal/day are at best rarely followed, and at worst, dangerous.

REFERENCES

1. National Institutes of Health: *Methods for voluntary weight loss and control,* Technology Assessment Conference Statement, Bethesda, Md, March 30-April 1, 1992 National Institute of Health.

2. Bray GA: Pathophysiology of obesity, *Am J Clin Nutr* 55(Suppl):488S, 1992.

3. Sjöström L: Impact of body weight, body composition, and adipose tissue distribution on morbidity and mortality. In Stunkard AJ, Wadden T, editors: *Obesity: theory and therapy,* New York, 1993, Raven Press.

4. Behavioral Risk Factor Surveillance System (BRFSS): Prevalence of overweight, *JAMA* 262:471, 1987.

5. Garn SM, Lavelle M: Two-decade follow-up of fatness in early childhood, *Am J Dis Child* 139:181, 1985.

6. Gibson RS: *Principles of nutritional assessment,* New York, 1990, Oxford University Press.

7. Garrow JS: Indices of adiposity, *Nutr Abstr Rev* 53:697, 1983.

8. Siri WE: Body composition from fluid spaces and density: analysis of methods. In National Academy of Sciences, National Research Council: *Techniques for measuring body composition,* Washington, DC, 1961, National Academy of Sciences Press.

9. Forbes GB, Gallup J, Hursh JB: Estimation of total body fat from potassium-40 content, *Science* 133:101, 1961.

10. Sjöström L: Methods for measurement of the visceral adipose tissue volume and relationship between visceral fat and disease in 1000 severely obese subjects. In Oomura Y and others, editors: *Progress in obesity research,* London, 1990, John Libbey.

11. Simopoulos A, Van Hallie T: Body weight, health and longevity, *Ann Intern Med* 100:285, 1984.

12. Fomon SJ: *Infant nutrition,* St Louis, 1993, Mosby.

13. Sjöström L: Mortality of severely obese subjects, *Am J Clin Nutr* 55(suppl):611S, 1992.

14. Wadden TA, Stunkard AJ: Psychosocial consequences of obesity and dieting. In Stunkard AS, Wadden TA, editors: *Obesity: theory and therapy,* New York, 1993, Raven Press.

15. National Institutes of Health Consensus Development Panel on the Health Implications of Obesity: Health complications of obesity, *Ann Intern Med* 103:1073, 1985.

16. Colditz GA: Economic costs of obesity, *Am J Clin Nutr* 55(suppl):503S, 1992.

17. Stunkard AJ and others: The body mass index of twins who have been reared apart, *N Engl J Med* 322:1483, 1990.

18. Bray GA: The nutrient balance approach to obesity, *Nutr Today* 28:13, 1993.

19. Lissner L, Brownell KD: Weight cycling, mortality, and cardiovascular disease: a review of epidemiologic findings. In Bjorntorp P, Brodoff BN, editors: *Obesity,* Philadelphia, 1992, JB Lippincott.

ADDITIONAL READINGS

Abrams M: The eating disorder inventory as a predictor of compliance in a behavioral weight-loss program, *Int J Eat Disord* 10(3):355, 1991.

American Dietetic Association Position Statement: Nutrition in the treatment of anorexia nervosa, bulimia nervosa, and binge eating, *J Am Diet Assoc* 94:902, 1994.

Andersson B and others: The effects of exercise, training on body composition, and metabolism in men and women, *Int J Obes* 15(1):75, 1991.

Astrup A, Vrist E, Quaade F: Dietary fibre added to very low calorie diet reduces hunger and alleviates constipation, *Int J Obes* 14(2):105, 1990.

Atkinson RL: Low and very low calorie diets, *Med Clin North Am* 73(1):203, 1989.

Bennett GA: Cognitive-behavioral treatments for obesity, *J Psychosom Res* 32(6):661, 1988.

Boyd MA: Living with overweight, *Perspect Psychiatr Care* 25(3-4): 48, 1990.

Bray GA: Obesity: a disorder of nutrient partitioning: the Mona Lisa hypothesis, *J Nutr* 121(8):1146, 1987.

Drewnowski A, Yee DK: Men and body image: are males satisfied with their body weight? *Psychosom Med* 49(6):626, 1987.

Durnin JVGA and others: How much food does man require? *Nature* 242:418, 1973.

Garrison RJ, Castelli WP: Weight and thirty-year mortality of men in the Framingham Study, *Ann Intern Med* 103:1006, 1985.

Garrow J: Importance of obesity, *Br Med J* 303(6804):704, 1991.

Keys A, Brozek J, Henschel A: *The biology of human starvation,* Minneapolis, Minn, 1950, University of Minnesota Press.

Landsberg L, Kruger D: Obesity, metabolism, and the sympathetic nervous system, *Am J Hypertens* 2:123S, 1989.

Lieber CS: Perspectives: do alcohol calories count? *Am J Clin Nutr* 54:976, 1991.

Kuczmarski RJ and others: Increasing prevalence of overweight among U.S. adults: The National Health and Nutrition Examination Surveys, 1960-1991, *JAMA* 272:207, 1994.

National Institutes of Health: Technology assessment conference statement: methods of voluntary weight loss and control, *Nutr Today* 27:27, 1992.

Pavlou KN, Krey S, Steffee WP: Exercise as an adjunct to weight loss and maintenance in moderately obese subjects, *Am J Clin Nutr* 49(suppl 5):1115, 1989.

Rosenbaum M, Leibel RL: Obesity in childhood, *Pediatr Rev* 11(2):43, 1989.

Simopoulos AP: The health implications of overweight and obesity, *Nutr Rev* 43(2):33, 1985.

Sjöström L: Mortality of severely obese subjects, *Am J Clin Nutr* 55:611S, 1992.

Willett WC and others: New weight guidelines for Americans: justified or injudicious? *Am J Clin Nutr* 53:1102, 1991.

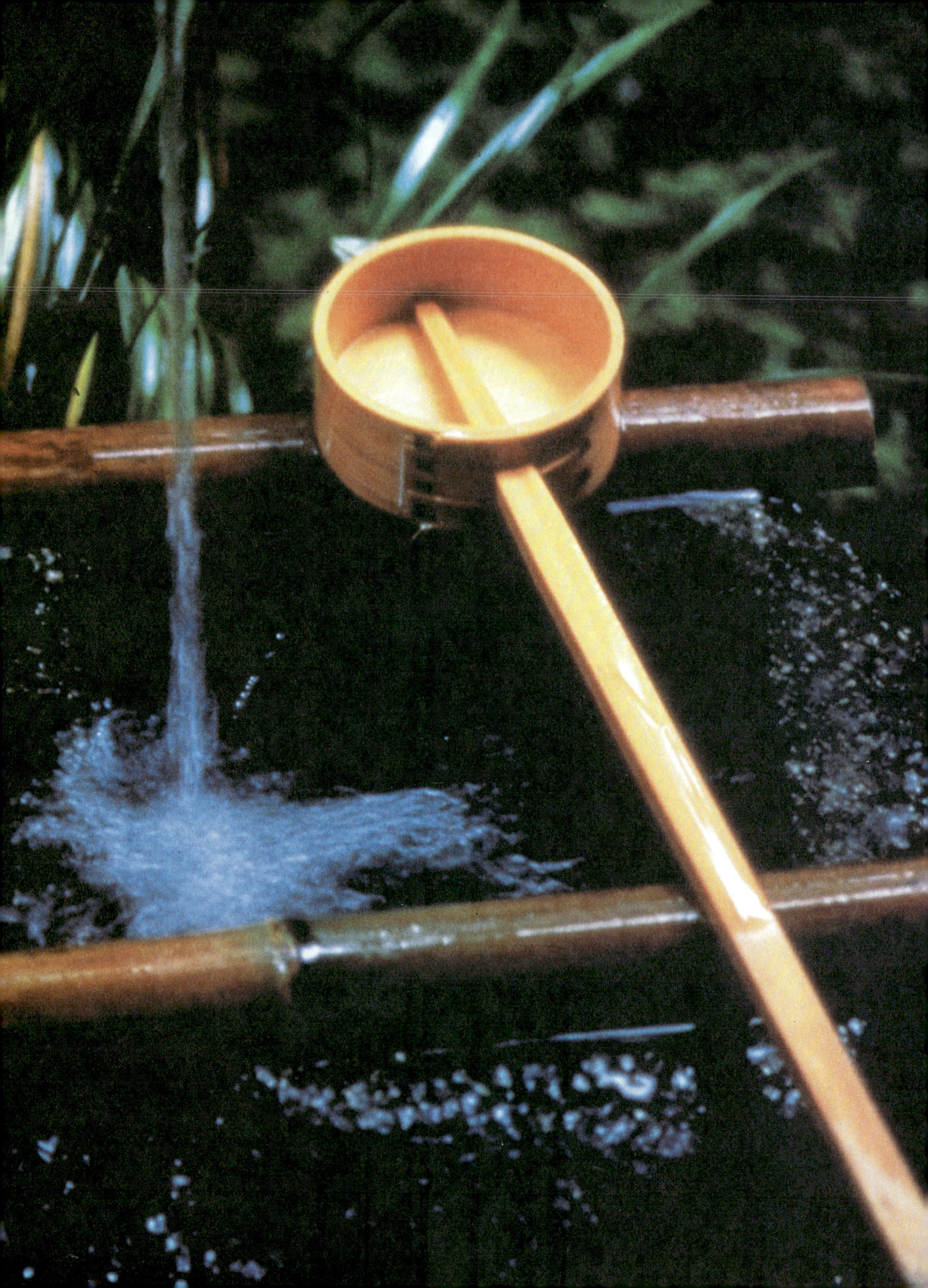

CHAPTER 8

WATER AND ELECTROLYTES

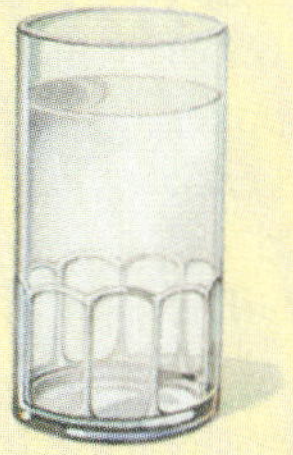

Water is the solvent in which most of the chemical reactions of life occur. It is the most essential of all the essential nutrients in the sense that the absence of water kills us more quickly than the absence of any other nutrient. In addition to the water consumed in the form of beverages, considerable supplies of water are received from our food. Some water is actually produced during the metabolism of the energy-yielding nutrients within food.

The distribution of water among the various intracellular and extracellular regions of the body depends to a large extent on the distribution of various mineral ions. Positively charged sodium and potassium ions and negatively charged chloride ions are the most significant of the many mineral ions in the body, commonly known as electrolytes. The physiological mechanisms that generate the sensation of thirst and eliminate excess water from the body usually ensure that the water content of the body is automatically maintained at the optimal level. In contrast, the level of one or more electrolytes in the body can stray far from the optimum before we become sufficiently aware of the problem to remedy it.

WATER

Water is the major essential chemical component of life, accounting for approximately half of the total weight of the adult body. Humans can survive only a few days without supplies of water. The longest known survival time without water is 17 days, but 2 or 3 days is a more common limit. In contrast, humans can survive for many weeks or even years without supplies of some other essential nutrients, with the actual time depending on which nutrient or combination of nutrients is absent.

For good health, water must be consumed every day to replace the continuous losses of water in urine, perspiration, exhaled air, and feces. In adults 4% to 6% of body water is excreted and replaced by fresh supplies each day, whereas in infants 15% of water is replaced each day. The quantities of water being consumed and excreted are subject to constant variation and control. The control mechanisms involve alterations in the functions of the kidneys, lungs, and skin and are integrated by the action of several hormones. Mechanisms in the body that act to prevent or at least minimize changes in the body's internal environment are called **homeostatic mechanisms.** The homeostatic mechanisms involved in regulating water intake and excretion normally maintain the water composition of tissues at a consistent optimal level. Although up to 4 qt (3.8 L) of water may be taken into the body each day and up to 4 qt lost each day, the homeostatic mechanisms are sufficiently sensitive to ensure that the variation in body weight resulting from changes in water content seldom exceeds ⅓ lb (150 g)/day, corresponding to a total gain or loss of just 0.16 qt (0.15 L) of water per day.

Water is an important constituent of every cell of the body, acting as the chemical medium or "solvent" in which most of the chemistry of life takes place. Considerable amounts of water are also found outside of the body's cells, and the amount of water in various tissues overall varies (Figure 8-1). The total amount of water in the body obviously depends on a person's total weight, but the *proportion* of water in the body varies in a regular way among individuals, depending mainly on age, gender, and body composition. Water accounts for about 74% of body weight at birth, 55% to 60% in adult males, and about 45% to 50% in adult females (Table 8-1). The steady fall in the proportion of body weight from water as we age is largely caused by a reduction in the amount of **extracellular water,** which is found outside of and therefore in-between the body's cells. In old age the body water of both males and females accounts for only 45% to 50% of total body weight. More muscular people contain a higher proportion of water than do less muscular people because muscle contains almost three times as much water as does adipose (fat) tissue. Males have a higher proportion of water in their bodies than do females because they have a higher proportion of lean tissue and a lower proportion of fat.

TABLE 8-1

Percentage total body water in infants, children, and adult males and females

SUBJECTS (YEARS OF AGE)	TOTAL BODY WATER (%)
Infants and children	
Birth	75
1	58
6-7	62
Adult males	
16-30	58.9
31-60	54.7
61-90	51.6
Adult females	
16-30	50.9
31-91	45.2

From Randall HT: Water, electrolytes and acid-base balance. In Shils ME, Young VR, editors: *Modern nutrition in health and disease,* Philadelphia, 1988, Lea & Febiger.

> Water accounts for about 55% to 60% of total body weight in adult males and about 45% to 50% in adult females.

DISTRIBUTION OF BODY WATER

Within the body, water is found in two major compartments: the **intracellular** compartment (*inside* cells) and the **extracellular** compartment (*outside* cells). The water in these compartments is part of complex and varied solutions of biochemicals known as the **intracellular fluid** and the **extracellular fluid.** The precise chemical composition of these fluid compartments varies from place to place in the body, depending on the types of cells the fluid is within or around. As indicated in Figure 8-2, the intracellular and extracellular fluid compartments are separated by the semipermeable membranes of the body's cells (represented schematically as one membrane but in reality, many trillions of membranes). These membranes allow water to pass through them but form a selective barrier to other chemicals, allowing some to diffuse or be carried through readily and restricting the passage of many others (Appendix A).

The extracellular fluid compartment is further subdivided into the **intravascular** fluid compartment and the **intercellular** (or **interstitial** or **extravascular**) fluid compartment. The intravascular compartment comprises all the fluid within the blood vessels of the "vascular"

FIGURE 8-1

Water content of various body tissues. The water content of adipose tissue varies between 20% and 35%.

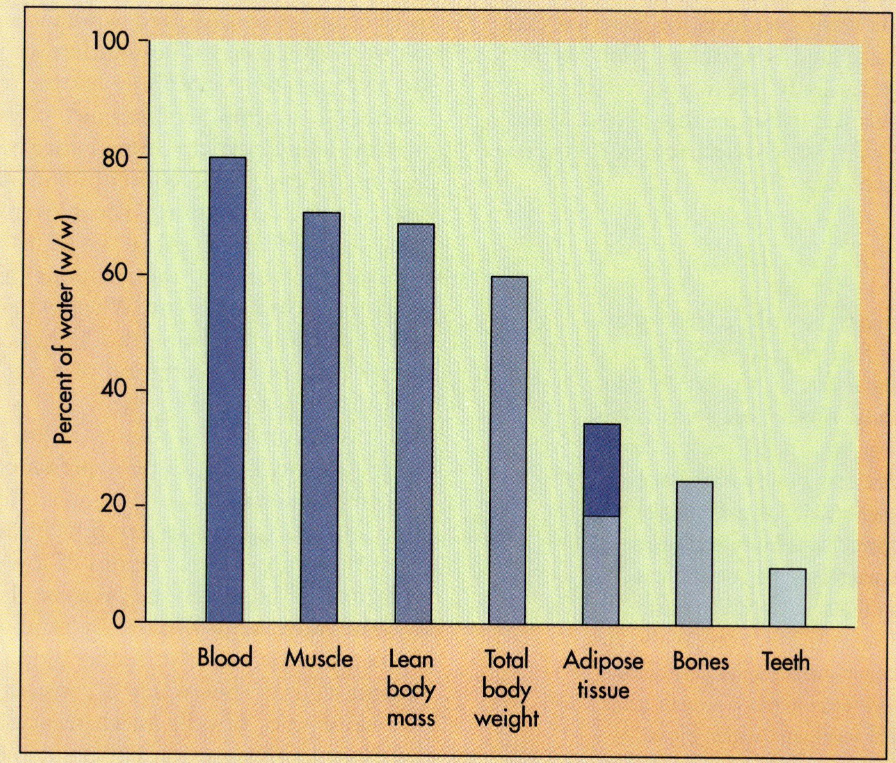

FIGURE 8-2

Diagrammatic representation of the two major fluid compartments of the body. The extracellular fluid compartment is subdivided into the intravascular fluid compartment (fluid within the blood vessels) and the intercellular, interstitial, or extravascular fluid compartment (fluid between the body cells but outside of the blood vessels).

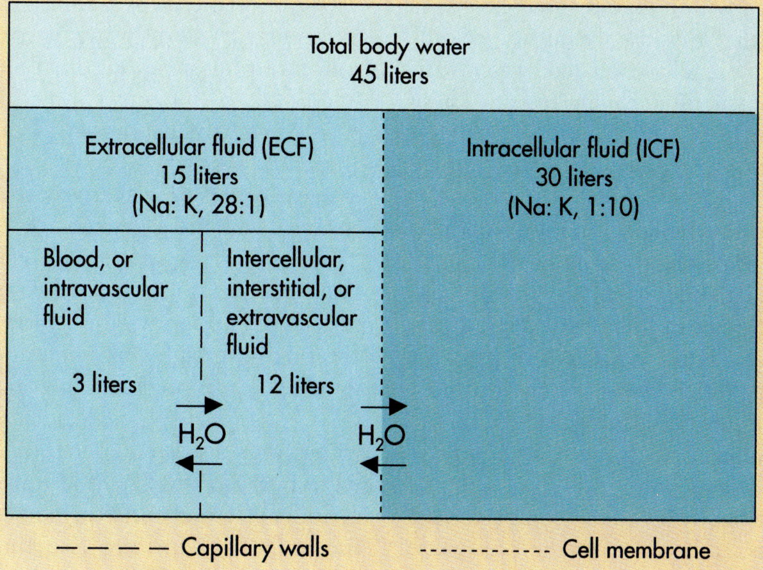

system—namely, the arteries, veins, and capillaries. The intercellular compartment contains the fluid around and between the cells of the body, which carries nutrients to the cells and collects waste products for eventual excretion. The intravascular fluid is separated from the intercellular fluid by the walls of the blood vessels, which again form a semipermeable barrier that allows water to pass through it but exerts strict selective control over the passage of other chemicals.

The water in the body is found in two main fluid compartments: the **intracellular fluid** within cells and the **extracellular fluid** outside of cells. The extracellular fluid compartment is further subdivided into the **intravascular** fluid compartment (within blood vessels) and the **intercellular** (or **interstitial** or **extravascular**) fluid compartment (between the body cells but outside of the blood vessels). The **transcellular** fluid compartment includes the fluids in the eyeball (vitreous humor), around joints (synovial fluid), and within digestive secretions, as well as a few other specialized fluids that do not readily exchange water with the bulk of the extracellular fluid compartment.

The fluids in the eyeball (vitreous humor), around joints (synovial fluid), and within digestive secretions, as well as a few other specialized fluids, are outside of cells (extracellular) but do not readily exchange water with the bulk of the extracellular fluid compartment. These fluids are labeled separately as a small, specialized, and relatively isolated compartment called the **transcellular fluid** compartment.

The volume of the intracellular and intravascular compartments remains relatively constant, whereas the volume of the intercellular fluid compartment can rise and fall in response to changes in the total water content of the body. In this way the intercellular compartment acts as a "buffer" region, which water can enter into or exit from in a way that prevents large changes in the volumes of the intracellular or intravascular compartments.

Water moves between the fluid compartments largely by passive diffusion because of the automatic movement of water molecules from regions of high water molecule concentration to regions of lower water molecule concentration. In other words, the water moves by the process known as *osmosis.* The direction in which water moves by osmosis depends on the total concentration of dissolved substances (solutes) in the solutions concerned. The solution with the highest solute concentration necessarily has the lowest water molecule concentration because much of its volume is occupied by solute particles, rather than water. Conversely, regions of low solute concentration have higher water molecule concentrations. The movement of water by osmosis is often described in terms of the differing **osmotic pressures** of the solutions on either side of a semipermeable membrane. When two solutions are compared, the solution with the highest concentration of solutes (lowest concentration of water) has the highest osmotic pressure. Conversely, the solution with the lowest concentration of solutes (highest concentration of water) has the lowest osmotic pressure. This means that the osmotic pressure of a solution is effectively a measure of its ability to *draw water into it.* So water tends to move by osmosis from regions of low osmotic pressure to regions of high osmotic pressure (Figure 8-3).

The movement of water by osmosis continues until the osmotic pressures on either side of the membrane become equal. Thus water is constantly moving across the membranes of cells in whatever direction equalizes the osmotic pressures on either side. This is one of the major automatic homeostatic processes of the body, constantly adjusting the distribution of water among the different cells and compartments of the body in a way that prevents any region of the body from becoming either too rich in solutes (or even dried out) or too dilute in solutes and waterlogged. The physiology of the body does exert some control over osmosis, however, by the selective movement of various solutes among cells and regions within the body.

One of the most significant factors controlling the movement of body water by osmosis is the combined concentration of various dissolved mineral ions on either side of cell membranes. Some of these mineral ions are positively charged (known as **cations** because they are attracted toward a negatively charged "cathode"), whereas others are negatively charged (known as **anions** because they are attracted toward a positively charged "anode"). These ions largely exist free within the solutions of the body, but when united into electrically neutral compounds, they form such salts as sodium chloride (composed of sodium ions [Na^+] and chloride ions [Cl^-] and potassium chloride (composed of potassium ions [K^+] and chloride ions). The mineral salts whose ions dissolve in water are also known as **electrolytes** because their mobile ions allow the solutions to conduct electricity. In nutrition and other health sciences the individual ions are also themselves commonly referred to as electrolytes, and the most important of these are discussed in a later section of this chapter.

FIGURE 8-3

A summary of the movement of water by osmosis.

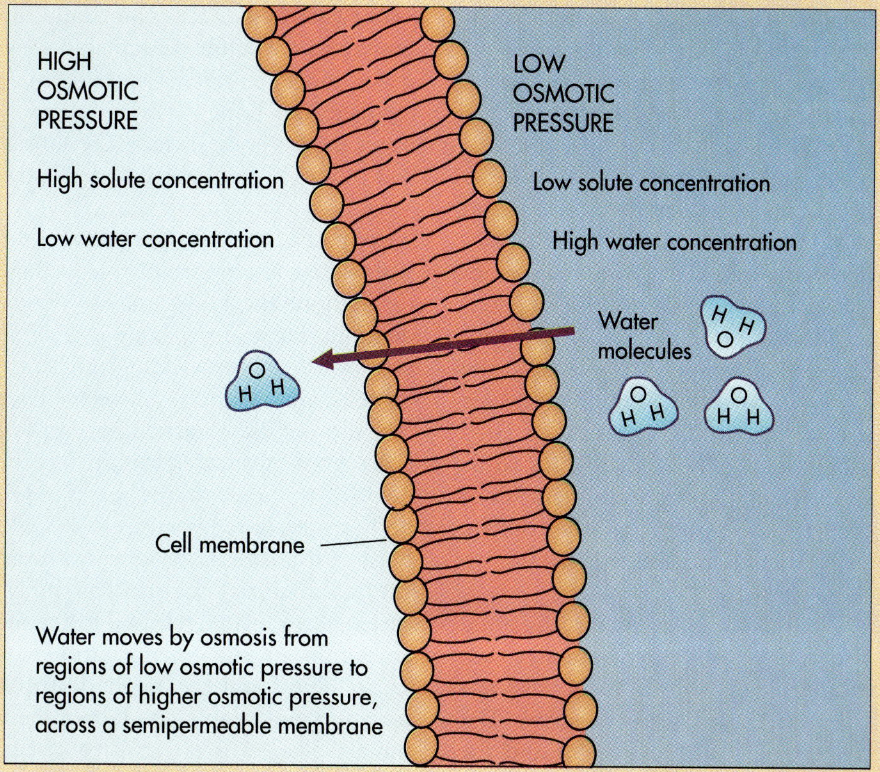

*E*lectrolytes are ionic compounds that dissolve in water and so release positive and negative ions that allow the solution to conduct electricity. The individual ions of electrolytes are also commonly referred to as electrolytes. Positively charged electrolyte ions are known as **cations** because they move to a negatively charged "cathode." Negatively charged electrolyte ions are known as **anions** because they move to a positively charged "anode."

FUNCTIONS IN THE BODY

Water performs five main functions within the body by acting as the following:

- The **solvent** in which most of the chemistry of life proceeds
- A chemical **reactant** participating in many biochemical reactions
- A **lubricant**
- A **temperature regulator**

Each of these functions is briefly examined.

Solvent

A solvent is a liquid in which other chemicals become dissolved, and water is the solvent of life. Without the presence of water as a solvent, few of the chemical reactions of life are able to proceed at any significant rate and the remaining chemicals certainly cannot react together to generate the integrated chemical complexity of a living body. By being dissolved in or otherwise exposed to intracellular and extracellular water, the chemistry of life gains the fluidity and flexibility that makes life possible.

When food enters the body, it is soon exposed to the watery secretions of saliva and the watery solutions in the stomach and intestine that allow the food to mix with and react with the chemicals responsible for digestion. The digested nutrients are then absorbed into the blood, which contains an average of about 3 L of water. It is this intravascular water that actually makes blood a fluid and allows absorbed nutrients to dissolve in blood and so be transported to every tissue of the body. The water of blood also acts as a solvent transporting many internally generated substances such as hormones and antibodies from their sites of manufacture in the body to the sites where they perform their function. Waste products of metabolism, such as carbon dioxide and urea, also dissolve in the intravascular water to be transported to the lungs or kidneys for excretion.

The 12 L or so of intercellular fluid, found in the spaces between cells, carry nutrients from the blood capillaries to the outer membranes of the body's cells, allowing them to be transported across the membranes and into the watery intracellular fluid within the cells. Waste products of cell metabolism, on the other hand, journey in the opposite direction. Within cells the intracellular water serves as a suitable medium for nutrients to be transformed into the chemicals needed to build and maintain cells. It allows metabolites to be transported between different regions and organelles of a cell, and in general it provides an appropriate chemical environment for the chemistry of life to proceed.

Some of the chemicals of the body are not dissolved in water, such as the lipid-based cell membranes, but water plays an important role in allowing such structures to form and maintain their structural integrity. The selective interactions between water molecules and the hydrophilic (water-loving) portions of membrane lipids, in concert with the forces that push the hydrophobic (water-hating) hydrocarbon chains of membrane lipids away from water, are directly responsible for the formation and maintenance of the structure of the membranes.

Reactant

Any chemical that participates in a chemical reaction is called a "reactant" of the reaction, and during the reaction the reactants are converted into products. Water is a reactant that participates directly in a variety of different reactions within the body. During these reactions the water molecules often split up, to donate hydrogen atoms (H), hydrogen ions (H^+), oxygen atoms (O), oxide ions (O^{2-}), hydroxyl groups (OH), or hydroxide ions (OH^-) to other reactants of the reactions concerned. Common examples of such reactions are the hydrolysis reactions in which large molecules such as polysaccharides, fats, and proteins are split into smaller molecules by reaction with water. During hydrolysis reactions a hydrogen atom derived from a water molecule ends up attached to one of the smaller products of the reaction, while a hydroxyl group containing the remaining atoms of the original water molecule becomes attached to the other product of the reaction (see Appendix A). Water is also *formed* as a product of many chemical reactions within the cell, such as the reversal of hydrolysis, known as *condensation*.

Lubricant

All fluids have lubricating properties because they make it easier for solid materials to slip over one another. Water-based fluids act as lubricants in various parts of the body, most notably within joints, where synovial fluid makes movement easier and minimizes wear and tear on cartilage and bone. The less obvious lubricant roles for water in the body include the lubricant action of saliva and mucus in the mouth and esophagus.

Temperature Regulator

Water plays an important role in the distribution of heat throughout the body and the regulation of body temperature. Heat in the body is generated by the metabolism of the energy-yielding nutrients (fat, carbohydrate, protein, and alcohol). All of the energy released by the oxidation of these nutrients is eventually released as heat, apart from any stored within the chemicals involved in net growth. Some of this heat is required to maintain the body's normal temperature of 98.6° F (37° C), but the body's total heat production normally exceeds the amount required to maintain body temperature. The excess heat must be released to the surroundings because any significant rise in temperature to above-normal levels causes illness and eventually death. Some heat is lost by radiation and simple conduction between the body and the air. The most effective route of heat loss from the body, however, is via the evaporation of the water as perspiration from the surface of the skin. As water evaporates from the liquid to the gas phase, it absorbs and carries away the heat energy needed to bring about the transition from liquid to gas. When perspiration evaporates, this heat energy is largely drawn from the body. The evaporation of 1 L (slightly more than 1 qt) of perspiration from the skin is accompanied by the loss of 600 kcal of heat energy from the body. Under normal circumstances the body is continuously cooled by the evaporation of perspiration from the surface of the skin, a process that accounts for about 25% of the body's basal energy expenditure. The accompanying water loss amounts to between 350 and 700 ml/day at normal environmental temperature and humidity and is known as **insensible perspiration.**

Subcutaneous fat, just beneath the skin, acts as an insulating material that reduces the speed at which heat can be lost from the body. This is advantageous in cold conditions but can be disadvantageous in hot conditions. The rate of heat loss can also be affected by how close the warm blood is to the surface of the skin and how great a volume of blood is circulating in the region just beneath the skin. When the body is too hot, the blood vessels just beneath the skin grow wider (dilate), increasing blood flow and accelerating heat loss. When the body is too cold, these blood vessels become thinner (constrict), reducing heat loss. In hot conditions obese people feel more discomfort than do nonobese people because of their thicker insulating layer of subcutaneous fat and also the associated tendency for most of their blood vessels to be farther from the surface of the skin.

WATER PROVIDES DIETARY MINERALS

Although water is composed of only the elements hydrogen and oxygen, the water we drink or use in food preparation can contain significant amounts of minerals, such as calcium, magnesium, sodium, zinc, copper, and fluoride. The actual amounts depend on the source of the water and any fluoridation of the water to prevent tooth decay. So-called hard water can contain up to 50 mg of calcium and 120 mg of magnesium per liter, whereas "soft" water contains much lower amounts of these minerals but up to 250 mg of sodium per liter. The minerals in water can be both advantageous and disadvantageous to health. Two liters of hard water can provide as much as 240 mg of magnesium, which is two thirds of the recommended daily intake of this essential mineral. The consumption of hard water has also been associated with a decreased risk of cardiovascular disease. Soft water, on the other hand, may contain up to 250 mg of sodium per liter, high intakes of which are associated with an increased risk of hypertension and cardiovascular disease. Because water is an effective solvent for many minerals and other chemicals, it may also carry significant quantities of toxic elements such as lead or cadmium, pesticides, herbicides, and industrial waste products. Constant monitoring of the water supply to check for such contamination is essential to safeguard public health.

SOURCES OF BODY WATER

Water can be ingested on its own, within beverages, or within foods, but unlike other nutrients it is also made available to the body as an end product of metabolism. The major sources of water are the fluids that are consumed as beverages, including tap water, which accounts for half of all beverages consumed. Infants generally consume more fluid per unit of body weight than do adults. People living in the tropics—where there are greater losses of water because of evaporation from the skin—consume more fluid than do those in temperate climates, and people who engage in strenuous physical activity drink more than do people who live sedentary life-styles. The amount of fluid consumed by adults each day varies from 3¾ cups to 6½ cups (900 ml to 1500 ml), with the average intake being 38 oz (approximately 4¾ cups, or 1100 ml) under normal circumstances. Intakes in excess of 3⅓ cups (800 ml)/hour exceed the rate at which water can be absorbed from the stomach. Alcoholic beverages, tea, and coffee are sources of water but also act as **diuretics,** meaning that they cause an increase in the rate of water loss via the kidneys as urine.

So-called solid foods, meaning all foods except beverages, are the second most important source of water for the body. They can contain any amount from no water to 96% water, although the majority contain more than 50% water. The water contents of various common solid foods and milk are shown in Figure 8-4. The solid food in a typical 2000-kcal diet containing food from all food groups provides around 500 to 800 ml of water.

Water of metabolism is the water that is released in the body as an end product of metabolism.[1] As discussed in earlier chapters the oxidation of carbohydrate, protein, fat, and alcohol generates carbon dioxide and water as end products. The carbon dioxide must be excreted as waste, but the water can either be used by the body or be released as waste, depending on prevailing needs. Table 8-2 indicates the constant amounts of water of metabolism released from each of the three main energy-yielding nutrients. Table 8-2 also shows the total amounts of water released from each nutrient and the dietary grand total provided by a 2000-kcal diet that reflects current dietary guidelines. The diet provides 55% of the 2000 kcal as carbohydrate, 30% as fat, and 15% as protein and generates 269 ml of water of metabolism per day (13.5 ml/100 kcal).

Two thirds of the weight of the glycogen stores in muscle and the liver is in fact a result of water embedded within the network of glycogen molecules. This water is made available to the body when the glycogen is used as a source of energy. In athletes using glycogen reserves during intense physical activity, this additional source of water may amount to as much as 3 cups (approximately ⅔ L) of water per 500 g of glycogen metabolized.

LOSS OF BODY WATER

Water is lost from the body in urine, through the skin in perspiration (sweat), through the lungs within exhaled air, and within the feces (Figure 8-5).

Urine

In the kidneys, water, specific waste products, and certain excess metabolites are filtered from the blood to produce urine, which is 97% water. Blood is continuously filtering through the kidneys at a rate of about 125 ml (½ cup)/min, amounting to up to 180 qt/day. Before urine leaves the kidneys, however, the kidneys can *reabsorb* a variable amount of water and various solutes, an ability that plays a major role in maintaining blood volume at normal levels. The eventual urine, produced after the reabsorption has occurred, is collected in the bladder and excreted periodically. A normal level of urine volume is between 1 and 2 L (approximately 1 to 2 qt)/day, but this rises if fluid intake is high and falls if fluid intake is low. When urine volume rises because of increased water intake, the concentration of wastes within the urine naturally falls. When increased reabsorp-

FIGURE 8-4

Water content of various solid foods and milk (percent of total weight).

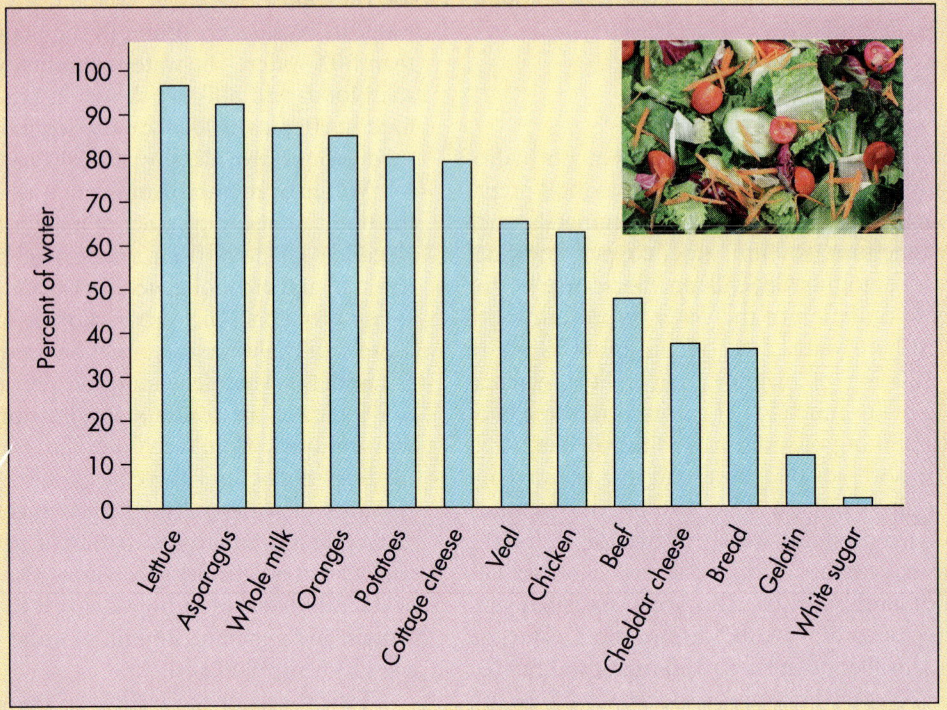

TABLE 8-2

Calculation of water of metabolism produced from a 2000-kcal diet

SOURCE OF kcal	kcal PROVIDED (%)	DISTRIBUTION IN 2000-kcal DIET (kcal)	WEIGHT OF NUTRIENT (g)*	WATER OF METABOLISM (ml/g)	TOTAL WATER OF METABOLISM (ml/2000 kcal)
Carbohydrate	55	1100	275	0.6	165
Fat	30	600	67	1.07	72
Protein	15	300	75	0.42	32
TOTAL					269

269 ml/2000 kcal = 13.5 ml/1000 kcal

* One gram of carbohydrate provides 4 kcal, 1 g of fat provides 9 kcal, and 1 g of protein provides 4 kcal.

tion of water by the kidneys causes a reduction in urine volume, the concentration of wastes within the urine rises. The specific gravity (density of any liquid divided by density of water) of urine rises as the concentration of wastes within it rises.

A certain minimal volume of urine is required to rid the body of its wastes because the ability of the kidneys to reabsorb water during the production of urine is limited. This minimal volume is between 300 and 500 ml/day, the exact figure depending on a factor known as the **solute load** of the body. The solute load is a measure of the total amount of dissolved substances (solutes) being produced by metabolism that must be excreted by the kidneys. The major contributors to the solute load are electrolyte ions and the nitrogen-containing waste material urea. If less than the minimal amount of water is available for urine production, some of the waste products of metabolism are retained within the blood and tissues where they may accumulate to harmful levels that interfere with the normal functioning of cells.

Under some circumstances, such as the aftermath of natural disasters or during spaceflight, available fluid may be limited and may need to be conserved. In such situations it is wise to limit the intake of certain foods

FIGURE 8-5

A summary of the flow of water through the body.

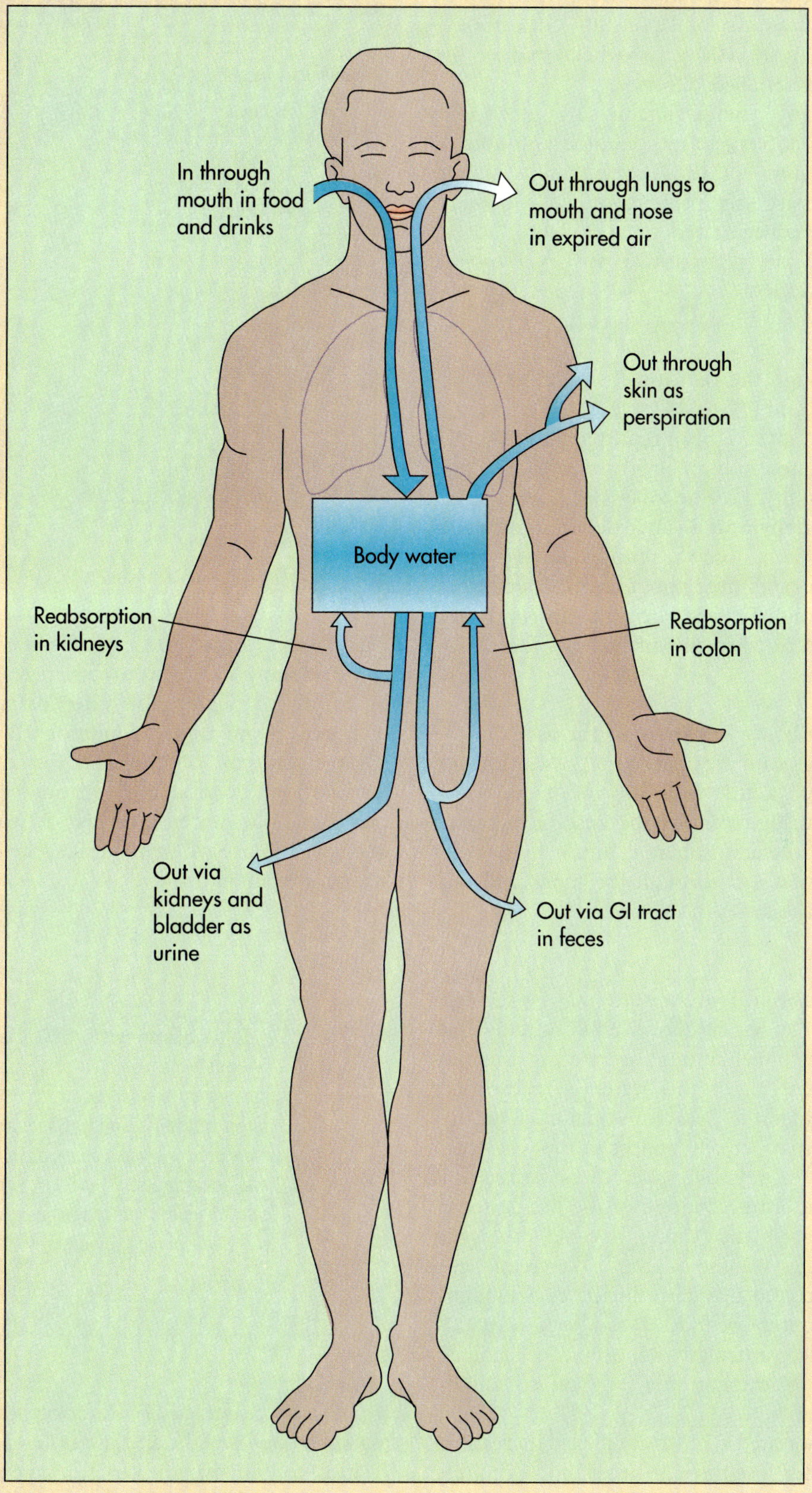

that normally produce large quantities of the waste products that must be excreted in urine. The easiest of such steps is to reduce the intake of protein (which generates urea) and salt. An intake of sufficient carbohydrate to prevent ketosis (100 g) also helps reduce the solute load from excretion of ketones.

The kidneys of young infants are not fully functional and so can excrete only limited amounts of electrolytes and water. For this reason infants should not be given excessive salt, protein, or fed a formula that is either too concentrated or too dilute. All of these things could put an excessive workload on the young, immature kidneys.[2]

Skin

Loss of water through the skin usually amounts to between 350 and 700 ml (12 to 14 oz)/day, but losses as high as 2500 ml/hour have been reported and 500 ml/hour is not uncommon in high environmental temperatures and low humidity. If these losses are not replaced, the body becomes **dehydrated** (discussed in more detail later). Because infants lose a proportionately large amount of water through their skin, they may need to be provided with additional fluids when the environmental temperature is high or when the infant has a fever.[2]

Lungs

Water is constantly being lost through the lungs in the form of water vapor within exhaled air. Losses through the lungs amount to a little over 300 ml (1 cup)/day, but they increase at high altitudes because of increased respiration rates. If the atmosphere is unusually dry, the total amount of water lost through the lungs and skin may be as high as the losses in urine.

Feces

Each day as much as 8 to 10 L of water may be secreted into the digestive tract within digestive juices, and 3.7 L is considered the minimal amount secreted in this way (Table 8-3). Almost all of this water is reabsorbed, however, further down the gastrointestinal tract, so that as little as 200 ml may actually be lost in the feces each day. The volume of the digestive juices secreted is influenced by the moisture content of food. The secretion of saliva is greatest when food is dry and least when the food is moist. The volume of gastric, pancreatic, and intestinal juices secreted may also fluctuate, depending on the moisture content of food. It is also known that the secretion of bile, particularly important in fat digestion, is stimulated by the ingestion of food containing large amounts of fat.

Diarrhea is associated with a significant increase in the amount of water lost through feces, and vomiting causes a large additional loss of water. Either condition results in dehydration, which can become a severe problem if lost water and sodium are not replaced quickly.

TABLE 8-3

Water balance in the gastrointestinal tract

	AMOUNT (ml)	
SOURCES		
Gastric secretions		8200
Saliva	1500	
Gastric juice	2500	
Bile	500	
Pancreatic juices	700	
Intestinal juices	3000	
Water intake		2000
TOTAL AVAILABLE		10,200
USES		
Reabsorbed	10,000	
Fecal loss	200	
TOTAL USED		10,200
Balance		0

REQUIREMENTS

Daily water intake must usually be at least 2 L, or approximately 2 qt, from beverages and foods combined, to compensate for water losses via all the routes discussed. Even under conditions of low solute load, minimal physical activity, and the absence of obvious perspiration, the total water provided by beverages, food, and metabolic water must be at least 1.5 L, or 1.5 qt/day. Table 8-4 summarizes typical water balance statistics in an adult.

> *O*ne **quart** equals 1.137 **liters (L)**. Because the volumes of a quart and a liter are so similar, quarts and liters are often treated as interchangeable units when approximate values of fluid volume are acceptable. So it is an acceptable "rule of thumb" to remember that 1 qt is *approximately* equal to 1 L.

The precise need for water obviously depends on a person's body weight and life-style. The requirement in relation to body weight varies in a general way with age: the younger the individual, the greater his or her requirement for water per unit of body weight. Specific water requirements (sometimes loosely called "fluid re-

TABLE 8-4

Typical water balance in adults

	AMOUNT (ml)
SOURCES OF WATER	
Beverages	1100
Solid food	500-1100
Water of oxidation	300-400
TOTAL	1900-2500
LOSS OF WATER	
Urine	900-1300
Insensible perspiration	500
Perspiration and evaporation from lungs	300-500
Feces	200
TOTAL	1900-2500

quirements") under various conditions of age and average environmental temperature are shown in Table 8-5.

As a general guide it is suggested that adults consume 1 L (approximately 1 qt) of water for every 1000 kcal in their diet. For infants, 1.5 L, or approximately 1.5 qt/1000 kcal is suggested. About two thirds of this amount usually comes from beverages, with the remainder being contained within solid foods.

> Adults should consume 1 L of water for every 1000 kcal in their diet; infants should consume 1.5 L/1000 kcal. About two thirds of the water consumed is usually supplied by beverages, with the remainder being contained within solid foods. Hence, adults should drink two thirds of a liter of fluids per 1000 kcal in their diet, whereas infants should consume 1 L of fluids per 1000 kcal in their diet.

REGULATION OF WATER BALANCE

The recommended minimal level of water intake is considerably less than the 4.7 to 17 L of water that can be cycled through the body each day. This makes it obvious that the body must have considerable capacity to control the amount of water—or more generally, fluid—it contains. **Water balance** (often called **fluid balance**) is achieved in two main ways: by the control of fluid intake through changes in thirst sensations and by the control of the rate of fluid loss through the kidneys.

TABLE 8-5

Water (fluid) requirement per kilogram of body weight

	REQUIREMENT (ml/kg)
Infants	110
10-year-old children	40
Young adults	40
Older adults	30
Elderly adults (>65 years of age)	25
Adults (by environmental temperature)	
22.2° C (75° F)	22
37.8° C (100° F)	38

When too much fluid is lost from the body, the concentration of electrolytes—particularly sodium—in the extracellular fluid increases. This causes water to be absorbed from saliva, creating a dry sensation in the mouth, which stimulates thirst and the intake of additional fluid. Also, the hypothalamus in the brain responds to the higher sodium content of blood in two ways: it generates an additional stimulus to the thirst sensation, and it stimulates the pituitary gland to release **antidiuretic hormone (ADH).** This hormone travels to the kidneys where it increases the reabsorption of water. Increases in blood sodium concentration of as little as 1% can stimulate thirst and the secretion of ADH, allowing the resulting combination of increased fluid intake and increased water reabsorption in the kidneys to quickly restore normal fluid balance (Figure 8-6).

When water intake is in excess of requirements, the concentration of electrolytes in extracellular fluid falls to below-normal values. In these circumstances there is no sensation of thirst and no stimulation of the release of ADH from the pituitary. The rate of water reabsorption by the kidneys falls, causing more water to be lost within urine. Thus by a combination of reduced water intake and increased water loss, fluid balance is soon restored to normal levels.

DISTURBANCES IN WATER BALANCE

The correct functioning of cells and tissues depends on appropriate concentrations of nutrients and metabolites; so any abnormal loss or accumulation of fluid can cause a variety of problems. These problems may be caused by water loss from diarrhea, nausea, excessive perspiration, or fever; by abnormal retention of fluid; by defects in intestinal absorption; or by undesirable changes in the distribution of fluid within the body.

Dehydration

Dehydration is defined simply as the excessive loss of body water. The fall in the level of total body water associated with dehydration is accompanied by a fall in

FIGURE 8-6

Rising electrolyte concentration in extracellular fluid stimulates increased water intake and increased water reabsorption by the kidneys.

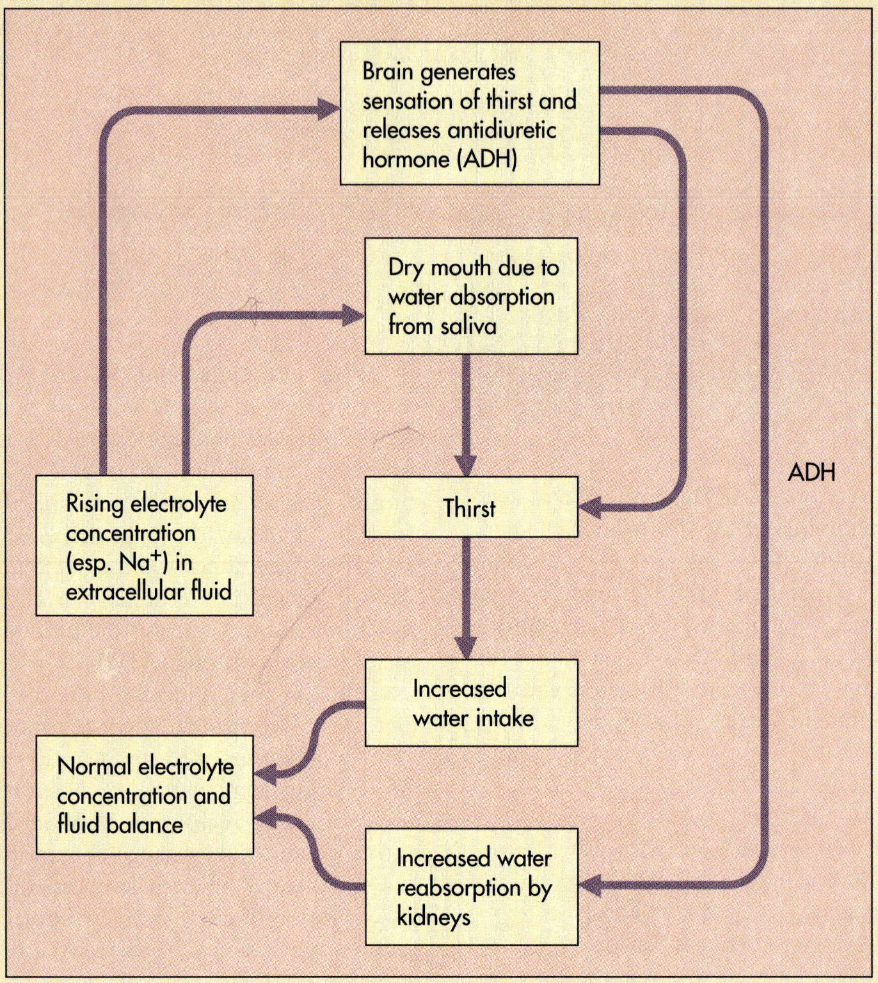

The main symptoms of dehydration are the following:

- Thirst
- Loss of appetite
- Decreased urination
- Impaired physical performance
- Nausea
- Impaired temperature regulation
- Muscle spasms
- Increased pulse rate
- Increased respiration rate
- General debilitation

both blood volume and blood pressure. Symptoms of severe dehydration appear when body fluid levels fall by more than 10%, whereas a 20% reduction is fatal. With water loss in excess of 10% of body weight there is a possibility of cardiovascular failure caused by a reduction in blood pressure and a compensating increase in heart rate.[3]

Athletes lose considerable amounts of water through the skin as a result of their strenuous physical activity. Losses of up to approximately 7 L of water in one afternoon have been recorded for football players. People who are in good condition tend to lose water but relatively little sodium during physical activity, whereas those in poor condition lose both water and sodium and so must replace both. People for whom water losses may be accompanied by significant sodium losses include those who engage in strenuous physical activity of any sort, those exposed to high environmental temperatures at work, and visitors to tropical regions who are unaccustomed to heat. Such people, and in general anyone losing in excess of 3 L of water per day, may need *small* amounts of table salt (sodium chloride) along with the fluid they drink to make up for their sodium losses. Too much salt, however, can be harmful. Salt tablets are rarely, if ever, required. If salt tablets are used, water is drawn into the gastrointestinal tract, which can cause bloating and cramping (see Chapter 18).

Athletes in good physical condition experience a reduction in athletic performance if they lose 3% of body water, although those in prime condition may be able to tolerate up to 5% water loss. These findings are especially significant for wrestlers, who sometimes purposely dehydrate themselves to lose the necessary weight to ensure that they are within the limits for their chosen weight class. It takes well over 5 hours to restore significant water losses, and so athletes who have purposely dehydrated themselves to meet a weight limit may enter a match at a competitive disadvantage.

Studies investigating the factors limiting our efficiency at work suggest that a lack of adequate water intake has a much more significant effect than does a lack of food. A reduction in body water amounting to approximately 2% of total body weight (about 5% of body water) causes a decline of 20% to 30% in efficiency at work.[4]

During starvation or a high-protein and low-carbohydrate diet, excessive amounts of body water, potassium, and sodium are lost in the urine. This accounts for the rapid initial weight loss and weakness often reported by people on starvation-like diets. The loss of water and weight peak after about 4 days, and by the ninth day a new level of water balance is usually established. As little as 60 g of carbohydrate per day can prevent the undesirable changes in body water balance and electrolyte levels by preventing the accumulation of ketones.

Overhydration

When a large amount of water is consumed quickly without sufficient intake of electrolytes, a condition known as **water intoxication** can result. In this condition the electrolyte concentration in extracellular fluids becomes dangerously low, causing water to enter cells from the watery extracellular fluid or causing potassium to leave cells. The resulting overhydration of cells can cause muscle cramps, and the decrease in the extracellular fluid volume can cause lowered blood pressure and a feeling of weakness. Water intoxication in brain cells can cause convulsions, leading eventually to coma and sometimes death from respiratory failure. Water intoxication can occur in infants fed large quantities of fluids low in electrolytes, as can happen when they are being treated for diarrhea or simply fed formula that is too dilute.[5]

An increase in body water for whatever reason to levels of 10% or more above normal results in edema, the abnormal infiltration of tissue by fluid. Localized edema of specific tissues accompanies a variety of injuries and diseases, particularly those affecting the circulation of blood and drainage of lymph.

FLUORIDE IN WATER

The element fluorine in the form of ionic compounds containing the fluoride ion (F^-) is commonly added to the public water supply as a means of preventing tooth decay. The ability of fluoride to give some protection against tooth decay is now well recognized, and there is some evidence that it might be required for proper growth and reproduction. There is still no general agreement, however, that fluoride is an essential mineral nutrient.

HISTORICAL BACKGROUND

Interest in the possible nutritional role of fluoride dates back to 1931, when it was shown that people living in some communities with a high level of fluoride in the water supply were also remarkably free of tooth decay. Unfortunately, these people also suffered from an undesirable brownish stain on the tooth surface caused by excessive fluoride deposition in their teeth now known as **dental fluorosis.** However, people in other communities with slightly less fluoride in the water supplies had a significantly reduced incidence of tooth decay while not suffering from fluorosis. By 1942 it had been well established that water supplies containing 1 part per million (ppm) of fluoride were associated with a 50% to 60% reduction in tooth decay among people habitually consuming the water. The problem of dental fluorosis occurred only when the fluoride content of the water was above 1.5 to 2 ppm.

In 1945 the U.S. Public Health Service recognized the possibility of reducing the prevalence of tooth decay by adding fluoride to the water supply. In a now classic study they added fluoride at a concentration of 1 ppm to the water supply in Newburgh, a city on the Hudson River in New York. The city of Kingston, across the river from Newburgh, was used as a control city that received no added fluoride. Tooth decay in the children of both cities was monitored using the **DMF index,** which is based on the number of decayed, missing, and filled teeth (without evaluating the *extent* of any decay). After 10 years of study it was found that children under age 10 in Newburgh had a DMF index that was 60% to 65%

lower than that of children of the same age in Kingston. Children in Newburgh aged 12 to 14 years who had drunk the fluoridated water since early childhood—but not since birth—had a 48% reduction in DMF index when compared with similar children in Kingston. Newburgh's 16-year-old residents showed only a 40% reduction. These results clearly indicated a protective effect of fluoride that was most effective if the fluoride had been administered since birth. Continued study of the two communities indicated that the protective effect of fluoride persisted and was not associated with any detectable adverse effects. Further confirmation of fluoride's protective abilities came from some communities that added fluoride to the water supply for a few years but then stopped the practice. In such communities tooth decay increased in the years after the addition of fluoride to the water was stopped.[6]

By 1974 over 80 million people in over 4000 communities throughout America, including Chicago and New York City, were consuming water containing added fluoride. Another 10 million people were drinking water in which the natural fluoride content was at the protective level. In 1985 over 50% of the population in 32 of the 50 states (mostly in the central and eastern United States) was served by public water supplies with added or natural fluoridation. The recent growth in community water fluoridation has slowed, however, to 1% to 2% of communities per year.

A little over a decade ago the National Institutes of Health described tooth decay as the leading chronic disease of childhood. Today, there is evidence that this once chronic disease is being successfully overcome by community water fluoridation programs, in combination with appropriate preventive dental health practice and services. In 1988, for example, the U.S. Public Health Service announced that preliminary results from a survey performed from 1986 to 1987 indicated that over 65% of American 9-year-old children had never had decay in their permanent teeth. A similar survey performed between 1979 and 1980 had found that only 51% of 9-year-old children were free from such decay.[7]

There are no adverse affects associated with the addition of fluoride to the water supply to provide the optimal fluoride content of 0.7 to 1.2 ppm. The optimal level is defined as the level that delivers to the population sufficient fluoride to protect against decay while causing no or negligible fluorosis. The precise value depends on location because of variations in the natural fluoride content of the water and also because a lower concentration is required in areas where water consumption is highest and vice versa.

In spite of the endorsement of fluoridation by every medical and dental group in the United States, the U.S. Public Health Service, and many European and Asian health authorities, the fluoridation of public water supplies remains a controversial issue because of concerns about its possible toxicity, which is discussed later.

DISTRIBUTION AND MODE OF ACTION OF FLUORIDE

Unlike most substances, fluoride is readily absorbed from the stomach, and most of the fluoride that escapes absorption in the stomach is absorbed from the intestine. Overall, about 80% to 90% of ingested fluoride is absorbed by the body. Approximately half of this absorbed fluoride, however, is then excreted, with the remaining half becoming incorporated into the structure of bones and teeth. Of the total fluoride present in the body at any time, 99% is associated with calcified tissue (tissue hardened by the deposition of calcium-containing salts), predominantly bones and teeth.[8] The level of fluoride in the blood remains fairly constant, even when the level ingested fluctuates. This reflects the ability of the rates of fluoride deposition into calcified tissue and of fluoride excretion through the kidneys to adjust according to the availability of fluoride in the blood. Small amounts of fluoride do appear in other tissues of the body, including most soft tissues, saliva, milk, and fetal blood. The amount in these noncalcified tissues is normally slightly lower than the level found in the blood, with the exception that the amount in saliva is greater than that found in blood.[9]

Fluoride becomes incorporated into the structure of developing teeth in the form of a chemical known as **fluorapatite,** which partially replaces the nonfluoridated chemical **hydroxyapatite** that is normally found in teeth. This process was once considered to be the main reason for the protective effect of fluoride against tooth decay because fluorapatite in tooth enamel is less soluble in acid than is hydroxyapatite and therefore less vulnerable to the cavity-producing action of acids in the mouth. As discussed in Chapter 3, tooth decay (dental caries) is produced by the action of acids formed in the mouth by cariogenic bacteria. Although the deposition of fluorapatite apparently offers some protection against decay,[10] it is no longer believed to be the main antidecay mechanism. It now appears that the dominant protective mechanism is a local effect of fluoride in saliva on the surface of teeth. The salivary fluoride decreases the rate at which teeth become demineralized, and therefore decay, in acidic (low pH) conditions and accelerates the rate of remineralization when the pH value rises.[11] Thus fluoride in saliva both reduces the rate of acid-induced tooth decay and increases the rate at which any damage can be repaired. Another protective mechanism of fluoride is its ability to inhibit the metabolism of polysaccharides by microorganisms normally present in the mouth, and thus inhibit the very processes that led to the formation of damaging acids in the first place.[12]

TABLE 8-6

Fluoride content of some representative foods

FOOD	CONTENT (mg/100 g)
Mackerel	2.70
Tea	0.47
Coffee	0.25
Rice	0.07
Buckwheat	0.17
Soybeans	0.40-0.67
Spinach	0.02
Onions	0.05
Lettuce	0.01
Wine	6.3 mg/L

From Gordenoff T, Member W: *World Rev Nutr Diet* 2:213, 1962.

VARIED SOURCES OF FLUORIDE

It has already been mentioned that fluoride is naturally present in the water supply in some areas, at concentrations that can be equal to or in excess of the optimal amount for dental health. With an optimal fluoride level of around 1 ppm in the water supply, adults usually ingest up to 1.5 mg of fluoride from that water each day. Fluoride in the water supply, however, whether natural or added, is not the only source of fluoride available to the body. The consumption of tea and solid foods usually provides a further 0.25 mg/day, and fish products—especially mackerel—is considered to be a particularly rich source (Table 8-6). Processed foods may contain two to three times more fluoride than the natural food has before processing, if fluoridated water is used in the manufacturing procedure. The fluoride content in vegetables reflects the level of fluoride naturally present in the area in which they are grown but may also be affected by fluoridation of the water supply if irrigation using water drawn from the public supply is widely used.

In areas where water naturally contains less than the optimal level of fluoride, the long-term intake of purposely fluoridated water has proved to be the most feasible way of protecting people against tooth decay. Some people, however, do not have access to the fluoridated public water supply, or they may live in areas that have not introduced the fluoridation of water. These people must rely on other methods of obtaining the optimal amount of fluoride. These methods include the use of sodium fluoride supplements, which are effective if taken consistently throughout an individual's growth period, and the use of fluoridated toothpastes, mouth rinses, and so on.

Before 1979 the recommended dosage of sodium fluoride supplements was 0.5 mg of fluoride ion per day from birth to 3 years of age and 1 mg/day thereafter. Of children exposed to this level of dosage, however, 33% have suffered from some fluorosis.[13] This has led the American Academy of Pediatrics to decrease the recommended dosage to 0.25 mg/day from 2 weeks to 2 years of age, 0.5 mg/day from 2 to 3 years, and 1 mg/day from 3 to 16 years.[14,15]

The recent dramatic reduction in tooth decay among people of all ages has been attributed to the extensive use of fluoridated toothpaste, mouth rinses, gels, and flosses. All such products contain high concentrations of fluoride. The average quantity of fluoride per single use of toothpaste or mouth rinse has been estimated at 1 mg. About 25% to 30% of that amount may be ingested,[9] although young children routinely ingest a larger proportion. It is estimated that the amount of fluoride ingested from such products each day can often equal or exceed the recommended daily dosage. Dentists are currently advising parents to instruct their children never to swallow toothpaste and to use only a pea-sized amount on the brush. The use of fluoride-containing mouth rinses is not recommended for children under 6 years of age or for anyone who may be liable to swallow some of the product. For people who regularly use fluoridated dental health products, the addition of fluoride to the water supply probably plays only a minor role in protection against tooth decay. For all others, fluoride in the public water supply remains by far their most significant source, and this is probably particularly applicable to low-income families less inclined to purchase the specifically fluoridated products.

TOXICITY OF FLUORIDE

There is some well-publicized concern about the possibility of harmful effects from the consumption of fluoride in the water supply or from other sources. The kidneys appear to excrete any excess fluoride, however, and there is no evidence that the levels of fluoride normally consumed present any threat to health. On examining the health records of 2 million people living in areas with artificial fluoridation of the water supply, the U.S. Public Health Service found no evidence of increased deposition of fluoride in soft tissues such as the kidneys and heart, no increase in morbidity or mortality rates, no abnormalities of or depression of growth; no increase in cancer or nephritis; and no increase in the births of mentally retarded children, all of which have been claimed by antifluoridation activists to be problems associated with fluoridation. However, there is a growing concern that the prevalence and (in some cases) severity of dental fluorosis are increasing. Such increases have recently been documented in both fluoridated and nonfluoridated regions of America and also in naturally low-fluoride areas of Denmark, where fluoride has not been added to the public water supply.[9] These data suggest, and it is now widely believed, that the increase in fluorosis is a result of the use of fluoridated toothpastes, mouth rinses, and other dental hygiene products, regardless of the level of fluoride in the water supply. It is significant that the difference between the daily level of fluoride intake recommended for dental health and the level known to cause fluorosis is small. The difference amounts to only about 0.25 mg/day, and we have seen that each application of toothpaste, mouth rinse, and so on contains about 1 mg of fluoride (although only a portion of that is likely to be ingested).

The U.S. Department of Health and Human Services recently assembled a panel of experts to review all current and past research relating to fluoride toxicity. The panel concluded that the levels of fluoride added to water supplies pose no risk to health. They did find, however, that there is a real risk of adverse effects, especially of fluorosis, in infants and young children who ingest more fluoride than is required for the prevention of tooth decay. If large quantities of fluoride are consumed, such as by a small infant eating a whole tube of toothpaste, acute toxicity becomes a problem.

A potentially toxic dose of fluoride is approximately 5 mg of fluoride per kilogram of body weight. This level may or may not in fact prove toxic, but it certainly signifies a medical emergency that requires immediate treatment and hospitalization. Such emergencies are rare. Chronic toxicity that involves lower levels of fluoride consumed over longer periods is also relatively rare. It is associated with fluoride intakes of around 20 to 80 mg/day and is usually the result of prolonged consumption of water with a high natural fluoride content or industrial contamination of water or food.

> Electrolytes are often measured in milliequivalents (mEq), rather than in weight (mg), to allow the relative osmotic effect of different electrolytes to be compared. Equal milliequivalent amounts of different electrolytes each have the same osmotic effect. To convert the weight of an electrolyte ion (in milligrams) into milliequivalents, divide the weight of an electrolyte by the numerical value of its atomic weight (for simple ions, such as Na^+, Cl^-, and so on) or by the formula weight of the ion (for "compound" ions containing more than one element, such as NH_4^+, HCO_3^-, and so on).

ELECTROLYTES

All mineral salts whose ions dissolve in water are electrolytes, and in nutrition and other health sciences the individual ions of these compounds are also commonly referred to as electrolytes. A wide variety of such electrolyte ions is found in the body, where they have a great influence on the flow of water between the various fluid compartments because of their effect on the osmotic pressure of the fluids of which they are a part. They also influence the contraction of muscles and the transmission of nerve impulses by the nervous system. Three of the most important electrolyte ions are the sodium (Na^+), potassium (K^+), and chloride (Cl^-) ions.

SODIUM (Na^+)

Sodium in food and in the body occurs in the form of positively charged sodium ions, either free in solution or bound within sodium salts. These ions must be counterbalanced by sufficient negatively charged ions to compensate for the positive charge on the sodium ions because all compounds—and therefore all foods—are electrically neutral overall. However, in solutions (and most of the chemistry of life takes place in solution), positive and negative ions follow a relatively independent existence. So any one type of ion can be discussed as an independent entity.

The major source of sodium in the diet is sodium chloride (NaCl), known as common table salt (or just salt). In solution, this separates into sodium ions and chloride ions. Sodium ions are also available as part of a wide variety of other sodium-containing compounds in food, and once these ions are released into solution, there is no way to distinguish which compounds they were once part of.

Because table salt is the major source of sodium in the diet, the terms *salt* and *sodium* are sometimes treated as equivalent in discussions of nutrition. This practice should be avoided, or at least used with great care, because sodium is present in a wide variety of natural and added chemicals in food. The preeminence of salt as a source of sodium, however, has given salt a major role in both political and economic history. Many of the major conquests of the world were motivated by the search for plentiful supplies of salt for use as both a preservative and a flavoring. In many countries salt can be mined from deposits of rock salt, whereas in others the evaporation of seawater is the only source of supply.

Absorption and Excretion

Each day, 3000 to 6000 mg of sodium is normally taken into the body. The actual amount varies greatly, however, largely because of the considerable variations in the amount of table salt that is added during cooking and at the table. A small portion of ingested sodium is absorbed in the stomach, but most of it is absorbed rapidly in the small intestine. The absorbed sodium is carried by the blood throughout the body. As blood passes through the kidneys, sodium is filtered out and then partially reabsorbed into the blood in the amounts needed to maintain blood sodium concentration at an appropriate level. The operation of this partial reabsorption usually results in between 90% and 98% of ingested sodium being excreted in urine.

The regulation of sodium reabsorption by the kidneys is controlled by the hormone aldosterone, which is secreted by the adrenal gland, and the enzyme renin, which is secreted by the kidney. When the concentration of sodium in the blood falls below optimal levels (usually as a result of restricted sodium intake), the secretion of aldosterone is stimulated and this hormone directly stimulates the reabsorption of sodium in the kidneys, causing more sodium to be retained in the blood and less to be excreted in urine. At the same time, specialized cells in the kidney are stimulated to secrete the enzyme renin into the blood. The renin catalyzes the conversion of a protein called angiotensinogen (in blood plasma) into angiotensin I. The angiotensin I is then split to form angiotensin II, which stimulates the secretion of more aldosterone from the adrenal gland, giving a further stimulus to the process of sodium reabsorption (Figure 8-7).

When blood sodium levels are high, the secretion of aldosterone and renin is diminished, causing less sodium to be reabsorbed by the kidneys and more to be excreted in urine. High levels of sodium in the blood also cause the hypothalamus of the brain to stimulate the sensation of thirst. This leads to increased fluid intake, providing the additional water needed to carry the excess sodium out of the body in urine.

In addition to the losses via urine, sodium is also lost from the body in perspiration. Each liter of perspiration usually contains about 200 mg of sodium. The total amount of sodium lost in this way is usually about 1000 mg/day but may rise to as much as 2400 mg/day when the rate of perspiration rises because of hot environmental temperatures, prolonged strenuous physical activity, or fever. Another hormone, atrial natriuretic peptide, secreted by the heart and the brain, interacts with the renin-angiotensin-aldosterone system to modulate sodium and water excretion.

Distribution

About half of the sodium in the body is found in the extracellular fluids, which includes the intravascular fluids within blood vessels and the intercellular fluids surrounding cells. Under normal conditions, as little as 10% of total body sodium is found within cells. The sodium constantly enters the cells, but it is also constantly pumped out of cells by specialized proteins embedded in the cell membranes. The rest of the sodium in the body is found in the skeleton, where it is bound to the surface of the bones. About half of this skeletal sodium acts as a reservoir of exchangeable sodium, which is available to the extracellular fluids when their levels of sodium fall because of reduced dietary intake or excessive excretion of sodium. Even when low dietary intake of sodium is combined with high levels of losses because of excretion, it takes a long time for these skeletal reserves to be depleted.

FIGURE 8-7

Falling blood sodium concentration stimulates increased reabsorption of sodium by the kidneys.

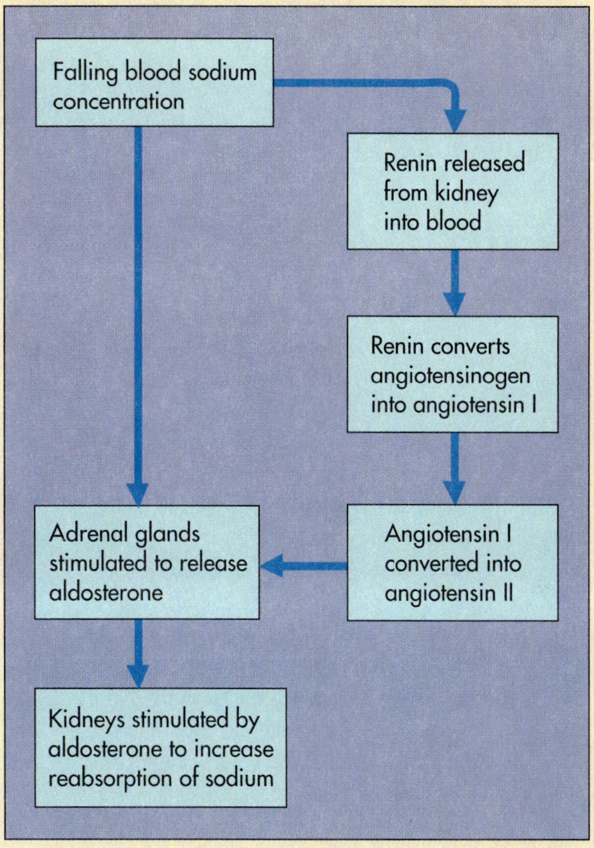

Functions

Sodium is the predominant positively charged ion in the extracellular fluid, and it accounts for much of the osmotic pressure of the fluid. In other words, sodium ions are one of the major types of dissolved particles that, in the absence of counterbalancing forces, cause water to move out from cells and into extracellular fluid by osmosis. The osmotic pressure of extracellular fluid, however, is opposed by the osmotic pressure of intracellular fluid. Inside the cell, potassium ions (K^+) are one of the major types of dissolved particles that cause water to move into cells from the extracellular fluid. Normally, the levels of extracellular sodium and intracellular potassium are maintained at the levels that allow the appropriate water balance between the extracellular and intracellular regions to be maintained.

If the amount of sodium within a cell rises, however, water enters the cell, causing it to swell. Such swollen cells are found in edematous tissue (tissue characterized by edema, i.e., increased water content). Water balance can also be upset when the level of sodium in extracellular fluid falls. In this case, water enters into cells by osmosis from the now more watery extracellular medium, causing a fall in the volume of extracellular fluid and an associated fall in blood pressure.

*I*ons and acid-base balance

- Acid conditions (low pH) result from the predominance of hydrogen ion (H^+) over hydroxide ion (OH^-) in a solution.
- Basic (alkaline) conditions (high pH) result from the predominance of hydroxide ions over hydrogen ions in a solution.
- Other types of ions can be referred to as "acid-forming" or "alkali-forming" ("base-forming"), depending on their relative tendency to combine with hydrogen or hydroxide ions and so remove them from solution.
- Positive ions that have *no* tendency to combine with, and so remove, the hydroxide ions that are directly responsible for a solution's alkalinity (basicity) can be referred to as alkali-forming ions.
- Positive ions that *do* combine with hydroxide ions, and so remove them from solution, can be referred to as acid-forming ions.
- Negative ions that have *no* tendency to combine with, and so remove, the hydrogen ions that are directly responsible for a solution's acidity can be referred to as acid-forming ions.
- Negative ions that *do* combine with hydrogen ions, and so remove them from solution, can be referred to as alkali-forming ions.
- It is important to remember that *only hydrogen ions and hydroxide ions influence a solution's pH (level of acidity or alkalinity) directly.* All other ions influence the pH *indirectly,* by altering the concentration of hydrogen or hydroxide ions.

Sodium ions also help to maintain the normal pH value of the extracellular fluids. They are regarded as alkali-forming in the sense that they have no tendency to combine with and so remove the hydroxide ions (OH^-) responsible for alkalinity. Such a substance as sodium bicarbonate, for example, is alkaline because the negative bicarbonate ions (HCO_3^-) combine with hydrogen ions (responsible for acidity) and remove some of them from solution, whereas the positive sodium ions do not combine with and remove any of the hydroxide ions responsible for alkalinity. Sodium compounds can be released from bone in a way that neutralizes undesirable extracellular acidity. Also, one of the major causes of **alkalosis,** a condition in which blood becomes too alkaline, is the ingestion of sodium-containing antacid preparations designed to combat acid indigestion.

Sodium is essential for the absorption of glucose and the transport of many other nutrients across membranes, particularly in intestinal cells. The sodium ions bind to carriers embedded in the membrane, along with nutrient molecules, and the nutrients are then taken into cells with the sodium ions as the sodium ions move down their concentration gradient.

Requirements

The dietary requirement for sodium has not yet been determined, but normal intakes usually provide far more sodium than is needed. This is reflected in the statistic, already mentioned, that 90% to 98% of ingested sodium is usually excreted. The body's requirement for sodium, whatever the actual value is, is based on the needs for growth added to the amount needed to replace sodium lost in perspiration and other secretions.[16] The minimal amount of sodium that must be replaced corresponds to what are known as the **obligatory losses** of sodium, the losses that cannot be avoided. These obligatory losses amount to about 115 mg/day, including unavoidable losses in urine and feces and both perspiration and nonperspiration losses from the skin.

In America the recommended minimal sodium allowance for adults is 500 mg/day, a little more than four times the 115 mg required to maintain sodium balance (Table 8-7). This allowance is equivalent to 1.25 g of sodium chloride (¼ tsp of table salt). Health and Welfare Canada estimates the sodium requirement of adults to be 80 mg/day.[17] Infants lose proportionately more sodium in feces than do adults and need some sodium for healthy growth; so they have a higher sodium need per unit of body weight than adults.

Because there is no known benefit associated with current levels of sodium consumption and there is a clear disadvantage to people susceptible to hypertension (discussed later), the Food and Nutrition Board Committee on Diet and Health recommends that daily intakes of sodium be limited to no more than 2.4 g/day (equivalent to 6 g of sodium chloride).[18]

TABLE 8-7

Estimated minimal requirements of sodium

SUBJECTS (AGE)	REQUIREMENT (mg)
0-5 months	120
6-11 months	200
1 year	225
2-5 years	300
6-9 years	400
10-18 years	500
>18 years	500

From National Academy of Sciences: *Recommended dietary allowances,* Washington, DC, 1989, National Academy of Sciences.

Food Sources

The sodium in food falls into three main categories: sodium naturally present in the food, sodium added during processing or cooking, and sodium in table salt that is added at the table.

Sodium is naturally present in widely varying amounts (Figure 8-8). In contrast to most minerals, more sodium is generally found in foods of animal origin than of plant origin. The total amount of sodium in a person's diet, however, is influenced at least as much by the amount of salt added during processing and preparation and at the table as it is by the amount of sodium occurring naturally within the food. Raw potatoes, for example, contain only 5 mg of sodium per 100 g, whereas the same amount of potato converted into potato chips provides 200 to 300 mg of sodium. Cured ham has 20 times as much sodium as does raw pork. Fresh peas have less than 1 mg of sodium per 100 g, whereas frozen peas have up to 85 mg of sodium per 100 g and canned peas have up to 220 mg of sodium per 100 g. These higher amounts of sodium in frozen or canned peas result if a salt solution is used as one method of sorting peas by size based on differences in specific gravity. The amounts quoted previously do not include any sodium in salt added at the table or within added butter or other toppings and dressings.

In many countries monosodium glutamate (MSG) is used as a flavor enhancer and can contribute considerable quantities of sodium to the diet. As can be seen from Table 8-8, many other sodium-containing chemicals are also added to food, often for reasons other than the enhancement of flavor.

In some areas the sodium content of the water supply may be high enough to make it a significant source of sodium. This is true for one fifth of the water sources in America, which yield water containing up to 250 mg of sodium per liter. Many of the ion-exchange units used as water softeners also produce water with a high sodium content (up to 100 mg/L) because they release sodium ions in exchange for the calcium and magnesium ions in hard water.

The amount of table salt each person adds to food is often referred to as his or her **discretionary salt** intake. This amount varies widely, but The National Health and Nutrition Examination Survey (NHANES) estimated discretionary salt intake at an average of 2700 mg/day. There is evidence that although salt preference is established early in life, it can be modified by a stepwise reduction in salt intake over a period.

In response to current health concerns about the overconsumption of sodium, many food processors are seeking ways to reduce the sodium content of their foods. In May 1994 it became mandatory to list the sodium content of foods on food labels in America. A product can be labeled as "sodium free" if it contains fewer than 5 mg of sodium per serving, as "very low sodium" if it contains no more than 35 mg of sodium per serving, as "low sodium" if it contains fewer than 140 mg of sodium per serving, as "less sodium" if it contains at least 25% less sodium than a corresponding reference food, and as "light in sodium" if the sodium content in a low-fat, low-calorie food has been reduced by 50%.

The following information indicates how to convert between various commonly used methods of quoting quantities of sodium and sodium chloride.

- To convert grams of sodium into milligrams of sodium, multiply weight in grams by 1000.
- To convert a weight of sodium (for example, grams or milligrams) into the equivalent weight of sodium chloride, multiply by 2.5.
- To convert a weight of sodium chloride into the equivalent weight of sodium, multiply by 0.4.
- To convert sodium in milligrams to sodium in milliequivalents (mEq), often used in dietary prescriptions, divide by 23.
- To convert milliequivalents of sodium to milligrams of sodium, multiply by 23.
- To convert milligrams of sodium chloride to milliequivalents of sodium, divide by 58.5.
- To convert milliequivalents of sodium to milligrams of sodium chloride, multiply by 58.5.
- One tsp of sodium chloride (5 g or 5000 mg) contains 2000 mg of sodium.

FIGURE 8-8

Sodium content of typical servings of various foods.

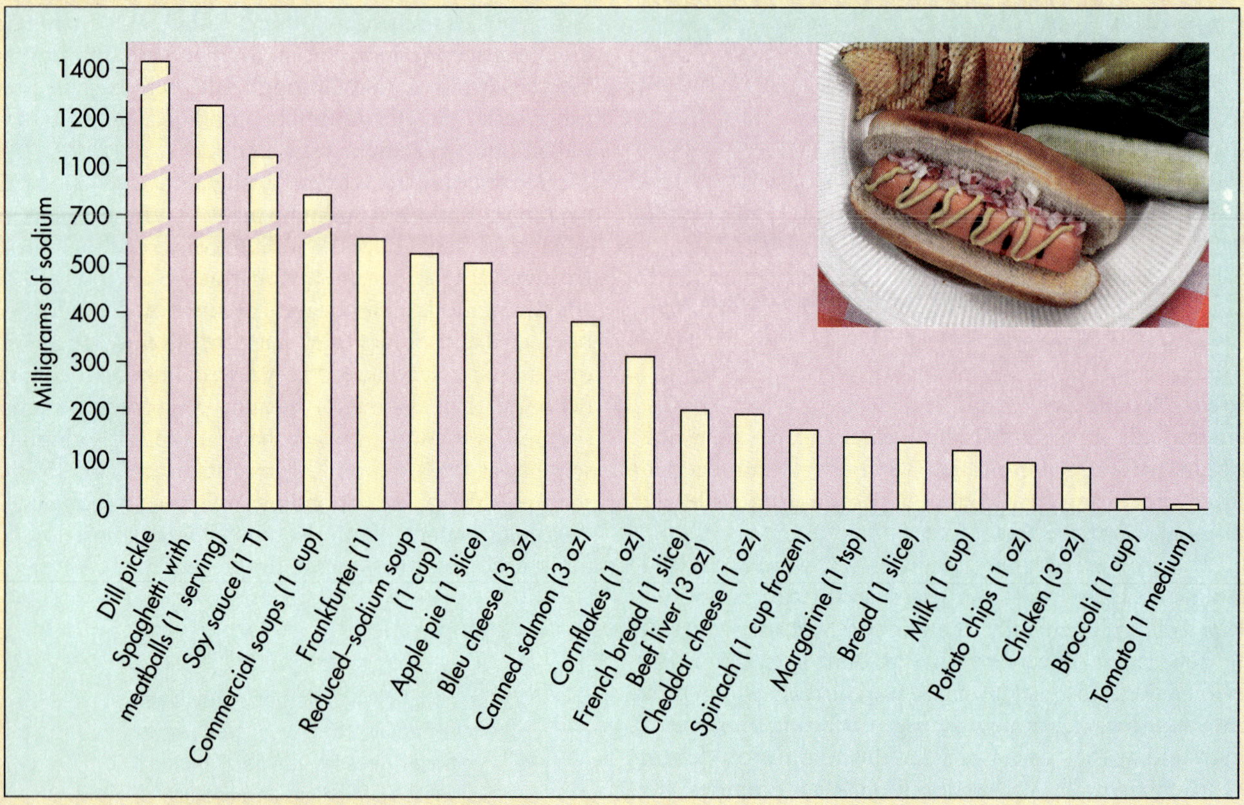

TABLE 8-8

Functions of sodium-containing compounds in processed food products

SODIUM-CONTAINING COMPOUNDS	FUNCTIONS
Baking powder	Leavening agent
Baking soda	Leavening agent; alkali
Monosodium glutamate	Flavor enhancer
Sodium benzoate	Preservative
Sodium caseinate	Thickener and binder
Sodium citrate	Buffer; used to control acidity in soft drinks and fruit drinks
Sodium nitrate	Curing agent in meat; provides color, prevents botulism (a food poisoning)
Sodium phosphate	Emulsifier, stabilizer, buffer
Sodium propionate	Mold inhibitor
Sodium saccharin	Artificial sweetener

Deficiency

The usual daily sodium intake of 3000 to 6000 mg clearly represents many times the minimal required intake. It is unlikely that anyone will have insufficient sodium intake in the long term because a diet providing only 100 to 150 mg of sodium is extremely unpalatable and practically impossible to achieve. If body stores of sodium are depleted rapidly, however, symptoms of lethargy, nausea, and vomiting result. The person also becomes irritable, confused, weak, and sometimes hostile. Low body stores of sodium are also reflected in low sodium levels in the blood, known as **hyponatremia.** Long-term severe sodium deficiency can lead to coma and ultimately death.

Hypernatremia = too much sodium in the blood
Hyponatremia = too little sodium in the blood
Hyperkalemia = too much potassium in the blood
Hypokalemia = too little potassium in the blood

Excess

Although sodium is an essential mineral, excessive amounts are not only unnecessary, but also harmful.

Excessive amounts in the body are associated with excessive sodium in the blood, known as **hypernatremia.** Most current interest in dietary sodium is focused on possible detrimental effects of excess sodium on health, leading to concern that its intake should be restricted. The major concern is not the toxicity of high doses of sodium (discussed later) but the link between chronically excessive sodium consumption and hypertension (high blood pressure). When sodium intake exceeds the capacity of the kidneys to excrete all of the excess, blood sodium levels rise and cause an increase in blood volume because of the extra water drawn into the blood by osmosis. This increase in blood volume in turn causes an increase in blood pressure and an increased workload on the heart, which must pump the greater volume of fluid at higher pressure. A large international epidemiological study, called the **INTERSALT study,** examined the link between sodium and hypertension. It involved the monitoring of urinary sodium excretion and blood pressure in 10,079 people by 52 centers in 23 countries. Urinary sodium excretion is a good measure of sodium intake because 90% to 98% of ingested sodium is excreted in urine. The study revealed that the level of sodium excretion was significantly and independently related to blood pressure. Thus the study confirmed that high sodium intake was correlated with high blood pressure in all countries and across all age-groups.[19]

Hypertension is the most common form of chronic disease in America, affecting between 17% and 25% of the population and as many as 75% of those in the 65- to 74-year-old age-group. The adverse results of hypertension include strokes, heart disease, and kidney failure, capable of causing either disability or death.[20] People with hypertension are routinely advised to take dietary measures aimed at restricting their sodium intake, a procedure that is considered in the following section.

Dietary Restriction

Restriction of sodium intake results in the lowering of blood pressure to normal levels in some, but unfortunately not all, people.[21] There is general agreement that the average levels of sodium intake in the United States and Canada are excessive, although in many cases the potential adverse effects in salt-responsive individuals (estimated at 20% of the population) are at least partially counteracted by a comparable increase in potassium and possibly calcium intake.[22,23] Governmental dietary guidelines now urge the public to restrict or decrease sodium intake, especially by control of the intake of table salt. Mild restriction of sodium intake to the 2500- to 3000-mg level can often be achieved simply by limiting the use of salt at the table.

The therapeutic level of sodium intake recommended for people with detected sodium-related problems such as hypertension is no more than 500 mg/day. It is not believed to be necessary, however, to recommend such a low level of intake for the general population. To achieve intakes as low as 500 mg, it is necessary to choose foods that are naturally low in sodium, to avoid all foods to which sodium is added during processing, and to use sodium-free salt substitutes and low-salt milk (from which most sodium has been removed by ion-exchange processes). Spices and herbs, with the exception of garlic salts and celery, contain virtually no sodium and so can be safely used to add flavor to low-sodium diets.

Low-sodium diets have long been used to treat hypertension induced by pregnancy, a major complication during late pregnancy. This is no longer recommended, however, because a series of clinical studies have shown that a moderate-sodium—rather than a low-sodium—diet is most appropriate during pregnancy. Pregnant women require an additional 70 mg of sodium per day because of the increase in their blood volume, the additional needs of the fetus, and the need for sodium in the amniotic fluid that surrounds the fetus.

There has been concern that infants whose diets are high in sodium are less able to excrete the excess than are adults and therefore develop a predisposition to hypertension. In response to this concern, manufacturers of baby foods have either eliminated all added sodium from their products or restricted it to 0.25%. They also advise parents not to add salt to make the food more acceptable to their adult tastes. It is well established that infants do not discriminate between salted and unsalted food.

Toxicity

Although sodium chloride is regularly added to food, doses of just a several grams per kilogram of body weight can be lethal for adults. Fortunately, these amounts are extremely unpalatable and are not normally taken voluntarily. Considerably smaller doses can be lethal for infants, however, because of the limited ability of their immature kidneys to excrete excess sodium. Because infants sometimes consume large quantities of unfamiliar foods and even nonfood substances, salt should be kept from their reach in the same way as is done for medicines and household chemicals.

POTASSIUM (K^+)

Potassium in food and in the body occurs in the form of positively charged potassium ions (K^+), either free in solution or bound within potassium salts. The chemical properties of potassium ions are similar to those of sodium ions. Both are regarded as alkali-forming ions because they have no tendency to combine with the hydroxide ions that are directly responsible for a solution's alkalinity. The one major physiological difference between potassium and sodium, however, is that sodium ions are most concentrated outside of cells and potassium ions are most concentrated inside of cells. The active and continuous pumping of sodium out of cells

FIGURE 8-9

Potassium is constantly pumped into cells, whereas sodium is constantly pumped out.

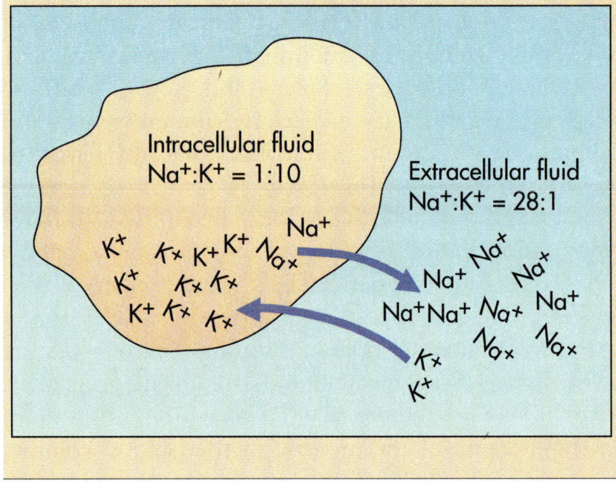

TABLE 8-9

Estimated minimal requirements of potassium (mg/d) and chloride (mg/d)

SUBJECTS (AGE)	POTASSIUM (mg/day)	CHLORIDE (mg/day)
0-1 year	500-700	180-300
1-5 years	1000-1400	350-500
6-9 years	1600	600
10-18 years	2000	750
Adult	2000	750

and potassium into cells maintains a Na^+/K^+ ratio of 1:10 in the intracellular fluid and 28:1 in the extracellular fluid (Figure 8-9).

The total amount of potassium in the body averages 250 g and because most of this is within cells, the level of potassium in the blood is not a good indicator of the body's potassium content. Instead, the potassium levels of the blood reflect changes in cellular metabolism. Blood potassium levels rise during the catabolic breakdown of body tissue and also in the condition of acidosis (abnormal acidity of the blood) associated with diarrhea, when potassium is drawn from cells to help restore normal acid-base balance. Blood potassium levels fall when the anabolic synthesis of proteins or glycogen within cells increases or during alkalosis, when potassium is drawn into cells to help restore acid-base balance.

Unusually high levels of potassium in the blood and other extracellular fluids, greater than 0.5 g/L, cause disturbances in muscular coordination and in severe cases can lead to cardiac arrest. Such high levels usually result from a failure of the kidneys to excrete excess potassium. Normally the kidneys excrete about 7% of the potassium in the blood they are filtering, because the kidneys reabsorb potassium less efficiently than most other substances in blood.

As was discussed in Chapter 7, estimation of the amount of potassium in the body can be used to determine the amount of lean tissue mass in body composition studies.

Functions

Potassium ions are an integral and essential part of every cell and are required for cell growth. To sustain every pound of weight gained, 1050 mg of potassium is required. Within the cell, potassium assists in many biochemical reactions, especially those involved in the release of energy from food and in the synthesis of glycogen and protein. As already considered, potassium ions are a major factor in influencing the osmotic pressure within cells and therefore in controlling the distribution of water between the intracellular and extracellular fluids. Potassium also plays an important role in maintaining acid-base balance by increasing in concentration in fluids that become too acidic and decreasing in concentration in fluids that become too alkaline. Potassium is also a crucial participant in the movements of ions across nerve cell membranes that form and sustain nerve impulses; and it is involved in the release of insulin from the pancreas. Potassium, along with magnesium ions (Mg^{2+}), acts as a muscle relaxant that opposes the muscle-contracting stimulus of calcium ions (Ca^{2+}).

Although sodium is usually considered to be the dietary factor most related to blood pressure, it appears that the sodium/potassium ratio is more important than the absolute amount of sodium. It is possible that maintaining potassium intake at a level equal to sodium intake (a Na^+/K^+ intake ratio of 1:1) may protect against the adverse effects of high sodium intake.[19]

Requirements

Although potassium is a dietary essential, there is little information about minimal requirements; however, they are estimated at about 2000 mg/day for adults.[16] Infants and children are estimated to need from 15 to 65 mg/day for growth, although their actual intake must be higher to cover losses in urine, feces, and perspiration (Table 8-9). The usual potassium content of the North American diet is estimated at 2 to 6 g/day, or 0.8 to 1.5 g/1000 kcal. Intakes are higher among people who eat large amounts of fruits and vegetables.

Food Sources

Potassium is found in a wide range of foods, although at particularly high levels in some fruits and vegetables. Figure 8-10 lists the potassium content of some common foods. Because potassium is found in significant quantities in such a wide range of foods, the content of potassium in the diet is usually roughly proportional to the diet's energy content. In addition to naturally occur-

FIGURE 8-10

Potassium content of some common foods.

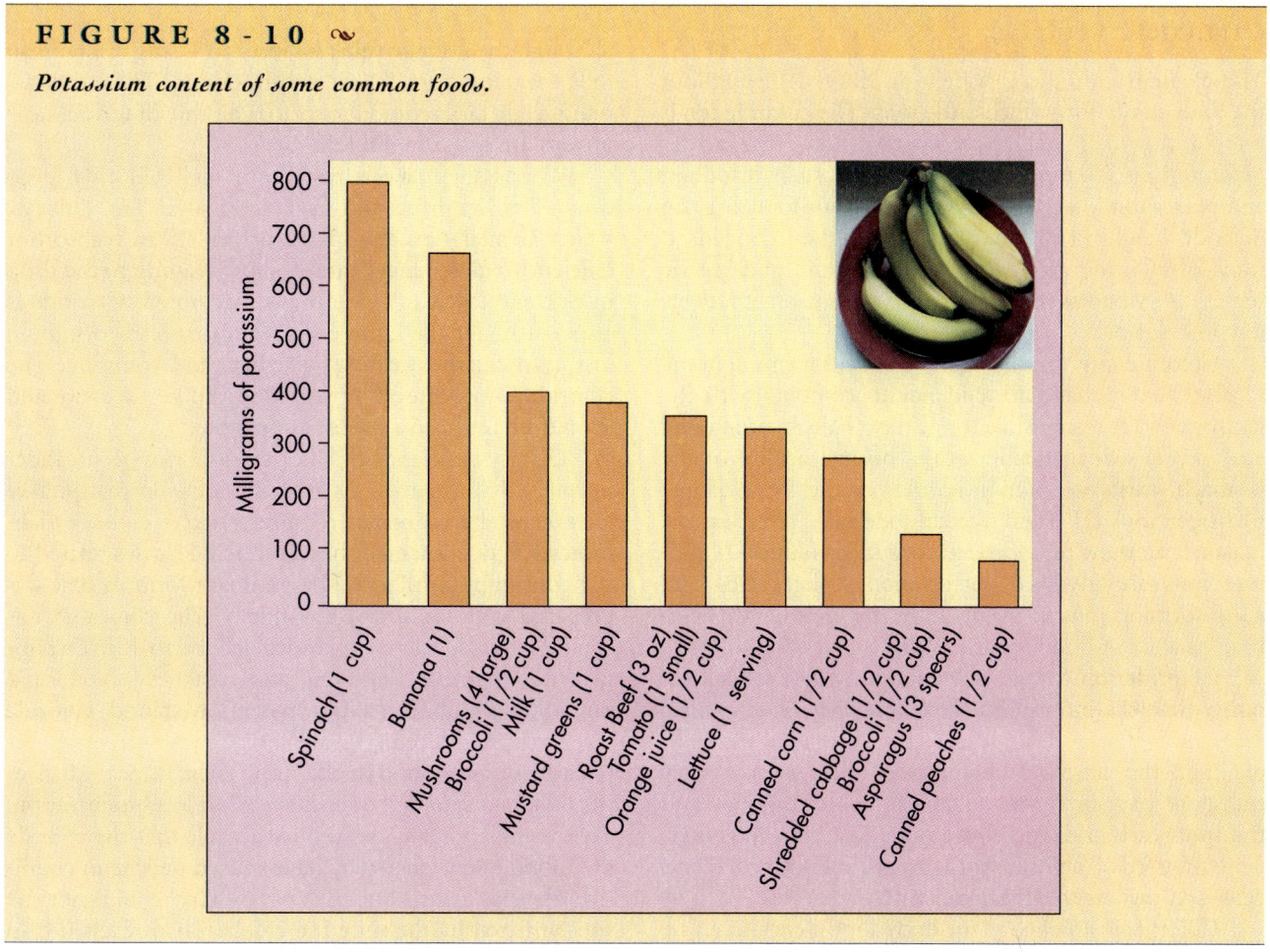

ring potassium, many foods contain potassium in the form of various food additives. Potassium alginate, for example, is used as a thickener and an emulsifying agent; potassium iodate, as a dough conditioner; and potassium nitrate, as a preservative. Potassium chloride can be used as a sodium-free salt substitute for people trying to restrict their sodium intake (as can lithium chloride).

The potassium in food is very soluble, and so a considerable amount of the potassium in a raw food may dissolve in cooking water and be lost to the diet (unless the water is used in some way, most probably as a stock for soup). Potassium is also lost in the whey discarded during cheese making.

Deficiency

Potassium deficiency seldom occurs as a result of dietary intake falling below accepted norms. It can occur, however, in infants with diarrhea. During diarrhea, any food in the gastrointestinal tract passes through so quickly that the absorption of potassium from it, and reabsorption of potassium from digestive secretions, is significantly decreased. Vomiting (including vomiting induced by people with bulimia), the use of diuretics (often taken to control hypertension), severe energy-protein malnutrition, and surgery may also lead to potassium depletion and perhaps deficiency. Having too little potassium in the blood is known as **hypokalemia.** The main symptoms of potassium deficiency are general muscle weakness, specific weakness of respiratory muscles, poor intestinal function with abdominal bloating, and heart abnormalities.

The best treatment for potassium deficiency is simply to replace potassium losses through normal dietary sources, thus minimizing the risk of excessive intake. Infants with potassium deficiency associated with the energy-protein deficiency disease kwashiorkor respond to treatment only when sufficient dietary potassium is accompanied by an increased intake of protein.

Excess

Excessive intake of potassium can lead to excessively high levels in the blood (**hyperkalemia**). Excessive potassium in the blood can cause cardiac arrest, as can too little. The proper functioning of the heart requires that blood potassium levels neither exceed nor fall below the optimal range. Hyperkalemia can present particular problems in elderly persons, who may have impaired kidney function and a resulting difficulty in excreting the excess potassium.

CHLORIDE (Cl^-)

The element chlorine is widely distributed throughout the body in the form of chloride ions. The chloride ion is one of the main negatively charged ions that act as "counterions" to positively charged ions, such as sodium and potassium ions. Chloride ions account for 1.5 g/kg of body weight (1500 mg/kg). The highest concentrations of chloride are in cerebrospinal fluid and gastric secretions, whereas muscle and nerve tissue are relatively low in chloride.

Chloride ions can be regarded as acid-forming in the sense that they have no tendency to combine with the hydrogen ions responsible for acidity. Thus hydrochloric acid (HCl), which maintains the normal acidity of the stomach, exists in solution entirely in the form of free hydrogen ions (H^+) and free chloride ions, releasing the maximal amount of hydrogen ions into solution. Chloride ions are involved with various other acid- and alkali-forming ions in maintaining the appropriate acid-base balance in body fluids.

Chloride ions are largely found in the extracellular rather than the intracellular fluid, but they readily move into and out of red blood cells in a way that serves to maintain the electrical neutrality of these cells as they transport oxygen from the lungs to body tissues and transport carbon dioxide from body tissues to the lungs. This transfer of chloride ions in and out of red blood cells is known as the **chloride shift.**

Chloride is supplied to the body almost exclusively by the sodium chloride (table salt) in the diet. Some water supplies, however, may provide as much as 300 mg/L, although the average value is closer to 42 mg/L. Human milk contains more chloride than sodium. The estimated minimal dietary requirements for chloride of various age-groups are listed in Table 8-9.

When salt intake is restricted, body chloride levels drop—first in urine and then in tissues. The kidneys, which normally excrete excess chloride, can reabsorb it efficiently when dietary intake is low, leading to the drop in chloride levels in urine previously noted. Chloride is also lost under the same conditions that lead to sodium loss, particularly sweating, diarrhea, and vomiting. The chloride losses caused by vomiting can be excessive and should be replaced as soon as possible.

Dietary deficiency of chloride does not occur under normal circumstances. As with sodium, normal intakes far exceed the estimated requirements. A chloride deficiency was documented, however, in 141 cases related to the consumption of a soy-based infant formula that was prepared without added chloride.[24] The clinical symptoms of the deficiency included failure to thrive (poor growth), anorexia, lethargy, and weakness. Associated physiological abnormalities were low blood chloride levels (hypochloremia), alkalosis, hyponatremia, hypokalemia, and blood in the urine (hematuria). Most of the infants responded quickly to chloride administration. Follow-up studies suggested for a while that the episode of chloride deficiency may have caused deficits in cognitive development, but this possibility could not be substantiated by the time the children had reached 8 to 10 years of age.[25]

ISSUES AND OPINIONS

Water: An Essential Nutrient and an Increasingly Popular Bottled Beverage

The importance of consuming sufficient water cannot be overemphasized. A reduction in the body's water content of as little as 3% to 5% and the resulting changes in electrolyte concentrations can dramatically reduce the body's ability to regulate its temperature, transport oxygen to tissues, and perform work.

Approximately half of the water consumed is provided by beverages, and the favored beverage in America is the soft drink, or soda. In 1992 the average American consumed 60 gallons of soft drink, an increase of 35% since 1982. During this same period consumption of the following beverages changed by the amounts shown in parentheses*

- Coffee and tea (down 2%)
- Milk (down 3%)
- Alcoholic beverages (down 8%)
- Powdered drinks (up 2%)
- Juice (up 0.1%)

Increasing numbers of Americans are now turning to bottled water as their preferred beverage. The average American drank 8.3 gallons of bottled water in 1992, three times more than a decade ago, although only one fourth as much as the average European.

*International Bottled Water Association: *Fact sheets*, 113 North, Henry Street, Alexandria, Va, 1993, Beverage Marketing Corporation.

According to the International Bottled Water Association the primary reason U.S. consumers choose bottled water is taste.† Bottled water is most commonly disinfected using ozone (O_3), a form of oxygen which leaves no residual taste, color, or odor in the water. Tap water, on the other hand, is disinfected with chlorine.

Some consumers choose bottled water because they are concerned about the chemical purity of their tap water. For example, lead pipes, well pumps, solder, or fixtures with a high lead content can all contaminate water as it sits in pipes or is drawn for use. In areas where the level of lead in the water is more than 15 parts per billion (ppb), pregnant women, infants, and children are advised to drink bottled water. The main justification for this advice is that even low levels of lead can seriously impair normal development.

Consumers are also turning to bottled water because it provides no kilocalories, caffeine, or alcohol. It is therefore compatible with attempts to adopt a healthy life-style, including improved nutrition and regular exercise.

Approximately 700 different brands of bottled water are now produced in the United States, and 75 imported brands are widely available. Many of these brands are carbonated mineral waters. The gas that bubbles out of carbonated water (or "sparkling" water) is carbon dioxide (CO_2), which is naturally present in water that has percolated through certain types of rock. Water and soft drinks can also be artificially carbonated at the bottling plant. The different types of bottled water on the market differ according to their initial source (a specific well, spring, or public water supply), their native mineral content, and whether they are naturally carbonated, artificially carbonated, or noncarbonated.

About 75% of American bottled water comes from protected wells or springs. The remainder is drawn from public water supplies but is then further processed by filtration, distillation, deionization, or reverse osmosis, principally to remove dissolved minerals. Bottled water may also contain added flavors, extracts, or essences derived from spices or fruits, but it should not contain any sweeteners.

Bottled water marketed in the United States must meet quality standards based on the "maximum contaminant levels" set by the Environmental Protection Agency (EPA) in the *Safe Drinking Water Act*. Bottled water is also considered a "food" by the Food and Drug Administration (FDA) and therefore must be processed and packaged in accordance with the FDA's *Good Manufacturing Prac-*

tices (see Chapter 19). It must also be described using an appropriate choice of the standardized labeling terms: "mineral," "spring," "artesian," "well," "distilled," and "purified." There are also official quality standards for 38 compounds found in drinking water. For example, the maximum contamination level for lead is 5 ppb for bottled water, whereas the current federal standard for tap water is 15 ppb. Seltzer water and club soda are considered to be soft drinks, not bottled waters, and are regulated separately.*

Bottled water and packaged ice are analyzed and certified by The National Sanitation Foundation (NSF). This is an independent, not-for-profit, international organization of scientists, engineers, educators, and analysts. It performs a voluntary program of testing, retesting, and unannounced plant site inspections to ensure adequate and consistent standards. A listing of NSF-certified bottled waters and packaged ices can be obtained by contacting the NSF directly at 3475 Plymouth Road, P.O. Box 130140, Ann Arbor, Mich, 48113-0140, USA.

*International Bottled Water Association, 113 North Henry Street, Alexandria, Va, 22314.

BY NOW YOU SHOULD KNOW

- Water is the most essential of all essential nutrients.
- Water is a constituent of every cell of the body.
- Water is found in the spaces between cells and within blood.
- A higher proportion of water is found in blood and lean tissue than in fat tissue.
- We lose body water as we age.
- Water is obtained from beverages and solid foods and is an end product of the metabolism of energy-yielding nutrients within the body.
- Water is eliminated from the body in urine, through the skin and lungs, and in feces.
- The water balance of the body is maintained by a variety of sensitive physiological control systems.
- Water serves as a solvent for the chemistry of life, a reactant in a variety of biochemical reactions, a lubricant, a temperature regulator, and a source of dietary minerals.
- It is recommended that we consume 1 L (approximately 1 qt) of fluid for every 1000 kcal in the diet, approximately two thirds of which come from beverages.
- A change in body water content of as little as 3% can have a profound effect on body function and performance.
- The addition of fluoride to the water supply is considered a safe and effective way to reduce the incidence of tooth decay.
- For those who do not have a fluoridated water supply, topical applications of fluoride-containing dental products or the use of fluoride supplements provides effective protection against tooth decay.
- Sodium, potassium, and chloride ions are three of the main electrolyte ions influencing the distribution of water within the body.
- Sodium and potassium are alkali-forming (base-forming) ions, whereas chloride is an acid-forming ion.

- The intake of sodium is usually many times the amount required by the body, leading to approximately 90% of ingested sodium being excreted.
- Sodium plays an important role in fluid balance, acid-base balance, and the transport of nutrients into cells.
- The estimated requirement for sodium for adults is 500 mg/day, but typical intakes are found to be well in excess of this, up to as much as 6000 mg/day.
- Information on sodium content is mandatory on food labels.
- People with a predisposition to hypertension should avoid high intakes of sodium.
- In sodium intake is recommended for everyone to reduce the risk of developing hypertension.
- Potassium, which is concentrated mainly within cells, is found in a wide variety of foods, particularly fruits and vegetables.
- Chloride is a part of hydrochloric acid, which serves to maintain the acidity of the stomach.

STUDY QUESTIONS

1. Name four functions of water in the body.
2. What foods would you choose if you were advised to increase your potassium intake?
3. How can a child who gets water from home be well protected against tooth decay?
4. What happens when the need for sodium in the body increases?
5. What happens when the intake of sodium exceeds the ability of the kidneys to excrete the excess?
6. What is the major dietary source of chloride?
7. What function do sodium and potassium have in common?
8. Name five foods high in sodium and five foods low in sodium.
9. What is dental fluorosis?
10. How is water involved in the regulation of body temperature?
11. How much water should be provided in a 2000-kcal diet?
12. A food recipe for Spanish green beans calls for 1 tsp of salt. The recipe will feed 15 people. How many milligrams of sodium will there be per serving? Also, using the salt and sodium conversions chart on p. 279, convert your answer to milliequivalents of sodium.
13. A patient is advised to follow a low-sodium diet with a dietary prescription of 43 mEq of sodium per day. How many milligrams of sodium does that correspond to?
14. What effect might changes in body potassium have on the heart?

CRITICAL ANALYSIS

1. Do you take in enough water? Deficiencies in electrolytes (sodium, potassium, and chloride) are uncommon. However, many people fail to take in adequate amounts of water or fluid, particularly in hot weather. Although 8 cups of water or fluids (64 oz or 1920 ml) is commonly recommended, more water is necessary if the weather is warm or if the activity level is higher than normal for the individual, to name two circumstances when this can be true. Here is an exercise to estimate your fluid intake for 1 day.

   Think back to the first beverage you drank yesterday and work through the end of that day, recording your total intake of beverages in the categories listed below. To help you assess serving size, here are some approximate volumes: coffee cup, 5 to 6 oz; coffee mug, 8 oz; tall hot drink cup, 12 to 20 oz; small juice glass, 4 oz; tumbler, 7 to 8 oz; tall glass, 8 oz; can of soft drink, 12 oz. Note that alcoholic beverages are not listed below. They do contain water but also stimulate urination to the extent that there is little, if any, fluid retained by the body. This effect is shared by coffees and teas that contain caffeine, but not to the same extent.

BEVERAGE	SERVING SIZE	NUMBER OF SERVINGS	TOTAL AMOUNT CONSUMED
Water (tap or bottled)	________	________	________
Coffee, any kind	________	________	________
Tea, any kind	________	________	________
Juice, any variety	________	________	________
Juice-like drinks (e.g., Kool Aid, Tang)	________	________	________
Soft drinks	________	________	________
Fluid replacement drinks (e.g., Gatorade, Exceed)	________	________	________
Other beverages	________	________	________
		Total fluid consumption =	________

REFERENCES

1. Roberts KE: Normal metabolic requirements. In Maxwell WH, Kleeman CR, editors: *Clinical disorders of fluid and electrolyte metabolism,* New York, 1962, McGraw-Hill.
2. Fomon SJ, Ziegler EE: Water and renal solute load. In Fomon SJ, editor: *Nutrition of normal infants,* St Louis, 1993, Mosby.
3. Adolph EI: *Physiology of man in the desert,* New York, 1947, Interscience.
4. Sawka MN, Pandolph KB: Effect of body water loss on exercise performance and physiological functions. In Gesolfi CV, Lamb DR, editors: *Perspectives in exercise science and sports medicine, vol 3, Fluid homeostasis during exercise,* Indianapolis, 1990, Benchmark Press.
5. Keating JP, Schears GJ, Dodge PR: Oral water intoxication in infants: an American epidemic. *Am J Dis Child* 145:985, 1991.
6. Klein H: Dental caries (DMF) experiences in relocated children exposed to water containing fluorine, *J Am Dent Assoc* 33:1136, 1946.
7. Schultz D: *Fluoride FDA consumer,* Washington, DC, 1992, The Food and Drug Administration.
8. Ekstrand J and others: Fluoride pharmacokinetics during acid-base balance changes in man, *Eur J Clin Pharmacol* 18:189, 1980.
9. Whitford GM: The physiological and toxicological characteristics of fluoride, *J Dent Res* 69:539, 1990.
10. Groeneveld A, Van Eck AAMJ, Dirks OB: Fluoride in caries prevention: is the effect pre- or post-eruptive? *J Dent Res* 69:751, 1990.
11. Ten Cate JM: *In vitro* studies on the effects of fluoride on de- and remineralization *J Dent Res* 69:614, 1990.
12. Hamilton I, Bowden G: Effect of fluoride on oral microorganisms. In Ekstrand Y, Fejerskov O, Silverstone LM, editors: *Fluoride in dentistry,* Capenhagen, Denmark, 1988, Munksgaar.
13. Aasenden R, Peebles TC: Effects of fluoride supplementation from birth on human deciduous and permanent teeth, *Arch Oral Biol* 19:321, 1974.

14. American Academy of Pediatrics, Committee on Nutrition: Fluoride supplementation: revised dosage schedule, *Pediatrics* 63:150, 1979.

15. American Academy of Pediatrics, Committee on Nutrition: Fluoride supplementation, *Pediatrics* 77:758, 1986.

16. National Research Council/Institute of Medicine: *Recommended dietary allowances,* Washington, DC, 1989, National Academy of Sciences Press.

17. Health and Welfare Canada: *Nutrition recommendations,* Ottawa, Canada, 1990, Canadian Government Publishing Centre.

18. National Research Council: *Diet and health: implications for reducing chronic disease risk. Report of the Committee on Diet and Health, Food and Nutrition Board,* Washington, DC, 1989, National Academy of Sciences Press.

19. Stamler J and others: Intersalt study findings: public health and medical care implications, *Hypertension* 14:570, 1989.

20. Haddy FJ: Sodium, potassium, and hypertension, *Cardiol Illustrated* 2:19, 1987.

21. Law MR, Frost CD, Wald NJ: Analyses of data from trials of salt restriction, *BMJ* 302:819, 1991.

22. Siani A and others: Increasing the dietary potassium intake reduces the need for antihypertension medication, *Ann Intern Med* 115:753, 1991.

23. Haddy FJ: Role of sodium, potassium, calcium, and natriuretic factors in hypertension, *Hypertension* 18(suppl 3):179, 1991.

24. Ray S: The chloride depletion syndrome, *Adv Pediatr* 31:235, 1984.

25. Malloy MH and others: Hypochloremic metabolic alkalosis from ingestion of a chloride deficient infant formula: outcome 9 and 10 years later, *Pediatrics* 87:811, 1991.

ADDITIONAL READINGS

Water

Adolph EI: *Physiology of man in the desert,* New York, 1947, Interscience.

Marriott BM, Rosemont C: *Fluid replacement and heat stress: proceedings of a workshop,* Washington, DC, 1991, National Academy Press.

Robinson JR: Water and life, *World Rev Nutr Diet* 12:172, 1970.

Walker JS and others: Water intake of normal children, *Science* 140:890, 1963.

Fluoride

Drummond BK, Curzon MEJ, Strong M: Estimation of fluoride absorption from swallowed fluoride toothpastes, *Caries Res* 24:211, 1990.

Szpunai SM, Burt BA: Trends in the development of dental fluorosis in the United States: a review, *J Public Health Dent* 47:71, 1987.

Whitford GM: Fluoride in dental products: safety considerations, *J Dent Res* 66:1056, 1987.

Sodium

Beilin LJ: Diet and hypertension—critical concepts and controversies, *J Hypertens* 5(suppl 5):S447, 1987.

Frost CD, Law MR, Wald NJ: By how much does dietary salt reduction lower blood pressure? II. Analysis of observational data within populations, *BMJ* 302:815, 1991.

Joossens JV, Geboers J: Dietary salt and risks to health, *Am J Clin Nutr* 45:1277, 1987.

Law MR, Frost CD, Wald NJ: By how much does dietary salt reduction lower blood pressure? I. Analysis of observational data among populations, *BMJ* 302:811, 1991.

Law MR, Frost CD, Wald NJ: By how much does dietary salt reduction lower blood pressure? III. Analysis of data from trials of salt reduction, *BMJ* 302:819, 1991.

Weinberger MH: Sodium chloride and blood pressures, *N Engl J Med* 317:1084, 1987.

Potassium

Cappuccio FP, MacGregor GA: Does potassium supplementation lower blood pressure? a meta-analysis of published trials, *J Hypertens* 9:465, 1991.

Siani AP and others: Increasing the dietary potassium intake reduces the need for antihypertensive medication, *Ann Intern Med* 115:753, 1991.

Tobian L: Potassium and hypertension, *Nutr Rev* 46:273, 1988.

O V E R V I E W

Minerals

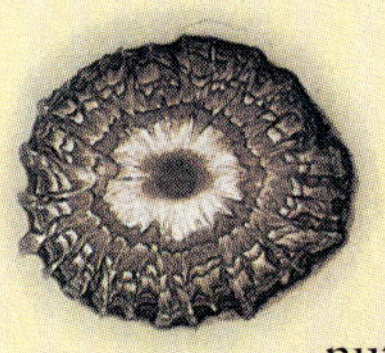

All of the chemicals on Earth, apart from the carbon-containing organic compounds made in living organisms, are known as **minerals**. Minerals are one of the six categories of nutrients essential for life. The key distinction between minerals and the other chemicals of life is that (apart from a few exceptions discussed below) minerals ***do not contain carbon atoms*** within their structure, although they often combine with carbon-containing organic chemicals when performing their functions in the body. The terminology in this area is not as clear-cut as it could be, however. Carbon dioxide (CO_2) contains carbon atoms and is formed as a waste product in the body from the metabolism of organic compounds, but it is normally considered a mineral compound rather than an organic compound. Crude oil, containing organic chemicals derived from ancient living things, is often referred to as ***mineral oil***. Such compounds as calcium carbonate ($CaCO_3$), which contain carbon atoms but are found largely in the form of natural rock deposits, are considered to be minerals rather than organic compounds. Also, water is a mineral compound but is traditionally listed as a distinct category of nutrient, considered separately from all other mineral nutrients because of its unique importance to life.

The element earth and the element air.
Wheatfield by Robert Zünd, painted in 1855.

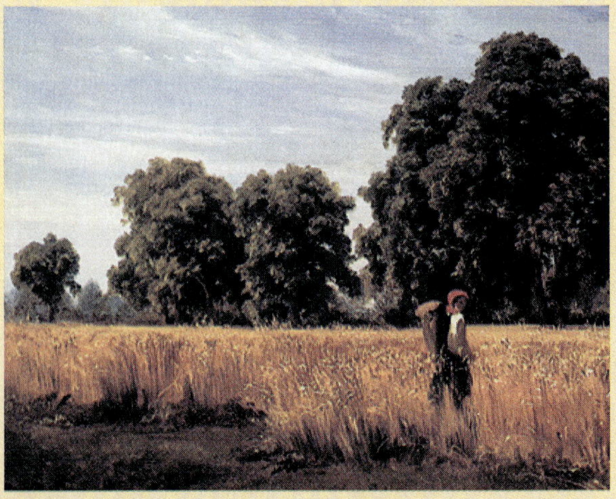

An enormous number of different minerals are found on earth, including all the various kinds of rocks that make up the solid structure of the planet. All minerals, however, are composed of various arrangements of just the 92 naturally occurring elements listed in the periodic table (see p. 3). Thus the mineral compound sodium chloride (NaCl) is composed of the mineral elements sodium and chlorine. The mineral compound magnesium sulfate ($MgSo_4$) is composed of the mineral elements magnesium and sulfur, along with oxygen, and so on. This greatly simplifies the consideration of minerals in nutrition because it allows us to focus attention on only the mineral *elements* required by the body without worrying too much about which compounds these elements are part of. It may be necessary to assess the chemical behavior of mineral compounds in food to determine how readily they are absorbed into the body and how readily their constituent minerals are made available to body metabolism, but the mineral elements themselves are the main objects of our attention.

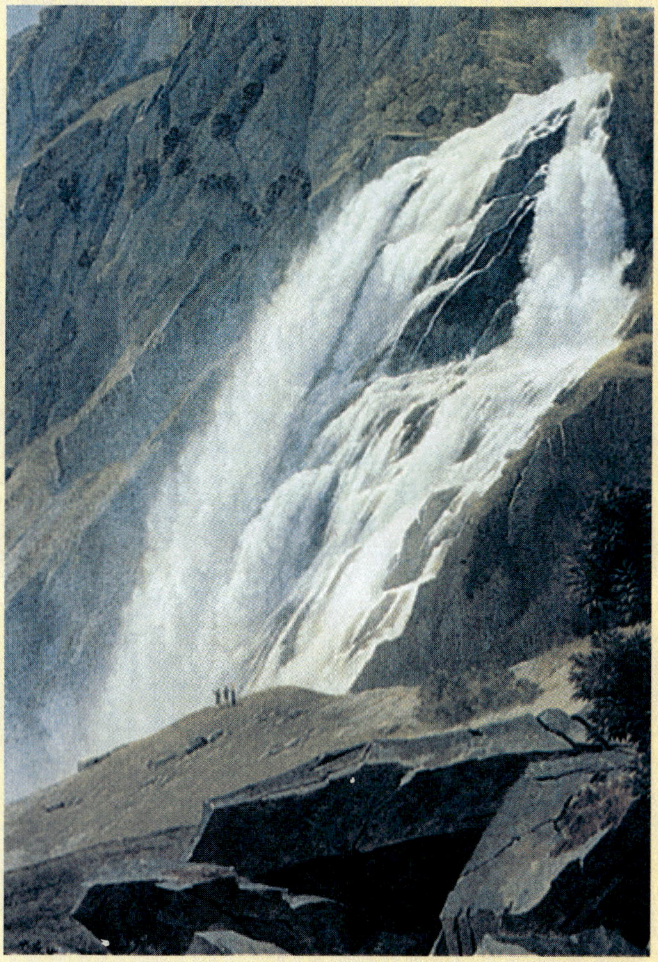

Essential water.
Cascade de Pissevache, detail
by Johann Jakob Biedermann, painted in 1815.

Each mineral element, of course, is composed of only one type of atom, although in food and in the body the mineral atoms have usually been converted into ions by the loss or gain of one or more electrons. Thus the element sodium consists solely of sodium atoms, although present in the body as Na^+ ions; the element chlorine contains only chlorine atoms, present in the body mostly as Cl^- ions; and so on.

Our knowledge of the importance of mineral elements dates from the middle of the nineteenth century. Scientists of that time fed mice a mixture of carbohydrate, fat, protein, and water, which they thought were the only essential nutrients, and were baffled to find that the animals died. This made it obvious that some other component or components of food must be essential for life. One clue was the small amount of ash left behind when food was burned. When this ash was added to the diet of the mice, however, they still died. We now know that the ash did indeed contain essential minerals, missing from the original diet, but the ash-supplemented diet was still lacking in vitamins, which did not become apparent until 1912. Subsequent research on the minerals essential for good nutrition has revealed that, although required in relatively small amounts, they play a wide variety of crucial roles within the living and growing body.

For a mineral to be considered essential, it must perform at least one function that is vital for life, growth, or reproduction. The following lines of evidence are all required to indicate that it performs some vital function:

- There must be an improvement in health or growth when, having previously been absent from or deficient in the diet, the mineral is included in the diet in amounts compatible with the normal operation of the body
- There must be evidence of a deterioration in health or growth when the mineral is removed from the diet or is present in reduced amounts.
- A detectable reduction in the levels of the mineral in blood or other tissues must be associated with the deterioration in health or growth noted previously.
- There should be good reason to believe that the normal function of the mineral cannot be adequately performed by some other component of the diet.

TABLE OV2-1

Classification of minerals found in the body

CLASSIFICATION	MINERALS*	BODY WEIGHT (%)	AMOUNT IN BODY BASED ON 80-kg (176-lb) MAN	RECOMMENDED DIETARY INTAKE FOR ADULTS
MACRONUTRIENT MINERALS				
(>0.005% body weight, or 50 ppm)				
Minerals essential for human nutrition	Calcium	1.5-2.2	1.2 kg	800 mg‡
	Phosphorus	0.8-1.2	0.64 kg	800 mg‡
	Potassium	0.35	0.28 kg	700 mg§
	Sulfur	0.25	0.20 kg	
	Sodium	0.15	0.12 kg	500 mg§
	Chlorine	0.15	0.12 kg	2000 mg§
	Magnesium (1950)	0.05	0.04 kg	300-350 mg‡
MICRONUTRIENT MINERALS				
(<0.005% body weight or 50 ppm)				
Minerals essential for human nutrition	Iron (17th century)	0.004	3.2 g	10-18 mg‡
	Zinc (1934)	0.002	1.6 g	15 mg‡
	Selenium (1957)	0.0003	0.24 g	0.05-0.07 mg‡
	Manganese (1931)	0.0002	0.16 g	2.0-5.0 mg‖
	Copper (1928)	0.00015	0.12 g	1.5-3.0 mg‖
	Iodine (1850)	0.00004	0.032 g	0.15 mg‡
	Molybdenum (1953)	0.0002	0.16 g	0.075-0.25 mg‖
	Cobalt (1935)	0.00003	0.024 g	0.15-0.5 mg
	Chromium (1959)	0.00003	0.024 g	0.05-0.2 mg‖
Minerals for which essentiality has not yet been established, although there is evidence of their participation in certain biological reactions	Silicon (1972)†			
	Vanadium (1971)†	0.00045	0.36 g	
	Nickel (1971)†	0.00023	0.18 g	
	Arsenic (1980)†			
	Boron (1987)†			
	Fluorine (1972)†			1.5-4.0 mg ‖
	Tin (1970)†			
	Barium			
	Bromine			
	Strontium	0.0006	0.48 g	
	Cadmium	0.0006	0.48 g	
Minerals found in the body that have not been assigned a metabolic role yet	Gold			
	Silver			
	Aluminum			
	Mercury			
	Bismuth			
	Gallium			
	Lead			
	Antimony			
	Lithium			
	+20 others			

* Dates in parentheses identify year in which essentiality was established.
† Essentiality almost certain or a health benefit established and essentiality being debated.
‡ Recommended dietary allowances established.
§ Estimated safe and adequate daily dietary intakes.
‖ Estimated minimal requirement.

From National Research Council/Food and Nutrition Board: *Recommended dietary allowances,* ed 10, Washington, DC, 1989, National Academy of Sciences.

Sixteen mineral elements are now known to meet these criteria and are therefore considered essential (Table Ov2-1). For eleven others (silicon, vandium, nickel, arsenic boron, fluoride, tin, barium, bromine, strontium, and cadmium), there is evidence that they participate in certain biological reactions, although it has not yet been established that any of them are actually essential. Of these minerals, tin is currently a strong candidate for essentiality, and even if not absolutely essential, it is certainly associated with some benefit to health. Similarly, while a health benefit can be demonstrated for fluoride, some authorities argue that it is not absolutely essential for maintenance of dental health and therefore is not an essential micronutrient element. An additional 29 minerals are found in the body, but no role for them in metabolism has yet been uncovered. It remains possible (and indeed probable) that further research will result in more additions to the list of minerals considered essential for optimal health. In general, a mineral is categorized as essential only when it has been established as essential by at least two independent research teams and in more than one species of animal.

Table Ov2 - 1 indicates that the essential minerals can be divided into two categories: the **macronutrient minerals,** which are present in the body in relatively large amounts (and therefore required in the diet in relatively large amounts), and the **micronutrient minerals,** which are present and required in relatively small amounts. It is important to realize, however, that the amounts of *all* minerals present in the body and required in the diet are small, when compared with the amounts of water, carbohydrate, fat, and protein in the body and in food. Thus a mineral is defined as a macronutrient mineral if present in the body at a concentration of more than 50 parts per million (ppm), or more than 0.005% of body weight. Most of the macronutrient minerals account for considerably less than 1% of body weight, and even the most abundant—calcium—accounts for only 1.5% to 2.2% of body weight. It follows from this definition that the micronutrient minerals are those present in the body at concentrations of less than 50 ppm, or less than 0.005% of body weight.

The terms **macroelements** and **microelements** are often used in place of *macronutrient minerals* and *micronutrient minerals,* respectively. The micronutrient minerals (or microelements) are also often known as **trace elements.** Although present only in small, or "trace," amounts, however, they are extremely important to health. For example, iodine represents only 1 part in 80 million of body weight, but iodine deficiency can be as debilitating as a deficiency of calcium, which represents about 2 parts per hundred (2%) of body weight.

Functions

Minerals are involved in a wide variety of biochemical processes within the body, many of which probably remain to be discovered. This section provides only a brief summary of the main categories of function known to be performed by minerals. Fuller details of specific examples are given where appropriate in Chapters 9 and 10.

Components of Essential Body Compounds

A wide variety of essential compounds in the body include mineral atoms or ions as part of their structure. Bones and teeth contain large concentrations of calcium- and phosphorus-containing compounds, playing largely structural roles. Chlorine, in the form of chloride ions, is required to form the hydrochloric acid within the stomach, which assists in digestion. The hormone thyroxin includes four iodine atoms within its molecular structure. The vitamin thiamine contains sulfur, vitamin B_{12} contains cobalt, and so on. Many specific examples are given in subsequent chapters, but the general point is that without minerals, many of the most essential compounds of the body could not be formed.

In many cases the minerals are permanently incorporated into the structure of the body compounds, but in other cases they form more loose and temporary associations. In all cases, however, the involvement of the minerals is essential for the compounds concerned to function properly.

Cofactors in Biological Reactions

Many mineral ions bind to specific enzymes and form key parts of the **active sites** of the enzymes, which are the regions of the enzymes at which the reactions they catalyze actually take place. The mineral ions are known as **cofactors** required by the enzymes. The mineral ions concerned are usually ions of metals—such as iron, zinc, and copper—and in such cases, the complexes they form with enzymes are known as **metalloenzymes.**

Because enzymes catalyze virtually every chemical reaction of life and because about one third of all known enzymes require the presence of mineral ions to function properly, this role of minerals alone is

FIGURE OV2-1

Minerals required for the key pathways of metabolism.

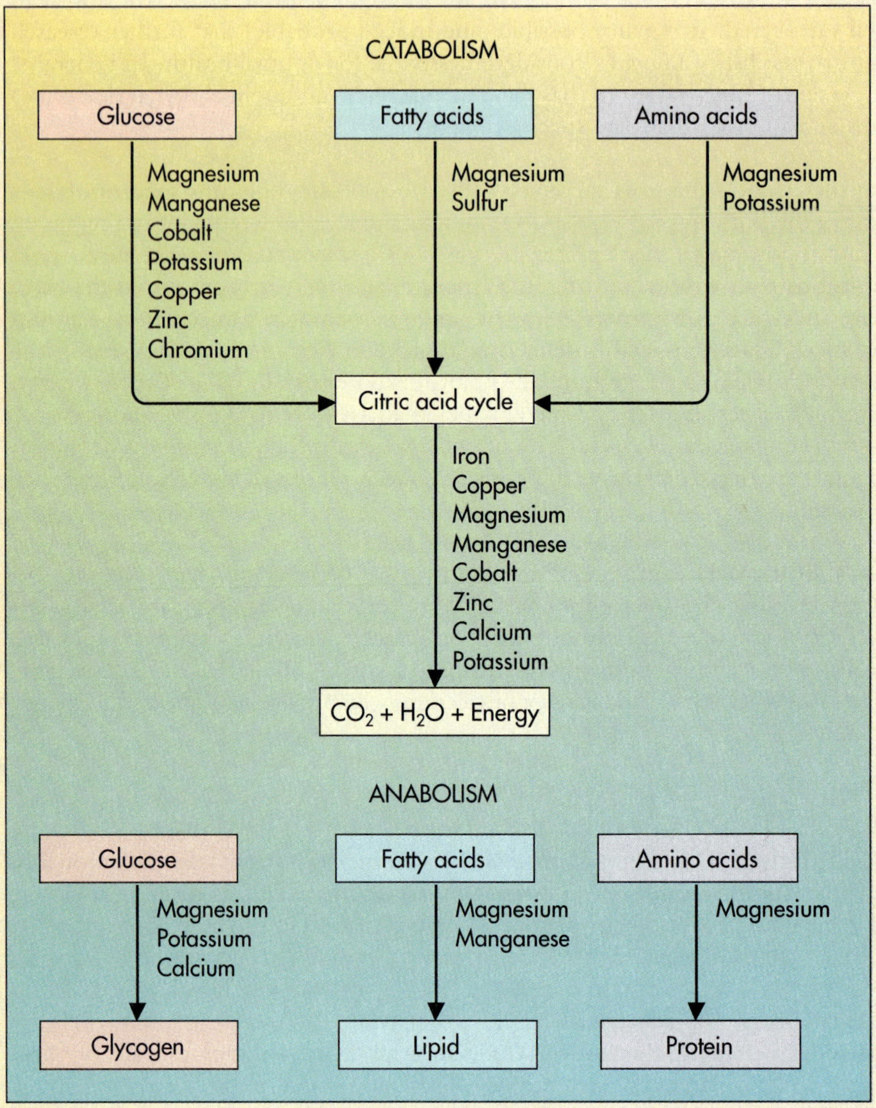

sufficient to make them essential for life. Figure Ov2 - 1 indicates the specific minerals required for the key pathways of anabolism and catabolism. Each of the enzymes concerned requires a specific mineral ion to operate, and so a deficiency of any one type of mineral causes a loss of function of only the particular enzymes that require it. This effect of particular mineral deficiencies lies behind many of the specific problems associated with them.

Mineral ions can also act as cofactors for proteins that are not enzymes, and some mineral atoms or groupings of atoms can become covalently bonded to such chemicals as proteins to influence their activities. Many proteins, for example, are activated ("switched on") by the process of phosphorylation in which a phosphate ion (PO_4^{3-}) becomes attached to a specific part of the protein via a covalent bond between the phosphorus atom of the phosphate ion and an oxygen atom of the protein. The protein hemoglobin, which transports oxygen in the body, incorporates ions of the mineral iron, which actually bind to the oxygen molecules and so attach them to the protein. The list of crucial biological reactions that depend on mineral cofactors is long and varied, but the general principle behind it is that the diverse chemical properties of mineral ions have been exploited during the course of evolution in ways that make many of the chemical processes of life possible.

Facilitation of Absorption, Digestion, and Transport
The absorption of some nutrients from the gastrointestinal tract and their transport across cell membranes within the body are dependent on a variety of minerals. How sodium facilitates the absorption of carbohydrates and their entry into various types of cell has already been discussed. Magnesium also facilitates carbohydrate absorption, whereas calcium facilitates the absorption of vitamin B_{12}. Also, several digestive enzymes are activated by minerals within the gastrointestinal tract.

Maintenance of Acid-Base Balance
Most of the biological reactions within the body can occur only when the pH value of the cell lies within a fairly narrow range. For most cells and body fluids the normal pH range is between pH 7.35 and 7.45, which is just slightly more alkaline than the neutral pH 7 of pure water. The most significant exception to this guideline is the gastric fluid in the stomach, which is maintained at an acidic pH of around 2. One major reason for the sensitivity of cell chemistry to the pH value is that the structure and function of the crucial enzyme molecules are sensitive to changes in the pH value.

The pH level of a fluid is determined directly by the relative concentrations of hydrogen ions (H^+) and hydroxide ions (OH^-) in the solution. As discussed in Chapter 8, however, other ions can have a strong influence on pH value because of their differing tendencies to combine with hydrogen or hydroxide ions and so remove them from solution. This means that the particular mixture of mineral ions in any region of the body or within any food has a strong influence on the prevailing pH level. Some major acid-forming minerals are chlorine (as the chloride ion), sulfur (often found within the sulfate ion [SO_4^{2-}]), and phosphorus (usually found within the phosphate ion [PO_4^{3-}]). Some major alkali-forming (or base forming) minerals are sodium (as Na^+ ions), potassium (K^+), magnesium (Mg^{2+}), and calcium (Ca^{2+}).

The acid-forming or alkali-forming properties of foods tend to be largely determined by the proportions in which these various minerals are present in them. Foods in which acid-forming minerals predominate are known as **acid-forming foods** and include most high-protein foods such as meat, fish, poultry, eggs, and cereals. Foods in which alkali-forming minerals predominate are known as **alkali-forming foods** (or **base-forming foods**) and include most fruits, vegetables, and nuts. Some foods are regarded as **neutral foods** because they contain few minerals or an even balance of acid- and alkali-forming minerals and thus have little effect on the pH level. Neutral foods include milk, sugar, starch, fats, and oils.

Most mixed diets contain a slight excess of acid-forming minerals, but the body has a variety of mechanisms to counteract their acid-forming effects. First, excess acid is removed from the body by the excretion of carbon dioxide (which forms an acid in solution) through the lungs and by the excretion of urine (which is slightly acidic). Also, blood and other body fluids contain a variety of chemicals that are able to stabilize pH at optimal levels by reducing the concentration of hydrogen ions in solution if the solution is too acidic or increasing the concentration of hydrogen ions in solution if the solution is too alkaline. Such chemicals are known as **buffers,** and they include various carbonates, phosphates, and protein molecules.

Two further mechanisms are available that cope with situations where excess acid or alkali threatens to overwhelm the buffers. If excess acidity is the problem, this can be neutralized by the trapping of some hydrogen ions within ammonium ions (NH_4^+), formed using nitrogen released by the deamination of proteins. If excess alkalinity is the problem, the alkali can be neutralized by reacting with carbonic acid (H_2CO_3), formed when carbon dioxide waste reacts with water. So the body is well equipped with mechanisms to maintain acid-base balance (or acid-alkali balance) and avoid the problems of acidosis (acidic blood) or alkalosis (alkaline blood). These mechanisms ensure that a disturbance in acid-base balance is seldom caused by the acid-forming or alkali-forming foods in our diet alone. When such disturbances do arise from a variety of medical problems, however, they can sometimes be complicated by the acidity or alkalinity of food.

Maintenance of Water Balance
As was discussed in Chapter 8, mineral ions have a great influence on the movement of water among the various fluid compartments of the body because of their effect on the osmotic pressure of the solutions

of which they are part. The physiological systems of the body exploit this effect of mineral ions by transporting them across cell membranes and secreting them into specific fluids in the body in a way that exerts considerable control over the process of water balance within the entire body.

Transmission of Nerve Impulses

Minerals play a central role in the transmission of nerve impulses along nerve fibers because a nerve impulse is essentially just a wave of mineral ion movement across the nerve cell membrane. When a nerve cell is induced to "fire"—or, in other words, to transmit an impulse—proteins in the membrane called ***sodium channels*** change to the "open" configuration. This allows sodium ions to flood into the cell from the extracellular fluid, where they are more abundant. This entry of positive ions changes the electrical balance of the membrane in a way that causes neighboring sodium channels to open. Thus a wave of sodium ion entry moves down the cell, but the entry of sodium is soon blocked by the closing of the sodium channels. Normality is then restored by membrane proteins that pump sodium ions and other ions (especially potassium ions) across the nerve cell membrane. When the nerve impulse reaches the end of the nerve cell, it induces proteins in the membrane to let calcium ions (Ca^{2+}) enter the cell. These calcium ions induce the cell to release neurotransmitter molecules, which can bind to the membrane of the next nerve cell in line and —if other circumstances allow—initiate it to fire and so cause the whole process to be repeated in another nerve cell. That is a brief summary of the foundations of a complex process, but it is sufficient to make it clear that mineral ions—especially sodium, potassium, and calcium ions—are essential for the normal functioning of the nervous system. Thus all of the activities of the brain; all of our senses such as sight, hearing, touch, and pain sensations; and the ability of the nervous system to control the movement of muscles, depend on an adequate supply of appropriate minerals in the diet.

Regulation of Muscle Contraction

The muscles of the body are bathed in the intercellular fluid, which contains some ions that encourage muscular contraction (such as calcium ions) and some that encourage muscular relaxation (such as sodium, potassium, and magnesium ions). For muscles to function normally, contracting when stimulated by the arrival of nerve signals and relaxing when not, the concentrations of these mineral ions must be maintained at appropriately balanced levels. Dietary variations in the supply of the minerals are usually compensated for automatically, however. So any disturbance in mineral levels that interferes with muscle contraction is usually caused by hormonal changes or various diseases, rather than by dietary factors.

Sources

Minerals are present in both drinking water and solid food. The kinds and amounts of minerals in drinking water depend on the type of rocks and soils to which the water is exposed on its way to the public supply (and any additional fluoridation of the supply). Some of the minerals listed in Table Ov2 - 1 as essential for humans are also required for plant growth and therefore must be found in the plants that humans eat. Other minerals that are essential for humans but not for plants, such as sodium and iodine, nevertheless occur in plants and therefore foods of plant origin.

Because minerals are essentially just atoms or ions, they cannot be synthesized by any form of life. So all of the minerals within humans and other animals have been taken in as minerals within food or water, and all of the minerals within plants have been absorbed through the plants' roots as minerals that were originally present in the soil or were added through organic or chemical fertilizers.

Requirements

Although plants—unlike animals—can take in minerals directly from the soil, minerals are actually present in a higher concentration in foods of animal origin than of plant origin. The animals we eat, however, have obtained these minerals largely by eating plants, although some minerals are present in the water animals drink. Another advantage of foods of animal origin is that the minerals they contain are often in a form that is more readily absorbed by the body. Such minerals are said to be more **bioavailable** than those in other forms. So foods of animal origin are often better sources of minerals than foods of plant origin because of a combination of greater mineral content and greater bioavailability of the minerals they contain.

TABLE OV2-2

Dietary factors influencing mineral absorption

Chemical form
Oxidation state
Amount in the diet
Other nutrients in the diet
Minerals
Carbohydrates
Lipids
Proteins
Vitamins
Nonnutritive components of the diet
Phytate
Fiber

Modified from Trunlund J: *Crit Rev Food Sci Nutr* 30:387, 1991.

The amount of a mineral needed each day for adequate nutrition varies from much less than a milligram to as much as 2000 mg (2g). Table Ov2-1 lists current estimates of the actual values for each mineral. The Recommended Dietary Allowances (RDAs) have been established for the macronutrient minerals calcium, phosphorus, and magnesium and for the micronutrient minerals iron, zinc, iodine, and selenium. Estimated Safe and Adequate Daily Dietary Intakes have also been established for copper, manganese, fluoride, chromium, and molybdenum, and Estimated Minimum Requirements have been established for sodium, potassium, and chloride.

When assessing a diet for mineral adequacy or excess, it is not sufficient simply to compare the total amount of each mineral in the diet with the estimated requirements listed in Table Ov2-1. It is important to also consider the *bioavailability* of each mineral. The proportion of an ingested mineral that is actually absorbed into the body can vary from less than 1% to more than 90%, depending on the mineral concerned and various other factors.[2] The main factors that can cause the bioavailability of any particular mineral to vary are listed in Table Ov2-2. Some minerals, including sodium and potassium, are well absorbed in most circumstances, regardless of the composition of the diet. Other minerals are poorly absorbed even under optimal conditions and can be even less effectively absorbed in certain chemical forms; or in the presence of such substances as fiber, which inhibit the absorption of some minerals.

The minerals present in grains are concentrated in the outer husk of the grain, which is rich in fiber and **phytic acid**; both tend to restrict the absorption of minerals into the body. This means that the difference in the amounts of minerals available from whole grain and refined cereals is not as great as might be expected. Although the refining process removes many of the minerals in the whole grain, it also removes the fiber and phytic acid, thus allowing the remaining minerals of the grain to be absorbed more effectively into the body.

Only about 3% of the iron in foods of plant origin is normally absorbed by the body. The protein hemoglobin in foods of animal origin, however, contains iron in a form that allows about 20% to 25% of it to be absorbed. This explains why red meats and liver are rich sources of iron for the body. Another example of bioavailability variation is provided by chromium. This mineral can be present in a wide variety of chemical forms, including natural chromium complexes, inorganic chromium salts, and the insoluble compound chromium chloride. The chromium of chromium chloride is not absorbed into the body at all, chromium within natural chromium complexes found within food is absorbed quite well, and the chromium of inorganic salts is absorbed at varying levels, depending on the particular salt concerned and the chemical form of the chromium.[3]

Deficiency and toxicity

The deficiency or absence of an essential mineral in the diet results in deficiency symptoms that become increasingly severe the greater the deficiency, perhaps leading to death in cases of extreme and prolonged deficiency. Deficiencies of most minerals become evident only after fairly prolonged dietary inadequacies and, in some cases, only when decreased absorption or other changes in the body lead to requirements

FIGURE OV2-2

A graphic representation of the concept of a safe range of mineral intake. The dotted line represents uncertainty about the point at which an intake becomes lethal.

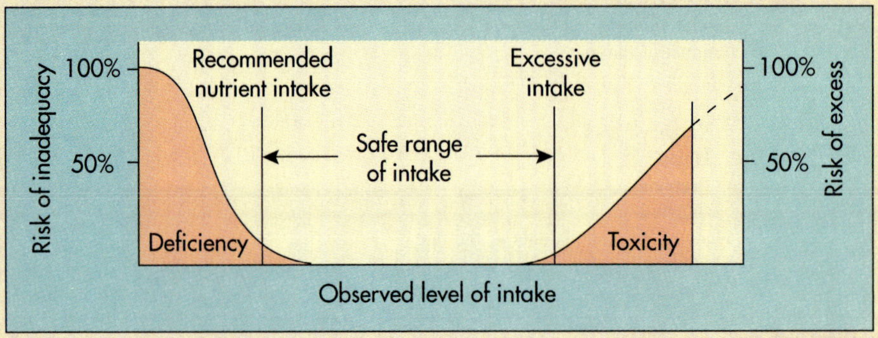

above normal. It is not appropriate to protect oneself against the dangers of mineral deficiency by consuming as much of the mineral as possible, however, because minerals can have toxic effects at excessive levels.

The dangers of both deficiency and excess have led to the concept of a "safe range" of mineral intake. (Figure Ov2-2). The actual quantities involved vary among minerals, but the general concept of the deficiency-toxicity curve of Figure Ov2-2 applies to all minerals. Consuming an amount of a mineral anywhere in the safe range should be sufficient to sustain good health while avoiding any of the toxic effects associated with the mineral. If intake falls into the deficiency range, symptoms appear, with the severity dependent on how far into the deficiency range the intake has fallen. Conversely, if intake rises into the toxicity range, symptoms of toxicity appear, with the severity dependent on how far into the toxicity range the intake has risen. Individuals also vary in their sensitivity to specific levels of toxicity or deficiency.

For some minerals a wide range of intakes can be regarded as safe. For others—such as iron, copper, selenium, and zinc—the safe range of intake is rather narrow. The fact that minerals are toxic in excess, combined with the fact that they are all required in only small quantities, raises considerable concern about the indiscriminate use of mineral supplements as supposed aids to good health. Such concerns apply particularly to those minerals whose safe range of intake is narrow.

Regulation of mineral content by the body

Because problems are caused by both deficiencies and excesses of minerals, it is not surprising that evolution has equipped the body with various mechanisms to regulate its essential mineral content in ways that tend to maintain optimal levels. Regulation can be achieved by alterations in both the amount of a mineral absorbed and the amount excreted. Excess minerals can be excreted in urine and feces and through the skin in perspiration; however, increased reabsorption by the kidneys can limit urinary losses in times of need (see Chapter 8). There appear to be no comparable mechanisms for regulating the amount of the nonessential minerals absorbed or excreted. This means that nutritionists must promote the use of food-processing procedures that avoid excessive introduction of nonessential minerals into the food supply, as well as ensuring that the processing methods retain essential minerals as much as possible.

Interactions between minerals

One of the major difficulties in getting information on the functions of many minerals is the extent to which some minerals can interact with one another in ways that modify the effects of the minerals and our requirements for them. Such interactions can be **synergistic** (each mineral enhancing the effects of the other) or **antagonistic** (each mineral working against some aspect of the other's metabolism or function).

For example, increased copper levels interfere with the metabolism of iron and zinc. High levels of manganese interfere with iron metabolism. High intakes of calcium can reduce the absorption of iron, whereas too much iron can reduce the absorption of zinc. An increase in the molybdenum content of the diet without a simultaneous increase in copper or sulfur content results in depressed growth and restricted hemoglobin production.

Various minerals can also offer some protection against the toxic effects of other minerals. Selenium, for example, protects the body to some extent against the toxic effects of mercury, whereas calcium offers some protection against the toxicity of lead. However, abnormally high levels of some minerals can cause these minerals to displace other required minerals from enzyme molecules, leading to a loss of enzyme activity.

Problems caused by mineral interactions are most likely to occur when there is a significant imbalance in the intakes of the minerals concerned. This is unlikely to occur when food is selected from a wide variety of sources, which is one of the basic guidelines of good nutrition. It can result, however, from the indiscriminate use of mineral supplements. Formulas for mineral supplements are too often developed to give the producer a competitive advantage, rather than to meet the nutritional needs of the consumer. Unbalanced mineral supplements, for example, one which provides 300% of the RDA of one mineral and only 15% of another, are without a doubt potentially harmful, yet it is now possible for the public to buy any amount of most minerals on the open market without a prescription.

~ BY NOW YOU SHOULD KNOW ~

- Minerals, elements essential in human nutrition, are found in the ash, or noncombustible portion, of food.
- Macronutrient minerals, or macroelements, are present in amounts of more than 50 parts per million (ppm), or 0.005% of body weight.
- Micronutrient elements, also known as *microelements* or *trace elements*, are present in amounts of less than 50 ppm, or 0.005% of body weight.
- The pH, or relative acidic and basic properties, of body fluids and tissues is influenced by the balance of acid- and base-forming elements.
- The body counteracts excess acid by excreting more acidic urine or exhaling more carbon dioxide. Excess base is counteracted by carbonic acid, formed from carbon dioxide and water. Buffers such as proteins, carbonates, and phosphates also help maintain the desirable pH level.
- Minerals in animal tissues are present in higher concentrations and are more readily absorbed or bioavailable than those in plant foods.
- For some minerals the range between adequate and toxic intakes is wide, whereas for others it is comparatively narrow.
- The mineral content of body fluids influences water balance, the transmission of nerve impulses, and the contraction of muscles.
- Many minerals interact with one another to influence the absorption of the other or the amount of each needed.

~ STUDY QUESTIONS ~

1. Name four macronutrient minerals and four micronutrient minerals.
2. How do minerals influence the pH level of body fluids?
3. How does the body counteract excess acid or excess base in body fluids or tissues?
4. Define the following terms as related to minerals: bioavailability, trace element, metalloenzymes, safe range of intake, synergistic reactions, and antagonistic reactions.
5. List factors that determine the amount of a mineral in a plant food.
6. Why are minerals present in higher concentrations in animal foods than in plant foods?
7. Identify four factors that influence the bioavailability of minerals from food.

~ REFERENCES ~

1. National Research Council/Food and Nutrition Board: *Recommended dietary allowances,* ed 10, Washington DC, 1989, National Academy of Sciences.
2. Trunlund JR: Bioavailability of dietary minerals to humans: the stable isotope approach, *Criti Rev Food Sci Nutr* 30:387, 1991.
3. Anderson RA: Chromium. In Mertz W, editor: *Trace elements in human and animal nutrition,* vol 1, San Diego, 1987, Academic Press.

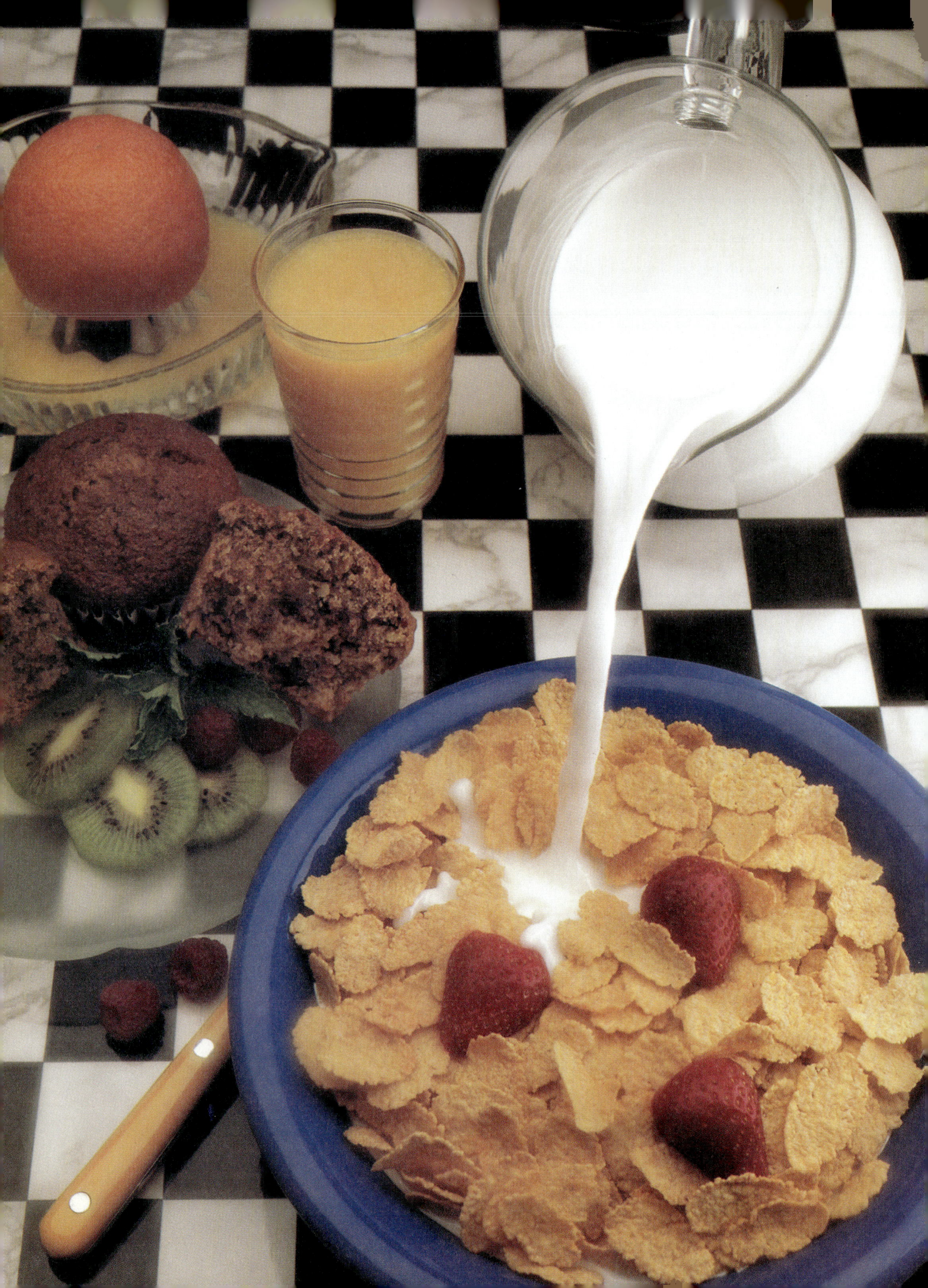

CHAPTER 9

MACRONUTRIENT MINERALS

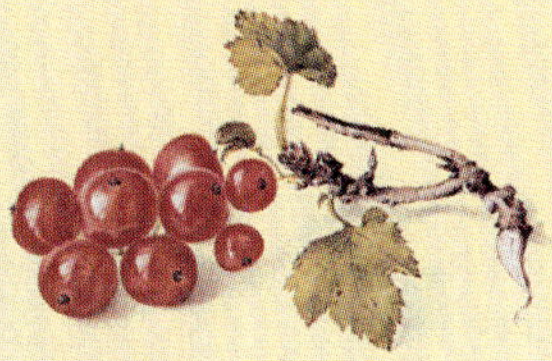

The macronutrient minerals, in order of their abundance in the body, and their percentages of body weight are as follows: calcium (1.5% to 2.2%), phosphorus (0.8% to 1.2%), potassium (0.35%), sulfur (0.25%), sodium (0.15%), chlorine (0.15%), and magnesium (0.05%). They each account for 0.05% or more of total body weight, satisfying the definition of a macronutrient mineral. Those minerals present at levels of less than 0.05% are defined as micronutrient minerals, and the most abundant micronutrient mineral (iron) accounts for a mere 0.004% of body weight, less than one tenth of the proportion accounted for by magnesium, the least abundant of the macronutrient minerals. Thus there is a clear separation between the macronutrient and micronutrient minerals.

The macronutrient minerals sodium, potassium, and chlorine are considered in detail in Chapter 8. The ions of these three minerals (Na^+, K^+, and Cl^-) are three of the main electrolyte ions of the body. As such, they are involved in regulating the flow of water by osmosis between the different regions of the body. These properties of sodium, potassium, and chloride are explored fully in Chapter 8, along with consideration of our dietary requirements for them, the dangers of deficiency, toxicity, and so on. This chapter, therefore, concentrates on the four macronutrient minerals not yet discussed in any detail: calcium, phosphorus, sulfur, and magnesium. It should be remembered, however, that there are seven macronutrient minerals in all, and that this class of minerals includes the three key electrolyte ions: sodium, potassium, and chloride.

CALCIUM (Ca)

Most people correctly associate calcium with bones, teeth, and milk. This presumably reflects widespread publicity on the importance of providing children with adequate calcium to support the growth of bones and teeth, with milk usually highlighted as one of the best dietary sources of calcium. The link between calcium and bones has been further emphasized by growing awareness of its role in preventing osteoporosis, a bone disease that most often affects women after menopause. In addition to its role in the development of bones and teeth, however, calcium also performs a variety of other functions in the body, particularly as a regulator of many of the body's biochemical processes.

DISTRIBUTION

Calcium makes up between 1.5% and 2% of body weight, accounting for 1200 to 1600 g (2.6 to 3.5 lb) of the typical adult male body (80 kg). Almost all (99%) of this calcium is found in the hard tissues of the body—namely, the bones and teeth. The rest is widely distributed throughout the blood and soft tissues, such as muscles, the liver, and the heart. Approximately half of the calcium in the blood exists in the form of free dissolved calcium ions (Ca^{2+}), about 40% is loosely bound to protein molecules, and the remaining 7% to 10% is "complexed" within low–molecular-weight ionic compounds, such as calcium citrate and calcium phosphate (Figure 9-1).

Although 99% of body calcium is within bones and teeth, the relatively small amount distributed throughout the body's cells is vital for the proper functioning of the cells. The importance of the calcium in soft tissues and blood is reflected in the fact that the calcium content of the blood plasma is maintained within a narrow range of 9 to 11 mg/dl, rarely varying by more than 3%. One of the main factors allowing plasma calcium levels to be maintained within such a narrow range is the body's ability to mobilize calcium from reserves in the bones when levels in the plasma begin to fall.

FIGURE 9-1

Distribution of calcium in blood plasma.

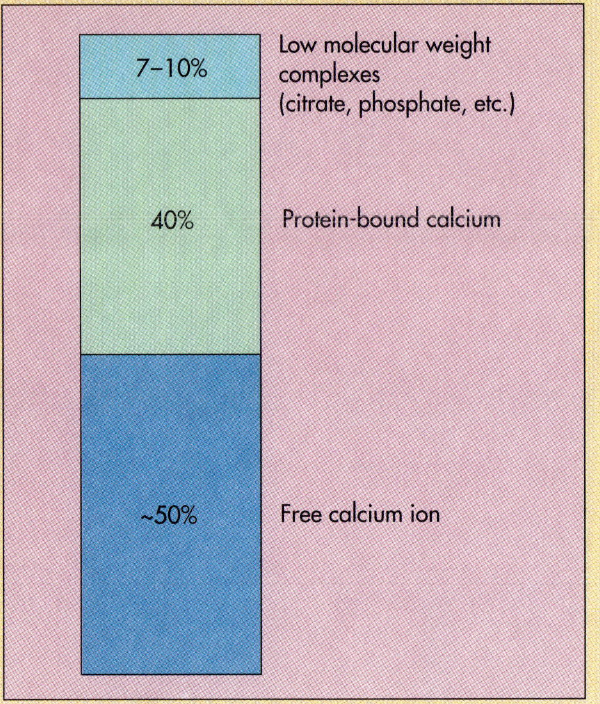

FUNCTIONS

Bone Formation

The formation of bone begins early in fetal development, with the laying down of a strong but flexible **matrix,** which forms the basic structure around which the rest of the bone is assembled. The matrix accounts for about one third of the structure of a bone and remains flexible until after birth, which may make the birth process easier for both the fetus and the mother. The matrix is composed of fibers of a protein called **collagen,** which is embedded in a gelatinous mixture of protein and polysaccharides called **ground substance.** Shortly after birth the matrix begins to gain strength and rigidity, largely because of the deposition of mineral crystals within it. This process is known as **ossification** or **calcification** because the matrix hardens and the minerals involved are calcium-containing compounds. By the time a child is ready to walk, calcification has made the bones strong enough and rigid enough to support the weight of the body.

The mineral crystals laid down during bone calcification are composed of calcium phosphate, $Ca_3(PO_4)_2$, known as **apatite**; or a mixture of calcium phosphate and calcium hydroxide ($Ca[OH]_2$), called **hydroxyapatite.** Because calcium and phosphorus are the predominant mineral elements in bone, an adequate supply of both must be present in the fluid surrounding the bone matrix during growth.

FIGURE 9-2

Diagrammatic representation of bone structure.

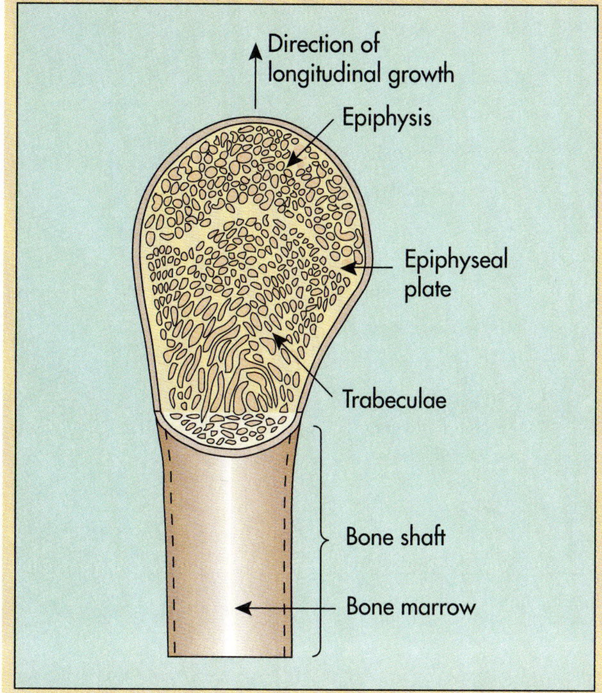

The general structure of a long bone of the body is shown in Figure 9-2. The bone shaft—which is the main and most rigid part of the bone—contains hydroxyapatite, calcium phosphate, and ions of magnesium (Mg^{2+}), zinc (Zn^{2+}), sodium (Na^{+}), carbonate (CO_3^{2-}), and fluoride (F^{-}). This part of a bone is reshaped throughout life as the body grows, or its weight distribution shifts, putting different stresses on the bones. At the end of a long bone is the **epiphysis,** a region that regulates bone growth. Beneath the epiphysis is a more porous region of bone, known as the **trabeculae.** The porosity of the trabeculae permits access to the blood supply, allowing this part of a bone to act as a reservoir of calcium, ready to supply calcium to the blood if plasma calcium levels begin to fall. Trabecular bone tissue also predominates in the vertebrae.

Tooth Formation

The outer and middle layers of a tooth—known as the **enamel** and **dentin,** respectively (Figure 9-3)—contain considerable amounts of hydroxyapatite. In teeth, however, the hydroxyapatite is present alongside a protein called **keratin,** in place of the collagen found in bones. Also, the hydroxyapatite crystals in teeth are more dense, having a lower water content than the hydroxyapatite in bone. The first teeth to "erupt" through the gums into the oral cavity are known as the **deciduous teeth** and are lost between the ages of 5 and 10 years, when they are replaced by a new set of permanent teeth. The calcification of deciduous teeth begins by the time a fetus is about 20 weeks old and is completed only shortly before they erupt, at about 6 months. Permanent teeth begin to calcify when the child is between 3 months and 3 years old, while they are still buried in the gums below the deciduous teeth. The wisdom teeth, which are the last to erupt, may not begin to calcify until a child is between 8 and 10 years old. The full complement of adult teeth contains about 1% of the total calcium found in the hard tissues of the body.

The slow exchange of calcium between the blood and a forming tooth occurs almost entirely in the dentin layer, although there may also be some exchange of calcium between saliva and the tooth enamel. A deficiency of calcium during tooth formation may result in an increased susceptibility to tooth decay. Despite the emphasis on the role of calcium in tooth formation, it should be remembered that—as with bone structure—the integrity of tooth structure also depends on many other nutrients.

Growth

Calcium is obviously required for growth because it forms such an important part of bones and teeth and is also required in much smaller amounts for the proper functioning of every cell in the body. Studies in Japan have revealed that people with a diet that is low in calcium are frequently shorter than those with adequate calcium in their diet. Diets low in calcium, however, are also low in protein, and protein is also required for growth, including the growth of bones. It is difficult to argue, therefore, that we have evidence to suggest that a lack of calcium is ever a primary cause of failure to grow. It may well, however, be a contributing factor.

Cofactor for and Regulator of Biochemical Reactions

The role of calcium in blood clotting is one of the best understood of its functions. When tissue has been injured by a cut, the enzyme **thromboplastin** is released from affected cells or blood platelets. Thromboplastin catalyzes the conversion of the protein **prothrombin** (present in the blood) into **thrombin,** a process that requires the presence of calcium ions. Thrombin is an enzyme that converts a soluble blood protein called **fibrinogen** into **fibrin,** which forms the insoluble network of fibrous protein that composes the basic structure of a blood clot. This process is summarized in Figure 9-4. Plasma calcium levels are normally maintained within a narrow range and permit clotting of the blood at most times. In people with sufficient calcium in their normal diet, no benefit is achieved by increasing dietary calcium before surgery.

The role of calcium in blood clotting is just one example of its wide variety of roles as a cofactor for and

FIGURE 9-3

Structure of a tooth.

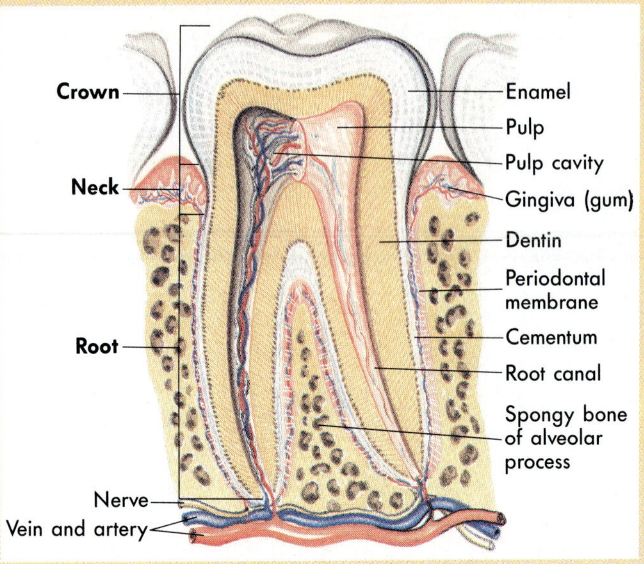

FIGURE 9-4

Schematic summary of the process of blood clotting.

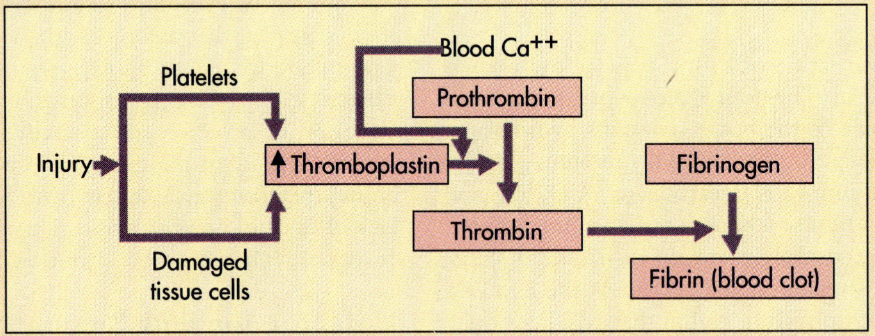

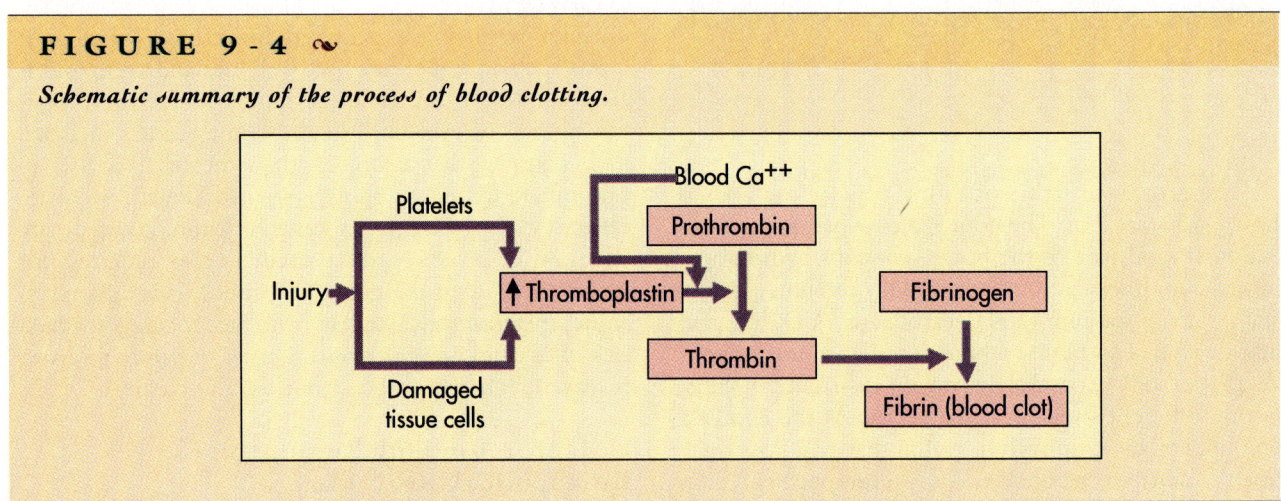

regulator of biochemical reactions. Another example is the involvement of calcium in initiating neurotransmitter release in the nervous system, mentioned in the Overview of Minerals. Among many other functions of calcium, some of particular relevance to nutrition are the involvement of calcium in the absorption of vitamin B_{12}, the action of the fat-digesting enzyme pancreatic lipase, the secretion of insulin from the pancreas, and the contraction of muscle fibers needed to power all physical activity. Literally dozens of other vital roles of calcium in biochemical processes are known, but changes in dietary calcium levels have little immediate effect on them because the level of calcium they require can be maintained by the release of calcium from the stores held in bone.

Absorption

The efficiency with which calcium is absorbed into the adult body varies from less than 10% to more than 60%.[1] In growing children, however, up to 75% of dietary calcium may be absorbed. Calcium absorption is a complex process that is influenced by a variety of factors, including the amount of calcium available in the diet, the prevailing need for calcium, a person's age and gender, the use of certain drugs, and the presence of certain other nutrients such as lactose, protein, and vitamin D. The proportion of calcium absorbed varies inversely with the amount in the diet. Women generally absorb less of their dietary calcium than do men, and absorption in both genders declines with age. For adults, who may absorb as little as 10% in some circumstances, an intake in excess of 1000 mg/day may be required to maintain calcium balance. The amount of calcium absorbed by people consuming the typical American diet is estimated at 20% to 40% on average, but there is considerable variation among individuals.

> *F*actors favoring calcium absorption
> - Adequate vitamin D in the body
> - Acidity of digestive mass
> - Presence of lactose in food
> - A need for calcium

Calcium is absorbed by two distinct mechanisms: passive diffusion and active transport.[2] The active process requires the expenditure of energy stored within adenosine triphosphate (ATP), is mediated by a carrier protein, and is "saturable," meaning it can occur no faster than at a maximal rate corresponding to the rate when all of the carrier molecules are carrying calcium all of the time. The active process also requires the presence of vitamin D. The passive process relies on simple nonsaturable diffusion of calcium down its concentration gradient, with no requirement for energy expenditure to make it happen.

The relative contribution of each absorption process depends on the concentration of calcium in the intestinal lumen and the plasma concentrations of the active form of vitamin D. Allen[3] estimated that in normal adults, 95% of the calcium absorbed from a low-calcium meal is absorbed by the active process, indicating that this vitamin D–dependent process normally predominates.

Factors Favoring Absorption

Vitamin D The importance of vitamin D in calcium absorption has been recognized since the early 1920s, but only recently have we discovered how it acts.[4] We now know that vitamin D is changed to an active form (the 1,-25 dihydroxy derivative of vitamin D), which directly affects the ability of intestinal cells to absorb calcium. Vitamin D regulates the synthesis of a calcium-binding protein that serves as a calcium carrier in the intestinal cell, transporting calcium across the intestinal cells for it to be released into the blood. The presence of the active form of vitamin D can result in a 10% to 30% increase in calcium absorption.

Acidity of the digestive mass Calcium is more soluble in acidic conditions and so is more readily absorbed from an acidic solution than from an alkaline one. Most calcium absorption occurs in the small intestine, in which the acidity of the digestive mass released from the stomach is soon neutralized. Anything that increases the acidity of the digestive mass before it enters the small intestine prolongs the time taken for this neutralization to occur and so increases the efficiency of calcium absorption. The normal decline in the efficiency of calcium absorption with age is at least partly caused by an associated decline in hydrochloric acid secretions into the stomach.

Lactose It has been known since 1926 that the absorption of calcium can be enhanced by lactose.[5] In a classic experiment, Bergeim[5] fed rats diets containing 25% lactose, glucose, sucrose, maltose, or starch. Lactose was found to increase calcium absorption, whereas the other carbohydrates did not. Since that first demonstration, numerous other studies on the effect of lactose have been performed on laboratory animals and humans. Unfortunately, the data from these studies are inconsistent but do suggest that in certain circumstances lactose does increase calcium absorption in humans.[6] In infants, for example, lactose can raise the proportion of dietary calcium absorbed from 33% to 48%.[7] A relatively high ratio of lactose to calcium is required to promote calcium absorption, and the mechanism of the effect is unknown.

Protein and phosphorus The extent to which protein intake affects calcium adsorption may depend on the amount of calcium in the diet. With a calcium intake of 500 mg/day, one study (of adult men) found that increasing protein intake from 50 to 150 g/day did not produce a significant effect on calcium absorption.[8] In another study, however, in which the daily calcium intake was 800 or 1400 mg/day, increased dietary protein was associated with increased calcium absorption.[9] This same study confirmed that protein had no effect when calcium intake was reduced to 500 mg/day.

Increased protein is reported to increase the excretion of calcium in urine. It has been estimated by Zemel[10] that a doubling of protein intake could lead to a 50% increase in urinary calcium excretion. An increase in the amount of phosphate in the diet has the opposite effect on calcium excretion, causing a reduction in the amount excreted. Fortunately, foods with a high protein content are also rich in phosphate; so the net effect of increased protein intake on calcium losses via urine is considerably less than is expected from the effect of the protein alone. Protein supplements composed of purified protein practically devoid of phosphate, however, may have an adverse effect on calcium balance if consumed in large amounts.

Need for calcium The efficiency with which calcium is absorbed may be influenced by the body's need for calcium. During pregnancy, lactation, and adolescence, when calcium needs are greatest, absorption efficiencies as high as 50% have been observed. Also, when calcium intakes are low, the body adapts by absorbing a greater proportion of the dietary calcium available and excreting less.

Factors Depressing Absorption or Increasing Losses

Oxalic acid Oxalic acid—which is found in some leafy green vegetables such as spinach, combines with calcium to form an insoluble complex of calcium oxalate. The calcium in this compound cannot be absorbed. Whether oxalic acid interferes with the absorption of calcium from other components of a meal depends on the calcium/oxalic acid ratio in the food that is the source of the oxalic acid. If that food contains sufficient calcium to form a complex with all of the oxalic acid, there is no free oxalic acid left to combine with calcium from other sources in a meal. Some leafy vegetables, however, do contain substantial amounts of free oxalic acid. Approximately 55% of the oxalic acid in spinach, for example, is in the form of free and soluble oxalic acid, rather than in the complexed and insoluble form calcium oxalate. The idea that free oxalic acid in such foods as spinach can reduce the absorption of calcium in other foods is supported by some documented evidence.[6]

Factors depressing calcium absorption
- Oxalic acid
- Phytic acid
- Steatorrhea
- Emotional instability
- Increased gastrointestinal motility
- Lack of exercise
- Dietary fiber
- Caffeine
- Drugs

The presence of free oxalic acid in lower grades of cocoa led to concern about the suitability of chocolate drinks for children. Studies on college women, however, showed that the amount of cocoa they could tolerate (1 oz) was insufficient to cause any depression of calcium absorption, regardless of whether their calcium intake was high or low. Comparable studies have not been done on children, but similar results are expected. This has led to the conclusion that there is no reason to discourage the consumption of chocolate drinks on the basis of any effect on calcium absorption.

Phytic acid Another organic acid—phytic acid—also binds to calcium, but this is of little consequence in most diets. Phytic acid is found primarily in the outer husk of whole grain cereals. Only when calcium-rich foods are eaten with such foods as oatmeal or whole grain pita bread, which are high in phytic acid, could this become a significant factor in calcium absorption.

Steatorrhea The effect of fat on calcium absorption is unclear. It is known that improved absorption results from slow passage of food through the digestive tract, and foods that are high in fat do move more slowly through the tract. On the other hand, high-fat diets promote the formation of insoluble salts of fatty acids combined with calcium (soaps), with a resulting reduction in calcium absorption. When high-fat diets result in steatorrhea (large, foul-smelling stools containing a large amount of unabsorbed fat), calcium absorption is certainly reduced.

Emotional instability The efficiency of calcium absorption can be influenced by the emotional stability of an individual. Stress, tension, anxiety, grief, and boredom can all interfere with calcium absorption. In one study, a group of emotionally distressed young women were found to require a higher intake of calcium to maintain calcium balance, when compared with a similar group of happy, relaxed women. Another study, of college men, found a decreased efficiency of absorption and increased excretion of calcium under conditions of stress, such as occurs during examinations.

Increased gastrointestinal motility Anything that increases the rate of passage of food through the intestinal tract decreases calcium absorption by reducing the time available for the absorption to occur. Laxatives and foods high in bulk may have this effect.

Lack of exercise People who do not engage in weight-bearing exercise, such as walking, and bedridden people, who are essentially immobile, can lose as much as 0.5% of bone calcium in a month and have a reduced ability to replace it. This may be a cause of, or at least a complicating factor associated with, the decalcification of bone found in many old people. Some evidence suggests that it is the lack of weight on the bones, rather than the actual immobility, that causes the loss of calcium during bed rest. Similarly, people whose main regular exercise is swimming may have a lower bone density than those who exercise by walking or running because of the much decreased load on the bones during swimming. Astronauts suffer from calcium loss during spaceflight because of either weightlessness or their relative immobility.

Dietary fiber Various types of dietary fiber reduce the efficiency with which calcium and other minerals are absorbed. This can be caused by a variety of factors: increased gastrointestinal motility, increased bulk of the

FIGURE 9-5

Absorption and excretion of calcium.

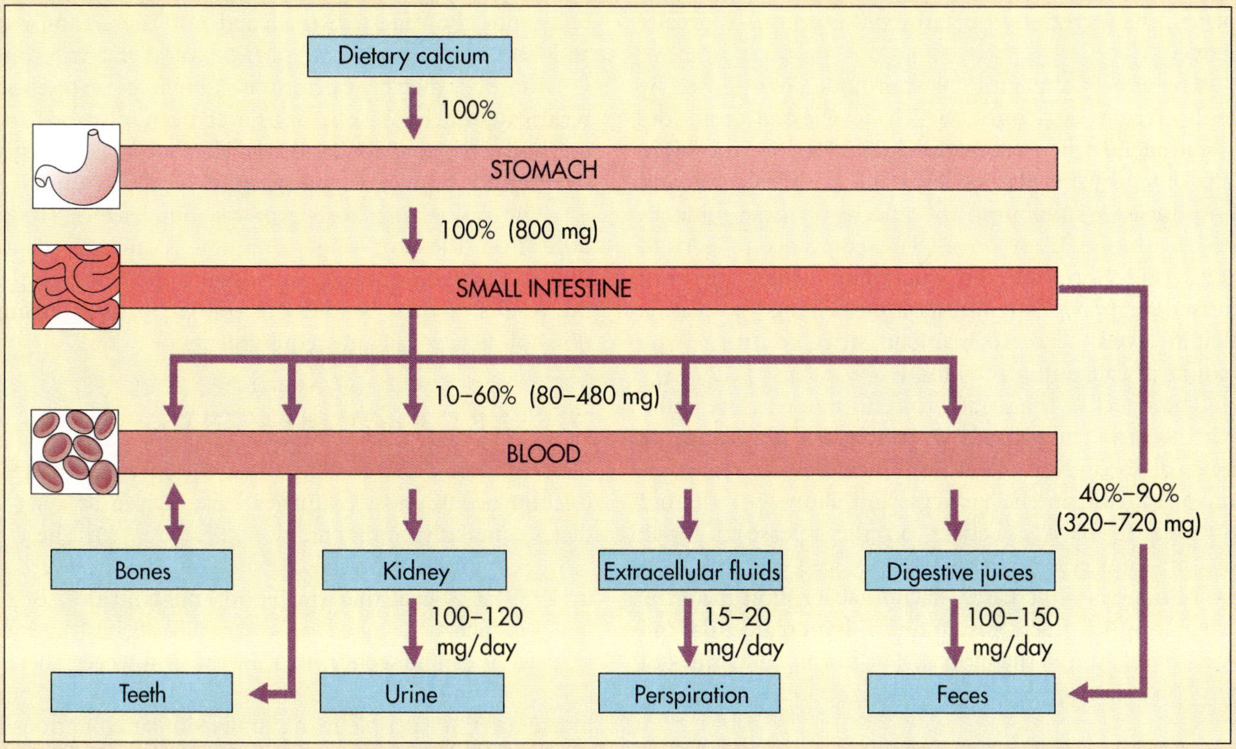

digestive mass, and the binding of minerals within the structure of fiber.

Caffeine High intakes of caffeine affect the bioavailability of calcium by increasing the loss of calcium in urine and stimulating the secretion of calcium into the gastrointestinal tract.

Drugs Some medications—including anticonvulsants, cortisone, thyroxine, and aluminum-containing antacids—are associated with reduced calcium absorption as a side effect.

METABOLISM

Once calcium has been absorbed, it is transported in the blood and released into the fluids bathing the tissues of the body. From these extracellular fluids the cells take up the amounts of calcium needed for their normal functioning and growth. As blood is filtered through the kidneys, about 99% of the calcium is reabsorbed into the blood. The remaining 1% (normally amounting to 100 to 120 mg/day) is excreted in urine. Some calcium is secreted within the digestive secretions of the stomach and intestine. Much of this calcium is reabsorbed, but the amount lost to the feces amounts to about 100 to 150 mg/day, regardless of dietary intake. Figure 9-5 summarizes the absorption and excretion of calcium.

Most of the calcium absorbed by the body is used in the calcification of bones, a process that is facilitated by vitamin D. About one third of the calcium in bone acts as a reservoir of calcium that can be drawn on to maintain blood plasma calcium levels when required. The parathyroid gland plays a major role in maintaining plasma calcium level (normal range, 9-11 mg/dl) which does not fluctuate by more than 3% during a day. If the plasma calcium level falls slightly, the parathyroid gland secretes a hormone known as **parathyroid hormone** (or **parathormone**). Within minutes of its release the parathyroid hormone stimulates the kidneys to reabsorb more of the calcium that would otherwise be excreted in urine and also to enhance phosphate excretion. Also, within hours of its release, the parathyroid hormone stimulates the release of bone calcium and phosphate into the blood. It achieves this effect on bone by stimulating the synthesis of carbonic acid by the enzyme carbonic anhydrase, generating the acid for the dissolution of bone. Parathyroid hormone also stimulates the absorption of calcium from the gastrointestinal tract. However, this effect only occurs several days after release of the hormone and is a result of formation of the active form of vitamin D required for the synthesis of the calcium-binding protein involved in calcium absorption. When the combination of these effects of parathyroid hormone has caused plasma calcium levels to return to normal, the secretion of parathyroid hormone is greatly reduced.

The effects of parathyroid hormone are opposed by the hormone **calcitonin,** which is released from the thyroid gland when plasma calcium levels rise too high. Calcitonin lowers plasma levels of both calcium and phosphorus by inhibiting the release of these minerals into the blood from bone. The combined effects of parathyroid hormone and calcitonin, which are both released as appropriate in response to changes in plasma calcium levels, serve to maintain strict control of the amount of calcium in the blood.

The effect of the parathyroid hormone is integrated with the action of vitamin D, which also stimulates the intestinal absorption of calcium, increases the reabsorption of calcium in the kidneys, and allows parathyroid hormone to have its effect on the release of bone calcium. An excess of vitamin D may lead to decalcification of bone and increased calcium absorption from the gastrointestinal tract, resulting in **hypercalcemia** (an excess of calcium in the blood). The hormonal control of the plasma calcium level is summarized in Figure 9-6.

CALCIUM BALANCE STUDIES

Estimates of calcium requirements are based on the results of **calcium balance studies,** which compare calcium intake with calcium excretion. If the results of a calcium balance study reveal calcium intake to be greater than calcium excretion (a situation known as **positive calcium balance),** the body is assumed to be building up its stores of calcium. If excretion exceeds intake (**negative calcium balance**), the net loss of calcium from the body presumably reflects the decalcification of bone tissue. If intake equals excretion (**calcium equilibrium**), the intake concerned is assumed to be adequate, because the body is neither gaining nor losing calcium.

Calcium balance studies are difficult to perform and involve the following:

- Careful analysis of calcium intake, including analysis of the calcium content of drinking water
- Gathering of information on the subject's history of calcium intake, phosphorus intake, and nitrogen balance, all of which influence calcium balance
- Collection and analysis of urinary and fecal excretions over several weeks
- Estimation of calcium losses in perspiration and tears

All of the calcium in urine comes from one source: blood calcium that has not been reabsorbed by the kidneys. Calcium lost through the skin and in tears is also ultimately derived from the blood. Fecal losses, on the other hand, comprise calcium secreted from the body into the digestive tract and not later reabsorbed and also the unabsorbed portion of dietary calcium. Unabsorbed dietary calcium is known as **exogenous fecal calcium** because it has never been absorbed into the body, whereas fecal calcium derived from digestive secretions is known as **endogenous fecal calcium.**

The results of short-term calcium balance studies differ from those of longer duration because of adaptation to changing intakes, but despite this complication the results of these studies are still the basis of estimations of dietary calcium requirements.

DIETARY REQUIREMENTS

Despite some disagreement about the best way to assess calcium needs, most countries have arrived at a set of dietary intake recommendations (Table 9-1). The current recommended intakes for the United States were set in 1989 at a level that the Food and Nutrition Board believes meets the needs of essentially all healthy individuals. As can be seen from Table 9-1, however, there is no general agreement on the optimal level of calcium intake, even for people living under similar conditions in developed countries.

The Food and Agriculture Organization's "Suggested Practical Allowances" are designed as intake levels that can be met in practice by a large proportion of the world's population, including people in developing countries who sometimes obtain little calcium because of the limited amount in their country's food supply. The Expert Committee maintained that there is no evidence of any harmful effects from diets containing only 300 mg of calcium per day, provided that the body's content of vitamin D—which facilitates calcium absorption—is adequate.

Infants

It is assumed that the breast-fed infant receives adequate calcium from its mother's milk. The amount received corresponds to about 50 mg of calcium per kilogram of body weight per day, of which two thirds is retained in the infant's body. Infants fed cow's milk formula receive 65 mg of calcium per kilogram of body weight per day but retain only half of this calcium. If undiluted whole cow's milk is fed to an infant, calcium absorption is greatly reduced because the relatively high fat content of the milk restricts calcium absorption.

The total amount of calcium taken in by an infant works out to be approximately the same, whether he or she is fed breast milk or formula. Vitamin D is essential for the body to absorb and use calcium at this stage of life.

FIGURE 9-6

Hormonal control of the plasma calcium level.

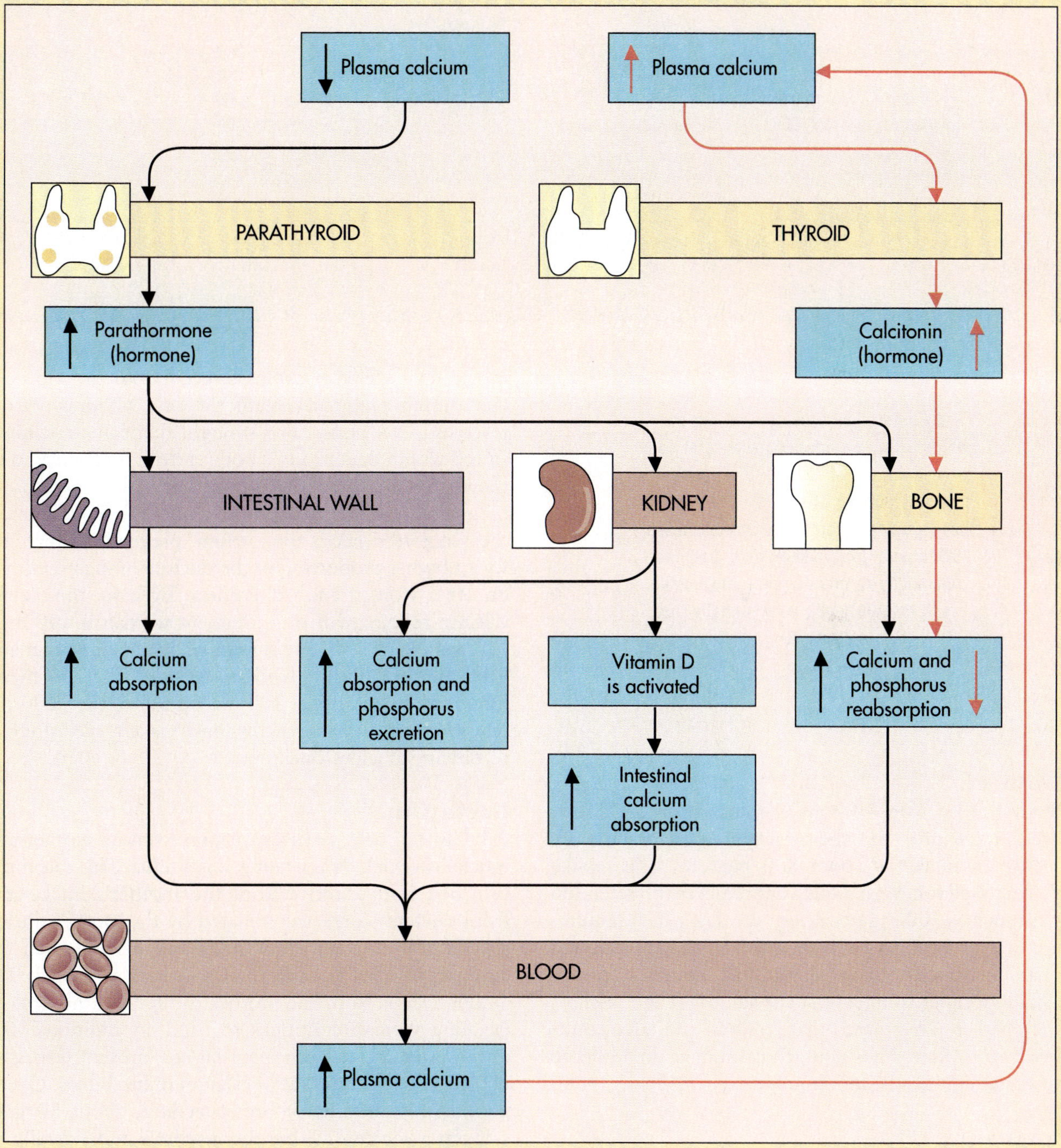

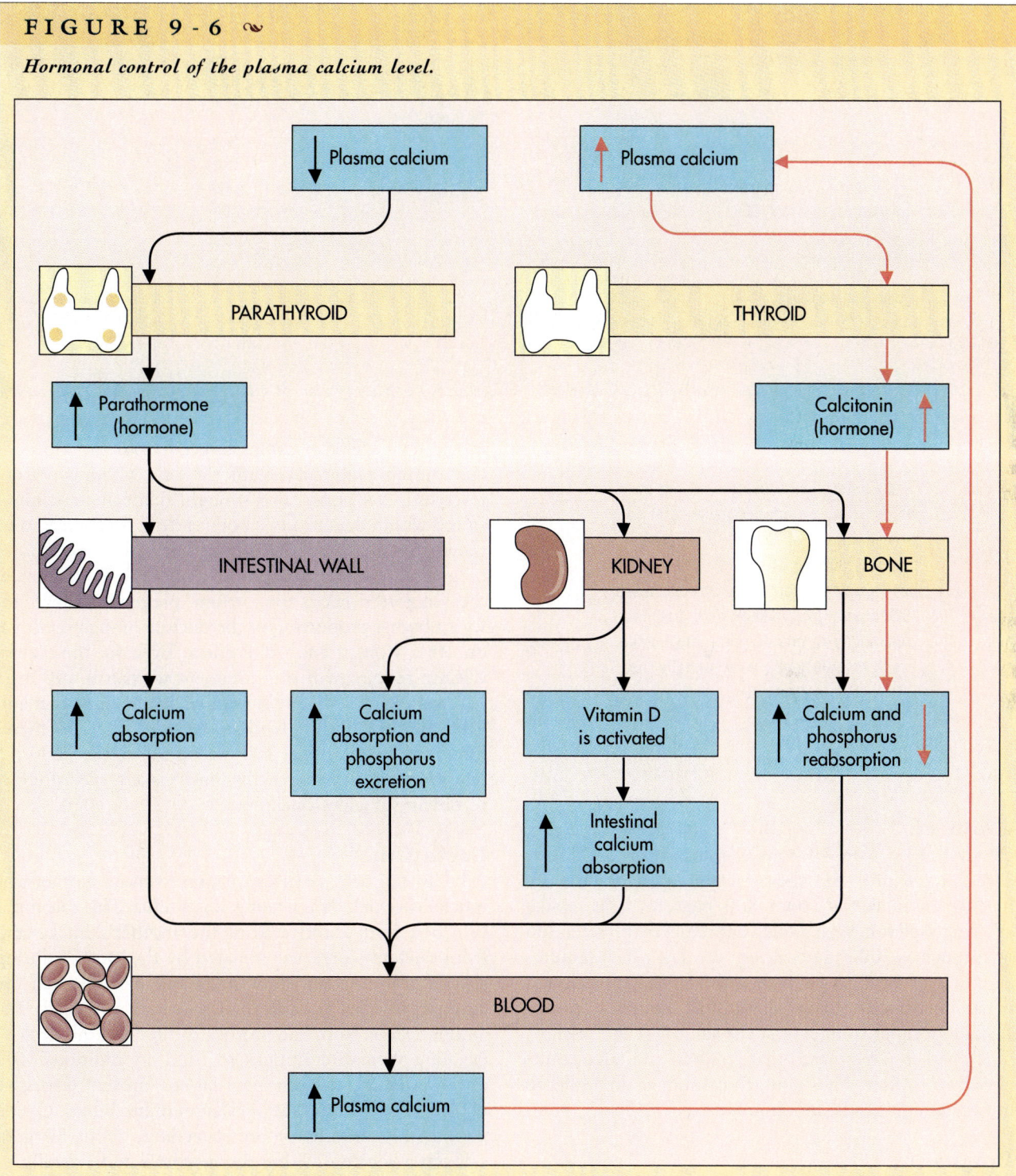

TABLE 9-1

Comparison of recommended calcium intakes (mg)

	AGE	RECOMMENDED NUTRIENT INTAKES, CANADA (1990)*	REFERENCE NUTRIENT INTAKES, UNITED KINGDOM (1991)†	NRC RECOMMENDED DIETARY ALLOWANCES (1989)‡	FAO/WHO SUGGESTED PRACTICAL ALLOWANCES§
Infants and children	7-12 mo	400	525	600	500-600
	1-10 yr	500-700	350-550	800	600-700
Males	11-19 yr	900-1100	1000	1200	500-600
	Adult	800	700	800	400-500
Females	11-19 yr	700-1100	800	1200	500-600
	Adult	700	700	800	400-500
	Pregnancy	1200	700	1200	1000-2000
	Lactating	1200	1250	1200	1000-2000

* From Scientific Review Committee. *Nutrition recommendations,* Ottawa, Canada, 1990, Canadian Government Printing Center.

† Deptartment of Health and Social Security: *Dietary Reference Values for food energy and nutrients for the United Kingdom: reports on health and social subjects,* London, 1991, Her Majesty's Stationery Office.

‡ National Academy of Sciences: National Research Council: *Recommended dietary allowances,* ed 10, Washington, DC, 1989, National Academy Press.

§ Report of Joint Food and Agricultural Organization/ World Health Organization Expert Committee: *Calcium requirements,* WHO Technical Report Series No 230, Geneva, Switzerland, 1962, World Health Organization .

> Human milk provides 210 mg of calcium from an infant's usual total daily milk intake of 750 ml. Cow's milk contains 300 mg of calcium per 750 ml, but because calcium is absorbed more effectively from human milk, calcium availability to infants when fed human milk or cow's milk is essentially the same.

Children

Children aged 1 to 10 years can absorb up to 75% of ingested calcium, and their calcium requirements are met by an intake of about 800 mg/day. The rapidly growing skeleton of an adolescent requires the retention of as much as 500 mg of calcium per day, which requires an intake of 1200 to 1500 mg/day. Unless complicated by an increase in body weight, the body's need for calcium declines from at least the age of 30 and possibly much earlier. This means that children and adolescents need two to four times as much calcium as do adults to meet the high needs during growth.

Pregnancy

Although a child is born with relatively poorly calcified bones, the full-term fetus contains approximately 30 g (1 oz) of calcium, two thirds of which is deposited during the last 3 months of pregnancy. Studies using stable isotopes of calcium show that up to 90% of the calcium in the fetal skeleton comes directly from the mother's diet during pregnancy, with the rest withdrawn from reserves in her bones. It is thought that some calcium is stored within the mother's body early in pregnancy to be transferred to the fetus during the last 3 months of pregnancy at a rate of about 300 mg/day. To help meet their increased needs for calcium, pregnant women absorb a higher proportion of the calcium in their diet than do other women and excrete less. Even so, the dietary calcium requirement of a pregnant woman is 400 mg/day greater than her requirement when not pregnant. Pregnant adolescents, who are still growing and therefore need an additional 400 mg on top of the 1200 mg required for normal growth, must make a special effort to obtain sufficient calcium.

Lactation

A breast-fed baby receives calcium from its mother at a much faster rate than when it was a fetus. This calcium is provided both directly from the mother's intake and from calcium stores accumulated by the mother during the sixth and seventh months of pregnancy (when the amount of calcium absorbed usually far exceeds the amount required by the mother and fetus combined). A lactating woman continues to need an additional 400 mg of dietary calcium per day to prevent excessive depletion of the reserves of calcium in her bones. Over a period of 6 months of breast-feeding, about 50 g of calcium is secreted within the mother's milk overall.

To ensure that they receive adequate supplies of calcium, lactating mothers should consume large amounts of dairy products and other calcium-rich foods. Even when they follow this advice, few women maintain calcium balance during lactation. Instead, they draw on existing reserves of calcium to provide some of the calcium required to produce their breast milk, and so they should continue with a high-calcium diet after lactation to help replenish their reserves.

Adults

As people grow old they generally lose bone mass, resulting in reduced bone strength and increasing vulnerability to fracture. There is considerable evidence, however, that the more bone mass a person acquires in the first 20 to 30 years of life, the more he or she is protected against loss of bone mass in later years. Calcium intake during early adulthood has a marked influence on the total amount of bone accumulated.

The RDA for calcium has been set at 800 mg/day for all adults over 35 years, based largely on the results of calcium balance studies and the assumption that 20% to 30% of dietary calcium is absorbed. There is some evidence, however, that higher levels of calcium may provide additional benefits to adult women. Before menopause, women are protected against bone loss by estrogen hormones, but the loss of this protection after menopause leaves them particularly prone to losing bone mass as they age. Heaney[11] has reevaluated the calcium balance studies on which the recommended dietary allowance (RDA) was based and has argued that the RDA should be 1500 mg/day for premenopausal women and 1000 mg/day for postmenopausal women. However, based on the advice of a panel of experts the National Institutes of Health recommend a daily calcium intake of 1000 mg for premenopausal and estrogen-treated postmenopausal women and 1500 mg for postmenopausal women who are not undergoing estrogen therapy. These levels are considerably greater than the average daily calcium intake of 500 to 600 mg reported by adult women in the most recent dietary surveys. To attain the recommended level requires a substantial change in food intake patterns or the use of supplements or calcium-fortified foods.

There is little evidence to suggest that the recommended level of calcium intake should be increased for men; thus 800 mg/day should be sufficient to meet calcium needs and minimize bone demineralization in adult men of all ages. A considerable amount of research is currently in progress to gain more information on which to base recommendations for dietary calcium intake.

ADEQUACY OF CALCIUM IN THE NORTH AMERICAN DIET

The Nationwide Food Consumption Study (1987-1988) of more than 25,000 people found average calcium intakes to range between 702 and 863 mg/day for adult males between 20 and 70 years of age and between 532 and 639 mg/day for adult females aged between 20 and 70 years.[12] The Health and Nutrition Examination Survey (HANES) III study found that men aged 20 to 59 years had average calcium intakes of 859 to 1075 mg/day and women aged 20 to 59 years had average calcium intakes of 747 to 924 mg/day. These figures indicate that consumption of calcium by adults can often be below recommended levels. Levels of calcium intake have fluctuated over the past 25 years, but in adolescents and adult women, they are generally between 200 and 400 mg/day less than the recommended levels. Median intakes by men are also below recommended levels, but by a smaller amount (Figure 9-7). The average reported intake for children under the age of 10, however, exceeds the RDA. For those over 12, diets of girls were less adequate than those of boys. From the ages of 18 to 30, which is the peak time for bone mass development, 66% of the women surveyed failed to consume the RDA of calcium. Although black women generally have a larger bone mass than do white women, their diets were less adequate in calcium than those of white women. Milk was the major source of calcium in all diets, providing about three fourths of the total amount of calcium consumed.

FOOD SOURCES

Calcium is present in significant amounts in only a limited number of foods. Milk and milk products are by far the most important dietary sources of calcium (Figure 9-8). The calcium content of the foods consumed most frequently in the United States and some recommended sources are shown in Table 9-2. The amount of calcium available in the U.S. food supply has declined from a peak of 1.07 g/person/day in 1945 to 0.88 g in 1988. The relative amount of calcium per serving of some representative foods is presented in Figure 9-9.

Milk and other dairy products serve as the most dependable sources of calcium because they are readily available, relatively low in cost, and exist in a wide variety of forms such as milk, cheese, yogurt, and ice cream. Also, the calcium in milk is readily absorbed because all milk contains lactose and is fortified with vitamin D, both of which are known to facilitate calcium absorption. Nondairy products are also a more expensive source of calcium than are dairy products. Nondairy foods that contain significant quantities of calcium such as sardines, almonds, and sesame seeds, also tend to be high in kilocalories, an especially important consideration for people on kilocalorie-restricted diets.

The calcium in chocolate milk is absorbed as efficiently as that in unflavored milk, despite the small amount of oxalic acid in cocoa. Nonfat milk and buttermilk, however, are slightly better sources of calcium than is whole-fat milk because the fat portion is replaced by the calcium-rich portion.

FIGURE 9-7

Adequacy of calcium intake in the North American diet base on data from NHANES II.

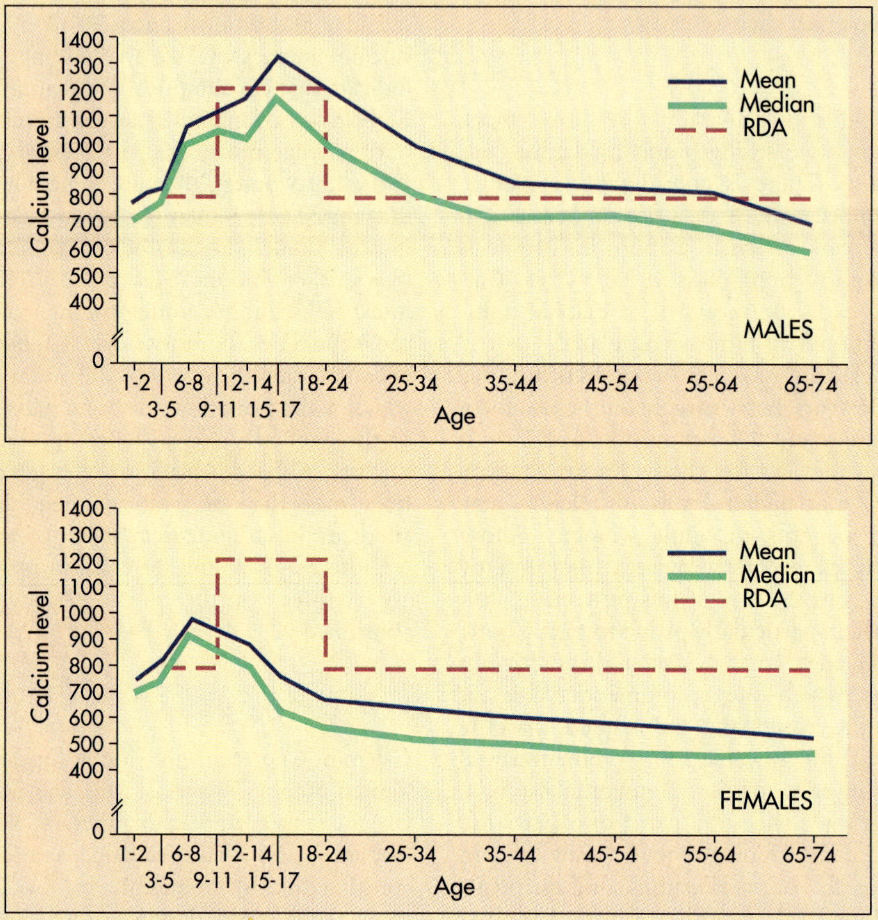

Many people find cheddar cheese to be a more palatable source of calcium than milk, although it is relatively high in both kilocalories and sodium. Cottage cheese is a less dependable source of calcium. During the preparation of cottage cheese, the required coagulation of milk can be brought about by use of the enzyme rennin, by treatment with acid, or by a combination of rennin and acid use. When rennin coagulation is used, more calcium is retained in the cheese curd than when either acid or acid and rennin coagulation is used. The consumer usually has no way of knowing which method was used. Cream cheese is a poor source of calcium because it is made from the fat portion of milk, which contains practically no calcium.

Goat's milk contains slightly more calcium than does cow's milk and is often given to children who are allergic to cow's milk. Calcium-enriched soybean milk preparations are also satisfactory.

Broccoli and such green leafy vegetables as turnip greens, which do not contain oxalic acid, contain an appreciable amount of available calcium but are not used often enough to be considered consistent sources of calcium. In general, the calcium in vegetables is not as well used by the body as that in dairy products because the bulk of the vegetables increases the rate at which food passes through the intestinal tract and hence reduces the time available for calcium to be absorbed. Also, the fiber in vegetables binds to some of the calcium, making it unavailable for absorption. Considerable calcium can also be lost during the preparation of vegetables if thick skins are removed or if dark green leaves are discarded.

Soybeans, which (if mature) contain 70 mg of calcium per ounce, become a significant source of calcium when consumed in large amounts, although their high fiber and phytic-acid contents reduce calcium absorption.

Although bread has not traditionally been considered a source of calcium, the use of dried milk solids and calcium-containing mold inhibitors now makes some breads significant sources. Many adults can receive up to one seventh of their daily calcium requirement from bread alone. The optional enrichment of flour with 500 to 1500 mg of calcium per pound also makes some

FIGURE 9-8

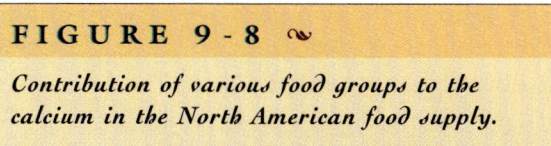

Contribution of various food groups to the calcium in the North American food supply.

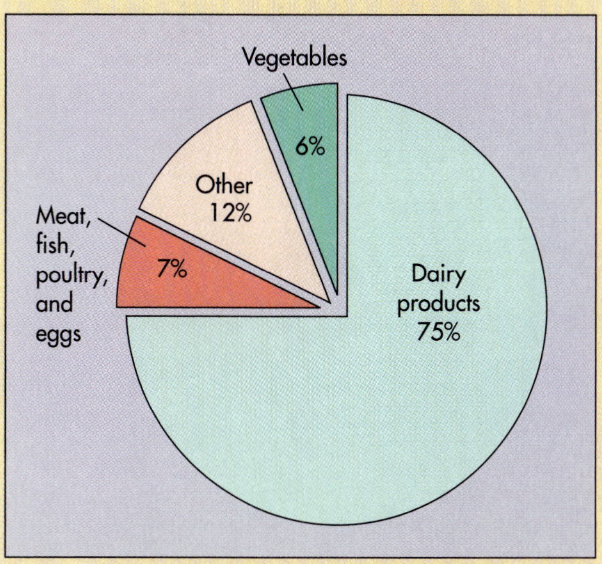

breads (with 20 to 60 mg of calcium per slice) a significant source of calcium for the 10% of the population who eat three or more slices each day. Similarly, the calcium content of baked products (such as muffins, waffles, and cakes) made with milk or calcium-enriched flour should not be overlooked.

People in developing countries in tropical areas, where milk products are generally unavailable, must rely on alternative sources of calcium. Because water consumption is high in the tropics, it can provide up to 200 mg of calcium per day in areas where the mineral content of the water is high. Other sources of calcium in such countries include small whole fish and fermented fish pastes; the mill powder used in grinding rice; soybean products such as tofu, saridele, and tempeh if calcium sulfate is used to coagulate the curd; the lime used in making tortillas in Mexico and by betel chewers; and a ground rock called **cal** that is used in porridges in Peru. Even such foods as sweet potatoes, a dietary staple in the Papuan highlands of New Guinea, and aged eggs, which are packed in lime in China, may contribute to the limited total of calcium consumed. In Malaya, pregnant women eat ground-up whole shellfish, which are rich in calcium. These examples are only some of the many different ways in which various populations throughout the world can acquire some dietary calcium, despite consuming practically no dairy products. There is, however, virtually no information available on how well calcium from such sources is absorbed by the body.

Because of the relative difficulty of getting adequate calcium, even in developed countries, many dietary supplements containing calcium are being promoted. These generally contain oyster shell, bonemeal, dolomite, or calcium salts, such as calcium carbonate, calcium lactate, or calcium gluconate. Some antacids, such as "Tums," contain up to 200 mg of calcium in the form of calcium carbonate. Supplements or antacids that dissolve in water can preclude any possible absorption problems associated with poor solubility. Some supplements—such as calcium citrate—are absorbed best on an empty stomach, whereas others—such as calcium carbonate—are absorbed best if taken with food. The percentage of calcium in the most common types of supplements is listed in Table 9-3.

About 12 years ago the U.S. Food and Drug Administration cautioned the public to limit consumption of calcium supplements because of the potentially high lead levels in some of them, particularly those produced from bonemeal and dolomite.[14] A recent analysis of 70 brands of nonprescription calcium supplements marketed in the United States and Canada found that 25% (17 out of 70) contained lead at a level exceeding the total daily tolerable intake (6 mg/day), when used at the suggested dosage.[15] The U.S. National Center for Health Statistics has reported that 25% of U.S. women and 8% of U.S. children aged 2 to 6 years consume nonprescribed calcium supplements each day.[16]

Sellers of special food-blending devices often promote the ingestion of pulverized egg shell as a way to achieve adequate calcium intake. An average egg shell does contain 2 g of calcium. There are no data on how effectively the body can use calcium from this source, however, and because there is a danger of contamination with Salmonella organisms, the consumption of crushed egg shells is risky.

HIGH CALCIUM INTAKE

In general, the body adapts to high calcium intakes by decreasing the proportion that is taken up by vitamin D–facilitated absorption. The portion of ingested calcium that is absorbed by passive diffusion (about 15%), however, is not subject to this adaptive response and so continues to be absorbed.

Regular consumption of calcium supplements and the deliberate use of calcium-fortified foods has become common only in the past few years; so we may not yet have had time to detect any side effects of high intakes. So far no evidence has emerged to suggest that high oral calcium intakes of more than 2 g/day have any effect on the level of calcium in the urine of normal subjects and hence on kidney stone formation or the deposition of calcium in other soft tissues.[17] Contrary to what conventional wisdom suggests, results from a recent study indicate that *low* calcium intakes, rather than high calcium intakes, are associated with increased risk of kidney stone formation. Any abnormal deposition of calcium in soft tissues is also believed to be more likely to result

TABLE 9-2

Calcium, phosphorus, and magnesium in average servings and per 100 kcal of the most frequently used foods and some recommended sources of calcium

			CALCIUM		PHOSPHORUS		MAGNESIUM	
FOOD	AMOUNT	kcal	mg PER SERVING	mg PER 100 kcal	mg PER SERVING	mg PER 100 kcal	mg PER SERVING	mg PER 100 kcal
MEAT, FISH, EGGS, POULTRY, NUTS								
Egg, fried	1 large	83	25	31	78	94	5	6
Beef roast	3 oz	318	11	4	202	63	22	7
Hamburger	3 oz	285	11	4	207	72	25	9
Chicken	3 oz	242	15	6	182	75	23	10
Tuna	3 oz	170	8	5	234	138	35	20
Peanut butter	2 Tbsp	178	18	10	114	64	59	33
Bacon	3 slices	89	12	13	188	211	21	24
Salmon, canned*	3 oz	120	167	133	243	200	81	134
Almonds*	1 oz (10)	165	75	45	147	90		
Pizza*	1/8 of a 12-in pie	145	86	59				
Tofu*	4 oz	114	102	90	145	120		
CEREAL PRODUCTS								
Cornflakes	1 cup	88	1	1	11	13	4	5
Shredded wheat	1 biscuit	83	13	16	388	467	4	48
Saltines	4 crackers	43	2	5	9	21	3	7
Rice	1 oz, dry	109	10	9	28	25	8	7
White bread	1 slice	81	28	34	22	27	5	6
Whole wheat bread	1 slice	73	28	39	52	71	18	25
DAIRY PRODUCTS								
Whole milk*	8 oz	157	91	182	223	142	31	20
2% fat milk*	8 oz	121	297	254	240	198	34	28
Cheddar cheese*	1 oz	114	204	190	154	135	8	7
Cottage cheese†	4 oz	103	75	73	340	330	6	6
Yogurt, plain*	8 oz	139	274	197	326	234	26	36
Ice cream*	8 oz	349	151	43	115	33	16	56
Nonfat milk*	8 oz	86	302	345	247	281	23	24
FRUITS								
Apple	1 medium	81	10	12	14	17	11	14
Banana	1 medium	105	7	9	32	30	41	39
Orange juice, frozen	4 oz	56	11	19	19	34	12	22
Peach	1 medium	37	4	24	19	51	10	27
VEGETABLES								
Corn, canned	4 oz (1/2 cup)	84	5	5	71	72	19	20
Green beans	4 oz (1/2 cup)	52	39	75	32	61	19	37
Green peas	4 oz (1/2 cup)	88	19	22	84	95	19	22
Lettuce	1/4 head	13	20	154	22	169	11	85
Tomato	1 medium	22	13	59	27	122	14	64
Potato, baked	1 medium	93	9	10	65	69	31	33
Broccoli*	3.5 oz, cooked	26	205	207	37	10	47	12
Turnip greens*	1/2 cup, cooked	15	99	15	21	3	16	2

* Recommended sources of calcium.

† Variable source of calcium, depending on manufacturing procedure.

Data from U.S. Department of Agriculture: *Handbooks 8-1 to 8-21: composition of foods raw, processed and prepared,* Washington, DC, 1972-1991, U.S. Government Printing Office.

FIGURE 9-9

Amount of calcium per serving in various foods.

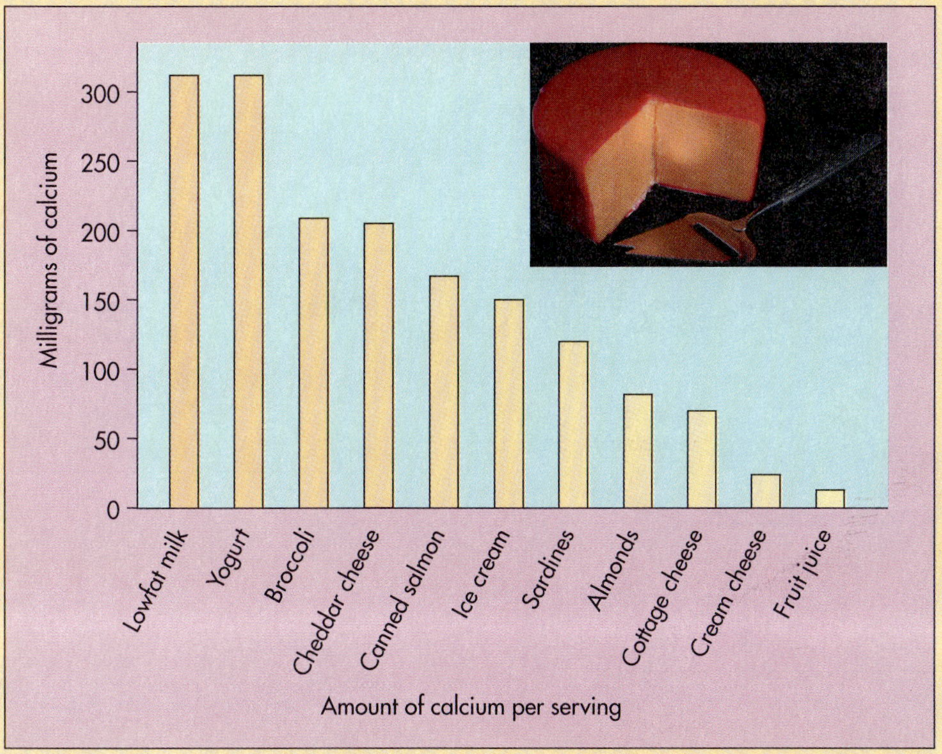

TABLE 9-3

Amount of calcium in various calcium supplements

SUPPLEMENT	CALCIUM (%)	MILLIGRAMS IN 1000-mg TABLET (1 g)
Calcium carbonate	40	400
Calcium lactate	13	130
Calcium gluconate	9	90
Calcium citrate	18	180
Dibasic calcium phosphate	23	230
Bonemeal	28-33	280-330
Dolomite	20	200
Tums	20	200

from a low magnesium intake rather than from a high calcium intake.

Studies in animals have suggested that excessively high intakes of calcium depress the use of some other mineral nutrients such as phosphorus, copper, iodine, zinc, and magnesium. The ratios of calcium to other minerals likely to result in this effect are well beyond those possible from a normal diet but may occur as a result of unwise consumption of calcium supplements.

ASSESSMENT OF CALCIUM STATUS

There is as yet no reliable method for determining a person's overall calcium status. The plasma calcium level is readily determined but is stabilized against change by the secretions of the parathyroid and thyroid glands, as considered earlier. This means that the plasma calcium level is not a good indicator of the calcium status of the whole body. Much work has been done to assess the usefulness of x-ray measurements of bone density as an indicator of bone mineralization and hence calcium status. It has been found that, in general, traditional x-ray methods are not sufficiently sensitive to variations in mineralization to be of any use in this area. The more sophisticated x-ray–based technique of **computed tomography** is showing more promise, however. Two other new techniques, known as **single photon absorptiometry** and **dual photon absorptiometry,** are also promising. These absorptiometry techniques involve focusing special light sources on the body and measuring the extent to which the light is absorbed.

CALCIUM-RELATED HEALTH PROBLEMS

Osteoporosis

Osteoporosis is a condition associated with a loss in bone density and bone mass and is primarily found in middle-

FIGURE 9-10

The bone remodeling cycle.

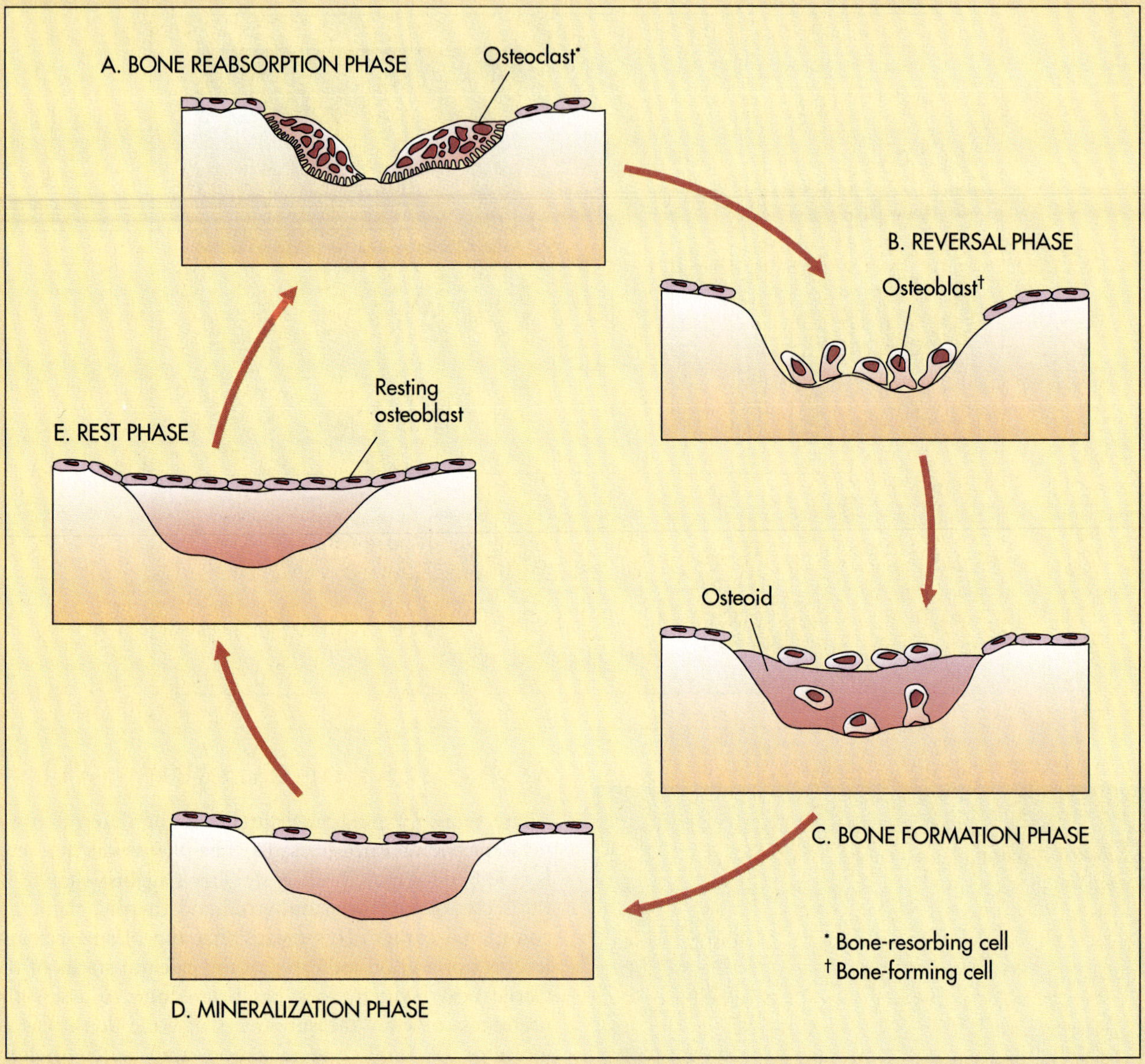

aged and elderly women. Its major symptom is an increased vulnerability to bone fractures. The most effective way of preventing or at least minimizing the extent of osteoporosis is an adequate calcium intake throughout life, combined with adequate exercise; thus the nutritionist's interest in osteoporosis is firmly focused on calcium.

The bones of the skeleton are "remodeled" throughout life, a process involving the breakdown of existing bone and formation of new bone in a perpetual cycle that affects 10% of the skeleton at any one time. When existing bone is being broken down, calcium is resorbed into the blood plasma; however, plasma calcium must be deposited in the new bone during its phase of mineralization (Figure 9-10). In young people in good health the rate of calcium reabsorption equals that of bone formation. As people age, however, reabsorption begins to predominate over bone formation, eventually resulting in osteoporosis. In osteoporosis the total amount of bone is reduced, but the remaining bone is of normal composition and quality.

> Some studies have suggested that many women do not consume even half of the recommended amount of calcium each day, greatly increasing their risk of osteoporosis.

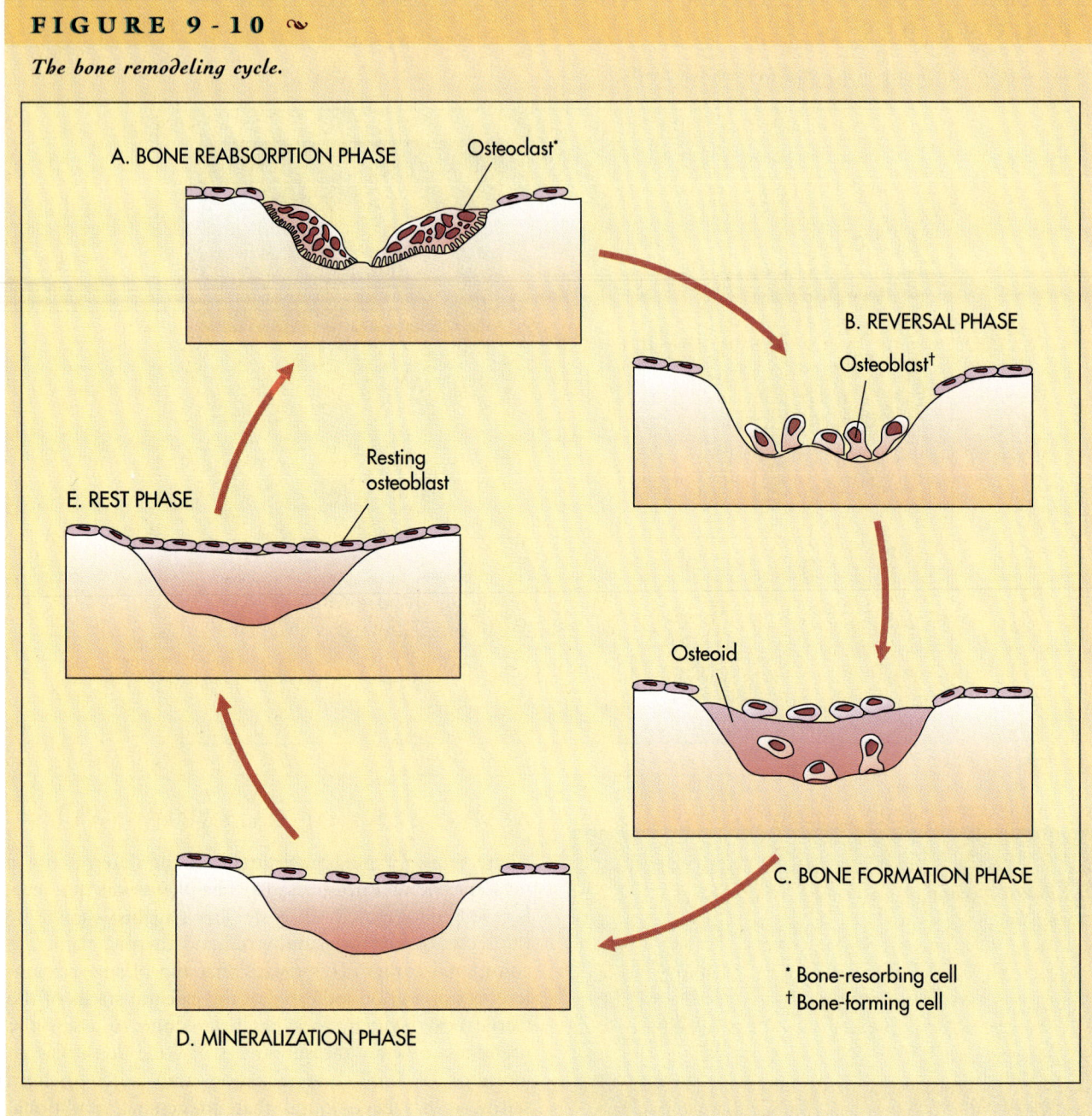

Although aging is one universal and unavoidable factor that brings a risk of osteoporosis, a variety of other factors—some unavoidable and some avoidable or controllable to some degree—contribute to a person's overall risk.

The main additional unavoidable factors are the following:

- **Gender:** Females are at considerably greater risk of osteoporosis than are males. They have approximately 25% less bone mass than do men and have an accelerated rate of bone loss after menopause because of the loss of hormones that act to maintain bone mass and density. Men tend to have higher levels of bone-preserving hormones to begin with and also do not live as long as women and so have less "opportunity" to develop osteoporosis. Overall, these factors combine to make women eight times more likely to be affected by osteoporosis than men. Up to half of all postmenopausal women can expect to develop some degree of osteoporosis.
- **Race:** People of white or Asian ancestry are more likely to develop osteoporosis than those with a black African ancestry. This is presumably related to the fact that black people have a greater bone density than do whites or Asians, giving them a total bone mass that averages 10% to 15% greater than that of fairer skinned people. One statistical consequence of this is that black women over 60 have only half as many hip fractures as do white women of the same age.
- **Body size:** Small-boned people are at greater risk of osteoporosis than those with larger bones. Also, their lower body weight puts less stress on their bones throughout life, which is a disadvantage—rather than an advantage—in terms of osteoporosis risk because such stress on the bones causes them to increase in density. This effect means that one health advantage, reduced risk of osteoporosis, is associated with the presence of a significant amount of body fat. Fat also helps produce the hormone estrogen, which has been proven to slow the loss of bone.
- **Family history:** A family history of osteoporosis puts a person at increased risk of developing osteoporosis.
- **Disease:** Some diseases known to reduce bone mass and density bring with them an increased risk of osteoporosis. These include overactivity of the thyroid gland, which can overstimulate the cells that destroy bone during bone remodeling; malfunctions of the parathyroid gland, which can disturb the calcium balance of blood plasma; gastrointestinal tract disorders, which may restrict the body's ability to absorb and use calcium and other nutrients needed for bone formation; liver diseases, which interfere with the absorption and use of minerals; and kidney diseases, which lead to increased acidity of blood and increased phosphate levels in the blood, with consequent damage to bones.
- **Drug therapy:** Some drugs can accelerate the loss of bone mass and density. Such drugs include anticonvulsants, some of which can cause vitamin D deficiency and an associated impairment of calcium absorption; thyroid hormones given to counteract malfunctions of the thyroid gland; and corticosteroids used to treat rheumatoid arthritis and asthma.

> Many adults of African and Asian ancestry produce only very small amounts of the enzyme lactase, which is necessary for the digestion of the carbohydrate lactose in milk. This state of lactase insufficiency causes lactose intolerance, associated with digestive discomfort when large amounts of milk are consumed. Milk cannot be the main source of calcium for people with lactase insufficiency, although cheeses in which the lactose has been converted to lactic acid are an acceptable alternative. Yogurt, made from partially fermented milk, is also acceptable. It still contains some lactose but also contains an enzyme that can convert the lactose into lactic acid in the intestine. Sweet acidophilus milk, designed to provide a source of microorganisms thought to be beneficial to the gastrointestinal tract, is not really useful for these persons because its lactose remains unchanged.

These unavoidable risk factors can be accompanied by various other risk factors that are all avoidable or at least controllable to some extent. The major risk factors in this category are the following:

- **Alcohol:** Drinking an average of three or more alcoholic drinks per day is clearly associated with an increased risk of osteoporosis. It has been well established that even small doses of alcohol interfere with the absorption and use of both calcium and vitamin D. Excessive alcohol consumption is the predominant avoidable risk factor promoting osteoporosis in men.

- **Caffeine:** Daily consumption of the amount of caffeine in 3½ cups of coffee or seven cups of tea has been shown to almost double the risk of developing osteoporosis. There is evidence to suggest that this is caused by caffeine's ability to interfere with the normal bone remodeling cycle, leading to increased loss of calcium in urine. The details are still being investigated, but the ability of caffeine to increase the risk of osteoporosis seems clear.
- **Smoking:** Many independent studies have found a greater incidence of osteoporosis among smokers than among nonsmokers. The precise mechanism of smoking's apparent effect on bone structure is still under investigation. Smokers tend to have less body fat than do nonsmokers of the same age, and as previously mentioned, low levels of body fat can increase the risk of osteoporosis because of decreased strain on the bones and reduced production of estrogen. Also, in women, smoking can bring forward the age of menopause by up to 5 years, leaving women who are smokers vulnerable to the postmenopausal risk of osteoporosis for a greater proportion of their lives.
- **Sedentary life-style:** It is now well established that regular exercise has a considerable beneficial effect on bone structure, leading to reduced risk of osteoporosis. As discussed already, bones subjected to the stresses and strains involved in exercise respond by becoming more dense and therefore stronger. For maximal beneficial effect the exercise should be undertaken regularly throughout a person's entire life, not just when he or she reaches the age at which the risk of osteoporosis begins to be a concern.
- **Emotional stress:** Emotional stress increases the secretion of hormones, such as adrenaline, known to increase the breakdown of bone tissue during bone remodeling, without causing any balancing increase in bone formation. Stress is also known to interfere with the body's ability to absorb minerals, including calcium. Thus for at least two reasons stress can lead to a deterioration in bone condition that brings an increased risk of osteoporosis.
- **Reproductive status:** Pregnancy and childbirth are known to improve the general bone condition of mothers for two main reasons. During pregnancy a woman's body weight is significantly increased and she produces greater quantities of the hormone estrogen—both factors known to increase bone mass. Women who never have children do not receive this beneficial stimulation of bone condition.
- **Inappropriate diet:** Finally, but of most relevance to nutritionists, various avoidable dietary factors can increase the risk of osteoporosis. The most obvious is a lack of sufficient calcium in the diet. Some studies have suggested that many women do not even consume half of the recommended amount of calcium each day and that taking additional calcium could cut their risk of suffering fractures by about 60%. As already discussed, fiber in the diet can reduce the efficiency with which calcium is absorbed. Although adequate fiber is required in the diet, it is important that it be accompanied by adequate calcium. Some studies have also found that excessive consumption of meat may be linked with an increased risk of osteoporosis. For this reason—along with others, such as the need to control animal fat intake—a healthful diet should probably contain no more than 6 oz of meat per day. Two other dietary factors that can adversely affect calcium balance are the consumption of carbonated beverages and excess salt. Carbonated beverages contain phosphate ions, which can bind to calcium in the gastrointestinal tract and so reduce its absorption. Many also contain some caffeine, whose adverse effect has already been considered. Excess salt, especially when taken by women after menopause, can lead to increased losses of calcium in urine.

The main risk factors for osteoporosis, both unavoidable and avoidable, are summarized in the box on p. 321. The number of people who develop osteoporosis because of some combination of these risk factors is considerable. Osteoporosis is the most common metabolic bone disorder in the United States and is responsible for many hundreds of thousands of fractures each year. All of these fractures are painful and at least temporarily disabling, but many of them can be life-threatening. Fractures of the hip are among the most serious, and in many old people, a hip fracture can cause a person to become bedridden and lead to complications that ultimately result in death.

There is no simple, safe, and effective treatment for osteoporosis once it has become established. The only agents presently approved by the Food and Drug Administration for the actual treatment of osteoporosis are calcitonin and the estrogen hormones. Calcitonin inhibits the reabsorption of bone calcium into the blood but has only a relatively short-lived beneficial effect for 1 to 2 years. Estrogen-replacement therapy for women after menopause has been shown to slow the rate of bone loss, although it does not stimulate new bone formation. It is much more effective as a *preventive* measure begun immediately after menopause than as a treatment of osteoporosis that has already developed. Long-term estrogen replacement therapy, however, may be associated with risks, as well as benefits, such as increased risks of

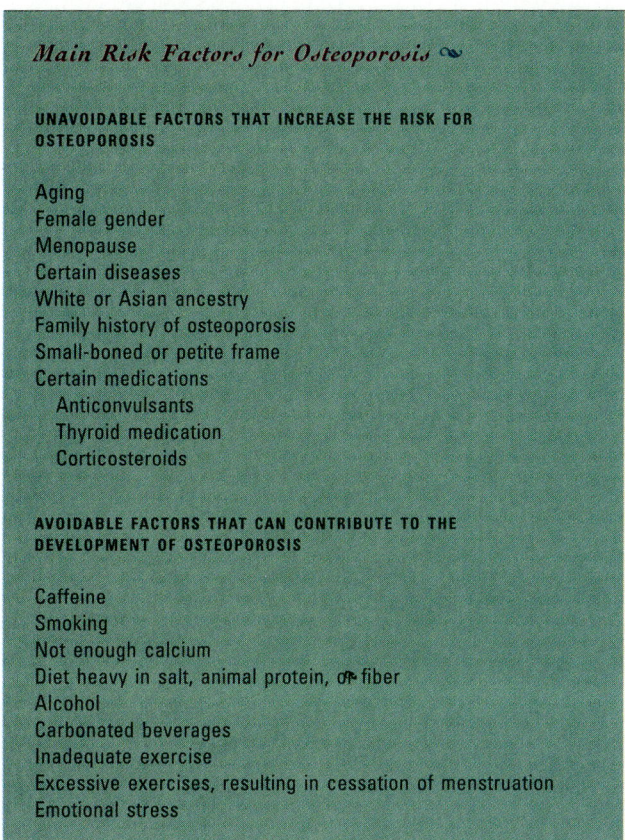

Main Risk Factors for Osteoporosis

UNAVOIDABLE FACTORS THAT INCREASE THE RISK FOR OSTEOPOROSIS

- Aging
- Female gender
- Menopause
- Certain diseases
- White or Asian ancestry
- Family history of osteoporosis
- Small-boned or petite frame
- Certain medications
  - Anticonvulsants
  - Thyroid medication
  - Corticosteroids

AVOIDABLE FACTORS THAT CAN CONTRIBUTE TO THE DEVELOPMENT OF OSTEOPOROSIS

- Caffeine
- Smoking
- Not enough calcium
- Diet heavy in salt, animal protein, or fiber
- Alcohol
- Carbonated beverages
- Inadequate exercise
- Excessive exercises, resulting in cessation of menstruation
- Emotional stress

FIGURE 9-11

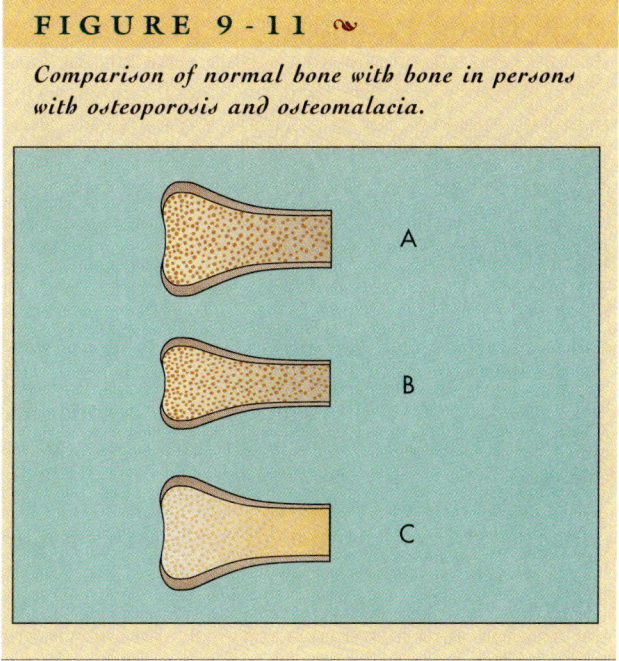

Comparison of normal bone with bone in persons with osteoporosis and osteomalacia.

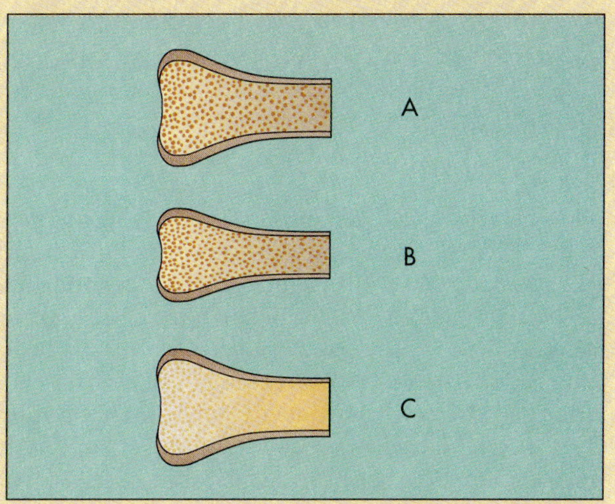

various cancers, liver disease, and circulatory problems. The potential value of estrogen replacement therapy must be assessed individually, in consultation with a qualified doctor.

With no simple remedy for osteoporosis available, the main focus of attention on the disease is on the many ways of preventing it or at least minimizing each person's risk of developing it. As already mentioned, the most effective preventive measures are ensuring that calcium intake is adequate *throughout* life and adopting a lifestyle that involves regular exercise. In addition, each person should try to minimize exposure to the various avoidable risk factors mentioned previously.

Only a limited amount of time is available for us to build up our bone mass to the optimal levels likely to protect us from osteoporosis. Bone mass reaches its peak between the ages of 35 and 40 and then begins a steady decline, which we can only hope to slow rather than prevent entirely.

Osteomalacia

Osteomalacia is a condition in which the quality of the bone is reduced, while the quantity of bone remains normal (Figure 9-11). It is characterized by the development of softness within the bones and associated pain. The most common cause of osteomalacia is low levels of calcium in the blood plasma, which is often itself caused by a deficiency of vitamin D. In addition to being a nutrient within food, vitamin D is synthesized in the body on exposure of the skin to sunshine. Osteomalacia is most commonly found in women who live in areas with limited sunshine, in people taking anticonvulsant drugs (which restrict calcium absorption), and in those with depleted mineral reserves because of the demands of successive pregnancies and prolonged lactation. Most people with osteomalacia respond well to vitamin D therapy, reflecting the common role of vitamin D deficiency as a primary cause of the condition. Osteomalacia can also, less commonly, be caused by a low phosphorus content of the body.

Hypercalcemia

Hypercalcemia, meaning too much calcium in the blood plasma, occurs in infants as a result of high intakes of vitamin D. It has been found when many different baby foods, each supplemented with vitamin D, are included in a baby's diet. It is best corrected by reducing the vitamin D content of the diet, rather than by reducing the dietary calcium intake.

Tetany and Calcium Rigor

When the amount of calcium in blood plasma (and therefore in all extracellular fluids) falls below a critical level, the appropriate stimulation of nerve cells is impaired, leading to increased excitability of affected nerves and hence spasmodic and uncontrolled contraction of muscles. This condition is known as **tetany.** Conversely, when plasma calcium levels rise too far above normal, muscle fibers maintain an inappropriate level of contraction known as **calcium rigor.** These conditions do not result from abnormal dietary intakes of calcium but are produced by malfunctions of the parathyroid gland, which—as we have seen—normally plays a key role in maintaining plasma calcium at an appropriate level.

High Blood Pressure

Recent research on the relationship between diet and blood pressure suggests that low calcium intakes (less than 100 mg/day) are associated with increased blood pressure.[18] Increasing the calcium intake in people with hypertension associated with low calcium intake has been found to lead to a marked decrease in blood pressure and hence in the incidence of hypertension.[19]

Colon Cancer

Colon cancer is one of the most common types of cancer in the United States and in other countries with Western-style diets.[20] Calcium supplementation has been found to reduce the proliferation of colon epithelial cells associated with these cancers in people at risk for "familial" colon cancer. Also, several studies have reported an inverse correlation between dietary calcium levels and the incidence of colon cancer. These results, which are supported by many animal studies, have led to the promotion of increased dietary calcium and vitamin D intakes as a means of reducing a person's risk of developing colon cancer.

PHOSPHORUS (P)

Phosphorus constitutes approximately 1% of the weight of the human body, largely in the form of phosphate (PO_4).

DISTRIBUTION

Up to 90% of the phosphorus in the body is found within calcium phosphate (apatite) crystals in the bones and teeth. The requirement for phosphorus to promote the development of healthy bones and teeth is well known and tends to draw attention away from its many lesser known but vital roles in the body, discussed below. The 10% of body phosphorus involved in these other roles is distributed throughout all the cells of the body, although about half of it is found in muscle.

FUNCTIONS

This section highlights only the major categories of function attributed to phosphorus in the body. The mineral is involved in such a wide variety of chemical processes that it is impossible to consider them all individually.

Mineralization of Bones and Teeth

As discussed already, the mineral crystals laid down during so-called bone calcification are actually composed of calcium phosphate, known as apatite, and a mixture of calcium phosphate and calcium hydroxide called hydroxyapatite. So although this process is called calcification, it actually involves the deposition of large quantities of phosphate in addition to calcium and is more accurately described as bone **mineralization.** Phosphorus in the form of phosphate is as important a part of bone as is calcium, and a failure of bone "calcification" is often in fact caused by an imbalance between calcium and phosphate levels in the blood plasma. If phosphate levels are low, a series of reactions are initiated that trigger vitamin D metabolism and ultimately raise the level of plasma phosphorus.

Facilitation of Energy Transactions

We saw in earlier chapters that energy released during the oxidation of carbohydrates, fats, proteins, and alcohol is stored by cells within the structure of the phosphate-containing compound adenosine triphosphate (ATP). The presence of phosphorus in ATP and also in adenosine diphosphate (ADP) and various coenzymes involved in energy transactions makes phosphorus essential for the capture and use of energy by all cells.

Absorption and Transport of Nutrients

Many nutrients must be combined with phosphate groups before they are able to be transported across cell membranes and hence absorbed into the body and distributed among its various cells and tissues. Thus the phosphorylation of nutrients and other biochemicals is essential for their proper distribution within the body.

Regulation of Protein Activity

Many proteins, including many enzymes, are "switched" between active and inactive forms, or—in other words—turned "on" and "off" by phosphorylation reactions that attach phosphate groups to particular amino acids within the proteins concerned. Among many other things, these phosphorylation reactions are involved in controlling the activities of proteins that in turn control the rate of cell growth and cell division and the extent to which the specific genes within cell nuclei are active.

Component of Essential Body Compounds

As previously mentioned, ATP, ADP, various coenzymes, and regulated proteins require phosphorus as part of their chemical structure. Many other vital chemicals can be added to the list of those essential body compounds, which contain phosphorus. For example, the DNA of our genes, the RNA that carries the genetic message from the nucleus to the cytoplasm, the phospholipids of cell membranes, and some vitamins contain phosphorus as a necessary part of their structure.

Regulation of Acid-Base Balance

Phosphate ions have the ability to combine with hydrogen ions, as do the phosphate groups that form part of various compounds in the body. Phosphate ions (PO_4^{3-}), hydrogen phosphate ions (HPO_4^{2-}), and bihydrogen phosphate ions ($H_2PO_4^{-}$) are the major anions (negatively charged ions) in blood plasma. This means that phosphate ions and phosphate-containing compounds have a role to play in maintaining the acid-base balance of the body. They can combine with excess hydrogen ions when conditions threaten to become too acidic and yet release hydrogen ions when conditions threaten to become too alkaline (or basic). In other words, phosphate ions and phosphate-containing compounds act as buffers against excessive variation in the pH level of fluids in the body.

ABSORPTION AND METABOLISM

Phosphorus can be released from phosphorus-containing chemicals in food by the action of intestinal enzymes known as **phosphatases** and is then absorbed into the blood plasma with the help of vitamin D. The level of phosphorus in the blood is regulated by the parathyroid gland, which interacts with vitamin D to control the amount of phosphorus absorbed, the amount retained by the kidneys, and the amount either released from or deposited in bone. The parathyroid gland is also involved in regulating calcium metabolism.

In healthy people the rates at which phosphorus is absorbed from the gastrointestinal tract and excreted via the kidneys are equal, maintaining total body phosphorus at a steady level.[21] Approximately 90% of ingested phosphorus is excreted via the kidneys, with the remaining 10% lost directly from the gastrointestinal tract without being absorbed. If plasma phosphorus levels decline for any reason, reabsorption of phosphorus by the kidneys increases to compensate, causing virtually no phosphorus to be excreted until normality is restored. On the other hand, if plasma phosphorus levels rise too high, no phosphorus is reabsorbed in the kidneys, causing all of the phosphorus filtered from the blood to be excreted until normality is restored.

Parathyroid hormone (parathormone) brings about a net loss of phosphorus from the body. Although the hormone stimulates phosphorus absorption from the gastrointestinal tract (by activation of vitamin D), phosphorus reabsorption into blood from bone, and phosphorus excretion via the kidneys, the increased excretion of phosphorus is the dominant effect.

If plasma phosphorus levels fall below 2.5 mg/100 ml, **hypophosphatemia** (low blood phosphorus level) results. This can result from either inadequate absorption of phosphorus from the gastrointestinal tract or increased excretion of phosphorus via the kidneys. Medical conditions that reduce phosphorus absorption include diarrhea, the use of laxatives, and the loss of intestinal tissue for any reason. Conditions that increase phosphorus excretion are generally those that lead to increased secretion of parathyroid hormone, such as hyperthyroidism, some forms of kidney disease, and some cancers.

DIETARY REQUIREMENTS

The RDA for phosphorus for children and adults corresponds to an intake that is at least equal to the calcium allowance during the growth period but no more than twice that amount. For infants less than 6 months old, the recommended intake of phosphorus is two thirds that of the recommended calcium intake, corresponding to the ratio in which these minerals occur in human milk.

> The North American diet provides ample amount of phosphorus because it is found in all food groups. The richest sources of dietary phosphorus are foods that are high in protein.

Most diets of children and adults provide much more phosphorus than calcium, and it is almost impossible to have a diet with a phosphorus/calcium ratio as low as 1:1. In diets with few dairy products and a high protein content, the ratio can be as high as 4:1. With most typical diets, however, there is little chance of the phosphorus content being high enough to cause a problem.

FOOD SOURCES

Phosphorus is not only present in every cell of the human body; it is also present in every cell of every form of life. This means that practically all foods contain significant amounts of phosphorus, although it is particularly abundant in protein-rich foods. Meat, fish, poultry, eggs, dairy products, and cereal products are the primary sources of phosphorus in the average diet. The phosphorus in foods of animal origin is more bioavailable than that in foods of plant origin. The actual amount of phosphorus in some of the most frequently eaten foods in the United States is given in Table 9-2. A significant amount of phosphorus can also be supplied in the form of phosphates within carbonated beverages (containing up to 75 mg of phosphorus per 12-oz can) and various phosphorus-containing substances found in processed foods. Figure 9-12 summarizes the contributions of various food groups to the phosphorus content of the North American food supply.

Overall, the U.S. food supply provides 1500 to 1600 mg of phosphorus per person per day. Food consumption

FIGURE 9-12

Contribution of various food groups to the phosphorus content of the North American food supply.

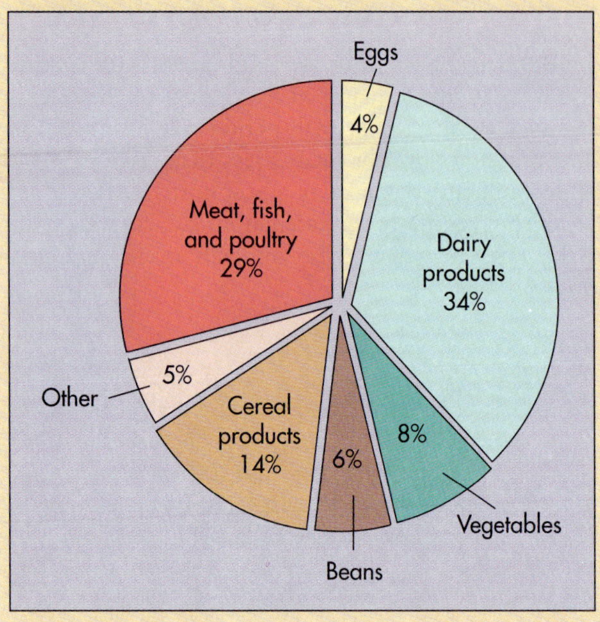

data show that men consume on average 1500 mg/day in both America and Canada, whereas women in these countries consume an average of 1000 mg/day. The amount of phosphorus in our diets has actually changed very little over the past 70 years, despite the many changes in our diet and food processing methods.

DEFICIENCY

Because of the wide distribution of phosphorus in almost all foods of both plant and animal origin, phosphorus deficiency is hardly ever found in humans. The rare exceptions include people who consume large amounts of antacids (especially aluminum hydroxide, which interferes with phosphorus absorption), people who suffer excessive losses in urine (such as those dependent on kidney dialysis), and prematurely born infants (who need more phosphorus than is naturally provided in human milk).

MAGNESIUM (Mg)

The presence of magnesium (as Mg^{2+} ions) in living organisms was first demonstrated in 1859. Even before that time, magnesium was used as a healing substance, an anesthetic, and an anticonvulsant. Magnesium was shown to be a dietary essential for mice in 1926 and for rats in 1932. Most of our information on its role in human nutrition was established after the 1950s. Considerable reserves of magnesium are stored in the bones of the human body, some of which can be released to help meet the needs of the soft tissues. This can make studies of magnesium deficiency in humans difficult because dietary deficiencies can take a long time to become apparent. Also, the kidneys are able to reabsorb magnesium when required. Despite these difficulties, magnesium is now fully recognized as an essential mineral in the human diet.

DISTRIBUTION

At birth the human infant contains approximately 0.5 g of magnesium, most of which is transferred into the fetus in the latter part of gestation. The adult male body contains a little more than 1 oz (approximately 40 g) of magnesium, 60% of which is found in bone. About one third of the magnesium in bone is closely bound with phosphate ions, whereas the remainder adheres to the bone surface, from where it can be readily released when required to maintain normal levels of magnesium in blood plasma. The blood plasma contains only 1% of body magnesium, although it is the second most common cation (after sodium) in plasma. Just over half of the plasma magnesium is in the form of free magnesium ions, about one third is bound to the protein "albumin," and the remainder forms part of a wide variety of compounds (Figure 9-13). Red blood cells contain more magnesium than is found in plasma, in amounts that rise and fall in response to excesses or deficiencies in the magnesium levels of the plasma surrounding the red blood cells. The magnesium in the soft tissues is concentrated (similar to potassium) within the cells, rather than in the extracellular fluids.

FUNCTIONS

Magnesium plays a vital role in facilitating the progress of several hundred biochemical reactions. These include key steps in the trapping and use of energy and the metabolism of carbohydrates, lipids, proteins, and nucleic acids. To meet the intracellular needs for magnesium, the mineral is found within cells at a concentration seven times greater than in the blood.

Although most magnesium is found within cells, the 1% of body magnesium outside of cells but within extracellular fluids also plays an important part in the normal functioning of the body. In particular, extracellular magnesium is vital for the conduction of nerve impulses and the contraction of muscles. In these contexts, magnesium plays an opposite—or "antagonistic"— role to that of calcium: calcium stimulates, and magnesium relaxes. This accounts for the anesthetic effect of rising levels of magnesium in the blood, which can eventually lead to coma

FIGURE 9-13

Distribution of magnesium in plasma.

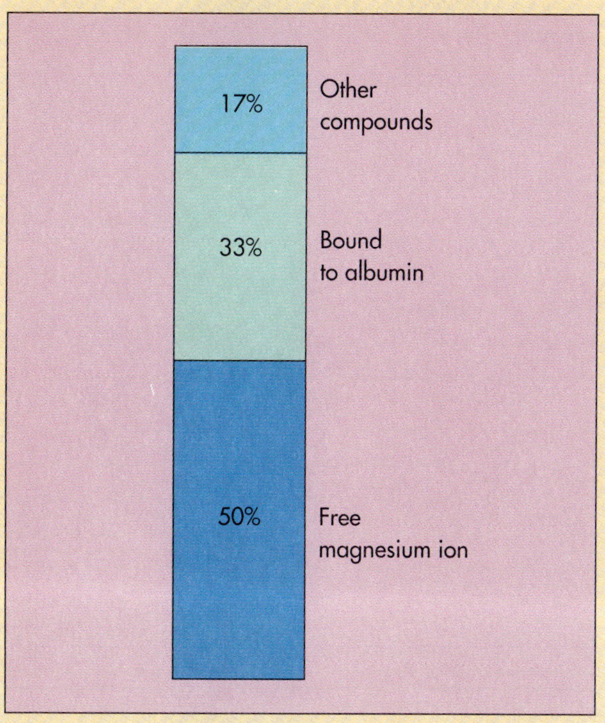

and heart failure. Such damagingly high levels of blood magnesium can result from kidney failure in which the excretion of excess magnesium via urine is stopped or is greatly reduced. The antagonism of calcium and magnesium is also evident when their rates of absorption and excretion are compared. If one of these ions is being absorbed or excreted in large amounts, there is usually a corresponding decrease in the rate at which the other is absorbed or excreted.

Magnesium is also required for the release of parathyroid hormone and its action on bone, the kidneys, and the intestine. It is also involved in the reactions that convert vitamin D into its active form.

ABSORPTION AND METABOLISM

Magnesium is absorbed primarily in the small intestine, probably with the help of a specific carrier. Approximately 35% to 40% of ingested magnesium is absorbed, with a lower proportion absorbed from diets providing high intakes and a higher proportion absorbed from diets with low intakes.[22] The efficiency of absorption is reduced by the presence of calcium, alcohol, phosphate, phytates, and fat but is increased by dietary vitamin D. The cellulose of fiber has little effect on magnesium absorption. A drop in plasma magnesium levels stimulates the secretion of parathyroid hormone, which in turn increases the efficiency of magnesium absorption. In addition to this role for parathyroid hormone, there is considerable evidence that magnesium metabolism is controlled by the thyroid gland.

The kidneys exert control over magnesium excretion, reabsorbing almost all magnesium when magnesium intake is low but excreting much of it when intakes exceed requirements. These variations in magnesium excretion, coupled with the ability of reserves in bone to be used when required, mean that variations in dietary magnesium intake seldom affect plasma levels of the mineral. Urinary losses of magnesium do increase in response to alcohol consumption or the use of diuretics.

Most of the magnesium within feces is unabsorbed dietary magnesium. A small amount of magnesium is lost within perspiration, but in high temperatures this loss can rise to account for 15% of magnesium losses overall.

DIETARY REQUIREMENTS

The Food and Nutrition Board recommends a magnesium intake of 280 mg/day for women and 350 mg/day for men. This corresponds to an intake of 5 mg/kg of body weight per day. These recommendations are based on data from magnesium balance studies and usual dietary intakes. A typical North American diet is estimated to provide around 12 mg of magnesium per 100 kcal, a level that barely provides the recommended intake. In one study of the effect of raising daily intake to 10 mg/kg of body weight, an initial period of increased magnesium retention occurred but then fell away, presumably once body reserves had been replenished to optimal levels.

There is an increased requirement for magnesium during pregnancy, so an additional 150 mg of magnesium per day is recommended for pregnant women. Similarly, an additional 150 mg/day is believed to be required to meet the additional needs during subsequent lactation. The recommended intake of magnesium for infants is 50 to 70 mg/day, a figure that is based on the level of magnesium found in human milk. The RDAs for magnesium in the United States and Recommended Nutrient Intakes applying to magnesium in Canada are shown in Table 9-4.

FOOD SOURCES

The magnesium content of the most frequently used foods is shown in Table 9-2. In terms of providing the most magnesium but the fewest kilocalories, vegetables are the best source of magnesium, followed by legumes, seafood, nuts, cereals, and dairy products. Magnesium is an essential component of chlorophyll, the green pigment of plants involved in trapping the sun's energy during photosynthesis. This makes green leafy vegetables major contributors to the magnesium content of the

TABLE 9-4

Recommended Dietary Allowances for magnesium in the United States and Recommended Nutrient Intakes for magnesium in Canada (mg/day).

AGE (YEARS)	UNITED STATES	CANADA
1-3	80	40-50
4-6	120	65
7-10	170	100
Boys, 10-12	270	130
Girls, 10-12	280	135
Men, 16-18	400	230
Women, 16-18	300	200
Men, 19-49	350	240-250
Women, 19-49	280	200
Men, 50-74	350	250
Women, 50-74	280	210

FIGURE 9-14

Contribution of various food groups to the magnesium content of the North American food supply.

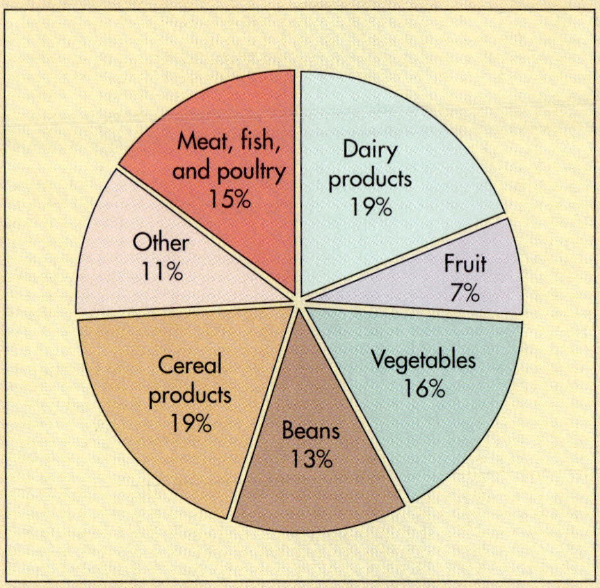

diet. Of the magnesium in cereal grains, 80% may be removed during the refining of flour and is not replaced in cereal enrichment.

Fresh water contains between 1 and 16 parts per million (ppm) of magnesium. Soft water contains amounts of magnesium at the bottom of this range, whereas hard water contains amounts at the top of the range. As much as one fifth of a person's magnesium intake can be provided by consumption of hard water. Seawater is sometimes promoted as a good source of magnesium, but although it is true that seawater contains about 1300 ppm of magnesium, it has little relevance to human nutrition because it is extremely unpalatable and has a high salt content. The relative contribution of various food groups to the magnesium content of the North American food supply is shown in Figure 9-14.

DEFICIENCY

Magnesium deficiency seldom occurs simply as a result of low dietary intake because of the efficiency with which the kidneys can reabsorb magnesium. Deficiency of magnesium can occur, however, as a result of starvation, persistent vomiting, the trauma of surgery, high calcium intake, or the rapid transit of food through the gastrointestinal tract.

The symptoms of low plasma magnesium levels are irritability, nervousness, and convulsions resulting from the overstimulation of nerves and increased muscular contraction. One well-recognized form of magnesium deficiency is **low magnesium tetany.** This is first diagnosed as uncontrolled neuromuscular tremors that progress until convulsive seizures occur. These symptoms often appear when a low dietary magnesium intake occurs, together with conditions that reduce magnesium absorption and increase magnesium excretion. In addition, alcohol and diuretics are capable of increasing the rate of magnesium excretion.

One of the less obvious effects of magnesium deficiency is the increased calcification of the soft tissues, including the formation of kidney stones. This may reflect the increased absorption of calcium that becomes possible when there is less magnesium available to compete with the calcium for absorption. At the same time, there is an increased mobilization of calcium from bone.

Inadequate magnesium also results in vasodilation, a widening of the blood vessels, and a consequent flushed appearance of the surface of the skin. It has been suggested that magnesium supplementation may be of value for the reduction of blood pressure.[23] Modern methods of measuring the magnesium content of body fluids have demonstrated that magnesium depletion occurs more often than had previously been assumed and may be linked to some cases of sudden death.[24]

ASSESSMENT OF MAGNESIUM RESERVES

Plasma magnesium levels do not provide an accurate indication of the amount of magnesium within cells because about 33% of plasma magnesium is bound to the albumin protein and is thus not detectable by standard clinical measurement techniques. Measuring the amount of magnesium within red blood cells gives an indication of the amount of magnesium available when the cells were formed, rather than at the time of measurement.

The most suitable method of assessing magnesium reserves, at least in children, is measurement of the amount excreted within urine after a large oral dose of magnesium. The higher the amount excreted, the greater the prevailing level of reserves is assumed to be. If less than 60% of the dietary dose is excreted, indicating that more than 40% has been retained, it is assumed that the body needs supplies of magnesium to correct a magnesium deficiency.

SULFUR (S)

Sulfur is present in every cell of the body and represents about 0.25% of body weight. The highest concentrations of sulfur are found in parts of the body that contain proteins rich in the sulfur-containing amino acids (cysteine and methionine), especially the skin, nails, and hair. The characteristic odor of sulfur dioxide is given off when these tissues are burned.

Sulfur is found in a variety of chemical forms within the body, as the "organic" sulfur within organic compounds, such as amino acids, and as "inorganic" sulfur within ions, such as the sulfate ion (SO_4^{2-}) and the sulfite ion (SO_3^{2-}). Any excess inorganic sulfur can be excreted in urine.

In addition to its role within two of the amino acids found in proteins, sulfur is present in compounds involved in the formation of blood clots and the transfer of energy. It is a part of at least three vitamins (thiamin, pantothenic acid, and biotin) and also the vitamin-like compound lipoic acid. Compounds containing sulfur act as detoxifying agents in the body, able to combine with toxic substances and convert them into harmless forms that are then excreted. Sulfur is also necessary for the formation of many mucopolysaccharides.

Interest in the sulfur present in the food supply has been heightened by the realization that "sulfiting agents," which have been used in salad bars to prevent the discoloration of such vegetables as mushrooms and lettuce, cause a severe reaction in many asthmatic people. In response to this discovery, the U.S. Food and Drug Administration decreed in 1987 that sulfite could no longer be used to preserve fresh fruits and vegetables and that its use in processed foods must be declared on the labels. The banning of some uses of sulfur in this way had little effect on the total dietary intake of sulfur. So far, however, there is insufficient information available on sulfur needs to form the basis of an RDA to be set.

ISSUES AND OPINIONS

Osteoporosis: A Pediatric Disease with a Geriatric Outcome

Dr. Tom Lloyd, Director of the Young Women's Health Study at the Pennsylvania State University M.S. Hershey Medical School, recently commented that "few 12-year-old girls care what happens to their bones when they are 70 years old." To a 12-year-old child, the age of 70 is literally a lifetime away. Yet research shows that dietary, exercise, and life-style habits between the ages of 10 and 20 significantly affect the accretion of bone mass and that the peak bone mass attained by premenopausal women is a major determinant of their risk of osteoporosis later in life.

Rapid increases in bone density and content occur during puberty, and peak bone density in the spine and hip of females (prime fracture sites in patients with osteoporosis) is achieved near the age of 20 years. It has recently been shown that additional calcium intake during childhood can have a positive influence on bone development. This was demonstrated by two well-controlled, double-blind clinical studies; one focused on identical twins* and the other focused on preadolescent girls.† Additional calcium, at levels of 700 mg/day or 250 mg/day, respectively, was shown to enhance total bone mineral content.

In both of these studies, mean calcium intake was about 900 mg/day (75% of the recommended dietary allowances [RDAs] of 1200 mg/day). The children receiving additional calcium from the researchers, however, had calcium intakes between 115% and 150% of the RDA. Other indices of childhood development were not influenced by the additional calcium intake. The participants' overall growth patterns (as assessed by height, weight, body mass index, and percentage body fat) were similar and unrelated to calcium intake. The rate at which the total body bone mineral density of young girls increased in response to additional intake of calcium was 1.5% per year, which achieved a 6% increase in bone density if maintained for 4 years. If the extra bone mass were retained into adulthood, the risk of bone fracture from osteoporosis would be reduced by 50%.

Clearly, early prevention holds the greatest promise in the prevention of osteoporosis (as with many chronic diseases afflicting modern society). So prevention strategies to reduce the incidence of osteoporosis should begin in childhood. Unfortunately, when children reach adolescence, their drive for independence is often expressed by disregard for parental advice on many matters, including nutrition. The calcium intake of female adolescents often falls dramatically during this critical period of bone development.

North Americans receive most of their dietary calcium from dairy products. An increasing number of calcium-enriched foods and beverages are also available for those who do not or cannot consume dairy products. A major U.S. health objective for the year 2000 is to "increase calcium intake so that at least 50% of youth aged 12 to 24 . . . consume three or more servings of foods rich in calcium." From 1985 to 1986 only 7% of U.S. females and 14% of males aged 19 to 24 years met this objective.

* Johnston CC Jr and others: *N Engl J Med* 327:82, 1992.
† Lloyd T and others: *JAMA* 270:841, 1993.

BY NOW YOU SHOULD KNOW

- Minerals are classified as macronutrient minerals or micronutrient minerals (trace elements), depending on how abundant they are in the body.
- In order of their abundance within the body, the macronutrient minerals are calcium, phosphorus, potassium, sulfur, sodium, chlorine, and magnesium.
- Sodium, potassium, and chloride ions (Na^+, K^+, and Cl^-, respectively) are three of the main electrolyte ions of the body and play a major role in regulating the flow of water (by osmosis) between the different regions of the body.
- Calcium is a component of bones and teeth, regulates many biochemical processes in the body, including the clotting of blood, and is involved in the transmission of nerve impulses and the contraction of muscles.
- Many different dietary factors influence the efficiency of calcium absorption.
- The use of calcium by the body is regulated by a variety of hormones.
- Calcium is provided by relatively few foods, with milk and other dairy products being the most dependable sources.
- Calcium deficiency in the diet results in depletion of the body's reserves of calcium within bones.
- Osteoporosis affects about 60% of postmenopausal women and is the major health problem that results from inadequate calcium intake. Women with osteoporosis are more likely to suffer from spontaneous fractures.
- Phosphorus performs many functions in the body, including facilitation of the absorption, transport, and metabolism of many other nutrients. It is a major component of bones and teeth.
- Phosphorus is found in all foods but is particularly abundant in protein-rich foods.
- Magnesium facilitates many biochemical processes.
- The typical North American diet provides adequate amounts of phosphorus but marginal amounts of magnesium and often inadequate amounts of calcium.
- The use of diuretics and the consumption of alcohol can increase the excretion of magnesium.
- Sulfur is found in all cells but is most concentrated in skin, hair, and nails.
- Sulfur occurs in the amino acids methionine and cysteine, as well as in a variety of other organic compounds of the body.

STUDY QUESTIONS

1. Describe the role of calcium in the formation of a blood clot.
2. List the reasons why milk is such a good source of calcium.
3. How can an individual with lactose intolerance obtain adequate calcium?
4. How can a postmenopausal woman plan a reasonable diet that includes as much as 800 mg of calcium per day and also supplies adequate amounts of all other nutrients and an energy intake of 2000 kcal or less?
5. What is the best strategy to reduce the risk of developing severe osteoporosis?
6. What hormones are involved in regulating calcium metabolism?
7. On the basis of nutrient density, what are the three best sources for calcium, phosphorus, and magnesium?
8. Discuss the influence of bone and of the kidneys on the body's levels of calcium, phosphorus, and magnesium.

CRITICAL ANALYSIS

1. Estimate your daily calcium intake.

This exercise employs a food frequency questionnaire (Appendix L) that was specifically developed to assess calcium intake. It takes about 5 minutes to fill out the questionnaire and calculate calcium intake. Although this food frequency questionnaire is not as accurate as the more work intensive 3-day food record, it has the advantages of being quick and easy to do and the results have been shown to be close to those obtained with the food record.

For the items you eat at least once a week, write the number of servings you typically eat per week in the column where you see the phrase "Every week" at the top. If you eat a food less than once a week, it does not make a large contribution to your daily calcium intake and does not need to be recorded.

For the items you eat every day, record the number of servings you typically eat per day in the column where you see the phrase "Every day" at the top.

After completing the two columns, calculate your daily intake using the following steps:

a. For items eaten daily, multiply the number of servings × 7 × score (the score is the number found in the column immediately before each food).
b. For items eaten weekly, multiply the number of servings × score.
c. Add the servings in both columns to get the total number of servings and divide this total by 7.
d. Add 100 to the number you obtained in step 3.
e. The number obtained in step 4 = the estimated milligrams of calcium consumed per day.

REFERENCES

1. Weaver CM: Calcium bioavailability and its relation to osteoporosis, *Proc Soc Exp Biol Med* 200:157, 1992.
2. Bronner F: Intestinal calcium absorption mechanisms and applications, *J Nutr* 117:1347, 1987.
3. Allen LH: Calcium bioavailability and absorption. A review, *Am J Clin Nutr* 35:783, 1982.
4. Wasserman RH: Calcium and phosphate entry into cells: a brief overview, *Prog Clin Biol Res* 252:3, 1988.
5. Bergeim O: Intestinal chemistry. v. Carbohydrates and calcium and phosphorus absorption, *J Biol Chem* 70:35, 1926.
6. Miller DD: Calcium in the diet: food sources, recommended intakes, and nutritional bioavailability, *Adv Food Nutr Res* 33:103, 1989.
7. Ziegler EE, Fomon SJ: Lactose enhances mineral absorption in infancy, *J Pediatr Gastroenterol Nutr* 2:288, 1983.
8. Hegsted MS and others: Urinary calcium and calcium balance in young men as affected by level of protein and phosphorus intake, *J Nutr* 111:553, 1981.
9. Linkswiler HM, Joyce CL, Anand R: Calcium retention of young adult males as affected by level of protein and calcium intake, *Trans N Y Acad Sci (series 2)* 36:333, 1974.
10. Zemel MB: Calcium utilization—effect of varying level and source of dietary proteins, *Am J Clin Nutr* 48:880, 1988.
11. Heaney RP: Effect of calcium on skeletal development, bone loss and risk of fractures, *Am J Med* 91(suppl 5B):23S, 1991.
12. Wright HS and others: The 1987-1988 Nationwide Food Consumption Survey: an update on the nutrient intake of respondents, *Nutr Today* 25:21, 1991.
13. National Center for Health Statistics: Nation Health and Nutrition Examination Survey (NHANES) III: *Vitamin and mineral intakes of persons aged 2 months and older in the United States: 1988-1991,* Hyattsville, Md, Advanced Data from Vital and Health Statistics, in press.
14. U.S. Food and Drug Administration: Advice on limiting intake of bonemeal, *1982 Food and Drug Administration Bull,* p 5, April, 1982.
15. Bourgoin BP and others: Lead content in 70 brands of dietary calcium supplements, *Am J Public Health* 83:1155, 1993.
16. Moss AJ and others: *Use of vitamin and mineral supplements in the United States: current users, types of products and nutrients,* Hyattsville, Md, Advanced Data from Vital and Health Statistics, in press.
17. Heaney RP: Calcium supplements: practical considerations, *Osteoporosis Int* 1:65, 1991.
18. McCarron DA: Is calcium more important than sodium in the pathogenesis of essential hypertension? *Hypertension* 7:604, 1985.

19. Belizan JM, Villar J, Pineda O: Reduction of blood pressure with calcium supplementation in young adults, *JAMA* 249:1161, 1983.

20. Newmark HL, Lipkin M: Calcium, vitamin D, and colon cancer, *Cancer Res* 52(suppl):2067S, 1992.

21. Pepper M, Geheb M, Desai T: Hypophosphatemia and hyperphosphatemia, *Crit Care Clin* 7:201, 1991.

22. Fine KD and others: Intestinal absorption of magnesium from food and supplements, *J Clin Invest* 88:396, 1991.

23. Whelton PK, Klag MJ: Magnesium and blood pressure: review of the epidemiological and clinical trial experience, *Am J Cardiol* 63:26G, 1989.

24. Eisenberg MJ: Magnesium deficiency and sudden death, *Am Heart J* 124:544, 1992.

~ ADDITIONAL READINGS ~

Calcium

Andon MB and others: Spinal bone density and calcium intake in healthy postmenopausal women, *Am J Clin Nutr* 54:927, 1991.

Baran D and others: Dietary modification with dairy products for preventing vertebral bone loss in premenopausal women: a three-year prospective study, *J Clin Endocrinol Metab* 70:264, 1990.

Bronner F: Nutrient bioavailability, with special reference to calcium, *J Nutr* 117:1347, 1987.

Cumming RG: Calcium intake and bone mass: a quantitative review of the evidence, *Calif Tiss Int* 47:194, 1990.

Dawson-Hughes B and others: A controlled trial on the effect of calcium supplementation on bone density in postmenopausal women, *N Engl J Med* 323:878, 1990.

Irwin MI, Kienholz EW: A conspectus of research on calcium requirements of man, *J Nutr* 103:1019, 1973.

Resnick LM: Dietary calcium and hypertension, *J Nutr* 117:1806, 1987.

Riggs BL, Melton LJ: The prevention and treatment of osteoporosis, *N Engl J Med* 327:620, 1992.

Simopolus A, Galli C, editors: Osteoporosis: nutrition aspects, *World Rev Nutr Diet* 73:1, 1993.

Spencer H, Kramer L, Osis D: Do protein and phosphorus cause calcium loss? *J Nutr* 118:666, 1988.

Toss G: Effect of calcium intake vs. other life-style factors on bone mass, *J Intern Med* 231:181, 1992.

Walden O: The relationship of dietary and supplemental calcium intake to bone loss and osteoporosis, *J Am Diet Assoc* 89:397, 1989.

Zimmerman J: Does dietary calcium supplementation reduce the risk of colon cancer? *Nutr Rev* 51:109, 1993.

Phosphorus

Anderson JJB, Barrett CJH: Dietary phosphorus, the benefits and problems, *Nutr Today* 29:29, 1994.

Gertner JM: Disorders of calcium and phosphorus homeostasis, *Pediatr Clin North Am* 37:1441, 1990.

Life Sciences Research Office: *Effects of dietary factors on skeletal integrity in adults: calcium, phosphorus, vitamin D and protein,* Bethesda, Md, 1981, Federation of American Societies for Experimental Biology.

Magnesium

Aikawa JK: *Magnesium: its biological significance,* Boca Raton, Fl, 1980, CRC Press.

Altura BM: Schematic heart disease and magnesium, *Magnesium* 7:57, 1988.

Quamme GA: Renal handling of magnesium: drug and hormone interactions, *Magnesium* 5:248, 1986.

Wester PO: Magnesium, *Am J Clin Nutr* 45:1305, 1987.

Sulfur

Expert Panel on Nutrition: Sulfites as food ingredients, *Food Technol* 40:47, 1986.

Ip C, Ganther HE: Comparison of selenium and sulfur analogs in cancer prevention, *Carcinogenesis* 13:1167, 1992.

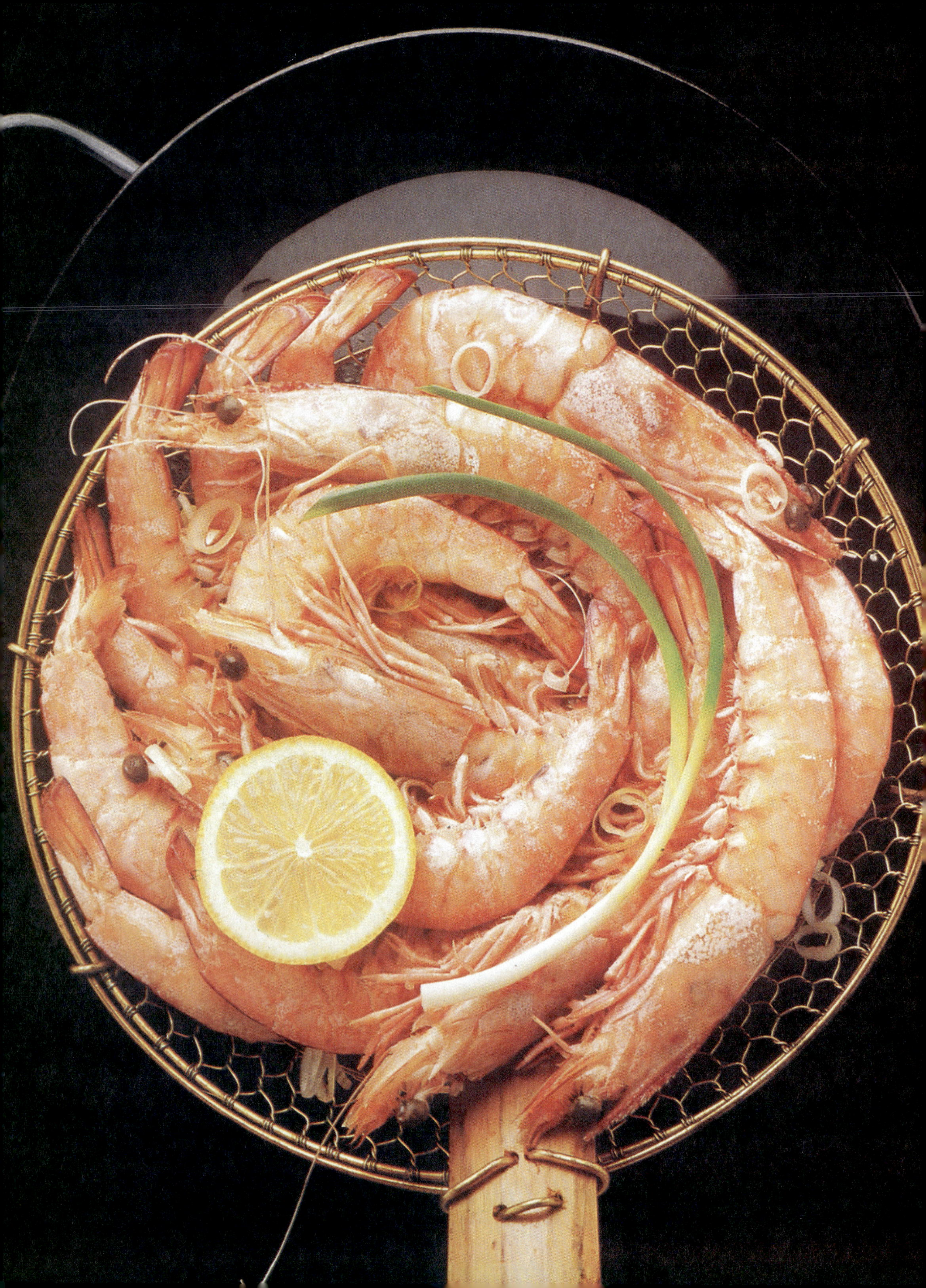

CHAPTER 10

MICRONUTRIENT MINERALS

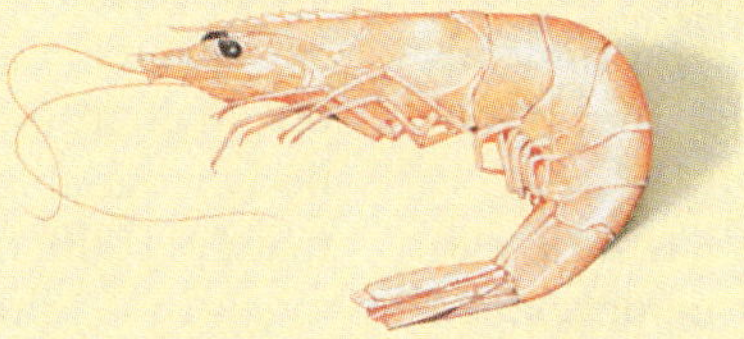

The micronutrient minerals are also known as the trace elements because they are mineral elements present in the body in small amounts. Some micronutrient minerals, such as iron and iodine, have been known for many years to be dietary essentials. Others have been detected in the body and established as dietary essentials only recently, thanks to the development of more sensitive techniques of chemical analysis. Nine of the trace elements (manganese, molybdenum, cobalt, chromium, silicon, vanadium, nickel, arsenic, and boron) are present in the body in such small amounts that they are also known as the ultratrace elements. Estimates of requirements for micronutrient minerals have raised some questions about the adequacy of the North American diet as a source of them. There is much information about some micronutrient minerals and little information about others. This imbalance in knowledge is reflected in the depth of coverage given to each mineral in this chapter, which does not imply that those minerals covered in less detail are any less important. Some essential micronutrient minerals have probably not been identified yet, and there are already several strong candidates for addition to the list.

The micronutrient minerals (or trace elements) that have been established as dietary essentials are the following:

Iron	**Iodine**	**Molybdenum**
Zinc	**Selenium**	**Cobalt**
Copper	**Manganese**	**Chromium**

The micronutient minerals that are *not* firmly established as dietary essentials are the following:

Silicon	**Nickel**	**Boron**
Vanadium	**Arsenic**	**Tin**

The most abundant of these minerals in the body is iron, which nevertheless accounts for a mere 0.004% of body weight. The tiny amounts of the micronutrient minerals in the body perform many essential chemical and physiological functions.

For most micronutrient minerals there is little evidence of naturally occurring deficiencies in developed nations of the world. More evidence of deficiencies can be found in less developed countries. Because of the rarity of deficiencies in the micronutrient minerals, it has often proved difficult to obtain experimental evidence of adequate dietary levels of them for human nutrition. Much of the evidence on the biological role of micronutrient minerals has thus come from animal studies.

IRON (Fe)

Iron is the fourth most abundant element on Earth, composing 4.7% of the Earth's crust. This great abundance of iron in nature makes it surprising that iron deficiency is the most common nutritional deficiency, both in the United States and worldwide.[1]

Iron was first recognized as a constituent of the body by Lérnery in 1713. In 1800 Lecanu identified iron in the metalloprotein hemoglobin, which is now known to bind to oxygen molecules to permit their transport in blood. It is also now known that virtually all of the iron in the body exists in combination with protein molecules. Overall, the body contains less than 1 tsp of iron (2.5 to 4 g), with the precise amount in any individual dependent on gender, age, size, nutritional status, general health, and level of iron stores.

DISTRIBUTION

Most of the iron in the body is found in the blood, but some is present in every cell, bound to iron-containing enzymes. The iron in the body can be divided into **functional iron,** which is iron actually participating in some biochemical function, and **nonfunctional iron,** which is iron either held in storage or in the act of being transported within the body (Table 10-1). Over two thirds of body iron is usually in the form of functional iron, and most of this iron is bound within the structure of hemoglobin. A small portion of the functional iron is bound within the structure of myoglobin, an iron-containing protein related to hemoglobin but found in muscle. The rest of the functional iron is part of various metalloenzymes that perform varied acts of catalysis in cells.[2]

Most of the nonfunctional iron of the body is held in iron storage compounds within the liver, spleen, and bone marrow. Some of the iron in these stores is held in a large internal cavity within the protein **ferritin,** each molecule of which can contain up to 4500 iron ions (as Fe^{3+}). Ferritin is a soluble iron-storage compound, but other stores of iron are in the form of an insoluble iron-protein complex called **hemosiderin,** which is up to one half iron. The amount of iron stored within the body is variable, generally being higher in men (approximately 1000 mg) than in women (approximately 400 mg). In addition to the iron held in stores, a small amount of nonfunctional iron is the iron being transported within the blood, either bound to the protein **transferrin** or within molecules of ferritin. Transported iron is exchanged rapidly with the iron in both functional forms and nonfunctional storage forms. Although only about 4 mg of iron is being transported within the blood at any time, a total of 40 mg passes through the transport stage each day.

FUNCTIONS

Transport and Storage of Oxygen

Iron (as Fe^{2+}) within the metalloproteins hemoglobin and myoglobin can bind to oxygen molecules (O_2) and transport them through the blood (in the case of hemoglobin) or store them within muscles (in the case of myoglobin).[3] The iron is not bound to these proteins directly but is instead bound within a **heme** group, which is itself bound to the protein chain (Figure 10-1). Hemoglobin is a multi-subunit protein comprising four subunits, each with one heme group and associated iron ion attached. This allows each hemoglobin molecule to bind to four oxygen molecules. Hemoglobin is found in the red blood cells and indeed is the chemical that is responsible for making these cells (and therefore blood) appear red. As red blood cells pass through the capillaries of the lungs, oxygen from the lungs becomes bound to the hemoglobin molecules in the cells. The red blood cells then transport their cargo of oxygen-bearing hemoglobin throughout the body. In tissues that require supplies of oxygen, the oxygen is released from the hemoglobin to diffuse out of the red blood cells, out of the blood, and into the tissue cells.

Myoglobin is a single-subunit protein that is structurally similar to the individual subunits of hemoglobin, and it too contains a heme group whose iron ion can bind to an oxygen molecule. Myoglobin is found only in

TABLE 10-1

Distribution of iron throughout the body

		APPROXIMATE AMOUNT (mg)	
	TOTAL (%)	MEN	WOMEN
FUNCTIONAL			
Hemoglobin	60-70	2100	1750
Myoglobin	3-4	100	100
Tissue iron (enzymes)	5-15	350	300
STORAGE AND TRANSPORT			
Storage iron (liver, spleen, and bone marrow)	15-30	1000	400
Transport iron (transferrin)	0.1	4	4
Serum ferritin	<1	0.3	0.1
TOTAL		3551.3	2554.1

FIGURE 10-1

Chemical structure of heme plus schematic three-dimensional diagram of hemoglobin showing the bound iron-containing groups.

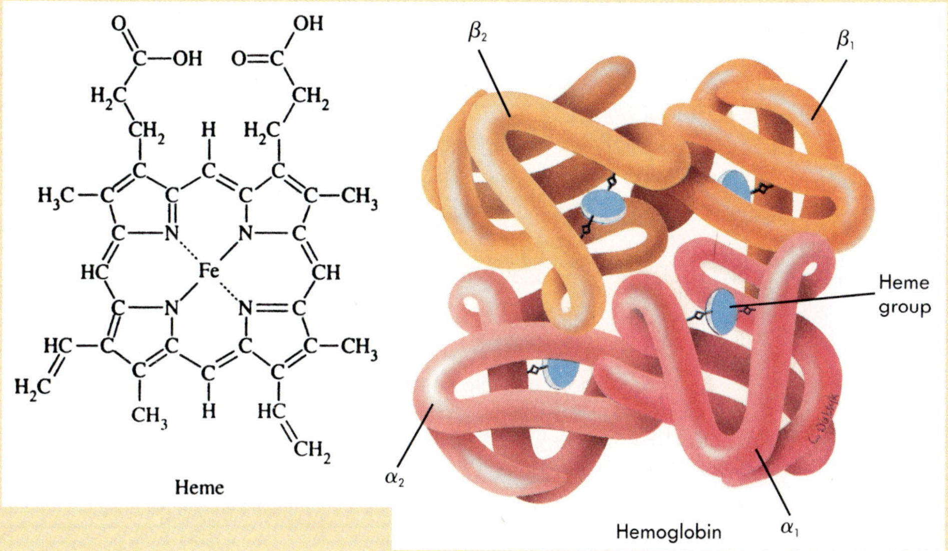

muscle, where it serves as a reservoir of oxygen. The oxygen is needed to combine with nutrient molecules to release the energy to power muscular contraction. The presence of considerable reserves of oxygen bound to myoglobin allows muscles to operate more effectively than they could if the only oxygen available was that being released from hemoglobin.

Cofactor of Enzymes and Other Proteins

The iron-containing heme group is also a part of several proteins involved in the release of energy during the oxidation of nutrients and the trapping of that energy within adenosine triphosphate (ATP). Also, iron on its own is a cofactor bound to several nonheme enzymes required for the proper functioning of cells.[3-5] Some of the other processes that depend on the activities of iron-containing enzymes are the following:

- Conversion of beta-carotene (a precursor of vitamin A) to the active form of vitamin A
- Synthesis of purines, which form an integral part of deoxyribonucleic acid (DNA) and ribonucleic acid (RNA)
- Synthesis of carnitine, a vitamin-like substance needed for the transport of fatty acids
- Synthesis of collagen, one of the major struuctural proteins of the body

FIGURE 10-2

Red blood cell formation (erythropoiesis).

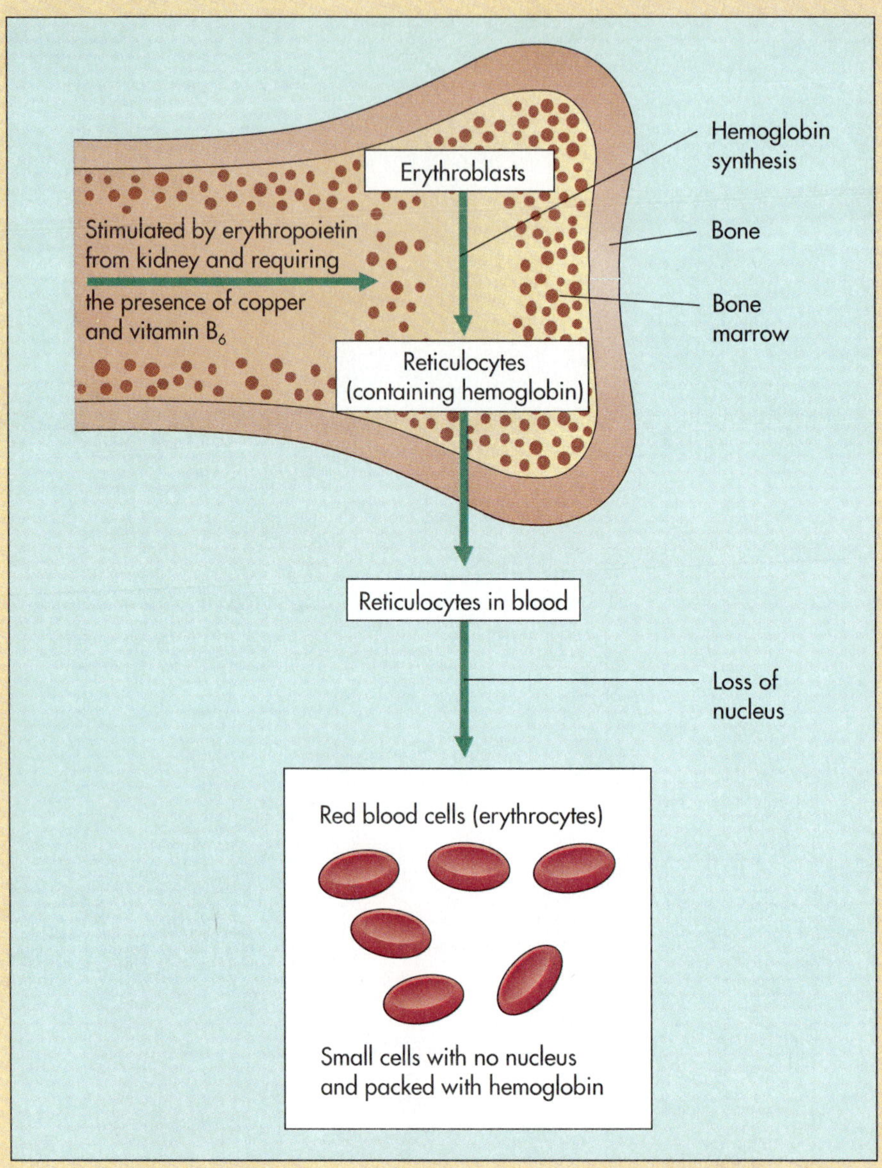

- Detoxification of drugs and other toxic compounds in the liver and intestine
- Synthesis of the neurotransmitters dopamine, serotonin, and norepinephrine

Formation of Red Blood Cells

Because the iron-containing protein hemoglobin is a major component of red blood cells (**erythrocytes**), iron is obviously required for the formation of red blood cells. Another way of expressing this is to say that iron is essential for the formation of blood. Red blood cells are formed in the bone marrow in a process known as **erythropoiesis** (Figure 10-2). Erythropoiesis is stimulated when the amount of oxygen reaching tissues from the blood begins to fall below normal levels. The first step mediating this effect of oxygen deficiency is the release from the kidneys of an enzyme called **renal erythropoietic factor** in direct response to the falling oxygen levels. The erythropoietic factor enters the blood, where it converts a protein called **erythropoietinogen** into **erythropoietin,** which in turn stimulates bone marrow cells to increase their production of red blood cells. When this results in increasing levels of circulating red blood cells, the oxygen deficiency subsides because of the new supplies carried by these new cells, and so the production of renal erythropoietic factor decreases, leading to a reduction in the rate of red blood cell production until a deficiency of oxygen sets in again.

The production of red blood cells begins with the production of immature cells in the bone marrow known as **erythroblasts,** each of which contains a nucleus, similar to a normal body cell. As the erythroblasts mature in the bone marrow, they synthesize the iron-containing heme groups in a process requiring the help of vitamin B_6 and the mineral copper. The heme groups become bound to **globin** molecules, also synthesized by the erythroblasts, to form completed hemoglobin molecules. The hemoglobin-containing cells are known as **reticulocytes** and are released from the bone marrow into the blood. Within 24 to 36 hours after their release the nuclei of the reticulocytes disintegrate and the cells become mature erythrocytes (red blood cells), ready to begin the transport of oxygen to the tissues and of carbon dioxide away from the tissues. Red blood cells are the only cells in the body that do not possess a nucleus.

> Over 100 million red blood cells are formed in an adult each minute of every day to replace the same number of cells that are destroyed each minute. Each of the red blood cells formed contains between 200 and 300 million molecules of hemoglobin, carrying a total of 800 to 1200 million iron ions. The hemoglobin molecules compose about 95% of the dry weight of each cell (that is, weight once water is removed).

Because a red blood cell has no nucleus, it cannot produce the enzymes and other proteins necessary for long-term survival. As a result, it survives only for as long as the enzymes originally present within it remain functional, which is usually about 120 days (4 months). When red blood cells die, they are removed from the blood by cells of the liver, bone marrow, and spleen, which are part of the **reticuloendothelial system.** In the spleen the iron and amino acids derived from hemoglobin are salvaged and recycled. The iron is stored as hemosiderin and ferritin in the liver and spleen or is returned to the bone marrow for incorporation into new hemoglobin molecules. In this way, iron is effectively conserved and reused. The amino acids are released to the blood, where they are available to all cells for the synthesis of new proteins or for the oxidative release of energy. The remaining portions of the hemoglobin molecule, its heme groups, are converted to a chemical called **bilirubin,** which is transported to the liver and then excreted in bile (Figure 10-3).

ABSORPTION

The absorption of iron occurs mainly in the duodenum and jejunum. Two distinct categories or "pools" of iron are available for absorption, and the absorption of iron from these two pools occurs by different mechanisms (Figure 10-4). The largest pool is **nonheme iron,** meaning iron that is not bound within the structure of heme. This consists largely of iron-containing salts within food, although the iron can be in the form of ferrous (Fe^{2+}) or ferric (Fe^{3+}) ions. The second, smaller pool of dietary iron is **heme iron,** meaning the iron that is combined within heme groups. Heme iron is largely derived from the hemoglobin and myoglobin molecules within foods of animal origin, although a little heme iron is also obtained from heme-containing enzymes within a wide variety of foods.

> Iron occurs within the body in the form of two types of iron ions:
> **Ferrous iron** consists of Fe^{2+} ions
> **Ferric iron** consists of Fe^{3+} ions
> One type of ion can be converted into the other type by the loss or gain of an electron. If an ion of ferrous iron loses an electron, it becomes an ion of ferric iron, whereas if an ion of ferric iron gains an electron, it becomes an ion of ferrous iron. Most of the iron within food is in the ferric (Fe^{3+}) form, but most of the iron within nutritional supplements is in the more soluble ferrous (Fe^{2+}) form.

Nonheme iron accounts for approximately 85% of the iron in the typical diet. To be available for absorption, the iron ions of nonheme iron (whether Fe^{2+} or Fe^{3+}) must be released within the duodenum and intestine in a free solubilized form. The dissolved iron ions then bind to transferrin-like iron-binding proteins, which are then carried into the cells of the gastrointestinal wall by specific transporters. The requirement for the nonheme iron within food to be released in soluble form before absorption means that its absorption can be inhibited by a large number of dietary factors able to bind to it and so prevent its release in soluble form.

The percentage of nonheme iron that is absorbed from a meal can vary from less than 1% to more than 50%.[6] The actual value is inversely related to the iron content of the meal. In one study, for example, the absorption of iron from a meal fell from 18% to 6.4% as the iron content of the meal was increased from 1.5 mg

FIGURE 10-3

The fate of hemoglobin during red blood cell destruction.

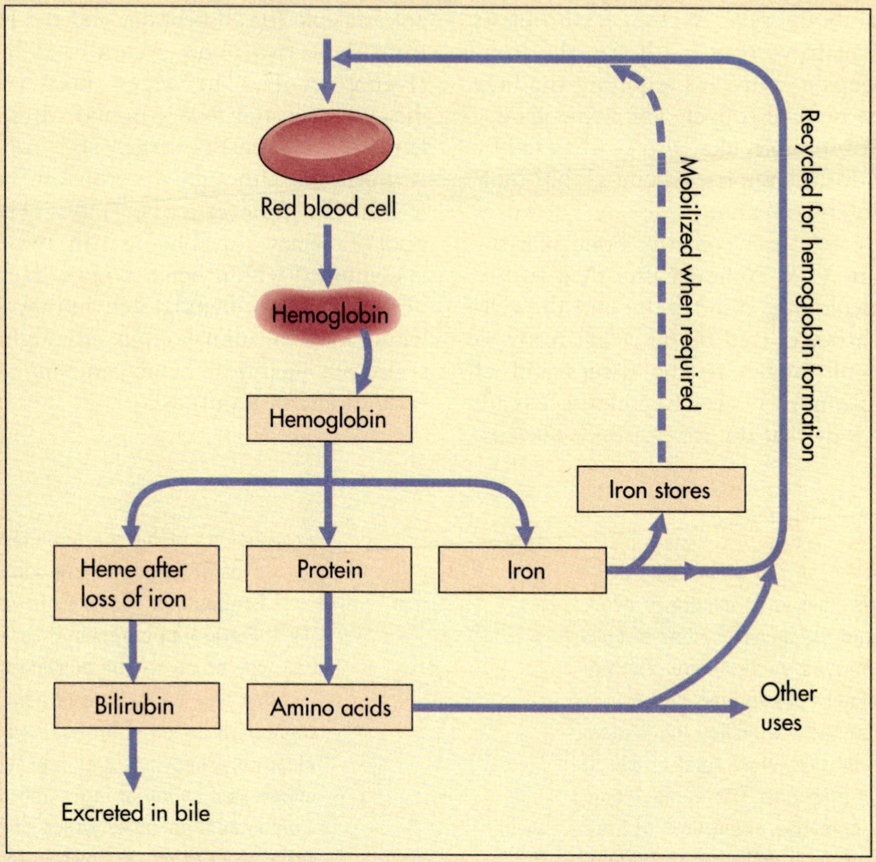

to 5.7 mg.[7] It is also known that iron is absorbed much more efficiently by people who are already deficient in iron than by those whose bodies contain sufficient iron.[8] This not only helps those who are deficient in iron (most children and premenopausal women) to absorb iron effectively, but also protects those with sufficient iron (most men and postmenopausal women) from the hazards associated with iron overload. Although it is clear that the factors mediating the control of iron absorption operate at the enterocyte cells lining the intestine and duodenum, many of the details are the subject of dispute.[5] Enterocytes are regularly sloughed off from the intestinal wall to be replaced by new ones, and any iron contained within the cells that are lost by sloughing never reaches the bloodstream. The proportion of iron that gets into enterocytes but never into the bloodstream because of this process of sloughing is unclear. It is also unclear exactly how the level of iron stores within the body is able to influence the efficiency with which iron absorption from the gastrointestinal tract occurs.

Heme iron is absorbed across the enterocyte cell membrane still embodied as part of the heme group.[9] Specific receptors mediating this process have been identified in laboratory animals but not yet in humans. Once the heme groups enter intestinal cells, they are rapidly degraded by the enzyme **heme oxygenase.** This releases the iron into the common intracellular pool. Because heme iron remains protected within the heme group before it is absorbed, the efficiency of its absorption is not influenced by most other dietary factors. The only known enhancer of heme iron absorption is protein from animal tissues. Calcium inhibits the delivery of ingested heme iron to the blood by inhibiting the transport of the iron through enterocytes, rather than by inhibiting the actual process of absorption into the cells.[10] The amount of heme iron in a meal has little effect on the percentage absorbed, which is usually between 20% and 25%.

Factors Affecting the Absorption of Nonheme Iron

Many different dietary factors can either enhance or inhibit the absorption of the nonheme iron within food; the major factors are as follows.

FIGURE 10-4

Proposed mechanisms of iron absorption.

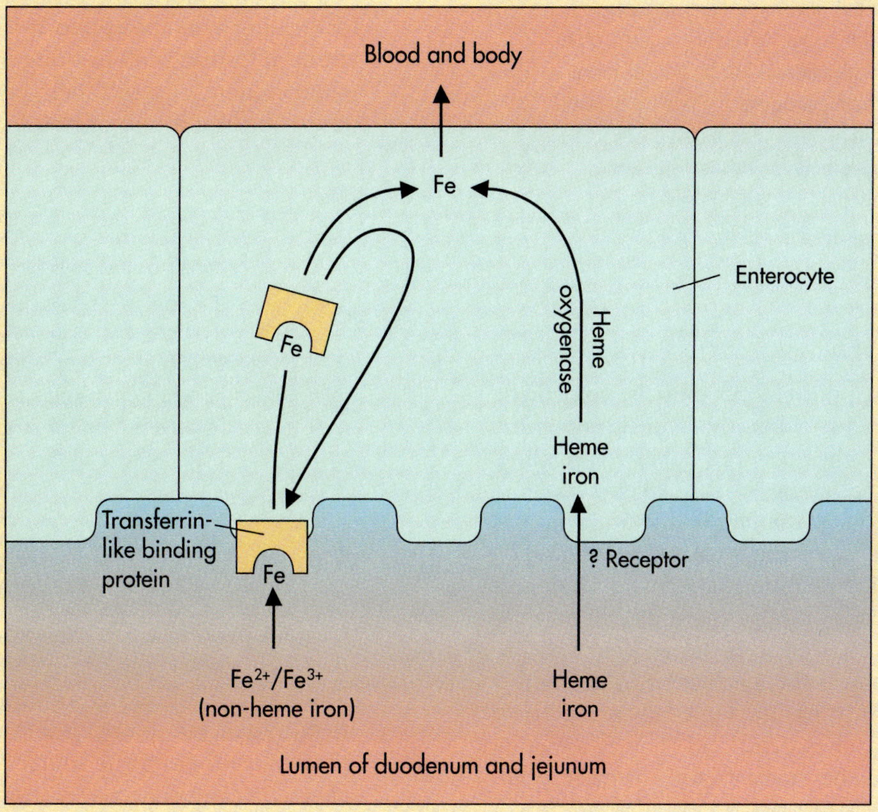

DIETARY FACTORS ENHANCING NONHEME IRON ABSORPTION

- Increased acidity (from ascorbic acid, organic acids, and so on)
- Animal tissue protein

DIETARY FACTORS INHIBITING NONHEME IRON ABSORPTION

- Low gastric acidity
- Dietary fiber
- High dietary calcium intakes
- High dietary phosphorus intakes
- Certain proteins
- Phytates and oxalates
- High manganese intakes
- Polyphenols

Enhancing factors Enhancing factors include the following:

- **Increased acidity** of food or gastric secretions promotes iron absorption by maintaining nonheme iron in the more soluble ferrous (Fe^{2+}) form or by forming soluble and readily absorbed complexes of iron and organic acids, known as iron **chelates.** Ascorbic acid (vitamin C), citric acid, lactic acid, malic acid, tartaric acid, hydrochloric acid, and the acidic amino acids all enhance the solubility and absorbability of iron. The most potent effect in humans is obtained from ascorbic acid. In adults, the inclusion of 25 to 30 mg of ascorbic acid in a meal enhances iron absorption by 85%. Enhancements by as much as 1500% (a 15-fold increase) can be achieved when large quantities of ascorbic acid (about 2 g) are taken with a meal. This amount of ascorbic acid could be obtained only from supplements, and such increases in iron absorption are potentially dangerous for the 6% to 10% of the population who are genetically susceptible to iron overload. Whatever amount is used, the effect of ascorbic acid is greatest in meals lacking meat, fish, or poultry.
- **Animal tissue protein** such as that contained within meat, fish, or poultry increases the absorption of iron from a meal two- to four-fold (by 200% to 400%).[11] The protein must not

> ***M**any mineral ions combine with larger chemical groups to form **chelates** in which the larger "chelating agent" often holds the mineral ion by two or more loose chemical bonds ("chela" = a claw). Chelated mineral ions may be absorbed more efficiently or less efficiently, depending on the mineral ion and "chelating agent" involved.*

only be animal protein but must be contained within animal tissue because animal protein in milk, cheese, and eggs does not have the same effect. The mechanism of this effect is unknown, but one possibility is that the amino acid cysteine, or cysteine-containing peptides, released during digestion of animal protein, may combine with iron to form soluble chelates, which allow the iron to be more effectively absorbed. Whatever the mechanism, it is found that 1 g of meat has the same enhancing effect as does 1 mg of ascorbic acid. This is sometimes referred to as the "meat factor" or meat, poultry, and fish (MFP) factor in iron absorption.

Inhibiting factors Inhibiting factors include the following:

- **Low gastric acidity** resulting from decreased secretion of hydrochloric acid into the stomach, overconsumption of antacids, or gastric surgery can lead to decreased absorption of nonheme iron. The secretion of hydrochloric acid into the stomach often decreases naturally with aging.
- **Dietary fiber** can inhibit the absorption of nonheme iron, although the effect is restricted to certain types of fiber. Cellulose, for example, has no effect, whereas hemicellulose causes a reduction in absorption. Fiber in general may also reduce iron absorption by increasing the speed at which the digestive mass moves through the gastrointestinal tract. Foods that are high in fiber are also high in phytates, which strongly inhibit nonheme iron absorption, as discussed below.
- **High dietary calcium and phosphorus intakes** can reduce nonheme iron absorption by as much as 50%. Dawson-Hughes and colleagues[12] have demonstrated that either calcium carbonate or hydroxyapatite (which contains both calcium and phosphorus) significantly reduces iron absorption. The inhibitory effect of calcium is dose-dependent up to a dose of 300 mg per meal,[10] with—for example—165 mg of calcium (as calcium chloride or within milk or cheeses) decreasing iron absorption by 50%. Adding calcium to human milk to bring it up to the calcium content of cow's milk, however, did not affect the absorption of iron from the milk.[13]

> ***B**ecause of the ability of calcium to interfere with iron absorption, calcium supplements should be taken several hours before or after a meal. If both calcium and iron supplements are used, they should not be taken at the same time of day.*

- **Certain proteins** that are not animal tissue proteins (known to enhance iron absorption) are found to inhibit iron absorption. This means that, in general, doubling the amount of dietary protein from nontissue sources such as milk, cheese, and eggs decreases iron absorption by 50%.
- **Phytates and oxalates** are salts derived from phytic and oxalic acid, and phytates and oxalates formed by combination with iron ions can convert the iron into an insoluble form that is unavailable for absorption. Phytic acid is a phosphorus-containing organic acid found in such foods as whole grains, bran, and soy products. Oxalic acid is an organic acid found in such foods as spinach, rhubarb, and chocolate.
- **A high manganese intake** can depress iron absorption because manganese and nonheme iron appear to share the same absorption pathway. Conversely, a high nonheme iron intake can depress the absorption of manganese because these two minerals effectively compete to follow the same entry route into the body.
- **Polyphenols** are organic compounds (including the well-known **tannins**) present in coffee, tea, cocoa, and some vegetables that are able to reduce the absorption of iron from a meal by as much as 70%. This is because of their ability to form insoluble complexes with iron.

TRANSPORT AND METABOLISM

Once iron is absorbed, it is transported through the blood bound to the protein transferrin. Each molecule of transferrin can bind to two Fe^{3+} ions, although under normal circumstances less than half of the binding sites available on the body's total pool of transferrin molecules are occupied. Blood also contains a small amount of the iron-storage protein ferritin, each molecule of which can contain up to 4500 Fe^{3+} ions. The iron ions transported by transferrin can be released to cells for the manufacture of iron-containing enzymes and other proteins, released to the bone marrow for use in hemoglobin synthesis, or deposited within the ferritin and hemosiderin in the iron-storage sites of the body. Most storage iron is held in the liver, bone marrow, and spleen, although (as stated already) a small quantity of ferritin occurs within the blood plasma.

The membranes of almost all cells of the body contain transferrin receptor molecules, which can each bind to two transferrin molecules and allow the transferrin to enter the cell and release its iron. If a cell is in need of iron, it produces more transferrin receptors and is thus able to collect more iron from the circulating supply. The placenta is particularly rich in transferrin receptors, allowing it to gain a good supply of iron to be transported into the developing fetus. The need for iron by the fetus is greatest during the last trimester of pregnancy.

Newly absorbed iron is only deposited in iron storage sites if the iron content of the body is in excess of the amount required to meet immediate needs. If the amount of iron absorbed from the diet and obtained from the breakdown of red blood cells is insufficient to meet the body's needs, iron is removed from the storage sites and transported to the sites of demand bound to transferrin molecules. Symptoms of iron deficiency appear only once the body's stores of iron have been depleted. In newborn infants these stores of iron can last for 3 to 6 months (90 to 180 days). Well-nourished adult women have sufficient stored iron to last about 500 days, whereas well-nourished men have enough for about 1000 days.

Key aspects of the absorption, transport, and metabolism of iron are summarized in Figure 10-5.

DIETARY REQUIREMENTS

The amounts of iron that must be absorbed each day to compensate for losses and meet the body's needs for good health and growth are summarized in Table 10-2. The data in the table reveal that adolescent girls and pregnant women need to absorb at least twice as much iron as do adult men each day. Absorbed iron goes to satisfy four general categories of need: iron to replace normal losses, to facilitate growth, to cope with the demands of pregnancy, and to replace unusual losses, such as those during blood donation or heavy bleeding.[14]

Iron Required to Replace Normal Losses

Because there is no mechanism for excreting iron, the iron in the body is generally well conserved. However, inevitable losses do occur. Some iron is lost in urine, perspiration, and feces; within dead cells shed from the skin; and in clippings of nails and hair. The greatest single loss is in feces, which contain iron derived from sloughed-off intestinal cells. Fecal losses of iron amount to about 0.7 mg/day. When these losses are added to the 0.2 to 0.5 mg/day lost in the various other ways, total daily iron losses rise to about 0.9 to 1.2 mg/day. This low level of loss represents the only iron that adult men must replace with dietary iron. Women, however, must also replace the significant amounts of iron lost in menstruation. Menstrual iron losses vary greatly among women but are fairly consistent from month to month in the same woman. Although menstrual losses occur only during menstruation, if they are averaged over the whole month, they usually amount to about 0.5 to 1 mg of iron per day. When the iron required to make up for menstrual losses is added to the amount required to replace other normal losses, it is found that adult women before menopause and who are not pregnant must absorb from 1.4 to 2.2 mg of iron per day (almost twice the amount required by men).

Iron Required to Facilitate Growth

Growth is accompanied by an increase in both tissue mass and blood volume, both of which require additional supplies of iron to make the necessary iron-containing compounds, especially the hemoglobin of red blood cells and the myoglobin of muscle tissue. From birth to adulthood the total amount of iron in the body increases from 0.5 to 5 g. Averaged over a 20-year growth period, this amounts to 225 mg/year, or 0.6 mg/day.

Iron Required During Pregnancy

Pregnant women need additional iron to allow for an increase in their red blood cell mass (requiring 450 mg of iron overall), to provide the iron needed by the fetus (270 mg) and the placenta (50 to 90 mg), and to replace the variable amount of blood lost during delivery. Hallberg[15] has estimated that the total amount of iron needed throughout a pregnancy is approximately 1040 mg, of which 840 mg are permanently lost from the body and 200 mg are retained to be added to the body's iron stores. Averaged over an entire 9-month pregnancy, the amount of iron that must be absorbed by the pregnant woman amounts to 3 mg/day.

Iron Required to Replace Losses from Blood Donation or Heavy Bleeding

The intentional donation or accidental loss of 1 pint (about 0.5 L) of blood brings about a total loss of about 25 mg of iron. This iron must be replaced from the

FIGURE 10-5

Absorption and metabolism of iron.

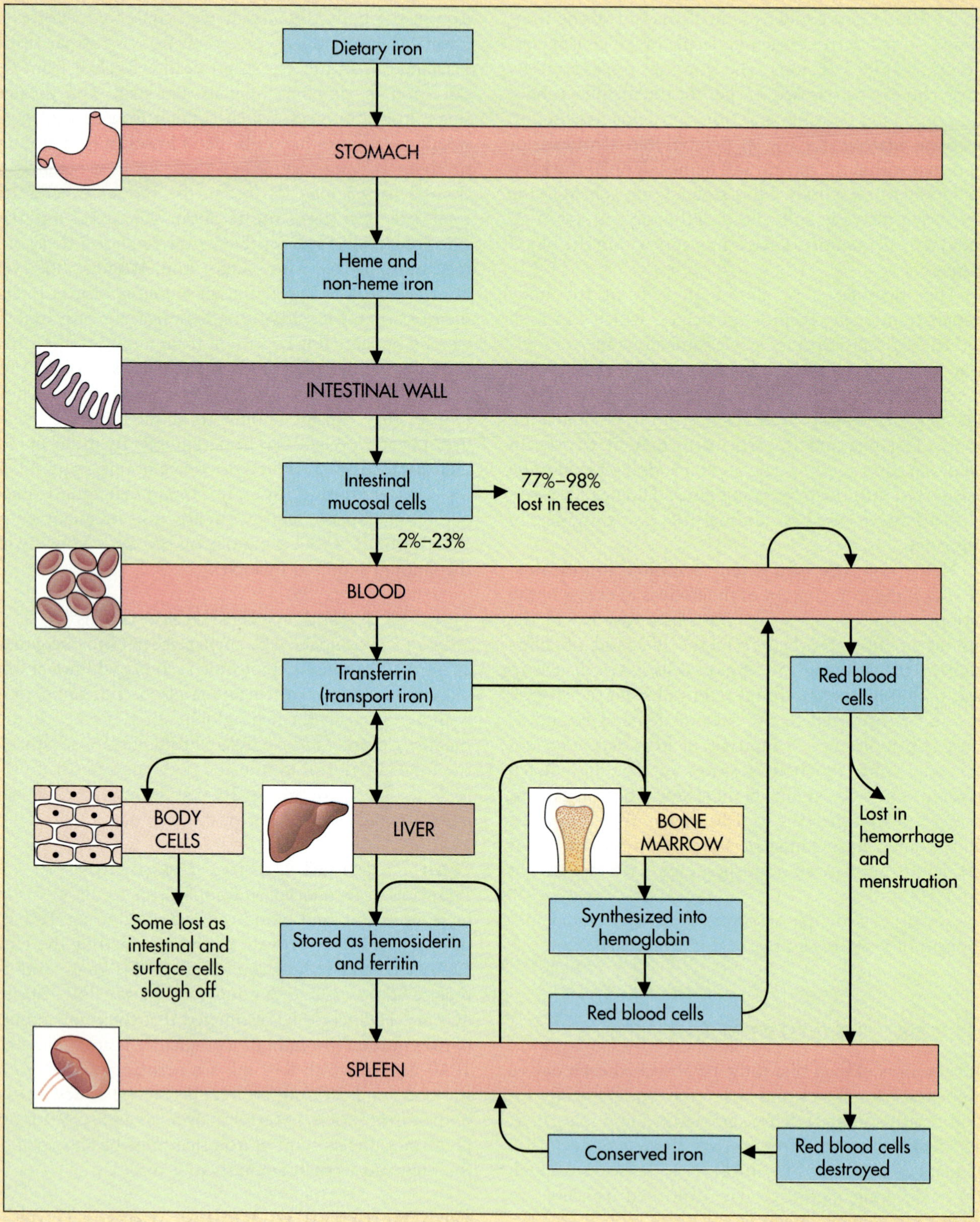

TABLE 10-2

Summary of requirements for absorbed iron (mg/day)

AGE-GROUP	LOSS IN FECES	LOSSES IN URINE, PERSPIRATION, AND DESQUAMATION	NEEDS FOR MENSTRUATION	NEEDS FOR GROWTH	NEEDS FOR PREGNANCY	TOTAL BODY NEEDS*
Adult men	0.7	0.2-0.5				0.9-1.2
Adult women	0.7	0.2-0.5	0.5-1.0			1.4-2.2
Pregnant women	0.7	0.2-0.5			1.9-2.2	2.8-3.2
Children	0.7	0.2-0.5		0.6		1.5-1.8
Adolescent girls	0.7	0.2-0.5	0.5-1.4	0.5-1.0		1.9-3.7

* Dietary needs are 3 to 10 times this amount, depending on the source of iron and the composition of the diet that ultimately determine the amount of iron absorbed.

TABLE 10-3

Recommended dietary allowances (United States) and recommended nutrient intakes (Canada) for iron (mg/day)

AGE (YEARS)	UNITED STATES	CANADA
Children		
0-6 mo	6	0.3*
6 mo-3	10	6
4-10	10	8
11-18	12	10
Males		
19+	10	9
Females		
19-50	15	13
51+	10	8
Pregnant	30†	23
Lactating	15	13

* Assumes human milk as source.

† A supplement to reach 30 mg iron is recommended.

dietary sources of blood donors and all victims of accidental bleeding who do not receive a blood transfusion. The volume of the blood and the number of cells in the blood return to normal relatively quickly, but the resynthesis of hemoglobin takes considerably longer. Averaged over a 3-month period the additional need for absorbed iron after the donation (or accidental loss) of 1 pint of blood is approximately 0.28 mg/day.

RECOMMENDED DIETARY ALLOWANCES

The Recommended Dietary Allowances (RDAs) for iron in the United States and comparable Canadian values are listed in Table 10-3. The rationale for the U.S. allowances is given in more detail below.

Adults

The National Research Council has recommended that adult allowances for iron be based on the assumption that an adult man must absorb approximately 1 mg of iron per day to replace normal losses and that an adult woman must absorb 1.5 to 2.2 mg/day to cover the additional losses of menstruation. Because an average of only 10% to 15% of ingested iron is absorbed, it is recommended that men consume 10 mg of iron per day, whereas women should consume 15 mg/day. This recommendation for women leaves a narrow margin of safety and may fail to meet the needs of women with high menstrual losses of iron (in excess of 32 mg/mo).

There is general agreement among the authorities of most countries that men need from 10 to 12 mg of dietary iron per day, but there is less agreement on the figure for women, which ranges from as little as 10 mg/day to as much as 20 mg/day.

Pregnant Women

During pregnancy, iron accumulates in the fetus at a rate of 0.5 mg/day in the first trimester, increasing to 3 to 4 mg/day in the last two trimesters. Iron is stored within the fetus during the latter half of pregnancy and continues to be transferred to the fetus, even if the mother's hemoglobin level drops. Despite the increased efficiency of the mother's absorption of iron during pregnancy and the reduced losses of iron from the absence of menstrual periods, it is virtually impossible for a pregnant woman to obtain the required amount of iron from her diet alone. As a result, the Food and Nutrition Board recommends that pregnant women, in addition to obtaining 15 mg of iron/day from dietary sources, take a supplement providing an additional 15 mg/day, to bring the total intake up to 30 mg/day. Because of the possible constipating effect of iron supplements, however, physicians have found that some women experience difficulty in complying with this recommendation. Supplementation to any greater extent than the recommended level (achieved either from medicinal products or highly fortified foods, i.e., cereals containing at least 100% RDA) should certainly not be used.

New mothers are encouraged to continue with iron supplementation for 2 to 3 months after delivery to help ensure that iron reserves, usually depleted in pregnancy, are adequately replenished. This replenishment is assisted by the fall in blood volume after pregnancy, which releases iron from the additional hemoglobin synthesized during pregnancy.

> In selecting an iron supplement, the amount of *elemental* iron—or in other words, the amount of iron ions—is the important factor, rather that the amount of the iron-containing compound present in the supplement. The amount of elemental iron in the iron-containing salts most commonly found in iron supplements can be calculated as follows:
>
> **Iron content in milligrams of iron per 100 mg of iron-containing compounds:**
> **20 mg—in ferrous sulfate**
> **33 mg—in ferrous fumarate**
> **12 mg—in ferrous gluconate**
> **16 mg—in ferroglycine sulfate**

Lactating Women

Human milk is a relatively poor source of iron, containing only 0.3 mg of iron per liter. The iron within the milk is highly bioavailable, however, with more than 50% of it usually absorbed by the breast-fed infant. The amount of iron in the milk is not influenced by the amount in the mother's diet but automatically adjusts to be greater at the end of the nursing period than at the beginning. Because the losses of iron within breast milk are relatively small, the recommended dietary intake of iron during lactation is the same as that recommended for the nonpregnant woman.

Infants and Children

The liver of a newborn infant contains sufficient iron stores to last for 3 to 6 months, during which time the infant doubles in weight. An infant's need for hemoglobin actually decreases after birth, when the infant moves from the uterine environment, where the oxygen concentration is low, to the normal atmosphere outside the uterus, with a much higher concentration of oxygen. This means that an inevitable drop in an infant's hemoglobin level occurs in the first 6 months of life from 18 g of hemoglobin per 100 ml of blood at birth to around 13 g/100 ml at 6 months. This level is then maintained throughout childhood, before rising in late adolescence to eventually reach the adult level. Because the blood volume increases during this time, of course, considerable new hemoglobin synthesis is needed to keep the amount per 100 ml constant.

Little iron is absorbed in early infancy, and giving an iron supplement from birth does not prevent the drop in hemoglobin levels. Iron supplementation may, however, provide some protection against anemia after 4 months of age, by which time dietary iron should be being absorbed for the synthesis of hemoglobin and the formation of new cells. Because the reserve of iron in twins is usually lower, it may be advantageous to give them an iron supplement from the age of 2 months.

Fomon[16] has estimated that an infant's requirement for absorbed iron is between 0.55 and 0.75 mg/day, depending on its weight. The RDA to deliver at least this amount of absorbed iron is set at 6 mg/day from birth to 6 months of age. From 6 months to 10 years, 10 mg/day is recommended, which is the same as the recommended intake for adult males. Between the ages of 11 and 18 years, the recommendation is 12 mg/day, which then falls back to 10 mg/day for adult males or rises to 15 mg/day for adult premenopausal females (Table 10-3).

FOOD SOURCES

The iron content of some frequently used foods in the North American diet is given in Table 10-4. Liver stands out as a particularly rich source of iron per typical serving, although green beans and lettuce are actually richer sources per 100 kcal. The iron content of beef liver is considerably lower than that of other livers, with the iron contents per 3-oz serving being 5.3 mg for beef liver, 7.6 mg for chicken liver, 12.8 mg for calf liver, 16.1 mg for lamb liver, and 27.2 mg for pork liver. Liver, however, has never been a popular dietary item in North America, where most people depend instead on a variety of moderately good alternative sources to meet their needs for iron. Liver has also fallen out of favor recently because of its high cholesterol content.

Figure 10-6 shows the contribution of various food groups to the iron content of the North American diet. The figure makes it clear that no single food group is responsible for a majority share of the iron in the diet but that cereal products, meat, fish, poultry, and vegetables make the greatest contributions. The amount of iron present in different foods within the diet, however, does not always give a true picture of where most of the iron *absorbed* by the body comes from because the bioavailability of iron varies widely among different sources. These variations are also illustrated in Table 10-4.

The iron in eggs is concentrated almost entirely in the yolk, but only 2% of this iron is absorbed by the body. In contrast, up to 30% of the iron in chicken is absorbed, whereas the absorption from other animal

TABLE 10-4

Iron available from various foods

HEME IRON SOURCES

FOOD (3 oz, COOKED, LEAN ONLY)		TOTAL IRON (mg)	AVAILABLE IRON (mg)*
BEEF	Liver, pan fried	5.34	0.60
	Chuck, arm pot roast, braised	3.22	0.48
	Tenderloin, roasted	3.05	0.46
	Sirloin, broiled	2.85	0.42
	Roundtip, roasted	2.50	0.38
	Top round, broiled	2.45	0.37
	Top loin, broiled	2.10	0.31
	Ground lean, broiled	1.79	0.27
	Eye round, roasted	1.65	0.25
PORK	Shoulder, blade, Boston, roasted	1.36	0.15
	Tenderloin, roasted	1.31	0.15
	Ham, boneless, 5% to 11% fat	1.19	0.14
	Loin chop, broiled	0.78	0.09
LAMB	Loin, roasted	2.07	o.31
	Leg, shank half, roasted	1.75	0.26
VEAL	Loin, roasted	0.93	0.14
	Cutlet, pan fried	0.74	0.11
CHICKEN	Liver, simmered	7.20	0.81
	Leg, roasted	1.11	0.17
	Breast, roasted	0.88	0.13
TURKEY	Leg, roasted	2.26	0.34
	Breast, roasted	0.99	0.14
FISH	Tuna, light meat, canned	2.72	0.31
	White meat, canned	0.51	0.06
	Halibut, dry heat	0.91	0.10
	Salmon, sockeye, dry heat	0.47	0.06
	Flounder/sole, dry heat	0.23	0.03
SHELLFISH	Oysters, 6 medium, raw	5.63	0.63
	Shrimp, moist heat	2.63	0.30
	Crab, Alaskan king, moist heat	0.65	0.07

NONHEME IRON SOURCES

FOOD		TOTAL IRON (mg)	AVAILABLE IRON (mg)†
CEREALS	Raisin bran (enriched), dry, ½ cup	4.5	0.23
	Corn flakes (enriched), dry, 1 oz	1.8	0.09
	Shredded wheat, dry, 1 oz	1.20	0.06
	Oatmeal, cooked, ½ cup	0.80	0.04
	Whole wheat hot cereal, ½ cup	0.75	0.04
GRAINS	Bagel, 1	1.8	0.09
	Bran muffin, home recipe, 1	1.4	0.07
	Whole wheat bread, 1 slice	1.0	0.05
	White rice (enriched), cooked, ½ cup	0.9	0.05
	White bread (enriched), 1 slice	0.7	0.04
	Brown rice, cooked, ½ cup	0.5	0.03
FRUITS	Apricots, dried, 7 halves	1.16	0.06
	Prunes, dried, 3 medium	0.84	0.04
	Raisins, 2 Tbsp	0.38	0.02
	Banana, 1 medium	0.35	0.02
	Apple, 1 medium	0.25	0.01
	Orange, 1 medium	0.13	0.01
VEGETABLES	Potato, baked w/skin, 1 medium	2.75	0.14
	Peas, cooked, ½ cup	1.26	0.06
	Spinach, raw, ½ cup	0.76	0.04
	Broccoli, raw, ½ cup	0.39	0.02
	Carrots, 1 medium	0.36	0.02
	Lettuce, iceberg, ⅛ head	0.34	0.02
	Corn, cooked, ½ cup	0.25	0.01
BEANS/ LEGUMES	Kidney beans, boiled, ½ cup	2.58	0.13
	Canned, ½ cup	1.57	0.08
	Chickpeas, boiled, ½ cup	2.37	0.12
	Canned, ½ cup	1.62	0.08
	Baked beans, canned, plain, ½ cup	0.37	0.02
MEAT SUBSTITUTES	Tofu, 2½ × 2¾ × 1 in.	2.3	0.12
	Egg, whole	1.0	0.05
	Yolk	0.95	0.05
	White	tr	—
	Peanut butter, 2 Tbsp	0.6	0.03
DAIRY	Milk, low-fat, 1 cup	0.12	0.01
	Yogurt, plain low-fat, 1 cup	0.18	0.01
	Cheese, cheddar, 1 oz	0.19	0.01
MOLASSES	Cane, blackstrap, 1 Tbsp	5.05	0.25

* Available iron for individuals with 500-mg iron stores = (heme iron × 23%) + (nonheme iron × 5%). For this calculation, a figure of 5% absorption for nonheme iron was used. The heme iron content of beef, lamb, and chicken was averaged as 55%, and the heme iron content of pork, liver, and fish as 35%.

† Available iron for individuals with 500-mg iron stores = nonheme iron × 5%. For this calculation, a figure of 5% absorption for nonheme iron was used.

From The National Live Stock and Meat Board: *Iron in human nutrition*, Chicago, 1990, The Education Department of the National Live Stock and Meat Board.

FIGURE 10-6

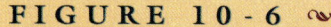

Contribution of various food groups to the iron content of the North American diet.

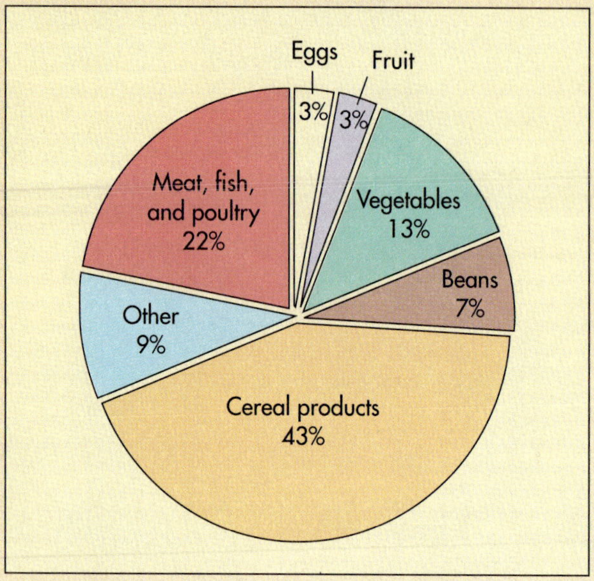

sources falls between these extremes. Soy products, often used as meat extenders, contain nonheme iron, which is poorly absorbed.

Vegetables can be fairly good sources of iron, but their iron is relatively poorly absorbed. Potatoes and green stalks and leaves are good sources, whereas legumes (peas and beans) are excellent sources. Vegetables provide three times as much iron in the North American diet as do fruits and fruit juices. The pulp of fruits contains twice as much iron as does the juice. Canned fruits and vegetables or acid foods cooked in an iron container pick up additional iron, which is just as available as the iron present in the foods before processing. This has led some people to propose a return to traditional iron cookware.

Although raisins and other dried fruits are often recommended as iron sources, they contain no more iron than they had in their original form. It should also be remembered that dried fruits are rich in kilocalories. For example, ¼ cup of raisins provides 0.7 mg of iron but also provides 109 kcal. Also, sticky raisins may contribute to dental problems.

Breads—either enriched or whole grain—provide a small amount of iron per unit weight, and only 5% of this iron is absorbed. Because bread is used in large amounts by adolescents and families on restricted budgets, however, it often makes a significant contribution to daily iron intake. Enriched bread, macaroni, and corn grits contain slightly less iron than does the whole grain cereal from which they are derived. Infant cereals and some prepared dry cereals are enriched with amounts of iron that allow one serving to provide a full day's allowance.

The only commonly used foods that, as a group, are regarded as poor sources of iron are milk and dairy products. Some foods are rich in iron but not of much nutritional significance because of the infrequency with which they are consumed. These foods include oysters (with 6.3 mg of iron per 3-oz serving), clams (6.1 mg/3-oz serving), and cocoa (1 mg/Tbsp).

Iron is present in drinking water, largely as ferric hydroxide ($Fe[OH]_3$), but water is a significant source of iron only when its iron content is more than 5 mg/L. Typical values in the United States are around 1 mg/L.

Blackstrap molasses, a by-product of the sugar refining process, contains about 2.5 mg of iron per tablespoon. Because of its bitter flavor, however, it cannot be considered a significant dietary item.

EFFECT OF FOOD PREPARATION METHODS ON CONTENT

The major causes of the loss of iron during food preparation are the discarding of iron-rich cooking water and the removal of vegetable peelings. Any cooking method that minimizes the possibility of iron's dissolving in cooking water increases the amount of iron available to the body. Suitable methods include cooking relatively large pieces of food, rather than finely chopped food; cooking food with any skin left on; steaming, rather than boiling; or cooking by microwave. Using vegetable stock in soups or gravies also provides some valuable iron that may otherwise be discarded. The use of iron cooking pots can increase the iron content of food two- to six-fold. During the past 70 years the total amount of dietary iron available to North Americans has increased from 15 to 17.6 mg/day, and yet the incidence of iron deficiency has increased. It is possible that this may be largely explained by the move away from iron cooking utensils.

FORTIFICATION OR ENRICHMENT OF FOOD WITH IRON

To try to ensure that people receive adequate iron in their diet, many countries purposely add iron to certain foods as part of **fortification** or **enrichment** programs. Fortification is the addition of a nutrient to a food to increase the nutrient content to above natural levels. Enrichment is the addition of a nutrient to a processed food to replace losses of the nutrient that occurred during processing. Food subjected to such treatments must be widely used by the general population but should be produced in relatively few centers to allow effective quality control. The iron added to the food must be in a soluble and biologically available form, and the food must be of a type that remains stable and palatable for a long time. Some foods become discolored by the addition of iron salts and so are not suitable for treatment. Bread and cereal are appropriate foods for fortification and enrichment in developed countries, whereas in developing countries, salt, sugar, and beverages may be more appropriate.

In the United States, certain foods such as bread, flour, macaroni, and corn grits have a **standard of identity** that permits them to be labeled as "enriched," in iron provided that the amount of iron and three vitamins (thiamin, riboflavin, and niacin) added lies between certain limits. For these and other foods with added nutrients, the actual amount of total nutrients such as iron must also be indicated on the label. Only 30 states in America have laws requiring the enrichment of flour, but about 90% of the flour and bread sold in America is enriched with at least iron and three vitamins.

EVALUATION OF IRON STATUS

There are many different indicators of the iron status of the human body. Only the four most commonly used indicators are discussed here.

Serum Ferritin Level

The serum ferritin test is the most sensitive indicator of iron status. Almost all of the ferritin in the body is stored within cells, but a small amount circulates within the blood and can be quantified by tests on blood serum. Each microgram (μg) of ferritin found per liter of serum indicates the presence in the body of 10 mg of stored iron. Thus a level of 10 μg/L indicates the presence of 100 mg of stored iron, and so on. Serum ferritin values below about 10 to 12 μg/L usually indicate that the body's iron stores have been depleted. People with a genetic predisposition to store iron should have their ferritin level determined before taking either iron or vitamin C supplements to ensure that they do not already have high amounts of iron stored.

Red Cell Protoporphyrin Level

Protoporphyrin is a chemical precursor of heme that accumulates within red blood cells if there is insufficient iron available to make heme. If the protoporphyrin content of red blood cells rises above 100 μg/100 ml of red blood cells, a depression of heme synthesis caused by a lack of iron is indicated.

Transferrin Saturation Level

The level of occupancy or "saturation" of the iron-binding sites on the protein transferrin is another indicator of the body's iron status. A decrease in the amount of iron bound to serum transferrin, corresponding to an increase in the "total iron-binding capacity" (TIBC) of serum, indicates that iron stores have been depleted. If the level of transferrin saturation falls below 10% to 16%, iron reserves are inadequate to meet the body's need for iron.

Hemoglobin Content of Blood

A widely used traditional method of assessing iron status is to determine the hemoglobin content of a blood sample. A person with low hemoglobin levels is said to be suffering from **anemia.** Despite widespread use, the measurement of hemoglobin levels as an indicator of overall iron status has several limitations and is the least sensitive of the four methods considered here. The first limitation is that there is no general agreement on the level of blood hemoglobin that indicates iron deficiency. For some people, a hemoglobin level of 12 g/dl of blood seems to be adequate, whereas in others this level results in a limited ability to exercise or undertake any strenuous activity. A second problem is that hemoglobin levels fluctuate over each 24-hour period; so a single determination of the blood hemoglobin level can give a misleading result. Third, hemoglobin levels fall only after the iron stores of the body have been depleted; so a low hemoglobin level arises at an advanced stage of iron deficiency, rather than providing any early warning of deficiency. Fourth, low hemoglobin levels can be caused by deficiencies of other nutrients besides iron, such as protein or vitamin B_6. Finally, depressed hemoglobin levels are a normal response to illness, making it difficult to judge the relevance of low levels to iron status in people who are ill. However, although the measurement of hemoglobin levels is not a good way to detect the early stages of iron deficiency, it is an effective way of assessing the severity of any existing anemia and of monitoring the course of recovery.

The relationship between the levels of the four indicators considered here and the level of the body's iron stores is summarized in Figure 10-7. Two different ways of assessing iron status using some *combination* of these and other factors, known as the **ferritin model** and the **mean corpuscular volume (MCV) model,** have been proposed. In the ferritin model, measurements are taken of the serum ferritin level, red blood cell protoporphyrin level, and transferrin saturation level. In the MCV model the measurements taken are of mean corpuscular volume (the average volume of blood cells), red blood cell protoporphyrin level, and transferrin saturation level. In both models, people with two out of three of the measures below the cutoff points indicated in Table 10-5 are described as having **impaired iron status.** Among this group, only those who also have hemoglobin levels below an acceptable standard for age and gender are considered to have **iron-deficiency anemia.** When these methods are used, a relatively small number of people are considered to be anemic, compared with the number deemed anemic on the basis of hemoglobin levels alone. The lower incidence of anemia produced by

FIGURE 10-7

Relationship between various indicators of iron status and the body's level of iron stores.

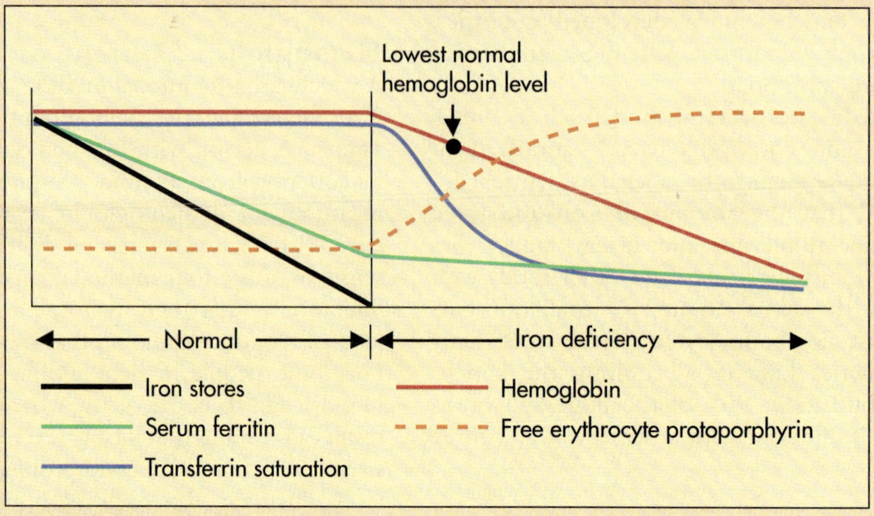

TABLE 10-5

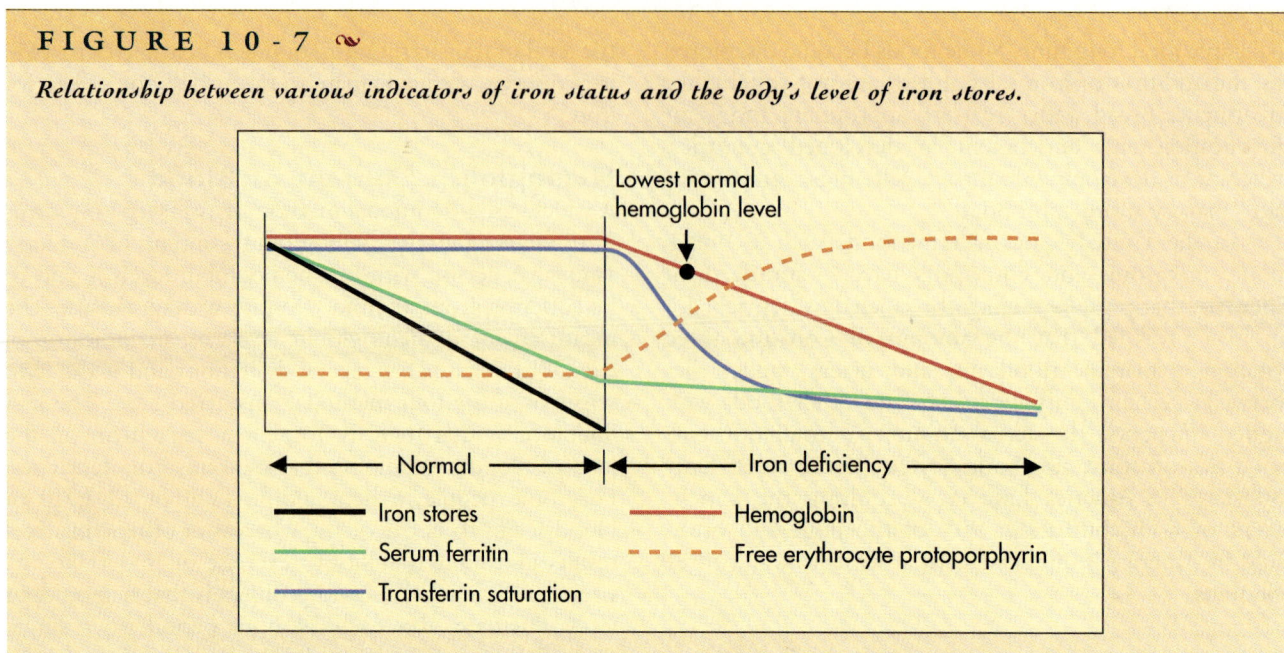

Criteria for assessment of iron status with levels indicative of deficiency

AGE (YEARS)	HEMOGLOBIN (g/dl)	SERUM FERRITIN (µg/ml)	TRANSFERRIN SATURATION (%)	ERYTHROCYTE PROTOPORPHYRIN (µg/dl RED BLOOD CELLS)	MEAN CORPUSCULAR VOLUME (cu µ)
1-2	<9	<10	<10	>100	<73
3-4	<10	<10	<14	>100	<75
5-10	<10	<10	<15	>100	<76
11-14	<12 (male)	<10	<16	>100	<78
	<10 (female)	<10	<10	>100	<78
15-74	<12 (male)	<12	<16	>100	<80
	<10 (female)	<12	<12	>100	<80

the more complex methods of assessment is more compatible with the best estimates of functional iron deficiency.

DEFICIENCY

Although the body conserves iron efficiently, iron deficiencies can arise when intake fails to meet needs, particularly during the growth period after loss of blood or in women who have gone through frequent pregnancies in rapid succession.

A typical diet that is adequate in most other nutrients provides only 6 mg of iron per 1000 kcal. This makes it difficult for adult women to obtain the recommended 15 mg of iron per day, especially if their caloric intake is below 2500 kcal. Data from the National Health and Nutrition Examination Survey (NHANES) II study showed an average iron intake of only 12.4 mg/day for women between the ages of 20 and 50, confirming that the recommended intake is difficult to achieve. A failure to achieve the recommended intake does not necessarily mean that a person is suffering from iron deficiency. It does mean, however, that he or she is at increased risk of iron deficiency. Although many people may fail to achieve the recommended intake of iron, the NHANES II study indicated that only a small proportion of the population (less than 2%) can be considered truly iron deficient. The condition of iron deficiency, however, can only be properly confirmed by biochemical tests.

Onset

The onset of iron deficiency involves a gradual and well-defined sequence of changes that ultimately result in anemia. In the first phase the body's iron stores are depleted (detected by a decrease in the serum ferritin

TABLE 10-6

Changes in measures of iron status indicative of developing iron deficiency

MEASURES OF IRON STATUS	NORMAL	IRON DEPLETION	IRON-DEFICIENT ERYTHROPOIESIS	IRON-DEFICIENT ANEMIA
Iron stores (bone marrow, liver, spleen)	Adequate	Very low	0	0
Erythron iron (iron in red blood cells)	Normal	Normal	Slightly reduced	Less than half of normal
TIBC (μg/dl)	330	360	390	410
Iron absorption	Normal	Increased	Increased	Increased
Plasma iron (μg/dl)	115-50	115	60	40
Transferrin saturation (%)	35	35	16	16
Red blood cell protoporphyrin (μg/dl in red blood cell)	30	30	100	100
Erythrocytes	Normal	Normal	Normal	Microcytic hypochromic
Hemoglobin (g/dl)	12	12	12	<12

TIBC, Total iron-binding capacity.

level), accompanied by an increase in iron absorption (resulting in increased iron-binding capacity, or in other words, low transferrin saturation levels). These changes lead into the next phase in which iron stores are exhausted and there is insufficient iron available for hemoglobin synthesis. This causes the heme precursor protoporphyrin to accumulate in red blood cells, detected by testing the red blood cell protoporphyrin level. In the third and final stage the hemoglobin concentration in red blood cells decreases and the red blood cells diminish in size, meaning that anemia sets in. Anemia resulting from iron deficiency is characterized as **microcytic, hypochromic anemia,** meaning anemia associated with small blood cells with little color (because the red color of the cells is from the hemoglobin they contain). The various phases of iron deficiency and the changes associated with them are summarized in Table 10-6.

Consequences

A considerable body of evidence indicates that iron deficiency leading to anemia results in functional impairment of the body to a degree that is related to the degree of iron depletion. Some of the impairments are a direct result of anemia, whereas others are a result of iron deficiency within the body's tissues or a combination of these factors.[17] Iron deficiency often develops slowly and insidiously. Many people affected by it experience no obvious problems, other than vague symptoms of tiredness, headache, irritability, or depression. The physical symptoms most frequently associated with iron-deficiency anemia are pallor, fatigue, dyspnea (difficult or labored breathing), palpitations, and a reduced capacity for work. Other physical effects are increased sensitivity to cold; gastrointestinal disturbances, such as a smooth or swollen tongue; achlorhydria (low levels of HCl in the stomach); constipation; and diarrhea. More recently, investigators have also found evidence that iron deficiency adversely affects intellectual performance and the health of the immune system. Some of these effects are considered in more detail below.

Reduced work capacity Studies in both animals and humans clearly indicate that significant reduction in work capacity can result from anemia caused by iron deficiency. Men working in Indonesian rubber plantations and women working in tea plantations in Sri Lanka exhibited decreased productivity when deficient in iron. Their productivity improved after supplementation with iron, most significantly among those with the most severe initial anemia. Although the impairment in productivity can be directly related to the degree of anemia, other tissue abnormalities resulting from iron deficiency may also be involved. Studies on animals show that the release and use of energy in muscles of iron-deficient animals are impaired, resulting in a reduced capacity for prolonged exercise. Several research teams have recently found that iron deficiency is common among athletes and is increasingly being associated with exercise training.[18] It is unknown, however, to what extent such deficiency is caused by increased iron losses via perspiration and feces, increased demands on the body, or redistribution of iron within the body.

Behavioral and intellectual impairment A growing body of evidence suggests that iron status is related to behavioral and intellectual performance.[19-21] Studies with infants and preschool-aged and school-aged children consistently show that iron-deficiency anemia is associated with poor mental and motor development, alterations in attention span, lower intelligence scores, and some degree of perceptual disturbances. The mechanism behind these effects is unknown, but several possibilities have been proposed. One possibility is that alterations in neurotransmitter metabolism developing early in iron deficiency may interfere with the normal operation of the brain. Alternatively, the changes may be caused by some more general effects of anemia on the whole body. Early studies suggested that the effects of iron deficiency on behavior and intellectual performance were not reversed when the deficiency was corrected. Later rigorous studies, however, clearly indicated that the changes were reversed once iron stores were replenished. The link between iron deficiency and behavioral and intellectual impairment is a strong argument in favor of public health programs aimed at preventing and correcting iron deficiency, especially in infants and children.

Reduced resistance to infection There is strong evidence from both human and animal studies that iron deficiency is associated with a decreased resistance to infection.[22] Abnormalities in the functioning of some of the white blood cells responsible for immunity (lymphocytes and neutrophils) have been found in children with iron deficiency. There is no convincing evidence indicating the way in which a deficiency in iron could directly cause increased rates of infections. Because iron is essential for the growth of microorganisms, their growth could be expected to be restricted when limited supplies of iron are available from the host. The iron within an infected individual is not readily available to infecting microorganisms in any case because it tends to be bound tightly by the iron-binding proteins of the host. This tight binding of iron within us probably explains why the administration of oral iron supplements or consumption of iron-fortified foods is not associated with increased risk or severity of infections, despite the fact that the microorganisms responsible require iron. However, the concern that iron supplementation might benefit infecting microorganisms, as well as the individual concerned, has led some investigators to suggest that supplemental iron should not be given to infants between 4 and 6 months of age. At this early age, infants have high transferrin saturation levels in excess of 50% and if supplementation were to raise these to saturation or near-saturation levels, there are fears that additional iron would be available for the benefit of infecting microorganisms.[23]

Impaired temperature regulation One of the most characteristic features of iron deficiency is an impaired ability to maintain body temperature in a cold environment. This appears to be caused by impaired functioning of the thyroid gland. Studies on women who were either anemic, iron depleted, or iron sufficient and of similar body fatness found that on exposure to water at 28° C for 100 minutes, the anemic women experienced a greater drop in core body temperature and a smaller increase in metabolic rate than did iron-sufficient women. Mean plasma thyroid hormone levels in the anemic women were found to be reduced by 50% at the start of the study and throughout the duration of the study.[24]

SUPPLEMENTATION

In many cases, supplementation may be the only way to treat people with iron deficiency. Any of over 30 different iron salts can be used in supplementation, although ferrous sulfate ($FeSO_4$) seems to be the most effective and is also the least expensive. Unfortunately, many common gastrointestinal problems, ranging from nausea and diarrhea to constipation, are associated with iron supplementation. Iron supplements should be taken without food because this enhances their absorption almost two-fold. Taking vitamin C with the supplement, however, enhances the effectiveness of the supplement by increasing its absorption into the body.

EXCESS

There used to be general agreement that it was impossible to absorb too much iron. This idea was first questioned when members of the Bantu tribe in Africa were found to suffer from a condition called **siderosis** or **hemosiderosis,** characterized by excessive storage of iron in the liver, largely as hemosiderin. In siderosis the excess iron accumulates in the normal storage sites for iron, the liver and spleen, and in the mitochondria within cells. Serum iron levels also increase, and the bone marrow develops more cells than normal or, in other words, becomes **hyperplastic.** The members of the Bantu tribe contained up to 30 times the normal 1 g of reserve iron as a result of absorbing as much as 200 mg/day from the iron kettles used to ferment beer. Since this first indication of problems caused by excess iron, acute iron toxicity has been reported among preschool children who accidentally consume large quantities of iron-containing nutritional supplements. This is actually one of the most common forms of poisoning in children. Iron-containing supplements should always be kept out of children's reach.

About 0.5% to 3.7% of the population have a genetic tendency toward iron overload because of a failure of the normal ability of the body to reduce iron absorption when high levels of iron are being consumed. The saturation level of transferrin in the blood of such people is three times the normal level, making the transferrin incapable of binding to all of the excess iron available. One effect of the increased levels of iron in the blood is to stimulate the growth of microorganisms, leading to increased risk of infection.

Another iron-storage disease, which occurs in less than 0.1% of the population (about 22,000 people in the United States), is **hemochromatosis.** This is caused by a genetic defect that causes affected individuals to absorb unusually high amounts of iron and store it in tissues that do not normally store iron. Opponents of iron-enrichment and fortification programs believe that the programs intensify the problems of people with hemochromatosis. Because the findings from the NHANES II study indicate that only a small proportion of the population (less than 2%) can be considered truly iron deficient, there is certainly little justification for increasing the levels of iron in enriched or fortified products to above present levels.

ZINC (Zn)

For more than 20 years it has been known that zinc is a dietary essential. Zinc deficiency is relatively rare. Zinc occurs within a great variety of foods in the form of Zn^{2+} ions, which become widely distributed throughout the body after absorption. Their major role is as components of as many as 60 metalloenzymes, which catalyze some steps in most of the central metabolic pathways of life. Zinc deficiency can impair growth, development, the onset of sexual maturity, and the functioning of the immune system.

DISTRIBUTION

Each adult contains between 1.5 and 2.5 g of zinc, making it the second most abundant mineral in the body. Zinc is present in all cells, tissues, organs, fluids, and secretions, although about 90% of the body's zinc is in muscle and bone (Table 10-7).[25] Over 95% of the body's zinc occurs bound within various metalloenzymes of cells and cell membranes. Blood plasma contains only 0.1% of the body's zinc, although the amount of zinc in the plasma can be used as a measure of the body's zinc status overall. The concentration of zinc in some tissues (including those of the blood, bones, skin, spleen, liver, and intestine) reflects variations in dietary intake, whereas in other tissues (such as those of the brain, lungs, heart, and muscles), zinc concentrations remain relatively constant, despite any variations in zinc intake.

Most of the zinc in the blood is found in the red blood cells, which contain significant amounts of the zinc-containing enzyme carbonic anhydrase, which converts carbon dioxide waste into bicarbonate ions (HCO_3^-). Of the blood's zinc, 12% to 22% is in the plasma, where it is distributed between three different pools: 60% to 80% loosely associated with the protein albumin, 20% to 40% tightly bound to the protein alpha-2-macroglobin, and a small fraction bound to a variety of other proteins and amino acids (about 3%). The zinc within plasma is available for transport into all other tissues. The level of zinc in plasma can vary with disease, pregnancy, or stress, in addition to responding to fluctuations in dietary intake.[26]

There are no permanent stores of zinc within the body. There is some evidence, however, that small amounts of the zinc in bone, liver, and plasma can move quickly to different tissues, if required.

TABLE 10-7

Zinc distribution in the body

TISSUE	PROPORTION OF TOTAL BODY ZINC (%)
Muscle	60
Bone	29
Liver	2
Gastrointestinal tract	1
Skin	1
Kidney	1
Brain	1
Lung	1
Prostate	1
Other organs	<1

TABLE 10-8

Selected zinc metalloenzymes

Alcohol dehydrogenase
Alkaline phosphatase
Carbonic anhydrase
Carboxypeptidase
Deoxynucleotidyl transferase
DNA polymerase
Glutamic acid dehydrogenase
Malic acid dehydrogenase
Nucleoside phosphorylase
RNA polymerase
Zinc-copper superoxide dismutase

FUNCTIONS

Zinc performs many functions as a part of every cell in the body, and so zinc is essential for normal growth, development, reproduction, and immunity. Zinc is also involved in maintaining a healthy appetite, assisting in the perception of taste, and maintaining our capacity for night vision. Zinc is involved in these functions not just as a component of metalloenzymes, but also as a result of specific interactions between zinc and various hormones.

Human and animal tissues contain about 200 enzymes whose activity depends on the presence of zinc.[26] The zinc of these enzymes plays a variety of roles, in many cases participating directly in the act of catalysis performed by the enzymes, but in other cases performing some role in shaping an enzyme's structure. A few of the zinc-containing metalloenzymes are listed in Table 10-8.

Zinc is essential for the maintenance of protein structure and for the metabolism of proteins and nucleic acids. The maintenance and replication of genetic material (DNA and RNA) and the use of genetic information to generate specific proteins are dependent on zinc. One major effect of zinc deficiency is an inability of cells to properly replicate their DNA, which is required for cells to multiply.[25] Zinc is also required for stabilizing the structure of certain DNA-binding ("zinc finger") proteins involved in the transcription of DNA to RNA.

Zinc forms an association with essential fatty acids, although the physiological relevance of this is unclear, and is also involved in cholesterol transport and in maintaining the stability of lipids within cell membranes. Zinc-dependent enzymes are involved in many other aspects of lipid metabolism, including the synthesis of long-chain fatty acids and various prostaglandins.

Zinc deficiency is associated with impaired glucose tolerance, implying a role for the mineral in carbohydrate metabolism. It is believed that zinc may interact with the hormone insulin in a way that influences the uptake of glucose by the cells of adipose (fat) tissue. In addition to this interaction with insulin, zinc is known to interact with a number of other hormones, including growth hormone, various sex hormones, thyroid hormones, prolactin, and corticosteroids. The interactions between zinc and hormones are double-edged because whereas zinc influences the synthesis and activities of hormones, various hormones also influence the absorption and metabolism of zinc. For example, changes in plasma zinc levels during pregnancy are probably mediated by hormones.

Zinc appears to be required for the normal development and maintenance of the immune system. An adequate content of zinc certainly helps the body resist infection.[27, 28] Even a mild deficiency of zinc in humans can lead to an increased risk of infection. This may make it especially important that elderly and sick persons receive adequate zinc because they are especially vulnerable to a wide variety of infections.

The functions of zinc within the body are so widespread and varied that only a broad impression of zinc's importance can be conveyed here. Further details of some of the most crucial functions of zinc are considered when we look at the effects of zinc deficiency later in this chapter.

ABSORPTION

Zinc is absorbed in the small intestine, although little is known about the precise mechanism involved. Zinc absorption is thought to be mediated by a combination of simple diffusion and the binding of zinc to specific carrier substances (ligands) able to take zinc along with them as they enter the cells of the intestinal wall.[29] Such ligands probably include amino acids (particularly histidine), citrate, and prostaglandins. Once inside the intestinal cells, much of the absorbed zinc becomes bound to **metallothionein,** a small metalloprotein able to bind to a variety of cations with a charge of 2+ (or in other words, a valency of 2). Metallothionein is responsible for key aspects of the homeostatic regulation of zinc absorption. The synthesis of metallothionein is stimulated by zinc within the cells of the intestinal wall cells. Another protein, cysteine-rich intestinal protein (CRIP) then binds to zinc within these cells and shuttles zinc to the blood. When the zinc content of the body is high, much of the zinc remains bound to metallothionein until the intestinal cells are shed from the intestinal wall and excreted, along with their zinc, in feces. When the zinc content of the body is low, the zinc ions are readily transferred to CRIP and transported to the blood to become bound to other proteins in the circulation that carry them throughout the body (Figure 10-8).

In general, about 20% of dietary zinc is absorbed, although the composition of the diet has a significant effect on the efficiency of absorption.[29] If zinc is taken in the form of a simple zinc salt in fasting conditions and without food, between 40% and 90% of the zinc is absorbed into the body. When the zinc consumed is a part of natural foods, however, absorption efficiencies are much lower. Zinc is absorbed most efficiently from meat, liver, eggs, and seafoods and less efficiently from vegetable and cereal foods containing large amounts of phytates and fiber. As much as 26% of the zinc in a high-meat, low-fiber meal is absorbed, compared with as little as 11% from a high-fiber meal with no meat.

Various specific chemicals in food are known to act as factors enhancing or inhibiting the absorption of zinc. The inhibiting factors include fiber, iron, copper, and possibly some other minerals, such as calcium, phosphorus, and folic acid. The situation on enhancing factors is less clear-cut, although protein, citric acid, and picolinic acid are believed to have an enhancing effect. Citric and picolinic acids are found in human milk and may be responsible for the fact that the bioavailability of zinc in human milk is greater than that of the zinc in cow's milk.

The absorption of zinc from the diet is subject to homeostatic control. When the dietary intake of zinc is low, the efficiency of zinc absorption is increased, and vice versa. These effects are probably vital for the body's ability to maintain relatively steady zinc levels, despite the fact that there are no specific storage sites for zinc within the body.

TRANSPORT AND METABOLISM

Zinc is transported within blood plasma bound to various carrier proteins such as albumin, alpha-2-macroglobulin, transferrin, and various amino acids. The inclusion of transferrin illustrates a general point about many micronutrient minerals: they often compete for binding to the same proteins during their absorption, transport, and sometimes storage. Most of the zinc in the blood is bound to the protein, albumin.

About 30% to 40% of absorbed zinc is taken up by the liver, with the remainder being distributed throughout the other organs and tissues of the body.

FIGURE 10-8

Role of metallothionein and cysteine-rich intestinal protein (CRIP) in regulating zinc absorption.

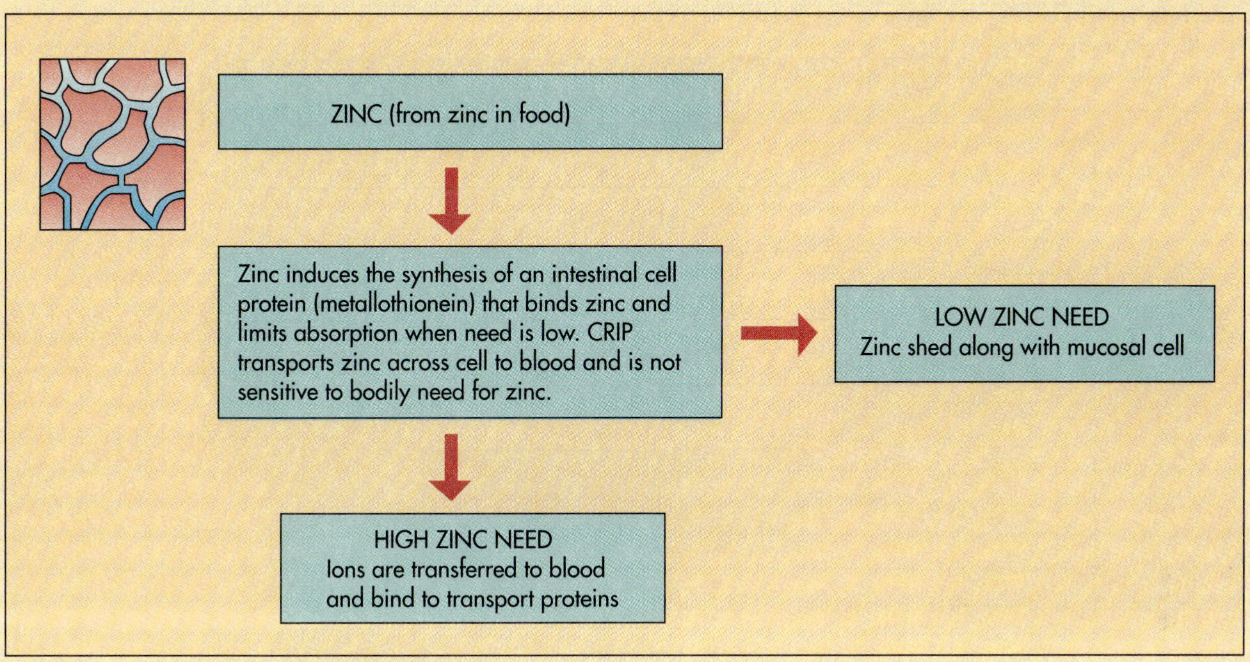

The main excretory route for zinc is the gastrointestinal tract, with between 1000 and 5000 μg of zinc excreted in the feces per day. About 300 to 500 μg of zinc is excreted from the kidneys each day, although the amount varies because the kidneys are another site at which homeostasis of body zinc is maintained.[30] When the body zinc level is low, excretion of zinc decreases, and vice versa. After severe burns, major surgery, or other physical trauma the amount of zinc lost in the urine can be significantly increased. Some zinc is also excreted within perspiration, although it has proved difficult to accurately measure how much. Key features of the flow of zinc through the body are summarized in Figure 10-9.

DIETARY REQUIREMENTS

The body's need for zinc is greatest during periods of growth, such as infancy, adolescence, and pregnancy, and during lactation. The U.S. RDA for zinc rises from 5 mg/day for newborn infants to 19 mg/day for females during their first 6 months of lactation. For adult males the RDA for zinc is set at 15 mg/day, whereas the figure for adult females who are neither pregnant nor lactating is 12 mg/day. All the values for different genders and age-groups, as well as for women during pregnancy or lactation, are given in Table 10-9. In Canada the Recommended Nutrient Intake (RNI) for zinc is set at 12 mg/day for adult males and 9 mg/day for adult females. An additional 4 mg/day is recommended during both pregnancy and lactation.

The zinc needs of infants appear to be fully met by the mother's milk, combined with zinc released from stores in the infant's liver. The zinc within human milk is more bioavailable than that of cow's milk. This is possibly because the action of ligands such as citric acid within human milk, which can bind to zinc and facilitate its absorption by the infant. Another possibility is that the iron-containing protein **lactoferrin** that is found in human milk may facilitate zinc absorption, whereas the protein **casein** in cow's milk may inhibit zinc absorption. The zinc of soy-based milk formulas is considerably less bioavailable than the zinc of cow's milk formula, probably because of the presence of considerable amounts of phytates in the soy-based formulas.

There has been some concern that the iron fortification of formulas and infant foods might result in less zinc being absorbed from the iron-fortified products. The American Academy of Pediatrics, however, has stated that there is no evidence to support any detrimental effect of iron-fortified formulas or infant foods on the zinc status of infants.

It is especially important for infants to obtain sufficient zinc during the weaning period, when an infant's stores of zinc are normally at a low level. There has been concern that the introduction of cereals to the infant's diet may reduce the bioavailability of the zinc supplied within the mother's milk or milk formula. Surveys across America, however, show that infants usually obtain sufficient zinc from their diet at all stages of infancy.

In contrast with the finding on zinc intake during infancy, intakes of zinc by American children are often

FIGURE 10-9

Flow of zinc through the body.

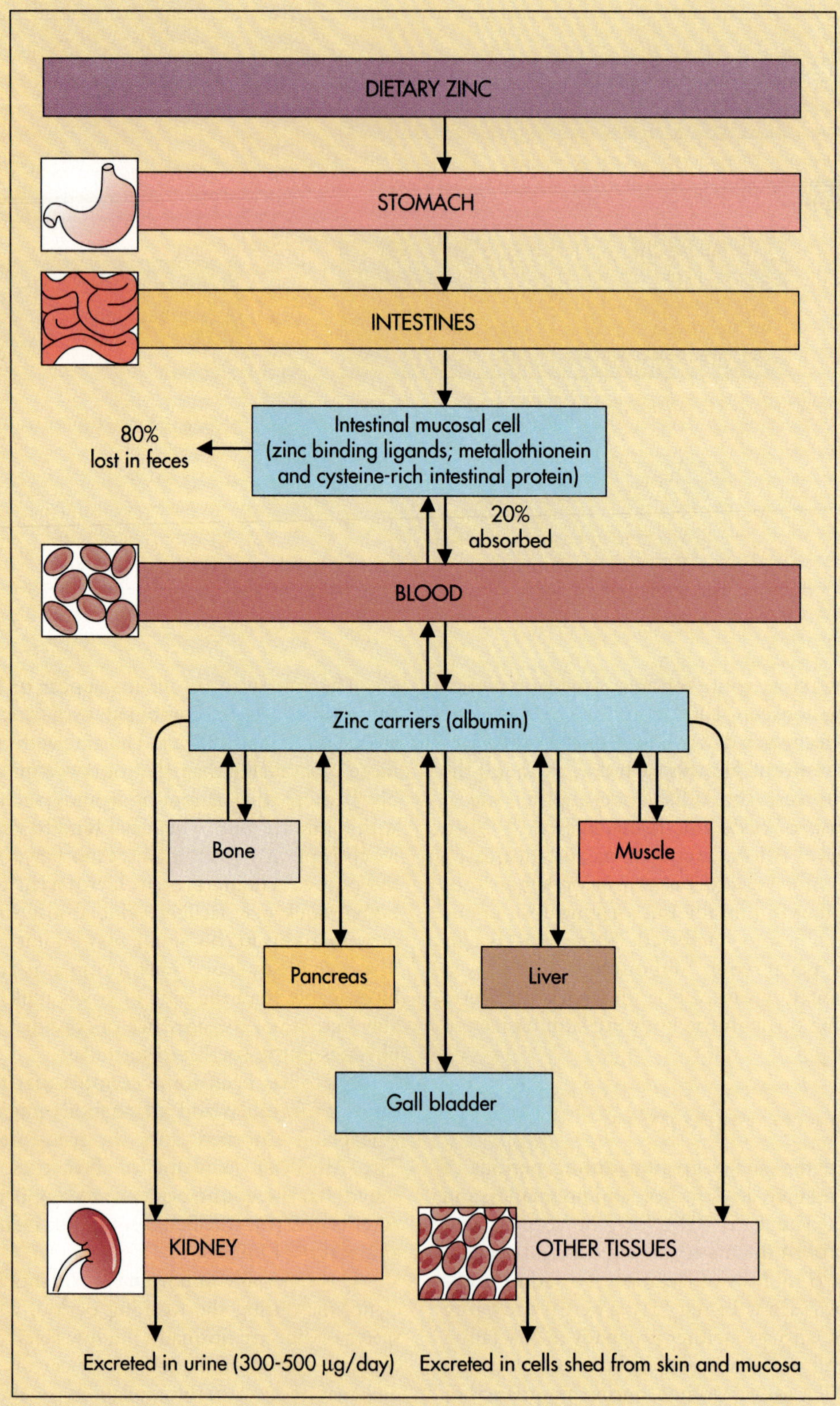

TABLE 10-9

Recommended dietary allowances (United States) and recommended nutrient intakes (Canada) for zinc (mg/day)

AGE (YEARS)	UNITED STATES	CANADA
Children		
0-1	5	3
1-10	10	4-7
Females		
11-51+	12	9
Males		
11-51+	15	12
Pregnant	15	15
Lactating		
First 6 months	19	15
Second 6 months	16	15

found to be below the RDA. This is of particular concern because of the role of zinc in promoting normal growth. Studies have suggested that the failure to meet zinc requirements may be causing poor growth in some children in the United States.

Adolescence is another period of rapid growth during which meeting zinc requirements is particularly important. There is evidence to suggest that most adolescent boys in America obtain the required amounts of zinc, whereas significant numbers of adolescent girls do not.

During adulthood, most American men appear to meet their zinc requirements, whereas significant numbers of women do not. Women need less zinc than do men, but their substantially lower kilocalorie intakes may make it difficult to obtain even the smaller amounts they require.

Pregnancy is a period in which vital processes of growth occur in both the fetus and the mother. Because zinc is crucially involved in promoting growth, zinc requirements increase during pregnancy. The total amount of additional zinc required during a typical pregnancy has been estimated at 100 mg, approximately 58 mg of which is used by the fetus, with the remainder being required by the mother's uterus (24 mg), placenta (about 6 mg), blood (about 6 mg), mammary tissue (about 5 mg), and amniotic fluid (0.5 mg).

In laboratory animals severe maternal zinc deficiency has been found to produce a range of adverse effects during pregnancy, including the death, malformation, or reduced growth of the fetus and prolonged labor. These effects all confirm the importance of adequate supplies of zinc during pregnancy. Iron supplements, which are routinely given during pregnancy, may inhibit the absorption of zinc by pregnant women. For this reason, no more than 30 mg of supplemental iron per day should be taken during pregnancy, and the iron should be provided by a supplement specifically intended for use by pregnant women.

FIGURE 10-10

Contributions of various food groups to zinc content of the U.S. food supply in 1988.

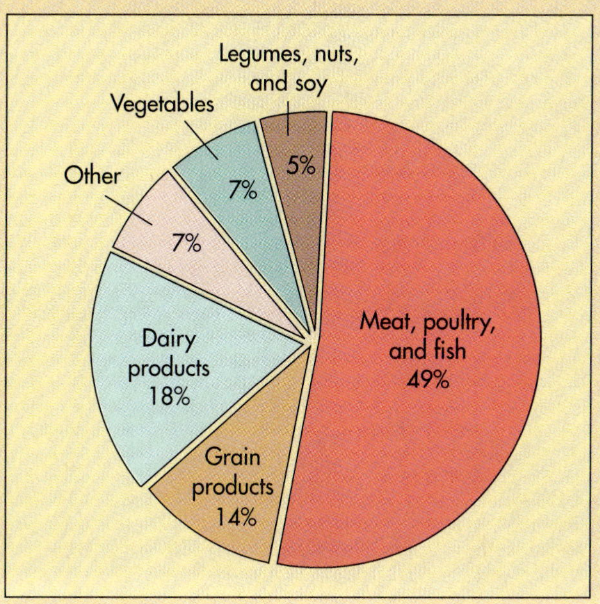

FOOD SOURCES

A wide variety of foods of both animal and plant origin contribute zinc to the diet. In general, however, the zinc within animal products is more readily absorbed than is the zinc within plant products. One of the best sources of zinc is oysters, but because these are rarely consumed by the general population, their zinc is of little dietary relevance overall. The best commonly consumed sources of zinc are meats, poultry, eggs, and dairy products. Of the plant-based sources of zinc, grains and grain products are the most significant. Zinc is found primarily in the outer layers of cereal grains; so considerable losses occur during any milling process. Fruits and most vegetables contain fairly small amounts of zinc, whereas drinking water provides us with hardly any zinc. Figure 10-10 shows sources of zinc in the U.S. food supply. Table 10-10 indicates the zinc content of a variety of common foods.

Overall, the U.S. food supply provides an average of just over 12 mg of zinc per person per day.[31] This amount has remained fairly stable since the turn of the century, indicating that all the changes in methods of food production and processing have had little overall impact on the level of zinc in our diets. Since the turn of the century, however, the percentage of zinc obtained from meat products has significantly increased, whereas

TABLE 10-10

Zinc content of selected common foods

FOOD	AMOUNT	kcal	ZINC PER SERVING (mg)
MEAT, FISH, EGGS, POULTRY, and NUTS			
Egg, fried	1 large	95	0.5
Roast beef*	3 oz	315	5.3
Ground beef*	3 oz	230	3.8
Chicken*	3 oz	140	2.5
Tuna	3 oz	165	0.9
Peanut butter	2 Tbsp	190	1.0
Bacon	3 slices	110	0.6
Lunch meat	3 oz	190	1.8
Oysters*	½ cup	80	8.2
Pork*	3 oz	275	3.2
CEREALS			
Cornflakes	1 cup	110	0.1
Shredded wheat	1 biscuit	100	0.8
Saltines	4 crackers	50	—
Rice, dry	1 oz	109	0.3
White bread	1 slice	65	0.2
Whole wheat bread	1 slice	70	0.51.8
DAIRY PRODUCTS			
Whole milk	8 oz	150	0.9
2% fat milk	8 oz	120	0.9
Cheddar cheese	1 oz	115	0.9
FRUITS			
Apple	1 medium	80	0.1
Banana	1 medium	105	0.2
Orange juice, frozen	4 oz	55	0.1
Peach	1 medium	35	0.1
VEGETABLES			
Corn, canned	4 oz (½ cup)	82	0.4
Green beans	4 oz (½ cup)	22	0.2
Green peas	4 oz (½ cup)	62	0.7
Lettuce	¼ head	20	0.4
Tomatoes	1 medium	25	0.2
Potato, baked	1 medium	130	0.4
Lima beans*	½ cup	95	1.7
Beans, dried (cooked)*	1 cup	210	1.8

* Sources of zinc usually included in recommended lists.

From Science and Education Administration: *United States Department of Agriculture composition of foods—raw, processed and prepared,* Agricultural Handbook No 8 (1-21), Washington, DC, 1978-1992, U.S. Government Printing Office.

the percentage obtained from grain-based products has fallen in a roughly compensating manner.

Zinc intake has been found to be closely related to calorie consumption because typical diets are found to contain almost identical amounts of zinc per 1000 kcal consumed (Table 10-11). This means that people on low-kilocalorie diets—such as elderly, ill, and poor persons or those trying to lose weight—are at a risk of zinc deficiency that is virtually directly related to any energy deficiency in their diet. Results of NHANES III showed that women had mean intakes of 9.5 mg/day, 2.5 mg below the RDA, whereas men had mean intakes of 16 mg/day, 1mg above the RDA.

TABLE 10-11

Dietary zinc intake

POPULATION	DIETARY ZINC* mg/DAY	DIETARY ZINC* mg/1000 kcal†
Men, 19 to 50 yr	14.1	5.6
Women, 19 to 50 yr	9.2	5.7
Children, 1 to 5 yr	8.2	5.8

* Dietary zinc (calculated from NHANES II data) intake is directly related to energy intake, because the amount of zinc provided per 1000 kcal is remarkably constant (at 5.6-5.8 mg/1000 kcal) for most diets.

† The zinc density (mg zinc/1000 kcal) of diets of men, women, and children is virtually the same. The lower intake of zinc by women and children is explained by their lower energy (kcal) intake, as compared with that of men.

> Zinc intake is closely related to energy consumption because typical diets contain almost identical amounts of zinc per 1000 kcal consumed. Thus people on low-kilocalorie diets—such as elderly, ill, and poor persons or those trying to lose weight—are at a risk of zinc deficiency that is directly related to any energy deficiency in their diet.

EVALUATION OF ZINC STATUS

The zinc status of the body can be measured in a variety of ways, especially by determination of the zinc content of blood plasma or serum, blood cells (red or white), saliva, sweat, skin, nails, hair, and urine. Table 10-12 lists the values expected from these tests in people with adequate amounts of zinc.

The most widely used test of zinc status is the level of zinc in blood plasma. The zinc content of plasma, however, does not decline immediately when inadequate intake of zinc begins to cause problems. Instead, growth rate (in periods of active growth) and the amount of zinc excreted in urine are reduced as a homeostatic response that serves to maintain plasma zinc levels near normal in the early stages of zinc deficiency. Only once the deficiency has become so great as to overwhelm this homeo-

TABLE 10-12

Test of zinc status and the levels of zinc associated with satisfactory zinc status

TISSUE OR FLUID	NORMAL VALUES
Serum	65-140 µg/dl
Red blood cells	40-44 µg/g hemoglobin
White blood cells	80-130 µg/10^{10} cells
Saliva (parotid)	23-79 µg/g
Sweat	0.55-1.75 mg/L
Skin	10-80 µg/g
Nails	100-400 µg/g
Hair	100-250 µg/g
24-hour urine	230-600 µg/g

static response do the plasma or serum zinc levels begin to fall.[32]

A relatively new way of assessing zinc status is to measure the plasma level of the metallothionein protein, which binds to zinc within the cells of the intestinal wall. It is possible that the plasma metallothionein level gives a more accurate guide to changes in the amount of zinc being absorbed from the diet. None of the traditional or new methods for evaluating zinc status are entirely satisfactory, however. The best way to assess a person's zinc status is to test for any improvement in health after a period of zinc supplementation, but such trials take a long time and must be carefully controlled to eliminate the possibility of changes in any other dietary or additional factors that might also affect general health.

DEFICIENCY

Many Americans reportedly consume less than the RDA for zinc, yet zinc deficiency does not appear to be a widespread problem in the United States. It is difficult, however, to detect clear-cut evidence of zinc deficiency because the mineral performs a wide variety of roles, none of which stands out clearly above the others. So it remains possible that many people may suffer from less than optimal health as a result of zinc deficiencies that are unrecognized.

In some other countries of the world, zinc deficiencies have been clearly identified, although only as recently as the 1960s. In Egypt and Iran, for example, zinc deficiencies have been found to result in retarded growth, delayed and impaired sexual development, rough skin, and anemia. Treatment with zinc supplementation was sufficient to reverse these symptoms. Other symptoms that have been associated with other cases of zinc deficiency include immune deficiency (mentioned earlier), loss of appetite, dermatitis, hair loss, reduced ability to experience taste, and reduced ability of wounds to heal. Although every organ in the body is susceptible to some damage because of zinc deficiency, growing tissues—with their need for rapid cell division (which requires zinc)—are most severely affected. This explains why young people during their periods of active growth are the population group at greatest risk of impaired body function caused by zinc deficiency. In addition to a basic inadequacy of zinc in the diet, many other factors can contribute to the seriousness of zinc deficiencies. Among such factors are excessive consumption of alcohol, medical conditions causing gastrointestinal problems, surgery, burns, and kidney diseases, which increase zinc excretion.

Most cases of zinc deficiency can be categorized as either mild or moderate. One form of more severe zinc deficiency, however, is **acrodermatitis enteropathica,** a rare genetic disease in which zinc absorption is significantly impaired for reasons that are not yet apparent. The symptoms of this condition, in particular, a severe dermatitis, usually appear in the first few months of an infant's life, particularly when the infant is switched from its mother's milk to cow's milk. It can be successfully treated by the administration of 30 to 50 mg of zinc per day. Some premature infants are also prone to symptoms of severe zinc deficiency, as are some people with energy-protein malnutrition.

TOXICITY

Zinc toxicity, either chronic or acute, is relatively uncommon but does occur for a variety of reasons. Chronic toxicity is more common than acute toxicity and is also more difficult to detect. It has been found in people who treat themselves with inappropriate doses of zinc supplements, raising their zinc consumption into the 100- to 300-mg/day range. The U.S. RDA Committee has recommended that zinc supplements providing more than 15 mg/day should never be taken without medical supervision. The adverse effects of chronic zinc toxicity include impairment of copper and iron status, anemia, and immune deficiency. Some findings have linked chronic zinc toxicity to the development of atherosclerosis because of a lowering of blood high-density lipoprotein (HDL) levels. This suggests that zinc toxicity might cause an increased risk of heart disease, but at present this possible link remains unproved.

Although much less common, cases of acute zinc toxicity have been reported in various circumstances. Some cases have been caused by the contamination of food and beverages with zinc from galvanized containers. Most other cases are caused by exposure to zinc within industrial pollutants, such as the inhalation of zinc oxide fumes. The symptoms of acute zinc poisoning include severe irritation of the gastrointestinal tract leading to nausea, vomiting, diarrhea, lethargy, muscle pains, and fever.

COPPER (Cu)

Copper was first recognized as a dietary essential in 1928, when it was discovered that anemia could be prevented only if both copper and iron were available in the diet. The first case of copper deficiency was reported in 1966. Since then, many metabolic roles for copper have been uncovered, although it has often been difficult to identify them because of the interaction of copper with other micronutrient minerals such as zinc, molybdenum, and sulfur.

FUNCTIONS

Copper ions have been identified as an essential component of many metalloproteins, including some vital enzymes.[33] The processes dependent on copper-containing enzymes include the release of energy during respiration and the synthesis of the structural proteins collagen and elastin, the neurotransmitter noradrenaline, and the pigment (melanin) in hair. As part of a multifunctional enzyme called **ceruloplasmin,** copper is involved in the oxidation of ferrous ions (Fe^{2+}) to ferric ions (Fe^{3+}). The role of copper in preventing anemia may be due to an ability to assist the absorption of iron, stimulate the synthesis of the nonprotein heme or protein globin parts of hemoglobin, or release stored iron from ferritin in the liver.

ABSORPTION AND METABOLISM

Typical diets provide about 1 mg of copper per day, about 25% to 40% of which is absorbed. Copper is absorbed from all parts of the gastrointestinal tract, including the stomach and large intestine. The mechanism of copper absorption is not clear but is certainly under homeostatic regulation. Once absorbed into the cells of the intestinal wall, most copper becomes bound to such proteins as metallothionein, which appears to act as a negative—rather than a positive—regulator of copper absorption, slowing absorption of the copper into the blood. High intakes of either iron or vitamin C are found to decrease the absorption of copper.

Absorbed copper can be detected in the blood plasma as quickly as 15 minutes after being consumed. Initially, it is loosely bound to the albumin protein or to amino acids within copper chelates. Copper within the chelates appears to pass more readily across cell membranes and into the cells of the body and accounts for 7% to 10% of the copper present in plasma.

Copper is removed from plasma by the liver, from where it is either excreted into bile, stored in a protein complex containing 2% copper, or used in the synthesis of the copper-containing enzyme ceruloplasmin, which is released back into the blood. Ceruloplasmin contains 90% of plasma copper. The total copper content of plasma is not a good indicator of the copper status of the body because plasma copper levels can be maintained at the expense of the copper stores in the liver. The release of copper from the liver is controlled by the adrenal gland.

TABLE 10-13

Estimated safe and adequate daily dietary intakes for copper

AGE (YEARS)	AMOUNT (mg/DAY)
1-3	1.0-1.5
4-6	1.5-2.0
6+	2.0-3.0

Some plasma copper enters the bone marrow, where it is used in the synthesis of the copper-containing enzyme **superoxide dismutase** (**SOD**) found in red blood cells and is responsible for protecting against the toxic effects of oxygen. New supplies of SOD cannot be made within mature red blood cells (which lack a nucleus); so the SOD content of red blood cells can be used as an indicator of long-standing copper status.

Copper is excreted in both feces and urine. The fecal copper accounts for more than 97% of copper losses and includes unabsorbed dietary copper, copper released in bile, and copper lost within cells sloughed from the intestinal wall.

The total copper content of the body is estimated at 75 to 150 mg, 40% of which is found in muscles. The liver, with 15% of body copper, is the major copper storage site. Newborn infants store 5 to 10 times as much copper in the liver as do adults, but these stores are depleted to adult levels within about the first 3 months of life.

REQUIREMENTS

Assuming 40% absorption, a dietary intake of 2 mg of copper per day is sufficient to replace all losses of copper and so should be sufficient to maintain copper balance in men, women, and elderly persons. The best estimates of actual copper intakes are often less than this amount, and it is possible that people are able to adapt to lower intakes without suffering from any evidence of copper deficiency. In the United States the average copper intake of women is 1.1 mg/day, whereas for men it is 1.6 mg/day, levels well below estimated requirements of 2 to 3 mg (NHANES III).

Pregnant women require approximately an extra 0.3 mg of copper per day to allow them to transfer a total of 20 mg to the developing fetus. During the first 6 months of breast-feeding the mother needs an extra 0.5 mg of copper each day; her extra need falls to 0.3 mg/day as both the copper content of the milk and the rate of milk

TABLE 10-14

Dietary sources of copper

RICH SOURCES (>8 ppm)	MODERATE SOURCES (2-8 ppm)	POOR SOURCES (<2 ppm)
Liver	Leafy vegetables	Milk
Shellfish (especially oysters)	Eggs	Butter
Nuts	Muscle meat	Cheese
Cocoa	Fish	Sugar
Mushrooms	Poultry	Fresh fruits and vegetables
Whole grain cereals	Peas	
Gelatin	Beans	
	Fresh fruit	
	Refined cereals	

ppm, Parts per million.

From Pennington JT, Calloway DH: *J Am Diet Assoc* 63:143, 1973.

production decrease. Infants require an exceptionally large amount of copper for their weight, estimated at 0.05 to 0.1 mg/kg of body weight, and the requirements of premature infants are even higher.

The Estimated Safe and Adequate Daily Dietary Intakes for copper are shown in Table 10-13.

FOOD SOURCES

Copper is widely distributed in foods, with the amount reflecting the copper content of the soil in or on which the food—plant or animal—was raised. An indication of the copper content of representative foods is given in Table 10-14. The use of copper pipes in water systems may provide an additional source of copper.

DEFICIENCY

Copper deficiency is rare in humans. It occurs mainly in infants, but only 51 cases have been reported since 1956.[34] The manifestations of copper deficiency in infants and young children include psychomotor retardation, hypotonia (low osmotic pressure of blood), hypopigmentation, pallor, anemia that proves resistant to iron therapy in infants, osteoporosis, and low concentrations of plasma copper and ceruloplasmin. Many afflicted children have been low–birth-weight infants who were nourished for a time by total parenteral nutrition and then fed cow's milk as a major part of their diet and who had been generally poorly nourished because of an inadequate diet, impaired absorption, or diarrhea.

Low serum copper and ceruloplasmin levels are also found in an inherited condition known as **Menkes' kinky hair syndrome.** This is characterized by slow growth, degeneration of brain tissue, hypothermia, seizures, defective arterial walls, depigmentation of skin and hair, and peculiarly stubby white hair (pili torti). The syndrome results from defective absorption of copper, abnormal transport of copper, and increased excretion of copper within urine. All the manifestations of the condition are probably caused by the reduced activity of various copper-containing enzymes.

TOXICITY

Copper is toxic to humans only when it exists in the form of unbound copper ions, rather than the more usual form of copper ions bound to molecules, such as proteins. In cases of acute toxicity, plasma copper levels can rise to 1450 μg/100 ml. The symptoms of acute copper toxicity are anemia associated with the destruction of red blood cells (hemolytic anemia), damage to the tubules of the kidney, and damage to the liver. Intakes of copper salts at levels 10 times higher than normal lead to nausea and vomiting.

Chronic copper toxicity is relatively rare but occurs in the hereditary condition called **Wilson's disease.** In this disease a failure to excrete copper in bile leads to the accumulation of copper in the liver, brain, kidneys, and cornea of the eyes (where it causes brown or green rings to appear). Penicillamine, a penicillin derivative that forms a chelate with copper in a way that promotes its excretion, has been used to help reduce the copper content of people with Wilson's disease.

There is no evidence of copper toxicity as a result of environmental contamination.

IODINE (I)

The essential trace mineral iodine is present in the body in a minute amount, accounting for approximately 0.00004% of body weight. The body contains a total of 15 to 23 mg of iodine, which is less than one hundredth of the amount of iron in the body.

FIGURE 10-11

Diagrammatic representation of the location of the thyroid and parathyroid glands in the neck area, on either side of the trachea (windpipe).

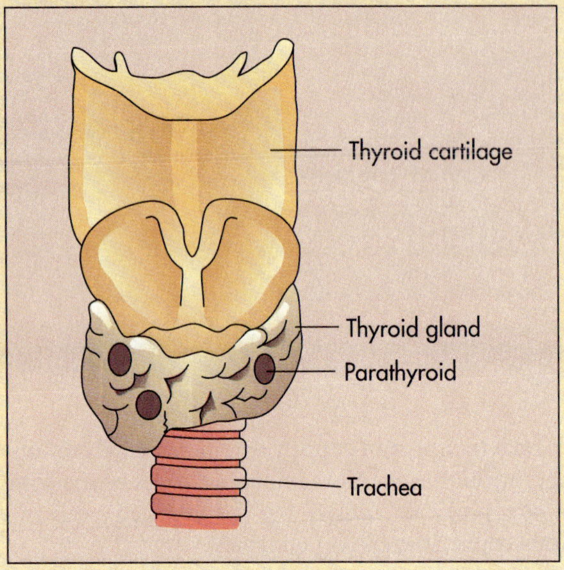

FIGURE 10-12

Chemical structure of triiodothyronine (T_3) and thyroxine (T_4).

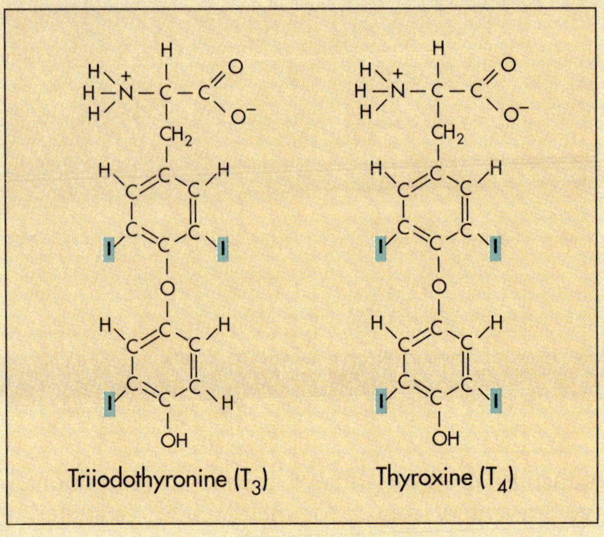

DISTRIBUTION

Over 75% of the iodine in the body is concentrated in a single location, the thyroid gland, where it is used in the synthesis of several thyroid hormones. The remainder is distributed throughout other tissues, particularly the salivary, mammary, and gastric glands and the kidneys. Within the circulation, iodine occurs either in the form of free iodide ions (I^-) or as protein-bound iodine (PBI).

The study of iodine is largely focused on its use in the thyroid gland. This gland consists of two lobes on either side of the windpipe, just below the voice box (Figure 10-11). Embedded within the thyroid gland are distinct, smaller glands known as the parathyroid glands.

FUNCTIONS

The function of iodine that attracts most attention is its role as part of the thyroid hormones **triiodothyronine** (**T_3**) and **thyroxine** (**T_4**). The presence of iodine atoms covalently bonded within the chemical structure of these hormones is illustrated in Figure 10-12. The thyroid hormones play a major role in regulating growth and development. They can stimulate the metabolic rate by as much as 30%, resulting in an increased rate of oxygen use and increased generation of heat.

The activities of the thyroid hormones are critical for the normal development of the brain. Anatomical studies have demonstrated that they increase the proliferation of brain cells and regulate other processes involved in brain function. The condition of **hypothyroidism** in which insufficient thyroid hormones are produced is associated with defective and disorganized development of the brain, resulting in serious impairment of brain function.[35]

Although the role of thyroid hormones in regulating the rate of general metabolism attracts most attention, an increasing number of other roles are becoming apparent. For example, the conversion of carotene (the precursor of vitamin A) into active vitamin A, the synthesis of protein, and the absorption of carbohydrate from the intestine all proceed less efficiently when thyroxine levels are below normal. Unusually high cholesterol levels are associated with hypothyroidism, whereas **hyperthyroidism** (oversecretion of thyroid hormones) leads to unusually low cholesterol levels. Thyroxine is also known to be essential for reproduction.

ABSORPTION AND METABOLISM

The absorption and metabolism of iodine provide further examples of the exquisite way in which the body controls the uptake and use of nutrients (Figure 10-13). Iodine occurs in food as iodide ions (I^-), as free inorganic iodine, or in the form of iodine atoms covalently bonded within organic compounds from which they must be freed before absorption. Iodide ions are absorbed rapidly, primarily in the small intestine, and then become distributed throughout the extracellular fluid. Free iodine is reduced to iodide ions, which are then absorbed. Some iodine is present in the air as a product of the combustion of fossil fuels, and some of this iodine may be absorbed through the skin and lungs.

Absorbed iodide travels quickly to the blood plasma, where one third of it is taken up by the thyroid gland.

FIGURE 10-13

Absorption and metabolism of iodine, including the synthesis of thyroxine and triiodothyronine.

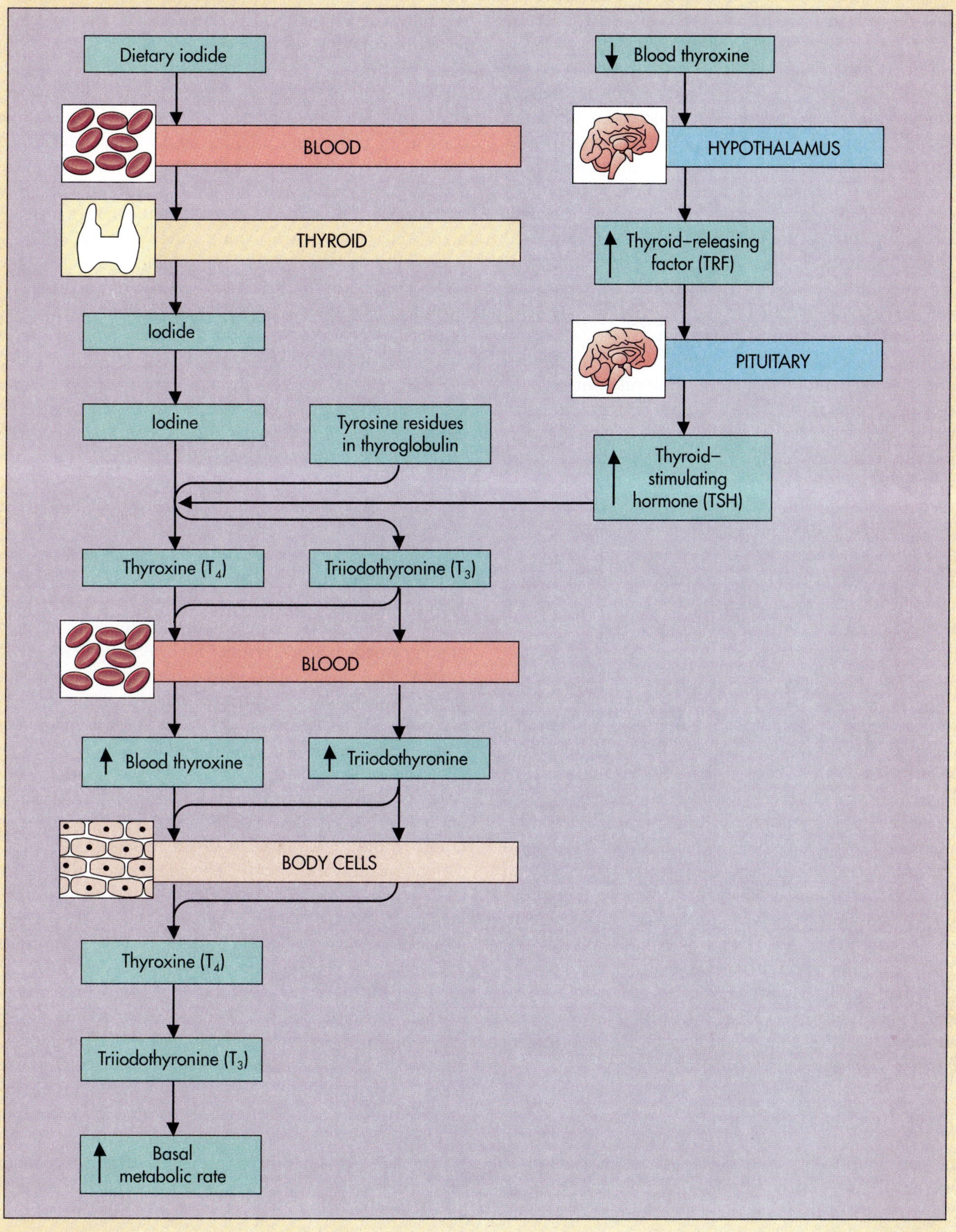

The remainder is removed as it passes through the kidneys to be excreted in urine. Small amounts of iodide are also lost in perspiration and feces. The excretion of iodide protects against the accumulation of toxic levels.

The iodide that enters the thyroid gland is oxidized back to iodine, which combines with residues of the amino acid tyrosine within the iodine-storage protein **thyroglobulin.** If the hypothalamus detects a fall in the blood thyroxine level, it releases a substance known as **thyroxine-releasing factor** (**TRF**) into the plasma. The TRF travels to the pituitary gland, where it stimulates the release into plasma of a hormone called **thyroid-stimulating hormone** (**TSH**). The TSH is transported to the thyroid gland, where it stimulates the production of an enzyme that acts on thyroglobulin to release the iodine-containing tyrosine residues from the protein. These residues are then converted into the two thyroid hormones, T_3 and T_4. These hormones are released into blood plasma in a ratio of four T_4 molecules for each T_3 molecule. They travel to every cell in the body to regulate the processes of energy release, which determine the overall metabolic rate of the body. T_3 is the more active of the two hormones, and there is some evidence to suggest that T_4 may be converted into T_3 by removal of one iodine atom after entry into a cell.

T_4 can be inactivated in the salivary gland by the removal of its iodine. The iodine removed in this way is secreted within saliva, allowing it to be reabsorbed in the gastrointestinal tract.

DIETARY REQUIREMENTS

The Food and Nutrition Board of the U.S. National Academy of Sciences has deemed that a daily iodine intake of 1 mg/kg of body weight is adequate for most adults. Growing children, especially adolescent females, may actually require more than this amount. To provide a margin of safety and to allow for individual variations in weight and needs, a total daily intake of 150 µg of iodine is recommended for men and women. For pregnant women, however, the recommended intake rises to 175 µg/day, and for lactating women it is 200 µg/day. Similar recommendations have been made for Canadians, at 160 µg/day for adults, with an additional 25 µg/day during pregnancy.[36] Most North Americans actually consume at least 300 µg of iodine each day, and intakes of up to 1000 µg (1 mg)/day are considered safe.

FOOD SOURCES

The contribution of various food groups to the iodine content of the North American diet is illustrated in Figure 10-14. Iodine is provided in the human diet by both food and water. The iodine in water occurs in the form of iodide ions in amounts that vary from region to region in line with variations in the iodine content of the soils. In the United States the iodine content of fresh water varies from 0.5 to 2 parts per billion (ppb), with the lowest levels being found in glacial rivers and lakes. Seawater contains higher levels of iodine, ranging from 17 to 50 ppb.

Variations in the iodine content of the soil in different regions are also reflected in variations in the iodine content of plants and animals raised on the soils. For example, the iodine content of carrots can vary five-fold, depending on where they are grown. Modern marketing practices mean that the food consumed in any one area is now likely to be drawn from a wide variety of different areas. This tends to ensure a more uniform and adequate level of iodine in food than was previously the case.

In general, the leaves of plants contain higher concentrations of iodine than do the roots. Spinach leaves contain up to 300 mg of iodine per serving. Various shellfish such as lobster, shrimp, and oysters are other rich sources of dietary iodine, with 15 to 150 µg of iodine per serving. These foods are consumed on relatively rare occasions, however, and so play only a minor role in contributing to the iodine content of most diets. Saltwater fish contain 10 to 100 times as much iodine as do freshwater fish.

An FDA analysis of the iodine content of foods found levels in whole milk ranging from 20 to 1300 µg/L. The study also found that a typical "market basket" diet, which is based on foods readily available in most grocery stores, provided from 550 to 850 µg of iodine in a 3000-kcal diet.[37] The iodine content of foods was found to vary not only with the iodine content of water and soil, but also with variations in the use of iodine-containing compounds for the sanitizing of processing equipment, particularly dairy equipment. Other substances contributing variable amounts of iodine, depending on their levels of use, were iodate (IO_3^-)–containing dough conditioners used in bread making and iodine-containing coloring agents. The FDA study also examined actual intakes of iodine and found that average intakes of women provided 180% of the RDA, whereas intakes by men averaged 350% of the RDA. These results suggest that it may no longer be appropriate to promote the use of **iodized salt** for cooking and table use except in areas where the soil is known to be low in iodine. The FDA study did not actually investigate the use of iodized salt, which, if consumed at an average level of 4.5 g/day, contributes an additional 340 µg of iodine to the daily diet. The iodine in iodized salt is provided in the form of iodide ions within the compound potassium iodide and provides 76 µg of iodide per gram of iodized salt. About 55% of the salt consumed in the United States is iodized at a cost of half a cent to 3 cents per person per year. Federal labeling laws require that iodized salt bear the following legend: "This salt contains added iodine, an

FIGURE 10-14

Contribution of various food groups to the iodine content of the North American diet.

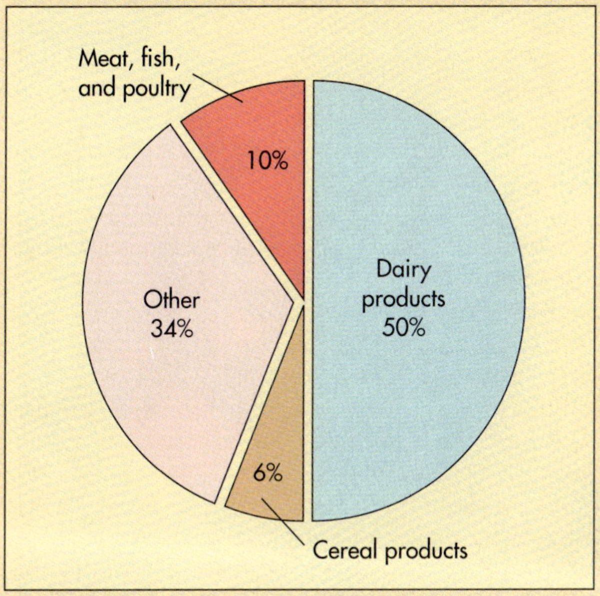

per gram of creatinine. When body iodine levels are high, urine contains about 50 μg of iodine per gram of creatinine. The uptake of a readily detectable stable isotope of iodine can also be used for the assessment of iodine status in people whose thyroid gland is functioning normally.

Relatively new **radioimmunoassay** techniques involving the binding of radioactive antibodies make it possible to measure the levels of thyroxine, triiodothyronine, and TSH in blood plasma, all of which are indicators of iodine status. Another method is the assessment of the amount of PBI in the blood. This value is found to change in parallel with both plasma thyroxine levels and the basal metabolic rate, which can itself be used as an indirect indicator of iodine status. PBI values of 4 to 8 μg/dl are normal; values greater than 11 μg/dl indicate hyperthyroidism, and values less than 3 μg/dl indicate hypothyroidism.

DEFICIENCY

A large proportion of the world's population is at risk of iodine deficiency, which is responsible for a variety of **iodine-deficiency disorders.** The problems associated with these disorders include goiter, hypothyroidism, impaired mental function, spontaneous abortions, stillbirths, congenital abnormalities, increased infant mortality, and cretinism.

essential nutrient," and noniodized salt must be labeled as follows: "This product does not contain iodine, an essential nutrient." Iodized salt is used in only 20% of processed foods because of technical and quality control problems associated with its use.

Contrary to popular opinion, sea salt is not a good source of iodine because iodine in seawater is lost as vapor when the seawater is evaporated and the salt dries. Seaweed is a good source of dietary iodine but only in cultures accustomed to its use.

> Approximately one sixth of the world's population is at risk of iodine deficiency, which is responsible for a variety of iodine-deficiency disorders. The most susceptible segments of the population are adolescent girls and pregnant women.

> Rich sources of iodine include spinach leaves and various shellfish such as shrimp, oysters, and lobster.

EVALUATION OF IODINE STATUS

The iodine status of the body is evaluated by comparing the amounts of iodine and **creatinine** excreted within a sample of urine. Creatinine is a nitrogen-containing compound that is excreted within urine in amounts proportional to the lean body mass. If iodine levels in the body are low, urine contains about 25 μg of iodine

Goiter

Iodine deficiency is responsible for simple goiter, a condition characterized by swelling in the neck caused by enlargement of the thyroid gland. The enlargement is apparently a compensatory adaptation to the lack of iodine required for the synthesis of thyroid hormones. The direct stimulus of the enlargement is an abnormally high level of TSH, itself brought about by low plasma levels of the thyroid hormones. The excessive TSH causes an increase in both the number and size of the cells of the thyroid gland.

FIGURE 10-15

Areas of the world where goiter is common because of low levels of iodine in soil or water.

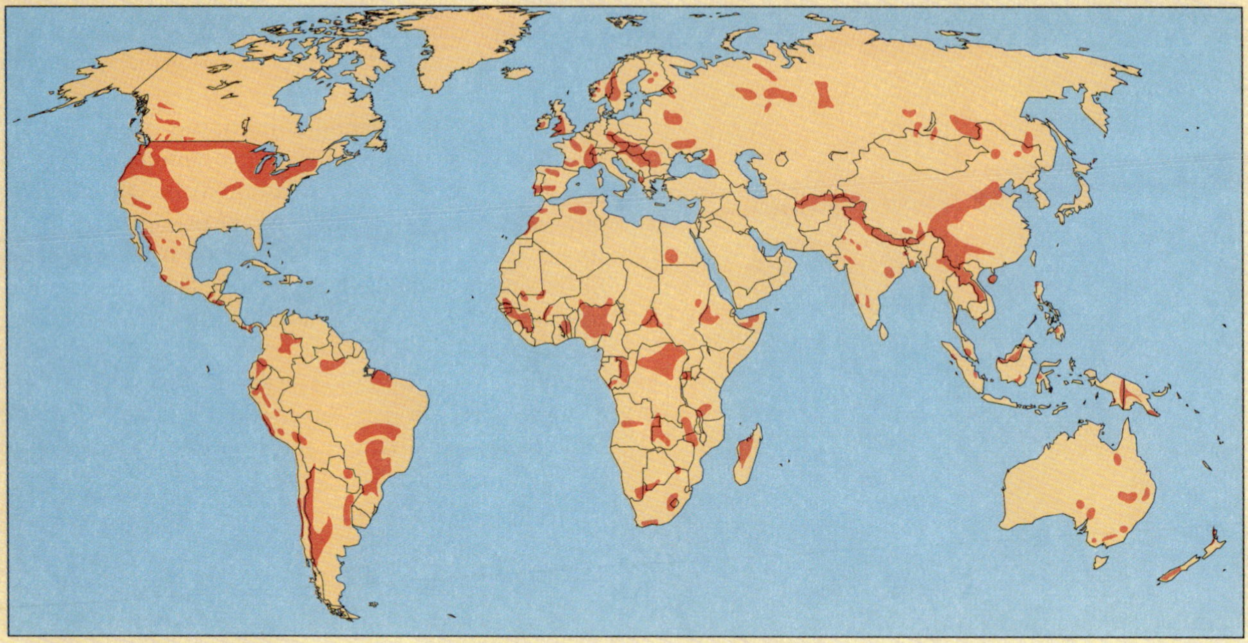

Simple goiter is a painless condition, but if uncorrected it can lead to pressure on the trachea, which may cause difficulty in breathing. Administration of appropriate doses of iodine results in a slow reduction in the size of the thyroid gland, although surgical removal of part of the gland may be required in the most severe cases. When surgery is necessary, it is complicated by the presence of the parathyroid glands, which are embedded in the thyroid gland.

Although iodine deficiency is the primary cause of simple goiter, it is not the only cause. Certain foods contain substances called **goitrogens,** which increase the susceptibility to goiter and play a decisive role in the onset of about 4% of all cases of goiter. The goitrogens act by blocking the absorption or use of iodine. They are found in peaches, almonds, soybeans, and cassava. Their presence in cassava is particularly significant because it is a dietary staple in many tropical countries.

Foods of the cabbage family such as cabbage, turnips, and rutabagas contain a heat-stable substance called **pregoitrin** and a heat-labile activator able to convert the pregoitrin into **goitrin,** which interferes with iodine use. Goitrin is found in raw foods but not in cooked foods. Ground nuts and peanuts contain a substance called **arachidoside,** which also interferes with iodine use.

The widely used **sulfonamide** antibiotics are potential causes of goiter because they reduce the conversion of iodine to iodide. At the levels commonly used to treat infection, however, they have little effect on thyroid activity. The vitamin-like substance paraaminobenzoic acid (PABA) has a similar potentially goitrogenic effect.

Goiter can also be caused by deficiencies or defects in the enzymes responsible for the synthesis and release of thyroid hormones.

Incidence Goiter occurs primarily in areas where the drinking water or soil contains little iodine. This occurs mainly where much of the water is of glacial origin or in areas in which tropical rainstorms and flooding have leached iodine from the soil (Figure 10-15). Goiter is almost nonexistent in areas where iodine-rich vapors from the sea condense and deposit iodine on the soil. This means that inhabitants of most coastal areas are relatively free of goiter.

In all areas the most susceptible sections of the population are adolescent girls and pregnant women. The incidence of goiter among females is about six times as high as that among males. Current estimates suggest that about one sixth of the world's population (1 billion people) is at risk of developing iodine deficiency and therefore goiter.[38] Most of the susceptible people live in developing countries, particularly within Africa and East Asia, although over 100 countries worldwide contain high-risk areas, including such developed countries as Germany and Italy. In 1970 a nutritional status survey in 10 states of America indicated that in some areas as much as 7.2% of the population was afflicted with goiter. A follow-up study, however, revealed that many of the people with enlarged thyroids were achieving recommended iodine intakes, suggesting a widespread prevalence of goiter unrelated to iodine deficiency. Since 1970 no evidence has been obtained to suggest any widespread iodine deficiency in the U.S.

Treatment When the United Nations and International Heads of State assembled at the Children's Summit in 1990, they pledged to strive for the virtual elimination of goiter by the year 2000. Such a bold aim is achievable because goiter is readily treated, and treatment of it in the Western world is already a significant public health success story. The use of iodine for treating goiter was first recognized around 1820, and 30 years later iodine deficiency was first linked with low levels of iodine in soil and water. The discovery that iodine was a normal constituent of the thyroid gland led to an upsurge in interest in and awareness of the use of iodine to treat goiter. Several investigations confirmed that endemic goiter (meaning goiter affecting many people within any particular region) could be controlled by raising the dietary iodine intake of the population in general. Many different methods of iodine administration were tried, but only the iodization of salt has proved consistently effective in reaching the majority of the population in developed countries. In developing countries intramuscular injections of **lipidoil,** an iodine-containing poppy seed oil, every 3 years have also proved successful. Most recently the oral administration of lipidoil has also met with success. Iodization of the water supply is another obvious strategy for the mass administration of iodine and has already been used in some situations.[39] Iodine deficiency, as well as iron and vitamin A deficiencies, is targetted in current major international efforts to reduce micronutrient deficiencies in developing countries, primarily by the enrichment of dietary staples.

Cretinism

The most severe problem associated with iodine deficiency is **cretinism,** a congenital defect of mental and physical development caused by iodine deficiency during development. Two types of cretinism are found: **neurological cretinism** and **myxedematous cretinism.** The key feature of neurological cretinism is mental retardation, but short stature, spasticity, rigidity of muscles and deaf mutism are also often found. The main organs affected are the inner ear, or cochlea, and the brain. The most significant stages in the development of these organs occur during the second trimester of pregnancy, and iodine deficiency during this critical time is believed to be responsible for the major manifestations of neurological cretinism. Myxedematous cretinism is also associated with mental retardation, but its victims are shorter in stature than neurological cretins and have clear hypothyroidism, but do not usually suffer from spasticity, goiter, or deaf mutism. This type of cretinism occurs mainly in Central Africa and, at least in its "pure" form, is relatively rare.

Neurological cretinism appears to be caused by an iodine deficiency in the patient's mother during the first and second trimesters of pregnancy. Myxedematous cretinism probably results from an iodine deficiency that developed later in the pregnancy, combined with continuing iodine deficiency throughout the infant's first few years of life.

In addition to being caused by iodine deficiency, cretinism can also result from congenital hypothyroidism, which causes a lack of thyroid hormones during the crucial phase of development. This is seen in about 1 in every 4000 births. In most developed countries screening programs based on measurements of plasma TSH level are in place to test for it. Early diagnosis and treatment can significantly reduce the risk of mental retardation and stunted growth.

HYPERTHYROIDISM

Hyperthyroidism, in which there is oversecretion of thyroid hormones and a resulting increase in basal metabolic rate, is also known as **Grave's disease** or **exophthalmic goiter.** People with this condition are commonly described as having an "overactive thyroid gland," and their basal metabolic rate may be as high as twice the normal value. The condition results in nervousness, lower-than-normal weight, reduced body fat (despite an increased appetite), intolerance to heat, tremors when the hand is outstretched, and noticeable protrusion of the eyeballs.

SELENIUM (Se)

Occasional reports of selenium deficiencies date back as far as from Marco Polo in 1295. Not until 1957, however, was selenium reported to have a specific nutritional function.[40] Difficulties have been encountered in producing a "pure" selenium deficiency condition in animals, but selenium is now considered an essential mineral for humans.[41]

DISTRIBUTION

Selenium reserves amounting to approximately 15 mg are believed to be concentrated in the liver. Plasma levels of 100 to 150 μg/L are considered normal in the United States. This is considerably higher than the 50-μg/L level found in New Zealand, where the soil is low in selenium, and considerably lower than the 355 to 800 μg/L level found in Venezuela. In New Zealand, however, signs of selenium deficiency among the population are not evident, and in Venezuela there are no signs of selenium toxicity.[42]

FUNCTIONS

For many years investigators were puzzled by an apparent overlap in functions between selenium and vitamin E. This puzzle was resolved in 1973, when selenium was found to be an integral part of the enzyme **glutathione peroxidase (Gpx),** which catalyzes the breakdown of toxic hydroperoxides. In this role, selenium is an essential component of the body's antioxidant defense system, as is vitamin E (see Chapter 11). Because of this overlap of functions, the body's need for selenium declines as the amount of vitamin E in the diet increases. Although the early interest in selenium was focused on its role in glutathione peroxidase, the mineral is now known to perform several important functions, as summarized below.

Several selenium-containing proteins, or selenoproteins, are now known. The first to be identified was Gpx, and it remains the best characterized of the selenium-containing proteins. As indicated previously, it protects cells from oxidative damage by catalyzing the reduction of lipid hydroperoxides and hydrogen peroxide, which are generated by the normal processes of metabolism. Evidence suggests that peroxides and other products of oxidative metabolism are involved in the onset of numerous diseases and also the natural aging process. In recent years it has been discovered that Gpx is also involved in the production of intercellular regulatory compounds and in the metabolism of the essential fatty acid arachidonic acid. The first RDA for selenium, set in 1989,[41] was established by determining the amount of selenium required to maintain maximal plasma Gpx activity.

A second, closely related selenoprotein is **phospholipid hydroperoxide glutathione peroxidase (Gpx II)**. This protein differs from Gpx in that it specifically reduces *membrane-bound* lipid hydroperoxides in phospholipids. In this role the enzyme is another component of the antioxidant defenses of the body.

Selenoprotein P is another selenoprotein, but its exact function remains unknown. It may be involved in selenium transport or may act as an extracellular antioxidant.[40] Plasma levels of selenoprotein P are particularly responsive to changes in dietary selenium intake. The concentration of selenoprotein P in the plasma of selenium-deficient animals is only 10% of that in animals with sufficient selenium. After repletion with selenium, selenoprotein P levels respond rapidly, increasing approximately eight-fold within 12 hours. During the same time, plasma Gpx activity increases only marginally.

A fourth selenoprotein is **Type 1 iodothyronine-5-deiodinase (ID-1)**, an enzyme required for the removal of iodine from thyroxine (T_4) to produce triiodothyronine (T_3). Selenium deficiency in animals causes abnormally high plasma T_4 levels and decreased plasma T_3 levels. The recent discovery of this function of selenium has important implications for the interpretation of the effects of selenium deficiency when vitamin E levels (and therefore antioxidant defenses) are adequate. In particular, decreased growth and susceptibility to cold stress during prolonged selenium deficiency may relate to altered thyroid hormone metabolism.[43]

Other functions of selenium that currently cannot be explained by its presence in the known selenoproteins include the metabolism of drugs, maintenance of plasma glutathione levels, an involvement in the function of the "neutrophil" white blood cells of the immune system, and some involvement in lipid and glucose metabolism.[44]

ABSORPTION AND METABOLISM

Selenium in food is primarily present in an organic form as two modified amino acids: **selenomethionine** (synthesized by plants) and **selenocysteine** (synthesized by animals).[45] Selenium in inorganic form is often supplied in experimental diets and in nutritional supplements. The absorption of all forms of selenium is efficient and estimated to be between 50% and 80% of intake. Selenium absorption does not appear to be subject to any regulatory control. Selenomethionine is known to be absorbed in the same way that the normal amino acid methionine is, but the mechanisms of absorption of selenocysteine and inorganic selenium are unknown. The body seems to be unable to distinguish between selenomethionine and methionine, and so selenomethionine is incorporated into proteins in amounts dependent on its availability from dietary sources. In sharp contrast, there is no evidence that selenocysteine can substitute for cysteine in proteins. Selenocysteine is the form of selenium that accounts for its biological activity. This means that selenocysteine is the form in which selenium is incorporated into *specific* sites to form the functional selenoproteins.

In blood plasma, most selenium is bound to proteins, probably the globulins and lipoproteins. Selenoprotein P may also be involved as a selenium transporter, but this has not yet been proven.

The excretion of selenium is primarily via urine and feces. In adults, 50% to 60% of excreted selenium is lost within urine.

REQUIREMENTS

Although several selenium balance studies have been conducted to investigate selenium requirements, homeostatic mechanisms appear to ensure that intakes of selenium are in balance with losses over a wide range of intakes, from 9 to 80 μg/day. Because of this, studies of selenium balance are not considered useful in determining our selenium requirements.

Another way to estimate requirements is to examine dietary intakes in areas both with and without selenium deficiency. Selenium deficiency is endemic in some areas of China in which intakes of selenium are as low as 10 μg/day. Comparison with intakes in nearby areas without selenium deficiency suggests that the minimal requirements for adult Chinese men and women are 19 and 13 μg/day, respectively. In New Zealand, intakes of 33 μg/day by men and 23 μg/day by women are not associated with deficiency. The administration of graded amounts of supplementary selenium to Chinese men with selenium deficiency demonstrated that 30 μg of additional selenium raised plasma glutathione peroxidase levels to a maximal plateau. Adding the supplemented amount to the amount previously taken in by these men produced a figure for the requirement for dietary selenium of 40 μg/day (0.67 μg/kg/day). The current U.S. RDAs for men and women are derived from this study, with upward adjustments for body size (assumed to be 79 kg for men and 63 kg for women in America) and an assumed 15% variation in selenium requirements. Thus the RDA for men is 70 μg/day and for women is 55 μg/day. Recommended intakes for children and adolescents are calculated with reference to these values on the basis of body weight and a factor to allow for growth. During pregnancy, assuming that 5 kg of lean tissue is accumulated, a total of 1.25 mg of additional absorbed selenium is required (5 to 6.5 μg/day, allowing for individual variability). With an assumed absorption rate of 80%, the average increase in dietary intake during pregnancy should be 10 μg/day. The selenium content of human milk is around 15 to 20 μg/L, causing a loss of about 13 μg/day during lactation. To compensate for these losses, the RDA during lactation includes an additional 20 μg/day.

The Recommended Dietary Intakes (RDIs) for selenium are summarized in Table 10-15. No Recommended Nutrient Intake (RNI) for selenium has yet been set in Canada.

TABLE 10-15

Recommended dietary intakes for selenium

AGE (YEARS)	AMOUNT (μg/DAY)
INFANTS	
<1.1	10-15
1.1-9	20
6-9.9	30
MALES	
10-11.9	40
12-17.9	50
18-51+	70
FEMALES	
11-14.9	45
15-18	50
19-51+	55

FOOD SOURCES

The selenium content of foods reflects the selenium content of the soil in which the plants consumed were grown or on which the animals consumed were raised. The relationship between soil content and a food's selenium content, however, is not always straightforward. Some plants are able to concentrate selenium, whereas others contain selenium at concentrations that are less than—but directly proportional to—the concentration of selenium in the soil. Large differences are found in the selenium content of foods from different regions of the world and different states of America, causing correspondingly large differences in the selenium intake of different populations. These variations in selenium intake lead, in turn, to the wide variations in plasma selenium levels considered already (from 50 μg/L in New Zealand to 800 μg/L in parts of Venezuela). Table 10-16 gives an indication of the range of variation in the selenium content of foods produced in various parts of the United States.

Market basket surveys suggest that the typical American diet provides 50 to 250 μg of selenium per day. The best sources of selenium, in descending order, are meats derived from organs, meats derived from muscle, cereals, and dairy products. In general, the more protein a food contains, the more selenium it contains. Selenium is lost from foods during milling in processing or during boiling in cooking.

> Rich sources of selenium include meats derived from organs, meats derived from muscle, cereals, and dairy products. In general, the more protein a food contains, the more selenium it contains.

The bioavailability of selenium derived from different foods varies widely, from 5% in mushrooms to 83% in wheat and up to as high as 97% in beef kidney.[46]

ASSESSMENT OF SELENIUM STATUS

The plasma or serum selenium concentration reflects recent dietary intake, whereas the selenium concentration of red blood cells reflects relatively long-term dietary intake over the preceding 120 days. This makes the red blood cell selenium level the best indicator of

TABLE 10-16

Typical values for the selenium content of foods

FOOD*	AMOUNT (µg/100 g)
Organ meats and seafood	40-150
Muscle meats	10-40
Cereals and grains	<10->80
Dairy products	<10-30
Fruits and vegetables	<10

* The selenium content of foods varies widely, depending on the amount of selenium in soil where plants were grown and amount in feed fed to animals.

selenium nutritional status. When selenium intake is low or moderate, plasma and red blood cell levels of selenium are correspondingly low or moderate and they show a good correlation with plasma and erythrocyte activity of Gpx. High plasma concentrations of selenium are not correlated with Gpx activity, presumably because a point is reached at which no further enzyme is synthesized when the concentration of selenium is raised further. The selenium concentration of hair and nails is directly related to plasma serum concentrations and has been used to determine selenium status in some epidemiological studies.

DEFICIENCY

Selenium deficiency is associated with **Keshan disease,** a heart muscle condition (a "cardiomyopathy") that affects children and women of child-bearing age in some parts of China. Diets in the areas where Keshan disease is found are low in selenium. Selenium supplementation has proved effective in controlling Keshan disease. Some aspects of the disease, however, such as its seasonal variation, suggest that it cannot be caused simply by selenium deficiency.

The best-documented cases of selenium deficiency involve children and adults who are undergoing long-term parenteral nutrition and receiving nutritional fluids containing no selenium. The clinical manifestations of selenium deficiency in these patients include muscle pain and weakness, cardiomyopathy, and a loss of pigmentation, described as **pseudoalbinism.** Decreased selenium concentrations and Gpx activity in plasma and various tissues were found in most cases. Treatment with selenium has proved effective in correcting the disorder.[45]

Epidemiological studies have demonstrated an increased incidence of several kinds of cancer in people living in areas with low selenium levels in the soil. Selenium intake and plasma selenium levels also appear to be inversely correlated with cancer mortality. This suggests that selenium may be a naturally occurring "anticarcinogen," able to give some protection against the development of cancer, a conclusion supported by some studies in laboratory animals. How selenium might act in this way is unknown, but it seems possible that selenium-containing enzymes may be involved in the detoxification of chemicals that can cause cancer (carcinogens).

It has also been suggested that low selenium intakes might be associated with increased death rates from age-related heart disease. Several epidemiological studies, however, have found no support for this idea.

TOXICITY

Selenium is toxic when consumed in excess, although the biochemical basis of its toxicity is unknown.[47] Selenium poisoning (**selenosis**) caused by the consumption of foods rich in selenium has been most widely reported in China, where plasma selenium levels as high as 3200 µg/L have been found.[42] The affected people had consumed an average of about 5 mg of selenium per day in a vegetable-based diet. The symptoms of selenium poisoning include loss of hair and nails, skin lesions, tooth decay, and abnormalities of the nervous system. The most acutely affected people had consumed as much as 38 mg of selenium per day and suffered complete loss of hair within a period of only 3 or 4 days.

In America, some cases of selenium poisoning resulted from the consumption of a so-called nutritional supplement that contained approximately 182 times the amount of selenium that was declared on the label. The total amount of selenium ingested by the victims was estimated at 27 to 2387 mg. The most common symptoms were nausea, vomiting, hair loss, nail changes, irritability, fatigue, and malfunctions of the peripheral nervous system.

Selenium toxicity is relatively uncommon when compared with the incidence of selenium deficiency in areas in which mainly traditional foods are consumed. Selenium poisoning in humans generally occurs only when abnormal intakes are forced on people because of the restricted range of foods available to them or when selenium-containing supplements are used unwisely.

An increased incidence of dental caries has been found among people living in areas where soils are high in selenium. Attempts to produce dental caries by selenium administration to laboratory animals have failed, however, so a causal link between selenium and caries remains to be proved. The restricted information available on the subject suggests that excessive—although nontoxic—levels of selenium intake may increase caries, although somewhat lower but still fairly high levels of selenium intake may offer some protection against caries. There is no information from studies on humans, however, to allow reliable correlations to be identified between specific levels of selenium intake by humans and their susceptibility to caries.

ULTRATRACE MINERALS

As explained in the Minerals Overview, the micronutrient minerals are also known as the trace elements because they are mineral elements required in the diet in only trace amounts. So far, this chapter has discussed the trace elements iron, zinc, copper, iodine, and selenium. Fluorine was discussed in Chapter 8. The remaining nine trace elements—manganese, molybdenum, cobalt, chromium, silicon, vanadium, nickel, arsenic, and boron—are present in the body in such small amounts that they are referred to as **ultratrace elements.** They are almost never found in free form within the body but occur bound to or within other compounds. Tin, although not yet officially recognized as essential in the human diet, is almost certainly another essential ultratrace element.

The ultratrace elements share some aspects of metabolism and are considered in this final section of the chapter as a group. Only brief details are given for each individual ultratrace element because they have not been subjected to such rigorous and long-standing analysis as have the other essential minerals.

MANGANESE (Mn)

Although manganese deficiency has never been demonstrated in humans, manganese is considered a dietary essential because it is known to play a variety of biochemical roles in the body. As a cofactor or component of various enzymes, it assists in the release of energy within mitochondria, the synthesis of fatty acids and cholesterol, the metabolism of carbohydrates, the formation of urea, and the release of lipid from the liver. It is also required for normal development of the skeleton and connective tissue. It must also be involved in aspects of metabolism crucial to the brain because both an excess and a deficiency (investigated in animal studies) of manganese can adversely affect brain function. The adult human body is estimated to contain 11 to 22 mg of manganese.

ABSORPTION AND METABOLISM

Manganese is absorbed by a mechanism similar to that involved in iron absorption, and in blood plasma the major manganese-binding protein is transferrin, best known for its binding to iron.[47] The efficiency of manganese absorption is low (at only 3% to 4% of dietary intake). High intakes of iron are known to depress the efficiency of manganese absorption, probably reflecting the shared mechanism of absorption for manganese and iron.

Most of the body's manganese is concentrated in the pancreas, bone, liver, and kidneys. Within cells, manganese is found mainly in the mitochondria. No storage site or storage protein for manganese has been identified.

The manganese content of the body is regulated by variations in the amount excreted in bile. Very little manganese is lost in urine. Newborn infants apparently lose manganese during the first few weeks of life but with no ill effects.

TABLE 10-17

Estimated Safe and Adequate Daily Dietary Intakes for manganese

AGE (YEARS)	AMOUNT (mg/DAY)
CHILDREN	
1-3	1.0-1.5
4-6	1.5-2.0
7-10	2.0-3.0
ADULTS	
11+	2.5-5.0

TABLE 10-18

Dietary sources of manganese

RICH SOURCES (>20 ppm)	MODERATE SOURCES (1-5 ppm)	POOR SOURCES (<1 ppm)
Nuts	Green leafy vegetables	Animal tissues
Whole grain cereals	Dried fruits	Poultry
Dried legumes	Fresh fruits	Dairy products
Tea	Nonleafy vegetables	Seafood

ppm, Parts per million.

DIETARY REQUIREMENTS AND FOOD SOURCES

A provisional recommended intake of manganese has been set at 2.0 to 5 mg/day (35 to 70 µg/kg of body weight) for adults (Table 10-17). Intakes lower than 0.7 µg/day are considered to be definitely inadequate. The typical North American diet provides 3.6 µg of manganese per day and is therefore adequate in manganese.

The best sources of manganese are derived from plants (Table 10-18), although the amount provided depends on the manganese content of the soil and water where the plants were grown. Whole grain cereals and green vegetables are the best sources among the most commonly eaten foods. Tea is extremely rich in manganese, and in British diets tea provides around 2.3 µg of manganese per day.

TABLE 10-19

Estimated Recommended Safe and Adequate Daily Dietary Intakes for molybdenum (mg/day)

AGE (YEARS)	AMOUNT (mg/DAY)
CHILDREN	
1-3	0.03-0.05
4-6	0.03-0.08
7+	0.05-0.15
ADULTS	
11+	0.075-0.25

TOXICITY

The accumulation of excessive amounts of manganese in the body is toxic but usually occurs as a result of the inhalation of industrial pollutants, rather than high dietary intake. Manganese poisoning is more likely in people with iron deficiency, whereas high intakes of protein offer some protection against it. The main manifestations of manganese poisoning are general weakness, impaired control of muscles, and psychological disturbances.

MOLYBDENUM (Mo)

Molybdenum has long been recognized as required for plant growth and is now also considered an essential nutrient for humans. Molybdenum deficiency has not been found in humans, but the mineral is believed to be particularly involved in early development. The body contains about 9 mg of molybdenum, concentrated mainly in the liver, kidneys, and skeleton.[48]

FUNCTIONS

Molybdenum is known to be an essential cofactor for three enzymes—xanthine oxidase, aldehyde oxidase, and sulfite oxidase—all of which catalyze oxidation-reduction reactions. A patient with an inborn error of molybdenum metabolism (lacking a functional molybdenum cofactor for the enzymes xanthine oxidase and sulfite oxidase) is reported to be severely retarded, suggesting an important role of molybdenum in human metabolism.[49]

ABSORPTION AND EXCRETION

Between 25% and 80% of dietary molybdenum is absorbed from both the stomach and the small intestine, and molybdenum is excreted in urine and bile. The amount excreted is influenced largely by the amount of sulfate ion (SO_4^{2-}) in the diet, with high-sulfate diets causing increased urinary excretion of molybdenum.

DIETARY REQUIREMENTS

The Estimated Recommended Safe and Adequate Daily Dietary Intake for molybdenum has been set at between 0.075 and 0.25 mg/day for adults (Table 10-19). Most diets supply between 0.5 and 1 mg of molybdenum per day, but daily intakes can range from 0.05 to 0.35 mg/day.[50] The apparent levels of intake typically ingested barely meet the lowest suggested safe and adequate level of intake. It is possible, however, that this may simply indicate that the safe and adequate levels of intake are set too high.

A spontaneous dietary deficiency of molybdenum in humans is unknown. There has been one report of molybdenum deficiency in a young man who received total parenteral nutrition for 18 months.[50] He experienced severe headache, tachycardia (rapid heart beat), nausea, vomiting, lethargy, disorientation, and coma. There was a low level of uric acid in his blood (hypouricemia), and the conversion of sulfite to sulfate was impaired, as indicated by low urinary sulfate excretion. The symptoms suggested a defect in sulfur metabolism at the level of sulfite oxidation to sulfate and a defect in uric acid production at the level of xanthine transformation to uric acid. The patient's condition was corrected by molybdenum supplementation. Most physicians do not add molybdenum to the feeding solution for patients receiving total parenteral nutrition until a definite need is demonstrated.

FOOD SOURCES

The best sources of molybdenum (containing 2 to 5 ppm) are milk and milk products; legumes, such as peas and beans; and meat. Whole grain cereals and bakery products are good sources (with at least 0.6 ppm), whereas fruits and vegetables are poor sources (containing less than 1 ppm).

TOXICITY

Evidence of molybdenum toxicity is rare. The symptoms of toxicity are known to include diarrhea, slow growth, and anemia associated with a failure of red blood cells to mature.

INTERRELATIONSHIPS BETWEEN MOLYBDENUM AND OTHER MINERALS

Most of the interest in molybdenum has been focused on its metabolic interrelationships with copper and sulfate. Depressed growth and low levels of hemoglobin production in animals with high levels of molybdenum are associated with high urinary losses of copper, and can be overcome by supplementation with copper. It is possible that high intakes of molybdenum can interfere with the removal of copper from plasma or the synthesis of ceruloplasmin or both.

COBALT (Co)

FUNCTIONS

The only known function of cobalt in humans is as an essential part of vitamin B_{12} (cobalamin), which is necessary to prevent pernicious anemia. The human requirement for cobalt is thus a part of the requirement for vitamin B_{12}. Apparently cobalt is not required in any other form. There is increasing evidence, however, that cobalt may also be involved in the functioning of some enzymes in humans.

ABSORPTION AND EXCRETION

Cobalt within vitamin B_{12} is absorbed primarily from the jejunum (upper small intestine). About 85% of absorbed cobalt is excreted in urine, and small amounts are excreted in feces and perspiration.

FOOD SOURCES

The average daily diet in North America contains about 300 mg of cobalt. The amount found in some representative foods is shown in Table 10-20. In spite of the large amount of cobalt consumed, only the 0.04 µg within the required daily amount of vitamin B_{12} is actually needed.

TABLE 10-20

Dietary sources of cobalt (mg/g of dry weight)

RICH SOURCES (>5 ppm)	MODERATE SOURCES (1.5-5 ppm)	POOR SOURCES (<0.5 ppm)
Liver	Lean beaf	Cereal grains
Kidney	Lamb	Leguminous seeds
Oysters	Veal	Grean leafy vegetables
Clams	Poultry	Yeast
	Saltwater fish	
	Milk	

ppm, Parts per million.

TOXICITY

High intakes of cobalt have been associated with toxic effects. One such effect is a goitrogenic influence of prolonged ingestion of cobalt chloride. The enlargement of the thyroid gland produced in this way is reversed when the consumption of this form of cobalt ceases. High cobalt intakes in animals have been known to cause **polycythemia,** an increase in the number of red blood cells, and an increase in the number of bone marrow cells. These effects are believed to be a result of the increased production of erythropoietin, the hormone that stimulates the production of red blood cells in the bone marrow.

Cobalt is added to beer to control foaming, and polycythemia is seen in cobalt toxicity associated with excessive beer drinking. Also related to the consumption of alcoholic beverages is a synergistic effect that is believed to exist between cobalt and ethanol (meaning that each increases the influence of the other). This effect is believed to contribute to cardiac problems found in people who consume large amounts of beer.

High dosages of cobalt are found to dilate the blood vessels, leading to its use in the treatment of human hypertension.

CHROMIUM (Cr)

Chromium was first identified as an essential mineral for mammals in 1959, and symptoms of chromium deficiency in humans were first detected in 1966. The amount of chromium in the body varies widely, with people in the United States having about 20% of the amount of chromium found in people in the Far East. Absorbed chromium tends to accumulate in the skin, muscle, and fat. The amount in hair is a sensitive indicator of the body's chromium content, but the level of chromium that indicates a deficiency is unknown. Chromium is excreted primarily in urine.

FUNCTIONS

The precise biochemical role of chromium in the body has not been identified, but it is required for the optimal use of glucose. Patients receiving chromium-free total parenteral nutrition have been found to develop an impaired glucose tolerance, which is corrected by the administration of chromium. Chromium's influence on glucose use may be a result of its ability to aid in the binding of insulin to the surface of cells, which allows glucose to enter the cells.

ABSORPTION AND METABOLISM

The percentage of dietary chromium that is absorbed into the body is low, varying from less than 1% to up to 3% at

TABLE 10-21

Estimated Safe and Adequate Daily Dietary Intakes for chromium

AGE (YEARS)	AMOUNT (mg/DAY)
CHILDREN	
1-3	0.02-0.08
4-6	0.03-0.12
7-10	0.05-0.20
ADULTS	
11+	0.05-0.20

most. Absorption is believed to occur most readily when the chromium is bound within organic complexes, rather than in its free ionic form as Cr^{3+}. Within the circulatory system, chromium occurs bound to the albumin, transferrin, and possibly globulin proteins.[51] The normal serum concentration of chromium is 10 to 30 mg/L, but as plasma insulin levels rise, chromium levels decline.[52]

DIETARY REQUIREMENTS

At present there is sufficient information to estimate chromium requirements (Table 10-21) but not to establish RDAs. A fetus obtains a generous supply of chromium from its mother, and the chromium concentration in the body then declines throughout life.

FOOD SOURCES

Meats and whole grains are some of the best sources of chromium. The amount of chromium in foods of plant origin varies with plant species, soil type, and season. Considerable losses of chromium occur during any milling process. Brown sugar and commercial syrups contain considerable amounts of chromium, whereas it is undetectable in raw sugar and white sugar. Fruits, vegetables, and milk are low in chromium.

Typical North American diets provide around 25 to 89 μg of chromium per day, amounts in the same region as the suggested adult intake of between 20 and 50 μg/day.

DEFICIENCY

Low intakes of chromium have been associated with a reduced tolerance to glucose and increased risk of diabetes, both of which tend to be more prevalent in older people. Many cases of mild glucose intolerance have reportedly been treated successfully with chromium.

Other symptoms of chromium deficiency include decreased glycogen reserves, retarded growth, disturbed amino acid metabolism, and an increased incidence of damage to the wall of the aorta. The damage to the aorta is associated with raised blood cholesterol levels.

TOXICITY

There is no evidence of chromium toxicity caused by excessive dietary intakes, but the ingestion of excess chromium as a contaminant of drinking water has resulted in some cases of chromium poisoning. Inhalation of chromium from industrial pollutants can also have toxic effects. The toxic effects of chromium are known to vary, depending on the compound of which the chromium is a part. Great uncertainty remains about the consequences of excessive amounts of chromium in the human body; so the use of chromium supplements should be discouraged.

SILICON (Si)

For a long time, most medical interest in silicon was focused on the damaging effects of **silicosis** because of the inhalation of silicon-containing dust. It is now known that silicon also performs a beneficial and normal role in the body because it is apparently required for the formation of cartilage, collagen, and bone.[54] Most of the evidence on silicon's role in metabolism has come from animal studies, but there is now general agreement that it is a dietary essential for humans. The amount required by humans is unknown, but average daily intakes are reported to be 19 mg/day for females and 40 mg/day for males.[55] Plant foods seem to be good sources of silicon, and animal foods are poor sources. Beer contains a relatively high concentration of silicon.

VANADIUM (V)

Studies on animals indicate that vanadium plays an essential role in growth; the metabolism of iron, glucose, and lipid; reproduction; and the development of bone. Some evidence suggests that vanadium may slow the development of dental caries when it takes the place of some of the phosphorus in the apatite crystals of tooth enamel.

Less than 5% of ingested vanadium is absorbed, and 60% of the amount absorbed is immediately excreted in urine. The adult human body is estimated to contain less than 1 mg of vanadium, mostly in liver, kidney, and bone.[56, 57] Bone is apparently the long-term storage compartment for vanadium, but some readily accessible vanadium is bound to ferritin and transferrin.

Particularly rich sources of vanadium are mushrooms, parsley, dill, and black pepper. Fresh fruits and vegetables are generally poor sources. The vanadium content of milk- and wheat-based products can be *increased* 10- to 20-fold from contamination during processing.

The average vanadium content of the North American diet is 6 to 20 μg of vanadium per day.

TABLE 10-22

Nickel content of selected foods

FOOD*	Ni (mg/g)
CEREAL AND CEREAL PRODUCTS	
Wheat germ	1.0
Plain flour	<0.06
Whole meal flour	0.16
White bread	<0.06
Whole meal bread	0.19
Rice	0.42
LEGUMINOUS FOODS	
Beans, kidney	0.45
Beans, frozen	0.55
Peas, frozen	0.35
Soy protein	4.30
NUTS	
Almond	1.3
Cashew	5.1
English walnut	3.6
Filbert	1.6
Pistachio	0.8
Peanut	1.6
FRUITS	
Apples	0.03
Cherry	0.08
Melon	0.12
Peach	0.16
Pear	0.07
Plum	0.07
VEGETABLES	
Bean, green	0.26
Carrot	0.14
Lettuce	0.17
Potato	0.11
Spinach	0.22
Tomato	0.08
DAIRY PRODUCTS	
Whole milk	0.06
Skim milk	0.08
Dried milk	<0.09
MEATS	
Beef	<0.05
Lamb	<0.09
Pork	<0.06
Chicken	<0.07
Fish	0.70
MISCELLANEOUS	
Cacoa powder	9.8
Bittersweet chocolate	2.6
Milk chocolate	1.2
Tea leaves	5.3
Tea, instant	15.5

* Fresh weight basis. One serving of cereal weighs approximately 30 g; that of fruits, vegetables, and meats, 90 to 120 g. One cup of fluid milk weighs 240 g.

NICKEL (Ni)

Nickel is present in all human tissues but is most concentrated in the lungs, adrenal glands, and thyroid glands. It seems possible that it functions as a cofactor or structural element of some metalloenzymes. In blood serum, nickel is found bound to the protein albumin, amino acids, and various other ligands. Less than 10% of ingested nickel is absorbed, and much of the absorbed nickel is excreted in the form of low–molecular-weight complexes within urine.

The adult human dietary requirement for nickel appears to be in the region of 150 μg/day. Plant foods are generally good sources of nickel, whereas animal foods are generally poor sources. The nickel content of selected foods is shown in Table 10-22.[57] There is little likelihood of any nickel deficiency in the human diet, although a diet completely lacking in fruits and vegetables contains marginal amounts.

Nickel is known to enhance the use of iron by the body when the iron content of the diet is adequate. When a diet is deficient in iron, the presence of nickel intensifies the symptoms of the resulting deficiency of iron in the body.

ARSENIC (As)

Arsenic is more commonly associated with doing humans harm rather than good. Its properties as a poison are well known, and it has also been implicated in the onset of some cancers. As early as 1937, however, arsenic in small doses was known to have some therapeutic properties. In 1976 conclusive evidence was finally obtained indicating that it was a nutritional essential. In experiments on animals, the first signs of arsenic deficiency were found to be restricted growth and abnormalities of reproduction. The precise biochemical functions of arsenic are still unknown, although recent studies suggest roles in the metabolism of phospholipids and methyl-group (CH_3) chemistry.

The estimated human dietary allowance for arsenic based on the results of animal studies is 12 to 15 mg/day. Fish, grains, and cereal products are among the best sources of arsenic.

The bioavailability of arsenic may be influenced by its interaction with other dietary factors, such as zinc and the amino acids arginine and methionine. Arsenic is also known to be an antagonist of selenium, allowing it to offer some protection against selenium toxicity. Oral arsenic has a relatively low toxicity.[48]

BORON (B)

Boron is the most recent addition to the list of possible essential mineral elements. In 1982 it was discovered that boron is required for the normal growth of bone in chicks. This involvement in bone integrity was confirmed by the discovery that postmenopausal women lost less calcium when their boron intake was raised from 0.25 to 3 mg/ day. Thus boron supplementation may be effective in minimizing the loss of bone mineral associated with the onset of osteoporosis.

Foods of plant origin are the richest sources of boron. Prunes, dates, raisins, and peanuts provide about 0.5 mg of boron per oz. Honey contains 0.2 mg of boron per oz, and wine contains 1 mg/4-oz glass. Soymeal is a rich source of boron but not one that could be readily incorporated into most diets. Survey data indicate that boron intakes in North America range from 0.5 to 3.1 mg/day.[48]

TIN (Sn)

Tin has not yet been officially recognized as a nutritionally essential mineral, but it probably will be soon. It has not been found in newborn infants, nor is it widespread in the animal kingdom. In 1970, however, a definite growth response to the presence of 1 ppm of tin was established. This implicates tin in optimal growth, and the symptoms of tin deficiency are believed to include poor growth, dermatitis, and hair loss.

Little information is available on the tin content of food. Estimates of typical dietary tin intakes vary from 3 to 17 µg/day. Our dietary requirements are estimated at between 3 and 6 µg/day. The most commonly available form of tin is **stannous sulfate** ($SnSO_4$), from which only a small proportion of tin can be absorbed.

Although the leaching of tin from unlaquered cans can produce tin levels as high as 114 ppm in some acidic juices, no evidence suggests any risks of toxic effects from the tin in food.

ISSUES AND OPINIONS

Is Iron Linked to Heart Disease?

Iron is well established as an essential nutrient that is required for proper growth and development, but does iron consumption also carry some risk? Some evidence suggests that high iron intake and the level of iron stores in the body may be associated with an increased risk of heart disease. The evidence is confused and conflicting, however.

Women who have not yet reached menopause have a lower incidence of coronary heart disease than either women after menopause or men. In 1981 it was suggested that this effect might be a result of the greater amount of iron stored in both postmeno/pausal women and men.*

The possibility that stored iron might be a risk factor for coronary heart disease is supported by some animal studies that have demonstrated a link between iron overload and damage to the heart muscle. A possible explanation for any damaging effect of iron on the circulatory system is the ability of iron to encourage the formation of oxygen-containing free radicals, which could attack and damage vulnerable tissues.

Further evidence linking iron to increased risk of coronary heart disease was provided in 1992 by a widely publicized study in Finland.† This study reported that serum ferritin levels higher than 200 μg/L were associated with a two-fold increase in the incidence of acute myocardial infarction (heart attacks). A Canadian study also reported that both men and women are at increased risk of myocardial infarction if they have high serum iron concentrations.‡ Recent studies in America and Iceland, however, have found no evidence of any link between serum ferritin levels and the risk of myocardial infarction. Also, results of a study published in 1994 of over 4500 American men and women indicate no evidence of a link between serum transferrin saturation levels and the risk of heart disease.§

It is difficult to interpret the true meaning of these conflicting results because the different studies used different methods of analysis and data collection. From a nutritional point of view the most significant question is whether there is an increased risk of heart disease caused by enhanced bodily iron storage as a result of current levels of dietary iron intake. In the Finnish study, dietary intakes of iron were assessed using food consumption records collected over 4 days. The Finnish results suggested a positive correlation between iron intake and the risk of myocardial infarction. In the Canadian and American studies, however, no link was found between dietary iron intake and the risk of heart disease. Further study is needed, and information about the particular food source and form of dietary iron may be important information to help resolve this controversy.

At present there is insufficient evidence to prove any link between iron status or dietary iron intake and any increased risk of heart disease. For this reason, current iron fortification practices remain unchanged because of their many proven benefits. It remains possible, however, that the undoubted benefits of good iron status may be counterbalanced by some significant risks of excess iron intake.

* Sullivan JL: *Lancet* 1:1293, 1981.

† Salonen JT and others: *Circulation* 86:803, 1992.

‡ Ascherio A, Willett WC: *N Engl J Med* 330:1152, 1994.

§ Stempos CT and others: *N Engl J Med* 330:1119, 1994.

BY NOW YOU SHOULD KNOW

- Iron, zinc, copper, iodine, selenium, manganese, molybdenum, cobalt, and chromium are all essential micronutrient minerals, also known as trace elements.
- Arsenic, boron, fluoride, nickel, silicon, and vanadium are micronutrient minerals that are not firmly established as dietary essentials.
- Some other minerals will probably be identified as essential micronutrient minerals in the future.
- Manganese, molybdenum, cobalt, chromium, silicon, vanadium, nickel, arsenic, and boron are present in the body in such small amounts that—in addition to being trace elements—they are often referred to separately as the ultratrace elements.
- Iron is an essential component of hemoglobin, the metalloprotein that transports oxygen from the lungs to the body's tissues and carbon dioxide from the tissues to the lungs.
- Iron-deficiency anemia is one of the most prevalent nutritional deficiencies in the United States.
- Iron-deficiency anemia can result from the consumption of a diet that is low in iron over a long period, from depressed iron absorption, from blood loss, or from some combination of these factors.
- Women during childbearing years have the highest recommended dietary allowance (RDA) for iron.
- Iron in food is found in two forms: heme iron and nonheme iron. Heme iron is found in the flesh of animal foods. Nonheme iron is found in other animal foods (such as eggs and milk products) and plants.
- Breads and cereals are usually enriched with iron.
- Iodine is an essential component of the thyroid hormones thyroxine and triiodothyronine, which play a major role in regulating the basal metabolic rate.
- Iodine deficiency results in goiter, the incidence of which has been greatly reduced by the iodization of salt.
- Zinc performs many functions in the body.
- Food processing may decrease the amount of many micronutrient minerals in food.
- Some micronutrient minerals may be introduced to food during processing, either purposely or as contaminants.
- A diet that is high in phytates reduces the bioavailability of both iron and zinc.
- It is difficult to make precise determinations of the amounts of micronutrient minerals required in the diet because of the wide variation in the content of food from various parts of the United States.
- There is evidence of toxicity for most micronutrient minerals if they are consumed in excessive amounts.
- The study of micronutrient minerals is difficult because of their rarity within the body and within food and the wide variety of interactions among them. Despite this, knowledge of their role in nutrition and in the body in general is steadily increasing.

~ STUDY QUESTIONS ~

1. Why have we only recently learned about many of the micronutrient minerals (trace elements)?
2. Name five commonly eaten foods that contain zinc.
3. How would you determine whether you had iron-deficiency anemia?
4. Why is salt iodized?
5. Outline the key features of the absorption and transportation of iron.
6. If the body has no mechanism to excrete iron, why does iron-deficiency anemia occur?
7. What is the role of hydrochloric acid in the absorption of iron?
8. List in sequence the things that occur when the oxygen-carrying capacity of the blood decreases.

~ CRITICAL ANALYSIS ~

1. How much iron did you have for lunch?

   There are really two parts to the answer to this question. The first part is how much iron was contained in the food you ate. The second part is how much iron was actually absorbed from the food. The first part can be answered by looking up the iron content of the foods we ate. Answering the second part requires that we also know how much of the iron in meat, fish, or poultry foods is heme iron; how much meat, poultry, or fish was consumed; and how much vitamin C (ascorbic acid) was contained in the food. This calculation is an estimate of the iron absorbed from the meal. Because the amount of iron absorbed from the meal varies depending on an individual's iron status (individuals with low iron stores absorb more iron, those with larger iron stores absorb less), we assume a level of 500 mg of stored iron, a reasonable level suggested by the authors of the method.[58]

   In the form below, record the foods and beverages you had for lunch today. You may carry out this exercise for any meal if lunch is not convenient. Estimate the amounts of each food or beverage as closely as possible. Then look up the iron content and ascorbic acid content of each food in the food tables in Appendix E. Remember to record the milligrams of iron contained in the amount of food eaten. For example, 3 oz of lean beef contains 2.7 mg of iron. If you had a sandwich that contained only 2 oz of roast beef, this amount of meat contained 1.8 mg of iron, ⅔ the amount in 3 oz. If you ate 6 oz of beef, multiply the iron content of 3 oz by 2. Then place the amounts of iron and ascorbic acid consumed in their respective columns.

   Only meat and fish contain heme iron. An average of 45% of the iron in meat and fish is heme iron (see Table 10-4). To calculate the amount of heme iron in the meats you ate, multiply the total iron in the meat by 0.45. For example, of the 2.7 mg of iron in 3 oz of beef, $0.45 \times 2.7 = 1.2$ mg is heme iron; the remainder, $2.7 - 1.2 = 1.5$ mg, is nonheme iron. Place these numbers in the appropriate columns. The iron content of all nonmeat foods is placed in the column for nonheme iron.

   Calculate the totals for the heme iron, nonheme iron, and ascorbic acid columns.

   For an adult with 500 mg of stored iron, the following calculations are made:

   a. Of total heme iron, 23% is absorbed. Multiply the total heme iron in the meal by 0.23 to calculate this amount.
   b. For nonheme iron,
      (1) If the amount of meat, poultry, or fish is *less* than 30 g (1 oz) or if the total ascorbic acid is *less* than 25 mg, multiply the total amount of nonheme iron by 0.03 (i.e., 3% is absorbed).
      (2) If the amount of meat, poultry, or fish is *between* 30 and 90 g (1 and 3 oz) *or* if the total ascorbic acid is *between* 25 and 75 mg, multiply the total amount of nonheme iron by 0.05 (i.e., 5% is absorbed).
      (3) If the amount of meat, poultry, or fish is *more* than 90 g (3 oz), the total ascorbic

acid is *more* than 75 mg, the amount of meat, poultry, or fish is 30 to 90 g (1 to 3 oz) *and* ascorbic acid is 25 to 75 mg, multiply the total amount of nonheme iron by 0.08 (i.e., 8% is absorbed).

Total heme iron ______ mg × 0.4 = _____ mg heme iron absorbed.

Total nonheme iron _____ mg × _____ = _____ mg nonheme iron absorbed.

_____ mg of heme iron absorbed + _______ mg nonheme iron absorbed = _______ mg total iron absorbed.

REFERENCES

1. Dallman PR: Iron. In Brown ML, editor: *Present knowledge in nutrition,* ed 6, Washington, DC, 1990, International Life Sciences Institute, Nutrition Foundation.
2. Bothwell TH, Finch CA: *Iron metabolism,* Boston, 1962, Little, Brown.
3. Dallman PR: Biochemical basis for the manifestations of iron deficiency, *Annu Rev Nutr* 6:13, 1986.
4. Bezkorovaen A: *Biochemistry of non-heme iron,* New York, 1980, Plenum Press.
5. Beard J, Dawson H: Iron. In O'Dell B, Sunde R, editors: *Handbook of nutritionally essential mineral elements,* New York, 1994, Marcel Dekker.
6. Charlton RW, Bothwell TH: Iron absorption, *Annu Rev Med* 34:55, 1983.
7. Bezwoda WR and others: The relative dietary importance of haem and non-haem iron, *South African Med J* 64:552, 1983.
8. Bothwell TH and others: *Iron metabolism in man,* Oxford, 1972, Blackwell.
9. Cook JD: Adaptation in iron metabolism, *Am J Clin Nutr* 51:301, 1990.
10. Hallberg L and others: Calcium: effect of different amounts on non-heme and heme iron absorption, *Am J Clin Nutr* 53:112, 1991.
11. Monsen ER: Iron nutrition and absorption: dietary factors which impact iron bioavailability, *J Am Diet Assoc* 88:786, 1988.
12. Dawson-Hughes B, Seligson FH, Hughes VS: Effect of calcium carbonate and hydroxyapatite on zinc and iron retention in postmenopausal women, *Am J Clin Nutr* 51:301, 1986.
13. Hallberg L and others: Bioavailability in man of iron in human milk and cow's milk in relation to their calcium contents, *Pediatr Res* 31:524, 1992.
14. Green R and others: Body iron excretion in man: a collaborative study, *Am J Med* 45:336, 1968.
15. Hallberg L: Iron balance in pregnancy. In Berger S, editor: *Vitamins and minerals in pregnancy and lactation,* New York, 1988, Raven Press.
16. Fomon SJ: Iron. In *Nutrition of normal infants,* St Louis, 1993, Mosby.
17. Dallman PR: Biochemical basis for the manifestations of iron deficiency, *Annu Rev Nutr* 6:13, 1986.
18. Weaver CM: Exercise and iron status, *J Nutr* 122:782, 1992.
19. Dobbing J, editor: *Brain, behavior, and iron in the infant diet,* London, 1990, Springer-Verlag.
20. Beard JL, Connor JR, Jones BC: Iron in the brain, *Nutr Rev* 51:157, 1993.
21. Pollitt E: Iron deficiency and cognitive function, *Annu Rev Nutr* 13:521, 1993.
22. Dallman PR: Iron deficiency and the immune response, *Am J Clin Nutr* 46:329, 1987.
23. Dallman PR: Upper limits of iron in infant formulas, *J Nutr* 119:1852, 1989.
24. Beard JL, Borel MJ, Derr J: Impaired thermoregulation and thyroid function in iron-deficiency anemia, *Am J Clin Nutr* 52:813, 1990.
25. Cunnane SC: *Zinc: clinical and biochemical significance,* Boca Raton, Fla, 1988, CRC Press.

26. Hambidge KM, Casey CE, Krebs NF: Zinc. In Mertz W, editor: *Trace elements in human and animal nutrition,* vol 2, ed 5, New York, 1986, Academic Press.

27. Fraker PJ and others: Interrelationships between zinc and immune function, *Fed Proc* 45:1474, 1986.

28. Keen CL, Gershwin ME: Zinc deficiency and immune function, *Annu Rev Nutr* 10:415, 1990.

29. Solomons NW: Zinc and copper. In Shils ME, Young VR, editor: *Modern nutrition in health & disease,* Philadelphia, 1988, Lea & Febiger.

30. Mills CF, editor: *Zinc in human biology,* New York, 1989, Springer-Verlag.

31. Moser-Veillon PB: Zinc: consumption patterns and dietary recommendations, *J Am Diet Assoc* 90:1089, 1990.

32. King JC: Assessment of zinc status, *J Nutr* 120:1474, 1990.

33. Danks DM: Copper deficiency in humans, *Annu Rev Nutr* 8:235, 1988.

34. Shaw JCL: Trace elements in term and preterm infants. In Fomon SJ, Zlotkin S, editors: *Nutritional anemias,* New York, 1992, Raven Press.

35. Dunn JT: Iodine supplementation and the prevention of cretinism, *Ann N Y Acad Sci* 678:158, 1991.

36. Health and Welfare Canada: *Nutritional recommendations,* Ottawa, Canada, 1990, Canadian Government Printing Centre.

37. Pennington JAT, Young BE, Wilson DB: Nutritional elements in US diets: results from the Total Diet Study, 1982 to 1986, *J Am Diet Assoc* 89:659, 1989.

38. Dann JT, van der Haar F: *A practical guide to the correction of iodine deficiency,* Amsterdam, The Netherlands, 1990, International Council for Control of Iodine Deficiency Disorders.

39. Fisch A and others: A new approach to combating iodine deficiency in developing countries: the controlled release of iodine in water by a silicon elastomer, *Am J Public Health* 83:540, 1993.

40. Burk RF: Recent developments in trace element metabolism and function: newer roles of selenium in nutrition, *J Nutr* 119:1051, 1989.

41. Levander OA: The scientific rationale for the 1989 recommended dietary allowances for selenium, *J Am Diet Assoc* 91:1572, 1991.

42. Diplock AT: Trace elements in human health with special reference to selenium, *Am J Clin Nutr* 45:1313, 1987.

43. Arthur JR, Nicol F, Beckett GJ: Selenium deficiency, thyroid hormone metabolism and thyroid hormone deiodinases, *Am J Clin Nutr Suppl* 57:236S, 1993.

44. Sunde RA: Molecular biology of selenoproteins, *Annu Rev Nutr* 10:451, 1990.

45. Lockitch B and others: Cardiomyopathy associated with nonendemic selenium deficiency in a Caucasian adolescent, *Am J Clin Nutr* 52:572, 1990.

46. Levander OA, Burke RF: Selenium. In Brown ML, editor: *Present knowledge in nutrition,* ed 6, Washington, DC, 1990, International Life Sciences Institute.

47. Keen CL, Zedenbert-Cheir S: Manganese. In Brown ML, editor: *Present knowledge in nutrition,* ed 6, Washington, DC, 1990, International Life Sciences Institute.

48. Nielsen FH: Other trace elements. In Brown ML, editor: *Present knowledge in nutrition,* ed 6, Washington DC, 1990, International Life Sciences Institute.

49. Johnson JL and others: Inborn error of molybdenum metabolism: combined deficiencies of sulfite oxidase and xanthine dehydrogenase in a patient lacking the molybdenum cofactor, *Proc Nat'l Acad Sci* 77(6):3715, 1980.

50. Pennington JAT, Jones JW: Molybdenum, nickel, cobalt, vanadium and strontium in total diets, *J Am Diet Assoc* 87:1644, 1987.

51. Rajagopalan KV: Molybdenum: an essential trace element in human nutrition, *Annu Rev Nutr* 8:401, 1988.

52. Stoecker BJ: Chromium. In Brown ML, editor: *Present knowledge in nutrition,* ed 6, Washington, DC, 1990, International Life Sciences Institute.

53. Morris BW and others: The trace element chromium—a role in glucose homeostasis, *Am J Clin Nutr* 55:989, 1992.

54. Seaborn CD, Nielsen FH: Silicon: a nutritional beneficence for bones, brains and blood vessels? *Nutr Today* 28:13, 1993.

55. Pennington JHT: Silicon in foods and diets, *Food Addit Contam* 8:97, 1991.

56. French RJ, Jones PJH: Role of vanadium in nutrition: metabolism essentiality and dietary considerations, *Life Sci* 52:339, 1992.

57. Nielsen FH, Uthus EO: The essentiality and metabolism of vanadium. In Chasteen ND, editor: *Vanadium in biological systems: physiology and biochemistry,* London, 1990, Kluwer Academia.

58. Nielsen FH: Is nickel nutritionally important? *Nutr Today* 28:14, 1993.

59. Monsen ER and others: Estimation of available dietary iron, *Am J Clin Nutr* 31:134, 1978.

ADDITIONAL READINGS

Apgar J: Zinc and reproduction, *Annu Rev Nutr* 5:43, 1985.

Apgar J: Zinc and reproduction: an update, *J Nutr Biochem* 3:266, 1992.

Cousins RJ: Metal elements and gene expression, *Annu Rev Nutr* 14:449, 1994.

Dobbing J, editor: *Brain, behavior, and iron in the infant diet,* London, 1992, Springer-Verlag.

Finch CA, Huebers HH: Perspectives in iron metabolism, *N Engl J Med* 306:1520, 1982.

Freeland-Graves JH: Manganese: an essential nutrient for humans, *Nutr Today* 23:15, 1988.

Greger JL: Aluminum metabolism, *Annu Rev Nutr* 13:43, 1993.

Helman AD: Vitamin and iron status in new Canadians, *Am J Clin Nutr* 45:785, 1987.

Herbert V and others: Most free-radical injury is iron related: it is promoted by iron, hemin, haloferritin, and vitamin C and inhibited by desferoxamine and apoferritin, *Stem Cell* 12:289, 1994.

Interaction of iron, copper, and zinc, *Nutr Rev* 45:167, 1987.

International Nutritional Anemia Consultative Group: *Iron deficiency in infancy and childhood,* Washington, DC, 1981, Nutrition Foundation.

International Nutritional Anemia Consultative Group: *Iron deficiency in women,* Washington, DC, 1981, Nutrition Foundation.

International Nutritional Anemia Consultative Group: *Measurements of iron status,* Washington, DC, 1987, Nutrition Foundation.

Johnson-Spear MA, Yip R: Hemoglobin differences between black and white women with comparable iron status: justification for race-specific anemia criteria, *Am J Clin Nutr* 60:117, 1994.

Loosli AR: Reversing sports-related iron and zinc deficiencies, *Physician Sports Med* 21:70, 1993.

Mills CF: Dietary interaction involving the trace elements, *Annu Rev Nutr* 5:173, 1985.

Nielson FH: Facts and fallicies about boron, *Nutr Today* 27:6, 1992.

O'Dell BL: Mineral interactions relevant to nutrient requirements, *J Nutr* 119:1832, 1989.

Pennington JAT: A review of iodine toxicity reports, *J Am Diet Assoc* 90:1571, 1990.

Proulx WR, Weaver CM: Ironing out heart disease: deplete or not deplete, *Nutr Today* 30:17, 1995.

Rajagopaian KV: Molybdenum—an essential trace element in human nutrition, *Annu Rev Nutr* 8:401, 1988.

Schubert A, Holden JM, Wolfe WR: Selenium content of a core group of foods based on a critical evaluation of published analytical data, *J Am Diet Assoc* 87:285, 1987.

Sokoloff L: Is chromium essential for humans? *Nutr Rev* 40:193, 1988.

Thompson PPH: Assessment of zinc status, *Proc Nutr Soc* 50:19, 1991.

Turner RJ, Finch JM: Selenium and the immune response, *Proc Nutr Soc* 50:275, 1991.

Vallee BL, Falchuk KH: The biochemical basis of zinc physiology, *Physiol Rev* 73:79, 1993.

O V E R V I E W

Vitamins

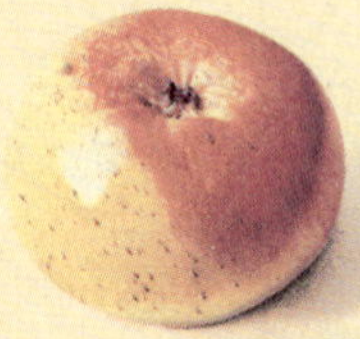

Vitamins were the last of the six categories of essential nutrients to be discovered. They are a group of organic chemicals with no general link between them, other than that they are needed by the body in small amounts because the body cannot make them for itself. Different animal species have different vitamin needs. Humans, for example, need vitamin C (ascorbic acid), but this chemical is not a vitamin for rabbits, whose cells can synthesize it from simpler compounds. All of the vitamins needed by humans are made in the plants or animals we eat.

Oranges in California. Detail from an orange growers carton label, painted around 1930.

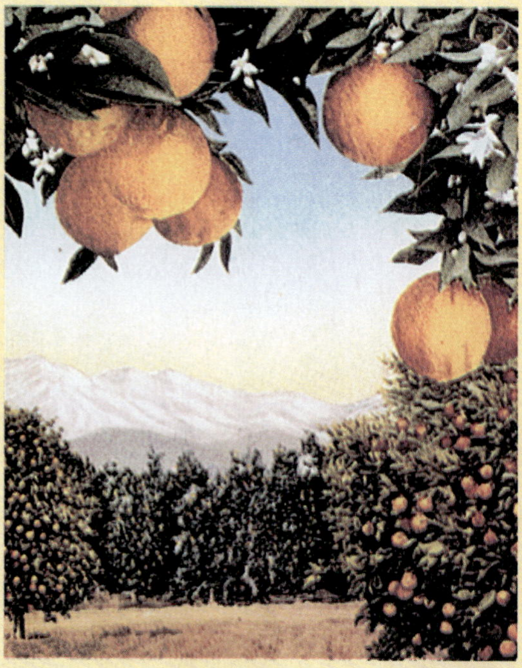

Vitamins have a high public profile. Most people are aware of vitamins in a general sense and could name a few of them (for example, vitamin C and vitamin A). In addition, many people know which types of foods are good sources of some specific vitamins. Many people also worry about the adequacy of their vitamin intake and consume vitamin supplements either as an aid to general health or with the intention of treating specific ailments. A large and growing industry supplies vitamin supplements to the public, despite the fact that ample amounts of vitamins for healthy people are supplied by a well-chosen diet.

The recommended daily adult intakes of the various vitamins range from just a few micrograms up to 95 mg. The amounts at even the top end of that range are small, but the small amounts required do not imply that vitamins play a minor role in health, when

FIGURE OV3-1

Phases in the development of our knowledge about vitamins.

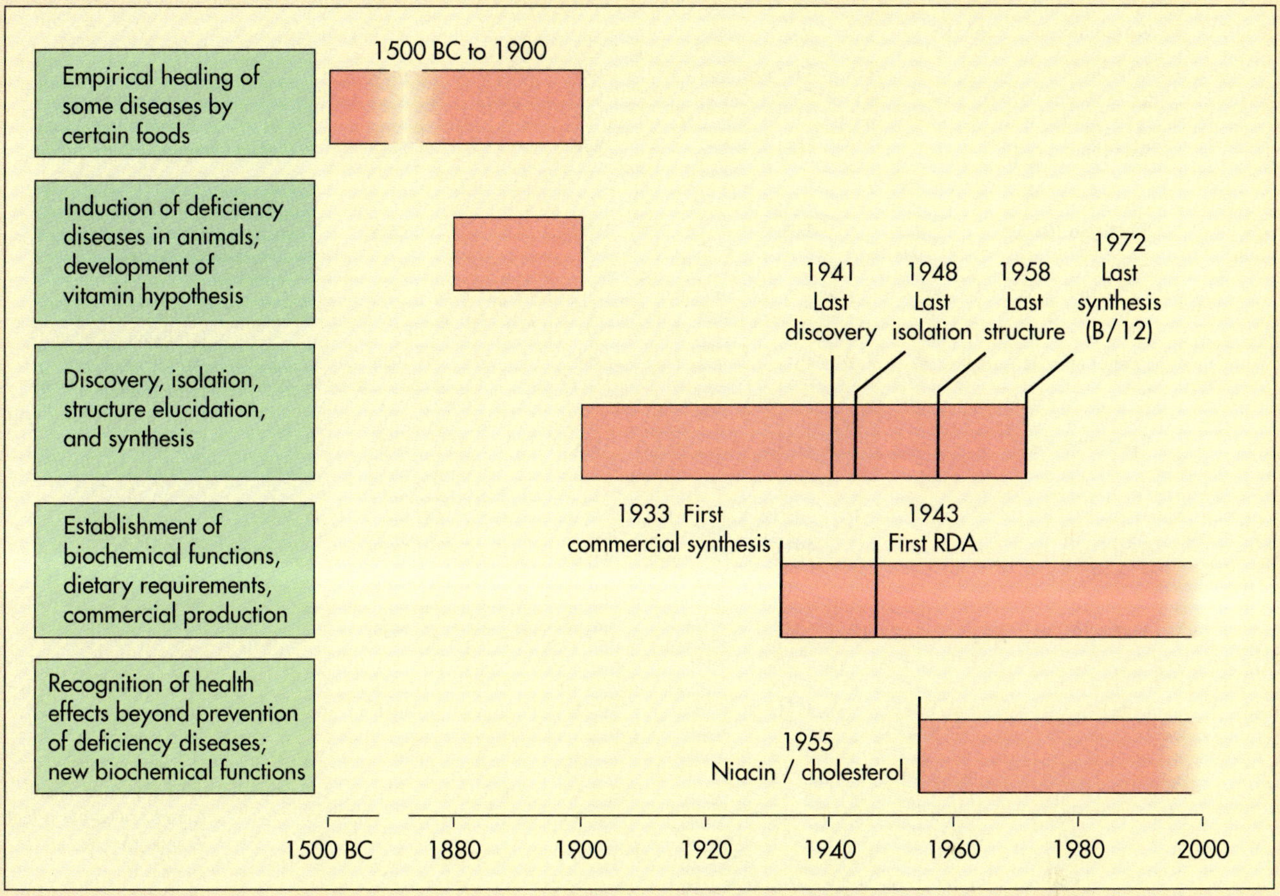

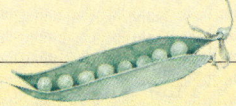

compared with other nutrients. All vitamins are essential for health, and the relative amounts of different vitamins required by the body do not reflect any differences in their nutritional importance.

The Development of Knowledge about Vitamins

The development of our knowledge about vitamins can be divided into five main phases (Figure Ov3-1). The first phase spanned over 3000 years, from around 1500 BC to 1880 AD. During this time there was no direct knowledge of vitamins as such, but it was known that various diseases (now known to be vitamin-deficiency diseases) could be treated with specific foods (now known to contain the required vitamins). The ancient Egyptians, for example, knew that night blindness (caused by vitamin A deficiency) could be prevented by eating liver (the major storage site of vitamin A). The American Indians knew that pine needle extracts (a source of vitamin C) could prevent scurvy caused by vitamin C deficiency. The classic work of Lind in treating scurvy with citrus juices (see Chapter 1) provides another example of this purely "empirical" phase in our knowledge of the effects of vitamins.

The second phase began around 1880, with the work of Christian Eijkman, a Dutch scientist who studied beriberi in Indonesia (then called the Dutch East Indies). Eijkman's crucial new step was to purposely produce a vitamin-deficiency condition in animals and then demonstrate the reversal of the con-

TABLE OV3-1

Discovery, isolation, synthesis, and nomenclature of vitamins essential for humans

	DISCOVERY	ISOLATION	SYNTHESIS	OTHER NAMES*
WATER-SOLUBLE VITAMINS				
Thiamin (B_1)	1897	1926	1936	Aneurin Antineuritic factor Antiberiberi factor
Ascorbic acid (C)	1912	1928	1933	Antiscorbutic factor Cevitamic acid Hexuronic acid
Riboflavin (B_2)	1920	1933	1935	Yellow enzyme Vitamin G Lactoflavin Hepatoflavin Ovoflavin
Pantothenic acid (B_5)	1931	1938	1940	Pantotheine Pantothenol Antichromotrichial factor
Pyridoxine (B_6)	1934	1938	1939	Pyridoxic acid Pyridoxal Pyridoxol Pyridoxamine
Biotin	1931	1935	1943	Anti–egg-white injury factor Bios II Vitamin H
Niacin (B_3)	1936	1912†	1894†	Nicotinic acid Nicotinamide or niacinamide Pellagra-preventive (p-p) factor
Folate	1941	1941	1946	Adermine Folic acid Citrovorum factor Pteroylglutamic acid *Lactobacillus casei* factor Vitamin M Vitamin B_c Factor U

dition by an appropriate feeding regimen. He was able to produce beriberi (now known to be caused by a deficiency of the vitamin thiamin) in chickens by feeding them polished rice. The disease disappeared when unpolished rice was supplied instead, and it is now known that the thiamin of the rice is concentrated in the outer husks, which are removed during polishing.

Such experiments as Eijkman's led the British biochemist Frederick Hopkins to make the explicit suggestion in 1906 that foods contained small amounts of "growth factors" required to sustain both growth and life itself. In 1912 Casimir Funk named these growth factors "vitamines" because they were required for life ("vita") and because he had discovered that the thiamin isolated from rice husks contained nitrogen ("amine").

Funk's original term *vitamine* was changed to "vitamin" during the third stage of research, when many scientists around the world identified, purified, and synthesized all the known vitamins and discovered that they did not all contain nitrogen. This third phase continued up until 1972, when vitamin B_{12} became the final vitamin to be synthesized by chemists. The last vitamin to actually be identified was vitamin B_{12} in 1948 (Table Ov3-1).

The fourth phase in our knowledge of the vitamins overlapped with the third and was the process of discovering the biochemical functions of the vitamins, establishing the body's requirements for them, and producing them commercially. The first step in this phase was taken in the early 1930s, when riboflavin was identified as a precursor of the cofactor of an enzyme known as "yellow enzyme." This led to the

TABLE OV3-1

Discovery, isolation, synthesis, and nomenclature of vitamins essential for humans (continued)

	DISCOVERY	ISOLATION	SYNTHESIS	OTHER NAMES*
WATER-SOLUBLE VITAMINS *(cont'd)*				
Cobalamin (B_{12})	1926	1948	1972	Anti–pernicious-anemia factor Cyanocobalamin Hydroxycobalamin Erythrocyte maturation factor Animal protein factor (APF)
FAT-SOLUBLE VITAMINS				
Vitamin A	1909	1931	1947	Axerophthol Retinoic acid Retinal Retinol Dehydroretinol
Vitamin D	1918	1932	1959	Antirachitic factor Cholecalciferol Ergocalciferol Calcitriol Calcidiol
Vitamin E	1922	1936	1938	Tocopherol Antisterility factor
Vitamin K	1929	1939	1939	Phytylquinone Multiprenylmenaquinone Farnoquinone Antihemorrhagic factor Menadione (synthetic) Synkayvite (synthetic) Hykinone (synthetic)

* Terms appearing in the literature, many of which are no longer recognized as correct terminology.

† Niacin was synthesized and isolated before it was recognized as a vitamin.

discovery that all of the B vitamins are precursors of coenzymes and that several other vitamins also act as coenzyme precursors. The laboratory synthesis of vitamin C in 1933 set in motion the commercial production of vitamins, which now supplies many vitamins at low cost for use in food fortification or enrichment and in "vitamin pills."

The fifth phase in vitamin history is the continuing process of research into new functions for known vitamins, some of which go beyond the simple prevention of deficiency diseases. The beginning of this phase is set at 1955,[1] when the vitamin niacin in pharmacological dose was found to lower blood cholesterol levels. This now well-recognized effect is clearly unrelated to the vitamin's major role as a coenzyme precursor, and it bestows an additional health benefit on top of its ability to prevent the niacin-deficiency disease pellagra. Subsequent studies have uncovered many roles for various vitamins that go far beyond their first recognized functions in preventing the traditional vitamin-deficiency diseases. For example, certain vitamins are now known to be involved in the regulation of gene expression, operation of the immune system, and secretion of various hormones.

Since the last vitamin was identified in 1948, there have been many claims of the discovery of new vitamins and vitamin-like compounds. None of these claims have yet been confirmed. There is, however, a small possibility that some vitamins required in small amounts remain to be discovered.

In 1940 the Food and Nutrition Board of the National Academy of Sciences was set up to advise on nutritional problems connected with national defense. The need for such a body had been demonstrated during World War I, when many young Americans entering the armed forces were found to have

TABLE OV3-2

General properties of fat-soluble and water-soluble vitamins

FAT-SOLUBLE VITAMINS	WATER-SOLUBLE VITAMINS
Soluble in fat and fat solvents (water-miscible derivatives available)	Soluble in water
Intake in excess of daily need stored in the body	Minimal storage of dietary excesses
Small amounts excreted in bile	Excreted in urine
Deficiency symptoms slow to develop	Deficiency symptoms often develop rapidly
Not absolutely necessary in diet every day	Must be supplied in diet every day
Have precursors or provitamins	Generally do not have precursors
Contain only the elements carbon, hydrogen, and oxygen	Contain the elements carbon, hydrogen, oxygen, and nitrogen and in some cases others, such as cobalt or sulfur
Absorbed into lymphatic system	Absorbed into blood through portal vein
Needed only by complex organisms	Needed by simple and complex organisms
Some are toxic at relatively low levels (6 to 10 times the recommended dietary allowances)	Toxic only at megadose levels (>10 times the recommended dietary allowances)

nutritional deficiencies. The board produced the first Recommended Dietary Allowances (RDAs) for six vitamins (vitamin A, thiamine, riboflavin, nicotinic acid, ascorbic acid, and vitamin D) in 1943.[2] The decision to choose the term *Recommended Allowances,* rather than *Standards,* to avoid the implication that the values set were the final word on the subject, has proved to be a wise one. As knowledge has advanced and the criteria used to establish the allowances have changed, the RDAs have been regularly modified and will no doubt continue to be modified.

Classification of Vitamins

The vitamins required for human health are divided into two distinct categories: the **fat-soluble vitamins** and the **water-soluble vitamins.** As the names imply, this subdivision is based on a physical characteristic of the vitamins—their solubility in fat or water, rather than on any functional link between the vitamins in each category. This categorization can be traced back to the early days of vitamin research, when the discovery by Funk of the water-soluble vitamin thiamin was followed by the discovery of the fat-soluble vitamin A. Vitamins discovered after these first two were naturally placed into either the water-soluble or fat-soluble category.

The distinction between vitamins on the basis of their solubility is still of relevance today, as recognized in the discussion of the fat-soluble vitamins in Chapter 11 and of the water-soluble vitamins in Chapter 12. As can be seen from Table Ov3-2, the separation of vitamins into fat-soluble and water-soluble vitamins also matches some distinctions between these groups on the basis of various other properties. As knowledge of the functions of vitamins increased, however, new terminology came into use. Such well-known names as vitamin A, vitamin B_{12}, vitamin C, and so on are now increasingly being replaced by more meaningful chemical names, such as retinoic acid (vitamin A), cobalamin (vitamin B_{12}), and ascorbic acid (vitamin C). It will undoubtedly be some time, however, before the older terminologies disappear (if they ever do). Table Ov3-1 lists the common alternative names in use for the vitamins and should be referred to whenever any confusion arises.

There are obvious gaps in the systems used to name vitamins by letter or number. There is no vitamin B_4, for example, or vitamin F. Such things are largely "accidents of history" because some substances that were initially labeled vitamins were later shown not to be vitamins or to be identical to previously known vitamins.

Functions of Vitamins

The single most common function of vitamins is to act as precursors to or components of a variety of coenzymes. Vitamins that are coenzyme precursors usually provide a major part of the coenzyme that is intimately involved in the chemical interactions required during the act of enzymatic catalysis. Some

FIGURE OV3-2

Examples of the reactions for which vitamins are essential in the metabolism of energy-yielding nutrients.

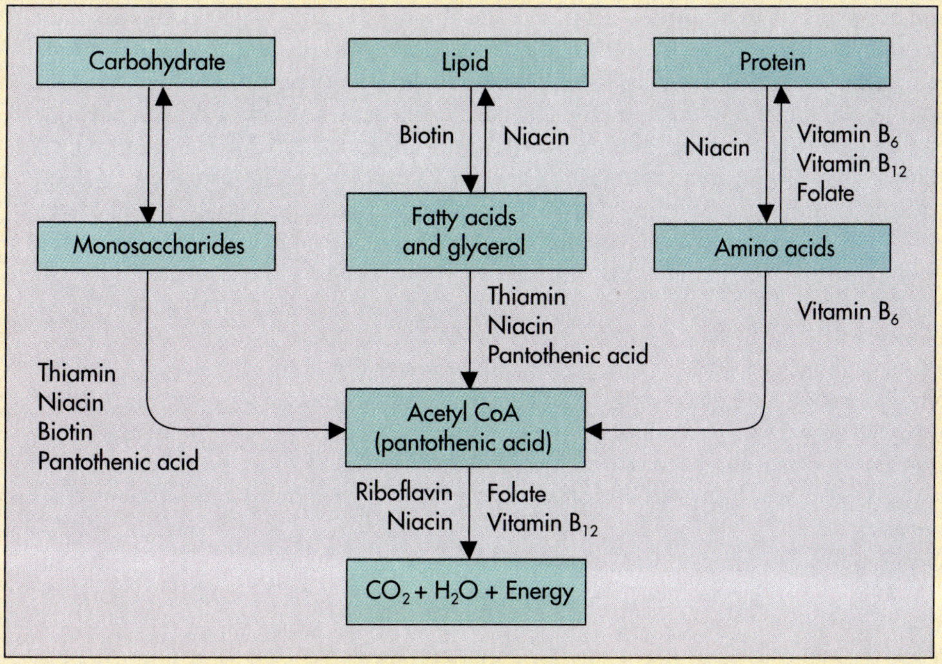

vitamins, however, are not coenzymes but perform some other chemical tasks required for the health of the body. Vitamin C, for example, is a reducing agent involved in a class of reactions known as hydroxylations in which the hydroxyl (OH) group is added to a range of chemicals within cells. Vitamin A is a precursor of the light-absorbing pigment of the eye, which is essential to our ability to see. Vitamin E protects lipid molecules from unwanted oxidation. The specific functions of each vitamin are considered fully in Chapters 11 to 13.

When the effects of all the vitamins are considered together, it is found that vitamins are required for many of the most fundamental pathways of metabolism, such as the central pathways involved in releasing energy from the energy-yielding nutrients: carbohydrate, lipid, and protein. Figure Ov3-2 summarizes the key points at which various vitamins are involved in these pathways. Although at least one function has been identified for each vitamin, additional functions of some vitamins almost certainly remain to be discovered, and the precise mechanisms behind even some of the known functions have not been fully explored.

Vitamins in Food

The amount of a vitamin in any specific food depends on two main factors: the amount originally present in the food when it was a living plant or animal and the amount of the vitamin that is destroyed or lost during harvesting of plants, slaughtering of animals, and subsequent storage, processing, and cooking. The original vitamin content of plant foods depends on various aspects of the plant's history, including the following:

- The type of soil in which the plant grew
- The rate at which the plant grew
- The amount of sunlight and moisture available during critical periods of growth
- The stage of maturity of the plant when it was harvested

Once a plant is harvested, the extent to which it retains its original vitamin content depends on the stability of the vitamins concerned and the conditions in which the harvest is stored. In general, vitamin losses of some vitamins increase with increased temperature or exposure to sunshine during storage, increased exposure to air, or increased length of storage.

Vitamin losses during processing and cooking are greatest when high temperatures are used; when large surface areas of the food are exposed to air, water, acid, or alkali during cooking; if the food is agitated during cooking; and if cooking water is discarded, rather than being consumed in some form. This means that practical measures to reduce vitamin losses include cooking at the lowest possible temperature for the shortest time feasible, cooking in a minimal amount of water, cooking at just below boiling point to reduce agitation of the food, cutting the food into pieces that are neither large (taking a long time to cook) nor small (exposing a large surface area), minimizing the food's exposure to air, using any cooking water for soups or gravies, and cutting food with a sharp knife to minimize damage to cells, which causes vitamins to be released. The vitamins lost in cooking water are, as can be expected, from the water-soluble category. The fat-soluble vitamins, like the water-soluble vitamins, are also susceptible to destruction by oxidation.

If food is to be stored for a significant length of time, its vitamin content can be maintained at a level as high as possible by storing in a cool, dark place, with as little exposure as possible to air, acids, and alkalis. Food that is grown at home but harvested and stored inappropriately can have a lower vitamin content than commercially produced food that has been stored longer and subjected to more processing. Fresh, home-produced fruits and vegetables, however, are often significantly higher in vitamin content than commercially bought equivalents.

Vitamin Deficiency

A dietary deficiency in any vitamin causes the particular deficiency condition associated with the vitamin, as explored in more detail in Chapters 11 to 13. The most common cause of vitamin deficiency is the simple lack of sufficient supplies of a vitamin in the diet. A second, less common cause is some impairment of the body's ability to absorb the vitamins available in food. Third, vitamin deficiency can result from an increased need for a vitamin that is not supplied by a person's normal diet.

Simple dietary deficiencies are rare in people who eat well-balanced diets (as exemplified by the Food Guide Pyramid) and are usually associated with diets that have an overreliance on a restricted range of foods, often with little or no fresh fruits and vegetables. Impaired absorption of fat-soluble vitamins can occur in people who secrete less bile than normal because bile is required for the efficient release of these vitamins during the digestion of fat. Reduced secretion of acid into the stomach inhibits the absorption of vitamin B_{12}. Also, the rapid passage of food through the gastrointestinal tract associated with high-fiber diets can significantly reduce the absorption of all vitamins and minerals from food.

Significantly increased needs for vitamins are found in people with certain illnesses and other altered physiological states. Alcoholics, for example, have an increased need for thiamin (vitamin B_1), whereas cigarette smokers and people with tuberculosis require more vitamin C (ascorbic acid). Recent findings suggest that pregnant women require increased amounts of folic acid (one of the B vitamins).[1] Other studies, however, provide a warning against overconsumption of vitamins during pregnancy. For example, if a pregnant woman consumes too much vitamin A, her infant may develop a birth defect.

Vitamin Supplements

Nutritionists and other health professionals have been successful in making the public aware of the importance of vitamins and the need to consume a well-chosen diet to obtain adequate supplies of vitamins. This success, however, has also resulted in some largely unjustified concern that food alone might not supply sufficient vitamins. Many of the commercial companies that sell vitamin supplements have exploited this concern to sell their supplements and have reinforced public doubts about the adequacy of food as a source of vitamins. This has resulted in many people routinely taking high levels of vitamin supplements, fortified foods, or both and so consuming vitamins in amounts that far exceed their daily requirements. This situation is compounded by the fact that many supplements contain far greater quantities of certain vitamins than anyone could possibly need.

Vitamin supplements are useful in certain circumstances, such as when a person's diet is low in vitamins because of illness (which might make him or her disinclined to eat), during adherence to strict weight-control diets, or in regions of the world that are chronically short of food and a variety of foods. The consumption of vitamin supplements by most people in industrialized countries, such as the United States, however, usually simply provides them with extra supplies of vitamins that are already available in adequate amounts from their normal diet. The extent to which vitamin supplements are consumed in the United States is suggested by a prospective study of 121,700 female registered nurses that began in 1976. This has revealed that vitamin supplements provide between 42% and 72% of the subjects' total daily intake of five selected vitamins.[3] Fortunately, the consumption of small amounts of vitamin supplements does little harm (apart from wasting money). As discussed in a later section, however, the consumption of large amounts of supplemental vitamins can have significant harmful effects. Many supplements contain vitamins and minerals.

Regulation of Vitamin Supplementation

In 1973 and 1976 the U.S. Food and Drug Administration (FDA) attempted to limit the nonprescription sale of vitamin supplements to those containing at least 50% but less than 150% of the U.S. RDAs (now known as the Daily Values [DVs]). The FDA believed there were no benefits associated with vitamin intakes of above the DVs and had considerable cause for concern about the indiscriminate and unsupervised consumption of large amounts of vitamins. The FDA's regulatory attempt was opposed by groups who believed it was an unwarranted infringement of individual rights, and in 1978 the proposed regulation was overruled. Thus it is currently permissible to sell vitamin and other nutrient supplements at any level to adults, provided that no unwarranted claims of health benefits are made on the labels or in advertising. The Nutritional Supplement Act of 1994 permits some of the same health claims on nutritional supplements as on food labels (see Chapter 2). It is recommended that supplements designed for children and pregnant or breast-feeding women should not contain more than 150% of the DVs for any nutrient. Also, multinutrient preparations must contain a specified number of nutrients at or above a specified minimal level. This is intended to ensure a reasonably balanced composition of such supplements and to prevent manufacturers from excluding some important nutrients because of their cost or the complexity of their production. Unfortunately, although these regulations exist, little is being done to enforce them.

Natural Versus Synthetic Vitamins

Naturally occurring vitamins are chemically identical to those produced synthetically in the laboratory. This means that natural and synthetic vitamins are absorbed and used by the body in exactly the same way. Despite some claims to the contrary, manufactured vitamins are just as beneficial as the same vitamins contained naturally within food. Advertisements claiming that certain products are more beneficial to health because they contain natural vitamins can be disregarded. Also, many products contain mostly synthetic vitamins but have small amounts of some natural product added to allow more favorable advertising. For example, synthetic vitamin C with added acerola or rose hips; synthetic vitamin E mixed with beta-, gamma-, and delta-tocopherol; and synthetic thiamin in a natural yeast base have all been promoted by advertisements that imply benefits due to their "natural" ingredients.

Toxicity of Vitamins

The water-soluble vitamins have not yet been associated with significant toxicity problems. Because these vitamins dissolve in water, excess amounts are readily excreted in urine or are converted into harmless substances within the body. In recent years, however, some people have purposely consumed extremely large **megadoses** of some water-soluble vitamins, such as vitamin C, in the belief that this brings significant health benefits. Instead, regular consumption of several vitamins in megadoses is more likely to cause a variety of health problems, but because it has become commonplace only recently, sufficient evidence is not yet available to quantify its risks. A megadose of a vitamin has been defined as a dose at least 10 times greater than the recommended intake. Such high doses are seldom, if ever, obtained from food alone. Because synthetic vitamins are low in cost, they are readily available in pills.

Despite warnings of possible health risks, the self-administration of megadoses of various water-soluble vitamins is still widespread; so evidence of any significant risks or genuine benefits of the practice can be expected to become available in the near future. The consumption of excessive amounts of the fat-soluble vitamins has been clearly linked to some toxicity hazards, presumably because these vitamins accumulate in fatty tissues, rather than being readily flushed out of the body. Excessive consumption of vitamin A by adults, for example, has been linked to headaches, drowsiness, nausea, loss of hair, dry skin, diarrhea, impaired bone condition, and the cessation of menstruation in women. Excessive vitamin D consumption has been associated with various symptoms of hypercalcemia (appetite loss, weight loss, nausea, and failure to thrive) because of the role of vitamin D in promoting the absorption of calcium into the blood.

Until more evidence emerges about the effect of vitamin supplements, nutritionists encourage people to obtain the vitamins they need from a well-chosen diet based on foods available in the grocery store. Despite frequent claims to the contrary, it is perfectly feasible to obtain all the vitamins needed by the body from normal food with no additional supplements. Only when the total kilocalorie content of the diet falls below about 1500 kcal/day is lack of vitamins in the diet likely to become a problem.

Related Substances

Two groups of compounds that are chemically related to vitamins are of nutritional importance: **provitamins** and **antivitamins.** Provitamins are vitamin precursors. In other words, they are chemicals that can be converted within the body into active vitamins. The conversion of provitamins into vitamins can occur in various parts of the body and with varying degrees of efficiency, depending on the vitamins concerned.

Antivitamins, also known as **antagonists** of vitamins, are substances that are chemically related to true vitamins but cannot perform the biological functions of the true vitamins. The body cannot discriminate between a vitamin antagonist and the corresponding true vitamins, so the presence of an antagonist can impair the ability of the true vitamins to perform their normal functions. Certain vitamin antagonists have been used to produce vitamin deficiencies under experimental conditions. They have also been used in medicine to retard the undesirable growth of some cancer cells, such as the rapidly growing and multiplying white blood cells found in leukemia. They must be used with extreme caution, however, because they also inhibit the growth of cells required to maintain normal health.

~ BY NOW YOU SHOULD KNOW ~

- Vitamins are essential nutrients needed in small amounts.
- The term *vitamine* was first introduced in 1912.
- Recommended Dietary Allowances (RDAs) for six vitamins were first proposed in 1943.
- RDAs now exist for 11 vitamins.
- Water-soluble and fat-soluble are two majors classes of vitamins.
- The most common function of vitamins involves their role as components of coenzymes.
- The vitamin content of plant foods is influenced by the conditions under which they are grown, harvested, and stored.
- Vitamin deficiencies may be caused by an inadequate dietary intake, poor absorption, or increased need.
- Provitamins or precursors of vitamins can be converted by the body into the active form of the vitamin.
- Several vitamins cause toxic reactions when consumed, primarily in supplements, in amounts many times their usual dietary intakes.
- Antivitamins and antagonists, which are chemically similar to vitamins, interfere with normal vitamin functions.

STUDY QUESTIONS

1. Identify all essential vitamins as either fat-soluble or water-soluble, and indicate the major functional differences between the two groups.
2. Summarize the scientific events that led to the discovery of vitamins.
3. Identify the following terms and indicate their relationship to vitamins: coenzymes, precursors, antivitamins, multinutrient supplements, and vitamin toxicity.
4. List the conditions that influence the retention of vitamins from harvest through consumption of plant foods.

REFERENCES

1. Machlin LR: Introduction. In Sauberlich HE, Machlin LR, editors: Beyond deficiencies: new views on the function and health effects of vitamins, *Ann N Y Acad Sci* 669:1, 1990.
2. Filer LJ: Recommended Dietary Allowances: how did we get where we are: *Nutr Today* 26:21, 1991.
3. Stryker WS and others: Contributions of specific foods to absolute intake and between person variation of nutrient consumption, *J Am Diet Assoc* 91:172, 1991.

ADDITIONAL READINGS

Combs GF Jr: *The vitamins: fundamental aspects in nutrition and health,* New York, 1992, Academic Press.

DeLuca H, Suttie JW, editors: *The fat soluble vitamins,* Madison, Wis, 1970, University of Wisconsin Press.

Eddy WH: *Vitaminology: the chemistry and function of the vitamins,* Baltimore, 1949, Williams & Wilkins.

Gyorgy P, Pearson WN, editors: *The vitamins: chemistry, physiology, pathology, methods,* vols 6 and 7, New York, 1973–1974, Academic Press.

Machlin LR, editor: *Handbook of vitamins,* ed 2, New York, 1991, Marcel Dekker.

Robinson FA: *The vitamin B complex,* New York, 1951, John Wiley.

Rosenberg HR: *Chemistry and physiology of the vitamins,* New York, 1942, Interscience Publications.

Sebrell WH Jr, Harris RS, editors: *The vitamins: chemistry, physiology, pathology, methods,* vols 1 to 5, New York, 1967–1972, Academic Press.

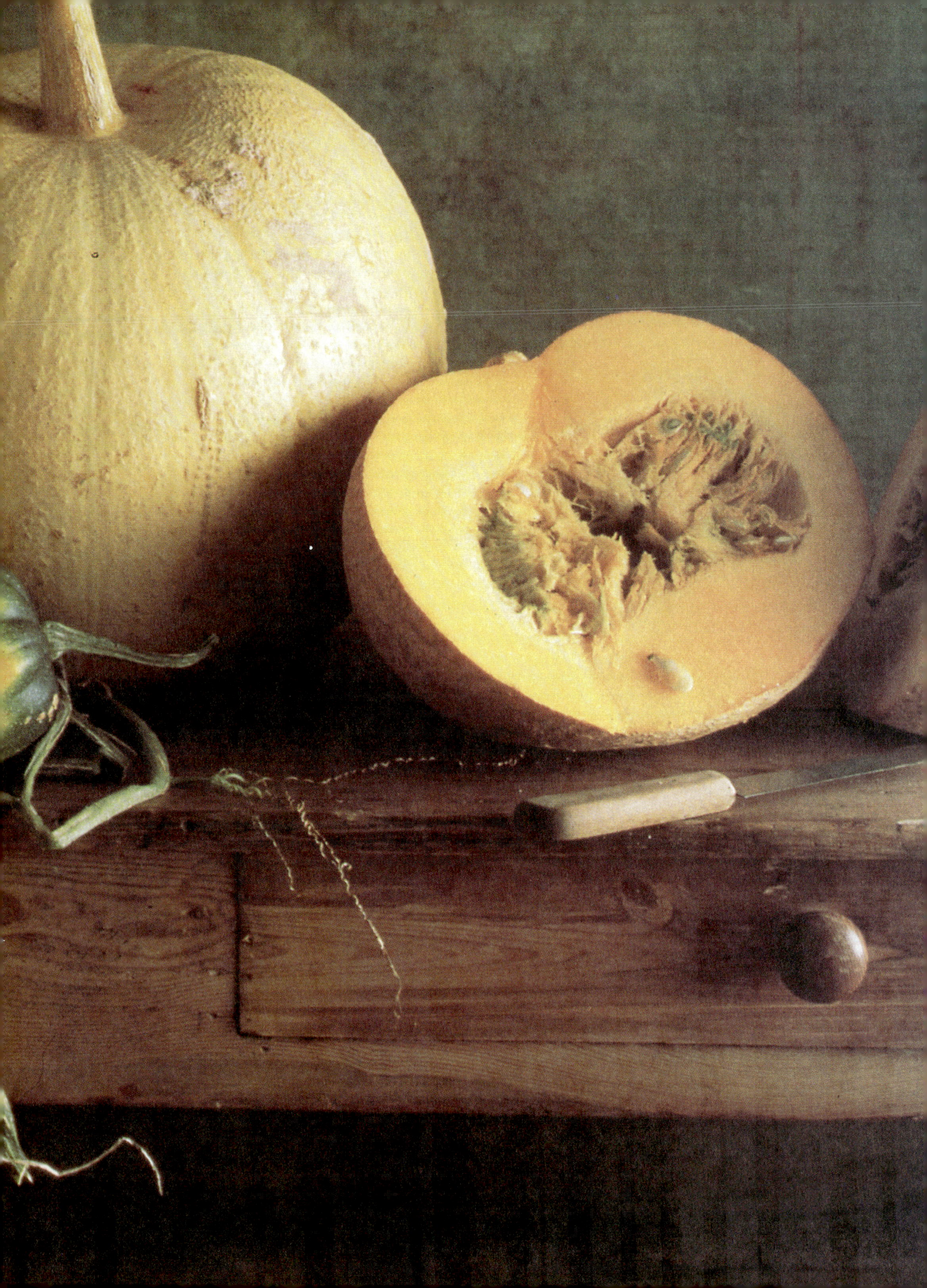

CHAPTER 11

FAT-SOLUBLE VITAMINS

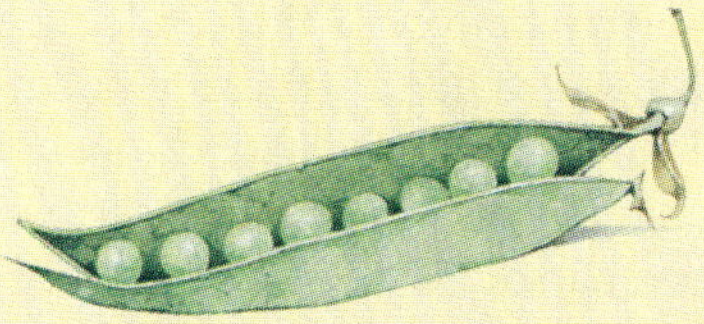

The four fat-soluble vitamins discussed in this chapter are vitamins A, D, E, and K. Of these four, vitamins A and D have been studied most extensively. Vitamin A is essential for normal vision, skin health, and immune function. Vitamin D is essential for normal bone and tooth formation. Beta-carotene, a precursor of vitamin A, and vitamin E act as antioxidants, protecting the other chemicals of the body from reacting with oxidizing agents. Vitamin K is essential for the normal clotting of blood and is involved in the mineralization of bone. The North American food supply provides ample amounts of vitamins A and D. Fat-soluble vitamins may have detrimental effects on health if excessive amounts are consumed. Although all vitamins have beneficial effects on health, claims of benefits resulting from consumption of high doses should be treated with great caution.

VITAMIN A

Vitamin A was discovered in 1909, when McCollum and Davis observed that a fat-soluble substance was necessary for the growth of animals. They had found that animals grew normally when fed diets containing milk fat but failed to grow if the milk fat was withdrawn. At the same time, another group had found that rats fed only lard as a source of fat failed to grow, whereas an extract of butter, cod liver oil, or egg yolk allowed the rats to grow normally. This group also correctly concluded that their results revealed the need for a fat-soluble vitamin in an animal's diet.

Several years later, dairy scientists reported better growth and improved fertility of cows fed yellow—rather than white—corn. By 1928 the compound carotene—a yellow pigment of various plants, including yellow corn—had been shown to be a potent precursor of vitamin A.

Although vitamin A was discovered as a vitamin in 1909, its chemical structure was not determined until 1931. Its correct chemical name is **retinol** and, as can be seen in Figure 11-1, it is an organic alcohol, with the hydroxyl (OH) group characteristic of alcohols being attached to a polyunsaturated hydrocarbon chain that ends in a hydrocarbon ring. In the body, vitamin A can also function in the slightly different aldehyde **(retinal)** or acid **(retinoic acid)** forms. Retinol and retinal (also known as retinaldehyde) can be readily interconverted, but retinoic acid cannot be converted back into either retinol or retinal. The two other members of the "vitamin A family" of compounds shown in Figure 11-1 are **retinyl esters** (produced when retinol combines with an organic acid, usually palmitic acid) and **β-carotene** (a precursor able to undergo oxidative cleavage to two molecules of retinal). Retinol can be converted into all major members of the vitamin A family, except β-carotene, and retinoic acid is a "terminal product" of vitamin A metabolism in the sense that it cannot be converted back into any other form of vitamin A. The irreversibility of the formation of retinoic acid explains why it can perform only some of the activities associated with vitamin A: it can support growth and allow most cells to differentiate, for example, but it cannot support vision (which requires retinal) or reproduction (which requires retinol). Important aspects of the structure, sources, and properties of the major members of the vitamin A family of compounds are summarized in Table 11-1.

Various compounds in food that have structures similar to vitamin A are known as the **retinoids.** Another class of compounds, the **carotenoids,** can serve as precursors (provitamins) of vitamin A. These are all structurally related to *β-carotene,* which is essentially composed of two molecules of vitamin A joined together but is not used as efficiently by the body as is vitamin A itself. It is commonplace to include vitamin A precursors within the general term "vitamin A" because eating the precursors of retinol within food ultimately has the same overall effect as eating retinol itself.

The biologically active forms of vitamin A (retinol and retinyl esters) are found only in foods of animal origin. Many plants, however, are rich in the carotenoid precursors of vitamin A. Over 400 related carotenoids have been discovered in plants, although only about 50 of them possess vitamin A activity in the sense that they can be converted into vitamin A. The most common carotenoids found in plant foods are β-carotene itself, **α-carotene, β-cryptoxanthin, lycopene, lutein**, and **zeaxanthin.** Of these, the most important as precursors of vitamin A are β-carotene, α-carotene, and β-cryptoxanthin. Some carotenoids, including some that do not act as vitamin A precursors, are biologically active antioxidants.

β-carotene is currently one of the few yellow pigments approved by the Food and Drug Administration (FDA) for the artificial coloring of food. It is used extensively in gelatin, margarine, soft drinks, cake mixes, and cereal products.

Until 1967 the vitamin A activity of plant and animal tissue was measured in International Units (IUs) or United States Pharmacopoeia (USP) units. In 1967 the Food and Agriculture Organization/World Health Organization (FAO/WHO) recommended that **retinol equivalents (REs)** be used instead, with 1 RE being equal to 3.3 IU of vitamin A. In 1974 REs were adopted as the standard units for quantifying vitamin A in the United States. Although recommended dietary allowances (RDAs), food composition tables, and labels on most food products continue to make use of both systems; it is important to remember the relationship between them.

1 Retinol equivalent (RE) =
- 1 μg of all-*trans* retinol
- 6 μg of all-*trans* β-carotene
- 12 μg of other provitamin A carotenoids
- 3.3 IU of vitamin A

Vitamin A was crystallized from halibut liver oil in 1937 and was chemically synthesized in 1947. Pure synthetic vitamin A contains about 1 million RE per gram (as is expected from the definition of 1 RE as 1 μg, meaning one millionth of a gram, of vitamin A). It is a pale yellow substance that is readily soluble in lipids (that is, fats and oils) or solvents in which lipids dissolve.

FIGURE 11-1

The chemical structure of vitamin A (retinol) and the relationship between retinol, retinal, retinoic acid, β-carotene, and retinyl esters.

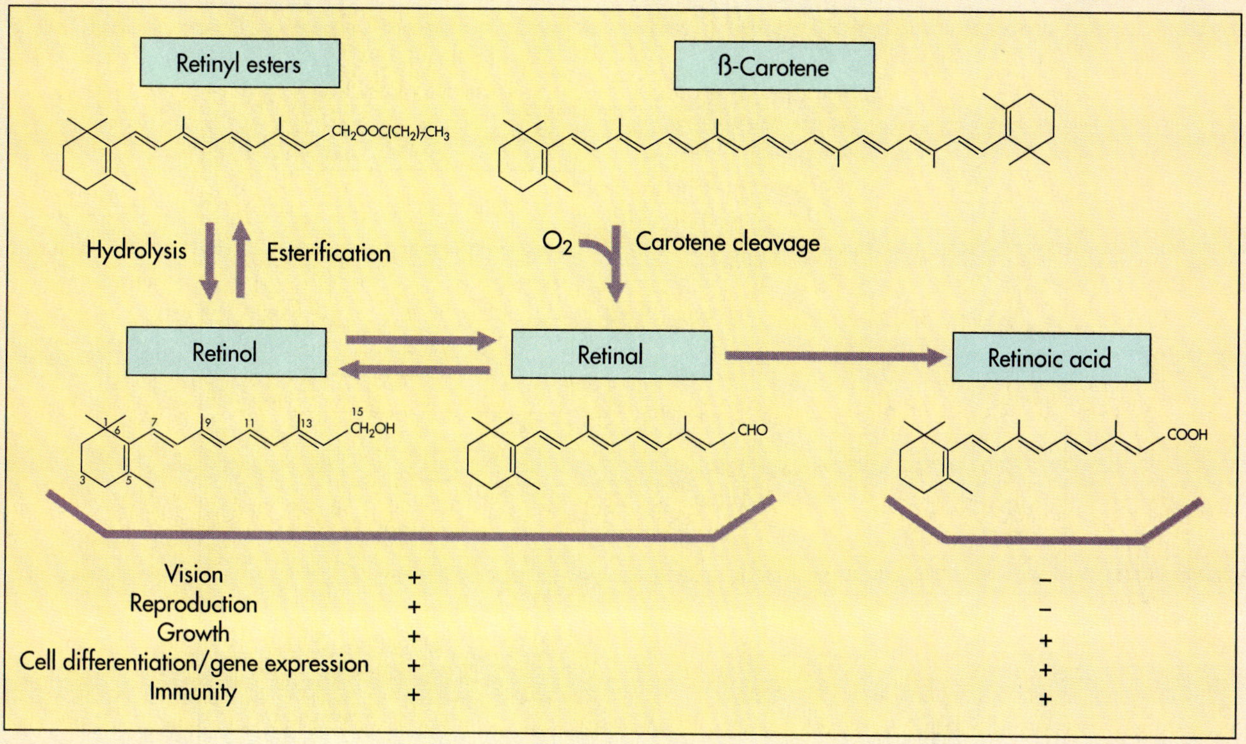

TABLE 11-1

Forms and properties of the major molecules in the vitamin A family

	RETINOL*	β-CAROTENE†	RETINAL	RETINOIC ACID
Chemistry	Hydrocarbon alcohol	Hydrocarbon	Aldehyde derivative of retinol	Carboxylic acid derivative of retinol
Dietary sources	Animal sources; supplements	Fruits and vegetables; dairy fats	Not significant	Not significant
Potential toxicity	Destabilizes membranes; teratogenic	Little, if any		Teratogenic
Transport	Bound to plasma RBP	Associated with plasma lipoproteins	Not significant	Low plasma concentration; bound to albumin
Cellular-binding proteins	CRBP-I, CRBP-II	None identified	CRABP (eye)	CRABP-I, CRABP-II
Antioxidant properties	Probably not significant	Quenches singlet oxygen		

* Includes retinyl ester.

† Other dietary carotenes, including α-carotene, also contribute provitamin A activity. However, most oxygenated carotenoids—e.g., xanthophylls, such as lutein—do not contribute to vitamin A.

RBP, Retinol-binding protein; *CRBP*, cellular retinol-binding protein; *CRABP*, cellular retinoic acid-binding protein.

From Ross AC: *J Nutr* 123:346, 1993.

FIGURE 11-2

Role of vitamin A in vision. As light splits rhodopsin (visual purple) to retinal and opsin, a nerve impulse is passed along the optic nerve to the brain.

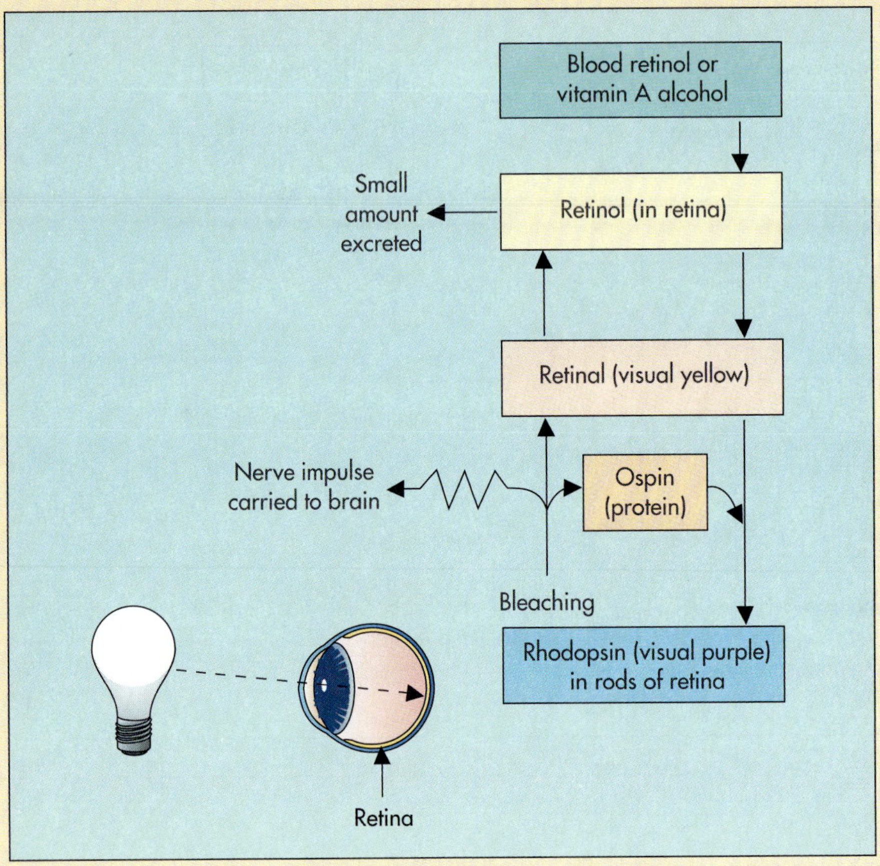

Synthetic vitamin A is used in the enrichment of many food products, such as milk. A modified, water-miscible form is also available for use in nonfat products, such as dried milk.

FUNCTIONS*

Although vitamin A was discovered as long ago as 1909 and chemically identified in 1931, it has been difficult to study its functions because it is needed only by complex organisms. It is best known for its role in vision, but several other important functions of the vitamin—as retinol, retinal, or retinoic acid—are now known. The general body processes supported by these functions are summarized in Figure 11-1, which shows that retinol and retinal are required for normal vision, reproduction, growth, cell differentiation, gene expression, and immune function, whereas retinoic acid is required for growth, cell differentiation, and immune function.

* The discussion for vitamin A function and metabolism is in greater depth than for other nutrients. The purpose is to sensitize the reader to the complexity of cellular metabolism and sophistication of advances in research.

Vision

The best-characterized function of vitamin A is its role in the **retina** of the eye.[1] Retinol, supplied to the retina in blood, is converted to retinal, which then combines with a protein called **opsin** to produce a purple pigment known as **rhodopsin.** Rhodopsin, also known as **visual purple,** is located in the light-sensitive **rod cells** of the retina. When light strikes the retina (11-cis-retinal is converted to all trans retinal), the rod cells are bleached as the rhodopsin splits to form retinal and opsin. As this occurs, a nerve stimulus is transmitted through the optic nerve fibers to the visual center of the brain, where the sensation of vision is created. Most of the retinal is rapidly converted to retinol. The retinol can then be converted to 11-cis-retinal that recombines with opsin to produce rhodopsin, ready to undergo the cycle again. At each "turn" of this cycle, however, a small amount of retinol is converted to retinoic acid or another inactive compound and is lost from the rod cells. This lost retinol must be continually replaced by fresh supplies of retinol brought by the blood (Figure 11-2). This means that the amount of retinol in the blood determines the rate at which rhodopsin is regenerated. If rhodopsin regeneration is slow, vision in dim light is poor.

The speed with which the eye recovers its full powers after exposure to bright light is directly related to the amount of vitamin A that is available to form rhodopsin. The recovery process is known as **dark adaptation** because it allows the eye to adapt to vision in dim light after exposure to bright light. The effects of vitamin A deficiency on the speed of dark adaptation are illustrated in Figure 11-3, which shows what a person with sufficient vitamin A and one with insufficient vitamin A see after exposure to a car's headlights on a dark road. The eyes of a person with sufficient vitamin A recover quickly after the car has passed, allowing him or her to gain a virtually normal view quickly (Figure 11-3, *B*). The eyes of someone who is deficient in vitamin A take much longer to recover because the reformation of the rhodopsin required for vision proceeds more slowly. As a result, vitamin A-deficient persons can barely see any of the dim scene before them for a considerable time after the car has passed (Figure 11-3, *C*). This effect of vitamin A deficiency is known as **night blindness.** Another common situation in which it becomes evident is on entering a dimly lit cinema or theater. In this situation, people with vitamin A deficiency may find it difficult to see the way to their seats, whereas those with sufficient vitamin A manage without difficulty. Although supplementation with vitamin A can correct night blindness, it cannot improve the vision of people who did not have a preexisting vitamin A deficiency.

The **dark adaptation test,** which measures the speed of recovery of vision in dim light, is considered to be an accurate and sensitive measure of vitamin A status. Unfortunately, it is a relatively complex and expensive test and is not very useful with children because it requires the subjects to describe accurately what they see.

In addition to the rod cells discussed already, the retina of the eye also contains **cone cells,** which are involved in the perception of color vision in good light. The light-sensitive opsins of the cone cells also contain vitamin A as part of their structure. The functioning of the cone cells, however, is not as sensitive to variations in available vitamin A as is the functioning of the rod cells.

Although the involvement of vitamin A in vision is the vitamin's best-known function, the eye contains only 0.01% of the vitamin A in the body.

FIGURE 11-3

Photographs simulating the effect of night blindness due to vitamin A deficiency (see text).

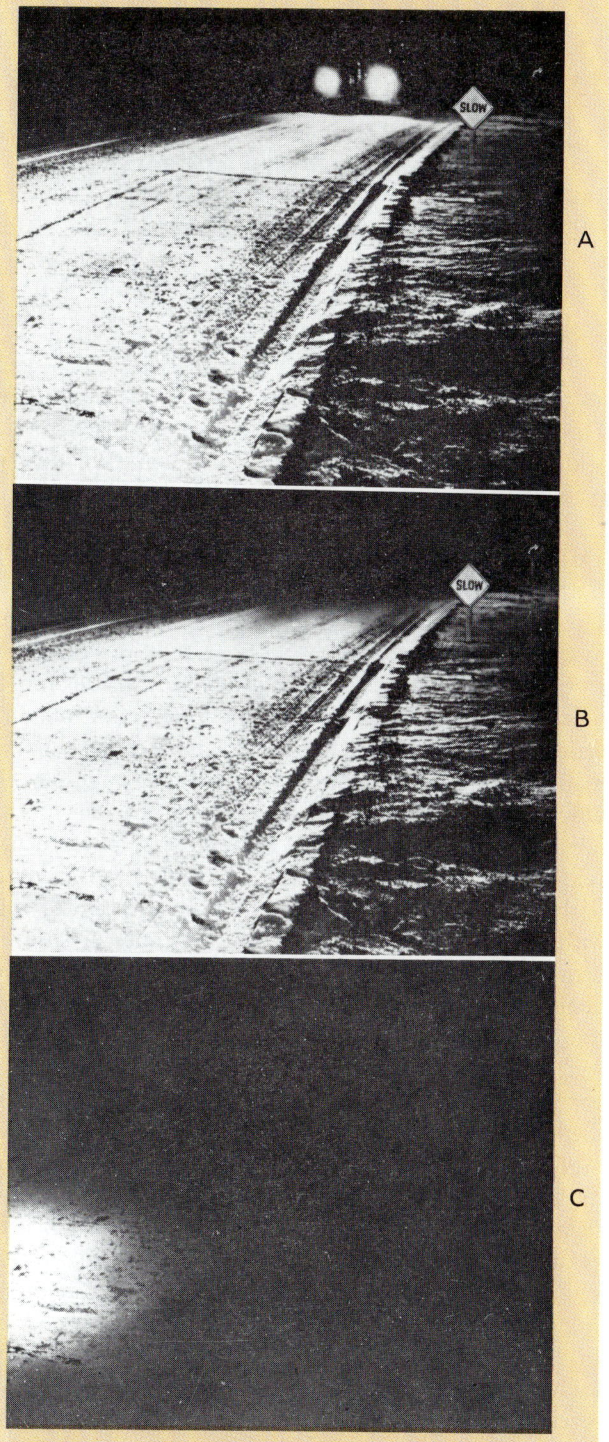

Growth

When animals are deprived of vitamin A, they stop growing once their reserves of the vitamin have been depleted. An early symptom of vitamin A deficiency is loss of appetite, followed by a cessation of growth (growth plateau), then rapid weight loss and ultimate death. It is well established that vitamin A is essential for the normal growth of bones. In vitamin A deficiency bones become weak, although thicker than normal. The cavities in the skull and the spinal column do not enlarge to make room for the growing nervous system. The precise function of vitamin A in bone growth is unclear, but deficiency may involve failure of immature bone cell to mature into osteoclasts (responsible for the breakdown of bone during bone remodeling). As a result of vitamin A deficiency, bone remodeling does not occur properly.

FIGURE 11-4

Changes in epithelial cells in vitamin A deficiency.

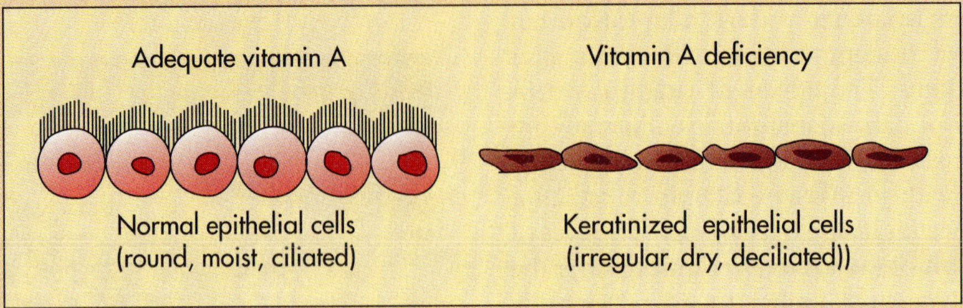

The facilitation of growth and the maintenance of normal vision are two distinct functions of vitamin A. This distinction is demonstrated by the fact that retinoic acid can support growth but will not maintain normal vision.

Cell Differentiation and Gene Expression

The likely involvement of vitamin A in the development or **differentiation** of immature bone cells into different types of mature cells is just one example of various forms of cell differentiation that depend on the vitamin. A variety of tissue changes within vitamin A–deficient animals, now known to be mostly related to changes in cell differentiation, was noted as early as 1925. The most obvious change is widespread keratinization of epithelial cells, which is associated with the drying and hardening of the cells caused by accumulation of the protein keratin within them. Epithelial cells are found in many locations, including the skin and the eye and in the lining of the genitourinary system and respiratory tract. Those within the body normally secrete mucus and are covered in hairlike **cilia.** The cilia on the lining of the respiratory system prevent the accumulation of foreign material on the surface of the epithelial cells by their constant motion. The action of the cilia is involved in protecting the body against infection by sweeping the cell surfaces clear of invading microorganisms. In vitamin A–deficient keratinized cells the cilia are lost (Figure 11-4). Because keratinization and the loss of cilia leave the body more vulnerable to infection, vitamin A has become known as an "antiinfective" vitamin. All of the changes in epithelial cells caused by vitamin A deficiency are rapidly reversed when vitamin A is returned to the diet in adequate amounts.

Epithelial cells are continually shed and replaced, and because vitamin A is required for their formation, a constant supply of vitamin A is required for normal health. The tissues that are most sensitive to vitamin A deficiency are the skin, trachea, salivary glands, cornea, and testes. Keratinization of the cornea can lead to its ulceration and eventual destruction and blindness. Keratinization of the cornea caused by vitamin A deficiency is the major cause of blindness in young children.[2]

The Regulatory Functions of Retinoic Acid

Studies in the 1970s demonstrated that retinoic acid could induce the differentiation of embryonic stem cells, meaning their conversion from immature precursor cells into mature specialized cells such as muscle, skin, and nerve cells.[3] This process of differentiation is mediated by changes in gene activity; so strong evidence suggests that retinoic acid is the active form of vitamin A involved in controlling cell development by influencing gene activity. This suggests a hormonelike activity of retinoic acid. At present, the specific functions of retinoic acid within the body are being discovered. It is certainly one of the signals switching on the specific genes that allow immature skin cells (keratinocytes) to develop into mature skin cells. The results of some studies also suggest that retinoic acid or synthetic derivatives of retinoic acid can delay or prevent the progression of certain epithelial cancers.

The search to uncover the mechanism by which retinoic acid can affect cell differentiation has revealed that there are specific receptor proteins for retinoic acid within the nuclei of cells. At least three main subtypes of **retinoic acid receptors (RARs)** have been identified; they are labeled **RAR-alpha, RAR-beta,** and **RAR-gamma.** A different class of receptors that binds only weakly to retinoic acid has also been identified. These **retinoid X receptors (RXRs)** are structurally unrelated to the RARs. The various subtypes of RARs appear to be regulated independently of both one another and the RXRs. In the mouse, for example, RAR-alpha is found to be present in the cells of all organs, RAR-beta is found only in specific tissues at specific times, and RAR-gamma is found only in skin and cartilage.

It is clear that the binding of retinoic acid to one of the RARs allows the RAR to then interact with specific regions of the DNA in the nucleus, presumably to control the transcription of specific genes into messenger ribonucleic acid (mRNA). In recognition of this activity the RARs have been described as **ligand-activated transcription factors,** with retinoic acid being the ligand that activates them. Which genes are controlled by RAR binding appears to be determined by the presence of a particular nucleotide sequence within the genes known as the **retinoic acid response element (RARE).** This is presumably the region of DNA to which an activated RAR protein can bind and so directly activate the transcription of the associated gene.[4]

Whatever the precise mechanisms and interactions of the RAR and RXR proteins, it is now clear that more than 1000 genes have the potential to interact with them. These genes include those that encode growth hormone and osteopontin, two hormones that are intimately involved in bone remodeling and growth.[5]

In addition to its effects on cell differentiation, retinoic acid appears to regulate several aspects of vitamin A metabolism in general. For example, the rate at which vitamin A is degraded slows as the body's reserves of the vitamin become depleted.[6] Also, if retinoic acid is added to the diet of a rat with vitamin A deficiency, the use of residual retinol in the rat is slowed. These observations suggest that some kind of feedback mechanism allows retinoic acid to inhibit the degradation of retinol. The metabolism of vitamin A within the liver is also influenced by the availability of dietary vitamin A or retinoic acid. In rats, for example, the activity of the liver enzyme **lecithin: retinol acyltransferase (LRAT)**, an enzyme that synthesizes retinyl esters, has been shown to be directly related to the vitamin A status of the animal. During vitamin A deficiency the esterification of retinol by liver LRAT was found to fall to negligible levels but returned to normal levels within hours of the administration of adequate retinol. If vitamin A sufficiency is mimicked by supplying only retinoic acid to the rat, the level of LRAT activity again rises, clearly implicating retinoic acid in the regulation of this enzyme's activity.

Reproduction

One of the first functions discovered for vitamin A was its promotion of animal fertility. Either retinol or retinal is required for normal reproduction in rats, for example, although in all animal species studied to date, retinoic acid *cannot* support reproduction. In the absence of sufficient retinol or retinal, male rats fail to produce sperm cells and any fetus within a female rat becomes reabsorbed into the body. The biochemical mechanism in the reproduction role of vitamin A remains unknown.

Immunity

Several features of the immune system are influenced by vitamin A. As previously mentioned, vitamin A is required to maintain the normal health and function of epithelial layers, which provide a first line of defense against invading microorganisms. Also, the role of retinoids in controlling cell differentiation is an important aspect of the differentiation of some cells of the immune system. The immune system comprises two main arms—the **humoral immune response,** which is mediated by the release of antibodies into blood, and the **cellular immune response,** which involves the direct killing of infected cells of the body or the cells of infectious pathogens themselves. Both types of immune response are regulated by vitamin A or its metabolites.[7]

ABSORPTION, TRANSPORT, AND METABOLISM

Retinol and retinyl esters (REs) account for virtually all of the preformed vitamin A available in the diet and are obtained exclusively from foods of animal origin. These are also the predominant forms in which vitamin A is available from supplements. β-carotene is widely available within fruits, vegetables, and dairy fats and is converted to retinol at a typical yield of 1 μg (or RE) of retinol per 6 μg of β-carotene. The proportion of dietary β-carotene that is actually cleaved to retinol varies with intake, with higher intakes being associated with proportionately lower levels of release of retinol. Other dietary factors that influence the bioavailability of retinol from β-carotene include the amount of protein and fat in the diet and variations in digestive function.

1 IU of vitamin A =
0.3 μg of all-*trans* retinol
1.8 μg of all-*trans* β-carotene
3.6 μg of other provitamin A carotenoids
0.3 RE

The common nutritional term *preformed retinol* includes both retinol itself and the retinyl esters from which retinol is readily released.[8] In the typical U.S. diet, preformed retinol (largely as retinyl ester) provides about two thirds of the total vitamin A. In typical diets in developing countries, however, β-carotene is the predominant dietary source of vitamin A.

Absorption

Retinol can be absorbed from food directly into the intestinal wall cells. Before retinyl esters can be absorbed, they must first be hydrolyzed to free retinol and an organic acid. This hydrolysis is catalyzed by enzymes within pancreatic juice, and the organic acid released is usually palmitic acid because **retinyl palmitate** is the predominant retinyl ester within food. Overall, approximately 75% of preformed dietary vitamin A is usually

FIGURE 11-5

Transport and metabolism of vitamin A. β-C, β-carotene; PL, phospholipid; LPL, lipoprotien lipase. (See text for other abbreviations.)

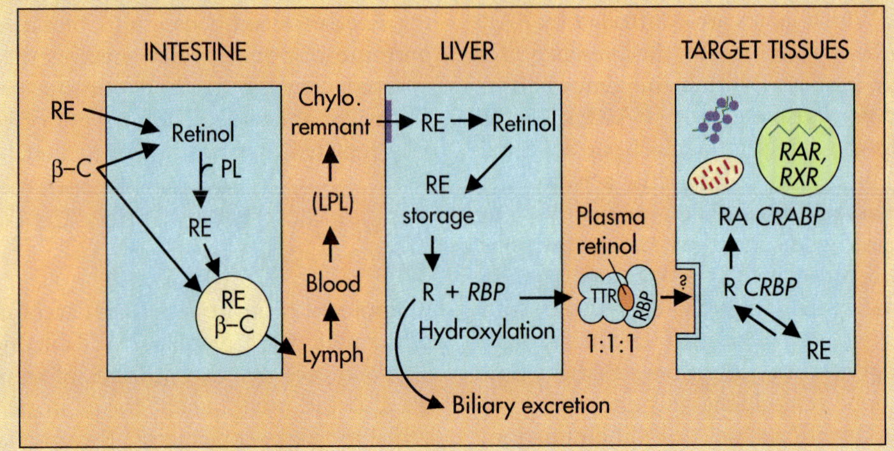

absorbed, compared with between 5% and 50% of dietary β-carotene and other carotenoids. Because vitamin A is a fat-soluble vitamin, its absorption is enhanced by factors that promote fat absorption and is diminished by those that inhibit fat absorption. The involvement of bile in facilitating fat absorption means that any condition that reduces the secretion of bile or obstructs the bile duct leads to diminished absorption of vitamin A from the diet.

> Retinyl palmitate is the predominant retinyl ester in food. It is hydrolyzed to retinol and palmitic acid before absorption into the body but is then reformed within intestinal cells before being incorporated into the chylomicrons released into the lymphatic system, which transports them to the blood.

Only small amounts of retinoic acid are found in food. β-carotene is hydrolyzed in the intestine to form retinal, and about 10% of the retinal is converted to retinoic acid.

Transport

Absorbed vitamin A in the form of retinol, retinyl esters, β-carotene, or the retinal produced from β-carotene is transported from the intestine within chylomicrons. For this to happen, much of the retinol must be reesterified back into the form of retinyl esters. The chylomicrons are released into the lymphatic system, which transports them to the blood. Most of the retinol and retinyl esters is transported to the liver (with some uncleaved β-carotene), and some enters adipose tissue and other tissues. In the liver, vitamin A is stored in lipid droplets, mostly in the form of retinyl palmitate within special fat-storing (stellate) cells of the liver.

The concentration of vitamin A in the liver (which holds 90% of body stores) reflects long-term dietary intake of vitamin A. The amount of vitamin A in the liver ranges from 100 to 1000 IU/g of liver tissue. A healthy person stores an estimated 500,000 IU in the liver, which is sufficient to meet the body's needs for several years. Autopsy data on the livers of Canadians, however, showed that 10% of those autopsied had no measurable reserves of vitamin A, whereas 20% had no more vitamin A than the amount normally present at birth.

When vitamin A is required by the rest of the body, it is released from the liver and transported to target tissues in the form of retinol bound to **retinol-binding protein (RBP).** The RBP within plasma itself, however, becomes bound to a protein called **transthyretin (TTR)** or **prealbumin** (also produced by the liver). The proteins RBP and transthyretin serve to make vitamin A more soluble in blood plasma, and by incorporating the vitamin into a much larger structure, they protect it from being filtered from blood and excreted via the kidneys. β-carotene, on the other hand, is released from the liver as part of the very–low-density lipoprotein (VLDL) complexes. Key features of the transport and metabolism of vitamin A are summarized in Figure 11-5.

Once delivered into a cell, vitamin A is picked up by various binding proteins, which are distinct from the proteins that serve to transport vitamin A within the blood.

FIGURE 11-6

Model of cellular retinoid metabolism.

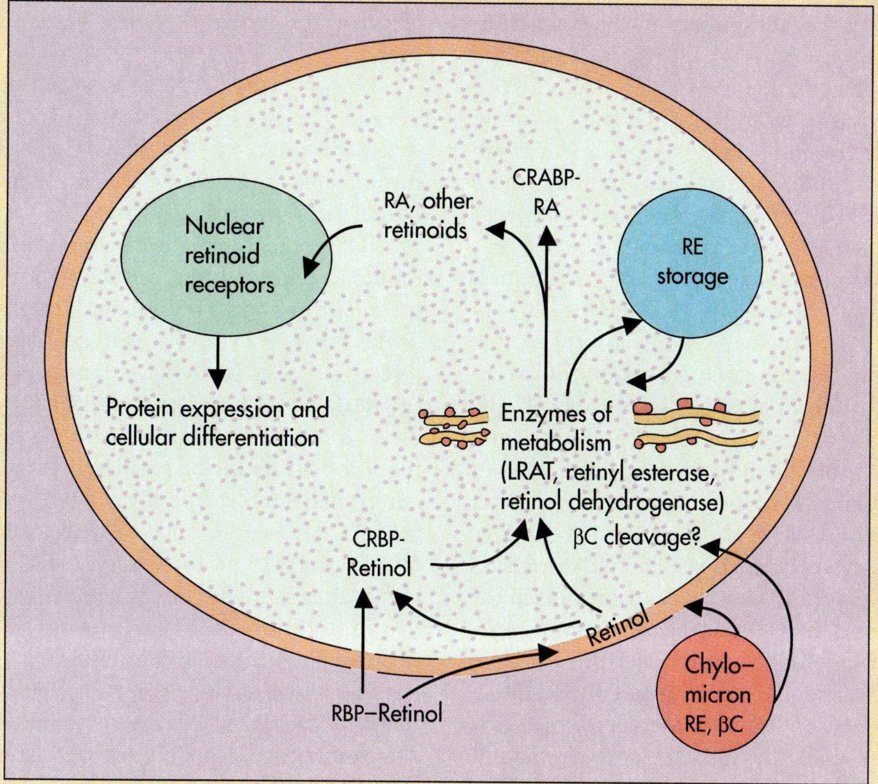

Vitamin A–binding Proteins

One major focus of vitamin A research is on the variety of RBPs to which various forms of vitamin A become bound at various stages in their metabolism. The first of such proteins to be characterized were RBP (mentioned previously), which transports retinol in the blood to various tissues, and two intracellular retinoid-binding proteins known as **cellular retinol-binding protein (CRBP)** and **cellular retinoic acid–binding protein (CRABP).** As their names suggest, CRBP binds to retinol and CRABP to retinoic acid.

It is now known that a much larger group of extracellular and intracellular RBPs is involved in the transport of the various forms of vitamin A and in the control of vitamin A metabolism. Many of these binding proteins are structurally similar ("homologous"), but they have different patterns of tissue distribution and are subject to different patterns of regulatory control during the course of the body's development.

Figure 11-6 summarizes the way in which these proteins are believed to be involved in the uptake of vitamin A by cells and the transport and metabolism of vitamin A within cells. Vitamin A is delivered to the cell either as retinol released from RBP or as retinol or β-carotene within chylomicrons. Once inside most cells, retinol becomes bound to one of the specific CRBPs available in the cell. In liver cells, at least, it is known that sufficient CRBP exists within the cells to bind to virtually all of the available retinol. Any retinoic acid can become bound to CRABP molecules, which are available in most cells.

After the cellular RBPs were discovered, research first focused on which types of cell contained them and whether they were regulated in any way by changes in vitamin A status. Most tissues were found to contain CRBP, although the highest concentrations are in the liver, kidneys, intestine, and male reproductive organs. Some of these tissues, especially the testis and skin, also contain CRABP. As an animal develops vitamin A deficiency, the concentration of retinol in the cytoplasms of the cells falls but no dramatic matching fall in CRBP concentration has been found.

It has become clear that the cellular RBPs act as both "buffer proteins," regulating the amount of free retinoids in the cell, and "guide proteins," delivering retinoids to specific enzymes of metabolism. Both CRBP and CRABP are likely to play important buffer roles in controlling and limiting the amount of free retinol and retinoic acid, respectively.

Retinol bound to CRBP is in chemical equilibrium with unbound retinol, so any rise in free retinol causes an immediate compensating increase in retinol binding to

CRBP, whereas any fall in free retinol causes an immediate compensating release of retinol from CRBP. The equilibrium "position," however, strongly favors the bound form, meaning that at equilibrium the concentration of retinol bound to CRBP is much greater than the concentration of free retinol. In a similar way, CRABP binds retinoic acid tightly, with the equilibrium position strongly favoring the bound form. In experiments with cultured cells it was found that manipulating the cells to give them high CRABP concentrations made the cells less sensitive to regulation by retinoic acid. This is taken as suggesting that one function of CRABP is to sequester retinoic acid within the cell.

The role of cellular RBPs as "guide proteins" has been demonstrated in three specific processes: the esterification of retinol to form retinyl esters in both the intestine and liver, the oxidation of retinol to retinal, and the hydrolysis of membrane-bound retinyl esters. For example, there are known to be two enzymes in liver cells that catalyze the esterification of retinol. One of them, LRAT, is likely to be involved in the storage of retinyl esters in the liver (and vitamin A absorption in the intestine). The second enzyme, **acyl-CoA:retinol acyltransferase (ARAT),** is found within liver cells in close proximity to LRAT. When retinol carried by CRBP is added in the presence of both of these enzymes, the retinol is esterified specifically and efficiently by LRAT. This discrimination is lost, however, when unbound retinol is added, with most of the unbound retinol following a less efficient pathway to esterification by ARAT. In the case of retinol oxidation to retinal, retinol molecules bound to CRBP appear to be directed specifically to the enzyme **retinol dehydrogenase.** So it seems certain that one function of the cellular RBPs is to direct retinol to specific enzymes in a way that discriminates between alternative metabolic processes.

The depressed use of vitamin A found in protein deficiency can be explained by the need for such a wide variety of proteins for the transport and metabolism of vitamin A. In addition to the wide range of binding proteins considered previously, many enzymes are required at various stages of vitamin A metabolism. In protein deficiency the synthesis of all these proteins is depressed. The need for protein to mobilize vitamin A reserves from the liver may explain why the low blood levels of vitamin A in people with kwashiorkor increase when protein alone is administered, that is, with no additional vitamin A being supplied along with the protein.

Carotene

After being released from plant cells during digestion, the carotene precursors of vitamin A are absorbed intact from the intestine in the presence of bile salts. Within the intestinal wall they are split to form retinol, which then enters the general retinol pool. The conversion of carotene to retinol is subject to regulation. Some carotene always survives intact to enter the general circulation. Blood carotene levels reflect the dietary availability of carotene, rather than the body's overall vitamin A status.

Unconverted carotene is stored in fat tissue and the adrenal glands, not the liver. It may be responsible for a yellowish tinge of the skin when large amounts are stored, but large doses of carotene have not been associated with any toxic effects.

Because β-carotene can be converted directly into retinal (Figure 11-1), it can clearly serve as a direct precursor of both retinol and retinoic acid. It seems likely, however, that β-carotene can also be converted directly to retinoic acid via compounds known as **apocarotenals** in a way that bypasses retinal as an intermediate. It is possible that this pathway for the formation of retinoic acid might be regulated independently from the better characterized pathway from retinal or retinol (via retinal). The significance of such an alternative pathway for the formation of retinoic acid remains unknown, although it is under investigation.

In addition to acting as a precursor of vitamin A, β-carotene and other carotenoids may perform a function as antioxidants, protecting the body from the potentially damaging effects of various oxidizing agents. The antioxidant capabilities of carotenoids have been clearly demonstrated under laboratory conditions and have been proposed as an explanation for the apparent ability of foods rich in carotenoids to protect against certain cancers and other degenerative diseases.

RECOMMENDED DIETARY ALLOWANCES

RDAs for vitamin A[9] are based on the assumption that two thirds of the vitamin A of a mixed diet comes from animal sources (retinol) and one third from plant sources (carotene). The U.S. RDAs and Canadian Recommended Nutrient Intakes (RNIs) are summarized in Table 11-2.

Studies on the amount of vitamin A required to maintain liver stores of at least 20 RE/g of liver, to restore plasma vitamin A levels to normal (greater than 30 μg/100 ml), and to correct abnormalities in dark adaptation suggest that vitamin A is used by adult men at an average rate of 910 μg/day. The Food and Nutrition Board of the U.S. National Academy of Sciences estimates that the adult male requirement for vitamin A actually varies considerably—from 570 to 1250 RE/day. The recommended intake is set at 1000 RE/day. For adult women the RDA for vitamin A is set at 800 RE, based on their lower body weight. Elderly people in good health appear to have no additional need for vitamin A; so their recommended intakes remain unchanged throughout adulthood.

TABLE 11-2

Recommended dietary allowances (United States) and recommended nutrient intakes (Canada) for vitamin A

	UNITED STATES		CANADA
AGE (YEARS)	RE	IU	RE
CHILDREN			
1-3	400	2000	400
4-6	500	2500	500
7-10	700	3300	700
ADULTS			
Male	1000	5000	1000
Female	800	4000	800
Pregnant	800	4000	800
Lactating	1200	6000	1200

RE, Retinol equivalent; *IU,* international units.

The RNIs for vitamin A established by Health and Welfare Canada[10] are similar to the U.S. RDAs. However, the United Kingdom's Committee on Medical Aspects of Food Policy[11] and the Food and Agricultural Organization/World Health Organization (FAO/WHO)[12] have both established daily recommended vitamin A intakes that are 25% to 30% lower than the U.S. or Canadian standards for adult males and females.

During the last trimester of pregnancy about 1.3 mg of retinol is transferred to the fetus. This can be provided by the mother without the consumption of any additional vitamin A, unless the mother's vitamin A reserves were depleted to begin with. For pregnant women with low reserves, an additional 200 RE of vitamin A per day is recommended. There is some danger that large doses of vitamin A, greater than 20,000 RE/day, may cause birth defects. It is important for pregnant women to avoid excessive intakes of vitamin A.

Human milk contains between 400 and 700 RE/L of vitamin A and 200 to 400 µg/L of carotenoids. These amounts could use up 50% of the mother's vitamin A reserves during 6 months of breast-feeding. To maintain maternal stores, it is recommended that an extra 500 RE/day of vitamin A be consumed during lactation, which provides about 350 to 500 RE/day to the infant. For older children, daily recommended intakes are extrapolated from the adult intakes because information is not available on the specific amounts needed by children.

If data on food composition are in IUs rather than REs, it is difficult to assess the adequacy of dietary intake relative to the RDA because these tables do not give sufficient information to make the necessary conversion. Fortunately, most tables now provide information on both units during the transition period.

FOOD SOURCES

The **vitamin A value** of food consists of preformed vitamin A that is found only in foods of animal origin, in addition to the vitamin A available from precursors found in plants and some foods of animal origin. Table 11-3 shows the vitamin A value of the most frequently used foods and some recommended sources of vitamin A.

Because liver is the organ in which vitamin A is stored, it is not surprising that liver is the richest food source of vitamin A. Pork liver contains 12,000 RE/100 g, whereas polar bear liver (the richest and, in fact, a toxic source) has 600,000 RE/100 g. The use of concentrates of fish liver oil, which were once widely used as therapeutic sources of vitamins A and D, has now been almost totally replaced by synthetic vitamin A in tablet or capsule form.

Egg yolk is a good source of vitamin A, with 310 IU or 94 RE per egg. Because preformed vitamin A in animal foods is colorless, the yellow color of egg yolk may be due to carotene and other carotenoids, rather than to vitamin A itself. The color of egg yolks also varies with the breed of hen and type of diet consumed by the hen, rather than reflecting its vitamin A value.

The vitamin A content of butter undergoes a definite seasonal variation. In winter the vitamin A content of butter averages 1900 IU/kg or 570 RE/kg. In summer, butter contains more yellow coloring due to unconverted carotene and has over 33,000 IU/kg. Margarine is usually fortified with vitamin A (usually as retinyl palmitate) to a level of 30,000 IU/kg, or 10,000 RE/kg.

Vitamin A is present in the fat portion of milk and so is absent from nonfat milk. Most fresh fluid nonfat milk and dried nonfat milk solids, however, are fortified with preformed vitamin A to an average of 500 IU (148 RE)/cup. Apart from milk products, egg yolks, and liver, other animal foods contain virtually no vitamin A.

Fruits and vegetables contain no preformed vitamin A, only precursors. Cereals and grain products generally supply little, if any, vitamin A.

The vitamin A values for foods of plant origin, for which carotenoid values are now included in some tables, depend on which precursors of vitamin A are present. In the past, carotenoids were considered primarily as vitamin A precursors, so interest in carotenoids was focused largely on those with provitamin A activity. Recent evidence, however, indicates that high carotenoid intakes from the consumption of fruits and vegetables—especially of carrots, tomatoes, and dark green vegetables—are associated with decreased risk of certain cancers and other chronic diseases. A carotenoid database has recently been compiled for the five most common carotenoids found in fruits and vegetables to enable researchers to further assess the correlation between fruit and vegetable intakes and disease risk in

TABLE 11-3

Vitamin A value of an average serving and per 100 kcal of foods frequently reported in dietary surveys, and some additional recommended sources

FOOD	AMOUNT	kcal	IU PER SERVING	IU PER 100 kcal	INQ*	RETINOL EQUIVALENT (RE)
MEAT, FISH, POULTRY, EGGS, NUTS						
Egg, fried	1 large	95	320	325	1.3	94
Beef, roast	3 oz	315	tr	tr		tr
Hamburger	3 oz	230	tr	tr		tr
Chicken	3 oz	140	20	14	0.5	5
Tuna	3 oz	165	70	42	0.2	20
Peanut butter	2 Tbsp	190	—	—	—	—
Bacon	3 slices	180	—	—	—	—
Beef liver†	3 oz	185	39,690	16,580	66	1920
CEREALS/BREAD						
Cornflakes	1 oz	110	—	—	—	—
Shredded wheat	1 biscuit	100	—	—	—	—
Saltines (10 g)	4 crackers	50	—	—	—	—
Rice (cooked)	½ cup	109	—	—	—	—
White bread	1 slice	65	tr	tr	—	—
Whole wheat bread	1 slice	70	tr	tr	—	—
DAIRY PRODUCTS						
Whole milk	8 oz	150	310	192	1.0	76
2% fat milk	8 oz	120	500	417	1.7	139
Cheddar cheese	1 oz	115	300	261	1.0	86
FRUITS						
Apple	1 medium	80	70	88	0.35	7
Banana	1 medium	105	90	86	0.34	9
Orange juice, frozen	4 oz	55	95	173	0.69	10
Peach	1 medium	35	470	1343	5.40	47
Cantaloupe†	½ of a 5″ melon	45	8610	9063	81.0	861
VEGETABLES						
Corn, canned	4 oz (½ cup)	83	255	310	1.2	26
Green beans	4 oz (½ cup)	22	235	1208	4.2	24
Green peas	4 oz (½ cup)	62	655	1129	4.5	65
Lettuce (100 g)	¼ head	20	446	2448	9.8	46
Tomatoes	1 medium	25	1390	5560	22.0	139
Potato, baked	1 medium	130	0	0	0	0
Broccoli†	½ cup	25	1090	4360	17	190
Spinach, cooked†	½ cup	20	7370	10,425	146	737
Carrots†	½ cup	35	19,150	54,714	219	1915

Tr, trace; —, none.

* Index of nutrient quality (INQ) based on daily value for vitamin A = 5000 international units (IU); energy need = 2000 kcal; INQ = % Daily value (5000 IU)/% Energy need (2000 kcal); INQ ≥ 2.0 = nutrient-dense source.

† Recommended sources in addition to most frequently mentioned foods in dietary surveys.

terms of specific intakes of various carotenoids.[13] Table 11-4 lists the carotenoid contents of selected fruits and vegetables.

The carotenoid database was used to estimate intakes of specific carotenoids for women aged 19 to 50 years old using dietary data collected as part of the U.S. Department of Agriculture Continuing Survey of Food Intake of Individuals, 1986. The per capita carotenoid (α-carotene, β-carotene, β-cryptoxanthin, lycopene, lutein, and zeaxanthin) consumption among the surveyed populations was 6 mg/day. Intakes of individual carotenoids ranged from 0.03 mg/day for

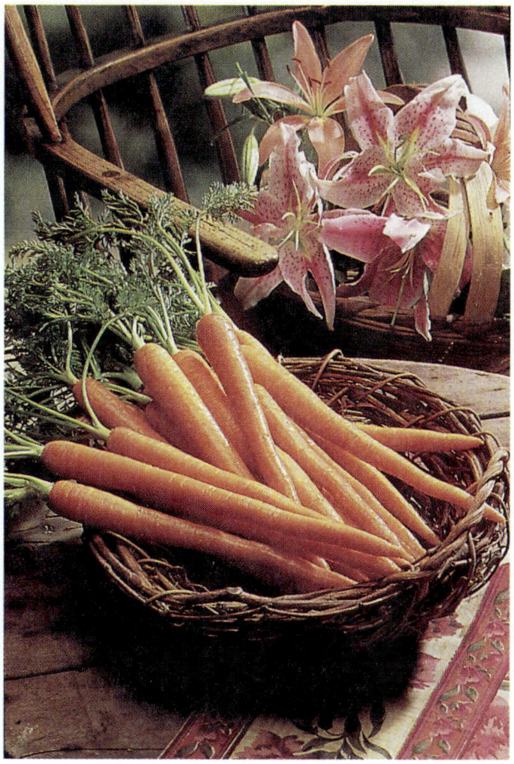

The deeper the color of vegetables, the higer the vitamin A content.

β-cryptoxanthin to 2.6 mg/day for lycopene. Mean intakes of α-carotene, β-carotene, and lutein were 0.4, 1.8, and 1.3 mg/day, respectively. The major food contributing to the α-carotene intake of women in this survey was carrots. Carrots, cantaloupe, and broccoli were the main sources of β-carotene. Orange juice, oranges, and tangerines were important contributors of β-cryptoxanthin. Tomatoes and tomato products provided most of the dietary lycopene. Contributors of lutein and zeaxanthin included spinach and broccoli. Foods particularly rich in carotenoids (such as mangoes, kale, and parsley) are not major contributors to intakes because they are infrequently consumed in the United States. HANES III data show that women have intakes of 400 to 600 RE of carotene. Comparable intakes for men are 550 to 600 RE.

The vitamin A value of fruits and vegetables is directly proportional to the color caused by either the carotene or chlorophyll in the food. So, in general, the deeper the orange, yellow, or green color of fruits and vegetables, the higher the vitamin A value. Also, in such vegetables as lettuce, which has bleached inner layers surrounded by increasingly green outer layers, the vitamin A value of the greenest parts can be 10 times greater than that of the most bleached parts. Unfortunately, a high concentration of chlorophyll is often accompanied by an astringent, bitter taste, as found in dark green romaine lettuce leaves. This means that some potentially rich sources of vitamin A are unpalatable to most tastes. In some fruits, such as mangoes, the vitamin A content increases with storage.

FIGURE 11-7

Contributions of various food groups to the vitamin A content of the North American food supply.

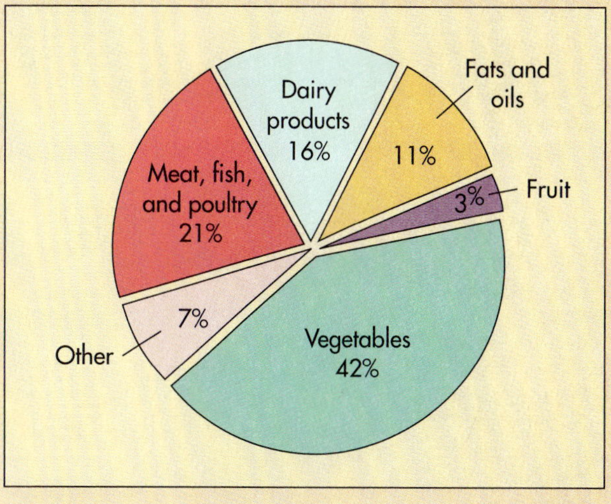

The pigments lycopene, found in watermelon and tomatoes, and zeaxanthin, found in corn, do not have vitamin A value. In countries where red palm oil (with 23 RE/g of vitamin A) is used in cooking, its carotene content is a major source of vitamin A activity.

Vitamin A and the carotenoids are stable on exposure to moderate heat and alkali but unstable in the presence of light, acids, and a variety of oxidizing agents. This means that little vitamin A is lost during most normal food preparation processes. Extremely hot frying oils may cause the destruction of a portion of the carotenoids present, as does the oxidation that occurs when fats turn rancid. The drying of fruits in sunlight, and any other form of dehydration, may lead to some loss of vitamin A activity. The small amount of yellow and green pigment that can leach into cooking water from fruits and vegetables represents an insignificant loss, if any, of vitamin A activity from the food.

The contributions of various food groups to the vitamin A content of the North American diet are shown in Figure 11-7. The relative amounts of vitamin A in typical servings of various foods are shown in Figure 11-8.

In the United States the average daily intake of vitamin A for adult men is about 1200 RE, one third of which comes from vegetable sources. In Canada the corresponding figure is 1500 RE, and in Britain it is 1800 RE. In all these countries the intakes of adult women average 75% to 85% of the adult male values.

DEFICIENCY

Deficiencies in vitamin A occur most often, but not exclusively, in preschool children. Vitamin A deficiency remains a major problem in large areas of the developing

TABLE 11-4

Carotenoid contents of selected fruits and vegetables (μg/g)

	β-CAROTENE	α-CAROTENE	LUTEIN AND ZEAXANTHIN	LYCOPENE	β-CRYPTOXANTHIN
Apricots, raw	3524	0	0	5	0
Cantaloupe, raw	3000	35	0	0	0
Grapefruit, pink, raw	1310	0	0	3362	0
Orange juice	7	6	74	0	24
Mango, raw	1300	0	0	0	54
Peach, raw	99	1	14	0	42
Papaya, raw	99	0	—	0	470
Tangerine, juice	8	5	135	—	214
Broccoli, cooked	1300	—	1800	—	—
Carrots, cooked, canned, frozen	9800	3700	—	0	—
Corn, yellow	51	50	780	0	—
Kale	4700	—	21,900	—	—
Romaine lettuce	1900	—	—	—	—
Parsley, not dried	5300	0	10,200	0	—
Peppers, green	230	11	700	0	—
Peppers, red	2200	60	—	—	—
Peppers, yellow	150	92	770	0	—
Pumpkin	3100	3800	1500	0	—
Spinach	5500	—	12,600	—	—
Squash, winter	2400	12	38	—	0
Sweet potato	8800	0	—	0	—
Swiss chard	3647	45	—	—	—
Tomato, raw	520	—	100	3100	—
Tomato sauce, canned	1000	—	—	—	—
Watermelon, raw	230	1	14	4100	—

0, Carotenoid not detected by analytical method employed; —, no acceptable analytical values found.

From Mangels AR and others: *J Am Diet Assoc* 93:284, 1993.

world and is estimated to affect 20 to 40 million children worldwide. In many cases the diet includes fruits and vegetables rich in vitamin A precursors, but the fat intake is so low (less than 10% of kilocalories) that the carotenoids are not absorbed. The symptoms begin to appear once the liver's reserves of vitamin A have been used up. Symptoms of vitamin A deficiency can also appear as a result of a deficiency of protein or zinc because a variety of proteins are involved in the transport and metabolism of vitamin A and zinc is required to mobilize vitamin A from the liver.

In general, the symptoms of vitamin A deficiency can result from low dietary intakes, interference with the absorption or storage of the vitamin, or interference with the conversion of precursors into vitamin A. Most of the symptoms (which have been mentioned already and are reviewed below) reflect the vitamin's role in maintaining the health of epithelial cells, with the eyes being particularly affected.

Visual Manifestations

One of the earliest symptoms of vitamin A deficiency is night blindness, which—as discussed previously—is an inability of the eye to see in dim lighting after exposure to bright lights. This is caused by insufficient supplies of vitamin A to reform the pigment rhodopsin in the retina.

The **cornea** of the eye (its outer transparent layer) is also affected early in the course of vitamin A deficiency. The tear glands fail to produce tears, leading to a drying out of the thin film of fluid that normally covers the cornea. This leads to keratinization of the epithelial cells of the cornea; the sloughing off of some of the cells; a developing opacity of the cornea, leading to defective vision; and the eventual rupture of the cornea. Infection then sets in, pus is released, and the eye begins to bleed (hemorrhages). These effects of vitamin A deficiency on the eye are known as **xerophthalmia.** In its mildest form, xerophthalmia produces what are known as **Bitot's spots** in the conjunctiva of the eye (Figure 11-9, *A*). In moderately severe form, a condition known as **xerosis conjunctiva** develops (Figure 11-9, *B*). The most severe, advanced stage of the effect of vitamin A deficiency on the eye is known as **keratomalacia**, in which irreversible scars occur in the cornea that can cause blindness.

Total blindness is a common outcome of vitamin A deficiency, especially in children, and is the leading cause of blindness in people under 21 years of age. Vitamin A deficiency is estimated to be responsible for 250,000 cases of permanent blindness per year in children in developing countries. Many children probably succumb to other manifestations of vitamin A deficiency before

FIGURE 11-8

Relative amounts of vitamin A in various food sources.

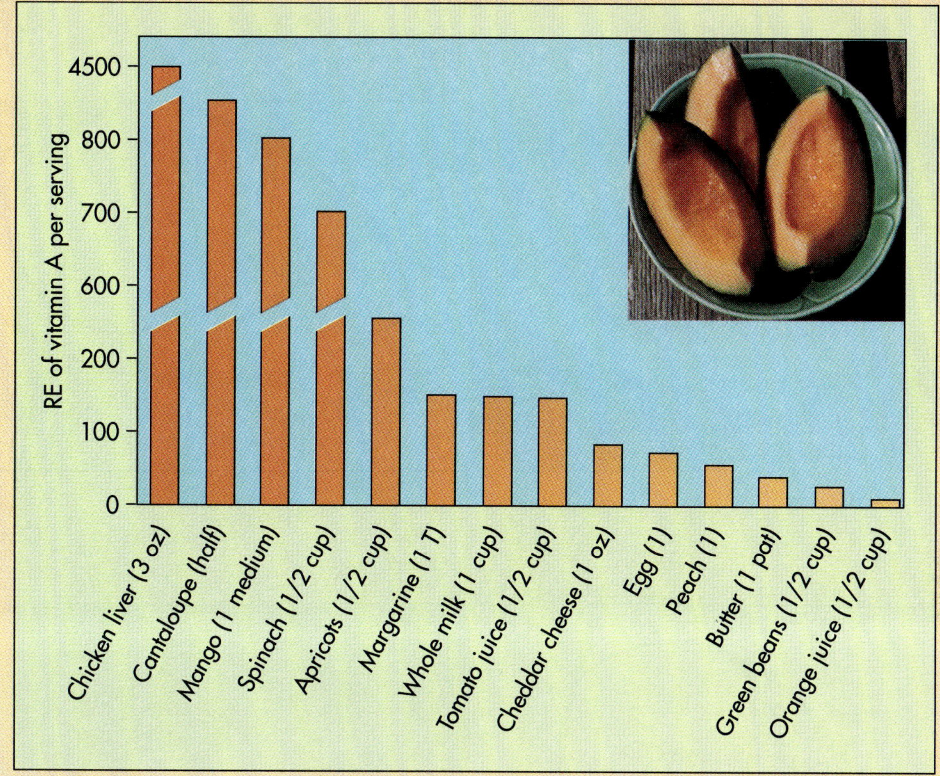

xerophthalmia develops. An infection, such as measles, usually precedes xerophthalmia, with the added stress of the infection making the child more susceptible to vitamin A deficiency and eventual blindness.

Nonvisual Manifestations

One of the most significant nonvisual manifestations of vitamin A deficiency is an increased susceptibility to infection. This is not surprising because vitamin A is known to be required for the proper activity of the immune system, which defends us against infection. Once an infection has taken hold, it can aggravate a preexisting vitamin A deficiency, placing the individual at even greater risk of further infections and perhaps eventual death. It has been shown that carotenoids can effectively stimulate the immune response in animals that are deficient in vitamin A, and this property is shared by both vitamin A–precursor carotenoids and those that are not precursors of vitamin A. This implies that the carotenoids do not need to act as a source of vitamin A to have their beneficial effect. Exactly *how* they stimulate the immune system is unknown, but it may well involve their role as antioxidants.

Children with mild xerophthalmia are known to be at increased risk of respiratory infections and diarrhea. Supplementation of vitamin A has been shown to reduce the prevalence of the infections and diarrhea and lead to increased growth rates.[14] It is also known that vitamin A deficiency is a significant factor in the course and severity of measles in developing countries. In these countries measles is a serious disease that causes about two million deaths every year. In Tanzania, controlled clinical trials have shown that giving extra vitamin A to infants and children with measles results in decreased severity of the disease and a decreased rate of death from it. The presence of a measles virus infection probably causes a depletion of the body's stores of vitamin A by increasing the use of vitamin A and so compounding the problems caused by decreased dietary intake and absorption of the vitamin. As mentioned previously, measles infections often precede the development of the effects on the eye of vitamin A deficiency.

The WHO and United Nations International Children's Emergency Fund (UNICEF) have jointly recommended that high oral doses of vitamin A should be given to all children suffering from measles in communities that are known to be at risk of vitamin A deficiency. Also, vitamin A should be given to all children with measles in countries where the death rate from measles is 1% or higher.[15]

In infants and laboratory animals vitamin A deficiency has been associated with increased concentrations

FIGURE 11-9

Development of symptoms of vitamin A deficiency affecting the eye. The first symptom is night blindness, followed by the occurrence of Bitot's spots on the conjunctiva (A). As the disease progresses, the conjunctiva becomes dry and rough, a condition known as xerosis conjunctiva (B), which can give way to keratomalacia and eventual blindness.

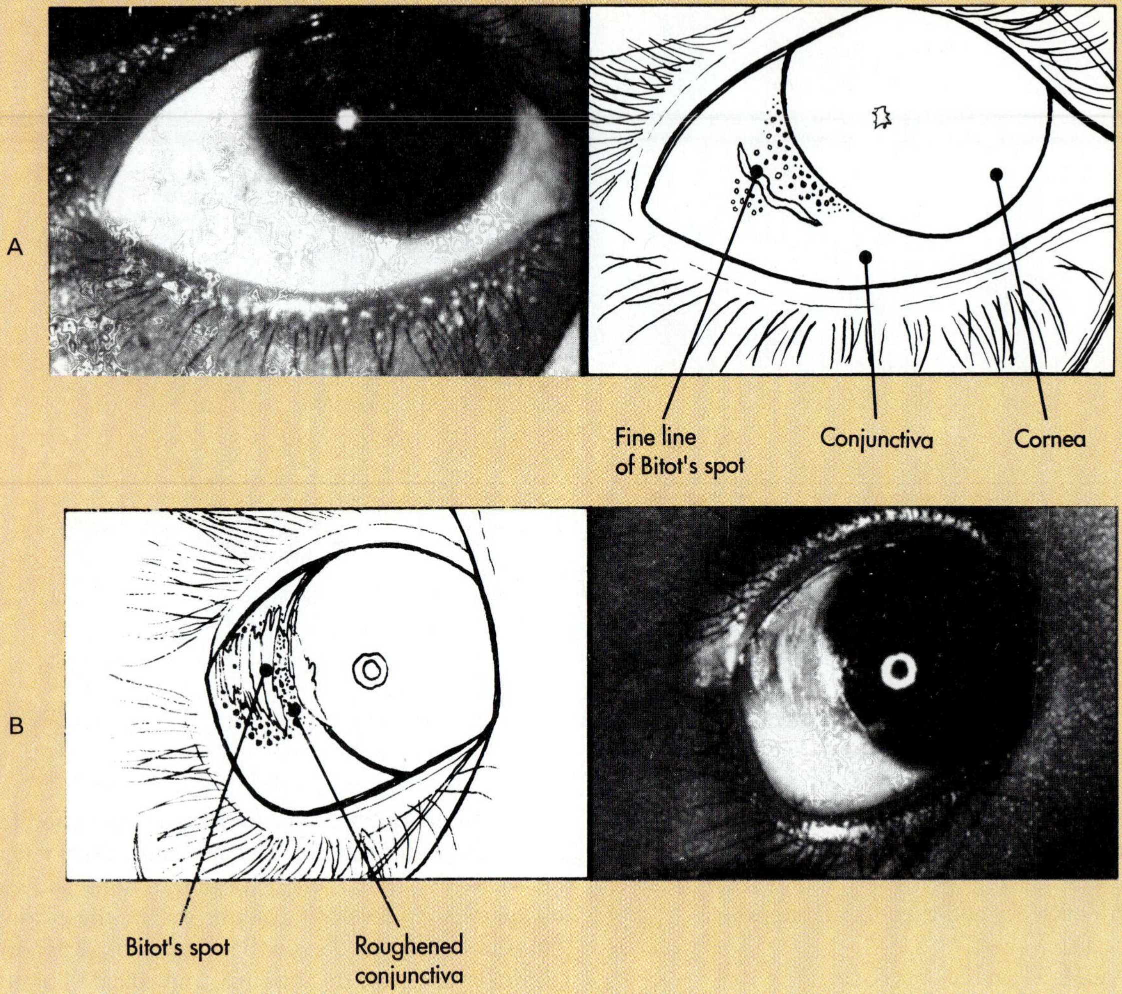

of iron in the liver and spleen. It is also known that administering vitamin A to individuals with a vitamin A deficiency is followed by a rise in serum iron levels, increased saturation of transferrin, and increased hemoglobin levels. The increase in the hemoglobin level occurs in children in as few as 2 weeks after a single large oral dose of vitamin A. The speed of this response suggests that increased absorption of iron is not the main explanation for it.[16] Instead, it is suggested that vitamin A deficiency may be associated with a failure to mobilize stored iron properly, although that may only be one of several ways in which vitamin A deficiency interferes with iron metabolism. Other possibilities are that vitamin A deficiency could directly prevent normal differentiation of red blood cells or that infections brought on by the impaired immunity of individuals with vitamin A deficiency could interfere with the normal functioning of the bone marrow tissue responsible for generating red blood cells.

In summary, vitamin A deficiency is a contributing factor in the deaths of large numbers of children in many parts of the developing world. Several studies have shown that death rates among infants and small children can be significantly reduced by the administration of vitamin A supplements.[17,18]

ADEQUACY OF DIETARY INTAKES

Data from the Nationwide Food Consumption Survey indicate that the average intake of vitamin A in the United States is 134% of the RDA. This is shown to be somewhat misleading, however, by the finding that only

50% of the individuals evaluated had dietary intakes meeting the RDA, and 30% had intakes below 70% of the RDA. Thus large intakes by a minority of the population produce an average intake figure that masks the fact that much of the population is failing to meet the RDA for vitamin A.

Data from the National Health and Nutrition Examination Survey (NHANES II) study found an average (mean) intake of 98% of the RDA but a median intake of only 3300 IU. A pattern of substantial inadequacy of dietary vitamin A was also found 10 years after the study in results from a survey of women, children, and men. NHANES III (1988-1991) data revealed that the average intakes of 700 to 900 RE (4600 to 6000 IU) for women and 1025 to 1245 RE (6600 to 7700 IU) for men exceeded the RDA of 800 RE and 1000 RE, respectively. The wide variation in intakes undoubtedly means that many people have vitamin A intakes below recommended levels.

There is little evidence of night blindness or other symptoms of vitamin A deficiency in the United States, but about 5% of U.S. children between the ages of 3 and 5 years have unacceptably low levels of vitamin A in blood serum or plasma. In the United States the minimal adequate level of serum or plasma vitamin A is set at 10 μg/100 ml. Values below this level indicate a state of **hypovitaminosis A** (too little vitamin A in the blood). Hypovitaminosis A is rarely found in U.S. citizens who are over 11 years of age.

> ***Hypovitaminosis*** is a general term for the condition in which the level of a vitamin in blood serum or plasma is too low. **Hypervitaminosis** is a general term for the condition in which the level of a vitamin in blood serum or plasma is too high. The specific vitamin involved in either condition can be specified by placing the letter identifying the vitamin after the general term, as in **hypovitaminosis A,** for example.

PROGRAMS FOR THE PREVENTION OF DEFICIENCY

Several countries in which vitamin A deficiency is common have supplementation programs to add vitamin A to a commercially processed staple food. In Central America the vitamin is added to white cane sugar, whereas in the Philippines it is added to monosodium glutamate. These programs have been effective in reducing the incidence of vitamin A deficiency. Programs to encourage the home production of fruits and vegetables rich in vitamin A or to promote the use of red palm oil in cooking have been considerably less successful.

India has a program that provides each child under 5 years of age with a single dose of 100,000 IU (30,000 RE) of vitamin A in oil dropped directly onto the tongue every 6 months by a health professional. This has produced an impressive reduction in the incidence of vitamin A deficiency. Unfortunately, however, about 35% of children are missed by this program because of difficulties in administering it within such a large population spread over a large area. An earlier program in India based on the administration of vitamin A in tablet form was considerably less successful.

EVALUATION OF VITAMIN A STATUS

Various methods for the evaluation of vitamin A status are available, of varying sensitivity and complexity.

Liver Vitamin A Concentration

The most sensitive indicator of vitamin A status is the measurement of vitamin A stores in the liver by analysis of a small piece of liver tissue removed by biopsy. This is not a feasible method for the evaluation of large numbers of people to obtain an estimate of the vitamin A status of communities or populations. Liver vitamin A concentrations in excess of 20 μg/g of wet liver are considered to indicate a sufficiency of vitamin A in the body as a whole. Concentrations lower than 5 μg/g of wet liver indicate that a person is at high risk of suffering the clinical consequences of vitamin A deficiency.

Serum Vitamin A

Serum vitamin A concentration can be used as an indicator of vitamin A status, although it is a less sensitive test than is the liver vitamin A concentration. The concentration of vitamin A in serum does not fall until the stores of the vitamin in the liver have been depleted. One factor making serum vitamin A concentration a useful test is that it is affected only slightly by day-to-day variations in dietary vitamin A intake. A serum vitamin A concentration below 10 μg/dl strongly suggests a state of vitamin A deficiency. Unfortunately, serum vitamin A concentrations considerably higher than this value can also be found in people who are suffering from vitamin A deficiency. For example, serum vitamin A concentrations as high as 20 μg/dl have occasionally been found in people whose liver vitamin A concentration has been less that 20 μg/g and who are therefore almost certainly deficient in vitamin A.

The Relative Dose Response Test

In the **relative dose response test,** a small amount of vitamin A is given by mouth or intravenously after a period of fasting and the change in serum vitamin A concentration that occurs in response to this dose is monitored over several hours before serum vitamin A returns to initial low levels. In people with adequate vitamin A status, only a modest and short-lived increase in serum vitamin A concentration occurs. In people with poor vitamin A status the increase in serum vitamin A concentration is significantly greater and a longer time elapses before the concentration returns to the initial level. The difference between the fasting serum vitamin A concentration and the concentration 5 hours after the dose of vitamin A is divided by the fasting concentration to obtain a value known as the **relative dose response.** It can be expressed as a percentage value by multiplying the result of this calculation by 100. The relative dose response gives an accurate indication of the concentration of vitamin A in the liver. A relative dose response of 20% or more suggests that a person's liver vitamin A concentration is less than 20 μg/g, indicating that he or she is probably suffering from vitamin A deficiency.

The vitamin A supplied in the relative dose response test has traditionally been in the form of the retinyl ester, retinyl acetate. A simplified modification of the traditional test uses an oral dose of the acetate ester of 3,4-didehydroretinol. Because this vitamin A derivative is not naturally present in the blood, only a single sample of serum need be taken 5 hours after the dose. The fasting concentration can be assumed to be zero without the need for an initial sample to be taken.

Conjunctival Impression Cytology

In **conjunctival impression cytology,** a piece of filter paper is brought briefly into contact with the conjunctiva of the eye and then removed. Some cells adhere to the paper, and these can be examined under the microscope after suitable fixing and staining. In this way the cell changes characteristic of **xerosis conjunctiva** can be identified before this symptom of vitamin A deficiency becomes apparent during a normal eye examination. Although this relatively new method shows some promise, it is difficult to obtain a suitable sample of cells from children younger than 3 years of age. Unfortunately, this is the group of people at high risk of vitamin A deficiency in developing countries.

CLINICAL USES OF VITAMIN A AND RELATED CAROTENOIDS

Treatment of Acne

Vitamin A has been widely used in attempts to treat acne, but until recently the results had been disappointing. The traditional approach has been the use of high oral doses or the topical application of retinol or retinal. More recently, however, treatments based on retinoic acid have met with considerable success. The topical application of retinoic acid (in the all-*trans* configuration) has proved effective in the treatment of some types of acne and in reducing wrinkling caused by overexposure to sunlight. Topical application and oral doses of a synthetic form of retinoic acid (13-cis-retinoic acid) have also met with dramatic success in the treatment of several common forms of acne. However, retinoic acid—whether naturally occurring or synthetic—should be used only under strict medical supervision. Because it may cause birth defects, it should not be used either by pregnant women or by women at any risk of pregnancy.

> Women taking oral doses of **cis-retinoic acid (Accutane)** to treat acne should stop taking it several months before they expect to become pregnant because its use is associated with developmental defects in infants. Similarly, pregnant women should not take supplements with more than 5000 IU of vitamin A.

Two synthetic analogs of vitamin A, **retinoyl-beta-glucuronide** and **hydroxyphenyl retinamide,** are currently being tested in clinical trials for the treatment of acne and other skin disorders. These conjugated derivatives of vitamin A retain their therapeutic action and show little or no toxicity.

Possible Health Benefits of β-carotene and Other Carotenoids

A large number of studies have suggested that β-carotene and other carotenoids offer protection against a variety of serious degenerative diseases, especially cancer, cardiovascular disease, and cataracts. β-carotene is found in a wide range of foods (Table 11-4), and in contrast to preformed vitamin A, high levels of consumption are not associated with toxicity. In the U.S. the National Cancer Institute (NCI) and the Department of Agriculture (USDA) recommend consumption of carotenoid-containing vegetables and fruits.[18] At present, it is uncertain whether the protective effects are from β-carotene alone, a combination of β-carotene and some other carotenoids that do not have vitamin A activity, or other factors in food rich in carotenoids. Future research should clarify this issue.

Cancer More than 50 epidemiological studies have found that a high intake of foods rich in β-carotene is correlated with a reduced risk of certain cancers. The most definite correlation is with reduced risk of lung cancer, but β-carotene has also been associated with reduced risk of cancers of the female reproductive system, gastrointestinal system, and mouth, gums, and trachea. These are all cancers of epithelial cells.

In clinical trials of the value of β-carotene, it has been shown to reverse "precancerous lesions" (the changes in cell growth known to precede the development of true cancers), especially those involved in the development of oral cancers. Preformed vitamin A, in contrast to β-carotene, has not been consistently found to offer protection against any types of cancer except at near toxic dosages.[18]

Although most attention has been focused on β-carotene, the beneficial effects attributed to β-carotene may in some cases be due to other carotenoids or may be shared by all carotenoids. It is relevant, however, that reduced risk of lung cancer correlates more strongly with the consumption of orange and yellow vegetables rich in β-carotene than with consumption of fruits and vegetables rich in other carotenoids. A continuing program of randomized clinical trials provides further evidence of the role of β-carotene and other carotenoids in the prevention of cancer. At this time, the preventative effects can be related only to the consumption of fruits and vegetables and not to any specific factor in fruits and vegetables.

Cardiovascular disease β-carotene may also be an important nutritional weapon in the fight against cardiovascular disease. Supplemental intake of β-carotene has been shown to reduce the incidence of angina in a small sample of men who had previously had heart attacks. Another study has found that women who consumed 15 to 20 mg/day of β-carotene had a significantly lower risk of stroke or heart attack than did women who reported consumption of less than 6 mg/day.

Cataracts Cataracts are areas of opacity in the lens of the eye. Their formation has been linked to damage by oxidizing agents and free radicals (highly reactive chemical species, including an unpaired electron). In one large study the risk of developing cataracts was found to be inversely related to serum carotenoid levels. Those people with low serum carotenoid levels had more than 5½ times the risk of developing cataracts than those with high serum carotenoid levels. Although the lens of the eye contains little β-carotene, it has been suggested that β-carotene may protect against cataracts simply by decreasing the level of oxidative damage in the body as a whole.

TOXICITY

The possibility that vitamin A may be toxic has been recognized for some time. Symptoms of vitamin A toxicity have been reported after the consumption of polar bear liver (with 6000 RE/g of vitamin A), after the treatment of adolescent skin disorders with vitamin A, and as a result of the administration of high levels of supplemental vitamin A to infants. In adults the symptoms of vitamin A toxicity are headaches, drowsiness, nausea, loss of hair, dry skin, diarrhea, rapid resorption of bone, and the cessation of menstruation in women. The symptoms in infants are scaly dermatitis, weight loss, anorexia, bulging of the head, hydrocephalus, hyperirritability, and skeletal pain.

The symptoms of toxicity set in within 6 to 15 months after the period of high vitamin A intake begins. Some adults exhibit symptoms of toxicity on receiving long-term dosages of 16,000 RE/day, whereas others do not suffer from any symptoms unless their intake is as high as 40,000 to 55,000 RE/day. Infants have exhibited bulging of the head, hydrocephalus, increased intracranial pressure, and hyperirritability after doses of 8000 RE/day for as few as 30 days.

Recovery from vitamin A toxicity proceeds rapidly after the vitamin is withdrawn. Symptoms often subside in as few as 72 hours. It is rare for an episode of vitamin A toxicity to cause permanent damage. There is some concern, however, that long-standing daily intakes of 25,000 RE or more of vitamin A by pregnant women may damage the fetus. In animal studies, single injections of vitamin A in pregnant females have produced cleft palates in their offspring.

Amounts of vitamin A sufficient to cause symptoms of toxicity in adults, children, and infants are readily available in over-the-counter supplements. This makes the possibility of vitamin A toxicity an ever-present danger, because of the tendency of many people to oversupplement their diet. The FDA is concerned about the effects of vitamin A toxicity but has been unsuccessful in its attempts to impose a ceiling of 25,000 RE for the amount of preformed vitamin A that can be included in a nonprescription multivitamin preparation.

Problems of toxicity occur only from the use of preformed vitamin A, not from the consumption of any vitamin A precursors. Consumption of carotene, for example, has never been associated with any problems, even at high levels of intake. A possible explanation may be that as intakes of β-carotene increase, percentage of absorption decreases. The storage of carotenes in subcutaneous fat can give the skin a yellow color, especially on the soles of the feet and palms of the hands. This condition is called **carotenodermia,** but it is completely harmless. It can be distressing, however, especially to the parents of young children who develop the condition.

VITAMIN D

Vitamin D is best known for its ability to cure **rickets,** a condition associated with defective bone formation, especially in infants (Figure 11-10). It has

FIGURE 11-10

Typical case of rickets in a young girl (right), as compared with a normal child.

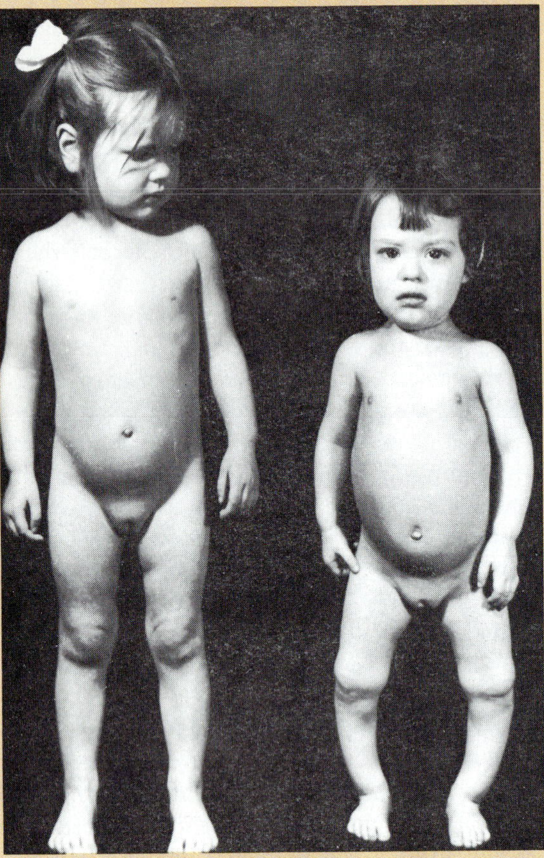

long been known that rickets can be avoided and treated by regular consumption of cod liver oil or by frequent exposure to sunlight. The active substance responsible for preventing or treating rickets was originally called vitamin D, although it is now known that—unlike other vitamins—it can be produced in the body on exposure to sufficient sunlight. For this reason, vitamin D also became known as "the sunshine vitamin." It has also been known as the **antirachitic factor,** or **rickets-preventive factor,** because of its ability to prevent rickets (*rachitic,* having rickets).

Vitamin D actually exists in two distinct forms in foods known as **cholecalciferol (vitamin D_3),** from animal products, and as **ergocalciferol (vitamin D_2),** mainly in vitamin D–fortified foods. Both forms are produced from precursors during the irradiation of animal or plant tissue by sunlight (Figure 11-11). Both forms of vitamin D can be described by the generic name **calciferol.**

Because vitamin D can be produced in the body, it is regarded by some scientists as a hormone. However, when vitamin D is supplied by the diet, it is technically a vitamin. Regardless of how it is classified, however, it is a substance that the body must have or that must be available in adequate amounts for the development of normal bones and teeth. It is also involved in the regulation of a variety of processes throughout the body.

DISCOVERY

In 1918 Sir Edward Mellanby presented evidence of a fat-soluble substance with antirachitic properties. Shortly afterward, the antirachitic properties of cod liver oil, which had been used as a folk remedy since the early nineteenth century, were properly recognized. Mellanby's fat-soluble substance and the active principle within cod liver oil were the same compound, which was soon designated as vitamin D by E.V. McCollum and associates at Johns Hopkins University. Unlike the earlier-discovered vitamin A, vitamin D was less susceptible to destruction by oxidation.

The precursors of vitamin D, 7-dehydrocholesterol in animals and ergosterol in plants, were discovered in 1922 (and are sometimes known as **provitamin D**). Vitamin D was isolated in crystalline form in 1932, and its chemical structure had been determined by 1936.

Most of the vitamin D used in supplements or in the fortification of food products is produced by the irradiation of vitamin D precursors. It is now possible, however, to synthesize two vitamin D derivatives that are even more effective in preventing several types of rickets than are the naturally occurring forms of the vitamin.

NOMENCLATURE AND VITAMIN D

The general terms *vitamin D* (with no subscript) and *calciferol* are used to refer to both vitamin D_2 (ergocalciferol) and vitamin D_3 (cholecalciferol) and to any combination of these two forms of the vitamin (Figure 11-11). When measurements are made of the concentration of vitamin D or calciferol within any food or tissue, they include the individual contributions of both vitamin D_2 and vitamin D_3 and also the contributions made by any active metabolites of vitamin D. Examples of such active metabolites are 25-hydroxyvitamin D; 24,25-dihydroxyvitamin D; and 1,25-dihydroxyvitamin D, which vary in the number and position of hydroxyl groups added to vitamin D.

The amount of vitamin D or one of its active metabolites is determined by measuring the amount required to elicit some biological response, such as intestinal calcium absorption or body growth. This has led to the standard IU of vitamin D being variously defined as follows:

1 IU OF VITAMIN D = 25 NANOGRAMS (25 NG) OF VITAMIN D
1 IU OF VITAMIN D = 5 NG OF 25-HYDROXYVITAMIN D
1 IU OF VITAMIN D = 5 NG OF 24,25-DIHYDROXYVITAMIN D
1 IU OF VITAMIN D = 1 NG OF 1,25-DIHYDROXYVITAMIN D

FIGURE 11-11

The structures and formation of vitamins D_2 and D_3 and their precursors.*

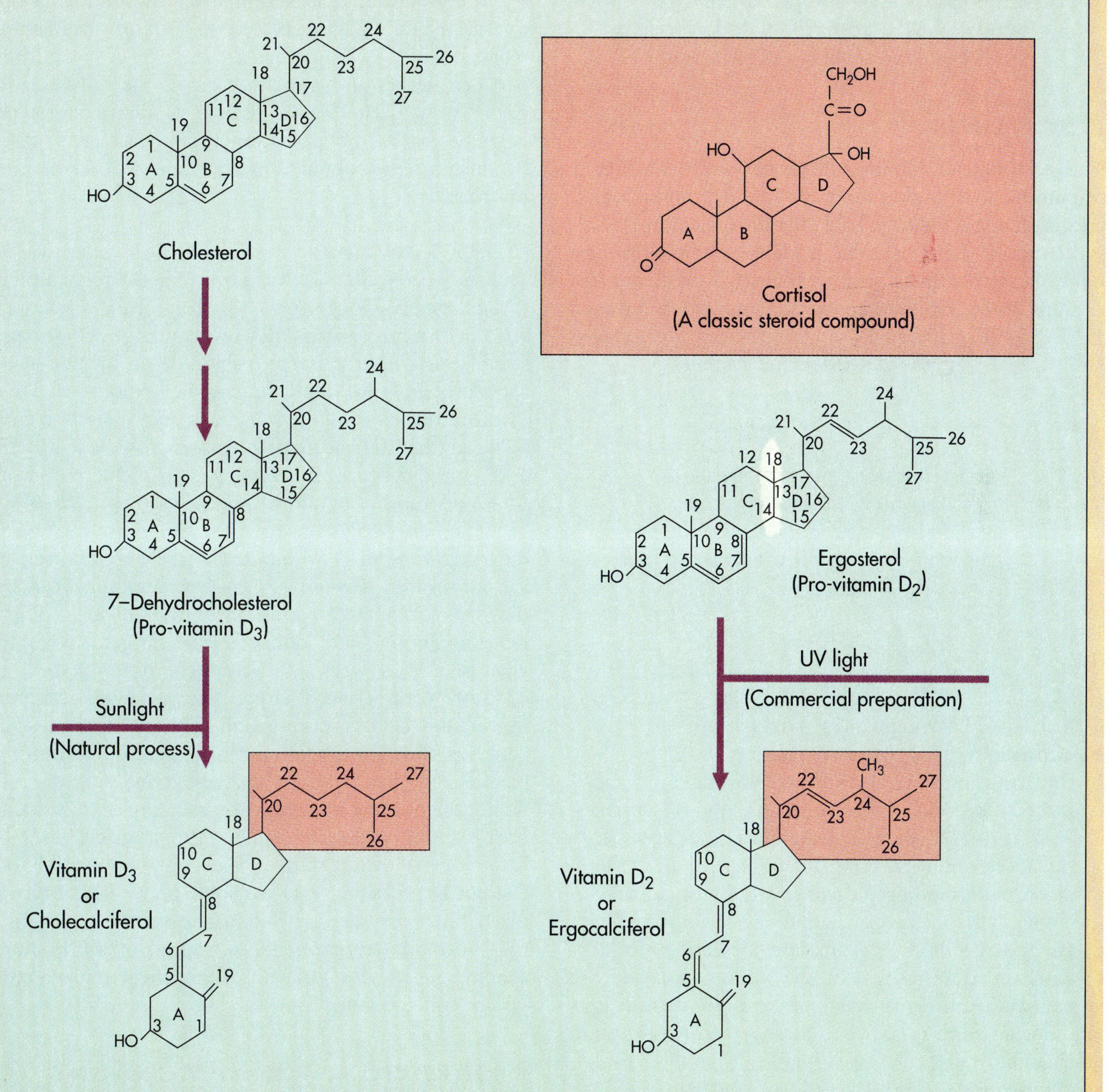

*The only structural differences between vitamin D_2 and D_3 are in the side chain: vitamin D_2 contains a double bond between carbons 22 and 23 and a methyl group at carbon 24 (see boxed areas).

Alternatively,

1 μg OF VITAMIN D = 40 IU OF VITAMIN D
1 μg OF 25-HYDROXYVITAMIN D = 200 IU OF VITAMIN D
1 μg OF 24,25-DIHYDROXYVITAMIN D = 200 IU OF VITAMIN D
1 μg OF 1,25-DIHYDROXYVITAMIN D = 1000 IU OF VITAMIN D

FUNCTIONS

The metabolite of vitamin D that is believed to be directly responsible for bringing about the vitamin's physiological effects on target tissues is 1,25-dihydroxyvitamin D. This is the specific metabolite that is often considered to be a hormone, rather than a vitamin. Indeed, the regulation of calcium homeostasis, involving the interaction between 1,25-dihydroxyvitamin D and parathyroid hormone, is known as **the vitamin D endocrine system.**[19]

> 1,25-dihydroxyvitamin D is the metabolite of vitamin D that is believed to be directly responsible for bringing about the vitamin's physiological effects on target tissues.

Calcium Homeostasis and Bone Formation and Maintenance

In the small intestine, 1,25-dihydroxyvitamin D facilitates the absorption of dietary calcium and phosphorus. This effect of 1,25-dihydroxyvitamin D is at least partly a result of its ability to stimulate an increase in the level of the calcium-binding protein in the intestinal cell. In the bone, 1,25-dihydroxyvitamin D acts together with parathyroid hormone to stimulate the mobilization of calcium and phosphorus. In the distal tubules of the kidney, 1,25-dihydroxyvitamin D and parathyroid hormone again work together to increase the reabsorption of calcium.

One major effect of 1,25-dihydroxyvitamin D in the body is to stimulate the mineralization of bone, probably mainly because of the stimulation of the absorption of dietary calcium and phosphorus. 1,25-dihydroxyvitamin D is not itself directly involved in bone mineralization, but it does have significant effects on osteoblasts (the bone-forming cells), which play an important role in bone formation. 1,25-dihydroxyvitamin D stimulates the role of the osteoblasts in the production of non-bone matrix proteins. It is involved in bone remodeling (essential for healthy bone condition) as an activator of the osteoclasts (bone-reabsorbing cells) and in facilitating the stimulating effect of parathyroid hormone on this bone reabsorption process.

The way in which 1,25-dihydroxyvitamin D and parathyroid hormone together regulate the concentration of calcium in blood plasma is summarized in Figure 11-12. As indicated, this is important not only for bone formation and maintenance, but also for maintaining blood calcium levels to facilitate the proper interactions between nerves and muscles. One of the most serious disorders associated with vitamin D deficiency is the convulsive state of **hypocalcemia tetany,** which is caused by insufficient supplies of calcium to nerves and muscles.[20]

Other Functions

1,25-dihydroxyvitamin D is involved in the regulation of specific genes. To perform this role, 1,25-dihydroxyvitamin D binds to a receptor protein in the cell nucleus, stimulating the protein (probably assisted by an "accessory protein") to bind to specific regions of DNA involved in controlling gene activity. It is currently believed that the accessory protein may be an RAR: RXR, some currently unknown protein, or perhaps both RXR and another unknown protein (see pp. 398-399).

The discovery of receptor proteins for 1,25-dihydroxyvitamin D within cell nuclei was followed by various studies demonstrating direct binding of 1,25-dihydroxyvitamin D within the nuclei of cells of the intestine, bone, and kidney (classic target tissues for vitamin D), as well as a variety of other tissues. In addition to the classical target tissues, nuclear receptors for vitamin D have been found in the islet cells of the pancreas, the parathyroid hormone–secreting cells of the parathyroid glands, bone marrow cells, specific cells within the ovaries, some brain cells, epithelial cells within breast tissue, endocrine cells of the stomach, and the keratinocytes of the skin. It is becoming apparent that vitamin D probably performs some previously unrecognized functions required for insulin secretion, parathyroid hormone secretion, the operation of the immune system, and the development of the female reproductive system and the skin.[20]

ABSORPTION, FORMATION, AND TRANSPORT

Absorption

Dietary vitamin D is absorbed in the small intestine with the aid of bile salts and is incorporated within chylomicrons, which take it through the lymph and then into the blood. The assistance of bile salts is also required for the absorption of active metabolites of vitamin D, such as 25-hydroxyvitamin D. If the secretion of bile salts is deficient for any reason, both ingested vitamin D and its active metabolites can be lost in feces, rather than being absorbed into the body.[21]

As a fat-soluble vitamin, the absorption of vitamin D is enhanced or depressed by the same factors that en-

FIGURE 11-12

Mechanism of plasma calcium regulation by vitamin D and parathyroid hormone.

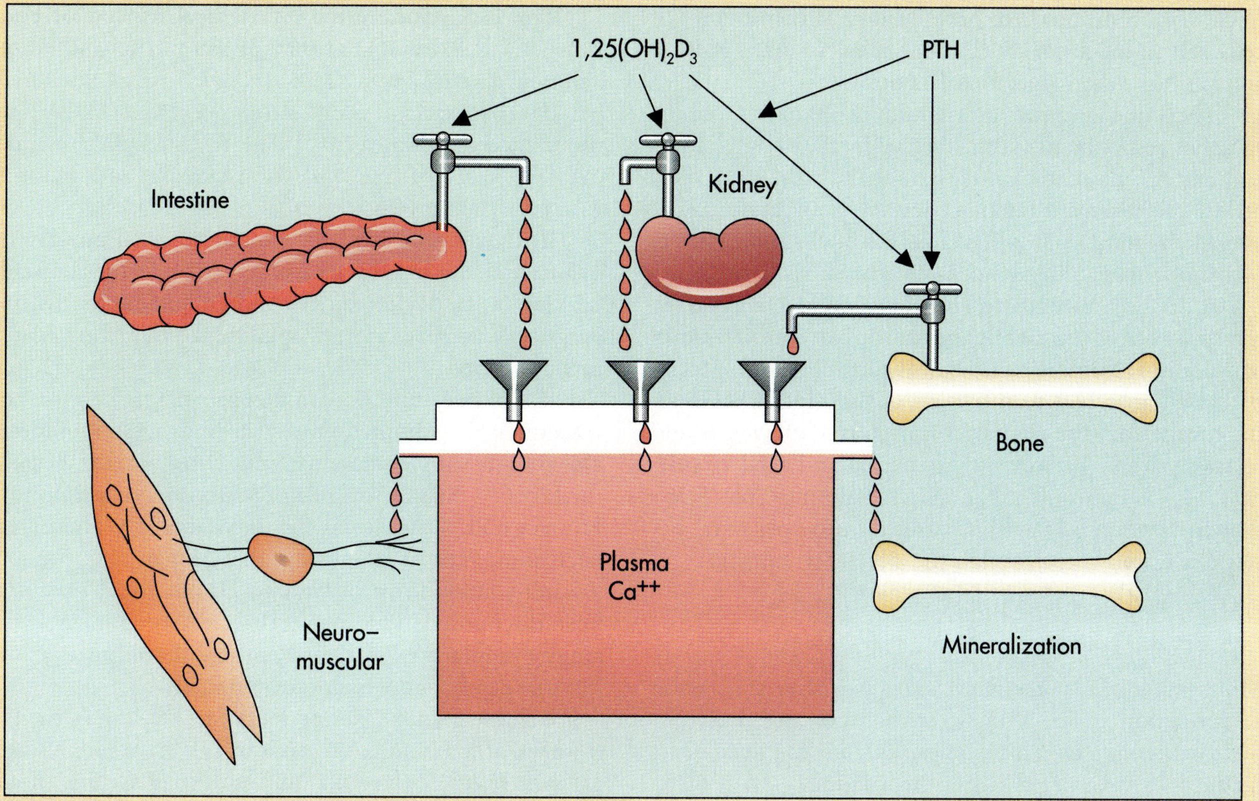

hance or depress the absorption of fats. An average of 80% of dietary vitamin D is absorbed by both infants and adults.

Formation

When the skin is exposed to ultraviolet radiation—most commonly, that in sunlight—7-dehydrocholesterol within the skin is converted into a compound known as provitamin D_3. This is then converted into vitamin D_3 (Figure 11-11) by a reaction that is greatly influenced by temperature. At normal body temperature, any provitamin D_3 produced by exposure to sunlight is converted into vitamin D within 2 to 3 days.

Provitamin D_3 is also sensitive to light, and the light-sensitive reactions can convert it to the biologically inactive compounds lumisterol and tachysterol. This probably explains why prolonged exposure to the sun is not associated with vitamin D toxicity. Although biologically inactive, lumisterol and tachysterol can be converted back into provitamin D_3 when the body's supplies of provitamin D_3 are low. This allows these compounds to serve as a form of vitamin D storage for as long as they remain in the skin.[22] If not converted back into previtamin D_3, they are eventually lost during the natural sloughing off of dead skin cells.

Obviously, the possibility for the synthesis of vitamin D within the body is greatest in areas of the world with most sunshine and at the sunniest times of the year. In Boston, for example, the average amount of sunlight is insufficient to produce significant vitamin D synthesis from November through February.[23] The degree of pigmentation of a person's skin is also an influence on the amount of vitamin D synthesized within him or her. Less vitamin D is synthesized in dark-skinned people exposed to the same amount of sunshine as fair-skinned people because the pigments within dark skin restrict the access of ultraviolet radiation. One consequence of this is that dark-skinned people living in northern industrialized cities are at particular risk of vitamin D deficiency.

In breast-fed infants the length of exposure to sunlight required to maintain normal serum concentrations of 25-hydroxyvitamin D has been estimated at 2 hours/week for the fully clothed but hatless infant and 30 minutes/week for an infant wearing only a diaper.[24]

Transport

Newly absorbed vitamin D is incorporated into chylomicrons and then transported into the lymphatic system. On release from lymph into the blood the vitamin D is removed from the chylomicrons and becomes bound to a specific **vitamin D–binding protein (DBP),** called **alpha-globulin$_2$.** This protein transports the vitamin D to the liver. DBP also binds to 1,25-dihydroxyvitamin D, as do various receptor proteins on the membranes of cells in the small intestine, distal tubules of the kidney, and various other organs and tissues.[19]

The concentration of vitamin D in blood plasma varies in response to recent dietary intake of vitamin D and any recent synthesis of vitamin D in the skin. This makes the plasma vitamin D level a poor indicator of overall vitamin D status. The half-life of vitamin D in the blood plasma is only about 24 hours.

A developing fetus receives its vitamin D largely by transport across the membranes of the placenta. The level of vitamin D within the umbilical cord blood appears to be closely matched to the levels in the mother's blood, suggesting that the vitamin is transported efficiently and relatively freely between the maternal and fetal circulation. It is possible that large amounts of 1,25-dihydroxyvitamin D are synthesized in the placenta, because it is known to contain the necessary enzymes.

METABOLISM

Most vitamin D is taken up by the liver after absorption or formation in the skin. It is then converted to 25-hydroxyvitamin D. This is released from the liver to be further hydroxylated in the kidney to 1,25-dihydroxyvitamin D and is the most biologically active forms of the vitamin, as can be seen by the relative amounts corresponding to 1 IU.

The most important point at which vitamin D metabolism is regulated is by control of the **vitamin D-1-hydroxylase** enzyme of the kidney, which converts 25-hydroxyvitamin D to 1,25-dihydroxyvitamin D. This point of control allows the production of 1,25-dihydroxyvitamin D to be modulated according to the calcium needs of the individual. The chief regulatory factors affecting the enzyme are 1,25-dihydroxyvitamin D itself, parathyroid hormone, and the serum concentration of calcium and phosphorus.

DIETARY REQUIREMENTS

Because variable amounts of vitamin D are made in the skin, it is difficult to estimate minimal dietary requirements for this vitamin. In general, however, 100 IU of vitamin D per day seems sufficient to protect against rickets and promote normal growth of the skeleton, provided that the diet also contains sufficient calcium and phosphorus. Daily vitamin D intakes between 300 and 400 IU (7.5 to 10 μg), however, seem to promote more effective calcium absorption. For this reason the RDA has been set at 10 μg/day for infants, children, adolescents, and pregnant and lactating women.[9] Intakes above 20 μg (800 IU)/day appear to provide no greater protection against rickets than does the recommended amount. For adults over 25 years of age, 5 μg/day is recommended.

The U.K. Committee on Medical Aspects of Food Policy has recommended that British infants and young children up to 2 years of age receive 7 μg of vitamin D per day but set no Daily Reference Value (DRV) for those aged 4 through 50.[11] The British DRV for those over 50 years of age and for pregnant and lactating women is 10 μg/day.

In Canada the RNI for vitamin D is 10 μg/day for infants and children up to 2 years old and varies between 2.5 and 5 μg/day for older children and adults. During pregnancy and lactation, a total intake of 7.5 μg/day is recommended.[10]

If fortified milk or commercial infant formulas are consumed, it is both unnecessary and possibly undesirable for any supplemental vitamin D to be taken because the fortified milk or formula provides adequate amounts. Human milk, however, is low in vitamin D. There have been some reports suggesting that human milk contains a water-soluble form of vitamin D, but these have now been discounted. This means that breast-fed infants who are not regularly exposed to sunshine should receive 5 to 7.5 μg/day of supplemental vitamin D.

Because a fetus takes up half of its calcium in the last 6 weeks of fetal life, premature infants have much lower calcium reserves than do full-term infants. This means that they need adequate vitamin D to ensure that they can quickly absorb the large amounts of calcium needed to promote rapid growth. Dosages of vitamin D as high as 400 IU/day have proved insufficient for breast-fed premature infants, but this may be because of the low calcium content of human milk, rather than an accurate indication of the premature infant's need for vitamin D.

During pregnancy and lactation the level of 1,25-dihydroxyvitamin D in a woman's blood plasma increases sharply. This increase results in an enhanced efficiency of absorption of calcium from the intestine and an increased mobilization of bone calcium to meet the needs of the developing fetus or breast-feeding infant.

FOOD SOURCES

In the temperate zone of the world the diet is the most reliable source of vitamin D, notably fortified foods. Foods of animal origin—such as eggs, milk, butter, and fish liver oils—are the major dietary sources of preformed vitamin D. Even the best food sources of vitamin D are somewhat unreliable sources, because their vitamin D content varies with the diets and breeds of the animals concerned. Most foods contain at least some cholecalciferol, and some also contain 25-hydroxycholecalciferol (that is, 25-hydroxyvitamin D), the metabolite of vitamin D that is normally formed in the liver. The vitamin D content of unfortified foods is listed in Table 11-5. Even

TABLE 11-5

Vitamin D content of unfortified foods

FOOD SOURCE	VITAMIN D (IU/100 g)
Beefsteak	13
Beet greens	0.2
Butter	35
Cabbage	0.2
Cheese	12
Cod	85
Cod liver oil	10,000
Corn oil	9
Cream	50
Egg yolk	25
Herring, canned	330
Herring liver oil	140,000
Liver, raw	
Beef	8-40
Calf	0-15
Pork	40
Chicken	50-65
Lamb	20
Mackerel	120
Milk	
Cow (100 ml)	0.3-4.0
Human (100 ml)	0-10
Salmon, canned	220-440
Sardines, canned	1500
Shrimp	150
Spinach	0.2

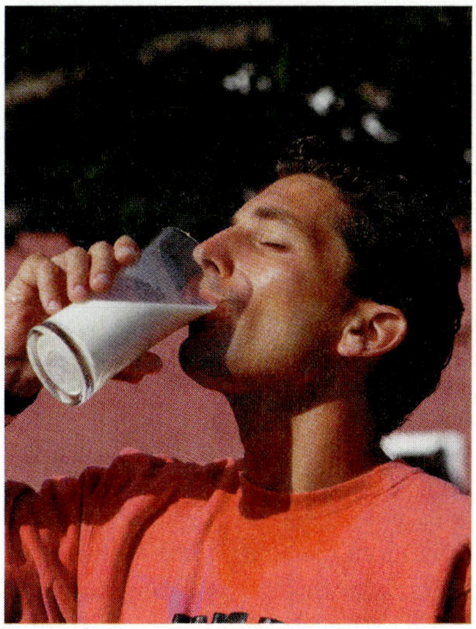

Fortified milk is a nutrient-dense source of vitamin D.

when all potential dietary sources of vitamin D are incorporated into a diet, it is possible to obtain only about 125 IU (3 μg) of dietary vitamin D per day. Because the RDA for vitamin D is set at 200-400 IU (5-10 μg), it is customary to rely on foods fortified in vitamin D or nutritional supplements to bring intakes up to the recommended level.

The food that is most commonly fortified with vitamin D is milk, a natural carrier of the calcium and phosphorus required for bone mineralization. Today 95% of homogenized milk, almost all nonfat milk, and a large proportion of dried nonfat milk solids contain added vitamin D (400 IU/qt). This means that most of the milk sold in North America is fortified with vitamin D at a level that allows the maximal use of the calcium and phosphorus within the milk. The cost of fortifying milk with vitamin D is relatively insignificant.

Although milk is the only product officially endorsed for fortification, vitamin D is also added by food manufacturers to many products, including infant cereals, prepared breakfast cereals, milk flavorings, bread, and some beverages. If a person consumed one serving of each of these products and 1 qt of fortified milk per day, his or her daily vitamin D intake could easily reach 1000 IU.

Assessing the amount of vitamin D actually present in a person's diet is difficult without access to the labels on the specific products consumed. In the United States, for example, flour producers can add between 250 and 1000 IU of vitamin D per pound (0.45 kg) of flour; so a person's vitamin D intake can vary considerably, depending on which manufacturer's flour is used in the bakery goods the person consumes. Although the addition of vitamin D to margarine is not allowed in the United States, in Britain it is required to be added at 1300 to 1600 IU/lb, and in Germany it must be added at 135 IU/lb.

In the temperate zone, pediatricians routinely introduce a supplementary source of vitamin D into the diet of infants. Cod liver oil, used since the early 1920s, has now been largely replaced by water-soluble vitamin D preparations (which also contain vitamin A and vitamin C). In 1965 in the United States, the Food and Drug Administration (FDA) imposed a mandatory limit of 400 IU per dose of any vitamin D supplement, although most manufacturers were voluntarily keeping to that limit by then. Labels of supplements usually carry a warning against excessive consumption of vitamin D.

EVALUATION OF VITAMIN D STATUS

The half-life of 25-hydroxyvitamin D in plasma is 3 to 7 weeks, and the plasma concentration of this metabolite of vitamin D appears to be a reliable indicator of the amount of vitamin D stored in the liver. Thus, the plasma 25-hydroxyvitamin D concentration is a good indicator of overall vitamin D status.

In infants with rickets caused by vitamin D deficiency, plasma 25-hydroxyvitamin D levels usually vary from less than 1 ng/ml to as much as 9 ng/ml. Normal levels are considered to be from 10 to 40 ng/ml.

Low plasma 25-hydroxyvitamin D levels are often found in institutionalized and homebound elderly persons. This suggests that the current RDA for vitamin D (5 μg/day) may be inadequate for these persons when they are deprived of exposure to sunlight. Calcium absorption decreases with age and loss of bone increases, and the effects of these changes could be at least partially offset by an increased intake of vitamin D. Levels of 1,25-dihydroxyvitamin D also fall with increasing age. All of these factors suggest that elderly persons may require greater amounts of dietary vitamin D than do young adults.[25, 26]

DEFICIENCY

The major problem associated with vitamin D deficiency is rickets. This condition has plagued infants in the temperate zone (where the climate changes through marked seasons) for centuries. It used to be so common in England that some writers referred to it as "the English disease" and believed it was caused by an environmental factor. The fact that rickets occurred frequently in people living in crowded, smoky, industrial areas of cities with poor sanitation led to the suggestion that it was caused by a bacterium. The children of the wealthy, however, were even more prone to rickets than those of the poor, which was evidence against the bacterial theory. From time to time it was suggested that exposure to sunshine could help prevent or treat rickets, but the truth of this relationship was not firmly established until the late 1920s.

As considered already, rickets is essentially a condition produced by defective bone formation and remodeling. Skeletal deformities develop when poorly mineralized bones prove insufficiently strong to perform their normal functions. The best-known deformity associated with rickets is the bowing of the legs that begins to develop as soon as a child begins to walk (Figure 11-12). The ends of the long bones also become enlarged, causing difficulties in movement. "Knock knees" can result from the flattening that occurs in the poorly mineralized ends of the bones. Deformities of the ribs produce a concave breast ("pigeon breast") that causes overcrowding of the chest cavity. The ribs also develop irregularly spaced swellings that look a bit like beads, sometimes described as "rachitic rosary." In infants, the **fontanel** (the gap between the bones at the top of the skull) fails to close in early life. This allows rapid enlargement of the head, which has sometimes been wrongly interpreted as a sign of good health, rather than of a nutritional problem. Teeth erupt later than normal, are less well formed, and are more susceptible to decay. General growth is retarded, although the severity of the other symptoms of the disease is often greatest in those affected children who have grown most quickly.

Rickets is primarily a disease of infancy and childhood. Many of the British and American cases of recurring rickets in the 1960s, for example, were identified in children aged 2 to 4 years when bowing of the legs and growth retardation became obvious. Deformities produced by rickets in childhood, however, can remain throughout adulthood.

Rickets was practically eradicated in the Western world by the mid-1920s, but it did reappear in the early 1960s. In Britain at that time, over 500 new cases of rickets were diagnosed and there were undoubtedly many more cases of less obvious "subclinical" rickets. Most of the people affected were immigrants whose dark skin pigmentation prevented sufficient ultraviolet light from penetrating their skin. The level of sunshine in their native countries would probably have produced sufficient vitamin D, but the amount available in Britain proved insufficient. In the United States an increased incidence of rickets has been reported during the past two decades. This is believed to be a result of the changing patterns of infant feeding and dietary preferences. In 56 of the 62 cases of rickets reported from 1980 to 1990, the patients belonged to vegetarian families. The vast majority of those vegetarians were on a macrobiotic diet devoid of meat products, milk products, fish, and eggs. In 26 of 27 infants in whom rickets was diagnosed in the first year of life, breast-feeding—rather than formula feeding—had been used.[27]

The term **adult rickets** is sometimes applied to the disease **osteomalacia,** which is associated with defective bone formation but not necessarily with vitamin D deficiency. Osteomalacia occurs most often in regions where cultural customs prevent women from exposing their skin to sunlight or where women bear and nurse children continuously throughout their fertile years.

Although most interest and research in vitamin D deficiency have been focused on rickets, one should remember that vitamin D deficiency can cause a variety of other problems. As stated earlier, for example, one of the most serious disorders associated with vitamin D deficiency is the convulsive state of **hypocalcemia tetany,** caused by insufficient supplies of calcium to nerves and muscles. Children and adults with vitamin D deficiency also experience bone pain, muscular tenderness, and weakness.

TOXICITY

Since the discovery, over 60 years ago, that cod liver oil was effective in the prevention of rickets, the disease has ceased to be of much public or professional concern. Today most health concerns related to vitamin D are centered on the harmful effects of overconsumption of the vitamin. Early studies on large intakes of vitamin D found no extra benefit from intakes in excess of 400 IU/day (10 μg), the currently recommended intake for infants, children, adolescents, and young adults. As more foods were fortified, especially those eaten by infants, reports of hypercalcemia in infants consuming high quantities of vitamin D from combined sources turned attention to possible toxicity.

Hypercalcemia can be associated with seriously damaging effects, such as the irreversible calcification of various soft tissues of the body, including the heart, lungs, and kidneys.[28] In infants, hypercalcemia can be caused by vitamin D intakes at or above 1000 μg (4000 IU)/day. Most cases of hypercalcemia in adults have been caused by vitamin D intakes of 25,000 to 60,000 IU/day continued over a period of 1 to 4 months. The first symptoms include loss of appetite, nausea, weight loss, and failure to thrive. These early symptoms all disappear quickly as soon as all sources of vitamin D are withdrawn from the diet. If the state of hypercalcemia is allowed to persist for a long period, however, the calcification of soft tissues can eventually cause death.

No adverse effect of hypervitaminosis D in human pregnancy has been established. Studies on pregnant rats, however, have found that excessive vitamin D can be associated with changes in the placenta and the impaired maturation of osteoblasts, resulting in defective bone formation.

There is no evidence that excessive vitamin D production ever becomes a problem simply as a result of overexposure to sunlight.

DRUG INTERACTIONS WITH VITAMIN D

The use of sedatives and tranquilizers, as well as anticonvulsive therapy in persons with epilepsy, has been associated with increases in the incidence of both rickets and osteomalacia. The mechanism of this effect may be a drug-induced increase in the catabolism (breakdown) of 1,25-dihydroxyvitamin D, leading to impaired absorption of calcium.

VITAMIN E

Among the general public, vitamin E is probably the best known of the fat-soluble vitamins. This is because of the widely publicized scientific interest in the possibility that vitamin E might help delay or prevent the onset of cancer, coronary heart disease, cataracts, and other major diseases. The key to these possible abilities of vitamin E is its action as an antioxidant.

Vitamin E was first recognized in 1922 by Evans and Bishop as a dietary factor obtained from plant-based foods that was essential for normal reproduction in rats. In 1933 it was identified as essential for humans and found to comprise a range of substances known as **tocopherols** and **tocotrienols.** What is called vitamin E in fact consists of at least eight naturally occurring tocopherols and tocotrienols, each of which makes a unique chemical contribution to the properties of vitamin E in food. The general structure of the family of compounds with vitamin E activity can be seen in Figure 11-13. The four tocopherols that have been identified are known as alpha-, beta-, gamma-, and delta-tocopherol, respectively, and are all oily yellow liquids. D-α-tocopherol (the D specifies its three-dimensional structure) is the most biologically active of the four.

FIGURE 11-13

The general structure of the family of compounds (tocopherols) with vitamin E activity, sites where they differ, and relative biological activity. **Me,** ***Methyl group;*** **TE,** ***tocopherol equivalents.***

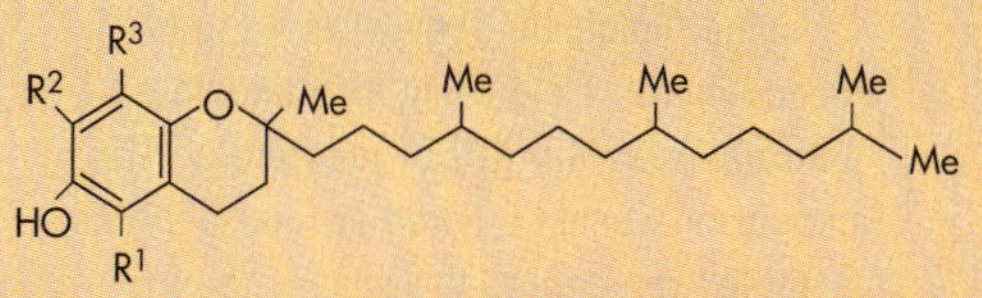

Compound	R1	R2	R3	TE
α–Tocopherol	Me	Me	Me	1 mg
β–Tocopherol	Me	H	Me	0.5 mg
γ–Tocopherol	H	Me	Me	0.1 mg
δ–Tocopherol	H	H	Me	0.02 mg

Vitamin E is a generic term that includes all compounds that exhibit the biological activity of α-tocopherol. Eight compounds with vitamin E activity (including α-tocopherol) are found in nature; four are tocopherols, and the other four are tocotrienols.

The amount of vitamin E present in any sample of food or tissue is quoted in terms of **tocopherol equivalents (TEs),** with 1 TE corresponding to 1 mg of α-tocopherol (also known as 1 IU of α-tocopherol). The TE value of any quantity of other members of the vitamin E group is determined by their biological activity relative to α-tocopherol. The amount of vitamin E listed in food analysis tables represents the sum of the TE values of all components of vitamin E that are present.

*T*he amount of vitamin E present in any sample of food or tissue is quoted in **tocopherol equivalents (TEs).** 1 mg TE = 1 mg of α-tocopherol, or whatever mass of any other form of vitamin E has the same biological activity as 1 mg of α-tocopherol. 1 mg TE is also known as 1 International Unit (IU) of tocopherol. The amount of vitamin E listed in food analysis tables represents the sum of the TE values of all components of vitamin E that are present.

The various forms of vitamin E differ only slightly from one another (Figure 11-13). These slight chemical differences, however, are sufficient to produce a fifty-fold difference in biological activity between the least active and the most active (α-tocopherol). Much of the vitamin E used in supplements is naturally occurring α-tocopherol concentrated from vegetable oils, but most of the vitamin E activity in such supplements is due to the derivatives vitamin E succinate and vitamin E acetate. These derivatives are more stable in light and during oxidation than are natural forms of vitamin E and so do not lose their biological activity when stored within pills or capsules. The synthetic form of vitamin E that is usually labeled as D-α-tocopherol acetate is in fact a mixture of eight "stereoisomers" (geometrically different forms), only one of which is equivalent to natural vitamin E.

Because of its role in preventing sterility in male animals, vitamin E was originally known as the *antisterility vitamin.* This term still persists to some extent, although sterility in animals is only one of many effects of vitamin E deficiency.

FUNCTIONS

The major clues to the functions of most vitamins are provided by the effects of deficiencies of the vitamins. In humans, deficiencies of vitamin E occur only in premature infants or in children and adults who exhibit some defect in fat absorption (associated with cystic fibrosis, for example). This means there is only limited direct knowledge of the functions of vitamin E in humans. Much of our knowledge is instead indirect knowledge based on the results of animal studies.

It is generally agreed that the main function of vitamin E within the body is to act as an **antioxidant.** Antioxidants are substances that protect other chemicals of the body from damaging oxidation reactions by reacting with oxidizing agents within the body. In the process the antioxidant is oxidized; so it acts in a "sacrificial" manner. Because vitamin E is a fat-soluble vitamin, it is able to mix with and protect lipid molecules from oxidation. It is considered to be the body's first line of defense against a specific form of lipid oxidation known as **lipid peroxidation,** which involves the formation of peroxide derivatives of lipids (see Chapter 4). In this role, vitamin E protects cell membranes against oxidizing free radicals.

The oxidizing agents that vitamin E and other antioxidants protect against are either produced within the body as part of its normal metabolic processes or enter the body from the atmosphere. For example, free radicals (highly reactive molecules carrying unpaired electrons) are produced during the normal oxidation of energy-yielding nutrients in the cell. Free radicals can also be produced by the presence in the body of various environmental pollutants (such as cigarette smoke, smog, and pesticides) and many drugs. When free radicals attack the lipids of cell membranes, they can initiate a highly damaging chain reaction, leading to widespread damage to the structure and therefore function of the membranes. Vitamin E is the main "chain-blocking" antioxidant in the body that is able to prevent these chain reactions from starting. Polyunsaturated lipids are the ones most prone to oxidation, and the change that occurs on oxidation is similar to what happens when a cooking fat becomes rancid during exposure to air.

In vitamin E deficiency the body is depleted in its major fat-soluble antioxidant defense against free radicals, and serious damage to various cells can result. The two types of cell that are most susceptible to damaging oxidation are red blood cells and the cells of the lungs. Oxidative damage to red blood cell membranes may cause the membranes to break, letting the cell contents escape in a process known as **hemolysis.**

The damage suffered by cells during vitamin E deficiency has been linked to the onset of several types of cancer,[29] the early stages of atherosclerosis,[30] premature aging, the formation of cataracts, and arthritis. Recent research also suggests that vitamin E may be required for the normal functioning of the immune system and, by regulating the production of prostaglandins, may control the aggregation of blood platelets during the formation of blood clots. Other suggested roles for vitamin E include some involvement in the metabolism of nucleic acids and proteins, the functioning of mitochondria, and the regulation of the production of various hormones.[31]

The antioxidant properties of vitamin E are believed to explain its role in inhibiting the formation of **lipofuscin,** a pigment that accumulates within tissues during aging. Brown spots in a variety of tissues caused by the accumulation of lipofuscin are one of the characteristic indicators of aging. Vitamin E is also involved in sparing the trace element selenium within the body and in protecting vitamin A against oxidative damage.

TABLE 11-6

Vitamin E content of human tissues (mg/100 g)

TISSUE	CONTENT OF VITAMIN E (D-α-TOCOPHEROL)
Adipose	150
Adrenal	132
Pituitary	40
Testis	40
Platelets	30
Heart	20
Muscle	19
Liver	13
Ovary	11
Uterus	9
Kidney	7

It should be clear from the foregoing discussion that vitamin E protects a wide variety of chemicals, cells, and tissues against oxidation. Attempts to fully characterize its protective actions, however, are complicated because many other substances also function as antioxidants and can perform some, but not all, of the roles of vitamin E. Other antioxidants within the body include vitamin C, β-carotene, and the enzymes superoxide dismutase, catalase, and glutathione peroxidase (which contain the trace minerals copper, iron, and selenium, respectively).

ABSORPTION, TRANSPORT, AND METABOLISM

Because vitamin E is a fat-soluble vitamin, it is absorbed best in the presence of fat and in the conditions that favor fat absorption. Between 40% and 60% of dietary vitamin E is absorbed, with the percentage absorbed decreasing as the dietary intake rises.

Most vitamin E is absorbed into lymph, carried within chylomicrons. When vitamin E reaches the blood plasma, it becomes associated with lipoproteins, primarily LDLs. It is exchanged rapidly between the LDL particles and lipid membranes, especially the membranes of red blood cells. The concentration of vitamin E in different tissues varies considerably (Table 11-6), with the highest concentrations being found in adipose tissue.

Plasma tocopherol concentrations are normally between 0.6 and 1.6 mg/100 ml, but they drop rapidly as soon as vitamin E is withdrawn from the diet. Most people have relatively abundant stores of vitamin E, sufficient to last for several months if no vitamin E is available from the diet.

Relatively little is known about the metabolism of vitamin E. Main routes for its excretion are the skin and the feces. Fecal vitamin E is a mixture of unabsorbed vitamin E and metabolites excreted within bile.

TABLE 11-7

Recommended dietary allowances (United States) and recommended nutrient intakes (Canada) for vitamin E (TE/day).

AGE (YEARS)	UNITED STATES	CANADA
Children (0–11)	6-7	3-7
Adults		
Males (>11)	10	8-10
Females (>11)	8	6-9
Pregnant	10	8-9
Lactating	12	9-10

TE, Tocopherol equivalents.

DIETARY REQUIREMENTS AND RECOMMENDED DIETARY ALLOWANCES

Studies in both humans and animals have clearly shown that the dietary requirement for vitamin E rises as the dietary intake of polyunsaturated fatty acids (PUFAs) rises. This effect can be associated with as much as a ten-fold variation in vitamin E requirements and is the result of two main influences of PUFA on the body. First, as the amount of PUFA in the body rises, so too does the need for vitamin E to protect these fatty acids against oxidation. One should remember that PUFAs are the lipids that are most prone to oxidative damage. Second, an increased proportion of PUFA within dietary lipid is known to impair the absorption of vitamin E from the intestine. It has proved difficult to devise a formula relating vitamin E requirement to PUFA intake, but a daily intake of 0.4 mg of vitamin E for each gram of PUFA in the diet has been proposed.[9]

Depending on the dietary intake of PUFA, the actual need for vitamin E may be as low as 5 mg/day or as high as 20 mg/day. The recommended allowance for vitamin E for adults, however, has been set at 10 mg TE (equivalent to 10 mg of α-tocopherol)/day for men and 8 mg TE/day for women (Table 11-7).[9] The RDAs of vitamin E maintain a blood level of the vitamin at about 0.5 mg/dl, which is considered adequate. The adult recommended intakes of vitamin E are readily obtained from the typical North American diet. The vitamin E/PUFA ratio in this diet is 0.6 mg vitamin E:1 mg PUFA, which is considered satisfactory.

During pregnancy, when the expectant mother's level of vitamin E need increases, an additional 2 mg TE/day is recommended. During lactation, a mother transfers 3 mg of vitamin E per day to her milk because an average of 750 ml of milk is produced with 0.4 mg of vitamin E per 100 ml. To make up for these losses, it is recommended that lactating women consume an additional 4 mg of vitamin E per day, on the assumption that

FIGURE 11-14

Relative amounts of vitamin E in various vegetable oils.

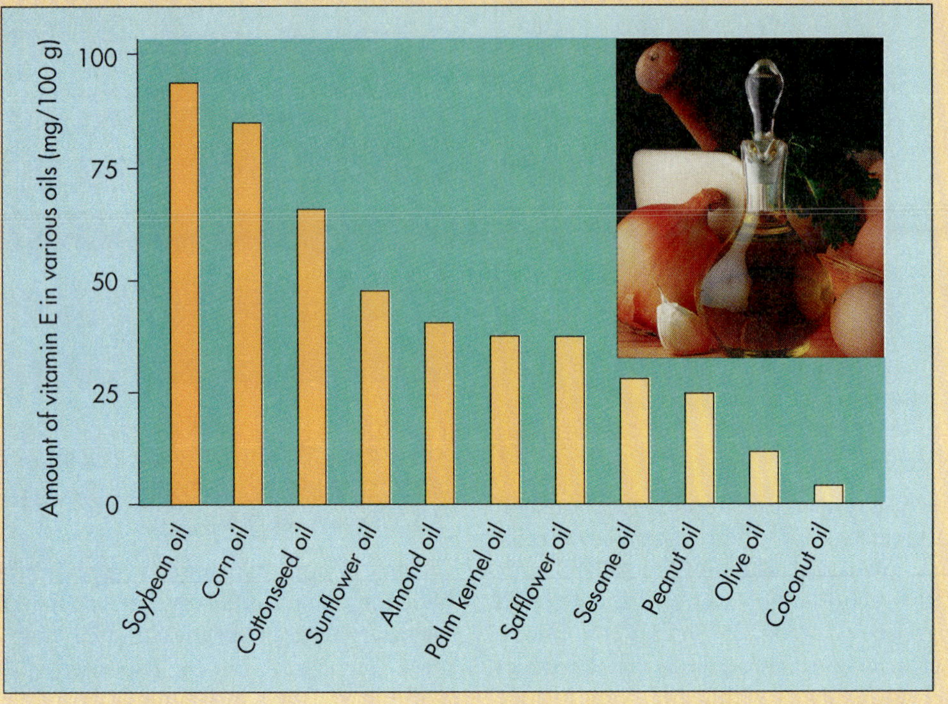

considerably less than 100% of the amount consumed is absorbed.

For infants, whose stores of vitamin E at birth are limited, the recommended intake of vitamin E is based on the amount supplied in human breast milk: approximately 2 mg/day. Human milk contains 10 times as much vitamin E as does cow's milk, and most infant formula includes added vitamin E sufficient to provide at least 1 mg/100 kcal, which is considerably greater than the concentration within human milk. A breast-fed infant, however, has the advantage of receiving extra vitamin E through the **colostrum,** the fluid secreted from the breast immediately after birth before mature milk is produced. Colostrum contains two to four times as much vitamin E (1.0 to 1.8 mg/100 ml) as does mature human milk (0.4 mg/100 ml).

Premature infants are born with low levels of vitamin E in their blood, undoubtedly because much of the vitamin E transferred to a fetus is transferred toward the end of pregnancy. To prevent the hemolysis of blood cells, the diet of premature infants is usually supplemented with up to 13 mg TE/kg of body weight for the first 3 months of life.

Recommended intakes of vitamin E for children range from 3 to 7 mg TE/day. The recommended amounts are higher for older children to reflect their needs for growth and increased weight.

The Committee on Medical Aspects of Food Policy of the United Kingdom decided it was not possible to set standards for vitamin E because requirements are so dependent on PUFA intake. They did conclude, however, that the range of acceptable intakes for pregnant and lactating women was 3.8 to 6.2 mg/day and that, for men and women in general, safe intakes were about 4 and 3 mg TE/day, respectively.[11] Health and Welfare Canada recommends vitamin E intakes of 6 to 10 mg/day for both men and women.[10]

FOOD SOURCES

The major source of vitamin E in the North American diet is vegetable oil, which accounts for about 67% of the estimated TE available. The vitamin E content of various oils ranges from 4 mg/100 g of coconut oil to 94 mg/100 g of soybean oil (Figure 11-14). In general, the vitamin E content of an oil increases in proportion to the amount of PUFA in the oil. Animal fats contain virtually no nutritionally significant amounts of vitamin E.

For most commercial purposes, corn, cottonseed, peanut, coconut, and soybean oils can be used interchangeably. This means that in the United States the use of any specific oil as a source of vitamin E is determined largely by considerations of price and availability. Current U.S. labeling laws require manufacturers to list every oil that might be present in a product on the label. Because the use of oils varies from time to time, this requires many manufacturers to put a long list of oils on their labels, even though only one or two oils in the list

TABLE 11-8

Vitamin E content per average portion size of major food sources of vitamin E in the U.S. diet

FOOD GROUP	VITAMIN E PER PORTION* (mg TE)	VITAMIN E PER 100 g* (mg TE)	VITAMIN E/ PUFA RATIO†
Superfortified cereals	33.5	137.5	254.4
Instant breakfast and diet bars	4.3	12.8	28.5
Shellfish	2.8	4.5	58.2
Mustard or turnip greens, kale, and collards	2.5	2.6	‡
Pies	2.5	2.5	1.9
Fried fish	2.1	2.3	0.8
French fries and fried potatoes	1.9	1.5	0.5
Spaghetti with tomato sauce	1.7	0.7	94.9
Chili	1.7	0.8	1.8
Peanuts and peanut butter	1.6	8.1	0.5
Mixed dishes with chicken	1.5	1.2	6.4
Pizza	1.4	0.9	1.0
Beef stew and pot pie	1.4	0.4	93.0
Coleslaw and cabbage	1.3	2.4	52.2
Fish, broiled, baked, or canned	1.3	1.4	21.7
Mayonnaise and salad dressings	1.3	11.3	0.4
Tuna, tuna salad, and tuna casserole	1.3	2.1	0.4
Spinach	1.2	1.9	95.1
Melons	1.2	0.4	‡
Salad and cooking oils	1.2	14.7	0.8
Salty snacks	1.0	4.8	0.5

* Vitamin E values are weighted, aggregate values of the individual foods within each category. Vitamin E content per usual portion size; data from National Health and Nutrition Examination Survey II, 1976-1980.

† Expressed in mg tocopherol equivalents (TE) per g polyunsaturated fatty acid (PUFA).

‡ These foods contain no PUFA, so a ratio cannot be calculated.

might be present in any particular batch of the product. Only when a product label lists one oil can the consumer be sure of which oil is actually present. At the time of writing, about 75% of the oil used in the United States is soybean oil. However, the success of commercial production of alternative oils, such as rapeseed oil (Canola) and sunflower seed oils, may cause that figure to fall significantly in the future.

The richest food sources of vitamin E per average portion (providing at least 1 mg per portion) are listed in Table 11-8, which also indicates the vitamin E/PUFA ratio of the chosen foods. The foods listed were selected from representative foods consumed by participants in the NHANES II survey. By far the most concentrated sources of vitamin E in the U.S. diet are the **superfortified cereals,** which contain at least 33.5 mg TE per serving. Next come instant breakfast diet bars and drinks, which are also fortified with vitamin E. Various foods that contain a high proportion of fats and oils (such as pies and fried foods) and foods that are usually consumed in large portions (such as vegetables and mixed dishes) are also major sources of vitamin E in the U.S. diet. Although salad oils and cooking oils are relatively rich sources of vitamin E, the average serving of them is relatively small, which explains their lowly twentieth place in the ranking of dietary vitamin E sources for U.S. citizens.

Many foods that are rich in vitamin E are also high in dietary fat. This means that following current dietary guidelines, which recommend a reduction in total fat intake, could also result in lowered vitamin E intake. There are, however, many low-fat sources of vitamin E listed in Table 11-8. Such low-fat sources should be exploited by people trying to reduce their fat intake while consuming a well-chosen diet.

Vitamin E is relatively stable at normal cooking temperatures, although a significant proportion of it is destroyed by the high temperatures used in deep fat frying. Foods stored frozen can lose a significant proportion of their original vitamin E, unless the storage temperature is very low. Vitamin E is also destroyed by exposure to light and oxygen.

TYPICAL DIETARY INTAKES

Murphy and associates[32] have used data from the NHANES II study to estimate typical dietary intakes of vitamin E and PUFA in the United States. Average ("mean") intakes of vitamin E by men (9.6 mg/day) and women (7.0 mg/day) were close to the recommended intakes of 10 and 8 mg/day, respectively. Median intakes, however, were considerably lower— 7.3 mg/day for men and 5.4 mg/day for women. This indicates that reasonable average intakes mask the fact that many people are consuming levels of vitamin E significantly below the recommended amount. Data from NHANES III were 5% to 10% higher for men and women (Appendix K).

The individual food categories that contributed the largest amounts of vitamin E to the diet were fats and oils (which provided 20% of total vitamin E) and vegetables (which provided an additional 20% of total vitamin E). The same study revealed that approximately 23% of men and 15% of women were consuming low ratios of vitamin E to PUFA, less than 0.4 mg of vitamin E per gram of PUFA.

EVALUATION OF VITAMIN E STATUS

Two main methods are used to assess the vitamin E status of the body: serum vitamin E concentrations and the erythrocyte hemolysis test.

Serum Vitamin E

The concentration of vitamin E in blood serum is not an accurate indicator of the amount of vitamin E in body tissues, but serum levels below 0.6 mg/dl suggest a state of vitamin E deficiency, whereas levels above 3.5 mg/dl may be associated with symptoms of vitamin E toxicity.[33] It has also been shown that the tocopherol concentration of serum is correlated to the lipoprotein concentration.

Erythrocyte Hemolysis Test

Weak solutions of hydrogen peroxide (H_2O_2) can be used to test the resistance of red blood cells (erythrocytes) to hemolysis. Because vitamin E offers protection against the peroxide-induced membrane damage responsible for hemolysis, the resistance of erythrocytes to hemolysis provides an indirect but useful indication of vitamin E status. A sample of blood is incubated in a 2% solution of hydrogen peroxide. If 5% or more of erythrocytes undergo hemolysis during a 3-hour incubation with the peroxide, vitamin E deficiency is indicated. Conversely, less than 5% hemolysis under these conditions can be used to rule out the possibility of vitamin E deficiency.[34]

DEFICIENCY

Vitamin E deficiency in humans occurs only in premature infants or in children and adults who have some defect in fat absorption. Steatorrhea in infants (fatty stools resulting from defective fat absorption) is a reliable indicator of those infants at risk of vitamin E deficiency. The defective fat absorption (in infants and others) is in turn usually associated with such conditions as cystic fibrosis of the pancreas, cholestasis (impaired production of bile), and celiac disease. In one study of patients with cystic fibrosis, serum vitamin E concentrations were less than 0.4 mg/dl in patients not receiving large doses of supplemental vitamin E. Vitamin E supplements were effective in raising serum vitamin E levels toward normal values (above 0.5 mg/dl).[35]

The symptoms of vitamin E deficiency include various neurological disorders, anemia caused by the hemolysis of red blood cells (hemolytic anemia), retinopathy, and abnormalities in the functioning of platelets and lymphocytes (white blood cells). These are considered individually below.

Neurological Disorders

The evidence associating neurological disorders with vitamin E deficiency has been reviewed by Sokol.[36] In animal studies vitamin E–deficient diets have been found to produce uncoordinated movement (ataxia), weakness, and sensory disturbances similar to those seen in humans who are deficient in vitamin E. A "pure" form of vitamin E deficiency in humans is caused by an inborn error of metabolism known as **isolated vitamin E deficiency,** and this produces neurological disorders similar to those found in people with vitamin E deficiency for other reasons, such as impaired absorption of fat. Also, the vitamin E content of nerves in the peripheral nervous system has been found to be reduced in some patients with vitamin E deficiency.

At least some of the neurological disorders associated with vitamin E deficiency are believed to be caused by the peroxidation of membrane lipids. In many cases these disturbances can be reduced or even corrected by the administration of sufficient vitamin E.

Hemolytic Anemia

Infant formula fed to premature infants in the 1960s and early 1970s often contained high levels of PUFA. The vitamin E to PUFA ratio of the formula was low, and the infants were often also given high doses of iron, which acts as an oxidant in the body. As a result of being fed formula with a low vitamin E/PUFA ratio in the presence of a powerful oxidant, some of the infants developed hemolytic anemia. The administration of vitamin E was found to readily correct this problem. This led to a modification of the formulas fed to premature infants, which now contain more vitamin E and less PUFA.

Retinopathy

Defective functioning of the retina of the eye (retinopathy), which can often cause permanent blindness, is a danger in premature infants. Large doses (30 mg) of vitamin E have been found to offer some protection against this risk. There are some concerns, however, about possible adverse side effects of the high doses of vitamin E required.

Platelet and Lymphocyte Malfunction

Vitamin E deficiency in children with severe liver disease or cystic fibrosis of the pancreas has been associated with increased aggregation of platelets in the blood. Studies in experimental animals have confirmed this effect.[37] In several species of animal, vitamin E deficiency has also been associated with a decreased ability of T and B lymphocytes to proliferate in an appropriate manner as part of the body's immune defenses. All these effects of vitamin E deficiency can be corrected by the administration of sufficient vitamin E.

TOXICITY

Because vitamin E is a fat-soluble vitamin that can be stored within the body, there has been much concern about possible adverse consequences caused by the consumption of large amounts without proper medical supervision. So far, however, there is only anecdotal evidence to suggest that the overconsumption of vitamin E by adults might be associated with any toxic effects. Daily intakes of as high as 200 to 1000 mg/day, which have been used in several intervention studies, produce no detectable adverse effects. However, because there is no scientific justification for the consumption of high doses of vitamin E, it seems unwise to consume **unphysiological levels** of more than 100 mg/day. The term *unphysiological levels* refers to amounts of a vitamin (or other nutrient) that exceed those that are required by the body and that the body could be reasonably expected to handle (arbitrarily considered about 10 times the RDA).

In infants, there is stronger evidence linking large oral or intravenous doses of vitamin E with possible toxicity. The intravenous administration of 15 to 30 mg of DL-α-tocopherol acetate (E-Ferol) to premature infants has been associated with liver and kidney failure, accumulation of fluid in the peritoneal cavity (ascites), decreased blood platelet numbers (thrombocytopenia), and eventual death. The concentrations of vitamin E in the plasma of some affected patients were higher than 10 mg/dl. Similar problems were produced in young animals given high doses of vitamin E.

VITAMIN E AND OTHER ANTIOXIDANTS IN HEALTH PROMOTION AND DISEASE RESISTANCE

A growing body of evidence suggests that damage caused by free radicals is involved in the development of a variety of degenerative diseases and that vitamin E and other antioxidant vitamins offer considerable protection against these diseases. Diseases linked to free radical damage include cancer, cardiovascular disease, and circulatory disorders. Free radicals are also believed to play a role in the aging process and to be responsible for some damaging effects of exposure to pollutants and regular participation in strenuous exercise.

Most of the evidence in this area comes from animal studies, but some revealing data from studies on humans are also available. For example, a large multinational study sponsored by WHO found that improved vitamin E status was strongly correlated with reduced death rates from coronary vascular diseases.[38] A "synergy" with the other antioxidants, vitamin C, and the carotenoids was also found, meaning that each antioxidant enhanced the others' effects. In general, as nutritional status for the antioxidant nutrients increases, death rates are found to decrease. There is also increasing evidence that vitamin E and other dietary antioxidants can decrease the risk of several kinds of cancer in humans.

Several investigations are currently underway to more fully document the precise roles and abilities of antioxidant nutrients in the prevention and treatment of diseases associated with peroxidative damage. In the meantime, given that few Americans consume adequate amounts of the fruits and vegetables that provide antioxidant nutrients, the population should be advised to increase their consumption of these foods.

VITAMIN K

Vitamin K was discovered in 1934 by a Danish scientist named Dam, who recognized the vitamin as the fat-soluble factor necessary for the coagulation of blood. The vitamin was designated as vitamin "K" after the Danish word *koagulation*. The term *vitamin K* now refers to several substances belonging to a group of chemicals known as **quinones.** These include naturally occurring **phylloquinone** in plant foods, several naturally occurring **menaquinones** found in animal tissues and synthesized by bacteria, and the synthetic substance **menadione** (Figure 11-15). These substances were once known as vitamins K_1, K_2, and K_3, respectively.

Phylloquinone is found primarily in green leafy plants and was first isolated from alfalfa meal in 1939 (which explains why alfalfa is a popular "health food"). Menaquinones are synthesized by bacteria in the gastrointestinal tract. The menaquinone family of vitamin K_2 includes several closely related compounds with unsaturated side chains that differ only in the number of "isoprenyl" units they contain (Figure 11-15). Although commonly known as the menaquinones (or sometimes just as menaquinone), their designated generic name is **menaquinone-n,** with a number in place of the "n" to specify a particular menaquinone on the basis of the number of isoprenyl groups in its side chain. Menaquinone-4, for example, is synthesized in some animals, whereas menaquinone-7 through menaquinone-13 are synthesized only in bacteria.

FIGURE 11-15

The chemical structure of quinones with vitamin K activity.

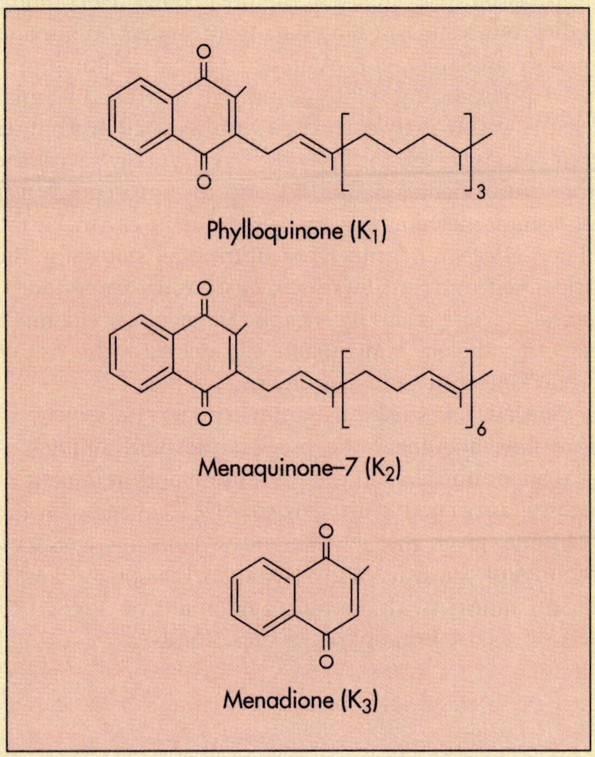

A synthetic water-soluble form of menadione is marketed as *Kappidione.* This form of the vitamin has been associated with the possibility of harmful side effects—namely, hemolytic anemia and hyperbilirubinemia (excess bilirubin in the blood). For this reason, phylloquinone is now the preferred form of vitamin K for clinical use. Phylloquinone is marketed as *AquaMEPHYTON, KanaKion, Mephyton,* and *Mono-Kay.*[39]

FUNCTIONS

The main function of vitamin K is to act as a cofactor in the enzymatic modification of residues of the amino acid glutamic acid within certain protein molecules. Prothrombin (also known as blood clotting factor II) and factors VII, IX, and X are proteins required for the appropriate formation of blood clots. During their synthesis in the liver, some of their glutamic acid residues must be modified to gamma-carboxyglutamic acid, and it is this process that requires vitamin K as a cofactor. The gamma-carboxyglutamic acid residues (Gla residues) are able to bind to calcium ions in a way that allows prothrombin, for example, to fulfill its proper role in blood clotting (see Chapter 9). Individuals who are deficient in vitamin K possess an abnormal form of prothrombin known as **PIVKA** (for protein induced by vitamin K absence or antagonism) or **PIVKA-II,** to specify that it is an abnormal form of factor II (prothrombin).

Two other Gla-containing vitamin K–dependent proteins found in the blood (known as proteins C and S) have *anticoagulant* properties, as opposed to the clot-forming "procoagulant" properties of prothrombin and factors VII, IX, and X. Thus vitamin K is involved in both stimulating and inhibiting coagulation and so in maintaining appropriate levels of coagulation to form clots in case of injury, while preventing the inappropriate formation of clots, which can lead to blockages of blood vessels **(thromboses).** Newborn infants with a deficiency of protein C have been found to suffer from multiple thromboses.

The anticoagulant drug **dicumarol** is chemically similar to vitamin K, and it blocks the conversion of vitamin K oxide to vitamin K, a step that is necessary for the regeneration of vitamin K, so a deficiency develops. The widespread use of anticoagulant drugs in treating phlebitis and thrombosis has made the use of vitamin K therapy important in counteracting any undesirable side effects of anticoagulants, such as hemorrhaging.

Two Gla-containing vitamin K–dependent proteins have also been found in bone. The most abundant of these proteins is called **osteocalcin** or **bone Gla protein,** whereas the other is known as **matrix Gla protein.** The precise functions of these proteins have not been characterized. Osteocalcin is known to have calcium-binding properties. It is synthesized in the osteoblasts of bone and may be involved in the mineralization of bone. Matrix Gla protein has been found in other tissues, and bone, but its function is unknown.

It was once believed that serum concentrations of osteocalcin could serve as a sensitive marker for the efficiency of bone formation in children and adolescents. It has been found, however, that serum osteocalcin levels are greater in breast-fed infants than in formula-fed infants, despite the fact that both groups of infants show similar rates of linear growth.

ABSORPTION TRANSPORT, AND METABOLISM

As with all fat-soluble vitamins, the absorption of vitamin K is affected by the same factors that affect fat absorption. Also, like all fat-soluble vitamins, the vitamin must be solubilized by incorporation into micelles before absorption. The absorption of vitamin K requires the action of both bile and pancreatic secretions. Phylloquinone is absorbed from the small intestine by active transport, whereas menaquinone-9 and probably other menaquinones are absorbed by passive transport.[39]

From 40% to 70% of dietary vitamin K is normally absorbed, and clinical signs of vitamin K deficiency are rarely found in humans. Any obstruction of the bile duct or the use of mineral oil as a laxative decreases the efficiency of vitamin K absorption. There is evidence to suggest that a proportion of the menaquinones synthesized by bacteria in the intestine is absorbed into the body and stored in the liver. No case of vitamin K deficiency is reported to result from use of antibiotics unless the person had a coexistent fat malabsorption problem. The absorption of bacterially synthesized vitamin K is insufficient to meet the body's requirements completely and must be supplemented by at least a little vitamin K from dietary sources. Restricting dietary vitamin K leads to an alteration in the clotting factors available in the blood.[40] However, in the 1960s some infants who were fed formulas low in vitamin K developed clinical signs of vitamin K deficiency, although they were not given broad-spectrum antibiotics.

Transport

Once absorbed into the intestinal wall cells, vitamin K is incorporated into chylomicrons, which are then passed into lymph. From the lymph the vitamin K moves into the veins and is taken up by cells of the liver. The transport of vitamin K across the placenta is limited, and the concentration of the vitamin in the cord blood of a fetus is normally considerably lower than in the mother's blood. Nevertheless, the consumption of supplemental vitamin K by a pregnant woman produces an increase in the vitamin K concentration of cord blood.

Storage and Metabolism

Vitamin K is stored in the liver but is turned over more quickly than are other fat-soluble vitamins. The half-life of phylloquinone in rats is approximately 10 to 12 hours, and that of menaquinones is about 24 hours. The concentration of vitamin K in the liver (determined in tests on adults dying from trauma) has been found to range between 7 and 42 mg/g.

The metabolism and excretion of vitamin K have not been well characterized. A portion of absorbed vitamin K is excreted in bile in the form of fat-soluble metabolites of the vitamin. Water-soluble metabolites of vitamin K are excreted efficiently in the urine, which also contains small amounts of fat-soluble metabolites.

DIETARY REQUIREMENTS

In the United States the Food and Nutrition Board recognizes vitamin K as a dietary essential and has established RDAs (Table 11-9). The needs for vitamin K in the first few days of life are of particular concern because of the danger of hemorrhagic disease of the newborn. The intestinal tract of a newborn infant is relatively sterile and so does not contain the bacteria that synthesize vitamin K. Also, little vitamin K is transferred to a fetus during pregnancy, unless the vitamin is given to the mother at the time of delivery. In addition, human milk is low in vitamin K (at 1.6 µg/L). Infant formulas are now routinely supplemented with vitamin K at a level of 1.5 µg/100 kcal. The American Academy of Pediatrics also recommends the routine intramuscular administration of phylloquinone to the infant at birth to prevent any risk of vitamin K deficiency.[41] In the absence of any administration of supplementary vitamin K, breast-fed infants have a significantly longer clotting time than do bottle-fed infants.

TABLE 11-9

Recommended dietary allowances for vitamin K

POPULATION	AMOUNT (µg/DAY)
Infants	5-10
Children	15-30
Adolescents	45-65
Adults	60-80

The newborn infant's need for vitamin K is estimated by the American Academy of Pediatrics and the Food and Nutrition Board to be between 5 and 30 µg/day, assuming 10% absorption of orally administered vitamin K. Adult requirements are estimated at 1 µg/kg of body weight on the assumption that half of the vitamin K needed by an adult comes from the diet and the other half is synthesized by intestinal bacteria.[9] No increase in vitamin K consumption is recommended during pregnancy or lactation, although there is some evidence that requirements increase during pregnancy.

The Committee on Medical Aspects of Food Policy of the United Kingdom concluded that 1 µg/kg/day of vitamin K is both safe and adequate for adults and recommended 10 µg/day as a safe intake for infants.[11] Health and Welfare Canada has not established an RNI for vitamin K for adults because vitamin K deficiency in healthy adults is rare.[10] To prevent hemorrhagic disease of the newborn, the Canadian Pediatric Society recommends that all healthy newborn infants be given a single dose of vitamin K, orally or intramuscularly, within 6 hours after birth.[42]

FOOD SOURCES

For most people, adequate amounts of vitamin K are provided both from the green leafy vegetables they consume and from the synthesis of the vitamin by intestinal bacteria. Because the average diet provides sufficient vitamin K, there is no need for the consumption of vitamin K supplements.

Vitamin K usually occurs in association with chlorophyll in the chloroplasts of plant cells. The highest concentrations of vitamin K are found in green leafy vegetables (with 120 to 750 µg/100 g), but it is also

TABLE 11-10

Approximate vitamin K (phylloquinone) content of selected fruits and vegetables

FOOD	AMOUNT (μg/100 g)*
Apples	5
Apple sauce	1
Avocado	20
Bananas	1
Broccoli	200
Brussels sprouts	220
Cabbage, Chinese	175
Cabbage, red	50
Cabbage, white	80
Carrots	10
Cauliflower	25
Celery	5
Corn	5
Cucumbers	25
Green beans	40
Green onions	60
Green pepper	5
Kale	750
Lettuce	120
Leeks	15
Oranges	1
Parsley	700
Parsnips	1
Peaches	5
Pears	1
Potatoes	1
Pumpkins	1
Spinach	350
Squash	5
Sweet potatoes	1
Tomatoes	10
Turnip greens	300
Watercress	200
Wheat flour	1
White rice	1

* In many cases, there is a wide variation in reported values for a single food by different investigators. Some foods listed as containing 1 μg/100 g actually contain much less.

From Suttie JW: *J Am Diet Assoc* 92:585, 1992.

found in fruits, tubers, seeds, eggs, and dairy and meat products (at between 1 and 50 μg/100 g).

The total dietary intake of vitamin K in North America is often estimated at 300 to 500 μg/day. One study of actual vitamin K intake by direct analysis, however, found a much lower average intake of only 77 μg/day for 10 young men but one that meets the recommended intake.[43] The phylloquinone content of common foods indicates that the actual intake is greatly influenced by the level of consumption of a few specific vegetables that are rich in vitamin K (Table 11-10). Although not listed in Table 11-10, alfalfa is an especially rich source of vitamin K, leading to its promotion by "health-food" advocates.

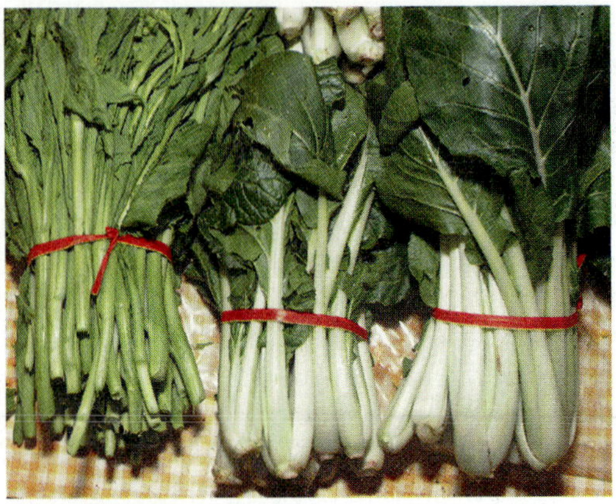

Green leafy vegetables are rich sources of vitamin K.

The amount of vitamin K synthesized by bacteria in the intestine obviously influences the amount absorbed by the body. Although only a small proportion of vitamin K from this source is actually absorbed, it provides approximately half of the vitamin K deposited in storage form in the liver. The amount of vitamin K synthesized in this way is reduced by the use of salicylic acid (an ingredient in most pain depressants of the aspirin type) and by certain antibiotics and sulfonamides.

Vitamin K is stable in heat and during oxidation but is destroyed by light, acid, alkali, oxidizing agents, and alcohol.

DEFICIENCY

The only known symptoms of vitamin K deficiency are a prolonged blood coagulation time and a consequent susceptibility to hemorrhage. Clotting time has been routinely used to assess the extent of any vitamin K deficiency, but it is a relatively insensitive method. The level of prothrombin in plasma can be reduced by 50% because of vitamin K deficiency, without producing any detectable prolongation of clotting time. It is now possible to assess vitamin K status with great sensitivity by directly measuring the ratio of active prothrombin to total prothrombin and hence the amount of abnormal prothrombin (PIVKA).

Because vitamin K is synthesized by bacteria in the intestines and is provided in adequate amounts by practically all diets, vitamin K deficiency in adults is almost always caused by a failure of the absorption of the vitamin. In one study of elderly people with vitamin K deficiency, the problem was attributed to poor absorption because of liver disease and the use of salicylates (salicylic acid derivatives) within aspirin preparations. Vitamin K deficiencies in adults also sometimes occur in people taking antibiotics for extended periods, although usually only if they also have difficulty absorbing fat or have a low dietary intake of the vitamin because of limited consumption of dark green, leafy vegetables.

In young infants, on the other hand, the lack of intestinal bacteria to synthesize vitamin K, the low levels of stored vitamin K at birth, and the small amount provided in human milk typically lead to low prothrombin levels and prolonged clotting time if supplementary vitamin K is not given. The initial attempts to reduce the risk of vitamin K deficiency in newborn infants involved the administration of over 5 mg of menadione (the synthetic form of vitamin K) either to the mother just before birth or to the infant in the first few days of life. Unfortunately the use of such a large quantity of menadione resulted in an increase in a hemolytic type of anemia, an accumulation of bilirubin in the blood, and a condition known as **kernicterus** in which bile pigment accumulates in the gray matter of the central nervous system. Kernicterus causes mental retardation, jaundice, hemorrhaging, and a variety of neurological symptoms. Fortunately, intramuscular injection of 0.5 to 1 mg of naturally occurring phylloquinone at birth has been found to significantly reduce the incidence of hemorrhage (to only 1 in 400 infants), with no undesirable side effects.

ISSUES AND OPINIONS

Are Antioxidant Supplements Beneficial or Harmful?

A large body of epidemiological evidence suggests that diets high in carotenoid-rich fruits and vegetables and high serum levels of beta-carotene (provitamin A) and vitamin E (alpha-tocopherol) are associated with a decreased risk of cancer (notably lung cancer) and cardiovascular disease. The underlying biological mechanism proposed to explain these observations is that antioxidant vitamins serve as scavengers of free radicals or highly reactive oxygen molecules. These reactive chemical species are normal products of oxidative metabolism that can cause damage to deoxyribonucleic acid (DNA) and convert a normal cell into a cancer cell. Antioxidant vitamins may also inhibit the oxidation of low-density lipoprotein (LDL) cholesterol, a particularly atherogenic form of cholesterol that can cause vascular damage.

Observational studies alone, however, do not establish cause and effect relationships. To determine the specific effects of antioxidant vitamins themselves, it is necessary to conduct randomized, double-blind, clinical trials. The results of the first major trial designed to assess the specific effects of supplemental beta-carotene and alpha-tocopherol were published recently and are surprising.*

The study examined 29,133 Finnish male smokers aged 50 to 69 years, who were given either beta-carotene (20 mg/day), alpha-tocopherol (50 mg/day), both supplements together, or a placebo (a supplement containing neither beta-carotene nor alpha-tocopherol). The intervention continued for 5 to 8 years (an average of 6.1 years).

Supplementation with beta-carotene was found to be associated with an 18% *increase* in lung cancer incidence and an 8% *increase* in total mortality. There was also more heart disease among participants who received beta-carotene. Vitamin E supplementation had no effect on lung cancer incidence or overall mortality. However, participants receiving supplemental vitamin E appeared to be at lower risk of heart disease, stroke, and prostate cancer and at increased risk of death from hemorrhagic stroke.

How can these findings be explained? The apparent beneficial effects of beta-carotene on cancer risk found in observational studies may result because of other substances that are present in the foods concerned. Also, serum levels of beta-carotene may only serve as a marker for the intake of other components of fruits and vegetables with true protective effects or for some other life-style variable that may reduce cancer risk. The authors of the Finnish study, however, express doubt that the suggestive adverse effect of beta-carotene supplementation was real. It may simply be a result of chance. This view was shared by other experts in the field in an accompanying editorial, who also point out that the risk of lung cancer and heart disease in the participants would have been dramatically reduced had they ceased smoking.† A short-term intervention may not be able to reverse the cumulative damaging effects of a lifetime of smoking.

The lack of an effect of vitamin E on overall mortality in this trial may be attributable to the low dose used and the apparently low bioavailability of the supplement.

Other clinical trials currently in progress are designed to assess the possible benefits of supplemental intakes of these antioxidant vitamins on cancer risk. Until the findings of such trials are available, it is impossible to state with confidence whether supplemental intakes of beta-carotene and vitamin E are beneficial, harmful, or without effect.‡ Although scientists continue to probe which constituents in fruits and vegetables account for the beneficial association of high intakes of these foods with reduced cancer risk, the judicious course of action is to increase consumption of fruits and vegetables as a disease prevention measure.

* The Alpha-Tocopherol, Beta-Carotene Cancer Prevention Study Group: *N Engl J Med 330*:1029, 1994.

† Hennekens CH, Buring JE, Peto R: *N Engl J Med 330*:1080, 1994.

‡ Herbert V: *Am J Clin Nutr* 60:157, 1994.

BY NOW YOU SHOULD KNOW

- Vitamins A, D, E, and K are fat-soluble vitamins that occur in a limited number of foods and are absorbed better in the presence of fat and in conditions that favor the absorption of fat.
- Vitamin A, also known as retinol, is required for normal vision, the maintenance of normal health of epithelial cells, and the remodeling of bone.
- Vitamin D, also known as calciferol, is involved in the absorption of calcium and the growth and remodeling of bone.
- Excessive intakes of vitamins A and D can lead to toxic symptoms, but excessive amounts are rarely obtained from food alone.
- Vitamin E, also known as α-tocopherol, functions as an antioxidant and is particularly important for protecting the polyunsaturated fatty acids in membrane lipids from oxidation.
- Vegetable oils are rich in vitamin E.
- Vitamin K is essential for the normal clotting of blood and for bone mineralization.
- Vitamin K is found primarily in dark green, leafy vegetables and is also provided by bacterial synthesis in the gastrointestinal tract.
- In general, fat-soluble vitamins are relatively stable to methods of preservation and preparation and are not soluble in water. As a result, losses during storage, food processing, and cooking are relatively small.
- The North American diet provides ample amounts of vitamins A and E.
- Supplementary vitamin D should be provided for infants, children, and the elderly in the temperate zone, who may not get sufficient exposure to the sun to synthesize enough of the vitamin in the skin.
- Supplementary vitamin K should be given orally or intramuscularly to newborn infants.

STUDY QUESTIONS

1. What groups of people are at risk of deficiency of each of the fat-soluble vitamins?
2. How do the factors that affect the absorption of fat affect the use of vitamins A and K?
3. Why are vitamins D and K of special concern in infant nutrition?
4. Why might vitamin A intakes be higher in summer than in winter?
5. Explain the role of vitamin K in blood clotting.
6. Explain why milk is a good source of vitamin D.
7. Explain the relationship between the skin and vitamin D, the small intestine and vitamin K, and the liver and vitamin A

CRITICAL ANALYSIS

1. List the deficiency symptoms for the vitamins below. Have you ever suffered two or more of these symptoms? What explanation can there be when your average daily intake is less than the RDA but when you do not experience deficiency symptoms?
2. The following exercise is a way to assess your intake of fat-soluble vitamins using a food frequency questionnaire. A food frequency questionnaire can be completed much faster than a 3-day food record and provides a less accurate, but often acceptable, estimate of dietary intake. Some food frequency questionnaires assess all aspects of the diet, and others focus on a single nutrient such as calcium or fat. The questionnaire below is incapable of providing a thorough estimate of vitamin intake, but it does allow you to assess your intake of many of the major food sources of the fat-soluble vitamins.

FOOD	SERVINGS PER WEEK
VITAMIN A	
Egg, 1 large	<1 2 3 4 5 6 7 >7
Milk, 2% fat, 8 oz	<1 2 3 4 5 6 7 >7
Cheddar cheese, 1 oz	<1 2 3 4 5 6 7 >7
Peach, 1 medium	<1 2 3 4 5 6 7 >7
Cantaloupe, ¼ of a 5-inch melon	<1 2 3 4 5 6 7 >7
Corn, canned, 4 oz	<1 2 3 4 5 6 7 >7
Green beans, 4 oz	<1 2 3 4 5 6 7 >7
Green peas, 4 oz	<1 2 3 4 5 6 7 >7
Tomato, 1 medium	<1 2 3 4 5 6 7 >7
Potato, baked, 1 medium	<1 2 3 4 5 6 7 >7
Broccoli, ½ cup	<1 2 3 4 5 6 7 >7
Carrots, ½ cup	<1 2 3 4 5 6 7 >7
Spinach, cooked, ½ cup	<1 2 3 4 5 6 7 >7
Total servings per week from these foods	______

FOOD	SERVINGS PER WEEK (3½ oz)
VITAMIN D	
Steak, beef	<1 2 3 4 5 6 7 >7
Butter	<1 2 3 4 5 6 7 >7
Cheese	<1 2 3 4 5 6 7 >7
Cod	<1 2 3 4 5 6 7 >7
Egg yolk	<1 2 3 4 5 6 7 >7
Shrimp	<1 2 3 4 5 6 7 >7
Salmon	<1 2 3 4 5 6 7 >7
Total servings per week from these foods	______

FOOD	SERVINGS PER WEEK
VITAMIN E	
Superfortified cereals	<1 2 3 4 5 6 7 >7
Instant breakfast or diet bar	<1 2 3 4 5 6 7 >7
Shellfish	<1 2 3 4 5 6 7 >7
Pie	<1 2 3 4 5 6 7 >7
Fried fish	<1 2 3 4 5 6 7 >7
French fries, fried potatoes	<1 2 3 4 5 6 7 >7
Spaghetti with tomato sauce	<1 2 3 4 5 6 7 >7
Pizza	<1 2 3 4 5 6 7 >7
Total servings per week from these foods	______

FOOD	SERVINGS PER WEEK (1 CUP RAW OR ½ CUP COOKED)
VITAMIN K	
Spinach	<1 2 3 4 5 6 7 >7
Kale	<1 2 3 4 5 6 7 >7
Parsley	<1 2 3 4 5 6 7 >7
Green onion	<1 2 3 4 5 6 7 >7
Green beans	<1 2 3 4 5 6 7 >7
Red cabbage	<1 2 3 4 5 6 7 >7
Cauliflower	<1 2 3 4 5 6 7 >7
Lettuce	<1 2 3 4 5 6 7 >7
Total servings per week from these foods	______

REFERENCES

1. Ovchinnikov YA editor: *Retinol proteins,* Utrecht, The Netherlands, 1987, VSP Press.
2. Summner A: *Nutritional blindness,* Oxford, England, 1982, Oxford University Press.
3. DeLuca LM: Retinoids and their receptors in differentiation, embryogenesis and neoplasia, *FASEB J* 5:2924, 1991.
4. Ross AC: Vitamin A: current understanding of the mechanism of action, *Nutr Today* 26:6, 1991.
5. Ross AC: Overview of retinoid metabolism, *J Nutr* 123:346, 1993.
6. Blomhoff R and others: Vitamin A metabolism: new perspectives on absorption, transport and storage, *Physiol Rev* 71:951, 1991.

7. Ross AC: Vitamin A and protective immunity, *Nutr Today* 27:18, 1992.
8. Ross AC, Termus ME: Vitamin A as a hormone: recent advances in understanding the actions of retinol, retinoic acid and beta carotene, *J Am Diet Assoc* 93:1285, 1993.
9. Food and Nutrition Board/National Academy of Sciences: *Recommended dietary allowances,* ed 10, Washington, DC, 1989, National Academy Press.
10. Health and Welfare Canada, Report of the Scientific Review Committee: *Nutrition recommendations,* Ottawa, Canada, 1990, Canadian Government Publishing Center.
11. Committee on Medical Aspects of Food Policy, Report of the Panel on Dietary Reference Values: *Dietary reference values for food energy and nutrients for the United Kingdom,* London, 1991, HMSO.
12. Food and Agriculture Organization/World Health Organization: *Requirement of vitamin A, iron, folate, and vitamin B_{12},* Food and Agriculture Organization Food and Nutrition Series No 23, Rome, 1988, The Food and Agricultural Organization.
13. Chug Ahuja JK and others: The development and application of a carotinoid database for fruits, vegetables, and selected multicomponent foods, *J Am Diet Assoc* 93:318, 1993.
14. Sommer A: New imperatives for an old vitamin (A), *J Nutr* 119:96, 1989.
15. WHO/UNICEF: Joint statement on vitamin A for measles, *Weekly Epidemiol Rec* 19:133, 1987.
16. Bloem MW and others: Vitamin A intervention: short-term effects of a single, oral, massive dose on iron metabolism, *Am J Clin Nutr* 51:76, 1990.
17. Underwood BA: Vitamin A prophylaxis programs in developing countries: past experiences and future prospects, *Nutr Rev* 48:265, 1990.
18. West KP Jr, Howard GR, Sommer A: Vitamin A and infection: public health implications, *Annu Rev Nutr* 9:63, 1989.
19. DeLuca HF: New concepts of vitamin D functions. In Machlin L, Sauberlich HE: Beyond deficiency: new views on the function and health effects of vitamins, *Ann N Y Acad Sci* 669:59, 1992.
20. DeLuca HD: Vitamin D: 1993, *Nutr Today* 28(6):6, 1993.
21. Alpers D: Absorption of vitamins and divalent minerals. In Sleisenger MH, Fordtran JS, editors: *Gastrointestinal disease: pathophysiology, diagnosis, and management,* ed 4, Philadelphia, 1989, WB Saunders.
22. Holick MF, MacLaughlin JA, Doppett SH: Regulation of cutaneous previtamin D, photosynthesis in man: skin pigment is not an essential regulation, *Science* 211:590, 1981.
23. Webb AR, Holick MF: The role of sunlight in the cutaneous production of vitamin D_3, *Annu Rev Nutr* 8:375, 1988.
24. Specker BL and others: Sunshine exposure and serum 25-hydroxyvitamin D concentrations in exclusively breast-fed infants, *J Pediatr* 107:372, 1985.
25. Webb AR and others: An evaluation of the relative contributions of exposure to sunlight and of diet to the circulating concentrations of 25-hydroxyvitamin D in an elderly nursing home population in Boston, *Am J Clin Nutr* 51:1075, 1990.
26. Gloth FM III and others: Is the Recommended Daily Allowance too low for the homebound elderly? *J Am Geriatr Soc* 39:137, 1992.
27. Key LL Jr: Nutritional rickets trends, *Endocrinol Metab* 2:81, 1991.
28. Collins ED, Norman AW: Vitamin D. In Machlin LJ, editor: *Handbook of vitamins,* ed 2, New York, 1991, Marcel Dekker.
29. Borek C: Vitamin E as an anticarcinogen, *Ann N Y Acad Sci* 570:417, 1990.
30. Ulbricht TLV, Southgate DAT: Coronary heart disease: seven dietary factors, *Lancet* 338:985, 1991.
31. Machlin LJ: Vitamin E. In Machlin LJ, editor: *Handbook of vitamins,* ed 2, New York, 1992, Marcel Dekker.
32. Murphy SP, Subar AF, Block G: Vitamin E intakes and sources in the U.S., *Am J Clin Nutr* 52:361, 1990.
33. Bell EF: Upper limit of vitamin E in infant formulas, *J Nutr* 119:1829, 1989.
34. Farrell PM: Vitamin E. In Shils ME, Young VR, editors: *Modern nutrition in health and disease,* Philadelphia, 1988, Lea & Febiger.
35. Bell EF: History of vitamin E in infant nutrition, *Am J Clin Nutr* 46:183, 1987.
36. Sokol RJ: Vitamin E deficiency and neurologic disease, *Annu Rev Nutr* 8:351, 1988.
37. Steiner M: Influence of vitamin E on platelet function in humans, *J Am Coll Nutr* 10:466, 1991.
38. Gey KF and others: Inverse correlation between plasma vitamin E and mortality from ischemic heart disease in cross-cultural epidemiology, *Am J Clin Nutr* 53:326S, 1991.
39. Suttie JW: Vitamin K. In Brown ML, editor: *Present knowledge in nutrition,* ed 6, Washington, DC, 1990, International Life Sciences Institute, Nutrition Foundation.
40. Suttie JW: Vitamin K and human nutrition, *J Am Diet Assoc* 92:585, 1992.
41. American Academy of Pediatrics: Controversies concerning vitamin K and the newborn, *Pediatrics* 91:1001, 1993.
42. Canadian Pediatric Society: The use of vitamin K in the perinatal period, *Can Med Assoc J* 139:127, 1988.
43. Suttie JW and others: Vitamin K deficiency from dietary vitamin K restriction in humans, *Am J Clin Nutr* 47:475, 1988.

ADDITIONAL READINGS

Allen RG, Venkatraj VS: Oxidants and antioxidants in development and differentiation, *J Nutr* 122(suppl):631S, 1992.

Bendich A: β-carotene and the immune response, *Proc Nutr Soc* 50:263, 1991.

Bendich A: Vitamin E status of U.S. children, *J Am Coll Nutr* 11:441, 1992.

Chesney RW: Vitamin D: can an upper limit be defined? *J Nutr* 119(suppl 12):1825, 1989.

Combs JF Jr: *The vitamins: fundamental aspects in nutrition and health,* San Diego, 1992, Academic Press.

Entrala BA, Lasuncion RMA: Antioxidant role of vitamin E, *Endocrinologia* 38:158, 1991.

Fifteenth Marabou Symposium: Vitamin A: from molecular biology to public health, *Nutr Rev* 52(2):1, 1994.

Hathcock JN and others: Evaluation of vitamin A toxicity, *Am J Clin Nutr* 52:183, 1990.

Holick MF: Vitamin D: biosynthesis, metabolism and mode of action. In De Groot LJ: *Endocrinology*, New York, 1989, Grune & Stratton.

Olson JA: Vitamin A. In Machlin L, editor: *The handbook of vitamins,* ed 2, New York, 1991, Marcel Dekker.

Pike JW: Vitamin D_3 receptors: structure and function in transcription, *Annu Rev Nutr* 11:189, 1991.

Rodrigues ME, Irwin MI: A conspectus of research on vitamin A requirement in man, *J Nutr* 102:909, 1972.

Ross AC, Ternus ME: Vitamin A as a hormone: recent advances in understanding the actions of retinol, retinoic acid and beta carotene, *J Am Diet Assoc* 93:1280, 1993.

Shearer MJ and others: Nutritional aspects of vitamin K in the human. In Suttie JW, editor: *Vitamin K metabolism and vitamin K–dependent proteins,* Baltimore, 1980, University Park Press.

Sies H, Stahl W, Sundquist AR: Antioxidant functions of vitamins: vitamins E and C, β-carotene, and other carotenoids, *Ann N Y Acad Sci* 669:7, 1992.

Suttie JW: Vitamin K. In Machlin LJ, editor: *Handbook of vitamins,* ed 2, New York, 1991, Marcel Dekker.

West CE and others: Vitamin A and immune function, *Proc Nutr Soc* 50:251, 1991.

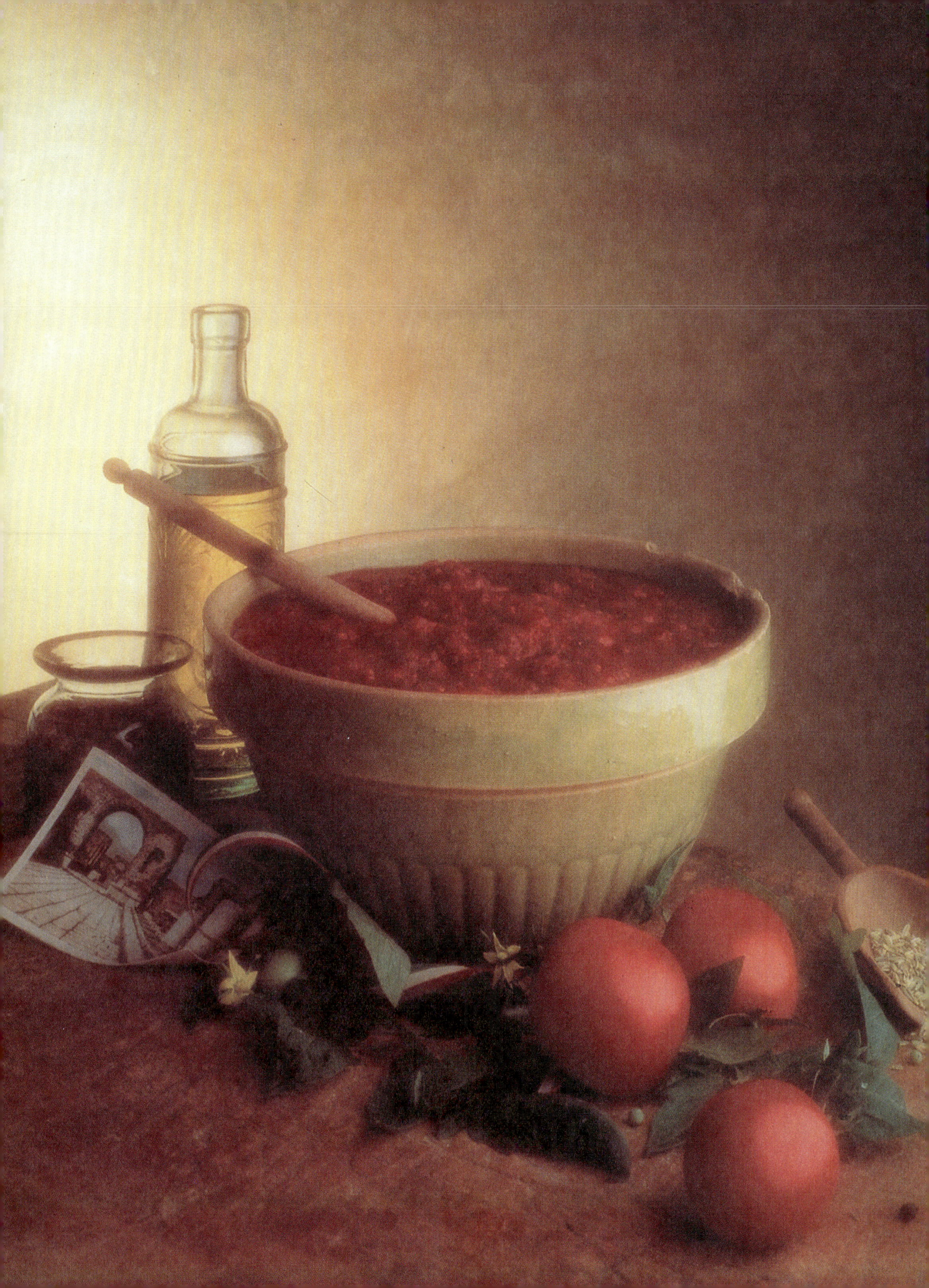

CHAPTER 12

WATER-SOLUBLE VITAMINS

PART 1

VITAMIN C, FOLIC ACID, VITAMIN B_{12}, & VITAMIN B_6

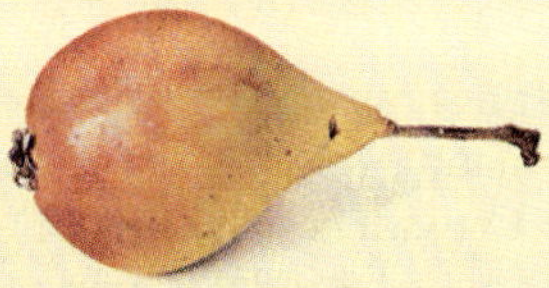

The nutrients discussed in this chapter are four water-soluble vitamins that are all involved directly or indirectly in blood formation, although each also performs at least one other unique role. Folic acid, vitamin B_{12}, and vitamin B_6 are regarded as components of the "B-complex" vitamins, which serve as coenzymes in many of the reactions of metabolism. Vitamin C (ascorbic acid), with unique metabolic roles, is the only water-soluble vitamin that is not considered a member of the "B-complex" vitamins and is not involved in either energy metabolism or protein synthesis. A deficiency of any of the four vitamins discussed here is associated with a unique pattern of symptoms.

VITAMIN C

Vitamin C is probably the most talked about vitamin and is certainly the one most widely used as a supplement. The chemical name for vitamin C is **ascorbic acid,** and vitamin C was once also known as **hexuronic acid** and **cevitamic acid.** Originally it was described as the **antiscorbutic** (scurvy-preventive) nutrient because of its ability to prevent scurvy. As early as the seventeenth century it was well known that scurvy could be controlled by eating certain foods, and we have known that it is a vitamin-deficiency disease since 1906. The search for the dietary substance responsible for preventing scurvy ended between 1928 and 1931, with the isolation of white crystals of the relatively simple compound vitamin C from lemons, oranges, paprika, cabbage, and adrenal glands.[1]

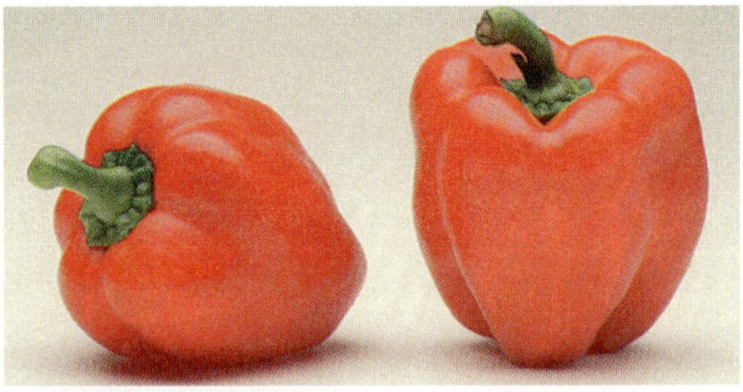

Sweet red peppers are a rich source of vitamin C.

The saga of the discovery of vitamin C is one of the longest and most interesting tales of nutritional history. Descriptions of illnesses that were unmistakably scurvy were reported in a papyrus from 1500 BC found at Thebes and in the writings of Hippocrates in 400 BC. Since that time and probably before, scurvy has been a major factor shaping the course of history. It has ravaged armies and navies and caused the death of many explorers and homesteaders. It was known to the Crusaders of the Middle Ages, who believed that those who could survive the pain that attacked feet and legs and the changes that occurred in their gums would usually be cured by the warm temperatures of spring, a time coinciding with the availability of fresh fruits and vegetables. When worldwide seafaring became commonplace, scurvy became known as the "scourge of the navy." Seamen embarked on long voyages in the knowledge that a significant proportion of them would either die of scurvy or be severely incapacitated by it. This was true for such celebrated explorers as Magellan, Vasco da Gama, and Jacques Cartier, whose vivid description of how the disease affected his men at Quebec in 1534 is a classic. Some of Cartier's men were saved by drinking a brew recommended by the Indians that was made by adding needles of coniferous trees, such as cedars, to hot water. Captain Cook's crew, on the other hand, was saved by his insistence that they eat a thick cabbage soup (similar to sauerkraut) that he called "sour krout." French and Spanish sailors did not succumb to scurvy because of the amount of onions and leeks in their rations, and sailors in the Mediterranean were rarely away from port long enough to use up their reserves of vitamin C–containing foods.

Although they were the most commonly affected, sailors were not the only people to suffer from scurvy. When a potato crop failed, even rural European populations were hit by outbreaks of the disease. Mormons making their way west to Utah were forced to winter in Nebraska, eating a diet of mush. Many of them succumbed to scurvy, as did many troops during the Civil War. One of the first tasks of the Spaniards after they landed in California was to search for a herb or plant that could cure scurvy. So, in many different ways, the deficiency of a nutrient needed in amounts of slightly more than 4 teaspoons per year has affected the course of history.

The first carefully conceived and controlled nutritional experiment on humans was conducted in an effort to cure scurvy among seamen. In 1747 the British physician Lind suggested that various "acidic principles" might have antiscorbutic properties. To test this, he divided sailors affected by scurvy into several groups of two and fed each group the basic ship's diet plus either oil of vitriol (sulfuric acid) in water, vinegar, seawater, oranges, or lemons. The results of this experiment are now legendary: both oranges and lemons were found to have miraculous curative powers, with the sailors given these treatments able to return to active duty within 6 days. Those sailors given the other treatments, however, showed no improvements. Lind not only demonstrated how to cure scurvy, but he also laid the foundations for the theory that the lack of an essential constituent of food could cause illness.

It took 50 years before the British navy recognized the importance of Lind's work and required every ship leaving a British port to carry sufficient lime juice for its crew throughout the entire voyage. This led to the term *limey* being applied to British seamen and later being extended to all British servicemen.

CHEMICAL PROPERTIES

Vitamin C is a generic term used to refer to all compounds that exhibit the biological activity of ascorbic acid. Ascorbic acid (AA) is a simple compound containing six carbon atoms, related to the monosaccharide glucose (Figure 12-1). It is stable to acid but easily destroyed by oxidation, light, alkali, and heat, especially in the presence of iron or copper. The oxidized form of ascorbic acid, known as *dehydroascorbic acid (DHAA),* also has vitamin C activity (Figure 12-1).

In food, vitamin C is largely present in the form of ascorbic acid, but smaller amounts of DHAA do occur and the total naturally occurring vitamin C activity of a food is the sum of its AA and DHAA contents. Both

FIGURE 12-1

Structures of related compounds with vitamin C activity (L-ascorbic acid and L-dehydroascorbic acid) and without vitamin C activity (D-erythrobic acid).

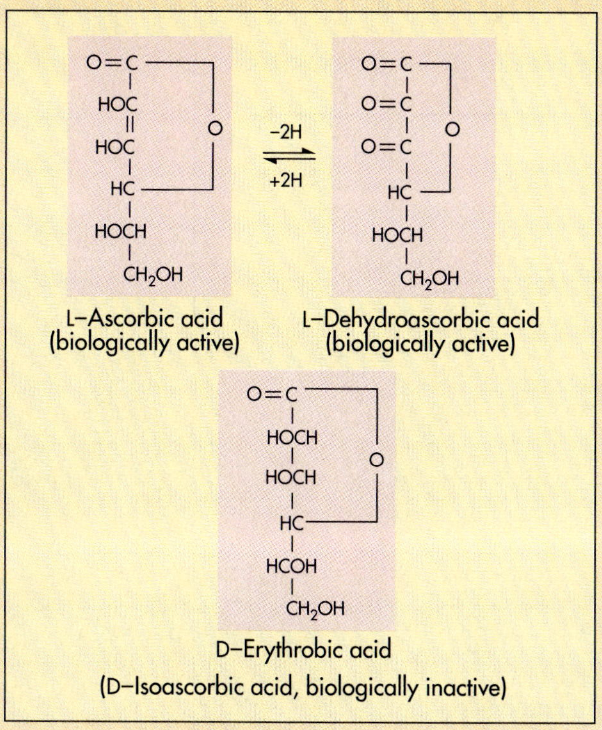

FIGURE 12-2

The oxidative degradation of ascorbic acid.

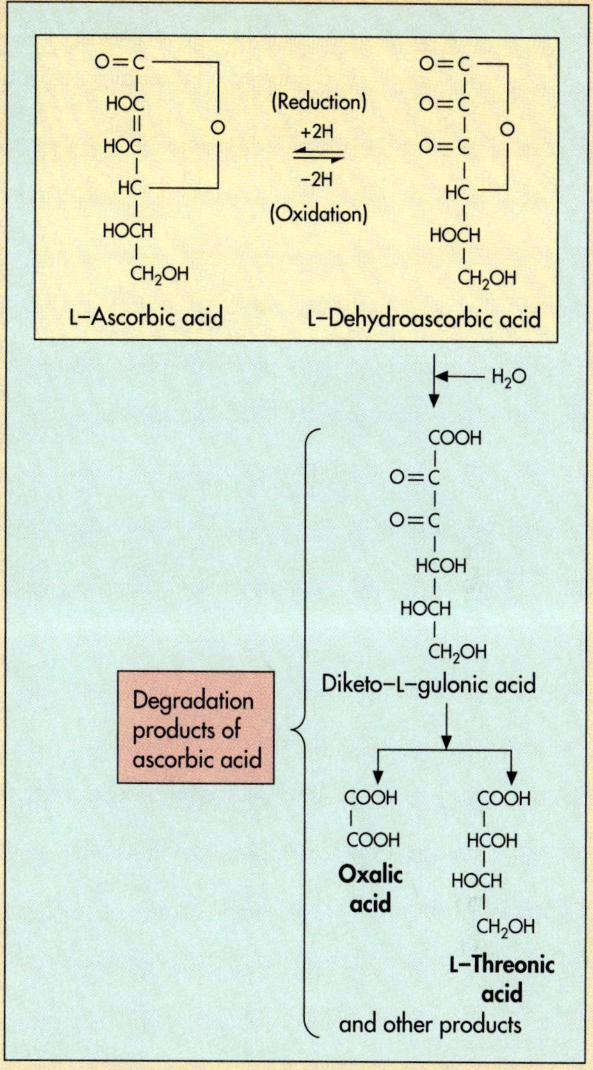

forms of vitamin C are susceptible to oxidation because they are reducing agents that function in the body as antioxidants. The first step in the oxidation of ascorbic acid is the formation of DHAA, which can then undergo further oxidation (Figure 12-2). Although the interconversion between AA and DHAA is reversible, the oxidation of DHAA is not, and the products of the oxidation of DHAA (diketo-L-gulonic acid, oxalic acid, and L-threonic acid) have no vitamin C activity.

Ascorbic acid occurs in the form of two geometrically different "stereoisomers": L-ascorbic acid and D-ascorbic acid. L-ascorbic acid predominates in food and is well used by humans, whereas the less common D-ascorbic acid is not. D-ascorbic acid is widely used as a preservative in processed meat and has been given the distinct name of **erythrobic acid** for use on food labels to avoid any implication that it contributes significant amounts of vitamin C activity to a food.

SYNTHESIS

Most mammals can synthesize vitamin C from glucose, but a few—including humans—lack the liver enzyme gulonolactone-oxidase, which is required to catalyze one step of this process. It is the lack of this enzyme that forces humans to obtain supplies of vitamin C from their food. Of the other animals that require a supply of dietary vitamin C, guinea pigs and monkeys have been most widely used in research, but fish are now proving increasingly useful also. In plants, vitamin C accumulates during the ripening process and is presumably synthesized within the plant cells from naturally occurring glucose.

Chemists learned how to produce synthetic vitamin C in 1933 from the monosaccharides glucose or galactose. Because the chemically synthesized and the natural forms extracted from plants are the same compound, the body cannot discriminate among them.

FUNCTIONS

Vitamin C is essential for the health of both animal and plant cells. Although it is a relatively simple compound that has been available in pure form for over 30 years, researchers have only recently been able to shed much light on its biochemical roles. Unlike most water-soluble

FIGURE 12-3

Examples of enzyme-mediated hydroxylations that require vitamin C and a metal ion (Fe^{2+} or Cu^{+}) as cofactors.

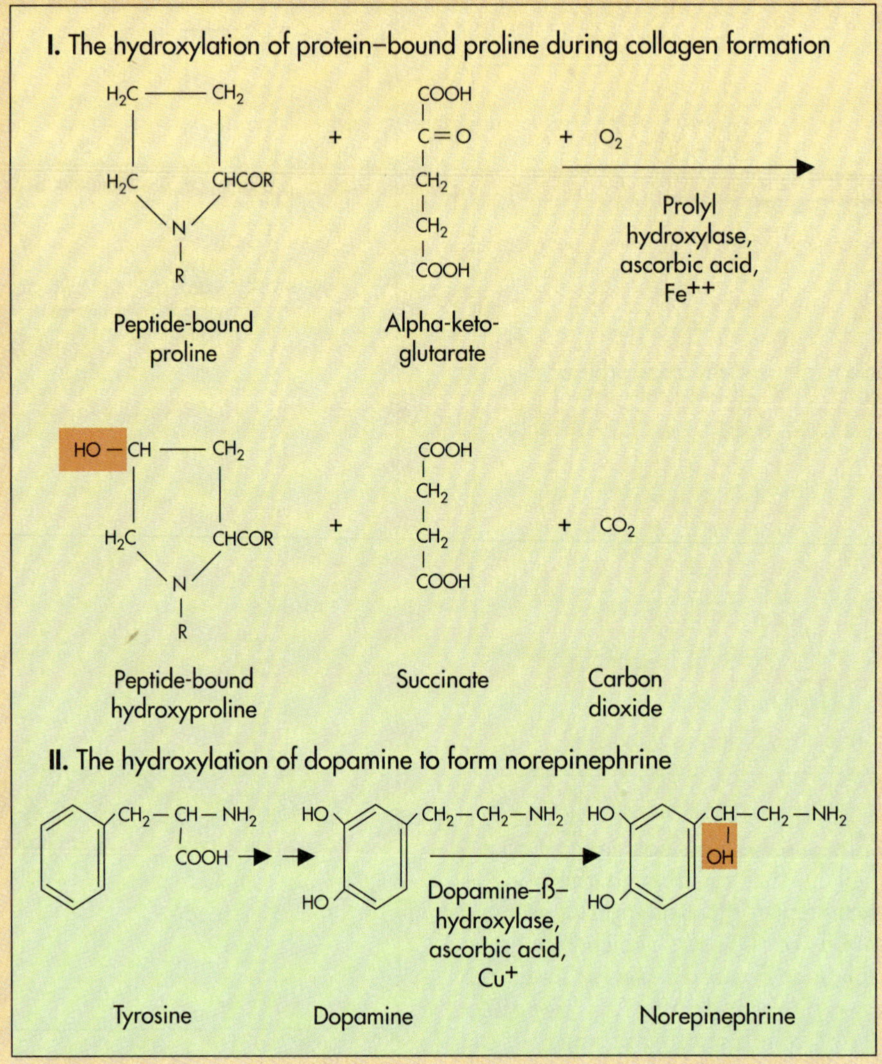

vitamins, vitamin C does not perform a clear-cut role as a coenzyme but rather as a substrate in the reaction. Vitamin C functions in a more general way as a biological reducing agent, especially during hydroxylation reactions, and as an antioxidant that protects the body against damaging oxidizing agents. When participating in hydroxylation reactions, vitamin C usually works in concert with metal ions, such as Fe^{2+} or Cu^{+} (Figure 12-3). Next, the range of specific roles of vitamin C are considered individually.

Collagen Formation

The best-characterized function of vitamin C is its role in the formation of the protein collagen. Collagen is a major structural protein of connective tissue (which binds cells and tissues together), bone, teeth, cartilage, skin, and scar tissue. Vitamin C is specifically required by the **fibroblast** cells of connective tissue (responsible for collagen synthesis) and the bone-forming osteoblasts within bone. It is estimated that collagen constitutes about one quarter of all the protein in the body.

Collagen is formed from a precursor protein known as tropocollagen by the hydroxylation of the amino acids proline and lysine within tropocollagen. Vitamin C is required to allow these essential hydroxylation reactions to proceed. The hydroxylation of proline residues in tropocollagen is essential to allow individual molecules of the protein to wind together to form strong and long triple-helical fibers, characteristic of mature collagen.[2] The hydroxylation of the lysine residues is required to allow the formation of strengthening cross-linkages within collagen.

The enzymes that catalyze these hydroxylation reactions (known as *prolyl* and *lysyl hydroxylases*) require the direct participation of ferrous iron (Fe^{2+} ions) and oxygen. The role of vitamin C is to act as a reducing agent that keeps the iron in the ferrous state, preventing its oxidation to the ferric (Fe^{3+}) state.

Any deficiency in vitamin C results in defective collagen synthesis, associated with impaired wound healing, disruption of capillaries, and faulty bone and tooth formation. One of the first effects of any impairment of collagen synthesis are small pinpoint hemorrhages, which result from weaknesses in the membranes that line the blood capillaries and in the fibers that hold cells together under the surface of the skin. These weaknesses allow blood to escape into the enlarged intercellular spaces, accounting for the capillary bleeding associated with scurvy. These subcutaneous hemorrhages appear most often in areas subjected to mechanical stress, such as the gums, which become soft, spongy, and prone to bleeding.

The bone matrix, which makes up one fifth of the weight of the bone shaft, is primarily collagen. If matrix formation is defective because of an impairment of collagen synthesis, it becomes less able to accumulate the calcium and phosphorus required for proper bone mineralization. As a result the bones become weakened and sometimes distorted. Bones sometimes become displaced from their joints when the supporting cartilage, which is also mainly collagen, becomes weakened.

The dentin layer of the tooth does not form normally during vitamin C deficiency. This results in teeth that are structurally weak and more prone to mechanical injury and decay.

The involvement of vitamin C in collagen formation during scar tissue formation has led some researchers to suggest that vitamin C intake should be increased to 50 times the RDA both before and after surgery. Others believe that such supplementation is unnecessary, provided that the patient's normal intake of vitamin C has been adequate. Skin grafts to repair burned tissue have been found to heal more quickly when adequate vitamin C is present.

TABLE 12-1

Vitamin C content of human tissues and fluids

TISSUE/FLUID	CONCENTRATION (mg/100 g OF WET TISSUE)
Pituitary gland	40-50
Adrenal glands	30-40
Eye lens	25-31
Brain	13-15
Liver	10-16
Spleen and pancreas	10-15
Kidneys	5-15
Heart muscle	5-15
Semen (whole)	4-11
Lungs	7
Skeletal muscle	3
Testes	3
Thyroid	2
Plasma/serum	0.3-1.5
Saliva	0.002-0.08

From Jacob RA: Vitamin C. In Shils ME, Olson JE, Shike M, editors: *Modern nutrition in health and disease,* vol 1, ed 8, Philadelphia, 1994, Lea & Febiger.

Carnitine Synthesis

Vitamin C is required for the activity of several other enzymes that catalyze hydroxylation reactions, including two ascorbic acid– and Fe^{2+}-dependent hydroxylations involved in the biosynthesis of carnitine. Carnitine is a small nitrogen-containing organic compound involved in the transport of fatty acids into mitochondria, where they can be oxidized to release energy for use by cells. The reduction in energy release because of limited carnitine biosynthesis has been proposed as the explanation for the fatigue and muscle weakness in those with vitamin C deficiency. However, this possibility has not yet been confirmed.[3]

Neurotransmitter Synthesis

Vitamin C is required to sustain the activity of the copper-containing enzyme **dopamine oxygenase,** which catalyzes the oxidation of dopamine to form the neurotransmitter norepinephrine. Vitamin C also appears to be involved in the hydroxylation of tryptophan during the biosynthesis of the neurotransmitter serotonin (5-hydroxytryptamine). It is also involved in the degradation of the amino acid tyrosine, although perhaps only as a nonspecific reducing agent. The involvement of vitamin C in the synthesis of neurotransmitters probably explains the high concentration of vitamin C found in brain and adrenal tissues (Table 12-1).

Activation of Hormones

Many peptide hormones and hormone-releasing factors are synthesized as precursor molecules that are enzymatically modified into their active forms. One such modification is the process of **α-amidation.** This is catalyzed by a copper-containing enzyme, **peptidyl glycine α-amidating monooxygenase,** which requires the presence of oxygen and a reducing agent for its activity. Ascorbic acid is the most effective of various reducing agents that have been studied and is found in high concentrations in the tissues in which α-amidation occurs. This suggests that vitamin C is the physiological reducing agent (or "reductant") for this reaction in the body.[2,4] The peptides that may be amidated in this vitamin C–dependent manner include bombesin (human gastrin-releasing peptide), calcitonin, gastrin, oxytocin, thyrotropin, corticotropin, vasopressin, and growth hormone–releasing factor.

Drug Detoxification

Vitamin C is required for the optimal activity of various drug-detoxifying metabolic systems within the body.

These include the **mixed-function oxidase** system and the **flavin-monooxygenase** system in the liver. These systems promote a series of modifications to drugs and other toxic molecules (such as those within environmental pollutants) to convert them into forms that can be excreted in urine. The modifications involved include hydroxylation and demethylation (the removal of CH_3 "methyl" groups).

General Antioxidant

Vitamin C is one of several compounds that form part of the body's antioxidant defensive system. As discussed in Chapter 11, a variety of damaging oxidizing agents occur in the body, as a result of both normal metabolic processes and exposure to drugs and environmental pollutants. A range of enzymes and antioxidant reducing agents (including vitamin E, β-carotene, and vitamin C) is able to convert these oxidizing agents to harmless substances that can be excreted. In particular, vitamin C can combine with and so "scavenge" many types of oxidizing free radicals. It can also regenerate the reduced form of vitamin E, converting that vitamin back into the form in which it can act as an antioxidant.

Vitamin C appears to be an important antioxidant in plasma, in other extracellular fluids, and within cells. Some investigators maintain that the primary function of vitamin C is its role as an antioxidant.[4]

Use of Iron, Calcium, and Folic Acid

Because vitamin C acts as a reducing agent that is able to keep iron ions in the more readily absorbed ferrous (Fe^{2+}) form, it facilitates the absorption of nonheme iron from the gastrointestinal tract. Vitamin C also assists the transfer of iron from blood plasma into ferritin for storage in the liver, as well as the release of iron from ferritin when required. Vitamin C also aids calcium absorption by preventing the calcium from becoming incorporated into insoluble complexes.

The conversion of the inactive form of the vitamin folic acid into its active forms, dihydrofolic acid and tetrahydrofolic acid, is also facilitated by vitamin C. In addition to assisting in their formation, vitamin C may also stabilize the active forms of folic acid, preventing their loss via urine.

Other Functions

Many other functions have been attributed to vitamin C, including roles in alleviating allergic reactions, enhancing immune function, stimulating formation of bile, and facilitating the release of some steroid hormones. Vitamin C is necessary for the conversion of cholesterol to bile acids and has been reported to be involved in the detoxification of many chemical carcinogens.[4]

ABSORPTION, TRANSPORT, AND METABOLISM

In humans, ascorbic acid is absorbed in the jejunum (distal part of the intestine), principally by a sodium-dependent active transport mechanism. As the name implies, this mechanism requires both the expenditure of energy and the presence of sodium ions. In addition to the active process, however, the vitamin is absorbed at a lower rate by simple diffusion. Evidence suggests that dehydroascorbic acid is passively absorbed and ascorbic acid is the form that is actively absorbed. There is a considerable quantity of dehydroascorbic acid in the intestine because ascorbic acid is rapidly oxidized in the presence of Fe^{+++}.

When consumed in small amounts of up to 100 mg, 80% to 90% of ingested vitamin C is absorbed. As intakes increase, the efficiency of absorption has been found to fall to 49%, 36%, and 16% for intakes of 1.5 g, 3.0 g, and 12 g, respectively. The presence of large amounts of unabsorbed vitamin C in the intestine has the same osmotic effect as do sugars, causing watery stools or diarrhea, accompanied by intestinal discomfort. These symptoms are often experienced by people consuming large amounts of vitamin C supplements.

The vitamin C content of blood serum rises to a maximal stable level of 1.2 to 1.5 mg/100 ml with an intake of 100 mg/day or more and falls to 0.2 to 0.1 mg/100 ml when the intake is less than 10 mg/day. If amounts of vitamin C of more than 100 mg/day are ingested, the vitamin C concentration in serum rises very high, but the excess is soon either picked up by tissue cells or excreted in urine. Within tissues the highest concentration of vitamin C is found in the pituitary and adrenal glands, with approximately 50 times the concentration found in serum. Other tissues such as the eye, brain, kidneys, lungs, and liver have between 5 and 30 times the concentration of vitamin C as found in serum. The concentration of vitamin C within muscle tissue is relatively low, but because of the large total mass of muscle in the body, as much as 600 mg of vitamin C can be stored in the muscles of a 70-kg person.

The total "pool" of vitamin C within the body can rise to a level of 1.2 to 2.0 g (or about 20 mg/kg) with an intake of 100 mg/day. This level of vitamin C content is sufficient to protect the body from severe scurvy for 90 days. On a diet free of vitamin C, the amount of the vitamin in the body declines at a rate of about 3% to 4%/day until reaching 300 mg, at which point the first signs of scurvy become apparent (Figure 12-4).

As previously mentioned, vitamin C is metabolized to diketo-L-gulonic acid and then oxalic acid and L-threonic acid, which are excreted in urine along with unmetabolized vitamin C (Figure 12-2). If large amounts of vitamin C are consumed, however, substantial amounts can be excreted unchanged. As any vitamin

TABLE 12-2

Comparison of dietary standards for vitamin C for selected age-groups (mg/day)

	UNITED STATES* (1989)	CANADA† (1990)	UNITED KINGDOM‡ (1991)	WHO/FAO§ (1988)
Children, 4-6 yr	45	25	25	20
Boys, 11-14 yr	45	20	35	30
Men 19+ yrs	60	40	40	30
Women 19+ yrs	60	30	40	30
Pregnant	70	40	50	50
Lactating				
First 6 mo	95	55	70	50
Second 6 mo	90			

* Food and Nutrition Board, National Research Council: *Recommended Dietary Allowances,* ed 10, Washington, DC, 1989, National Academy Press.

† Health and Welfare Canada: *Nutrition recommendations,* The Report of the Scientific Review Committee, Ottawa, Canada, 1990, Canadian Government Publishing Centre.

‡ *Dietary reference values for food energy and nutrients for the United Kingdom,* Report of the Panel on Dietary Reference Values of the Committee on Medical Aspects of Food Policy, Report on Health and Social Subjects No 41, London, 1991, Her Majesty's Stationery Office.

§ Food and Agriculture Organization: *Requirements of vitamin A, iron, folate, and vitamin B_{12}:* report of a Joint Food and Agriculture Organization/World Health Organization Expert Consultation, FAO Food and Nutrition Series No 23, Rome, 1988, The Organization.

FIGURE 12-4

Depletion of vitamin C from body stores over time with a vitamin C–deficient diet.

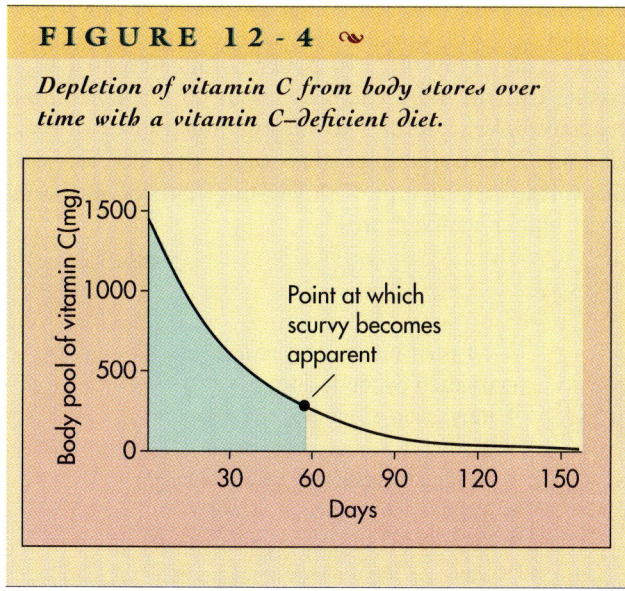

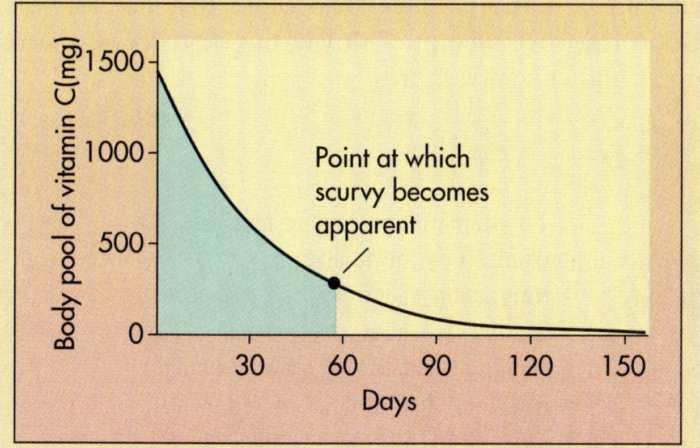

C is filtered through the kidneys, enough is reabsorbed to maintain a plasma concentration of 1.2 to 1.5 mg/100 ml and a total body pool of 1.2 to 2.0 g. All vitamin C in excess of the amounts needed to maintain these plasma and body levels is excreted in urine.

Because vitamin C is metabolized to oxalic acid, it has been suggested that high intakes may contribute to the development of oxalate-containing kidney stones. The amount metabolized to oxalic acid is limited, however, regardless of the level of intake. Nevertheless, patients with kidney stones or renal insufficiency are currently advised to avoid excessive intakes of vitamin C.

RECOMMENDED INTAKES

There has been considerable controversy about the appropriate criteria to use in setting recommended dietary allowances (RDAs) for vitamin C. Some nutritionists believe that the recommended allowance need not be too much greater than the amount that prevents scurvy (10 to 12 mg/day). Others recommend 60 mg/day or more to ensure that tissues become saturated with vitamin C (that is, contain the maximal concentration of the vitamin) without introducing any potential hazards as a result of overconsumption. This 60 mg/day figure is in line with the **urinary excretion threshold** of 60 to 80 mg/day, so called because any vitamin C consumed in excess of this threshold is excreted unused in urine. Recent evidence, however, indicates that saturation of the tissues of young men with vitamin C requires an intake of about 138 mg/day.[5]

The RDAs for vitamin C that have actually been set by the Food and Nutrition Board[6] are listed in Table 12-2 and considered in more detail as follows.

Adults

The current standards for adults reflect the philosophy that vitamin C intakes that allow tissue levels to approach the saturation level are desirable. This results in recommended intakes (varying from 30 to 100 mg/day in different countries) that are many times the 10 to 12 mg/day known to prevent or cure scurvy. The extent of disagreement between the authorities in different countries about appropriate levels of vitamin C intake is apparent from Table 12-2.

It is clear that vitamin C performs many functions in the body in addition to those required merely to prevent scurvy. It is assumed that vitamin C intakes in excess of the amounts required to prevent scurvy bring additional benefits to health, but the level of intake at which these additional benefits are maximized (with the least risk of problems as a result of overconsumption) has not been established. Recent studies suggest that the vitamin C needs of nonpregnant, nonlactating women may be met by an intake at the recommended level of 60 mg/day.[7] The consumption of the recommended five servings of fruits and vegetables each day provides vitamin C in excess of the amounts currently recommended.

Pregnancy

It is currently recommended that pregnant women should consume an additional 10 mg of vitamin C per day in addition to the normal adult recommended intake. The concentration of vitamin C in the serum of a fetus is 50% higher than in the maternal serum, and a high concentration of the vitamin is also found in the placenta.

Lactation

The vitamin C content of human milk usually varies from 3 to 10 mg/100 ml. The RDA Committee assumed a concentration of 3 mg/100 ml in its calculations, which results in a mother's losing 22 mg of vitamin C per day during the first 6 months of lactation (assuming a daily milk production of 700 ml/day) and 18 mg/day during the second 6 months of lactation (when milk production is assumed to be 600 ml/day). During early lactation it is recommended that a mother consume an additional 35 mg/day of vitamin C, falling to an additional 30 mg/day during late lactation.

Infants

Based on the amount of vitamin C in human milk, a breast-fed infant receives 22 to 85 mg of vitamin C per day and has a plasma vitamin C level of 0.5 to 1.5 mg/100 ml. The RDA committee recommends that an infant's intake of vitamin C be 30 mg/day, based on the average intake of breast-fed infants. Premature infants may require greater amounts of vitamin C, up to as much as twice the amount required by term infants. Most infant formulas have sufficient vitamin C added to provide 5 to 6 mg of vitamin C per 100 ml, which is similar to the concentration in human milk.

Children

For children the RDA for vitamin C increases only slightly beyond the infant level, to 40 mg/day for children of 4 to 10 years of age and 50 mg/day for those aged 11 to 14. On reaching the age of 15, children enter the adult band of recommended vitamin C intake (60 mg/day).

Cigarette Smokers

Serum vitamin C levels are lower in cigarette smokers than in nonsmokers. The biochemical mechanism behind this effect is unknown, but there is evidence of an increased rate of metabolic turnover and decreased efficiency of absorption of vitamin C in smokers. Thus it is recommended that the RDA for vitamin C for both male and female smokers should be 100 mg/day, rather than 60 mg/day. Some investigators estimate that the actual requirement for vitamin C among smokers may be as high as 140 mg/day.[8]

FOOD SOURCES

Vitamin C occurs almost exclusively in foods of plant origin. Among animal-based foods, only liver and kidney can be considered significant sources of vitamin C. There is a small amount of vitamin C present in fresh milk, but it can be destroyed by heat during processing. The amount of vitamin C in plant-based foods depends on many factors, as follows.

Part and Type of Plant

The head of broccoli has more vitamin C than the stem, but tests have shown that stems retain 82% of their vitamin C during 10 minutes of cooking, whereas the heads retain only 60%. In general, thin-stemmed vegetables contain more vitamin C than do thick-stemmed vegetables. Vegetables that wilt lose much more of their vitamin C during storage than those that do not wilt. Roots lose their vitamin C slowly, but this process speeds up at higher temperatures.

The vitamin C content of food is maximized by the following:

- Harvesting at the peak of maturity
- Storing in a cool, moist place
- Limiting exposure to air and sunlight
- Avoiding soaking food in water
- Cooking food in the minimal amount of water or, even better, cooking by microwave
- Cooking the food in pieces as large as possible

Stage of Maturity

Because vitamin C accumulates in fruit throughout the maturing and ripening process, the highest levels of the vitamin are found in fruits that have been left for the longest times on the tree or vine. In contrast, seeds such as peas and beans contain some vitamin C when immature but lose it as they reach maturity. Allowing the peas or beans to sprout, however, causes the buildup of significant amounts of vitamin C within them.

FIGURE 12-5

Contribution of various food groups to the vitamin C in the North American food supply.

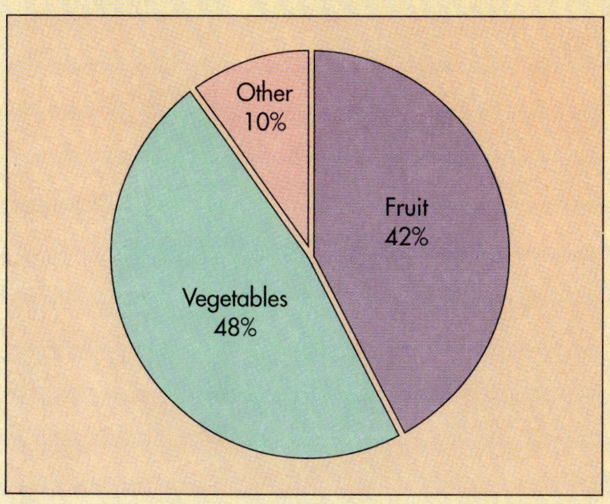

Conditions of Storage

The vitamin C content of foods declines as they are stored, but the losses are kept to a minimum by storing the foods at refrigerator temperatures in high humidity and with a minimum of air movement around the food. The amount of vitamin C in vegetables bought in the temperate zone in the winter months depends on the storage conditions during harvesting, shipping, and display in stores before selling.

Season of the Year

The vitamin C content of vegetables such as broccoli fluctuates widely, reflecting variations in weather and conditions of growing, harvesting, transporting, and storing, in addition to variations among different types of plant.

Method of Processing

Any method of food processing that involves the use of heat is likely to reduce the vitamin C content of the food. If the processing is done in the absence of air, however, the losses are much lower. Blanching of vegetables before freezing is required to destroy certain enzymes that otherwise catalyze the destruction of vitamin C. The irradiation of potatoes causes no immediate decrease in vitamin C content, but a 50% loss is found after 1 week. The freeze-drying of fruit causes little or no loss of vitamin C. When frozen and canned foods have been picked at the peak of maturity and processed immediately under optimal conditions, they may contain more vitamin C than does the fresh product that has endured a relatively long period between harvesting and consumption, possibly under conditions of poor temperature and humidity control.

Method of Preparation

Fortunately, many of the best sources of vitamin C are normally consumed raw. In cooked foods, most losses of vitamin C occur in the early stages of cooking. For example, broccoli heads lose 40% of their vitamin C content during the first 10 minutes of cooking because of destruction by heat and leaching into the cooking water. Cabbage is known to lose more by heat destruction than by leaching. In general, the amount of vitamin C lost by leaching depends more on the amount of water used and on the surface area of the food exposed to water than on the total cooking time. Tests have shown that the losses of vitamin C from broccoli cooked by microwaving, pressure cooking, steaming, and boiling were 15%, 20%, 30%, and 55%, respectively.

ADEQUACY OF VITAMIN C CONTENT OF THE FOOD SUPPLY AND THE DIET

Figure 12-5 shows the contribution of various food groups to the vitamin C available in the North American food supply. Fruits and vegetables provide 90% of the available vitamin C, with the remaining 10% coming from the relatively small amounts in meat, fish, eggs, poultry, and dairy products. The major individual contributors of vitamin C in the American diet are orange juice (contributing 26.5% of the total), grapefruit (7.2%), tomatoes and tomato juice (6.1%), and potatoes (4.2%). Although cereal products—such as grains—do not naturally provide much vitamin C, some of them are fortified with ascorbic acid and therefore can make a significant contribution to the daily intake of vitamin C. Enriched beverages, usually fruit drinks, can also be an important source of dietary vitamin C.

Results of The Nationwide Food Consumption Study (NFCS) 1987-1988 and the National Health and Nutrition Examination Survey (NHANES III, 1988-1991) indicate that mean vitamin C intake in the United States is approximately 90 to 120 mg/day for adult males and females.[9,10] Little change in vitamin C intake has been reported in national survey data over the past 20 years.[9] Throughout that time, reported mean intakes of vitamin C by all age-groups have either met or exceeded the recommended levels.

Food composition tables, such as the one in Appendix E, are reported to list the content of only the reduced form of vitamin C (ascorbic acid) within food, whereas the oxidized form (dehydroascorbic acid) can also be used by humans. Theoretically then, food composition tables should underestimate the actual vitamin C content of foods. Recent state of the art chemical analyses, however, which determine both the AA and DHAA content of foods, have provided values for the vitamin C content of some foods that are lower than those in commonly used food composition tables.[11]

TABLE 12-3

Vitamin C content of foods (mg/100g)

	USDA HANDBOOK #8 (REDUCED AA)	RECENT ANALYSIS*		
		REDUCED AA	DHAA	TOTAL
VEGETABLES				
String beans, green beans (boiled)	9.7	6.7	1.3	8
Tomatoes, tomato juice (raw)	18	10.6	3	13.6
Broccoli (boiled)	62.8	37	2.6	39.6
Cauliflower or brussel sprouts (raw)	71.5	54	8.7	62.7
Spinach (raw)	28.1	52.4	—	52.4
Spinach (cooked)	9.8	15.1	—	15.1
Mustard greens, turnip greens, collards (boiled); cabbage, sauerkraut	25.3	4.8	—	4.8
Carrots or mixed vegetables	32.7	20.7	9.6	30.3
Mixed green salad	—†	7.9	2.8	10.7
Sweet red pepper	128	151	4	155
French fries (fast food)	10.3	14.3	9	23.3
Other potatoes (boiled, baked, potato salad)	10.7	7	1.3	8.3
FRUITS				
Bananas	9.1	15.3	3.3	18.6
Cantaloupe	42.2	28	2.7	30.7
Grapefruit	33.3	21.3	2.3	23.6
Orange	52.2	58.7	5.6	64.3
Watermelon	9.6	8	1.7	9.7
JUICES				
Orange juice or grapefruit juice (1 day old, reconstituted)	36.3	33	4.3	37.3
Tang, Start breakfast drink	—	57.3	2	59.3
OTHER FOODS				
Pizza (fast food)	2	0.9	0.3	1.2
Spaghetti (with tomato sauce), lasagne, other pasta	—	1	0.5	1.5
Highly fortified cereals (e.g., Product 19) (without milk)	212	226	38	264
Other cold cereals (e.g., Corn Flakes) (without milk)	53	59.7	2.5	62.2
Hot dogs‡	0.1	18	3	21

AA, Ascorbic acid; *DHAA,* dehydroascorbic acid; *USDA,* United States Department of Agriculture.

* Analyzed by Vanderslice JT and others: *J Food Compos Anal* 3:105, 1990.

† Where no values are listed, the concentration was less than 1 mg/100 g sample.

‡ Hot dog analyzed in USDA Handbook No 8 is with a bun, whereas the recent analysis is for hot dog without a bun.

From Sinha R, Block G, Taylor PR: *Am J Clin Nutr* 57:547, 1993.

Table 12-3 gives a comparison of the vitamin C content of foods identified as common sources of the vitamin in the United States, as listed in the United States Department of Agriculture (USDA) Handbook No. 8 (AA content only) and as obtained from recent analysis of both AA and DHAA content. Large discrepancies are apparent in the vitamin C values listed for broccoli, red pepper, and cooked greens, such as mustard, turnip, and collard greens. These differences may be an important source of error when estimating the vitamin C intakes of individuals or groups of people who obtain much of their vitamin C from these sources. This may be the case for African-Americans, who reportedly obtain more than 10% of their vitamin C from cooked greens.[11] Recalculation of vitamin C intakes using the results of the most recent analyses of the vitamin C content of foods suggests that past national surveys may have overestimated total vitamin C intake by approximately 10% to 24%.

The most frequently used sources of vitamin C are citrus fruits and their juices, broccoli, spinach, and melon in season, but several other rich sources are available. Parsley has a high vitamin C content (175 mg/100 g) but is used in such small quantities that it is not an important source. Many of the earliest concentrates of vitamin C that were made before the synthetic

FIGURE 12-6

Relative amounts of vitamin C in various juices.

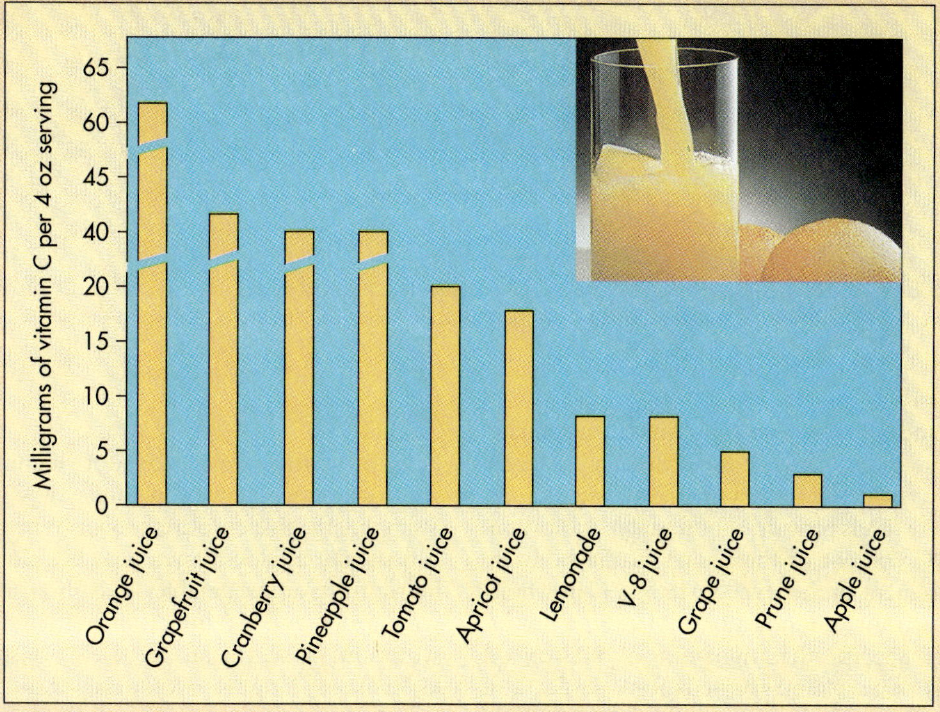

vitamin was readily available were made from rose hips gathered mainly by Indians in northern Alberta, Canada. The acerola cherry, native to the tropics, is also an extremely rich source (1500 mg/100 g), and although it is unpalatable on its own, it is used to fortify juices that are less rich in vitamin C, especially for infant feeding. Camucamu, a fruit native to South America, contains even more vitamin C, at an average level of 2000 mg/ 100 g. Today, supplements labeled "with acerola," "with rose hips," or "with natural vitamin C" usually contain little vitamin C from these identified sources, with the bulk of the vitamin C coming from less expensive synthetic sources.

The relative amounts of vitamin C in various juices are shown in Figure 12-6, which makes it clear that citrus juices are clearly better sources than are other commonly consumed juices. In the processing of noncitrus fruit juices, however, vitamin C is usually added at a level of about 30 mg/4-oz serving. This is a commendable practice of benefit to those who are not aware of the differences in vitamin C content among different fruit juices. The actual amounts of vitamin C found in fruit juices by analysis are usually higher than the amounts listed on the labels. The values on the labels are set low to ensure that the vitamin C content of a product at least matches the value on the label after losses during processing and storage. In Canada the enrichment of apple juice with vitamin C is approved by government agencies because it puts a native product in a better competitive position with respect to imported orange juice.

Vitamin C is often added to dehydrated potatoes. This is of questionable value, however, because of the likelihood that much of the added vitamin C is destroyed by heat and oxidation during preparation of the food. The enrichment of milk and carbonated beverages with vitamin C is widely practiced but has not been officially endorsed in the United States.

During the processing of frozen fruits, such as peaches and apples, vitamin C is often added as a reducing agent to help prevent discoloration of the fruit. Vitamin C is also used as a preservative in jams and jellies, a color stabilizer in fruit cocktail, a dough conditioner in white flour, and an acidulant in frozen desserts. It is also added to wines and beers to prevent darkening and deterioration of flavor. Although the amounts of vitamin C consumed because of these uses of the vitamin are small, they do make some contribution to the overall intake of vitamin C.

EVALUATION OF VITAMIN C STATUS

Measurements of vitamin C levels in blood plasma and within leukocytes (white blood cells) are currently the

TABLE 12-4

Guidelines for interpreting biochemical measures of vitamin C status

	PLASMA (mg/100 ml)	BODY POOL (mg)	MIXED LEUKOCYTES (μg/10⁸ CELLS)	MONONUCLEAR LEUKOCYTES (μg/10⁸ CELLS)
Adequate	>0.4	>600	>20	>25
Low	0.2-0.4	300-600	10-20	20-25
Deficient	<0.2	<300	<10	<20
Normal range*	0.4-1.5	500-1500 (10-22 mg/kg)	20-53	25-40

* Upper end of range may be higher in individuals taking vitamin C supplements.

From Jacob RA: Vitamin C. In Shils ME, Olson JA, Shike M, editors: *Modern nutrition in health and disease,* ed 8, Philadelphia, 1994, Lea & Febiger.

most practical and reliable tests with which to evaluate vitamin C status in humans. Plasma vitamin C levels respond quickly to recent dietary intake of vitamin C, whereas leukocyte levels provide a more stable indication of the vitamin C content of the tissues of the body in general. Measurement of the level of vitamin C in whole blood is not as sensitive an indicator of vitamin C status as is the more specific determination of plasma or leukocyte levels. The plasma or leukocyte levels, for example, fall more quickly as vitamin C deficiency sets in than does the vitamin C level of whole blood. Guidelines for interpreting four different biochemical measures of vitamin C status are presented in Table 12-4.

The interpretation of leukocyte vitamin C levels is complicated because there are different types of leukocytes, which contain different concentrations of vitamin C. Table 12-4, for example, lists values for "mixed leukocytes" (a sample of all types) and for a specific category of leukocytes known as the *mononuclear leukocytes.* These mononuclear leukocytes are known to contain two to three times the amount of vitamin C as do those leukocytes within a category known as *polymorphonuclear leukocytes.* It has been suggested that the vitamin C level in the mononuclear leukocytes may be the best functional indicator of vitamin C status because of their ability to concentrate the vitamin within them, their importance to the status of the immune system, and their relative resistance to vitamin C depletion as a deficiency of the vitamin develops. However, which category of leukocytes is the most useful for determining vitamin C status is the subject of continuing research.[12]

No relationship has been detected between age and vitamin C status in adults. Earlier reports of decreasing vitamin C levels with age have now been attributed to differences in vitamin C intake among the people studied, rather than their age as such. Throughout life, women have consistently higher vitamin C levels than do men with similar intakes. As already mentioned, smokers have poorer vitamin C status than do nonsmokers, and lower dietary intakes of the vitamin by smokers cannot account for all of the difference.

DEFICIENCY

Scurvy, the most severe form of vitamin C deficiency, is relatively rare, especially in adults, now that its cause and a simple effective cure are known. When it does develop, it is usually in elderly men who live alone and eat a diet low in fruits and vegetables. It is also sometimes found in young men and alcoholics on restricted diets. The early symptoms of scurvy are relatively nonspecific, including listlessness; fatigue; weakness; shortness of breath; muscle cramps; aching bones, joints, and muscles; and a loss of appetite. The skin then becomes dry, feverish, rough, and covered with reddish-blue spots. Hemorrhaging of the gums can often lead to secondary infections. Delayed or incomplete wound healing is a frequent sign of vitamin C deficiency, and anemia invariably occurs after 2 months on a restricted vitamin C intake because of the loss of blood caused by hemorrhaging.

One study of experimentally induced scurvy in men found that the clinical symptoms included enlargement (hypertrophy) of the cornea, congestion of follicles and ducts, swollen joints, bleeding gums, muscular aches and pains, fatigue, and difficulty in breathing.[13] Pinpoint hemorrhages under the skin causing the reddish-blue spots (**petechiae**) occurred when the total vitamin C reserves in the body fell to below 300 mg. The first signs of these petechial hemorrhages appeared after 29 days of a vitamin C–free diet, at the time when all urinary excretion of vitamin C and its metabolites had ceased. All subjects showed severe symptoms of scurvy after 90 days, by which time their plasma and whole blood vitamin C levels had fallen to almost zero. Intakes of 6.5 to 10 mg of ascorbic acid per day were effective in eliminating the clinical symptoms of scurvy.

Scurvy in infants was first reported in the late nineteenth century, at a time when the practice of wet nursing was being replaced by the use of preserved milk. It then reappeared when the pasteurization of milk (with its resultant destruction of vitamin C) became mandatory. It appeared yet again in the 1960s and 1970s in infants given home-prepared formula that had been subjected to prolonged heating. There have also been a few reports of scurvy in infants born to mothers who had consumed megadoses of vitamin C during pregnancy. It was presumed that the large amount of vitamin C available to such infants while in the womb conditioned them to require more vitamin C than is provided by human milk or infant formula. Controlled studies in guinea pigs and humans, however, have failed to reproduce such conditioning.[14]

Infant scurvy is now almost unknown in developed countries, but when it does occur, it is most likely to develop during the period of rapid growth between 6 and 24 months of age. Scurvy develops rapidly in infants, with irritability, anorexia, growth failure, tenderness of the hips, and anemia progressing quickly to the point at which the infant may be at risk of death. When treated with vitamin C, the recovery of infants is equally dramatic.

Breast-fed infants never have scurvy. So the most effective way to ensure that infants receive sufficient vitamin C is to encourage breast-feeding. Properly prepared infant formula and the use of vitamin C supplements can readily provide the vitamin C needed by infants who are not breast-fed.

ADDITIONAL PROPOSED BENEFITS OF HIGH DOSES

A number of investigators have suggested that higher amounts of vitamin C than those currently recommended can bring additional health benefits and prevent some common and, in some cases, serious diseases. If these additional benefits prove to be genuine, they may involve actions of vitamin C that could more appropriately be described as those of a pharmacological agent, rather than a vitamin. At present, the available information on such additional health benefits is not considered sufficiently persuasive to justify any increase in the RDAs. Nevertheless, the three main benefits claimed to be provided by higher-than-recommended intakes of vitamin C, involving protection against the common cold, cancer, and cardiovascular disease, are briefly considered.

Vitamin C and the Common Cold

Over 20 years ago Linus Pauling[15] wrote a book aimed at the lay public entitled *Vitamin C and the Common Cold* in which he claimed that vitamin C offered protection against the common cold and relief from its symptoms. This book provoked considerable controversy within the scientific community, and its conclusions were not generally accepted. As a result of its publication, several controlled trials were performed to investigate the effect of vitamin C on the common cold. At least 17 such studies have been carried out since 1970, studying the effects of dosages of 1 g of vitamin C per day. Pauling's book has also prompted the publication of more than 100 articles in the scientific literature on the possible role of vitamin C in the treatment of the common cold.[16] The bulk of the evidence accumulated does not support the theory that vitamin C can decrease the incidence of the common cold. It has been found, however, that the administration of supplemental vitamin C can significantly decrease the duration of an episode of the cold and reduce the severity of the symptoms. The biochemical explanation for this beneficial effect may involve the general antioxidant properties of vitamin C. During an infection, cells known as *phagocytes* become activated to fight the infection and produce free radicals, which are released from the cells. By combining with these free radicals, vitamin C may decrease their inflammatory effects.

Vitamin C and Cancer

Some evidence from epidemiological studies suggests that vitamin C may play a role in the prevention of cancer, an idea that is also supported by the results of some animal studies.[17] Of 46 studies that have investigated the relationship between the intake of vitamin C or fruits rich in vitamin C and the risk of developing non–hormone-dependent cancers, 33 found that high vitamin C intakes offered a statistically significant protective effect. In 29 other studies that specifically assessed fruit intake, 21 revealed that high intakes of fruit offered significant protection against the development of cancer. The protective associations were stronger for cancers of the esophagus, larynx, oral cavity, and pancreas than for cancers of the stomach, rectum, breast, and cervix. No evidence of any protective effect was found for cancers of the ovary and prostate gland.

The biochemical mechanism behind the anticancer properties of vitamin C is believed to be a combination of its general antioxidant abilities (especially against free radicals) and its involvement in the detoxification of some known carcinogens. Other nutrients present in foods rich in vitamin C probably also play a role because many of the studies have looked at the intake of such foods, rather than actual vitamin C intake. Other nutrients contributing to the anticancer effect probably include vitamin E, carotenoids, vitamin A, and folic acid.

Recent survey data in the United States indicate that 41% of those surveyed had no fruit on the survey day, and only 25% consumed one fruit or vegetable rich in vitamin C or vitamin A.[18] This suggests that whatever the mechanism, an increase in the consumption of vitamin C–rich foods by the U.S. population could lead to a considerable reduction in the incidence of several types of cancer.

Vitamin C and Cardiovascular Disease

Some epidemiological and experimental evidence suggests that high vitamin C intakes may help prevent the onset of cardiovascular disease. Vitamin C is known to be involved in regulating cholesterol metabolism and in maintaining the structure of blood vessels, and the antioxidant effects of the vitamin might prevent the tissue damage that leads to cardiovascular disease. Vitamin C deficiency has been shown to encourage atherosclerosis in guinea pigs. There is some evidence to suggest that patients with coronary artery disease and apoplexy (stroke) have lowered serum and leukocyte vitamin C levels. To prove that lowered vitamin C levels can cause such conditions or that high intakes of vitamin C can prevent them, however, requires a more rigorous series of trials than have currently been performed. New information is expected in this area in the future.

TOXICITY OF VITAMIN C

Because there is considerable interest in possible beneficial effects of high doses of vitamin C, it is obviously relevant to consider whether high doses are associated with any risks to health. This is particularly important because 20% to 25% of the U.S. population takes daily vitamin C supplements of between 100 and 10,000 mg. The relative scarcity of reports of harmful effects of vitamin C, however, despite the large numbers of people taking doses well in excess of the RDAs, suggests that the vitamin must be relatively nontoxic.

Many people who ingest large doses of vitamin C develop nausea and diarrhea, which are believed to result from the osmotic effect of vitamin C, drawing water into the gastrointestinal tract. Because vitamin C is known to enhance iron absorption, there is some concern that regular consumption of high levels of the vitamin might increase the risk of iron overload in men, 6% of whom have a genetic predisposition to absorb excess iron. This possibility is currently under active investigation. Also, large doses of vitamin C may interfere with anticoagulant therapy and are known to interfere with the results of many laboratory tests that rely on oxidation or reduction reactions (such as estimations of cholesterol or glucose levels).

FOLIC ACID

Folic acid was discovered in 1945 during the search for the nutritional factor that gives liver the ability to cure **pernicious anemia.** It is now known that vitamin B_{12}, rather than folic acid, is the nutrient that cures pernicious anemia. Folic acid, however, has also proved to be a vitamin because it plays a role in a variety of essential biological processes.

Folic acid has been known by many names. It is the active ingredient of the **Wills factor,** which was isolated from yeast and liver in the 1930s and found to cure an anemia of pregnancy characterized by large red blood cells. It is also the active ingredient of nutritional factors that were once known as **vitamin M, vitamin B_c, factor U,** and the ***Lactobacillus casei*** factor. Folic acid is actually a generic term for the chemical **pteroylglutamic acid (PGA)** and related chemicals with the same biological activities as PGA. PGA itself is rarely found in significant amounts either in food or in the human body. Instead, food contains a variety of chemically related substances that all have the biological activities of folic acid. The term **folate** is commonly used to describe any compound or mixture of compounds with the activities of folic acid.

CHEMICAL COMPOSITION

The chemical structures of PGA and a variety of naturally occurring compounds that have folic acid activity are shown in Figure 12-7. PGA itself is formed when **pteroic acid** (made when pterin combines with para-amino-benzoic acid) combines with one molecule of glutamic acid. Other components of the mixtures that are referred to as folic acid or folate include compounds with up to 11 additional glutamic acid molecules added to the basic PGA structure. These are known as **polyglutamate** forms of folate, whereas PGA is a **monoglutamate** form. Naturally occurring folate also contains reduced (dihydro and tetrahydro) forms of the vitamin and forms with a variety of one-carbon "substituent" groups added at various sites. Naturally occurring folate includes a large number of such compounds (Figure 12-7).

FUNCTIONS OF FOLATE

Shortly after its discovery, folate was found to cure **megaloblastic anemia** (or macrocytic anemia). This is a form of anemia characterized by large red blood cells that continue to grow because they do not lose their nucleus as do normal red blood cells. Although effective in curing this type of anemia, folate could not cure the neurological symptoms of pernicious anemia and so the initial view that it was the anti–pernicious anemia factor was abandoned. Folate is now known to be required for the normal growth and division of all cells—not only human cells, but also all animal, plant, and microbial cells.

The specific biochemical function of folate is to act as a coenzyme in reactions involving the transfer of one-carbon units, such as the methyl group (CH_3) from one compound to another.[19] Examples of processes requiring the presence of folate are the following:

- The synthesis of the amino acids methionine, histidine, and serine
- The conversion of the amino acid phenylalanine into the amino acid tyrosine
- The formation of the heme group of hemoglobin
- The synthesis of the purine and pyrimidine

FIGURE 12-7

Chemical structure of pteroylglutamic acid and related components of the mixture of compounds referred to collectively as folic acid or folate.

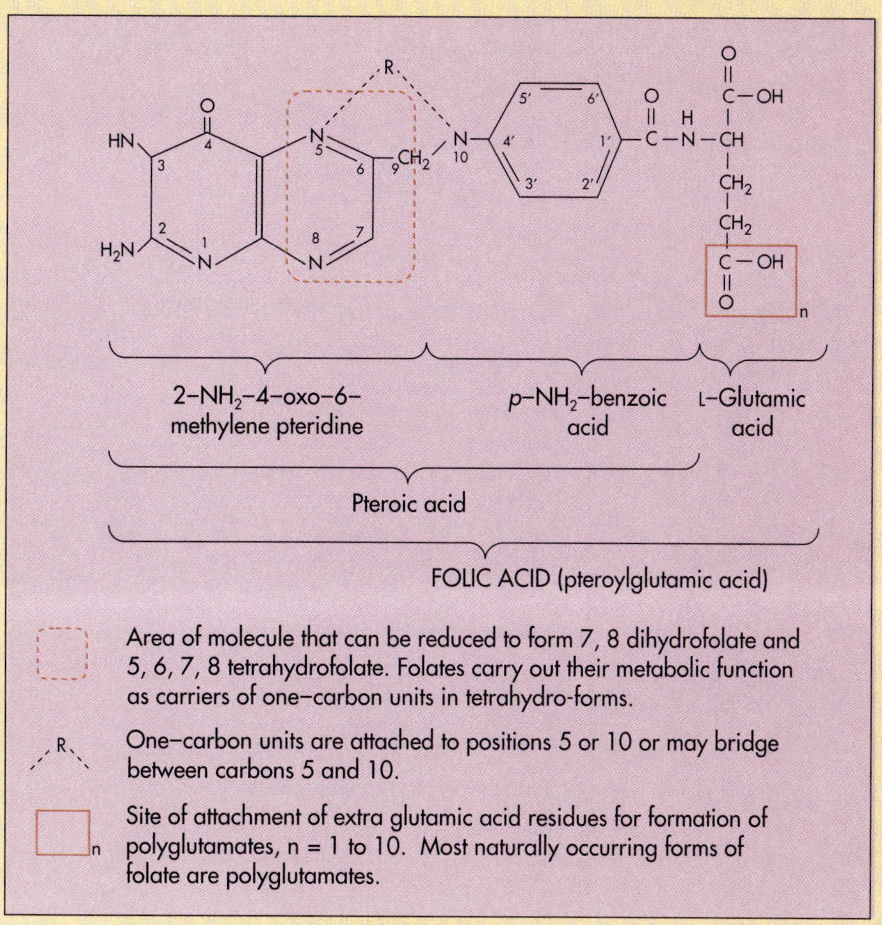
2-NH2-4-oxo-6-methylene pteridine
p-NH2-benzoic acid
L-Glutamic acid
Pteroic acid
FOLIC ACID (pteroylglutamic acid)
Area of molecule that can be reduced to form 7, 8 dihydrofolate and 5, 6, 7, 8 tetrahydrofolate. Folates carry out their metabolic function as carriers of one-carbon units in tetrahydro-forms.
One-carbon units are attached to positions 5 or 10 or may bridge between carbons 5 and 10.
Site of attachment of extra glutamic acid residues for formation of polyglutamates, n = 1 to 10. Most naturally occurring forms of folate are polyglutamates.

bases needed for the synthesis of deoxyribonucleic acid (DNA) and ribonucleic acid (RNA)
- The formation of the vitamin-like compound choline from ethanolamine
- The conversion of the vitamin niacin to N-methyl nicotinamide, the form in which it is excreted

Cells whose normal activities require rapid cell growth and division are particularly sensitive to folate deficiency because folate is required for the formation of amino acids (and therefore proteins) and nucleic acids, some of the key compounds of the cell. Examples of such cells are red blood cells and the cells lining the gastrointestinal tract. The involvement of folate in hemoglobin synthesis is another factor that makes red blood cell formation particularly sensitive to folate deficiency. A substantial interrelationship exists between folate and vitamin B_{12} that is discussed later in this chapter (see *Function of Vitamin* B_{12}).

ABSORPTION, TRANSPORT, AND METABOLISM

Before the folate in food can be absorbed, any additional glutamic acid residues must be split off to produce a monoglutamic acid form (that is, containing only one glutamic acid residue). This conversion occurs in the intestinal lumen, catalyzed by the brush border enzyme **folate hydrolase** (also known as **conjugase**). Certain foods, such as cabbage and legumes, contain conjugase inhibitors that can impede the absorption of folate from a meal.

Absorption of folate occurs by both active transport and diffusion along the entire length of the small intestine (although mainly in the upper third). Recent evidence suggests that folate in milk is absorbed by a different mechanism than is folate from other sources. The vitamin within milk is bound to **folate-binding proteins,** which are absorbed—along with their bound folate—in the lower third of the small intestine.[20] Studies in adults have shown that 70% of the monoglutamate

FIGURE 12-8

Summary of key features of the absorption, transport, and metabolism of folate.

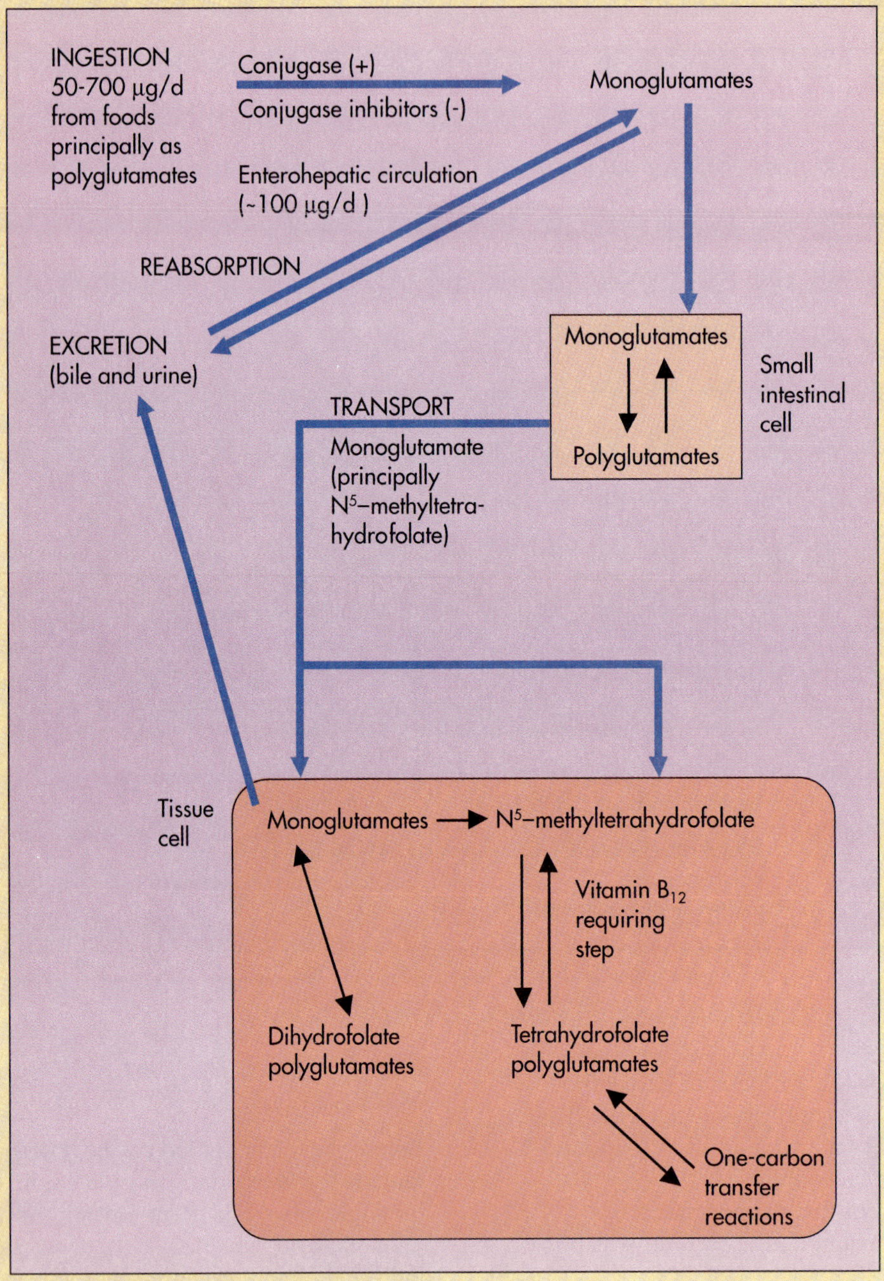

form of folate and approximately 50% of the polyglutamate forms are absorbed.[21] When synthetic folate monoglutamate is added to rice, maize, or bread, it is 45% less bioavailable than when taken in tablet form with water.[22]

Once absorbed into the intestinal wall cells, folate is transported in the blood to all cells of the body, with any excess being stored in the liver. The main form in which folate is transported around the body is **N^5-methyltetrahydrofolate**. The mechanism by which folate is transported from intestinal cells into the circulation is not well understood.

The total amount of folate in the body is normally between 5 and 10 mg, 50% of which is stored in the liver.[23] Within cells folate is found mainly in polyglutamate forms with three or more glutamic acid residues, although to cross cell membranes, the vitamin must be converted into a monoglutamate form with all but one glutamic acid residue removed. Polyglutamate forms are more active as coenzymes because of their

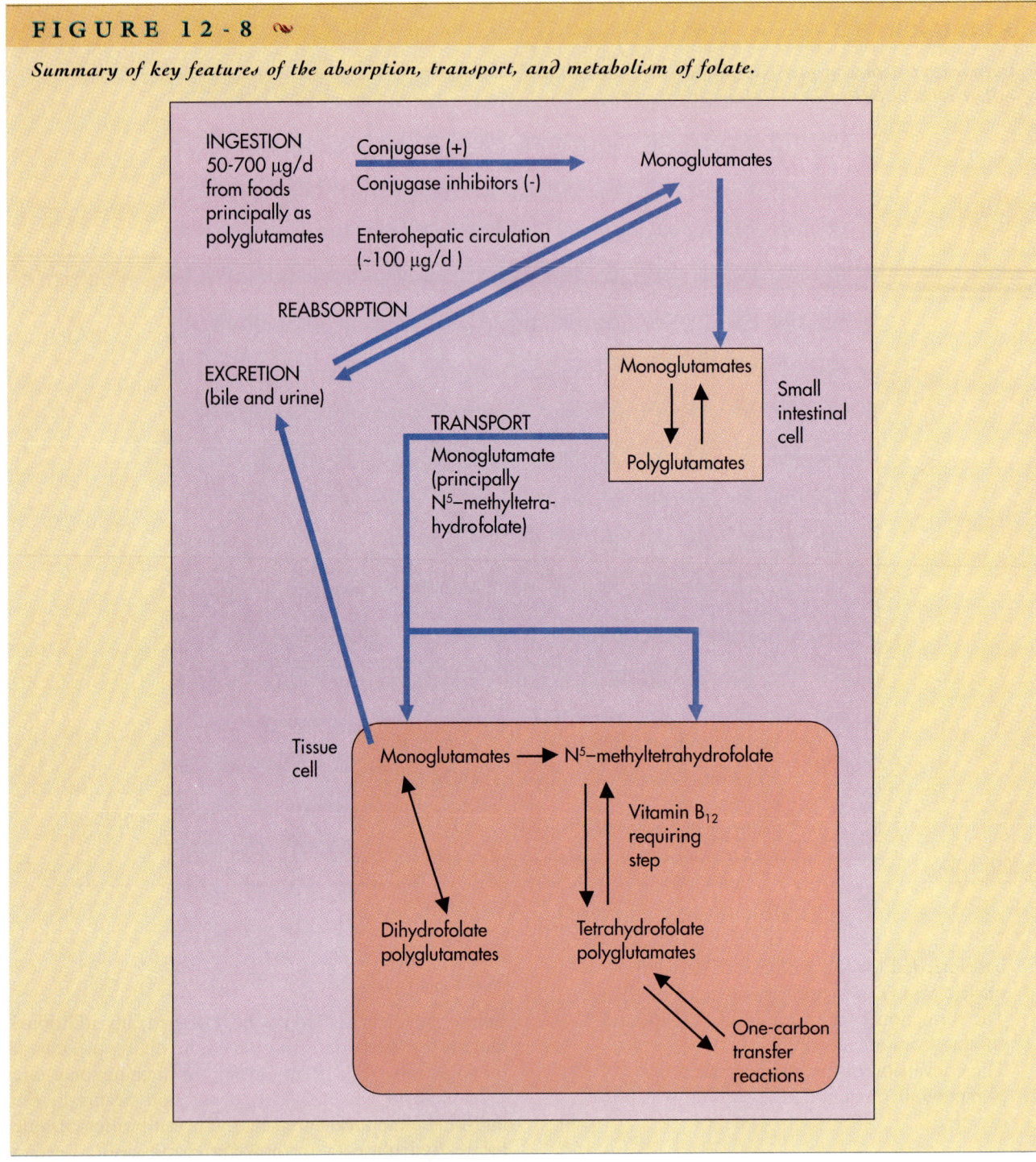

TABLE 12-5

Comparison of recommended intakes of folate in different countries (μg/day)

	UNITED STATES*	CANADA†	GREAT BRITAIN‡	FAO/WHO§
Children, 5-8 yr	75-100	90-125	100	102
Girls, 12-14 yr	150	145	200	170
Women, 19-34 yr	180	175	200	170
Boys, 12-14 yr	200	150	200	170
Men, 18-34 yr	200	210-220	200	200
Pregnant women	400	+300	+100	370-470
Lactating women	+100	+100	+60	+100

* Food and Nutrition Board, National Research Council: *Recommended Dietary Allowances,* ed 10, Washington, DC, 1989, National Academy Press.

† Health and Welfare Canada: *Nutrition recommendations,* The Report of the Scientific Review Committee, Ottawa, Canada, 1990, Canadian Government Publishing Centre.

‡ *Dietary reference values for food energy and nutrients for the United Kingdom,* Report of the Panel on Dietary Reference Values of the Committee on Medical Aspects of Food Policy, Report on Health and Social Subjects No 41, London, 1991, Her Majesty's Stationery Office.

§ Food and Agriculture Organization: *Requirements of vitamin A, iron, folate,* and vitamin B_{12}, Report of a Joint Food and Agriculture Organization/World Health Organization (FAO/WHO) Expert Consultation, FAO Food and Nutrition Series No 23, Rome, 1988, World Health Organization.

greater binding affinity for the enzymes involved. The key features of the absorption, transport, and metabolism of folate are summarized in Figure 12-8.

Folate can be excreted in urine and bile in active or inactive forms. As much as 100 μg of folate may be excreted within bile and then reabsorbed each day. Most adults excrete up to 40 μg of folate in their urine each day. Losses in feces amount to about 200 μg/day. This total includes folate synthesized by bacteria in the large intestine and so can often be higher than the total dietary intake of folate. When pregnant, women have been found to excrete increased quantities of an inactive form of folate, requiring an additional 200 to 300 μg of folate to be consumed each day to compensate for this increased loss.[24] This may explain why pregnant women are at increased risk of folate deficiency.

RECOMMENDED DIETARY ALLOWANCES

The amount of folate required for optimal health has not been clearly established. It is believed, however, that 3 μg/kg of body weight meets the needs of most adults.[25] This figure was used in the United States by the Food and Nutrition Board to set the RDAs for folate listed in Table 12-5. It was estimated in two separate ways.[6] One method involved estimating a minimal requirement for pure folate (as PGA) and then increasing the figure to allow for the bioavailability of folate within foods, individual variation in requirements, and the need for the body to build up adequate stores of the vitamin. The second method was based on examining the average intake of folate in people with adequate folate status.

The 3 μg/kg figure and the current RDAs are called into question by one depletion-repletion study that found that 200 to 250 μg of dietary folate meets the daily requirements of normal adult females, whereas 300 μg/day allows some storage of folate to occur.[26] For a typical 63-kg woman, 300 μg/day is equivalent to 4.8 μg/kg.

As can be seen from Table 12-5, the recommended intakes for folate do not vary much from one country to another. For example, the recommended intakes for adult women vary only within a 170 to 200 μg/day range.

The amount of folate required by an individual may be influenced by metabolic rate. The amount required is also known to increase with increased consumption of alcohol (which inhibits folate absorption) and with any physiological condition that leads to increased metabolism of one-carbon units. Such conditions include pregnancy, hyperthyroidism, and hemolytic anemia. The use of many drugs can also increase folate requirements.

The average amount of folate consumed by U.S. and Canadian adults ranges from 180 to 250 μg/day, corresponding to about 3 μg/kg/day. NHANES III dietary data (1988-1991) show intakes for women that range from 230 to 280 μg/day and for men that range from 300 to 390 μg/day. Data from the NHANES II survey indicate that less than 10% of U.S. adults show biochemical evidence of folate deficiency. However, 21.2% of non-Hispanic white women and 40.7% of non-Hispanic black women had low red blood cell folate levels, reflecting depleted stores of the vitamin. The corresponding figure for Hispanic women was 8% to 11%.

Studies on infants have shown that stores of folate are relatively low at birth. To meet an infant's needs, 3.6 μg/kg of folate per day is recommended. Some researchers, however, recommend 5 to 8 μg/kg/day during infancy.[27] Infants fed only by breast-feeding receive approximately 10 to 12 μg/kg/day when the mother's folate status is adequate.

The RDA for children aged 1 to 10 years is based on their need for 3.7 μg/kg of body weight. Their need per kilogram of body weight is estimated to be greater than that of adults because of the role of folate in facilitating cell growth and division.

During pregnancy, when folate needs are markedly increased, 400 μg/day is recommended. Because it is not always possible to obtain this amount from food alone, the use of a folate supplement is often recommended during pregnancy. Most prenatal nutritional supplements marketed in the United States contain between 800 and 1000 μg of folate.

Evidence is accumulating to suggest that insufficient folate intake during pregnancy, especially in the periconceptual period, plays a role in a variety of fetal problems, including low birth weight and neural tube defects.[28] The generic term *neural tube defect* covers a range of conditions resulting from malformation of the embryonic neural tube, including spina bifida, anencephaly, and encephalocoele. In spina bifida the neural tube has failed to close properly, which can lead to a variety of physical disabilities, including paralysis and hydrocephalus. In anencephaly, the cranial vault and cerebral hemisphere of the brain are missing and an affected fetus cannot survive. Encephalocoele is a defect of the cranium that causes the brain to protrude outside of the skull. Each year about 400,000 infants throughout the world are born with neural tube defects. The detailed causes of these defects are believed to involve both genetic and environmental factors. A number of international trials, however, have shown that folate supplementation (at between 800 and 4000 μg/day) before and during early pregnancy is exceedingly effective in preventing their occurrence.

Although it is now clear that supplementary folate can offer significant protection against neural tube defects, little information on the relationship between dietary folate intakes and the incidence of neural tube defects is available. Nevertheless, the U.S. Department of Health and Human Services now recommends that all women of childbearing age should consume 0.4 mg (400 μg) of folate per day. At present, the typical intakes of this group of people are about 200 μg/day. The enrichment of food with folate is currently being evaluated by various U.S. government agencies. Proposed regulations for the addition of folate to grain products at the level of 70 μg/100 g of food have been issued by the FDA as a public health solution to the problem.

During lactation, it is recommended that mothers consume an additional 100 μg of folate per day to allow for the amount lost in milk. This recommendation, however, was based on a presumed folate content of human milk of between 2 and 5 μg/100 ml and a 50% efficiency of absorption of the additional folate consumed by the mothers. It has since been found that the folate content of the milk of U.S. lactating women is approximately 10 μg/100 ml.[29] This indicates that the current recommended additional allowance for lactating women is too low.

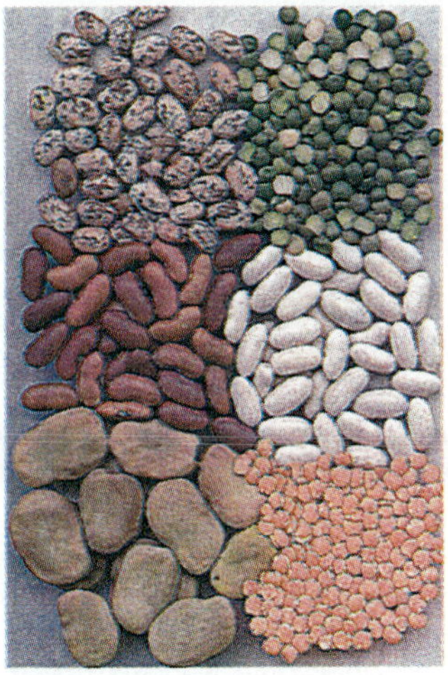

FOOD SOURCES

Unlike many nutrients, folate is found in practically all foods. Data are now available on the folate content of a sufficient number of foods to allow the folate content of diets to be estimated. Most diets are estimated to provide from 200 to 400 μg of folate per day. One difficulty in estimating the folate content of foods as they are consumed is the susceptibility of the vitamin to destruction by heat, ultraviolet light, or oxidation. Losses during cooking or processing are often as high as 50% to 90% and can reach 100% when high temperatures and large amounts of water are used.

Food sources of folate are ranked as "excellent" if they provide at least 55 μg per serving, "good" (33 to 54 μg per serving), or simply as "sources" (11 to 32 μg per serving). Wheat germ, with 178 μg/100 g, is one of the most concentrated sources of folate, along with liver, kidney, and yeast. Because these foods are a relatively insignificant part of most diets, however, fruits and vegetables make a much greater total contribution to the dietary intake of folate. Oranges and orange juice—with 40 and 20 μg per serving, respectively—are dependable sources whose acidity helps protect the folate from destruction. Asparagus, brussels sprouts, greens, and spinach are excellent vegetable sources of folate, whereas avocado, strawberries, and melon are good fruit sources. Many legumes, nuts, and seeds are also excellent sources. Milk contains a modest amount of folate (6 μg/100 ml). The contribution of various food groups to the total folate available in the North American food supply is shown in Figure 12-9. The folate content of a wide variety of foods is shown in Table 12-6.

Of the folate in a mixed North American diet, 75% is present as polyglutamates, but 35% of the folate in orange juice, 53% in soybeans, and 60% in milk occur in the monoglutamate form. The monoglutamate form of

FIGURE 12-9

Contributions of various food groups to the folate content of the North American food supply.

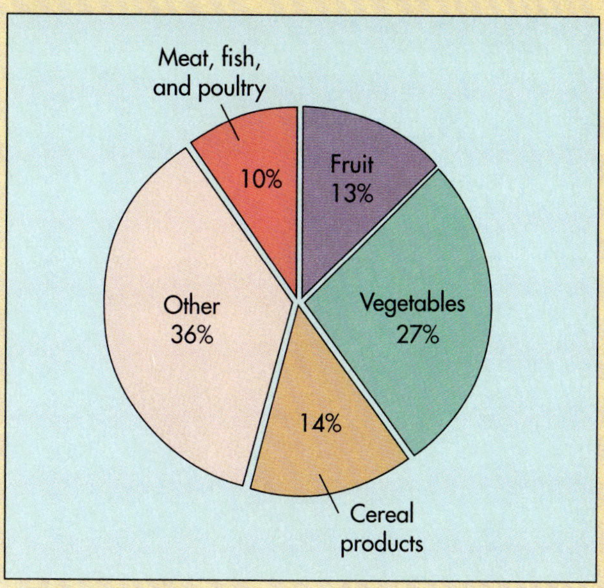

the vitamin is somewhat more bioavailable than are the polyglutamate forms.

DEFICIENCY

A variety of surveys suggest that approximately 10% of the American population have low stores of folate. Many nutritionists and other scientists believe that folate deficiency will eventually be recognized as the most prevalent of all vitamin deficiencies. Folate deficiency produces its first effects in tissues with a high rate of cell division, such as intestinal cells and red blood cells. It has also been implicated in **pregnancy-induced hypertension,** a condition of late pregnancy whose symptoms include high blood pressure, proteinurea, and edema. As previously discussed, folate deficiency during pregnancy has been firmly linked to various forms of damage to the developing fetus. In addition to its well-characterized effect on red blood cells, folate deficiency may also reduce the production of leukocytes (white blood cells) and thus impair the ability of the immune system to fight infection.

> Many nutritionists and other health professionals believe that folate deficiency will eventually be recognized as the most prevalent of all vitamin deficiencies.

The reserves of folate within a woman's body become severely depleted during pregnancy. They also fall constantly in lactating women because of the need to maintain the folate content of secreted milk at 10 µg/ 100 ml.

> The following people are most at risk of folate deficiency:
> - Pregnant women
> - Elderly people
> - Alcoholics
> - People taking certain drugs, including oral contraceptives and anticonvulsants

A number of drugs—such as aspirin, antacids, antibacterial agents, and chemotherapeutic agents—are known to interfere with folate use and so may cause a deficiency to develop.[30] The overall effect of any drug on folate status depends on the dosage taken and the duration of its use.

About 50% of all people from low-income communities who are admitted to hospitals show evidence of folate deficiency, compared with 20% to 30% of those admitted from other communities. In general, folate deficiency occurs more often among poor, elderly, and lonely persons, all of whom tend to consume diets of limited variety. Folate absorption is impaired in alcoholics, 50% of whom are found to have folate deficiency. Alcoholics often also have both liver damage, which interferes with the storage and metabolism of folate, and excessive losses of the vitamin in urine and feces. In one experimental study of folate deficiency, symptoms developed over a period of 5 months to the final stage of megaloblastic anemia. Infants, who have lower reserves and greater needs, developed deficiency symptoms in only 8 weeks.

Localized Deficiency

An important new concept in nutrition is that there can be a localized or selective deficiency in one cell line or tissue but not another in the same patient. Certain tissues of the body can develop symptoms of folate deficiency, which can be cured by supplementation with the vitamin, despite the fact that plasma and red blood cell folate levels are normal. The first such localized folate deficiency to be observed involved megaloblastic changes in the cervix in women taking oral contraceptives. Other localized folate deficiencies have since been found in the bronchial and oral tissues of smokers and the colonic tissue of patients with ulcerative colitis. These localized deficiencies in folate may be caused by

TABLE 12-6

Folate content of foods

DESCRIPTION	FOLATE PER USUAL (μg)* SERVING	FOLATE (μg/100 g)†
Liver	383	428
Superfortified cereals	242	991
Cold cereals (not bran or superfortified)	112	275
Pinto, navy, and other dried beans (cooked)	84	100
Asparagus	82	101
Spinach	70	128
Instant breakfast, diet bars, supplements	65	112
Bran and granola cereals	58	236
Broccoli	53	65
Avocados	49	62
Okra	49	84
Brussels sprouts	47	60
Orange juice	43	41
Artichokes	43	46
Chili	36	19
Mustard or turnip greens, kale, collards	36	54
Corn	35	43
Oranges, tangerines	33	26
Cantaloupe	33	17
Eggs	31	43
Edible seeds	29	163
Cooked cereals	29	15
Cauliflower	28	53
Green peas	27	46
Beets	27	37
Dressings, stuffings	26	28
Winter squash	26	18
Beef stew, potpie	26	10
Peanuts, peanut butter	25	92
Plantains	25	22
Spaghetti with tomato sauce	24	14
Veal, lamb	24	15
Pizza	24	16
Grapefruit, grapefruit juice	23	10
Papaya, mangos	21	32
Mixed dishes with pork, veal or lamb	21	23
Blackberries, raspberries	21	27
Green beans	21	28
Tomatoes, tomato juice	21	10
Vegetable, tomato, and minestrone soups	20	6
2% fat milk	20	5
Green salad	20	48
Bananas	19	19
Honeydew and other melons (except cantaloupe)	19	17
Mixed vegetables	19	19
Strawberries	19	17
Yogurt	18	10
Meat substitutes	17	108
Mixed dishes with beef	17	8
Sweet potatoes	17	17

* Usual serving is the median portion size observed for a food or foods in the National Health and Nutrition Examination Survey II data for all adults aged 19 to 74 years, male and female. Values should be considered approximate, because portion sizes vary by age and gender.

† Folate values are weighted: aggregate values for individual food codes comprise each food or foods.

From Subar AF, Block G, James LD: *Am J Clin Nutr* 50:508, 1989.

increased turnover of the vitamin brought about by the rapid proliferation of the tissue. Alternatively, they may be caused by the inactivation or alteration of folate metabolism by oral contraceptives, cigarette smoke, or drugs. It has been suggested that localized folate deficiencies may have a **cocarcinogenic** effect, meaning that affected tissues are at increased risk of cancers produced by specific carcinogens.

EVALUATION OF FOLATE STATUS

The most common result of severe folate deficiency in humans is megaloblastic anemia, which is associated with the development of abnormally large red blood cells. These enlarged cells can be readily identified under the microscope and with the aid of electronic sizing devices. Megaloblastic anemia is also characterized by a fall in total red blood cell number as the size of the individual cells increases. However, megaloblastic anemia appears only in people with an advanced state of folate deficiency. It is estimated that over half of all cases of folate deficiency are missed by tests that rely solely on the sizing and counting of red blood cells.

Determination of folate levels in serum or plasma is a more sensitive indicator of folate status, which can identify a deficiency condition long before clinical symptoms appear. Diets that are low in folate cause a fall in serum or plasma levels of the vitamin within 1 week. This contrasts with the 15 to 17 weeks that must pass before changes in red blood cell number or size are noted. Serum or plasma levels of folate offer the best first indication of folate deficiency, whereas changes in red blood cell size and number give the best indication of the amount of folate retained within the body's stores.

Another biochemical change associated with folate deficiency is the excretion within urine of **formiminoglutamic acid (FIGLU),** a metabolite of the amino acid histidine. Testing urine for FIGLU is done by performing a **histidine load test** in which a large dose of histidine is given before the test to increase the sensitivity with which it can detect a developing folate deficiency. The most recent development in this area has been the discovery that plasma homocysteine levels vary inversely with plasma folate levels, and so the homocysteine levels offer an alternative indicator of folate status. In fact, recent evidence indicates that elevated plasma homocysteine is a very sensitive marker of functional folate deficiency and that current standards for normal plasma folate values (greater than or equal to 3 ng/ml) may be set too low.[30a] Criteria used to evaluate folate nutritional status in the absence of vitamin B_{12} deficiency are listed in Table 12-7.

TABLE 12-7

Criteria used to evaluate folate status in the absence of vitamin B_{12} deficiency

CRITERION	VALUES INDICATIVE OF DEFICIENCY
Megaloblastic anemia	Positive
Plasma folates	<3 ng/ml
Red blood cell folates	<160 ng/ml
Formiminoglutamic (FIGLU) acid excretion	Elevated after histidine load
Neutrophil hypersegmentation	>3.5%
Plasma homocysteine	Elevated (> 16 μmol/L)

TOXICITY

No toxic effects of folate have been clearly established. Up to 15 mg of the vitamin can be taken each day for a month with no adverse effects. However, folate may cause neurological damage if given to patients with undiagnosed pernicious anemia because it can mask some of the symptoms of this disease. Amounts of folate in excess of 20 mg/day may promote the development of certain cancers and interfere with the action of some drugs, including anticonvulsants. Excessive consumption of folate has been implicated in the impairment of zinc absorption, but at present the data supporting this possibility are not convincing.

VITAMIN B_{12} (COBALAMIN)

Until 1926, pernicious anemia was a fatal disease of unknown origin with an unknown cure. In 1926 Minot and Murphy found that pernicious anemia could be cured by feeding a patient at least ⅔ lb (0.3 kg) of raw liver per day. In 1934, with Whipple, they were awarded the Nobel Prize in medicine for this discovery.

Also in 1926 Castle noted that patients with pernicious anemia had a low level of gastric secretions. He suggested that the anti–pernicious anemia factor able to cure the disease had two components: an **extrinsic factor** found in food (especially liver) and an **intrinsic factor** within normal gastric secretions. The search for the extrinsic factor proposed by Castle led to the discovery in 1946 that it was the compound now known as vitamin B_{12}.

Attempts to identify the anti–pernicious anemia factor were hampered because no animal other than humans had been found to need the substance. This meant that experimental work to identify the factor had to be done on human subjects with pernicious anemia. Through a series of careful experiments, medical researchers were able to produce progressively more concentrated extracts of the anti–pernicious anemia factor within liver. Although the rate of progress was slow, each increasingly pure concentrate brought additional benefits to the subjects. Eventually, it was discovered that

FIGURE 12-10

The chemical structure of cobalamin—vitamin B_{12}.

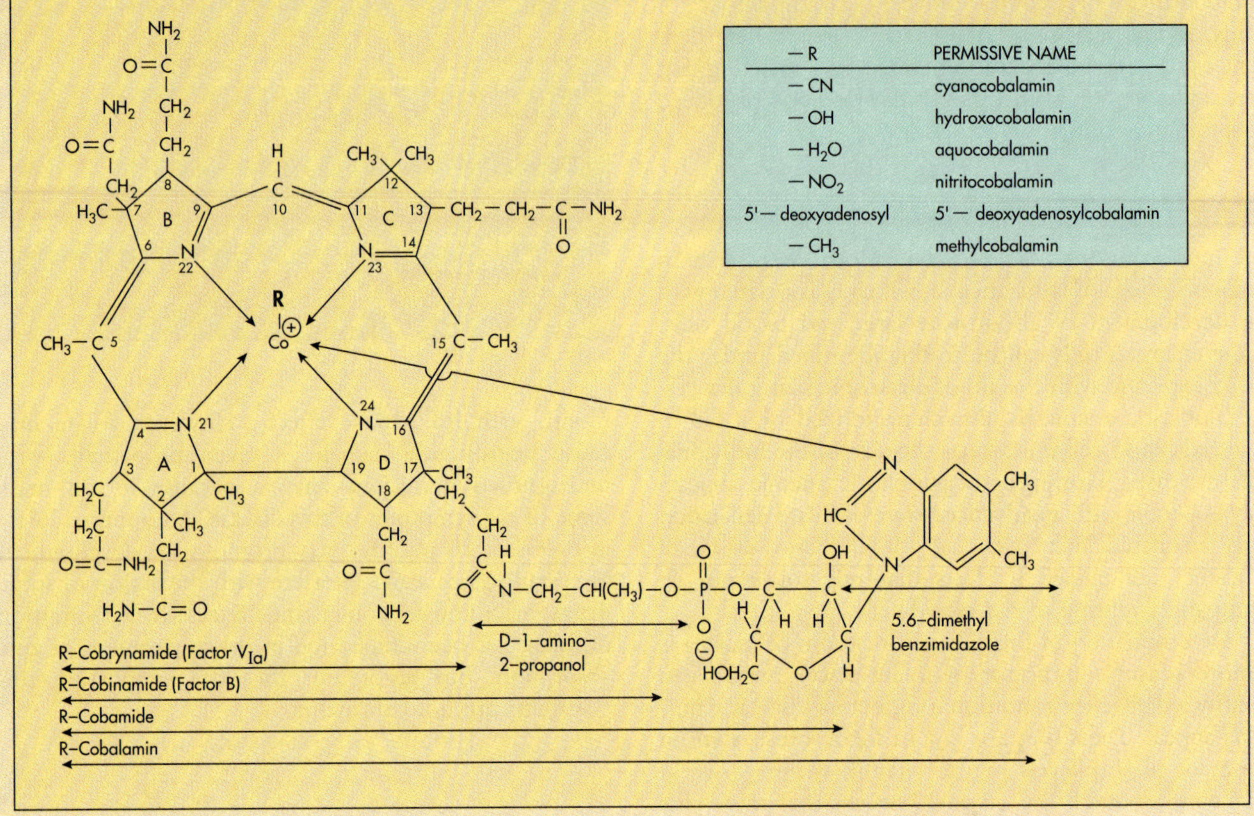

—R	PERMISSIVE NAME
—CN	cyanocobalamin
—OH	hydroxocobalamin
—H_2O	aquocobalamin
—NO_2	nitritocobalamin
5'—deoxyadenosyl	5'—deoxyadenosylcobalamin
—CH_3	methylcobalamin

the microorganism *Lactobacillus lactisi* also needed the anti–pernicious anemia factor for growth. This allowed the more extensive experimental work that eventually led to the isolation of pure vitamin B_{12}, now known as **cobalamin.** It was later found that an intrinsic factor (in fact, a mucoprotein molecule) secreted by the gastric mucosal cells was indeed required to facilitate the absorption of ingested vitamin B_{12}. Patients with pernicious anemia have a deficiency of this intrinsic factor, but a small proportion of ingested vitamin B_{12} can be absorbed without its assistance by simple diffusion. This explains why the large amounts of vitamin B_{12} in the raw liver or liver extracts used in the early experiments allowed enough of the vitamin to be absorbed for the subjects to be cured. It is interesting to note that, in contrast to other vitamin deficiencies, most deficiencies of vitamin B_{12} are primarily caused by a failure of the absorption of the vitamin, rather than from insufficient dietary intake.

In 1972 vitamin B_{12} was first synthesized by chemists. Even though it is now possible to synthetically produce vitamin B_{12} in a chemical laboratory, it is more economically made by microorganisms and by fungi. This naturally produced vitamin B_{12} is the most common commercial source of the vitamin today.

CHEMICAL COMPOSITION

In 1948 small red crystals of pure vitamin B_{12} were first obtained. Chemical analysis indicated that about 4% of the weight of the vitamin was accounted for by the mineral cobalt. It was later found that the cobalt was held at the center of a complex organic molecule known as a corrinoid (or corrin ring), which closely resembles the organic portions of the heme group and the "head region" of a chlorophyll molecule. It was the discovery that cobalt played a central role in the structure of vitamin B_{12} that led to the vitamin's being renamed cobalamin. There are actually a variety of different cobalamins with vitamin B_{12} activity. Their chemical structures are indicated in Figure 12-10.

The term *vitamin B_{12}* is now used as a generic term to describe the full range of cobalt-containing corrinoids (cobalamins) that have the biological activity of vitamin B_{12} in humans. The predominant forms of vitamin B_{12} in plasma and within tissues are **methylcobalamin, 5-deoxyadenosylcobalamin** (also called coenzyme vitamin B_{12}), and **hydroxocobalamin.** The role of vitamin B_{12} is to function as a coenzyme in a variety of important biochemical reactions, but only methylcobalamin and 5-deoxyadenosylcobalamin are known to function as

FIGURE 12-11

The interrelationship of vitamin B_{12}, folate, and DNA synthesis.

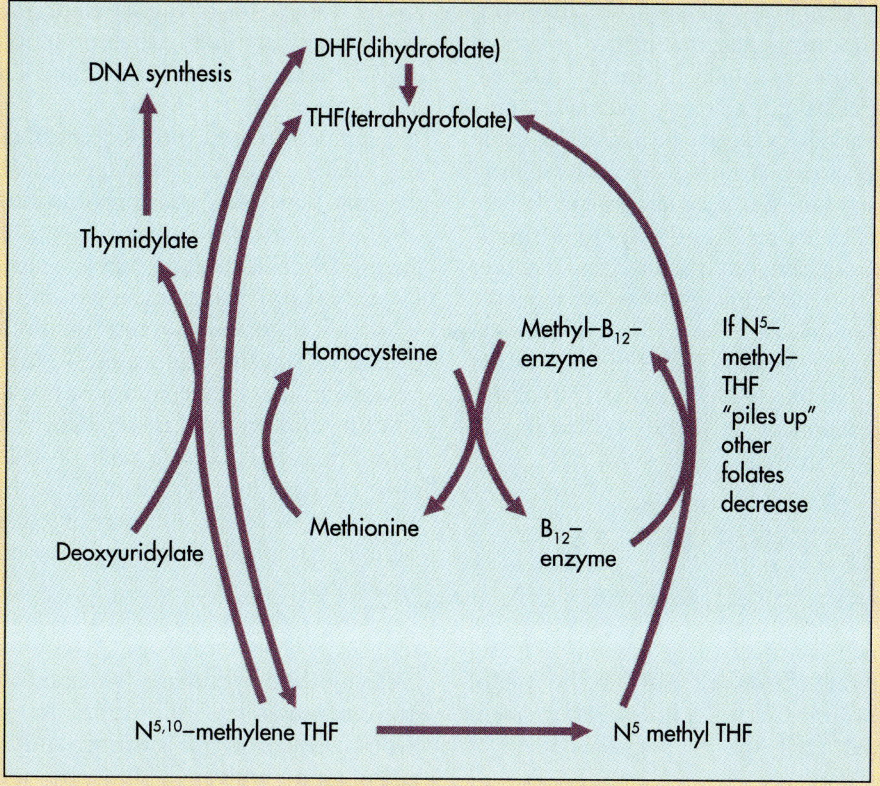

coenzymes in humans in their native form. The other cobalamins included within the generic term *vitamin B_{12}* must be converted into methylcobalamin or 5-deoxyadenosylcobalamin before they can become biologically active. The common pharmaceutical form of vitamin B_{12}, used widely in supplements, is **cyanocobalamin**. This is a heat-stable form of the vitamin and is converted into an active form by removal of the cyano (CN) group.

FUNCTIONS

Vitamin B_{12}, like folate, is involved in biochemical processes essential for DNA synthesis and therefore for the growth and division of cells. As illustrated in Figure 12-11, vitamin B_{12} acts as a coenzyme mediating the conversion of homocysteine to the amino acid methionine. In achieving this conversion the vitamin B_{12}–assisted reaction involves the transfer of a methyl group (CH_3) from N^5-methyl tetrahydrofolate (THF) onto homocysteine, regenerating THF in the process. N^5-methyl THF is the predominant form in which folate is found within the liver, but another form—$N^{5,10}$-methylene THF—is required for the synthesis of DNA. The only way in which N^5-methyl THF returns to the body's folate pool is via the vitamin B_{12}–mediated reaction illustrated in Figure 12-11. This means that vitamin B_{12} deficiency causes folate to accumulate in the "trapped" form of N^5-methyl THF, reducing the availability of other forms of folate for DNA synthesis and its other metabolic functions.

In the bone marrow, where the erythroblast precursors of red blood cells are formed, both vitamin B_{12} and folate are needed for $N^{5,10}$-methylene THF to provide the methyl groups needed for the synthesis of DNA. If DNA cannot be produced in adequate amounts, the erythroblasts cannot divide and mature properly. Instead, they simply grow in size to produce the abnormally large red blood cells characteristic of the anemia found both in pernicious anemia and when folate is merely deficient. Although vitamin B_{12} is required for the synthesis of DNA in all human cells, the erythroblasts are particularly vulnerable to vitamin B_{12} deficiency because of the extremely rapid rate at which they normally divide. New red blood cells are normally produced at a rate of at least 200 million per minute.

The interrelationship between vitamin B_{12} and folate explains the similar effects on red blood cell production of deficiencies of folate or vitamin B_{12}. It also explains why supplemental folate can mask the effects of vitamin B_{12} deficiency.[31]

Vitamin B_{12} is also required for the synthesis of myelin, the white sheath of lipoprotein that surrounds many nerve fibers. During vitamin B_{12} deficiency, progressive demyelination of nerve fibers occurs, leading to a variety of neurological symptoms. The biochemical basis of this effect of vitamin B_{12} deficiency is unknown. There is some evidence to suggest that it may be caused by a generalized lack of availability of methyl groups, which is a result of the inability to synthesize methionine (Figure 12-11). Alternatively, it may be a result of some toxic effect of homocysteine (which accumulates during vitamin B_{12} deficiency) on the nervous system. People with vitamin B_{12} deficiency are found to possess abnormal fatty acids in their myelin, but it is uncertain whether these play a role in the demyelination that these people exhibit. It may be relevant that the only other reaction known to be mediated by vitamin B_{12} is the conversion of methylmalonyl-CoA to succinyl-CoA, which is involved in the degradation of fatty acids containing an odd number of carbon atoms.

ABSORPTION, TRANSPORT, AND METABOLISM

The absorption of vitamin B_{12} is mediated by the intrinsic factor, which is a heat-labile mucoprotein secreted from specific cells ("parietal cells") in the wall of the stomach. The intrinsic factor is a normal component of gastric juice, and each species possesses its own version of it.

As food passes through the digestive tract, the acidity of gastric juice and the proteases in pancreatic juice cause vitamin B_{12} to be released from the protein complexes in which it occurs within many foods. The freed vitamin B_{12} then binds to a salivary polypeptide called the **R-binder,** but is then released again when this polypeptide is digested by the enzyme trypsin. Vitamin B_{12} then binds to the intrinsic factor, which assists in the binding of the vitamin to a receptor protein on the surface of the mucosal cells lining the ileum. This process is catalyzed by calcium ions. The vitamin B_{12}-intrinsic factor complex is absorbed into the intestinal cells intact. A failure of any stage of this process results in all or some dietary vitamin B_{12} not being absorbed. For example, one third of people over 60 years of age no longer secrete adequate gastric acid and so cannot absorb sufficient vitamin B_{12} from food because it is not completely released from the protein complex. Also, about 1% of elderly people secrete less intrinsic factor than normal and so are less able to reabsorb the vitamin B_{12} that is released in bile.

The proportion of dietary vitamin B_{12} that is absorbed decreases as the amount consumed increases. The efficiency of absorption has been found to be 56% for intakes of 1 µg and 28% for intakes of 5 µg, and it declines progressively for higher intakes. When more than 10 µg of pure crystalline vitamin B_{12} is consumed, only 1% of the vitamin is absorbed, casting doubt on the value of large oral intakes of supplementary vitamin B_{12}. When a test dose of vitamin B_{12} is given to normal subjects under standardized conditions, they usually absorb about 30% of the dose and then excrete most of the absorbed amount in their urine. When the same dose is given to people with pernicious anemia, only about 2% of it is absorbed.

If a person lacks intrinsic factor, none of the vitamin B_{12} available from a normal diet is absorbed. However, if the same person is given approximately 1000 times more of the vitamin than is normally available in food in the form of liver extracts or supplements, sufficient vitamin B_{12} for his or her needs can pass into the intestinal cells by simple diffusion. Because the intrinsic factor in hog stomach is similar to human intrinsic factor, it has proved possible to use a concentrate of hog's stomach to facilitate the absorption of the vitamin from food or supplements by people lacking their own intrinsic factor. The most effective way of administering vitamin B_{12} to such people, however, is by intramuscular injection of the vitamin, completely bypassing their defective absorption mechanism.

The efficiency with which vitamin B_{12} is absorbed appears to decline with age. Absorption is also decreased in people with pyridoxine (vitamin B_6) deficiency (which decreases the release of intrinsic factor), iron deficiency, hyperthyroidism, and gastritis, and in people who are taking some anticonvulsants and antibiotics. The efficiency of absorption increases, on the other hand, during pregnancy or when an intrinsic factor concentrate is fed with vitamin B_{12}.

After absorption, vitamin B_{12} passes into the circulation, where it becomes bound to one of three transport proteins known as **transcobalamins I, II,** and **III.** These proteins carry the vitamin B_{12} to the various tissues of the body, particularly the liver and bone marrow. When combined within a large vitamin-protein complex, vitamin B_{12} is not lost to urine as blood is filtered through the kidneys. This means that when sufficient transport proteins are produced, the body loses little of its existing supply of vitamin B_{12}. Some vitamin B_{12} is excreted in bile each day, but much of this is reabsorbed, along with new supplies provided by the diet. Some analogs of vitamin B_{12} are also excreted in bile, but these are not reabsorbed. The total daily loss of vitamin B_{12} is estimated at between 1 and 2.6 µg.[6]

Excess vitamin B_{12} is stored in the liver, largely bound within a vitamin B_{12}–protein complex. The total amount stored in the liver can be as high as 2000 to 2500 µg, which is sufficient to last for 6 to 10 years in the absence of further supplies from the diet. Smaller amounts of the vitamin also accumulate in the kidneys, heart, spleen, and brain, amounting to about 20 to 30 µg in total. The amount of vitamin B_{12} stored in the liver increases with age. Appreciably higher amounts of stored vitamin B_{12} are found in citizens of the United States, when compared

TABLE 12-8

Recommended dietary allowances (United States) and recommended nutrient intakes (Canada) for cobalamin (vitamin B_{12}) (μg/day)

AGE (YEARS)	UNITED STATES	CANADA
CHILDREN		
1-3	0.7	0.5
4-6	1.0	0.8
7+	1.4	1.0
ADULTS	2.0	1.0
Pregnant	2.2	1.2
Lactating	2.6	1.2

to citizens of Great Britain, reflecting higher dietary intakes in the United States. The major form of vitamin B_{12} found in all tissues is adenosylcobalamin, which constitutes about 60% to 70% of the vitamin in the liver and 50% in other tissues.

RECOMMENDED DIETARY ALLOWANCES

The amount of vitamin B_{12} needed by humans is extremely small and has proved difficult to determine. It is estimated to be between 0.6 and 1.0 μg/day. Intakes below this may still prove adequate, however, because low intakes cause the body to conserve vitamin B_{12} by reabsorbing more from bile. Injections of as little as 0.5 to 1.0 μg of vitamin B_{12} per day have proved sufficient to maintain DNA synthesis and other biochemical functions in patients with pernicious anemia. The RDAs for vitamin B_{12} are shown in Table 12-8.

Because it is desirable to build up and maintain substantial stores of vitamin B_{12} in the body, an intake of 2 μg/day is suggested for adults. The stores built up on such an intake provide protection against any harmful effects of the impaired absorption of vitamin B_{12} that occurs in some people when they reach the age of about 60 years.

During the last half of pregnancy a fetus draws approximately 0.2 μg of vitamin B_{12} from its mother each day, which serves as the basis for the RDA during pregnancy being set at 2.2 μg/day. During lactation an additional 0.6 μg/day is recommended to compensate for the amount lost in milk.

Breast-fed infants normally receive 0.2 to 0.8 μg of vitamin B_{12} per day and show no evidence of deficiency in the vitamin, even when the mother's stores are marginal. The only exceptions are some breast-fed infants whose mothers are strict vegetarians. Pregnant and lactating women who avoid all animal foods are advised to take a vitamin B_{12} supplement to provide them with the RDA. Formula-fed infants should receive 0.15 μg of vitamin B_{12} per 100 kcal.

The RDAs for children increase progressively in line with body weight until the adult RDA is reached. The Food and Agricultural Organization/World Health Organization (FAO/WHO) recommend 0.1 μg/day during the first year of life and 1μg/day at all other ages, except during pregnancy (1.4 μg/day) and lactation (1.3 μg/day).[32] In Canada the Recommended Nutrient Intakes (RNIs) for vitamin B_{12} are 0.3 to 0.4 μg/day during the first year of life, progressively increasing to 1.0 μg/day from age 10 onward, except during pregnancy and lactation, when 1.2 μg/day is recommended.[33] The British Reference Nutrient Intakes for vitamin B_{12} lie between the U.S. and Canadian levels, with 1.5 μg/day recommended for adults.[34]

FOOD SOURCES

All of the vitamin B_{12} within food has been made by microorganisms; neither animals nor plants can make it for themselves. No vitamin B_{12} is present in foods of plant origin, apart from minute amounts as a contaminant of poorly washed root vegetables or synthesized by bacteria within the nodules on the roots of legumes. So the only nutritionally significant sources of vitamin B_{12} are foods of animal origin. Some of the animals we eat contain vitamin B_{12} because they absorb it after it has been synthesized by bacteria living in their gastrointestinal tract. Excess vitamin B_{12} is stored within the tissues of these animals, especially the liver, and so is available to us when we eat the animal tissues. Microorganisms in the gastrointestinal tract of humans can also synthesize vitamin B_{12}, but they live too far down the gastrointestinal tract for useful amounts to be absorbed. Thus humans are dependent on foods of animal origin, or manufactured supplements, for their supplies of vitamin B_{12}.[35]

> All of the vitamin B_{12} within food is made by microorganisms. No animals or plants can manufacture this vitamin.

The average North American diet provides 3 to 5 μg of vitamin B_{12} per day, which is considerably more than the recommended adult intake of 2 μg/day. People who eat a lot of liver can consume up to 100 μg/day. True vegetarians (vegans) may have intakes well below 1 μg/day, largely supplied by tiny quantities of soil and microorganisms on their food. The contribution of

TABLE 12-9

Cobalamin (vitamin B_{12}) content in average servings per 100 kcal of foods frequently consumed and other recommended sources

FOOD*	AMOUNT	kcal	PER SERVING (μg)	PER 100 kcal (μg)
EGGS, BEEF, POULTRY, FISH, AND NUTS				
Egg, fried	1 large	95	0.57	0.61
Beef, roast	3 oz	315	1.54	0.49
Ground beef	3 oz	230	1.52	0.66
Chicken	3 oz	140	0.3	0.21
Tuna	3 oz	165	2.2	1.3
Peanut butter	2 Tbsp	190	—	—
Bacon	3 slices	110	0.83	0.75
Oysters†	3 oz	80	16.2	20.3
Ham†	3 oz	229	0.72	0.31
Liver†	3 oz	85	87	100
DAIRY PRODUCTS				
Milk, whole	8 oz	150	0.86	0.57
Milk, 2% fat	8 oz	120	0.91	0.76
Cheddar cheese	1 oz	115	0.25	0.22

* Foods of vegetable origin provide no vitamin B_{12}; therefore they are not included in this table.

† Recommended sources.

FIGURE 12-12

Contribution of various food groups to the vitamin B_{12} in the North American food supply.

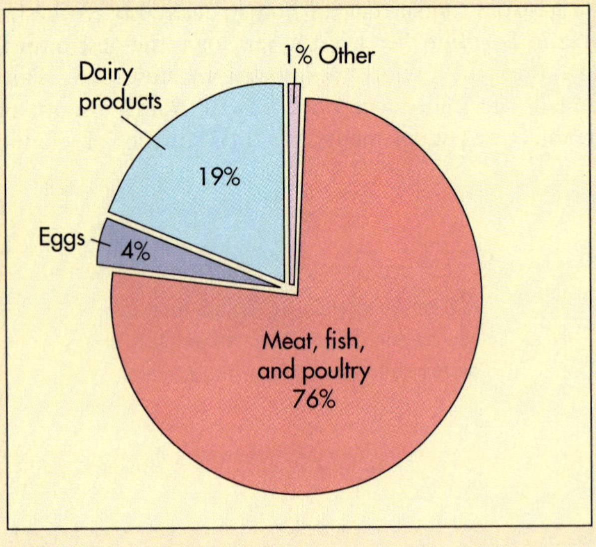

various food groups to the vitamin B_{12} content of the North American diet is shown in Figure 12-12.

The best sources of vitamin B_{12} are liver from various sources, followed by kidneys and muscle (meat) (Table 12-9). In these foods it occurs complexed with protein, predominantly in the form of adenosylcobalamin and hydroxycobalamin. In dairy products and milk it occurs mainly as methylcobalamin and hydroxycobalamin. Some manufacturers add vitamin B_{12} to cereals, but this is hard to rationalize, especially because cereals are usually consumed with milk, which is itself a source of the vitamin.

Over half of the cobalamin in food is in an unstable form that is destroyed by processing and most methods of food preparation. Little of the remaining portion is lost, unless high temperatures are used. When milk is pasteurized, it loses only 7% of its available vitamin B_{12}. Boiling milk for 2 to 3 minutes destroys 30% of its vitamin B_{12}, sterilizing for 13 minutes at 120° C destroys 70%, but rapid sterilization at 134° C for 3 to 4 seconds destroys only 10%.[36]

Almost all of the vitamin B_{12} produced commercially, and so available in supplements, is in the heat-stable form of cyanocobalamin, produced by bacterial fermentation.

DEFICIENCY

Vitamin B_{12} deficiency resulting strictly from a low dietary intake of the vitamin is virtually unknown, except in strict vegans. It takes years to develop in adults who turn to a vegan diet after many years on a mixed diet because the stores of the vitamin in the body can last for a long time (8 to 10 years). Some infants born to vegans, however, can develop vitamin B_{12} deficiency in their first year of life because they have no stores at birth.

The major cause of vitamin B_{12} deficiency is pernicious anemia, caused by failure of absorption of the vitamin, rather than lack of a dietary source of it. Although traditionally caused by lack of intrinsic factor, symptoms of pernicious anemia can also develop because of surgical removal of the stomach, a lack of the proteins that transport cobalamin in blood, a lack of the substance that releases cobalamin from intestinal cells into the blood, or degeneration of gastric mucosal cells (caused by aging, genetic factors, alcoholism, iron deficiency, or dysfunction of the thyroid gland).

Over the past several decades it has become increasingly apparent that elderly people are at great risk for the development of vitamin B_{12} deficiency. The reasons are not firmly established. Gastric dysfunction develops as part of the aging process and impairs the secretion of hydrochloric acid and pepsin that is necessary to liberate vitamin B_{12} from foods. Although some elderly people with low serum vitamin B_{12} values show evidence of gastric dysfunction, others show normal gastric function. It has been suggested that gastric and intestinal bacterial overgrowth may contribute to the development of vitamin B_{12} deficiency in elderly people by competing with their host for available vitamin B_{12}. The prevalence of vitamin B_{12} deficiency in surviving members aged 67 to 96 years of the original Framingham Study (see Chapter 4) was recently reported to be greater than 12%.[36a] Intestinal infestation with a tapeworm, which avidly absorbs the available vitamin B_{12}, can also result in deficiency symptoms.

During the development of vitamin B_{12} deficiency the bone marrow cells become abnormally enlarged (megaloblastic), the blood cells called *neutrophils* become hypersegmented (the cell nuclei develop multiple lobes because division of the nuclei continues while cell division is slowed), and eventually macrocytic anemia develops, as in folate deficiency. One of the reactions facilitated by vitamin B_{12}, the conversion of methylmalonyl-CoA to succinyl-CoA, is particularly sensitive to a developing deficiency of the vitamin. Methylmalonic acid accumulates when this conversion is blocked, and the high levels of methylmalonic acid in serum and urine can be used to confirm a vitamin B_{12} deficiency.

Vitamin B_{12} deficiency eventually results in defective or inadequate myelin synthesis, and a vast array of neurological signs and symptoms such as unsteadiness, poor muscular coordination, mental slowness, confusion, delusions, and even psychosis can develop.[23]

Vitamin B_{12} deficiency is usually first diagnosed by determining the level of the vitamin in blood. This is done either microbiologically or by radioimmunoassay. Normal serum levels of 200 to 900 ng of vitamin B_{12} per liter fall to below 80 ng/100 L in persons with pernicious anemia or any other form of vitamin B_{12} deficiency.

Recent evidence shows that elderly people with serum values of vitamin B_{12} conventionally defined as normal (200 to 900 ng/L) have metabolic evidence of vitamin B_{12} deficiency (elevated serum methylmalonic acid). Similarly, elderly people are reported to develop neurological disorders associated with vitamin B_{12} deficiency even though they have not developed megaloblastic anemia.[36b]

Once any deficiency has been detected, it is easily treated with injections of vitamin B_{12}. About 1000 µg is usually given twice in the first week of treatment, followed by 100 µg every month thereafter. The most crucial aspect of the medical handling of vitamin B_{12} deficiency is early diagnosis, allowing this simple and effective therapy to be given before irreversible nerve damage has occurred. It is also important that patients with pernicious anemia be made fully aware that they need this treatment regularly for the rest of their life.

CLINICAL USES

Over the years vitamin B_{12} has been promoted for the treatment of a wide range of conditions, including night blindness, psoriasis, warts, menopausal problems, and general malaise. There is no clinical evidence that vitamin B_{12} deficiency causes any of these problems or that vitamin B_{12} can effectively treat them. Fortunately, there is also no evidence to suggest that the amounts of vitamin B_{12} used in such "therapies" cause any detrimental effects. If the widespread administration of large doses of vitamin B_{12} continues, however, evidence of harmful effects may emerge. At present the only medically justified use of vitamin B_{12} is for the treatment of people with pernicious anemia or one of the other physiological defects in vitamin B_{12} absorption, as in elderly people, or for those who develop vitamin B_{12} deficiency because of their vegan diet.

VITAMIN B_6 (PYRIDOXINE)

Vitamin B_6, or **pyridoxine**, functions primarily in protein metabolism. A deficiency of this vitamin was first identified in 1951 in infants who had been fed an overprocessed infant formula.

CHEMICAL COMPOSITION

Vitamin B_6 and *pyridoxine* are generic terms used to denote a range of related chemicals that function as the vitamin for all animals. The three basic members of the vitamin B_6 family are **pyridoxine** itself (also known as **pyridoxol**), **pyridoxal,** and **pyridoxamine,** whose chemical structures are shown in Figure 12-13. As indicated in Figure 12-13, the vitamin can also occur with a phosphate or glucose group attached to it and all forms can be degraded in the body to pyridoxic acid.

Within the body's tissues the vitamin exists largely in

FIGURE 12-13

The chemical structure of the major naturally occurring forms of vitamin B_6 and the major metabolite into which they are degraded, pyridoxic acid.

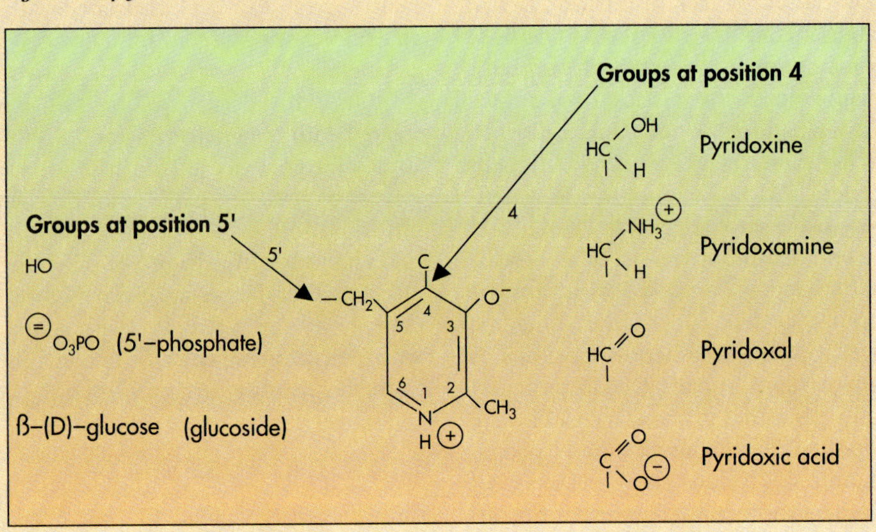

TABLE 12-10

Cellular processes affected by pyridoxal-5'-phosphate

CELLULAR PROCESS OR ENZYME	FUNCTION/SYSTEM INFLUENCED
One-carbon metabolism, hormone modulation	Immune function
Glycogen phosphorylase, transamination	Gluconeogenesis
Tryptophan metabolism	Niacin formation
Heme synthesis, transamination, O_2 affinity	Red blood cell metabolism and formation
Neurotransmitter synthesis, lipid metabolism	Nervous system
Hormone modulation, binding of PLP to lysine on hormone receptor	Hormone modulation

PLP, Pyridoxal phosphate.

the phosphorylated forms pyridoxal phosphate and pyridoxamine phosphate. Plant foods contain variable amounts of the glucoside derivatives (carrying a glucose group), and the proportion present in the glucoside form influences the bioavailability of the vitamin in plant foods.[37]

Pyridoxine was first identified in 1934 as a substance capable of curing a characteristic dermatitis in rats. It was isolated in pure form in 1938. Its structure was determined in 1939, and the vitamin was first chemically synthesized that same year.

FUNCTIONS

Vitamin B_6 in the form of pyridoxal phosphate (PLP) functions as a coenzyme in more than 60 biochemical reactions, including almost all aspects of the metabolism of amino acids and proteins. Some of the known functions of PLP and the systems affected by them are listed in Table 12-10. The key categories of reaction in which the vitamin acts as a coenzyme are the following:

- Transamination reactions, in which an amino group (NH_2) is transferred from one compound to another
- Deamination reactions, in which an amino group is removed from a compound
- Decarboxylation reactions, in which a carboxyl group (COOH or COO^-) is removed from a compound

These reactions are involved in the formation of certain neurotransmitters and other physiological regulators, including serotonin, norepinephrine, taurine, dopamine, gamma-amino butyric acid (GABA), and histamine. They are also involved in the formation of one of the precursors of DNA and RNA, the synthesis of the heme group of hemoglobin, and the process of gluconeogenesis, which is essential for the maintenance of blood glucose levels during fasting. A complex and incompletely understood interrelationship between vitamin B_6 and the receptors for steroid hormones makes the vitamin capable of modulating the actions of estrogens, androgens, and progesterone.

ABSORPTION, TRANSPORT, AND METABOLISM

In the lumen of the small intestine the phosphorylated forms of vitamin B_6 are dephosphorylated by the enzyme alkaline phosphatase and then absorbed by the intestinal cells with any nonphosphorylated forms present in food. The absorption proceeds by passive diffusion, mainly in the jejunum.

Vitamin B_6 is transported through the circulation bound to plasma proteins (mainly albumin) and made available to all cells.[38] Most absorbed vitamin B_6 is taken up by the liver, where the various forms are converted back into their phosphorylated derivatives. To readily cross any cell membrane, vitamin B_6 must be in a nonphosphorylated form. This means that the phosphorylation of the vitamin within cells effectively traps the affected molecules within the cells concerned. This "trapping" reaction is catalyzed by the enzyme **pyridoxine kinase.**

> To readily cross any cell membrane, vitamin B_6 must be in a nonphosphorylated form. This means that the phosphorylation of the vitamin within cells effectively traps the affected molecules within the cells. This "trapping" reaction is catalyzed by the enzyme **pyridoxine kinase.**

In addition to pyridoxine kinase, most cells possess the enzyme **pyridoxine oxidase,** which converts both pyridoxine phosphate and pyridoxamine phosphate into PLP. This enzyme requires the presence of riboflavin, a deficiency of which can cause many of the characteristic symptoms of vitamin B_6 deficiency, because of this metabolic interrelationship.[38] The metabolic interconversions of various forms of vitamin B_6 are summarized in Figure 12-14.

The total body pool of vitamin B_6 is estimated to be about 250 mg, with about 80% to 90% of the total present in muscle in the form of PLP coenzyme bound to the enzyme glycogen phosphorylase. When excess vitamin B_6 is absorbed, it is oxidized to pyridoxic acid, a metabolically inert substance that is excreted in urine.

TABLE 12-11

Recommended dietary allowances for vitamin B_6 *

AGE (YEARS)	AMOUNT (mg/DAY)
CHILDREN	
1-3	1
4-6	1.1
7-10	1.4
MALES	
11-14	1.7
15+	2
FEMALES	
11-14	1.4
15-18	1.5
19+	1.6
Pregnant	2.2
Lactating	2.1

*Canada has not set recommended daily intake levels for vitamin B_6.

Pyridoxine, pyridoxal, pyridoxamine, and pyridoxol phosphate also appear in urine and can be measured as indicators of vitamin B_6 status. Some pyridoxine is excreted in feces, but this has largely been produced by microorganisms in the intestine and so does not indicate any loss of dietary pyridoxine.

RECOMMENDED DIETARY ALLOWANCES

Because vitamin B_6 is required for many of the transformations of protein metabolism, the body's need for vitamin B_6 varies in direct proportion with the amount of protein in the diet. Because the typical North American diet contains more than the recommended amount of protein, the requirement for vitamin B_6 is set proportionately high. The current recommended intakes are listed in Table 12-11. They are based on a requirement of 0.016 mg of vitamin B_6 per gram of dietary protein and average daily protein intakes of 100 g for women and 126 g for men. This results in adult RDAs of 1.6 and 2 mg/day, respectively.

Pregnant women require an extra 0.6 mg/day in addition to the normal female requirement. During pregnancy the level of vitamin B_6 in fetal blood is three times as high as its level in the maternal blood.

The amount of vitamin B_6 in human milk is directly related to the amount in the mother's diet. Women estimated to ingest 2.5 mg of vitamin B_6 per day secrete milk with 192 μg of the vitamin per liter, whereas those estimated to consume 2.0 mg secrete milk containing only 93 μg/L. Infants consuming milk with only 88 μg of vitamin B_6 per liter have been found to display abnormal behavior in standard assessment tests.[39] Any large

FIGURE 12-14

Key metabolic interconversions of various forms of vitamin B_6

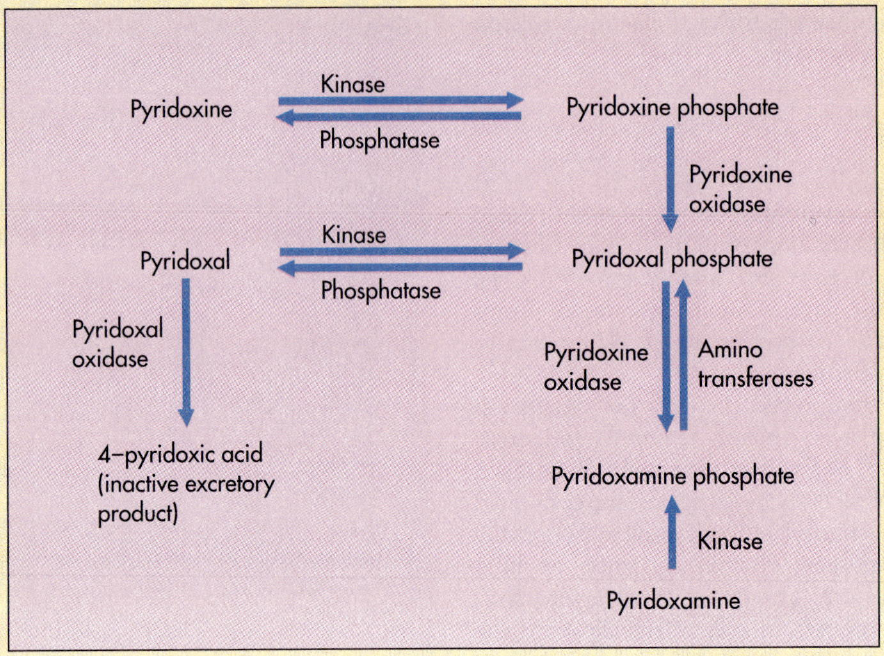

dietary intake produces an increase in the amount in milk within 4 hours. The RDA during lactation is 2.1 mg/day, but supplements may be recommended on top of this amount to ensure that an adequate level of the vitamin is always present in the milk.

The RDAs for infants are 0.3 mg/day for the first 2 months of life and 0.6 mg/day for the next 6 months. Adequate supplies in infants are required both to sustain normal metabolism and to permit the proper development of the nervous system. The RDAs for infants are somewhat generous, however, because they are not achieved by most breast-fed infants whose mothers were consuming plentiful supplies of vitamin B_6. For older infants and children, from 1.0 to 1.4 mg/day are recommended, whereas adolescents should consume from 1.5 to 2 mg/day.

The need for vitamin B_6 may be increased in older people. About one fourth of a test group of people over 60 years of age showed signs of a subclinical deficiency of vitamin B_6.

No recommendations on vitamin B_6 intakes are made for Canadian citizens.[33] The British recommendations are 25% to 40% lower than those in the United States.[34]

More than 40 drugs can increase the body's need for vitamin B_6, making it appropriate to consume more than the RDA. Examples of such drugs include oral contraceptives; isoniazid (isonicotinic acid hydrazide), which is chemically related to pyridoxine and is used to treat tuberculosis; and penicillamine, used to treat Wilson's disease, cystinuria, and rheumatoid arthritis.

FOOD SOURCES

A biochemical analysis of some representative diets suggests that adults consume around 1.2 mg of vitamin B_6 per day. The amount found in different foods tends to vary with the protein content of the foods. The vitamin is found in a wide variety of foods. Among the richest sources are chicken, fish, liver, whole grain cereals, and egg yolks. Bananas, avocados, and potatoes are the main good vegetable sources, whereas citrus fruits, milk, and cheese are poor sources. Figure 12-15 shows the sources of vitamin B_6 in the North American food supply.

The 1987-1988 Nationwide Food Consumption Survey revealed that women of all age-groups consume an average of 75% to 85% of their RDA, whereas men over 25 years of age average 85% to 95% of their RDA.[9] The NHANES III data (1988–1991) show vitamin B_6 intakes for women ranging from 1.5 to 1.6 mg/day and for men ranging from 2.1 to 2.3 mg/day, values closer to RDAs. Because the RDAs for vitamin B_6 are based on estimated protein intake, however, it is possible that analysis of actual protein intake would make the average amounts obtained by men and women appear more satisfactory.

Vitamin B_6 is relatively stable to heat but is destroyed by oxidation and ultraviolet light. Pyridoxal is unstable in alkali. Freezing vegetables causes a 15% to 70% reduction in their vitamin B_6 content, the milling of cereals causes losses of between 50% and 90%, and the processing of meat and fish causes a 40% to 60% loss. At present the addition of vitamin B_6 to enriched bread and

FIGURE 12-15

Contributions of various food groups to the vitamin B_6 in the North American food supply.

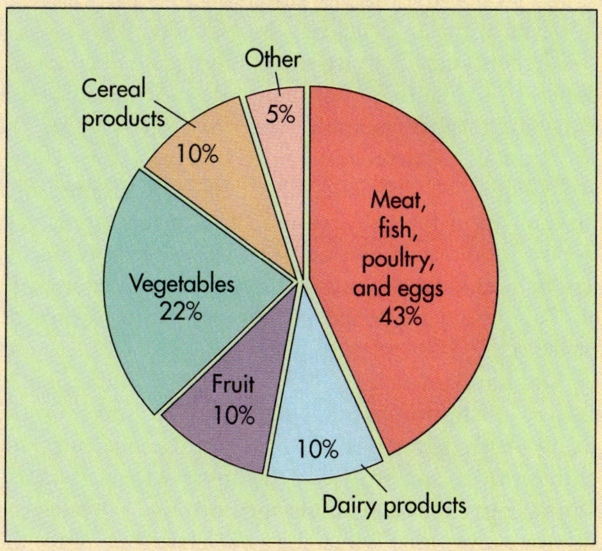

cereals is not mandatory. It is added to many cereals, however, and when added must be declared on the product's label.

The bioavailability of the vitamin B_6 in foods varies between 50% and 75%.[40] The more pyridoxine glucoside (PNG) present in a food, the lower the proportion of vitamin B_6 absorbed from the food. The vitamin B_6 and pyridoxine glucoside contents of commonly consumed foods are shown in Table 12-12. Other factors that may limit bioavailability are food processing (especially involving lysine) and the presence of fiber. Like many nutrients, vitamin B_6 binds to fiber, and it also binds to the amino acid lysine.

EVALUATION OF VITAMIN B_6 STATUS

Vitamin B_6 status can be assessed by a variety of biochemical tests. Direct measurement of the amount of PLP in the blood is one option, but a variety of other, more complex methods exist. For example, vitamin B_6 is required in several biochemical steps in the conversion of the amino acid tryptophan into the vitamin niacin. If a person has a vitamin B_6 deficiency, the results of one of these steps is that the intermediate kynurenine is shunted into xanthurenic acid rather than converted to niacin. This compound not normally produced is excreted in urine. In the **tryptophan load test** a subject is fed a 2-g dose and then the urine is analyzed for the presence of xanthurenic acid. If no xanthurenic acid appears in the urine, the subject's vitamin B_6 status is assumed to be adequate. Conversely, the appearance of xanthurenic acid in the urine indicates vitamin B_6 deficiency. Unfortunately, the tryptophan load test gives positive results (indicating a vitamin B_6 deficiency) for pregnant women and women receiving estrogens and who are riboflavin deficient. For these reasons, the tryptophan load test does not provide a very specific measure of vitamin B_6. Other tests include measurements of the amount of

TABLE 12-12

Vitamin B_6 and pyridoxine glucoside (PNG) content of commonly consumed foods

FOOD*	VITAMIN B_6 (mg/100 g)	PNG (mg/100 g)
VEGETABLES		
Carrots, raw	0.170	0.087
Cauliflower, frozen	0.084	0.069
Broccoli, frozen	0.119	0.078
Spinach, frozen	0.208	0.104
Cabbage, raw	0.140	0.065
Sprouts, alfalfa	0.250	0.105
Potatoes, cooked	0.394	0.165
BEANS/LEGUMES		
Soybeans, cooked	0.627	0.357
Beans, navy, cooked	0.381	0.159
Beans, lima, frozen	0.106	0.039
Peas, frozen	0.122	0.018
Peanut butter	0.302	0.054
Beans, garbanzo	0.653	0.111
Lentils	0.289	0.134
ANIMAL PRODUCTS		
Beef, ground, cooked	0.263	nd
Tuna, canned	0.316	nd
Chicken breast, raw	0.7	nd
Milk, skim	0.005	nd
NUTS/SEEDS		
Walnuts	0.535	0.038
Cashews, raw	0.351	0.046
Sunflower seeds	0.997	0.046
Almonds	0.086	0
FRUITS		
Orange juice, fresh	0.043	0.016
Tomato juice, canned	0.097	0.045
Blueberries, frozen	0.046	0.019
Banana	0.313	0.01
Pineapple, canned	0.079	0.017
Peaches, canned	0.009	0.002
Avocado	0.443	0.015
Raisins, seedless	0.23	0.154
CEREALS/GRAINS		
Wheat bran	0.903	0.326
Shredded wheat, cereal	0.313	0.087
Rice, brown	0.237	0.055

nd, none detected.

* All values given as milligrams of pyridoxine per 100 g of food. 1 mg of vitamin B_6 = 5.91 μmol.

From Leklem JE: Vitamin B_6. In Shils ME, Olson JA, Shike M, editors: *Modern nutrition in health and disease,* ed 8, Philadelphia, 1994, Lea & Febiger.

Factors That May Lead to Pyridoxine (Vitamin B_6) Deficiency or Dependency.

Inadequate dietary intake
Impaired delivery of vitamin (intake adequate)
- Defective intestinal absorption
- Defective cellular and intracellular transport
- Impaired oxidation of pyridoxine
- Impaired phosphorylation to form active coenzyme

Excessive loss of vitamin
- Through kidneys
- Through oxidation
- Inactivation by drugs

Relative deficiency (primary intake inadequate relative to demand)
- Increased metabolic activity (pregnancy, fever, and so on)
- Increased protein intake

Metabolic defects that alter use

pyridoxic acid in urine and measuring the amounts of various vitamin B_6–dependent enzymes in the blood. The recommended method of obtaining the most meaningful assessment of vitamin B_6 status involves a combination of the tryptophan load test and direct measurement of the level of PLP in blood.

DEFICIENCY

Vitamin B_6 deficiency produces a large number of abnormalities in amino acid and protein metabolism, producing a range of clinical symptoms, including poor growth, convulsions, anemia, decreased antibody formation, and skin lesions. Infants being fed a formula that provides less than 0.1 mg of vitamin B_6 per day became hyperirritable and then prone to convulsive seizures. These symptoms disappeared as soon as sufficient vitamin B_6 was added to the infants' diet. Other symptoms of vitamin B_6 deficiency in infants include rigidity of the body and a high, piercing cry.

The ability of vitamin B_6 deficiency to induce seizures has led to considerable interest in the role of the vitamin in the central nervous system. Changes in electroencephalogram readings (recording the electrical activity of the brain using electrodes attached to the scalp) can be detected in mild vitamin B_6 deficiency well before the stage at which seizures begin. If vitamin B_6 is deficient or absent during critical periods of brain growth in the first few months of life, the development of the brain and its ability to transmit nervous impulses can be permanently impaired.

In adults the only symptoms attributed to a lack of vitamin B_6 have been **microcytic hypochromic anemia** (anemia characterized by small red blood cells deficient in hemoglobin), depression, and confusion. Insufficient intakes of the vitamin have been associated with less specific symptoms, including weakness, nervousness, irritability, insomnia, and difficulty in walking.

Consumption of a vitamin B_6 antagonist (a substance that counteracts the effects of the vitamin) called **deoxypyridoxine** causes skin changes (glossitis, cheilosis, and stomatitis) that are different from those seen in riboflavin or niacin deficiency (see Chapter 13).

The amount of citrate excreted in urine decreases in people with vitamin B_6 deficiency. Because citrate assists in making oxalates soluble, this may account for the formation of oxalate-containing kidney stones. However, vitamin B_6 deficiency also decreases the rate of a transamination reaction required to convert oxalic acid into the amino acid glycine; so this may be the mechanism behind kidney stone formation. If both vitamin B_6 and magnesium are deficient, however, kidney stones do not form.

Vitamin B_6 deficiency can occur for a wide variety of reasons, in addition to inadequate dietary intake. Of the various drugs that may lead to vitamin B_6 deficiency, oral contraceptives are probably the most widely relevant. Contraceptive pills containing the hormone estrogen can lead to depression, which has been attributed to the failure to convert sufficient tryptophan into the neurotransmitter serotonin in the brain. This outward sign is accompanied by elevated levels of products of tryptophan metabolism in the urine. Both the depression and the urinary abnormalities can be corrected by taking supplements to provide 10 mg of vitamin B_6 per day.

CLINICAL USES

Vitamin B_6 has been used with some, although variable, success in the treatment of a variety of other conditions not obviously associated with vitamin B_6 deficiency. Such conditions include carpal tunnel syndrome, which causes paralysis of the fingers; nausea during pregnancy; premenstrual syndrome (PMS); and anemia. In all such conditions, however, it is essential that the vitamin be prescribed after proper medical diagnosis and that no more than 50 mg/day be consumed.

TOXICITY

Vitamin B_6 had long been considered nontoxic, but when self-medication with readily available megadoses came into practice, cases of toxicity began to appear. The first report of vitamin B_6 toxicity came in 1983 as a result of the consumption of 2 to 6 g over a 6-month period, corresponding to between 1000 and 3000 times the RDA.[41] The symptoms included loss of neuromotor coordination and were reversed when the vitamin B_6 supplementation was stopped. Dosages of up to 500 mg/day (250 times the RDA) have been taken by some people for as long as 2 years with no apparent damaging effects. However, intakes of 100 mg/day for 2 years have produced toxic symptoms (neurological damage), and 4 years were required for individuals to return to normal following cessation of vitamin B_6 supplementation.

ISSUES AND OPINIONS

The Future of Recommended Dietary Allowances

On June 28 and 29, 1993, the Food and Nutrition Board of The Institute Of Medicine/ National Academy Of Sciences sponsored a two-day workshop and public hearing in Washington, DC, to address the question, "Should the Recommended Dietary Allowances be revised?" The meeting was widely publicized to encourage broad participation of scientists, advocates, and individuals at all levels of the population. Twenty invited speakers gave prepared talks, 20 individuals and organizations gave oral testimony, and 19 gave written testimony. The Food and Nutrition Board reviewed all of the information and came up with the following conclusions:

- Sufficient new knowledge has accumulated to support a review of the current recommended dietary allowances (RDAs) for selected nutrients, especially energy and several vitamins and minerals.
- Future RDAs should incorporate the concept of reducing the risk of chronic disease where sufficient data for safety and efficacy exist.
- Serious consideration must be given to developing a new format for future RDAs.

The Food and Nutrition Board recognizes that it has to be more flexible to address multiple needs of users of the RDAs. To meet the broad range of needs, the Board proposes to develop a series of three publications. One publication will be the eleventh edition of the RDAs. This will review what is known about essential nutrients and important food components with respect to **four new proposed reference points:**

- **Deficient:** The level of intake below which almost all healthy people can be expected, over time, to experience deficiency symptoms of a clinical, physical, or functional nature.
- **Average requirement:** The mean level of intake of a nutrient or food component that appears, on the basis of experimental evidence, sufficient to maintain the desired biochemical and physiological function in a population.
- **Recommended Dietary Allowance:** The level of intake of an essential nutrient or food component considered, on the basis of available scientific knowledge, to be adequate to meet the needs of practically all healthy persons.
- **Upper safe:** The level of intake of a nutrient or food component that appears to be safe for most healthy people and beyond which there is concern that some people experience symptoms of toxicity over time.

The second publication will describe how the new RDAs could be used for a variety of purposes. A third publication will be developed for the lay public to explain what the RDAs are, how they were derived, and how they should be used. This publication will include dietary patterns designed to meet the RDAs for persons at various physiological stages of the life cycle and in population subgroups based on age, race, and ethnic dietary preferences.

The Food and Nutrition Board maintains that the main purpose of the RDAs remains as valid today as when first established. In 1941 the first RDA committee stated that the main purpose was "to provide standards to serve as goals for good nutrition." The Board recognizes, however, that future RDA documents must be broader in scope than their predecessors. The new RDA committee will be charged with the dual responsibility of providing the scientific basis for each RDA and providing explicit guidance on appropriate ways in which the RDAs can be used to develop food policy and to evaluate the nutrient needs of individuals.

From the Food and Nutrition Board/Institute of Medicine: *How should the Recommended Dietary Allowances be revised?* Washington, DC, 1994, National Academy Press.

~ BY NOW YOU SHOULD KNOW ~

- Vitamin C, folic acid (folate), vitamin B_{12}, and vitamin B_6 are water-soluble vitamins that directly or indirectly function in blood formation.
- Vitamin C (ascorbic acid) has long been known as the antiscorbutic (antiscurvy) vitamin and is found mainly in fruits and vegetables.
- Scurvy can be prevented with vitamin C intakes of 10 mg/day. Adequate reserves can be maintained with intakes of 60 mg/day.
- Large doses of vitamin C (from 250 to 12,000 mg/day) have been promoted for curing or protecting against a variety of conditions, including the common cold, cancer, and heart disease. Evidence in support of these claims is inconclusive.
- Because vitamin C is destroyed by heat, oxidation, and alkali, it is important to store and prepare foods rich in vitamin C in the ways that minimize loss of the vitamin.
- Life-style factors such as smoking, drinking alcohol, and stress can influence the body's need for several water-soluble vitamins.
- Folate and vitamin B_{12} are involved in growth and blood formation and are needed for the synthesis of DNA.
- Because DNA synthesis is essential for cell division, a deficiency of folate or vitamin B_{12} can result in poor growth and the failure of normal blood formation.
- High intakes of folate can mask a deficiency of vitamin B_{12}.
- Because vitamin B_{12} is found only in foods of animal origin, people who choose not to eat meat must find alternative sources of the vitamin.
- In contrast to other water-soluble vitamins, vitamin B_6 is required for almost all aspects of protein metabolism.
- Although vitamin B_6 was once considered nontoxic, reports dating from 1983 suggest that toxic effects may result from the popular practice of self-medication with large doses of the vitamin.
- Vitamin B_{12} and vitamin B_6 are important for maintaining normal function of the nervous system. Neurological problems develop as symptoms of a deficiency of either of these vitamins.

~ STUDY QUESTIONS ~

1. Under what circumstances or in what groups of people do you expect deficiencies in each of the water-soluble vitamins discussed in this chapter to appear?
2. What role has an inadequate vitamin C intake played in history?
3. Why is the body's need for vitamin B_6 related to protein intake?
4. List the most important food sources in the North American diet of each of the water-soluble vitamins discussed in this chapter.
5. Explain the function of intrinsic factor in the absorption of vitamin B_{12}.
6. Explain why vitamin preparations should not contain excessive amounts of folate.

~ CRITICAL ANALYSIS ~

1. Beginning with the first food or beverage you had after waking up yesterday, recall the fruits and vegetables you ate yesterday, including fruit or vegetable juices. Add the servings in each column below, then add the total servings from fruits and vegetables below.

How does your diet rate? Was at least 1 serving from a good source of vitamin C? Did you have 3 to 5 servings for the day? If you answered yes to both questions (and if those results are typical of your daily intake), you have done well in meeting the current dietary recommendations for fruit and vegetable consumption and for many vitamins they contain.

FRUITS		VEGETABLES		
Item	Servings	Item	Servings	
________	________	________	________	
________	________	________	________	
________	________	________	________	
________	________	________	________	
________	________	________	________	
________	________	________	________	
Total	________ +	Total	________	= Total servings ________

2. Below are listed some of the best sources and some of the more commonly eaten sources of the water soluble vitamins. Write the number of servings you ate yesterday next to each of the foods.

FOOD	TOTAL VITAMIN C (mg PER 3.5 OZ)	SERVINGS EATEN
Cauliflower	62.7	________
Broccoli	39.6	________
Spinach	52.4	________
Carrots or mixed vegetables	30.3	________
Sweet red pepper	155.0	________
Banana	18.6	________
Cantaloupe	30.7	________
Grapefruit	23.6	________
Orange	64.3	________
Orange juice (reconstituted)	37.3	________
Vitamin-fortified cereals	62.2	________
		________

RDA = ________ mg Intake from foods above = ________ mg

FOOD	FOLIC ACID (μg PER SERVING)	SERVINGS EATEN
Liver	383	________
Superfortified cereals (e.g., Product 19)	242	________
Cold cereals	112	________
Pinto, navy, or other dried beans	84	________
Spinach	70	________
Instant breakfast, diet bars, supplements	65	________
Bran, granola cereals	58	________
Broccoli	53	________
Orange juice	43	________
Chili	36	________
Corn	35	________
Oranges, tangerines	33	________

RDA = ________ μg Intake from foods above = ________ μg

FOOD	VITAMIN B_{12} (μg PER SERVING)	SERVINGS EATEN
Egg, fried	0.57	________
Beef, roast	1.54	________
Ground beef	1.52	________
Tuna	2.2	________
Oysters	16.2	________
Liver	87.0	________
Milk, whole	0.86	________
Milk, 2% fat	0.91	________
Ham	0.72	________
Chicken	0.3	________
		________

RDA = ________ μg Intake from foods above = ________ μg

FOOD	VITAMIN B_6 (mg PER 3.5 OZ)	SERVINGS EATEN
Potatoes, cooked	0.39	________
Soybeans, cooked	0.62	________
Garbanzo beans	0.65	________
Navy beans, cooked	0.38	________
Tuna, canned	0.31	________
Chicken breast	0.70	________
Walnuts	0.53	________
Sunflower seeds	0.99	________
Banana	0.31	________
Avocado	0.44	________
Wheat bran	0.90	________

RDA = ________ mg Intake from foods above = ________ mg

A point to note: Although a few foods such as tuna, broccoli, and bananas appear on more than one list, the lists differ with respect to many foods. This illustrates the need for a variety of foods in the diet. Because few individuals can eat the same foods meal after meal and day after day, the intake of adequate amounts of many nutrients, notably vitamins, is dependent on the selection of a variety of good sources of each nutrient over a period of time.

REFERENCES

1. Sauberlich HE: Ascorbic acid. In Brown ML, editor: *Present knowledge in nutrition,* ed 6, Washington, DC, 1990, International Life Sciences Institute.

2. Englard S, Seifter S: The biochemical functions of ascorbic acid, *Annu Rev Nutr* 6:365, 1986.

3. Jacob RA: Vitamin C. In Shils ME, Olson JE, Shike M, editors: *Modern nutrition in health and disease,* vol 1, ed 8, Philadelphia, 1994, Lea & Febiger.

4. Padh H: Vitamin C: newer insights into its biochemical functions, *Nutr Rev* 49:65, 1991.

5. Jacob RA, Skala JH, Omaye ST: Biochemical indices of human vitamin C status, *Am J Clin Nutr* 46:818, 1987.

6. Food and Nutrition Board: *Recommended Dietary Allowances,* ed 10, Washington, DC, 1989, National Academy Press.

7. Sauberlich HE and others: Ascorbic acid and erythorbic metabolism in nonpregnant women, *Am J Clin Nutr* 50:1039, 1989.

8. Kallner AB, Hartmann D, Homig DH: On the requirements of ascorbic acid in man: steady-state turnover and body pool in smokers, *Am J Clin Nutr* 34:1347, 1981.

9. Wright HS and others: The 1987-1988 Nationwide Food Consumption Survey: an update on the nutrient intake of respondents, *Nutr Today* 25:21, 1991.

10. Advanced Data from Vital and Health Statistics: *Vitamin and mineral intakes of persons aged 2 months and older in the U.S.: 1988-1991,* Hyattsville, Md, 1994, (in press).

11. Sinha R, Block G, Taylor PR: Problems with estimating vitamin C intakes, *Am J Clin Nutr* 57:547, 1993.

12. Jacob RA: Assessment of human vitamin C status, *J Nutr* 120:1480, 1990.

13. Hodges RE and others: Clinical manifestations of ascorbic acid deficiency in man, *Am J Clin Nutr* 24:432, 1971.

14. Moser U, Bendich A: Vitamin C. In Machlin LJ, editor: *Handbook of vitamins,* ed 2, New York, 1991, Marcel Dekker.

15. Pauling L: *Vitamin C and the common cold.* San Francisco, 1970, Freeman.

16. Hemilä H: Vitamin C and the common cold, *Br J Nutr* 67:3, 1992.

17. Block G: Vitamin C and cancer prevention: the epidemiological evidence, *Am J Clin Nutr* 53(suppl):270S, 1991.

18. Block G: Dietary guidelines and the results of food consumption surveys, *Am J Clin Nutr* 53(suppl):356S, 1991.

19. Shane B: Folate metabolism. In Picciano MF, Stokstad ELR, Gregory JF, editors: *Folic acid metabolism in health and disease,* New York, 1990, Wiley-Liss.

20. Mason J: Intestinal transport of monoglutamyl folates in mammalian systems. In Picciano MF, Stokstad ELR, Gregory JF, editors: *Folic acid metabolism in health and disease,* New York, 1990, Wiley-Liss.

21. Halstead CH and others: Clinical studies of intestinal folate conjugases, *J Lab Clin Med* 107:228, 1986.

22. Coleman N and others: Prevention of folate deficiency by food fortification, *Am J Clin Nutr* 27:339, *28*:465, *28*:471, 1974-1975.

23. Herbert V, Das KC: Folic acid and vitamin B_{12}. In Shils ME, Olson JE, Shike M, editors: *Modern nutrition in health and disease,* ed 8, Philadelphia, 1994, Lea & Febiger.

24. McPartlin J and others: Accelerated folate breakdowns in pregnancy, *Lancet* 341:148, 1993.

25. Herbert V: Recommended dietary intakes (RDI) of folate in humans, *Am J Clin Nutr* 45:661, 1987.

26. Sauberlich HE and others: Folate requirement and metabolism in non-pregnant women, *Am J Clin Nutr* 46:1016, 1987.

27. Fomon SJ, McCormick DB: B-vitamins and choline. In Fomon SJ, editor: *Nutrition of normal infants,* St. Louis, 1993, Mosby.

28. Center for Disease Control: Use of folic acid for prevention of spina bifida and other neural tube defects—1983-1991, *MMWR* 40:513, 1991.

29. O'Connor, DL, Tamura T, Picciano MF: Pteroylpolyglutamates in human milk, *Am J Clin Nutr* 53:930, 1991.

30. Sauberlich HE: Evaluation of folate nutrition in population groups. In Picciano MF, Stokstad ELR, Gregory JF, editors: *Folic acid metabolism in health and disease,* New York, 1990, Wiley-Liss.

30a. Jacob RA and others: Homocysteine increases as folate decreases in plasma of healthy men during short-term dietary folate and methyl group restriction, *J Nutr* 124:1072, 1994.

31. Herbert V: Vitamin B_{12}. In Brown ML, editor: *Present knowledge in nutrition,* ed 6, Washington DC, 1990, International Life Sciences Institute.

32. Report of a World Health Organization Study Group: *Diet, nutrition and the prevention of chronic diseases,* Technical Report Series No 797, Geneva, Switzerland, 1990, World Health Organization.

33. Health and Welfare Canada: *Nutrition recommendations,* Ottawa, Canada, 1990, Canadian Government Publishing Centre.

34. *Dietary references values for food energy and nutrients for the United Kingdoms, Report of the Panel on Dietary Reference Values of the Committee on Medical Aspects of Food Policy,* Report on Health and Social Subjects No 41, London, 1991, Her Majesty's Stationery Office.

35. Herbert V: Vitamin B_{12}: plant sources, requirement and assay, *Am J Clin Nutr* 48:852, 1988.

36. Ellenbogen L, Cooper BA: Vitamin B_{12}. In Machlin LJ, editor: *Handbook of vitamins,* ed 2, New York, 1991, Marcel Dekker.

36a. Lindenbaum J and others: Prevalence of cobalamin deficiency in the Framingham elderly population, *Am J Clin Nutr* 60:2, 1994.

36b. Lindenbaum J and others: Neuropsychiatric disorders caused by cobalamin deficiency in the absence of anemic or macrocytosis, *N Engl J Med* 318:1720, 1988.

37. Merrill AH, Burnham FS: Vitamin B_6. In Brown ML, editor: *Present knowledge in nutrition,* ed 6, Washington, DC, 1990, International Life Sciences Institute.

38. McCormick DB: Two interconnected B vitamins: riboflavin and pyridoxine, *Physiol Rev* 69:1170, 1987.

39. McCullough AL and others: Vitamin B_6 status of Egyptian mothers: relation to infant behavior and maternal-infant interactions, *Am J Clin Nutr* 51:1067, 1990.

40. Leklem JE: Vitamin B_6. In Shils ME, Olson JA, Shike M, editors: *Modern nutrition in health and disease,* ed 8, Philadelphia, 1994, Lea & Febiger.

41. Schaumberg HJ and others: Sensory neuropathy from pyridoxine abuse: a new megavitamin syndrome, *N Engl J Med* 309:445, 1983.

ADDITIONAL READINGS

Bailey L: Folate nutrition in adolescents and adults. In Picciano MF, Stokstad ELR, Gregory JF, editors: *Folic acid metabolism in health and disease,* New York, 1990, Wiley-Liss.

Carpenter KJ: *The history of scurvy and vitamin C,* New York, 1986, Cambridge University Press.

Dakshinamurti K, editor: Vitamin B_6, *Ann N Y Acad Sci* 585:1, 1990.

Gershoff SN: Vitamin C (ascorbic acid): new roles, new requirements? *Nutr Rev* 51:313, 1993.

Hanck AB: Vitamin C and cancer, *Prog Clin Biol Res* 259:307, 1987.

Herbert V: Experimental nutritional folate deficiency in man, *Trans Assoc Am Physicians* 75:307, 1962.

Herbert V: The 1986 Herman Award Lecture: nutrition science as a continually unfolding story: the folate and vitamin B_{12} paradigm, *Am J Clin Nutr* 46:387, 1987.

Merrill AH, Henderson JM: Diseases associated with defects in vitamin B_6 metabolism or utilization, *Annu Rev Nutr* 7:137, 1987.

Moss RW: *Free Radical: Albert Szent-Györgyi and the battle over vitamin C,* New York, 1987, Paragon House.

Reynolds RD, Leklem JE, editors: *Vitamin B_6: its role in health and disease,* New York, 1985, AR Liss.

Shane B: Folypolyglutamate synthesis and role in the regulation of one-carbon metabolism, *Vitam Horm* 45:263, 1989.

Woodson RD, editor: Symposium on new frontiers in vitamin B_{12} metabolism, *Am J Hematol* 34:81, 1990.

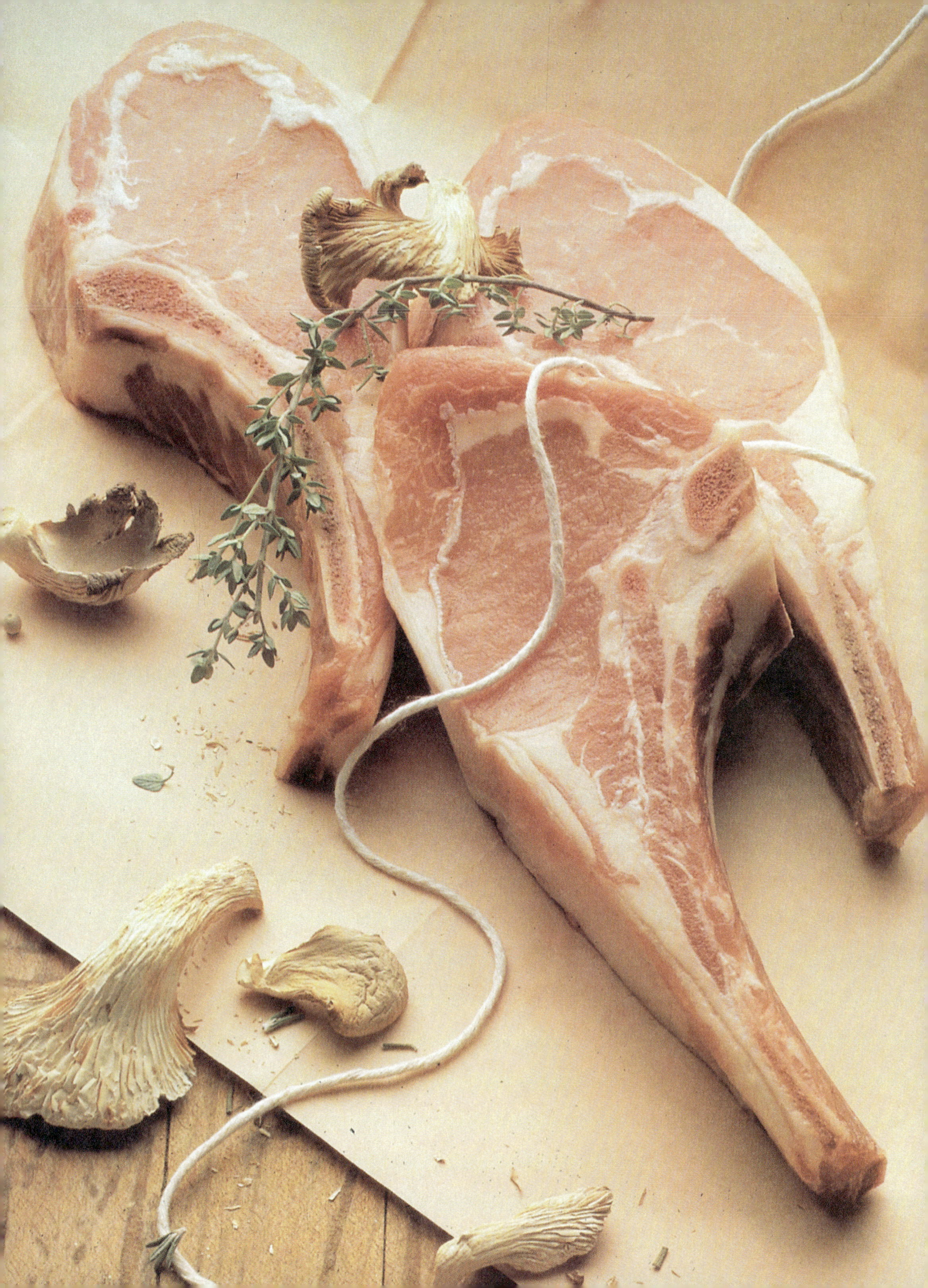

CHAPTER 13

WATER-SOLUBLE VITAMINS

PART 2

THIAMIN, RIBOFLAVIN, NIACIN, PANTOTHENIC ACID, & BIOTIN

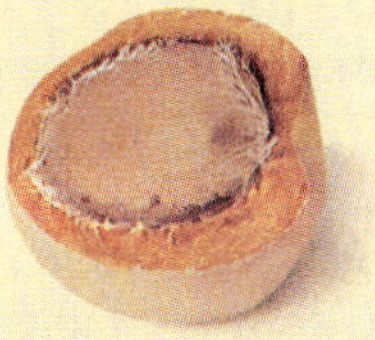

Many people tend to equate vitamins with energy largely because of misleading coverage of nutrition by the popular press. However, although vitamins are never a source of energy for the body, the vitamins discussed in this chapter are involved in facilitating the release of energy from the energy-yielding nutrients. They form essential parts of various coenzymes required to allow enzymes to catalyze the energy-releasing reactions of the body. Three of the vitamins discussed here—thiamin, riboflavin, and niacin—were discovered as cures for serious deficiency diseases. These diseases have now been almost eliminated from the Western world partly because of enrichment of cereal products. Deficiencies still occur, however, especially in developing countries. Some other vitamin-like substances and claimed nutrients are also discussed in this final chapter devoted to the analysis of the various nutrients required for health.

THIAMIN

Thiamin, also known as vitamin B_1, is widely known for its role in preventing the deficiency disease **beriberi.** The Philippine word *beriberi* means "I can't, I can't" and probably refers to the lack of neuromotor coordination in persons with the disease. Records of beriberi are found in Chinese writings from 2600 BC, but it remained virtually unknown until the middle of the nineteenth century. At that time it became a major health problem because of the increasing use of highly refined cereals. The countries most affected were those in which cereals, such as rice, provided as much as 80% of the kilocalories in the diet.

In 1855 Takaki had cured beriberi in the Japanese navy by using meat and milk to supplement the men's regular diet. At about the turn of the century, physicians in the Philippines and Indonesia recognized that consuming the rice bran extract called *tikitiki* brought about full recovery. It became obvious that a deficiency of some substance within rice bran, which was removed during milling, was the cause of beriberi.

By the mid-1920s scientists had isolated the substance able to cure beriberi from rice bran in the form of pure crystals of what is now known as thiamin. In 1936 the chemical structure of thiamin was fully established, and chemists learned how to synthesize it. Swiss and American firms immediately began commercial production of thiamin, and more than 300 tons are now made every year. Thiamin has also been known as the **antineuritis factor** because of its role in preventing the inflammation of nerves, known as *neuritis.*

Even though we now know what foods quickly cure beriberi and synthetic thiamin is available at low cost, beriberi still occurs in many parts of the world. In the Philippines it causes 75 infant deaths per 100,000 births and is that country's fourth leading cause of death. In addition to those who die from beriberi, an estimated 1.5 million people in the Philippines suffer from less severe deficiency of thiamin. The incidence of such is caused by the fact that the small rice mills—which produce 95% of the rice consumed—produce a highly polished rice that is low in thiamin and because a tax related to the amount of enrichment used discourages millers from enriching rice. The practice of repeatedly washing the milled rice causes further loss of thiamin. After the milling, washing, and cooking of rice and other foods, the typical Filipino diet provides less than the 0.27 mg of thiamin per 1000 kcal that is required to protect against beriberi.

CHEMICAL PROPERTIES

The chemical structure of thiamin is shown in Figure 13-1. The name "thiamin" indicates that it contains both sulfur ("thio") and nitrogen ("amine"). It is easily destroyed by heat or oxidation, especially in the presence of an alkali, such as baking soda. The commercially produced form of thiamin is **thiamin hydrochloride,** which is readily soluble in water and somewhat more stable than other forms.

FIGURE 13-1

The chemical structure of thiamin and thiamin pyrophosphate (TPP).

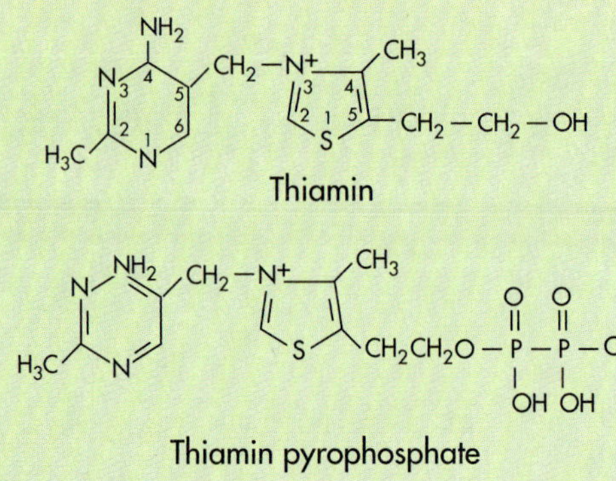

> ***B**aking soda and other alkalis have the following effects on food:*
> - Softening of cellulose
> - Reduction of cooking time
> - Destruction of some thiamin
> - Destruction of some vitamin C
> - Intensification of existing green color
>
> It is important to assess the balance of negative and positive effects of using alkali in cooking.

FUNCTIONS

Thiamin is converted into the coenzyme **thiamin pyrophosphate (TPP)** when two phosphate are added to the basic thiamin structure. This active coenzyme form of the vitamin has also been known as **thiamin diphosphate** and **cocarboxylase.**

TPP acts as a coenzyme in two types of reactions: oxidative decarboxylation and transketolation. In oxidative decarboxylation reactions, carbon dioxide (CO_2) is removed from some substrate molecule. In transketolation reactions, a ketone group is transferred from one molecule to another. These categories of reaction are important in carbohydrate metabolism, specifically in the citric acid cycle and the hexose monophosphate shunt or

FIGURE 13-2

Summary of metabolic pathways in which thiamin pyrophosphate (TPP) functions as a coenzyme.

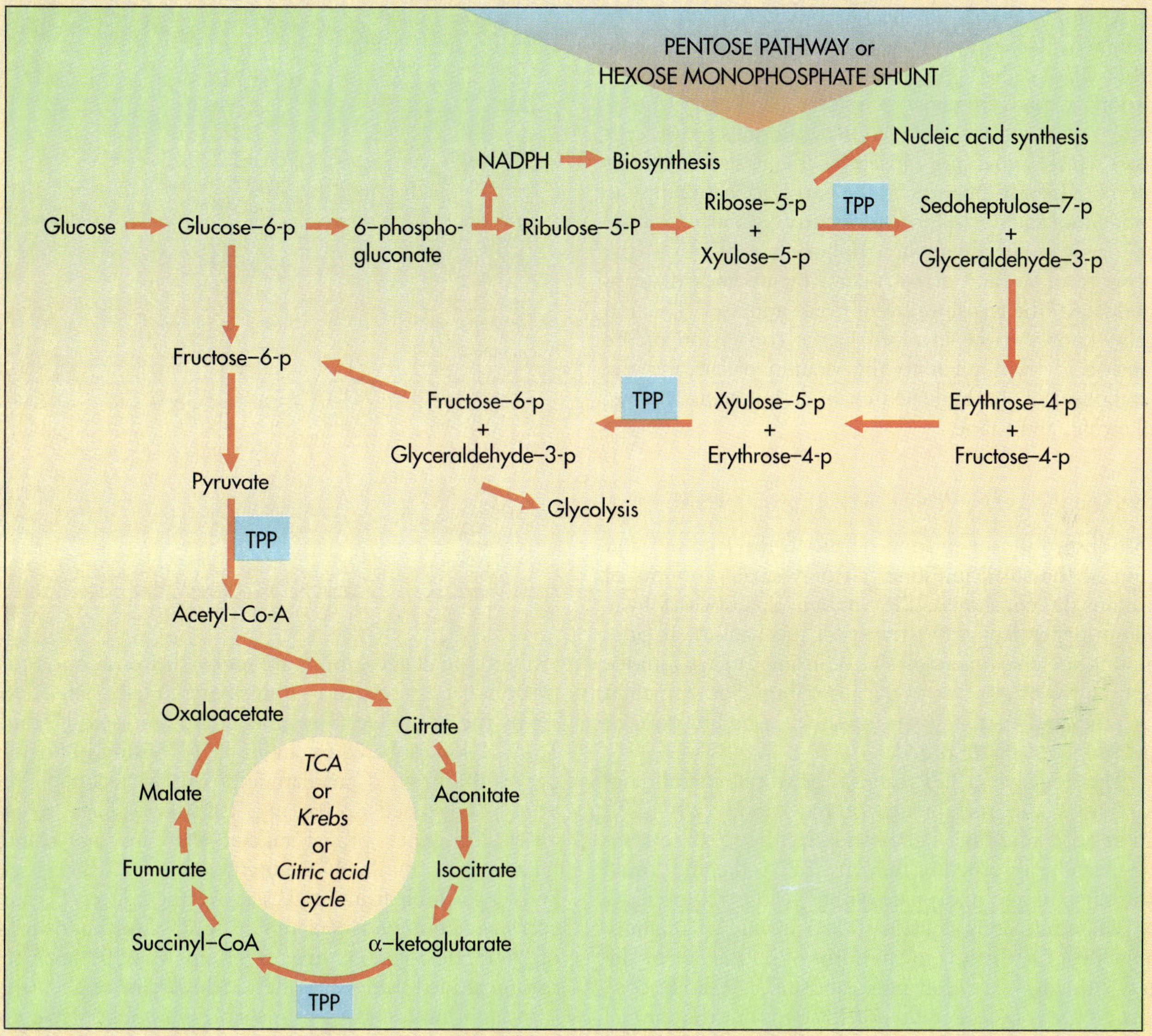

pentose pathway (Figure 13-2). In thiamin deficiency, metabolic intermediates whose further conversion depends on TPP tend to accumulate, causing the typical symptoms of thiamin deficiency.

TPP is needed for the decarboxylation of pyruvate (pyruvic acid) to form the acetyl-coenzyme A (acetyl-CoA) that enters the citric acid cycle and for the decarboxylation of α-ketoglutarate to succinyl-CoA within the citric acid cycle. These defects cause pyruvic acid and α-ketoglutarate to accumulate in those with thiamin deficiency.

A third vital role of TPP is as a coenzyme of the enzyme **transketolase**, which is required for the metabolism of glucose via the hexose monophosphate shunt or pentose pathway. Although only 10% of glucose is metabolized along this pathway, it is a vital process. In the liver and the adrenal gland, however, as much as 60% of glucose can be used via the hexose monophosphate shunt. It is the only way in which the body can produce the ribose and deoxyribose sugars needed for the synthesis of ribonucleic acid (RNA), deoxyribonucleic acid (DNA), and other coenzymes such as the reduced nicotinamide adenine dinucleotide phosphate (NADPH) needed, for example, in fatty acid synthesis. In the adult brain the pentose pathway metabolizes only a small amount of glucose, but in the developing brain of young persons, as much as 50% of glucose metabolism may follow this route. This is probably related to the need for NADPH for many synthetic processes during development and the need for ribose and deoxyribose sugars in the synthesis of RNA and DNA.[1] The most significant but certainly not all of the aspects of metabolism dependent on TPP have been mentioned.

Attempts to explain the neurological symptoms of thiamin deficiency have led to investigation of its role within nerve cells. It is apparently involved in the transmission of high-frequency impulses across nerve synapses, the junctions between neighboring nerve cells across which signals are carried by chemical neurotransmitters. Thiamin appears to be involved either in the production and release of the neurotransmitter acetylcholine or as the thymidine triphosphate (TTP) in the transport of sodium across neural membranes that are essential for the transmission of nerve impulses. Thiamin is also known to be involved in the conversion of the amino acid tryptophan to the vitamin niacin and the metabolism of the branched-chain amino acids leucine, isoleucine, and valine.

ABSORPTION AND METABOLISM

Most absorption of thiamin occurs in the jejunum and ileum of the small intestine.[2] If only small amounts of thiamin are consumed, the vitamin is absorbed by a sodium-dependent active transport mechanism. If large amounts are consumed, passive diffusion can account for a substantial proportion of the absorption. Some thiamin is synthesized in the gastrointestinal tract but too far down for it to be absorbed.

The coenzyme TPP cannot cross cell membranes apart from the membranes of red blood cells. TPP within food must be dephosphorylated to thiamin before it can be absorbed by humans. TPP is then reformed from thiamin and phosphate within cells as required.

The adult body contains 30 to 70 mg of thiamin, about 80% of which is in the form of TPP. Half of the body's thiamin is within muscle tissue. The body contains no specific storage site for thiamin, but the normal levels in the muscles, brain, liver, and kidneys can be doubled by thiamin therapy. During thiamin depletion the levels in these tissues soon drop to half of normal, except in the brain. Thiamin is excreted from the body as thiamin-acetic acid and as various other metabolites produced by its degradation.

RECOMMENDED DIETARY ALLOWANCES

Studies of the relationship between dietary intake and urinary excretion of thiamin have been used to try to establish our minimal and optimal needs. These are based on the assumption that any thiamin in excess of needs is excreted. An intake that leads to small (but not zero) levels of excreted thiamin is believed to correspond to minimal needs.

Because the coenzyme TPP is required for carbohydrate metabolism, the recommended dietary allowances (RDAs) for all age-groups are set on the assumption that thiamin need is related to total energy intake. The RDAs set by the Food and Nutrition Board are listed in Table 13-1. They are based on an intake of 0.5 mg of thiamin per 1000 kcal.[3] Canadian and British recommendations[4,5] are based on 0.4 mg/1000 kcal. These allowances represent optimal intakes that are significantly higher than minimal requirements. No benefits are known to result from intakes above these levels because excessive amounts are excreted. Because of the low cost of synthetic thiamin, intakes of up to 200 times the recommended values are often included in supplements. Although unnecessary, even such high intakes have not been linked to any harmful effects.

TABLE 13-1

Recommended dietary allowances (United States) and recommended nutrient intakes (Canada) for thiamin

AGE (YEARS)	UNITED STATES (mg/DAY)	CANADA (mg/DAY)
CHILDREN		
1-3	0.7	0.6
4-6	0.9	0.7
7-10	1	0.9
MALES		
11-14	1.3	1
15-24	1.5	1.3
25-50	1.5	1.1
50+	1.2	0.8-0.9
FEMALES		
11-50	1.1	0.8-0.9
50+	1	0.8
Pregnant	1.5	0.9
Lactating	1.6	1

Research has shown that the thiamin needs of older people are relatively high. They are found to excrete less thiamin than do others at all levels of intake, they react more rapidly to moderate depletion of thiamin, and they respond more slowly to the addition of thiamin to the diet.

The need for thiamin increases with increased consumption of alcohol because the vitamin is necessary for the metabolism of acetaldehyde, an intermediary product of alcohol metabolism. Also, a defect in the intestinal mucosal cells of alcoholics causes decreased absorption of thiamin.

As the amount of fat in the diet increases, the need for thiamin declines. For this reason, dietary fat has often been referred to as a "thiamin sparer." This effect occurs because only one of the reactions involved in the metabolism of fatty acids require thiamin, as opposed to several key reactions of carbohydrate metabolism. When

FIGURE 13-3

Contribution of various food groups to the thiamin in the North American food supply.

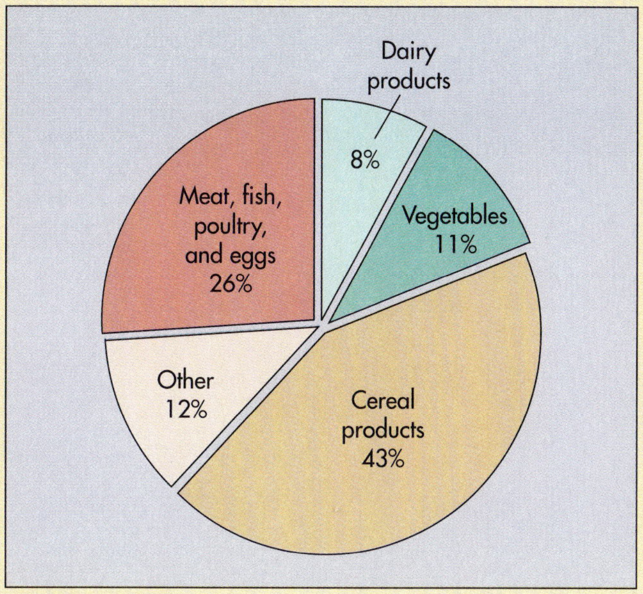

the amount of fat in the diet increases, the amount of carbohydrate usually decreases. People who develop beriberi are almost always eating a high-carbohydrate diet, with carbohydrates providing more than 80% of total kilocalories.

The need for thiamin is increased by some sulfonamide drugs and other antibiotics. The origin of this effect is unknown, although a variety of theories have been proposed.

FOOD SOURCES

As shown in Figure 13-3, cereal products (most of which are enriched in thiamin) provide almost half of the thiamin available in the North American food supply. Meat, fish, and poultry provide about one fourth, whereas dairy products and vegetables each provide about one tenth. Overall, the U.S. food supply makes about 2.2 mg of thiamin available per day. This is higher than the amount that was available at the turn of the century largely because of the practice of adding thiamin to most cereal-based products.

The richest sources of thiamin are pork products (Figure 13-4). People who do not eat pork, however, can readily obtain adequate amounts from other sources. The thiamin content of the most frequently used foods are listed in Table 13-2. Peas and other legumes are good sources of thiamin, and the amount of thiamin they contain increases with increasing maturity of the seed. The amount of thiamin obtained from dried legumes is reduced if they are soaked for a long time in water that is then discarded. It is also reduced if baking soda is used to soften the cellulose and reduce cooking time. Nevertheless, the use of minute amounts of baking soda (1/16 teaspoon per cup of beans) is acceptable because the shortened cooking time reduces the losses of thiamin during cooking by an amount that compensates for the increased losses caused by the alkalinity of the baking soda.

About 94% of the thiamin within whole grain cereals is in the outer husks and the germ, both of which are removed during milling. Although enriched and whole wheat bread may seem to contain modest amounts of thiamin per slice, they are consumed in such large quantities—especially by low-income families—that they can ensure an adequate intake from diets whose thiamin content is otherwise marginal. The enrichment of bread with thiamin is mandatory in 35 states. This is believed to be the reason for a decrease in the incidence of beriberi among alcoholics, many of whom eat large quantities of bread and bread products because they are an inexpensive source of kilocalories. Of the bread and flour marketed in the United States, 90% is now enriched in thiamin. The dietary significance of the enrichment of bread and other cereal products such as rice, macaroni, corn grits, and flour obviously depends on the extent to which these products are consumed as staple foods. The amount of thiamin added is regulated by **Standards of Identity** for enriched foods shipped in interstate trade.

Dried brewer's yeast and wheat germ both are rich in thiamin and are widely promoted in health food stores. In general, however, because people make little use of them, they are of little significance in the North American diet. Live yeast cells—found in compressed yeast cakes—are rich in thiamin, but because yeasts need thiamin to grow, they can deprive the body of thiamin

FIGURE 13-4

Amount of thiamin per serving of various foods.

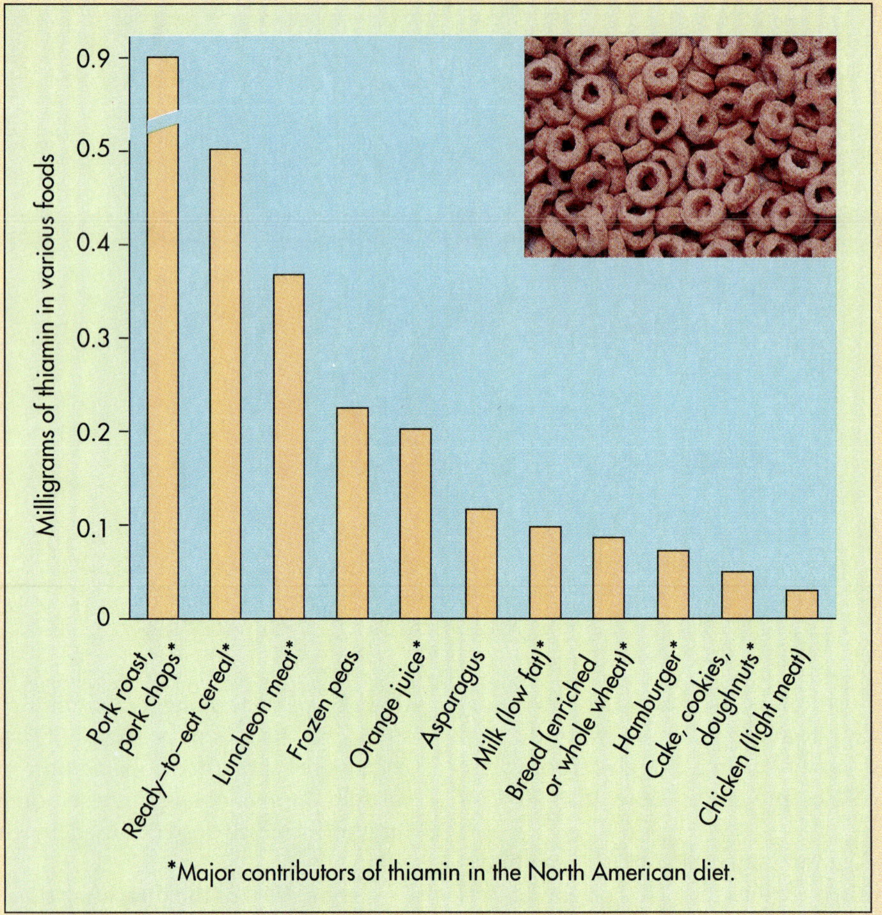

and actually cause thiamin deficiency. Cooking kills yeast cells, however, so the problem occurs only when live yeast in uncooked products is consumed. The consumption of live yeast was once common as a supposed cure for acne and other skin conditions.

Some freshwater fish; a few saltwater fish; some shellfish, such as clams, shrimps, and mussels; and bracken ferns contain a thiamin-splitting enzyme called **thiaminase.** Fortunately, because this is a heat-labile enzyme that is readily destroyed by the heat of cooking, it is a cause for concern only in diets containing significant amounts of raw fish. Tea, however, contains either a thiamin antagonist or a heat-stable thiaminase enzyme. This can have a significant effect on the availability of thiamin in food eaten with the tea, if about eight or more cups of tea are consumed per day.

DIETARY ADEQUACY OF THIAMIN INTAKES

Participants in the Nationwide Food Consumption Surveys (1977-1978 and 1987-1988) of all ages and genders had average thiamin intakes that either met or exceeded the RDAs. Also, Health and Nutritive Examination Surveys (HANES I and HANES II) have found that thiamin intake was at least 0.4 mg/1000 kcal for all economic, age, gender, and racial groups and averaged 0.6 mg/1000 kcal. Adult males surveyed in NHANES III (1988-1991) reported food intakes providing 2.0 mg, and adult females reported intakes providing 1.6 mg, both well above 0.5 mg/1000 kg.

EVALUATION OF THIAMIN STATUS

The most sensitive test available to determine thiamin status measures the activity of the **transketolase** enzyme of red blood cells (erythrocytes). This enzyme requires TPP as a coenzyme, and so its activity declines with declining thiamin status. Results from this test are found to reflect a decrease in dietary intake before any other signs of thiamin deficiency become detectable.

Another test measures the amount of thiamin excreted in urine after a "load" dose several times the daily requirement is given. People with low thiamin status

TABLE 13-2

Thiamin, riboflavin, and niacin contents in average servings and per 100 kcal of foods most frequently reported in surveys and recommended sources

			THIAMIN		RIBOFLAVIN		NIACIN	
FOOD	AMOUNT	Kcal	PER SERVING (mg)	PER 100 kcal	PER SERVING (mg)	PER 100 kcal	PER SERVING (mg)	PER 100 kcal
MEAT, FISH, EGGS, POULTRY, NUTS								
Egg, fried	1 large	95	0.03	0.03	0.14	0.15	tr	tr
Beef, roast	3 oz	315	0.07	0.02	0.19	0.06	4	1.2
Ground beef	3 oz	230	0.04	0.02	0.09	0.04	4.4	1.9
Chicken	3 oz	140	0.06	0.04	0.1	0.07	11.8	8.4
Tuna	3 oz	165	0.04	0.02	0.09	0.05	10.1	6.1
Peanut butter	2 Tbsp	190	0.04	0.02	0.04	0.02	—	—
Bacon	3 slices	110	0.13	0.13	0.05	0.04	1.4	1.2
Ham	3 oz	205	0.51	0.12	0.19	0.09	3.8	1.8
Beef liver	3 oz	185	0.18	0.09	3.52	1.9	12.3	6.6
CEREAL PRODUCTS								
Cornflakes	1 cup	110	0.37	0.34	0.43	0.39	5	4.5
Shredded wheat	1 biscuit	100	0.07	0.08	0.08	0.1	1.5	1.5
Saltines	4 crackers	50	0.06	0.12	0.05	0.12	0.6	1.2
Rice	1 oz, dry	109	0.11	0.1	0.01	0.009	0.9	0.8
White bread, enriched	1 slice	65	0.12	0.18	0.08	0.12	0.9	1.3
Whole wheat bread	1 slice	70	0.1	0.14	0.06	0.09	1.1	1.5
DAIRY PRODUCTS								
Whole milk	8 oz	150	0.1	0.06	0.38	0.24	0.21	0.14
2% fat milk	8 oz	120	0.1	0.08	0.41	0.34	0.21	0.17
Cheddar cheese	1 oz	115	0.01	0.01	0.11	0.1	0.02	0.02
Cottage cheese, low-fat (2%)	4 oz	102	0.05	0.05	0.42	0.2	0.3	0.3
FRUITS								
Apple	1 medium	80	0.02	0.05	0.02	0.03	0.11	0.13
Banana	1 medium	105	0.06	0.06	0.11	0.07	0.62	0.6
Orange juice, frozen	4 oz	56	0.11	0.2	0.01	0.02	0.06	1.1
Peach	1 medium	37	0.02	0.05	0.05	0.14	0.5	2.3
VEGETABLES								
Corn, canned	½ cup	82	0.04	0.05	0.07	0.08	1.2	1.5
Green beans	½ cup	22	0.04	0.18	0.06	0.27	0.4	1.8
Green peas	½ cup	88	0.26	0.3	0.08	0.09	0.7	0.8
Lettuce	¼ head	20	0.06	0.3	0.04	0.2	0.3	1.5
Tomato	1 medium	25	0.07	0.27	0.06	0.24	0.7	2.8
Potato, baked	1 medium	93	0.1	0.11	0.04	0.04	0.8	0.9
Asparagus	½ cup	22	0.18	0.6	0.11	0.5	0.9	4.1
Broccoli	½ cup	22	0.13	0.59	0.16	0.5	0.5	2.2

—, None; *tr*, trace.

retain more of the load dose and therefore excrete less of it than do people with adequate thiamin status. However, because many other factors influence the amount of thiamin excreted, these load tests are not regarded as reliable.

DEFICIENCY

Thiamin deficiency caused by a low dietary intake of the vitamin can occur in diets that are low in energy or limited in variety. Thiamin deficiency can also result from the following:

- Poor absorption of the vitamin because of some abnormality of the gastrointestinal tract
- The inability of tissues to accumulate adequate supplies of thiamin
- Failure of the tissues to use available thiamin properly
- An increased requirement for thiamin caused by, for example, diets high in carbohydrate or alcohol because thiamin is required for the metabolism of both

Infantile beriberi occurs most frequently in infants between 2 and 5 months of age. The condition develops frighteningly quickly, and unless treated in a matter of hours, it often causes death. The affected baby develops **cyanosis,** in which the lack of oxygen or accumulation of carbon dioxide in the blood causes the skin to turn blue, a fast heartbeat (**tachycardia**), and a loud, piercing cry that changes to a thin, weak, and almost inaudible one. These symptoms are sometimes accompanied by vomiting and convulsions. The administration of thiamin brings dramatic relief of the symptoms within a few hours.

> *I*nfantile beriberi is more common in breast-fed than in bottle-fed infants because a lactating mother's thiamin intake may be too low for her to secrete a sufficient amount in her milk.

Beriberi occurs more often in breast-fed than in bottle-fed infants because a lactating mother's intake of thiamin may be too low to allow a sufficient amount to enter her milk. The situation is complicated by the transfer into the milk of **pyruvic aldehyde,** a toxic product of carbohydrate metabolism that accumulates in thiamin deficiency.

In adults beriberi takes two distinct forms. In **wet (edematous) beriberi** the patient exhibits swelling of the limbs, usually starting at the feet and progressing upward through the body to cause a difficulty in walking. The accumulation of fluid in heart muscle then leads to heart failure and death. In **dry (wasting) beriberi** there is a gradual loss of body tissue and the patient becomes thin and emaciated. In both forms the symptoms include numbness in the legs, irritability, vague uneasiness, disorderly thinking, and nausea. These all suggest the involvement of the nervous system in their onset. In the Western societies, alcoholics are virtually the only group of adults found to suffer from beriberi.

The various symptoms of thiamin deficiency are presumably caused by the accumulation of intermediary products of metabolism, whose further conversion is blocked at a stage requiring TPP as a coenzyme. Because thiamin deficiency usually occurs with deficiencies of other B-complex vitamins, it is difficult to attribute symptoms specifically to a lack of thiamin. However, the following symptoms are believed to be specific results of thiamin deficiency.

Loss of Appetite

Loss of appetite, or **anorexia,** caused by thiamin deficiency has been clearly demonstrated in humans and other animals. Anorexia accompanied by vomiting was the first sign of thiamin deficiency in one group of normal men in whom the deficiency was experimentally induced. Even with intakes of 0.2 mg/1000 kcal, which did not cause any other symptoms, loss of appetite, nausea, and constipation were found. Increased intake of thiamin restores the appetite of people who have been deficient in thiamin, but it does not stimulate appetite beyond a normal level.

Decreased Muscle Tone

The loss of *tonus* (muscle tone) in the wall of the gastrointestinal tract results in decreased gastric motility, a distended colon, and constipation. Thiamin has been used in attempts to treat constipation caused by loss of muscle tone in elderly people, although the results have been variable.

Depression

Mental depression and confusion have sometimes been alleviated by the use of thiamin. This has led to the somewhat misleading name of "morale vitamin" being given to thiamin. People with low thiamin intakes do show pronounced mood changes, vague feelings of uneasiness, fear, disorderly thinking, and other signs of mental depression, which respond well to thiamin administration. For example, in a study of 10 elderly women limited to 0.33 mg of thiamin per day, all showed irritability, complained of fatigue and headaches, and voluntarily restricted their social engagements. In parallel with these symptoms the level of thiamin excreted in urine dropped dramatically. The symptoms could then be alleviated by a single dose of 1.4 mg of thiamin. Similar results have been obtained in men.

Neurological Changes

Thiamin levels in the brain can be reduced by 50% without any noticeable symptoms. Further reduction to 30% of normal levels leads to development of a slow and unsteady gait. At 20% of normal levels, severe disturbances of posture and equilibrium occur, and neuromuscular coordination in general becomes impaired, leading to deterioration in speed of movements (motor speed) and hand-eye coordination. The most acute symptom of thiamin deficiency is the mental confusion that precedes coma.

FIGURE 13-5

Chemical structure of riboflavin, flavin adenine dinucleotide, and flavin mononucleotide.

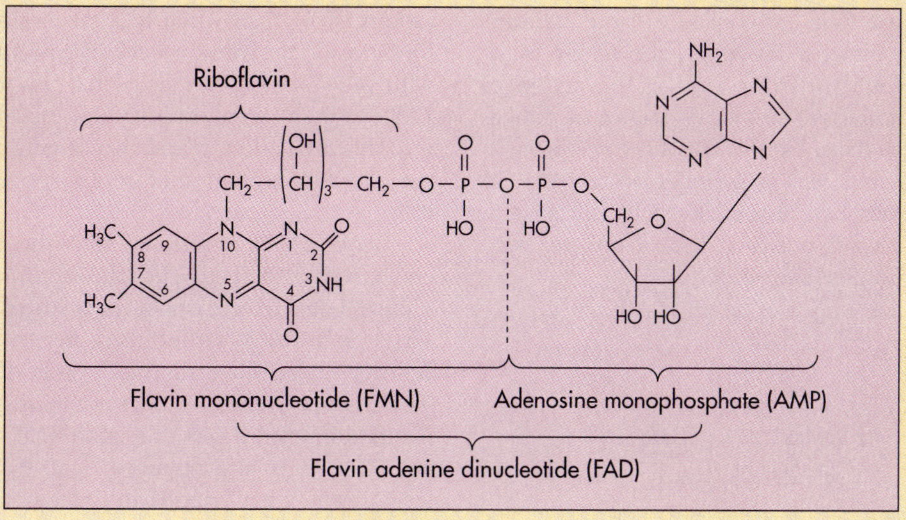

The most common form of thiamin deficiency in developed countries, particularly in the United States, is the well-known **Wernicke-Korsakoff syndrome** associated with alcohol abuse.[2] The manifestations of this syndrome range from mild confusion to coma and include involuntary rapid eye movement **(nystagmus)** and severe impairment of memory and cognitive function. All of these problems are quickly reversed by the administration of thiamin.

CLINICAL USES

Thiamin has been used to treat a wide variety of medical conditions, in addition to straightforward thiamin deficiency. One survey of the literature found that it had been tried as a therapy in 230 different conditions including neuritis, neuralgia, pain of various origins, diseases of the central nervous system, and cardiovascular conditions. The results of such trials have generally been inconclusive. There is no evidence of adverse effects from intakes of up to 100 mg of thiamin per day; so the use of thiamin in attempts to treat such conditions is probably safe, although of unknown or questionable effectiveness.

> Although thiamin has been used to treat a variety of medical conditions in addition to thiamin deficiency, the results of such trials have generally been proven to be inconclusive.

RIBOFLAVIN

What is now known as riboflavin—which has also been called vitamin B_2, vitamin G, and "the yellow enzyme"—was recognized as a vitamin in 1917. At that time it became clear that what was then known as vitamin B retained some growth-promoting properties even after its antiberiberi properties (from thiamin) had been destroyed by heat. The heat-labile and heat-stable components of vitamin B were named vitamin B_1 and vitamin B_2, respectively, and were eventually identified as thiamin and riboflavin.

Around the time that riboflavin was being identified, there were reports of four substances required for growth known as heptoflavin, lactoflavin, ovoflavin, and verdoflavin. These were all compounds containing the **flavin** chemical group (Figure 13-5), isolated from liver, milk, eggs, and grass, respectively. In 1933 it became evident that the active factor was the same in all of them and was composed of a protein plus a flavin pigment. Flavins produce an intense yellow-green fluorescence in water. The four substances became recognized as riboflavin. Originally the name *riboflavine* was used, but the final "e" was soon dropped in all countries except Britain. Riboflavin is now known to be essential for growth and tissue repair in all animals. So far no specific deficiency disease has been associated with this vitamin, although deficiency does cause a variety of general symptoms.

CHEMICAL PROPERTIES

The chemical structure of riboflavin is shown in Figure 13-5.[6] It is a relatively stable vitamin that is resistant to acid, heat, and oxidation. It is unstable, however, in the presence of alkali and light. Because it is slightly soluble in water, some losses occur when small pieces of riboflavin-containing food are cooked in large amounts of water for long periods. However, the major factor causing loss of riboflavin from food is the action of sunlight on milk, which is a significant source of riboflavin in most Western diets. Up to 70% of the riboflavin in milk can be destroyed during 4 hours of exposure to sunlight. Such losses have essentially been eliminated, however, by the almost universal use of opaque wax-lined cardboard containers for milk.

> *U*p to 70% of the riboflavin in milk can be destroyed during 4 hours of exposure to sunlight.

FUNCTIONS

Riboflavin is used to produce two coenzymes, **flavin mononucleotide (FMN)** and **flavin adenine dinucleotide (FAD)** (Figure 13-5). These coenzymes function primarily in oxidation-reduction reactions, because of their ability to accept and transfer hydrogen atoms. The proteins to which they become attached are known as **flavoproteins.**

Reactions dependent on the coenzymes derived from riboflavin include some required for the release of energy from glucose, fatty acids, and amino acids. Riboflavin is also required for the conversion of the amino acid tryptophan into the active form of the vitamin niacin and for the conversion of vitamin B_6 and folate into their active coenzyme and storage forms. Because vitamin B_6 and folate are required for DNA synthesis, riboflavin has an indirect effect on cell division and therefore growth.

Other biochemical roles of riboflavin include involvement in the production of hormones in the adrenal gland, the formation of red blood cells in bone marrow, the synthesis of glycogen (glycogenesis), and the catabolism of fatty acids.

ABSORPTION, TRANSPORT, AND METABOLISM

Riboflavin occurs in food in three forms: riboflavin itself and the FMN and FAD coenzyme forms of the vitamin. All three forms can be used to meet the body's need.[7] In the intestinal lumen, FMN and FAD are converted into free riboflavin before absorption. The riboflavin is then absorbed by a regulated active transport mechanism, largely in the upper portion of the gastrointestinal tract. More riboflavin is absorbed when it is taken with meals (about 70%) than when it is taken alone (about 15%). Once inside the intestinal cells the riboflavin is combined with phosphate (phosphorylated) to form FMN. Both FMN and any unphosphorylated riboflavin are released into the circulation, where they largely become bound to the albumin protein and are transported to the body's cells.

Most FMN is released into the liver, where it is converted into FAD by the addition of adenosine diphosphate. Excess riboflavin is stored within tissues as FMN and FAD, rather than free riboflavin. Overall, however, relatively little riboflavin is stored in the body. The amount in the liver does not increase above a certain maximum, even if plentiful additional supplies are available. The liver also retains at least 50% of its maximal level, even when riboflavin intakes are low. Thyroid hormone appears to stimulate the absorption and storage of riboflavin and the synthesis of FMN and FAD.

Riboflavin is excreted mainly in urine, after the kidneys have reabsorbed enough of the vitamin to maintain tissue saturation. Typical urinary excretion levels of riboflavin are 200 μg/24 hr, although in riboflavin deficiency, this falls to 40 to 70 μg/24 hr. Riboflavin excreted in feces is either unabsorbed dietary riboflavin or some of the riboflavin secreted in bile and not reabsorbed.

RECOMMENDED DIETARY ALLOWANCES

In different editions of the *Recommended Dietary Allowances,* riboflavin requirements have been based on total energy intake, protein allowances, or metabolic body size.[3] The allowances derived in these ways do not differ significantly. When related to energy intake, 0.6 mg of riboflavin/1000 kcal is recommended (with a minimum of 1.6 mg/day) to ensure tissue saturation of the vitamin. This estimate is based on studies of the amount of riboflavin excreted in response to various levels of intake.

The current RDAs for riboflavin are listed in Table 13-3. During pregnancy and lactation an additional 0.3 mg and 0.5 mg, respectively, is recommended, based on the assumption of 70% absorption. The need for riboflavin relative to energy intake is the same in older adults as in young men and women.[9] The lower RDAs for men and women over 51 years of age reflect their decreased energy requirements. There are some indications that riboflavin needs are greater in women who undertake regular exercise.[8] In the United States, RDAs for riboflavin are slightly higher than the recommended intakes in Canada[4] and Britain.[5] There are no known problems associated with high intakes of riboflavin.

TABLE 13-3

Recommended dietary allowances (United States) and recommended nutrient intakes (Canada) for riboflavin

AGE (YEARS)	UNITED STATES (mg/DAY)	CANADA (mg/DAY)
CHILDREN		
1-3	0.8	0.6-0.7
4-6	1.1	0.9
7-10	1.2	1-1.3
MALES		
11-14	1.5	1.3-1.4
15-18	1.8	1.6
19-50	1.7	1.4-1.5
51+	1.4	1-1.2
FEMALES		
11-50	1.3	1-1.1
51+	1.2	1
Pregnant	1.6	1.3
Lactating	1.8	1.4

FOOD SOURCES

Riboflavin is widely distributed in both animal and vegetable foods. The amounts present in various foods are listed in Table 13-2. Figure 13-6 shows the relative contributions of the major food groups to the riboflavin available in the North American food supply. Protein-rich foods provide about one third of the riboflavin in the North American diet.

Nationwide surveys in the United States conducted by the United States Department of Agriculture (USDA) found in 1986 to 1987 that adult men consumed an average of 2.08 mg of riboflavin per day, adult women consumed 1.34 mg/day, and their children aged 1 to 5 years consumed 1.57 mg/day.[10] NHANES III (1988-1991) recorded intakes of 2.2 to 2.5 mg for men and 1.5 to 1.7 mg for women.

About 60% to 90% of the riboflavin in fruits and vegetables remains after cooking. The milling of cereal, on the other hand, causes losses of riboflavin that can be as high as 60%. Because of its intense yellow color, riboflavin often is not used when fortifying cereals, such as rice. It is always added to flour and bread, however, to bring their riboflavin content up to a higher level than found in whole wheat products. These high enrichment standards as originally set reflected errors made in estimating the amount of riboflavin in whole wheat; they have been retained as a means of preventing riboflavin deficiency.

The riboflavin in milk makes a significant contribution to the total dietary intake. One quart of milk provides at least the entire recommended allowance for people of all ages, whereas 2 cups provides enough to meet our minimal needs for riboflavin. Cheese retains about one fourth of the riboflavin in the milk from which it was made. Liver and kidney are good sources of riboflavin, but other meats are only fair sources.

Riboflavin is synthesized by bacteria in the human gastrointestinal tract, but little evidence suggests that significant amounts of this riboflavin are absorbed.

There have been no reports of riboflavin toxicity, either in human beings or in other animals. This is probably because the absorption of riboflavin is a saturable process, meaning that it cannot rise beyond a certain saturation level. This level, our "maximal absorptive capacity" for riboflavin, is about 20 mg/day.

EVALUATION OF RIBOFLAVIN STATUS

Riboflavin status is determined by measuring the increase in activity of the enzyme **glutathione reductase** in red blood cells in response to the addition of FAD, which is required for the enzyme's activity. The activity of glutathione reductase in red blood cells of people with normal riboflavin status rises by less than 20% in response to the addition of FAD. In riboflavin deficiency, an activation of more than 40% is produced.[11] Neither urinary riboflavin levels nor red blood cell riboflavin levels are considered sensitive enough indicators of riboflavin status.

DEFICIENCY

Riboflavin deficiency appears to be more common than was previously suspected. In one study of 431 high school students, glutathione reductase activation measurements indicated that 16% of the girls and 6% of the boys had inadequate riboflavin intakes. Their riboflavin status was corrected by consumption of 0.5 mg of supplementary riboflavin per day for 1 week. Other studies found deficiencies in 11% of a group of children and in 26% of a group of girls, all aged 13 to 19 years and of low socioeconomic status. These deficiencies were all associated with milk intakes of less than 1 cup/day.[12]

Riboflavin deficiency is associated with a broad range of symptoms. An early symptom of what is known as **ariboflavinosis** (lack of riboflavin) is a condition known as **cheilosis** in which cracks appear at the corners of the mouth and the lips become inflamed. Another common symptom is a dermatitis around the nose and mouth and **glossitis** (inflammation of the tongue). For such symptoms to appear, intakes of riboflavin must be low for several months.

As with any vitamin deficiency, riboflavin deficiency can lead to growth retardation. In animal studies ribo-

FIGURE 13-6

Contributions of various food groups to the riboflavin content of the North American food supply.

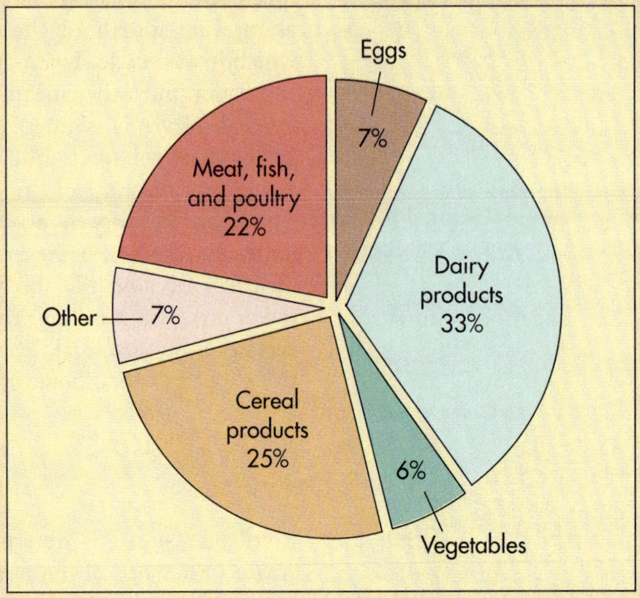

flavin deficiency at a crucial stage of fetal development has been shown to lead to congenital malformations such as cleft lip, cataracts, and skeletal deformities, but such a relationship has not been established in human pregnancy and humans and other animals certainly differ in their responses to riboflavin deficiency. For example, hair loss is seen in riboflavin-deficient animals but never in humans.

In one study of experimentally induced severe riboflavin deficiency in humans, six men consumed less than 0.07 mg of riboflavin per day for 39 to 56 days. The symptoms that developed included such personality changes as hypochondria, depression, and hysteria and reduced hand-grip strength. Clinically obvious riboflavin deficiency seldom occurs in isolation but tends to develop with deficiencies of other water-soluble vitamins.

NIACIN

Niacin, formerly known as *nicotinic acid* and occasionally as vitamin B_3, was originally obtained by the oxidation of nicotine in 1867. By 1912 it had been found in association with the antiberiberi substance in rice polishings and had been isolated in crystalline form. It took until 1937, however, for it to be recognized as the nutrient able to prevent or cure **pellagra** in humans and **blacktongue** in dogs. It has since been discovered that some derivatives of niacin have the same biological effects, so niacin is now used as a generic term that includes such derivatives, the principal one being **nicotinamide.**

DISCOVERY

The disease known as pellagra in Italy and "mal del sol" or "mal de la rosa" in Spain was first described in the eighteenth century. It occurred mainly among poor persons, who used corn (maize) produced in the New World as their dietary staple. The fact that pellagra occurred in people whose diets contained large amounts of highly refined maize led to the theory that it was caused by a mold or a toxic or infectious substance in spoiled corn. Later, a lack of nitrogen was implicated. It was also noted that corn diets were lacking in the essential amino acids lysine and tryptophan but were rich in another essential amino acid, leucine. This led to speculation that an amino acid imbalance was the cause. The skin symptoms of pellagra are aggravated by exposure to sunlight, which led to the belief that it resulted from "sun poisoning" (hence the Spanish name, "mal del sol"). Because the diets that caused pellagra were generally consumed by poor people living in crowded and unsanitary conditions, the idea that pellagra might be caused by an infectious agent or parasite received some support. The fact that several members of the same family often developed the disease led some people to suspect hereditary factors were involved. In 1917 a physician named Goldberger working for the United States Public Health Service demonstrated that pellagra was associated with the absence of a specific dietary factor.

Goldberger conducted a series of now-classic experiments on a group of male prisoners who were promised a reprieve in return for their cooperation. They were put on a diet typical of the areas in which pellagra was prevalent. After about 5 months the men began to develop the classic symptoms of pellagra: dermatitis, diarrhea, and depression. Other inmates eating the normal prison diet remained healthy. These results provided a strong argument against the idea that pellagra was an infectious condition and instead clearly implicated the lack of some unknown dietary factor. That factor, niacin, was not properly identified until 20 years later.

In 1918, the year after Goldberger's experiments, pellagra caused an estimated 10,000 deaths in the United States, out of a total of 110,000 reported cases. These cases were primarily confined to small cotton-mill towns in the southern states, where the diet was composed predominantly of corn. Because the factor that was lacking from these diets was unknown, the most effective means of preventing the disease was to encourage the increased consumption of meat and milk products.

The efforts to isolate the dietary factor that could prevent pellagra were complicated because many other dietary deficiencies produced similar skin conditions. However, in 1937 Elvehjem, at the University of Wisconsin, finally demonstrated that nicotinic acid (that is, niacin) could cure blacktongue in dogs. This led to the use of nicotinic acid to treat pellagra in humans, with dramatic results. The number of pellagra patients in southern hospitals and mental institutions soon dropped sharply. Several recent reports have suggested that niacin deficiency is still prevalent in some areas of the United States, usually in alcoholics or in people with an infection of the pancreas.

Pellagra is still found in countries where corn is a major staple, such as Romania, the former Yugoslavia, some parts of Egypt, and parts of India where sorghum is a major staple. The ability of diets containing a lot of sorghum to cause pellagra has been linked to the high proportion of the amino acid leucine in such diets. In people developing pellagra because of a sorghum-based diet, the addition of isoleucine to the diet can correct the condition. This suggests that the leucine-isoleucine balance of a diet can be an additional factor contributing to the onset of pellagra.

Pellagra is not found in Central America, despite the fact that corn provides 80% of kilocalories in this region. This is attributed to the use of alkalis (usually soda lime) in corn preparation, which liberate niacin that is bound to proteins and so make it available for absorption.

TRYPTOPHAN-NIACIN RELATIONSHIP

Some foods, such as milk, that are effective in curing or preventing pellagra actually have a rather low niacin content. Also, diets that are low in niacin do not always lead to pellagra. These discrepancies were explained in 1945, when it was discovered that the amino acid tryptophan could also cure pellagra. It has since been established that tryptophan is a chemical precursor of niacin and so can cure pellagra when converted into niacin within the body's cells.

Sixty milligrams of dietary tryptophan generally lead to the formation of 1 mg of niacin or one **niacin equivalent (NE).** Because protein is approximately 1% tryptophan, 60 g of protein (60,000 mg) provides about 600 mg of tryptophan, which can give rise to 10 mg of niacin. Thus 600 mg of tryptophan in excess of that needed for protein synthesis can be converted to 10 NE. These figures allow us to calculate the amount of niacin that can be produced by consuming specified amounts of protein or tryptophan. Interestingly, however, the conversion of tryptophan to niacin may be three times more efficient than normal during pregnancy.

The NE value of a food, found by adding its preformed niacin content (in milligrams) to the number of milligrams obtained from tryptophan, gives a more accurate indication of the food's value as a source of niacin than does the preformed niacin content alone. The food tables currently in use, however, list only the preformed niacin content of foods. Dietary requirements for niacin, on the other hand, are expressed in niacin equivalents, which include the contribution made by the tryptophan in food. This discrepancy means that a calculation of dietary niacin intake based on the values in food tables produces an underestimate of the amount of niacin actually available from the food. A result from such a calculation that is lower than the dietary requirement does not necessarily mean that the requirement cannot be met by the food consumed. Approximately two thirds of the niacin available to adults may be derived from dietary tryptophan.

> Tryptophan is a chemical precursor of niacin and so can cure pellagra by being converted into niacin within the body's cells.
> 60 mg tryptophan = 1 NE (niacin equivalent)
> 60 g of protein provides 600 mg of tryptophan

One complication of the tryptophan-niacin relationship is that the conversion of tryptophan into the body requires the presence of at least three other vitamins: thiamin, pyridoxine, and riboflavin. It is possible that biotin may also be required. This means that a deficiency

FIGURE 13-7

Chemical structure of niacin (as nicotinic acid and nicotinamide), the niacin precursor tryptophan, and the biologically active niacin coenzymes (NAD and NADP).

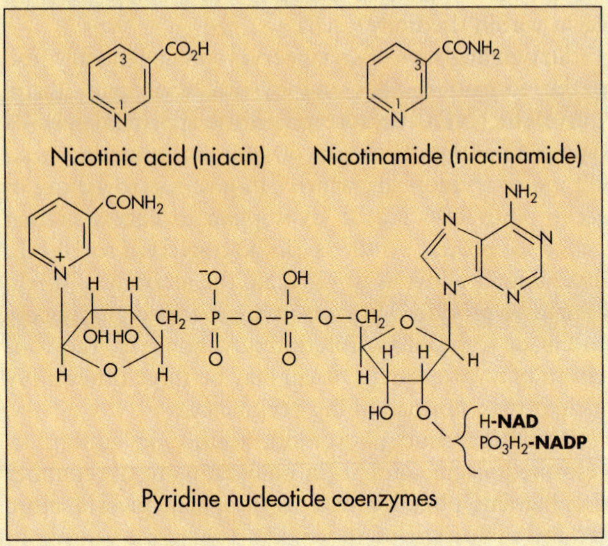

in any of these vitamins reduces the total amount of niacin available to the body from the diet, perhaps leading to symptoms of niacin deficiency, in addition to symptoms of the deficiency in the other vitamin concerned. This also explains why symptoms of pellagra can appear when the vitamin B_6 antagonist isonicotinic acid hydrazide (INH or isoniazid) is used in the treatment of tuberculosis.

CHEMICAL PROPERTIES

The chemical structure of niacin (as nicotinic acid or nicotinamide) is shown in Figure 13-7,[13] which also shows the structure of the biologically active niacin coenzyme (see the next section) and the niacin precursor tryptophan. Although both the acid and amide forms of niacin can be used by humans, the amide form is preferred for use in therapeutic doses of the vitamin. A large amount of the acid form can act as a vasodilator, widening the blood vessels and sometimes leading to flushed skin and uncomfortable tingling and burning sensations. Niacin is stable to heat, light, acid, alkali, and oxidation. This stability means that little niacin is lost during the processing or preparation of food.

FUNCTIONS

Niacin is required by all cells. Like thiamin and riboflavin, it plays a vital role in the release of energy from all the energy-yielding nutrients: carbohydrate, fat, protein, and alcohol. It is also required for the synthesis of protein, fat, and the five-carbon sugars (pentoses) needed for the formation of DNA and RNA. The biochemical role of niacin is to form part of the coenzymes **nicotinamide adenine dinucleotide (NAD)** and **nicotinamide adenine dinucleotide phosphate (NADP).** These coenzymes are required by many of the key pathways of metabolism, with NAD being primarily involved in catabolic reactions and NADP functioning mainly in anabolic reactions.

ABSORPTION AND METABOLISM

Niacin is readily absorbed from the stomach and small intestine. It is converted into the coenzymes NAD and NADP within cells, and limited stores of these coenzymes are held in the kidneys, liver, and brain. Any excess niacin is excreted in urine in the forms of methyl nicotinamide (accounting for 20% to 30% of total excretion) and methyl-carboxamido-pyridone (40% to 60% of total excretion). As niacin deficiency develops, the excretion of methyl-carboxamido-pyridone decreases more rapidly than that of methyl nicotinamide.

RECOMMENDED DIETARY ALLOWANCES

Because niacin is required for the release of energy from nutrients, the RDAs for niacin are based on kilocalorie intake. The minimal amount of niacin needed to prevent pellagra has been established at 4.4 NE/1000 kcal. A 50% margin of safety to take into account individual variations was added to derive RDAs based on 6.6 NE/100 kcal (Table 13-4). Regardless of their energy intake, adults are recommended to consume at least 13 NE/day.[14] Recommendations for British citizens are essentially the same,[5] whereas the Canadians have set their standard about 10% higher, based on 7.2 NE/1000 kcal.[4]

On the basis of the amount of niacin and tryptophan in human milk, the recommended intake for infants has been set at 8 NE/1000 kcal. No firm data are available on the niacin requirements of children and adolescents, but it is estimated that 6.6 mg/1000 kcal and a minimum of 8 NE/day should meet their needs.

Although tryptophan is converted into niacin more efficiently in pregnant women, an additional 2 NE/day is recommended for them. Human milk contains about 0.2 mg of preformed niacin and 16 mg of tryptophan per 100 ml (or 70 kcal). To cover this extra demand, lactating women are encouraged to consume an additional 5 NE/day. By consuming his or her mother's milk, a breast-fed infant receives about 3.5 NE/day, about two thirds of which is derived from tryptophan. Formula-fed infants almost always have a higher intake than this.

TABLE 13-4

Recommended dietary allowances (United States) and recommended nutrient intakes (Canada) for niacin

AGE (YEARS)	UNITED STATES (mg NE/DAY)	CANADA (mg NE/DAY)
CHILDREN		
1-3	9	8-9
4-6	12	13
7-10	13	14-16
MALES		
11-14	17	18-20
15-18	20	20-23
19-24	19	22
25-50	19	19
51+	15	14-16
FEMALES		
11-14	15	16
15-50	15	14-16
51+	13	14
Pregnant	17	16
Lactating	20	17

FIGURE 13-8

Contributions of various food groups to the preformed niacin content of the North American food supply.

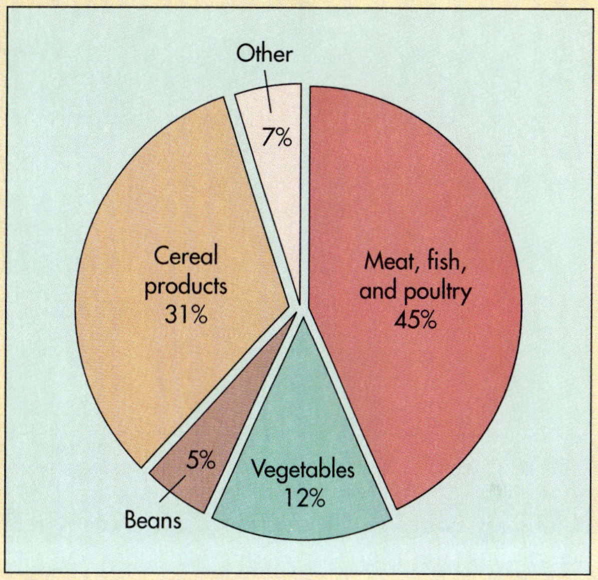

FOOD SOURCES

The amount of niacin in the most frequently used foods is shown in Table 13-2. Liver, meat, poultry, and legumes are the richest sources. Milk, eggs, and peanut butter, although low in preformed niacin, contain high amounts of tryptophan and so have a high NE value. Figure 13-8 shows the contributions of various food groups to the preformed niacin in the North American food supply. The major sources of preformed niacin in the diet of U.S. adults are bakery goods, meats, cereals, tea, coffee, and beer.[15]

Much of the niacin in cereals, such as rice and corn, occurs as niacinogen, a peptide containing at least 17 amino acids that binds niacin. The niacin in these foods has low biological value and provides little free niacin, unless the foods are prepared with alkali, which releases the bound niacin, as in the preparation of corn tortillas. In wheat bran, niacin occurs as the compound **niacytin,** which cannot usually be used by the body and is simply excreted in urine. As much as 90% of the niacin in cereals is in the outer husk, which is removed in the milling process. The addition of niacin to enriched cereal products has done much to compensate for this loss at low cost.

Most North American diets are adequate in protein and so supply sufficient niacin from the conversion of tryptophan in excess of growth and maintenance needs. Animal protein contains 1.4% tryptophan, and vegetable protein, 1%. This means that a diet with 60 g of protein provides at least 600 mg of tryptophan, which can yield 10 mg of niacin. Any tryptophan needed for the synthesis of protein, however, is not available for the formation of niacin.

In most North American diets, preformed niacin could meet the body's needs for the vitamin alone without any of the niacin produced from tryptophan. National dietary survey data collected by the USDA indicate that the average intake of preformed niacin exceeds the RDAs. Preformed niacin intakes below the RDAs were found, however, in approximately one third of those surveyed, who consumed less than 70% of their recommended kilocalorie intake. In such people the niacin provided by the conversion of tryptophan is vital. NHANES III (1988-1991) data showed preformed niacin intakes of 27 to 30 mg for men and 18 to 20 mg for women, intakes well in excess of the 6.6 mg/1000 kcal standard. These figures for preformed niacin intakes, combined with the high consumption of protein, suggest that the typical North American diet is a plentiful source of niacin overall.

EVALUATION OF NIACIN STATUS

Niacin status is evaluated by testing for excretory metabolites of niacin in urine after administration of a test dose of the vitamin. If niacin status is poor, less of the

FIGURE 13-9

Severe dermatosis of the legs in a patient suffering from pellagra.

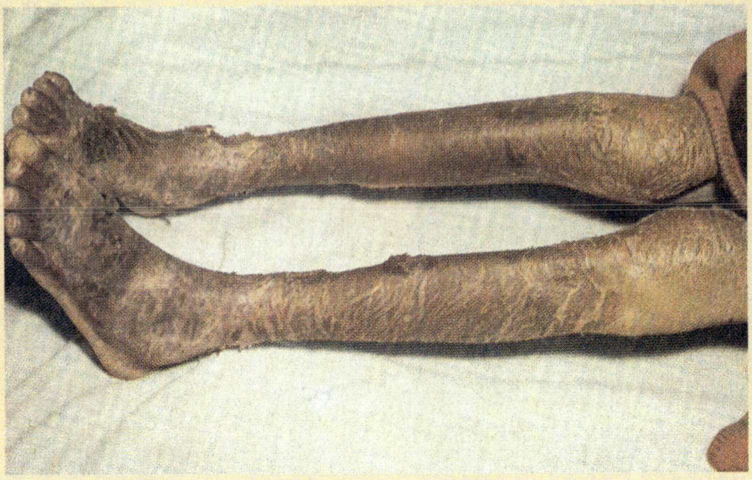

test dose is converted to excretory metabolites than when niacin status is good. Measurement of two urinary metabolites, methyl-carboxamido-pyridone and methyl nicotinamide, and their ratio have been used to measure niacin status. Urinary excretion of less than 0.8 mg/day of methyl nicotinamide is indicative of niacin deficiency. A ratio of less than 1 suggests latent niacin deficiency. Clinical symptoms, however, do not appear until the pyridone has been absent from the urine for several weeks.

DEFICIENCY

Niacin deficiency affects the skin, gastrointestinal tract, and central nervous system. The main symptoms of pellagra, sometimes called the "four Ds of pellagra," are dermatitis, diarrhea, depression, and eventually death. The dermatitis of pellagra is often complicated by symptoms of other B-vitamin deficiencies. When a niacin deficiency occurs, however, there is a characteristic skin inflammation almost exclusively on areas of the body exposed to sunlight and in a symmetrical pattern on both sides of the body (Figure 13-9). There is also a clear transition point between the affected and unaffected areas of the skin.

The main symptoms of pellagra—sometimes called the "four Ds of pellagra"—are dermatitis, diarrhea, depression, and eventually death.

As the mucous linings of the gastrointestinal tract become affected by niacin deficiency, the patient begins to suffer from diarrhea and other signs of infection. The irritability, headaches, and sleeplessness of the early stages are soon followed by more severe mental symptoms, such as loss of memory, hallucinations, delusions of persecution, and finally a severe depression that is almost inevitably followed by death.

MEGAVITAMIN THERAPY

Large pharmacological doses of niacin have been used in attempts to reduce high blood cholesterol levels and to treat schizophrenia. Under strict medical supervision, doses of 1.5 to 3 g of niacin (as nicotinic acid) three times a day may reduce total and low-density lipoprotein cholesterol levels and increase high-density lipoprotein cholesterol levels in plasma. This may be beneficial in protecting against recurrent nonfatal heart attacks.

Niacin is just one of several vitamins that have been used in extremely large amounts to try to treat psychiatric problems. This strategy is sometimes known as **orthomolecular therapy.** Using up to 4 to 5 g of niacin per day to treat schizophrenia has proved controversial. At the moment there is little scientific evidence to support its effectiveness.[16]

The use of nicotinic acid in oral doses of 50 mg or more leads to severe flushing of the skin within from a few minutes to half an hour. These symptoms persist for up to 1½ hours. Some people find them merely inconvenient, whereas they make others stop taking the nicotinic acid. Other reported symptoms of high doses of nicotinic acid include gastrointestinal distress, unusual nervousness, recurring ulcers, increased uric acid excre-

FIGURE 13-10

Chemical structure of pantothenic acid and coenzyme A.

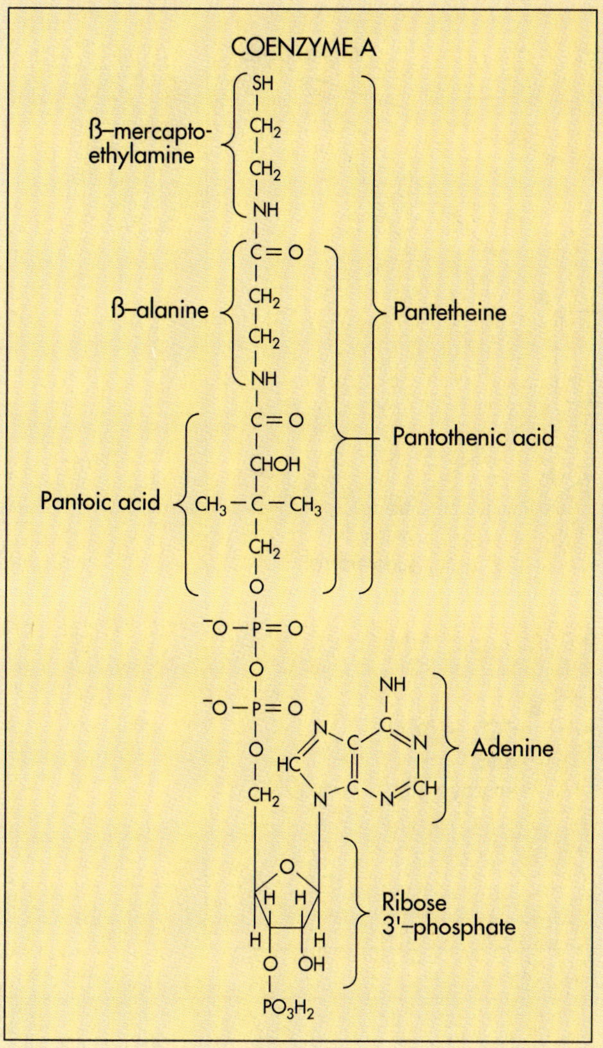

tion, and glucose intolerance. Intakes of as much as 3 to 9 g of the nicotinamide form of niacin produces no flushing of the skin but may produce other symptoms, since animal data show that nicotinamide is much more toxic than nicotinic acid.

PANTOTHENIC ACID

Pantothenic acid gets its name from its presence in a wide variety of foods ("pantos" means "everywhere"). When first identified, it was called vitamin B_5 and was known to be a growth factor in yeast and to be able to cure or prevent dermatitis in chicks and the graying of hair in rats. Pantothenic acid was isolated in 1938, and its chemical structure was identified in 1940.

CHEMICAL PROPERTIES

The chemical structure of pantothenic acid is shown in Figure 13-10, which also shows the structure of coenzyme A, which incorporates pantothenic acid within its structure.

Pantothenic acid is soluble in water and stable in moist heat and in neutral solutions, but it is relatively unstable in dry heat, acid, and alkali. There is little loss of pantothenic acid during cooking at normal temperatures. Pure pantothenic acid is a yellow oil that has never been crystallized. A synthetic derivative, **calcium pantothenate,** is available in crystalline form and is the form of pantothenic acid used in most nutritional supplements. The small amount of calcium in calcium pantothenate makes no significant contribution to calcium intake.

The alcohol derivative of pantothenic acid, **panthenol,** is used in cosmetics. Most of the pantothenic acid within tissues is found incorporated within the structure of coenzyme A (CoA).

FUNCTIONS

Most of the known biological functions of pantothenic acid are due to its role as one of the precursors of CoA, although pantothenic acid is also found combined within the structure of **acyl carrier protein,** a protein involved in the metabolism of fatty acids. CoA acts as a carrier of **acetyl** groups. It can be involved in the removal of acetyl groups, forming **acetyl-CoA,** which can then donate its acetyl group to another compound. Such reactions are involved in the metabolism of carbohydrate, fat, and protein and in the synthesis of many hormones, neurotransmitters, and other essential compounds of the body. Some of these key "acetylation" reactions are summarized in Figure 13-11. It is of particular relevance to nutrition to note that acetyl-CoA, and therefore pantothenic acid, is required for the following:

- The release of energy from carbohydrate, fat, and protein
- The synthesis of fat
- The formation of the heme group of hemoglobin
- The synthesis of cholesterol and other steroid hormones
- The synthesis of acetylcholine, required for the transmission of nerve impulses in many parts of the nervous system

Because acetyl-CoA is vital to all aspects of energy-yielding metabolism, as well as performing many other vital roles, it is fortunate that pantothenic acid is present

FIGURE 13-11

Acetylation reactions for which acetyl coenzyme A (CoA), and therefore pantothenic acid, is required.

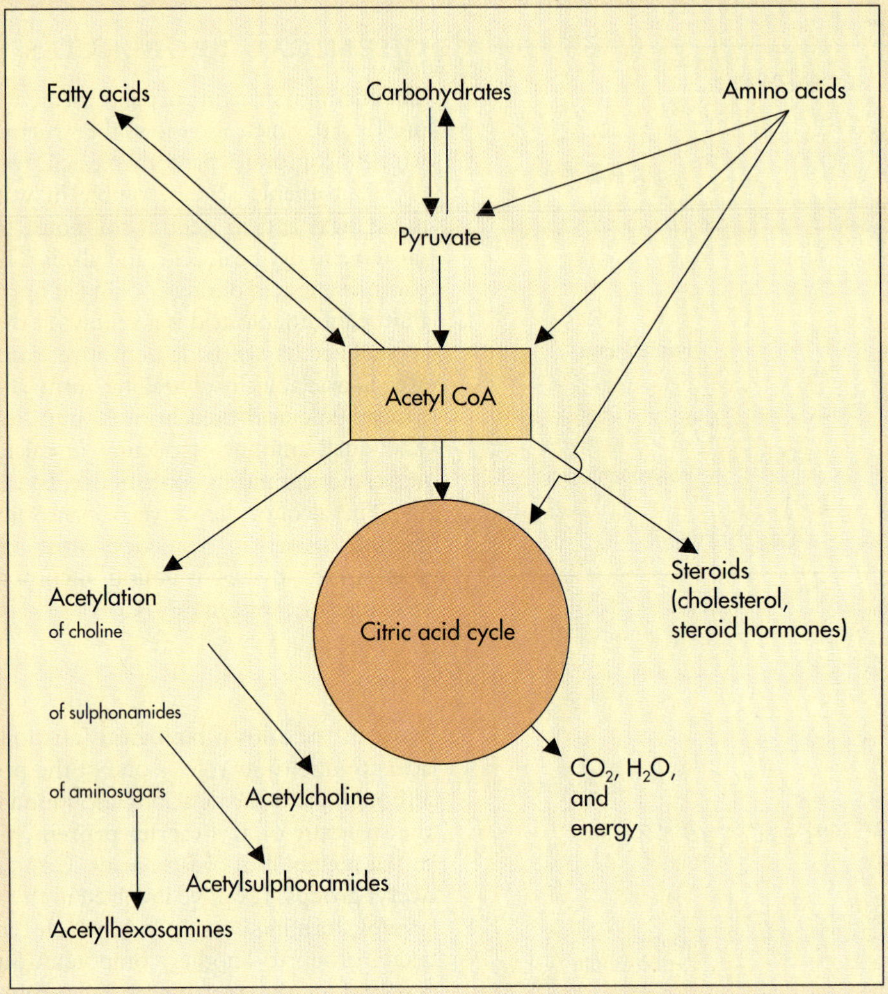

in almost all foods. Any excess free pantothenic acid can be excreted in urine.[17]

RECOMMENDED DIETARY ALLOWANCES

The precise amount of pantothenic acid needed by humans is not yet known. A 3000-kcal diet usually provides from 10 to 20 mg of pantothenic acid, of which 3 to 9 mg is excreted (2 to 7 mg in urine and 1 to 2 mg in feces), suggesting that 7 to 11 mg is retained. The wide variation in intakes, blood values, and urinary excretion levels found in people showing no evidence of deficiency makes it difficult to determine the minimal requirements. The estimated safe and adequate daily dietary intakes of pantothenic acid are shown in Table 13-5. Because pantothenic acid is so widely available, most diets provide adequate amounts, even when the body's need is high.

FOOD SOURCES

Pantothenic acid is present in significant amounts in almost all foods because it is present in all animal and plant cells. Although all food groups contribute some pantothenic acid to the diet (Table 13-6), excellent sources are avocados, broccoli, bran, organ meats, and whole grain cereals. The richest sources found so far are royal jelly (from queen bees) and fish ovaries just before spawning, which are rare and nonessential items in the everyday diet but are heavily promoted in health food stores. Human milk contains an average of 2.6 mg of pantothenic acid per liter, whereas cow's milk contains 3.2 mg/L.

TABLE 13-5

Estimated safe and adequate daily dietary intakes of pantothenic acid

POPULATION	AMOUNT (mg/DAY)
Infants	2-3
Children and adolescents	3-7
Adults	4-7

TABLE 13-6

Pantothenic acid content of foods

FOOD	mg/SERVING	AMOUNT (mg/100 g EDIBLE PORTION)
Avocados, raw	1.0	1.0
Beef, raw	0.6	0.6
Brains	2.6	2.6
Broccoli, raw	1.1	1.1
Cashew nuts	0.4	1.3
Egg yolk	0.6	4.4
Eggs, whole	1.0	1.6
Heart, raw	2.5	2.5
Kidneys, raw	2.5	3.8
Lentils, dry	0.4	1.3
Liver, raw	2.5	7.7
Milk, dry	1.3	3.6
Peanuts, raw	0.4	2.8
Rice, brown	0.4	1.1
Soybeans, raw	0.5	1.7
Tongue, raw	2.0	2.0
Bran, 100%	1.0	2.9
Yeast, baker's	0.3	11.0

From Fox H: Pantothenic acid. In Machlin LJ, editor: *Handbook of vitamins,* ed 2, New York, 1991, Marcel Dekker.

Foods subjected to dry heat during processing are relatively poor sources of pantothenic acid. In canning, up to one third of the pantothenic acid is lost from animal foods and three fourths from vegetable foods. About 50% of the pantothenic acid in wheat is lost when it is refined.

DEFICIENCY

Pantothenic acid deficiency causes a variety of biochemical disturbances in different tissues, presumably reflecting the wide range of biochemical processes for which this vitamin is required. Humans fed a diet deficient in pantothenic acid for 9 weeks became listless and complained of fatigue. Lowered resistance to infection is another well-documented symptom. Pantothenic acid deficiency was also reported to be the cause of "burning feet syndrome" among prisoners in Japan and the Philippines during World War II.[18] Increasing the pantothenic acid intake of people with a deficiency seems to improve their ability to withstand stress.

CLINICAL USES

Pantothenic acid has been used successfully to treat paralysis of the gastrointestinal tract after surgery, which causes the accumulation of gas and extreme pain. The vitamin appears to stimulate gastrointestinal motility, although large quantities (from 10 to 20 g) cause diarrhea. Although pantothenic acid has been promoted as able to prevent or reverse the graying of hair, there is no evidence to support such claims.

BIOTIN

Biotin was recognized as a dietary essential in 1924, when it was identified as "bios II," one of three factors necessary for the growth of microorganisms. As scientists tried to learn more about bios II and two other substances they had named "vitamin H" and "coenzyme R," it became clear that all three were the same sulfur-containing, water-soluble vitamin. It was given the unified name of *biotin* and was synthesized in 1943.

FIGURE 13-12

The chemical structure of biotin and biocytin.

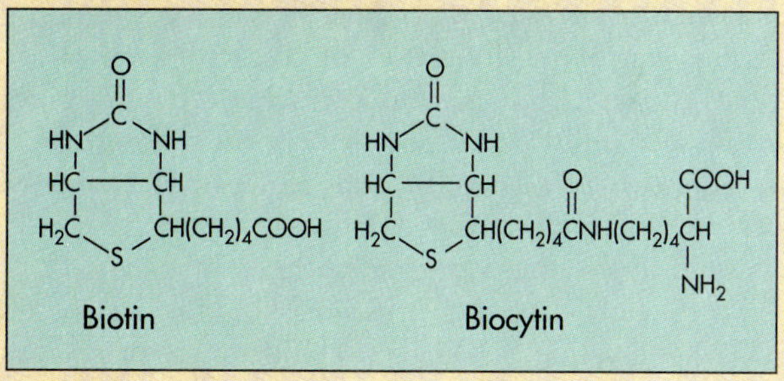

CHEMICAL PROPERTIES

The chemical structure of biotin is shown in Figure 13-12,[19] which also shows the structure of **biocytin,** a biologically active derivative of biotin in which biotin is chemically combined with the amino acid lysine. When biotin is performing its biological functions, it is bound to peptides and proteins via an amide bond to the amino group on the side chain of the amino acid lysine. When biotin-containing peptides and proteins within food are digested, biocytin is released into the gastrointestinal tract.

Both biotin and biocytin are relatively stable to exposure to air, daylight, or heat. They are slowly destroyed on exposure to ultraviolet light.[20]

FUNCTIONS

At least four enzymes in the human body require a bound biotin molecule to assist in their acts of catalysis. The main activity of these enzymes is to function as **carboxylases,** which transfer carbon dioxide groups between compounds. Carboxylation reactions occur throughout metabolism, and so biotin is involved in a variety of metabolic pathways, including the synthesis and oxidation of fatty acids and the oxidation of carbohydrates. Biotin is also required for the metabolism of at least five amino acids (valine, leucine, isoleucine, methionine, and threonine); the synthesis of nicotinic acid, purines, and prostaglandins; the activity of the digestive enzyme pancreatic amylase; and the normal functioning of the cells of the immune system.[20]

RECOMMENDED DIETARY ALLOWANCES

The Food and Nutrition Board made its first recommendations on dietary biotin intake for Americans in 1980 (Table 13-7). These were based on studies of usual biotin intakes and fecal and urinary excretions of biotin. It is unclear what proportion of dietary biotin is absorbed, and some evidence indicates that the synthesis of biotin in the intestine can supplement the amount available from the diet. There are wide variations in reported biotin levels in whole blood, plasma, and urine largely because of difficulties with the methods of analysis.[21]

Fortunately, there is no evidence of biotin deficiency in the U.S. population, whose diet is estimated to provide an average of 20 to 30 μg of biotin per day. The Food and Nutrition Board recommends 30 to 100 μg/day for adults, 20 to 100 μg/day for children, and 10 to 15 μg/day for infants. Infants consuming human milk (with 5 μg of biotin per liter) or infant formula (30 μg/L) have shown no signs of biotin deficiency. Intakes of as low as 2 to 4 μg/day, considerably less than the RDA, are apparently sufficient to meet the needs of young infants.[22]

TABLE 13-7

Estimated safe and adequate daily dietary intakes of biotin

POPULATION	AMOUNT (μg/DAY)
Infants	10-15
Children	20-100
Adolescents and adults	30-100

TABLE 13-8

Biotin content of foods

FOOD	AMOUNT (μg/100 g)
Cereals, legumes, and nuts	10-40
Eggs	20-25
Liver (beef, chicken, pork)	100-210
Oatmeal	15-30
Peanut butter	38
Poultry	10-11
Vegetables	2-4
Wheat germ	22-38

FOOD SOURCES

Biotin is present in almost all foods, mostly bound to protein, from which it is readily released. The richest food sources of biotin are liver, kidney, peanut butter, egg yolk, and yeast. Some vegetables such as cauliflower, nuts, and legumes are good sources, but all other meats, fruits, dairy products, and cereals are considered to be poor sources. Typical values for the biotin content of selected foods are shown in Table 13-8. Most of the best sources of biotin are the foods that are often eliminated from low-cholesterol diets, leading to concern that following such diets may significantly reduce biotin intake.[23]

Dietary biotin is supplemented by the synthesis of biotin by bacteria in the gastrointestinal tract, a process that is stimulated by dietary sucrose. Antibiotics, including sulfonamides and tetracyclines, are known to reduce the numbers of the biotin-producing bacteria.

Because there is no evidence of biotin deficiency in people eating a typical North American diet, there is no reason to include biotin in multivitamin supplements. Large doses of biotin have been promoted by their suppliers for the relief of stress and to enhance physical performance. There is no evidence to support these claims.

DEFICIENCY

Symptoms of biotin deficiency can result from prolonged dependence on total parenteral nutrition (TPN), the consumption of a diet that is low in biotin and includes many raw egg whites, or an inherited deficiency in biotinidase or carboxylase enzymes. Biotin deficiency in infants (Figure 13-13) and adults receiving TPN is readily corrected by the addition of biotin to the TPN mixture.

Egg whites contain a glycoprotein called **avidin,** which binds to biotin and retains it within a complex

FIGURE 13-13

***An infant with biotin deficiency before treatment,* (A), *and 15 days after treatment was started,* (B).**

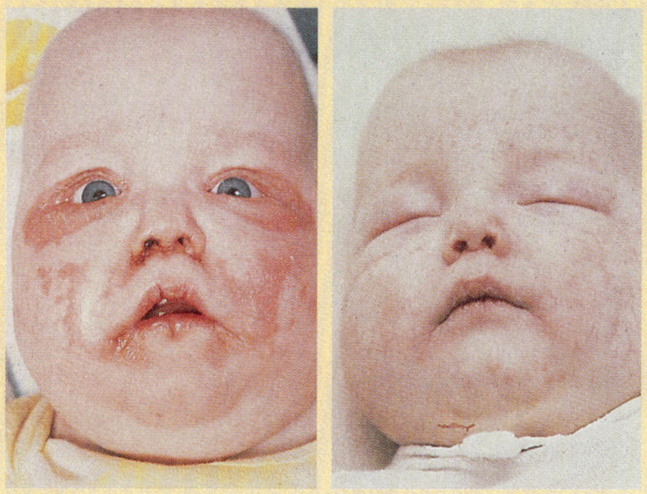

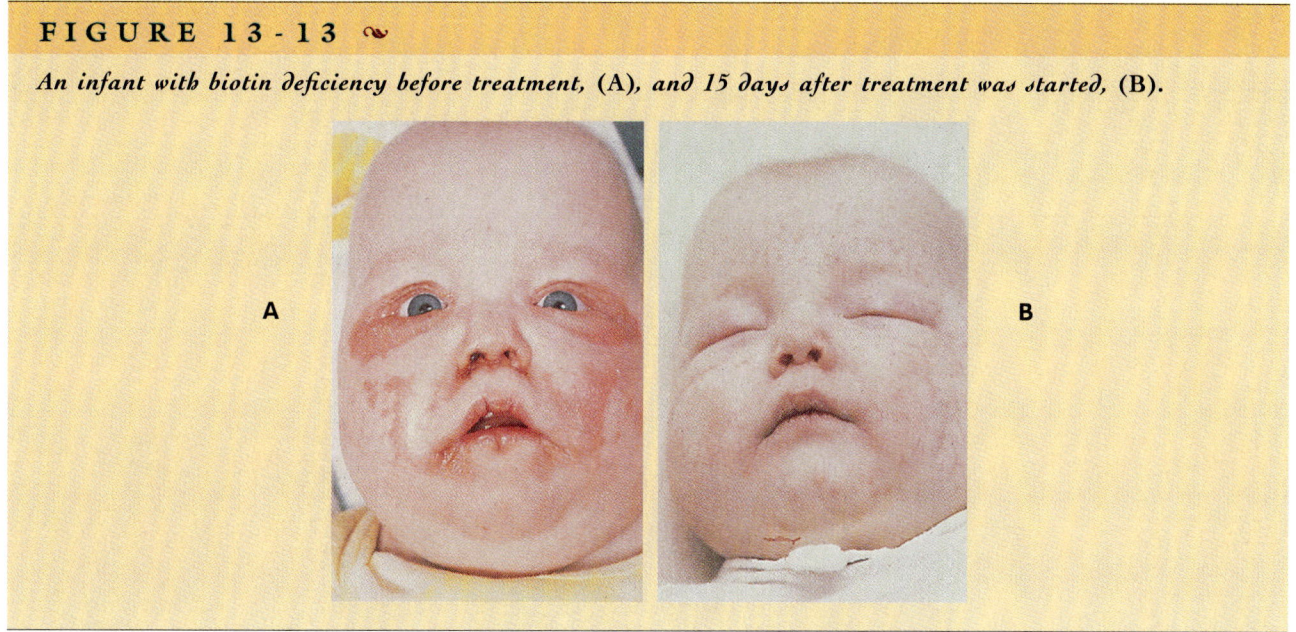

that is too big to be absorbed and is unaffected by digestive enzymes. Avidin is denatured by cooking, however, so cooked egg whites pose no threat to biotin status. For avidin to induce biotin deficiency, 30% of dietary energy must be supplied by raw egg whites, requiring the consumption of about 12 such egg whites per day. This is an unusual diet, and the consumption of the occasional raw egg white is clearly no threat to biotin status.

Inherited biotinidase deficiency and multiple carboxylase deficiency syndrome are life-threatening conditions in which the body fails to absorb biotin and manufacture completely functional carboxylase enzymes, respectively. They both can be successfully treated, however, by the administration of large amounts of biotin (10 mg/day).

Natural biotin deficiency in human adults on a normal diet is unknown, but the symptoms have been studied experimentally. In one study, four adults developed biotin deficiency on a diet that was both low in biotin and high in avidin. Their symptoms included a scaly, red skin rash; hair loss; loss of appetite; depression; and glossitis.[23]

VITAMIN-LIKE SUBSTANCES AND OTHER CLAIMED NUTRIENTS

The considerable and growing interest in nutrition among all segments of the population has been accompanied by many claims that other substances, in addition to the acknowledged vitamins, have vitamin-like effects. This has resulted in considerable confusion about whether certain components of food are essential, helpful, unnecessary but harmless, or harmful. The substances discussed in this section are among the many supposed vitamin-like substances or other supposed nutrients whose public profiles rise and fall with passing trends. Some of them share some characteristics with vitamins but do not meet all the criteria required for them to be classed as vitamins. Some are present in typical diets in larger amounts than are the true vitamins. Some can be synthesized by the body in amounts that meet the needs of most people. Some of them have not been linked to any definite biological role, even though they appear in both food and the tissues of the body. In the future, some of the vitamin-like substances may be established definitely as vitamins, whereas others will definitely be shown to have no true vitamin or vitamin-like effects.

MYOINOSITOL

Myoinositol—also known as muscle sugar, inositol, and mesoinositol—is a six-carbon compound chemically related to glucose. In 1928 it was recognized as a growth-promoting factor for yeast and as a cure for alopecia (hair loss) in mice.

Myoinositol is present in practically all animal and plant tissues in concentrations higher than those normally associated with vitamins. In animal cells it is found largely incorporated into the structure of a phospholipid. In grains it is present as part of the water-soluble compound phytic acid (inositol hexaphosphate), the organic acid of grain husks that binds calcium, zinc, and iron and so decreases their absorption.

A mixed American diet provides about 1 g of myoinositol per day.[24] Fruits, meat, milk, nuts, veg-

TABLE 13-9

Choline content of some common foods

	CHOLINE CONCENTRATION (mg/100 g)*		
FOOD	CHOLINE	PHOSPHATIDYLCHOLINE	SPHINGOMYELIN
Apple	0.3	2.9	0.2
Banana	2.5	0.4	0.2
Beef liver	61	453	19
Beef steak	0.8	63	5.3
Butter	0.4	18	4.8
Cauliflower	14	29	1.9
Corn oil	0.03	0.1	0.05
Coffee	10	0.2	0.2
Cucumber	2.3	0.8	0.3
Egg	0.4	542	23
Ginger ale	0.02	0.04	0.03
Grape juice	4.9	0.2	0.05
Iceburg lettuce	30	1.4	0.5
Margarine	0.3	4.7	0.2
Milk (bovine, whole)	1.6	1.5	0.8
Orange	2.1	5.1	0.2
Peanut butter	41	41	0.1
Peanuts	47	52	0.8
Potato	5.3	3.1	0.3
Tomato	4.5	0.5	0.3
Whole wheat bread	10	3.5	0.1

* Dietary choline is provided by free choline plus that in phosphatidylcholine (lecithin) and in sphingomyelin.

From Zeisel SH: Choline. In Shils ME, Olson JA, Shike M, editors: *Modern nutrition in health and disease,* ed 8, Philadelphia, 1994, Lea & Febiger.

etables, and whole grain cereals are the best food sources of myoinositol. Our kidneys are estimated to synthesize about 4 g of myoinositol per day, considerably more than is ingested from typical diets. Small and variable amounts are excreted in urine, ranging between 8 and 144 mg/day.

The biological significance of myoinositol in human nutrition is unknown, although it is widely distributed in the body, especially in heart, brain, liver, kidney, and skeletal muscle. Inositol phospholipids form an integral part of cellular and intracellular membranes, and myoinositol appears to regulate some aspects of membrane-related metabolism. In some species of animal, myoinositol has been found essential for prevention of fatty livers.

CHOLINE

Choline was identified in 1937 as a dietary factor that prevents the accumulation of fat in the liver of dogs. Since then we have learned that choline can act as a methyl group (CH_3) donor in a wide variety of biological reactions. Choline can be synthesized in the body from the nonessential amino acid serine, provided that another suitable source of methyl groups is available, together with vitamin B_6 to help catalyze the reaction. The required methyl groups are provided by the amino acid methionine. So, in most circumstances, humans are not solely dependent on a dietary source of either choline or its direct precursor.

Choline is required for the synthesis of the choline-containing phospholipids (phosphatidylcholine, lysophosphatidylcholine, choline plasmogen, and sphingomyelin), which are essential components of all membranes.[25] Choline is also a component of the neurotransmitter acetylcholine.

Choline is not considered to be an essential nutrient because it can be synthesized in the body, and no choline deficiency syndrome has been recognized. In a recent study, however, healthy adult males were fed a liquid diet devoid of choline but otherwise nutritionally adequate. These subjects showed evidence of liver damage, together with decreased plasma choline and erythrocyte membrane phosphatidylcholine levels. This study suggests that choline may be a dietary essential.

Choline is found in a wide variety of foods (Table 13-9) and is present in relatively large amounts in all foods that contain fat. The major food sources of choline are eggs, liver, nuts, beans, oatmeal, and fish. The average North American diet provides 600 to 1000 mg of choline per day.[26] Infants and children probably have the greatest need for dietary choline per kilogram of body weight because of the large amounts that must be incorporated into cellular membranes during growth.

Although choline deficiency has not been associated with any specific disease in humans, choline has been found to offer some protection against cirrhosis of the liver in alcoholics. It is also being used to stimulate the synthesis within the body of the neurotransmitter acetylcholine. Reports of its ability to reduce blood pressure and blood cholesterol levels have not been verified. It appears safe to consume up to 5 g of choline or 15 g of lecithin (phosphatidylcholine) per day.

Lecithin is the trivial name for phosphatidylcholine. It occurs in eggs and is used as an emulsifying agent in many processed foods.

TABLE 13-10

Carnitine content of selected foods

FOOD	AMOUNT (mg/100 g)
DAIRY PRODUCTS	
Whole milk	3.3
Butter	0.5
American cheese	3.7
Cottage cheese	1.1
Ice cream	3.7
MEAT PRODUCTS	
Beef steak	95 ± 42
Ground beef	94 ± 5.1
Chicken breast	3.9 ± 1.3
Cod fish	5.6 ± 1.9
Pork	28 ± 5.1
Bacon	23 ± 3.9

COENZYME Q (UBIQUINONE)

Coenzyme Q is a generic name for a range of lipidlike substances that are somewhat similar in chemical composition to both vitamin K and vitamin E. They are all members of the group of compounds known as **ubiquinones,** and the biologically important forms of coenzyme Q appear to have long hydrocarbon side chains containing from 30 to 50 carbon atoms.

Coenzyme Q is found in practically all cells and appears to be synthesized and concentrated in mitochondria. Within mitochondria it plays a role in the respiratory chain, in which the energy released from nutrients is trapped within adenosine triphosphate (ATP).

Coenzyme Q is probably synthesized readily by cells, with niacin, folate, vitamin B_{12}, pyridoxine, and pantothenic acid all being involved in its synthesis. Coenzyme Q–type ubiquinones are found in soybeans, vegetable oils, and a wide variety of animal tissues.

LIPOIC ACID

Lipoic acid has been isolated from liver and yeast and is essential for the growth of several microorganisms. It has not yet been shown to be a dietary essential for humans or other mammals. It does participate in certain biochemical reactions, but the amounts required are probably readily synthesized by the body. The reactions requiring lipoic acid include the steps in carbohydrate metabolism that convert pyruvic acid to acetyl-CoA (for which thiamin is also required).

Six other names for lipoic acid are in use. A protein-bound form is known as **factor 11,** whereas the other names are **factor 11A,** the **pyruvic oxidation factor, thioctic acid, thiocytin,** and **protogen.** The most commonly used names at present are lipoic acid (the official name) and thiocytin (which indicates that the molecule contains sulfur—"thio"). Lipoic acid is readily oxidized from its native fat-soluble form to the water-soluble form of β-lipoic acid.

CARNITINE

Carnitine is an essential substance in the body that is required for the transport of long-chain fatty acids into the mitochondria of cells, where they are oxidized to provide energy. If carnitine is not present, triglycerides accumulate in the blood. Carnitine's role in the metabolism of fatty acids makes it vital for the development and survival of young infants, particularly premature infants.[27] Carnitine is considered to be a dietary essential for infants but is provided in adequate amounts in human milk and cow's milk–based infant formulas. In the United States carnitine is also added to milk-free infant formulas.

Carnitine is normally synthesized in the liver and kidneys from the essential amino acids lysine and methionine via reactions that require the presence of iron. Some people are unable to synthesize their own carnitine, leading to several reports of carnitine deficiency, which was first recognized in 1973.

The major sources of carnitine in the North American diet are meat (especially dark red meat) and dairy products. A typical nonvegetarian diet provides about 100 to 300 mg of carnitine per day. Vegetarians have low intakes of carnitine because of the exceedingly low levels of the compound in vegetables, fruits, and grains. The carnitine content of some foods is listed in Table 13-10.

The natural form of carnitine is the L-form, but for

a time carnitine supplements contained both D- and L-forms. When it was found that these supplements are not only unnecessary, but also cause changes in skeletal and heart muscle, the Food and Drug Administration (FDA) ruled that D-carnitine (which is the cheaper form) cannot be used in supplements. Supplemental carnitine should be used only with strict medical supervision.

TAURINE

Taurine, or β-amino sulfonic acid, is a sulfur-containing amino acid but has a different chemical structure from that of the familiar amino acids that become incorporated into proteins.[28] Its acidic group is centered on a sulfur atom, rather than a carbon atom. Taurine never becomes part of a peptide or protein chain.

Taurine is derived from the amino acid cysteine, and it accounts for 10% of the sulfur in the body. It is found in a wide variety of tissues and at particularly high concentrations in heart, brain, and muscle. Taurine plays an important role in regulating the activity of the nervous system, most notably in the retina of the eye, and is the most abundant amino acid in the nervous system.

Taurine is involved in the absorption of fat. The infant body is able to form conjugates between bile salts and both taurine and glycine, which aid in fat absorption. The taurine conjugate is the main conjugate formed when abundant taurine is available, as it is when infants are being fed human milk or taurine-supplemented formula. In the United States taurine is added to commercially prepared infant formulas.[29] The taurine-conjugated bile salts are more soluble in water than those conjugated with glycine. Adding supplementary taurine to the diet of small, preterm infants increases the efficiency with which they absorb fat.

Results from animal studies suggest that taurine deficiency leads to growth retardation, impaired functioning of the nervous system, and impaired conjugation of bile acids. Human milk contains a relatively high amount of taurine, suggesting that taurine may be important in development, especially the development of the nervous system.

Taurine is found in large amounts in meat and fish but is almost absent from fruit, vegetables, and grains. Vegetarians maintain normal plasma concentrations of taurine and show no abnormalities that could be linked with low taurine intakes. Because they must consume little taurine, this suggests that adults probably do not require a dietary supply of taurine.[30] Table 13-11 lists the taurine content of selected foods.

TABLE 13-11

Taurine content of selected foods

DIETARY SOURCE	AMOUNT (mg/100 g)*
MEAT	
Beef (lean round)	36
Beef (liver)	19
Pork (loin)	50
Pork (liver)	17
Lamb (leg)	47
Chicken (leg)	34
SEAFOOD	
Cod (frozen)	31
Clams (fresh)	240
Clams (minced, canned)	152
Oysters (fresh)	70
Tuna fish (canned)	70

	AMOUNT (mg/L)
COW'S MILK	
Colostrum (1-3 days)	70
Early lactation (15-40 days)	12
Mid-lactation (over 100 days)	4
Pasteurized milk	6
HUMAN MILK	54

* 1 mg taurine equals 8 μmol.

From Roe DA, Weston, MO: *Nature* 205:287, 1965, and Erbersdobler HF, Braasch S, Trautwein EA: *J Anim Physiol Anim Nutr* 63:1, 1990.

PYRROLOQUINOLINE QUINONE

Pyrroloquinoline quinone (PQQ) has recently been identified as a potent growth factor and antioxidant in experimental studies on animals.[31] Also, animals deprived of PQQ either fail to reproduce or show low rates of reproduction. Other signs of PQQ deprivation are abnormalities of the skin, impaired immune response, and impaired maturation of connective tissue.

PQQ may be synthesized in humans from the amino acids glutamic acid and tyrosine. It is present in both human and cow's milk. In animal studies, the greatest dietary need for PQQ has been in the newborn. PQQ, taurine, and carnitine may all be "conditionally essential" nutrients, meaning that they are dietary essentials only in specific circumstances, such as during infant development.

Pyrroloquinoline quinone (PQQ), taurine, and carnitine may be **conditionally essential** nutrients, required in the diet only in specific circumstances, such as during infant development.

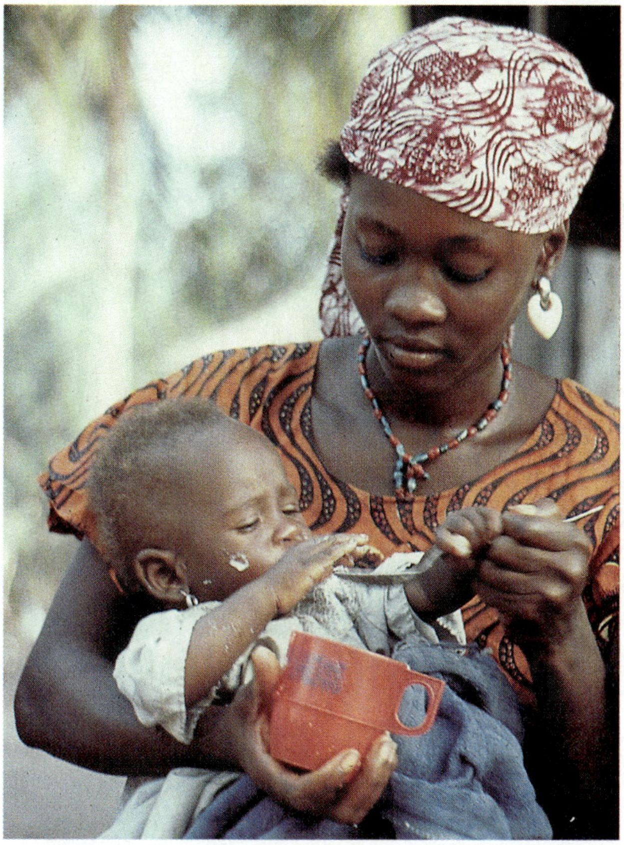

Carnitine, taurine, and PQQ are essential to infant development.

OTHER SUBSTANCES CLAIMED TO BE NUTRIENTS

Many other dietary factors have been reported to have beneficial effects on health, often by the people who are trying to sell them to confused members of the public looking for a simple panacea for their health problems. We will consider a few for which the most vociferous and persistent claims have been made. In general, however, it is best to be very skeptical about nutritional claims advertised to the public by people selling the products concerned, rather than presented in the scientific literature.

> It is advisable to be skeptical about nutritional claims advertised to the public by people selling the products concerned, rather than presented in the scientific literature.

Bioflavonoids

The bioflavonoids hesperidin and rutin were first suggested as beneficial dietary factors in 1936, when extracts of red pepper and lemons containing them were found to increase the antiscurvy effect of vitamin C. The bioflavonoids were also believed to reduce capillary bleeding and for a while were designated as "vitamin P." It is now known that they do not enhance the use of synthetic vitamin C, and no clinical uses of the bioflavonoids are known, although in large doses they may have some pharmacological effects. There is no justification for their addition to nutritional supplements, although several bioflavonoids are being investigated as possible low-calorie sweeteners.

Laetrile

Laetrile, also known as vitamin B_{17}, is a cyanide-containing, potentially toxic substance. It belongs to the amygdalin group of chemicals and is derived from the pits of apricots, peaches, and bitter almonds and from apple seeds. It has been widely promoted as a substance that can prevent and cure cancer, but there is no evidence to support these claims. The FDA has prohibited the promotion of laetrile as an anticancer agent. In response to this ban, promoters of laetrile have marketed it under such names as "bitter food tablets" and "Seventeen," without making any specific claims of beneficial effects. The sale of laetrile is currently legal in only 16 states in America.

Some of those who support the claims made for laetrile say that it seeks out cancer cells and releases hydrocyanic acid, which kills the cells. Alternatively, some say that cancer is caused by a deficiency of laetrile. At present there is no scientific evidence to suggest that laetrile is a vitamin or an anticancer agent or plays any positive role in metabolism.

Pangamic Acid

Pangamic acid was introduced to the public as "vitamin B_{15}" in 1978. Its promoters claim that it helps alleviate such diverse problems as indigestion, alcoholism, hepatitis, heart disease, and schizophrenia. Although pangamic acid was patented in 1949, there is no scientific evidence to suggest that it has any physiological function or that lack of it causes any adverse effects. It is marketed in the United States under many different names and in a great variety of forms. Although the majority of products that contain pangamic acid also contain calcium gluconate and a derivative of the amino acid glycine, the FDA has ruled that these are unidentifiable substances. The Canadian government has banned the sale of pangamic acid because there is no proof that it has any therapeutic effects. In the absence of anything but anecdotal evidence in support of its supposed benefits, pangamic acid should be regarded as a nutritionally worthless substance that is misleadingly labeled as a vitamin.

Spirulina

In 1981 a new entry into the field of "miracle nutrients" was spirulina. It is derived from microorganisms and is

FIGURE 13-14

Caffeine content of various beverages.

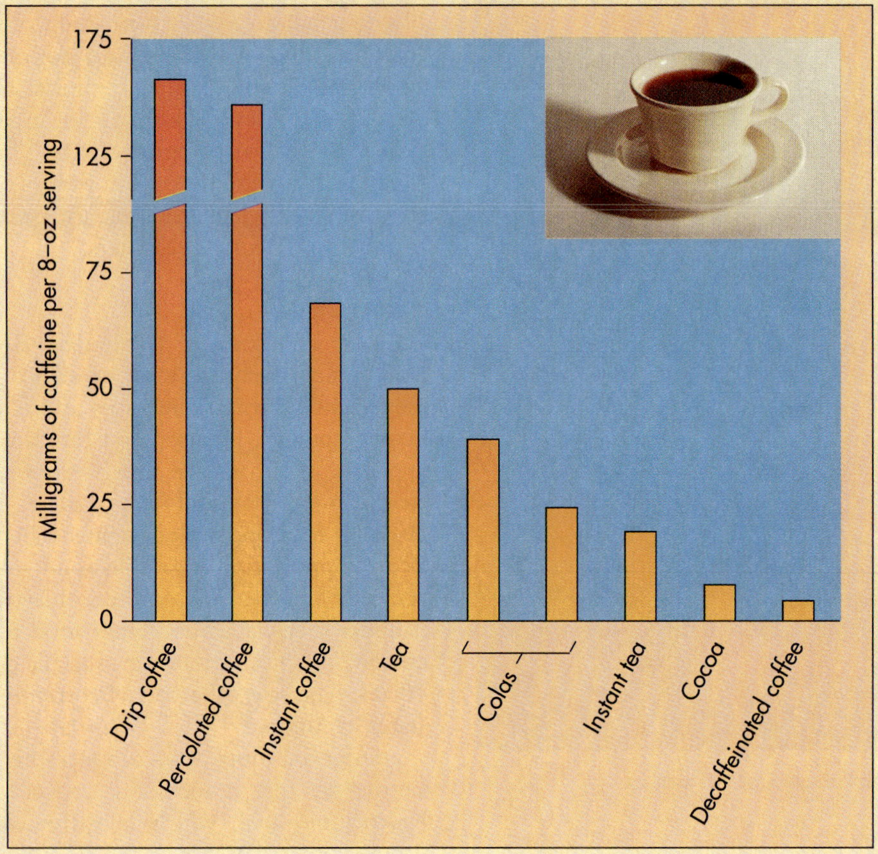

promoted as a rich protein source. It is indeed mostly composed of protein and provides a reasonable balance of amino acids. However, the few milligrams that constitute one dose are hardly significant, especially at a price of about $5.00 to $10.00 for 20 g of protein (an amount provided in one serving of meat or three eggs). Spirulina is an unnecessary purchase because adequate protein is readily obtained from other foods at a fraction of the cost and accompanied by other nutrients as a bonus.

Caffeine

Caffeine is a common dietary item obtained from coffee, tea, and cocoa (Figure 13-14). It has no nutritional significance, but it does have some physiological effects and is considered one of the most widely used drugs. Because 80% of the adult population regularly consumes caffeine, it is appropriate to consider it a component of the diet. The caffeine content of common beverages ranges from 6 to 85 mg per serving. Average consumption of caffeine in the United States is estimated at 2.6 mg/kg of body weight, or 150 to 200 mg/day. About 60% of this caffeine comes from coffee, 30% from tea, and 10% from cola beverages, chocolate, and medications. Caffeine consumption in Canada is estimated at 450 mg/day.

In addition to its well-known role as a stimulant of the central nervous system, caffeine acts as a diuretic (increasing urine production), relaxes smooth muscles, stimulates the heart muscle, stimulates gastric secretions, increases oxygen consumption, increases the levels of free fatty acids and glucose in blood plasma, and apparently depresses the absorption of iron. Caffeine is absorbed completely and quickly to become distributed throughout various tissues. It is excreted in the form of xanthines and uric acid 3 to 6 hours after ingestion. Daily intakes of between 65 and 130 mg of caffeine have beneficial effects on both motor and mental performance, whereas daily intakes of 400 mg or more cause insomnia and poor performance. It has been alleged that caffeine may be involved in the onset of cancer, cardiovascular disease, and birth defects. At present there is no conclusive evidence of any relationship between caffeine consumption and health, but pregnant women are advised to use caffeine in moderation.

Two compounds related to caffeine are theophylline and theobromine. Theophylline is found in tea and is also a stimulant of the central nervous system. Theobromine is found in cocoa. Neither theophylline nor theobromine has any nutritional benefit.

ISSUES AND OPINIONS

The Nutrient Enhancement of Foods—Policies and Practices

Various terms have been used for the addition of nutrients to food, whether to replace nutrients lost in processing or to correct a recognized inadequacy in the food supply. These terms include the following:

- *Restoration:* applied when the added nutrients replace those lost in processing
- *Enrichment:* usually used to describe the addition of nutrients (within specified limits) to staple cereals or flour
- *Nutrification, nutrient enhancement, and fortification:* all used for the addition of nutrients to a wide range of food products for a wide range of purposes

The addition of nutrients to the food supply only became appropriate and possible once scientists had identified the essential nutrients, the amount needed, and the amount readily available in the diet. The nutrients had to be relatively inexpensive and stable under food processing and storage conditions and had to have little or no effect on the appearance and palatability of the food to which they were added. In general, they were available through chemical or microbial synthesis or concentrated from naturally rich sources. Mineral elements or salts of minerals can be purified from natural sources before being added to foods.

One of the earliest examples of enhancing the nutritional quality of foods was the addition of potassium iodide to table salt to control the incidence of simple goiter. The irradiation of evaporated milk was also widely used to prepare infant feeding formulas that provide the vitamin D needed to prevent rickets.

Assessment of the health status of service recruits in World War II led the U.S. government to rule (in 1943) that the existing voluntary program to enrich white flour and bread with thiamin, riboflavin, niacin, and iron be mandated throughout the country. Vitamin D and calcium, which were not normally found in these products, were permitted as optional enrichment nutrients. Health problems had been attributed to the loss of nutrients associated with the practice of substituting refined white bread and flour for the more nutrient-dense whole grain cereal products. Once the wartime emergency passed, the individual states assumed responsibility for the programs. As a result, only 35 states now require the enrichment of bread and flour. However, because of the centralization of the milling industry, over 90% of all flour and bread and much of the pasta, corn grits, and cornmeal sold is now enriched with thiamin, riboflavin, niacin, and iron. Similarly, much rice has thiamin, niacin, and iron added to it.

The evidence that folate intake before pregnancy prevents neural tube defects in infants has led the Food and Drug Administration (FDA) to rule that folate should be added to enriched cereals. The Food and Nutrition Board of the National Research Council in 1974 recommended that certain other nutrients (vitamin B_6, vitamin A, calcium, magnesium, and zinc) should also be part of the required enrichment mix for products based on wheat, corn, and rice. As of 1994, however, for a variety of scientific, technical, and policy considerations, these recommendations have not been implemented.

The impetus for a comparable program instituted in Canada in 1952 came from the results of a study in the mid-1940s in Newfoundland. This demonstrated the effectiveness of fortifying margarine with vitamin A and bread and flour with thiamin, riboflavin, niacin, iron, and bonemeal (calcium) in alleviating the widespread malnutrition on the island. In addition to requiring the inclusion of thiamin, riboflavin, niacin, and iron, the Canadian government permits and encourages the addition of vitamin B_6, folate, pantothenic acid, magnesium, and calcium.

The health benefits of the addition of nutrients to

food to restore the nutritional quality of processed foods to that of the unprocessed foods or to levels designed to correct known nutrient shortfalls have been well documented. There is concern, however, about the practice of adding nutrients simply to enhance the marketability of the product. This is most common in, but not confined to, the dry cereal industry. It began with the addition of a wide variety of nutrients to raise the content of one serving to 25% of the Daily Value (DV) for 8 to 14 nutrients. Further competition for a trade advantage has led many companies to market at least one product that contains 100% of the DV for a similar list of nutrients. The long-term impact of such a "fortification race" is cause for concern because of our lack of information on the consequence of the use of several highly fortified foods in addition to high levels of intakes from foods naturally rich in the nutrients added to the fortified products. Because the cost of these cereals is usually considerably greater than the cost of the cereal and a multinutrient supplement of the "one-a-day" type, there is also concern about the economic consequences of their use.

The FDA, which is responsible for the safety and quality of the food supply, does not have the authority to limit the amounts of nutrients that can be added to a food, provided the amount is truthfully presented on the label and the level is considered safe. It has, however, issued voluntary guidelines on *"Nutritional Quality of Foods: Addition of Nutrients,"* based on the premise that food fortification should provide a reasonable benefit without contributing to a nutritional imbalance in the diet and without misleading the consumer to believe that the consumption of the fortified food necessarily ensures a complete and nutritionally sound diet. It states that food fortification is appropriate for the following reasons:

- To correct a dietary insufficiency recognized by the scientific community to exist and to result in a nutritional deficiency disease
- To restore such nutrient(s) to level(s) representative of the food before storage, handling, and processing
- To balance the vitamin, mineral, and protein content of a food in proportion to its total caloric content (nutrient density)
- To avoid nutritional inferiority in a food that replaces a traditional food in the diet.

The FDA policy neither encourages the indiscriminate addition of nutrients to foods nor considers it appropriate to fortify fresh produce; meat, poultry, or fish products; sugars; or snack foods.

The Food and Nutrition Board endorses the addition of nutrients to foods when all of the following conditions are met:

- The nutrient under consideration for addition to food is judged to be significantly below the RDA in the diets of a substantial segment of the population.
- The food that is to carry the nutrient is consumed by most individuals in the segment of the population in need.
- The amount of nutrient added makes an important contribution to the total diet.
- The addition of the specific nutrient does not create a nutrient imbalance.
- The nutrient added is physiologically available and sufficiently stable so that its value is retained during the normal shelf-life of the product. Reasonable excess is permitted to compensate for storage losses.
- There is reasonable assurance that excessive intake (to a level that may be harmful) will not occur.
- Any additional cost is affordable for the intended population.

Several multilateral trade agreements now govern the sale of food among various countries, requiring standardizing of fortification levels and labeling requirements. This standardization will inevitably lead to some compromising of policies.

A comparison of the standards for the enrichment of flour in the United States and Canada exemplifies the problem, especially in regard to nutrients permitted and prohibited in the two countries.

The addition of vitamin D to all milk, vitamin A to reduced and nonfat milk, and vitamin A to margarine are almost universal practices. Fortification of various fruit juices with vitamin C, orange juice with calcium, and infant formula with iron are some other examples of widespread uses of the addition of nutrients to individual foods. There will undoubtedly be others appearing on the market, targeted at specific segments of the population for whom a potential nutrient deficiency has been identified or postulated.

As the nutrient enhancement of food escalates not only in terms of the foods involved, but also in the number of nutrients and the level of fortification, it will be necessary to monitor the health impact of the individual foods and the cumulative effect of all potential sources of added nutrients. Any such assessment must also take into account the current dietary practices of the target population because it is the cumulative contribution of nutrients naturally present in food and those added that is important in determining both nutrient adequacy and possible problems of toxicity.

On an international level the main nutrients targeted in intervention programs are the micronutrients iodine, iron, and vitamin A. Primary efforts are directed toward finding the most appropriate food to serve as a vehicle for fortification. Currently, salt, sugar, and monosodium glutamate appear to have the most promise.

Standards for the addition of nutrients to flour in the United States and Canada

	UNITED STATES (mg/kg)	CANADA (mg/kg)
MANDATORY		
Thiamin	6.4	4.4-7.7
Riboflavin	4.0	2.7-4.8
Niacin	5.5	35-64
Iron	4.4	29-43
Folate	0.7†	—
OPTIONAL		
Calcium	1200	1100-1400
Vitamin B_6	*	25-31
Folate	—	0.40-0.50
Pantothenic acid	*	10-130
Magnesium	*	1500-1900

* Not permitted.
† Amount proposed by the Food and Drug Administration.

Food and Drug Administration: *Fed Reg* 45(18):6314, 1980.
Health and Welfare, Canada: *Health protection and food laws,* Ottawa, Canada, 1987, Health Protection Branch.
Position Statement of the American Dietetic Association: *J Am Diet Assoc* 94:661, 1994.

BY NOW YOU SHOULD KNOW

- Thiamin, riboflavin, niacin, pantothenic acid, and biotin are essential parts of coenzymes needed for the cell to release energy from carbohydrate, fat, protein, and alcohol.
- The recommended dietary allowances for thiamin, riboflavin, and niacin are based on energy intake.
- The classic thiamin deficiency is known as *beriberi.* The classic niacin deficiency is known as *pellagra.*
- Although the severe deficiency diseases beriberi and pellagra are now seldom seen in the developed world, many people suffer from marginal deficiencies of thiamin and niacin, which may produce symptoms when they experience physical or emotional stress.
- Thiamin, riboflavin, niacin, biotin, and pantothenic acid can be obtained in adequate amounts from a typical North American diet.
- Thiamin, riboflavin, and niacin are added to cereal and grain products.
- Sixty milligrams of the essential amino acid tryptophan can give rise to 1 mg of niacin.
- Pantothenic acid deficiency has not been documented in humans, except when produced experimentally.
- Pantothenic acid is found in all foods.
- Biotin deficiency has been documented in people receiving total parenteral nutrition but not in people who ingest food.
- Such substances as myoinositol, choline, carnitine, and taurine are essential for the functioning of the body but can be synthesized by the body or are normally ingested in adequate amounts.
- Many other substances have vitamin-like properties in certain conditions.
- A wide variety of substances that are not recognized as essential nutrients are promoted as valuable dietary supplements. Some of these substances have no effect, others have some physiological effect but are not essential, and others are useful at low levels of intake but may have undesirable, druglike effects at higher levels. Some are fraudulently represented as being of benefit to health, although—fortunately—they are mostly harmless.

STUDY QUESTIONS

1. Under what circumstances and in what groups of people would you expect deficiencies of each of the water-soluble vitamins to appear?
2. Which of the water-soluble vitamins are sensitive to heat, light, alkali, acid, and oxidation?
3. What part have inadequate intakes of the water-soluble vitamins played in the nutritional history of America and of the world?
4. Why are the RDAs for some vitamins related to energy intake, whereas the RDAs for other vitamins are related to protein intake?
5. List the three most important food sources of each of the water-soluble vitamins in the North American diet.
6. Plan meals for an adult female with a lactose intolerance, making sure they meet the RDA for riboflavin.

CRITICAL ANALYSIS

1. The content of thiamin, riboflavin, and niacin in some foods (the foods include both recommended sources of those vitamins and sources that people report eating most often) is listed in Table 13-2. The spaces below are arranged to allow estimation of your own intake of these vitamins from the sources listed in Table 13-2. In the spaces under the heading "Foods," is a list of foods from any of the food groups in Table 13-2 that are commonly eaten. The key is to identify foods that you eat (or like) that supply 20% or more of your RDA per serving. List the content of thiamin, riboflavin, or niacin for each serving in the appropriate space. Then estimate how many times per week you eat that food according to the following scale: less than once a week, 1 to 2 times per week, 3 to 4 times a week, 5 to 6 times a week, 7 or more times a week. If each serving of the foods you listed provides 20% of your RDA, then a good goal is 35 servings/week, or 7 servings/day, from any of the foods listed. Some foods may supply 50% or more of your RDA per serving. Including a number of these foods in your diet could reduce your goal to approximately 14 servings/week, or 2 servings/day. In addition, you obtain some of your vitamin intake from foods that you did not list or did not have room to list (for example, a ready-to-eat cereal that is fortified with these vitamins). If you could not list at least 2 or 3 sources for each vitamin, or if the total number of servings for sources of any one vitamin is less than 7 per week, it might be time to think about factors that may be limiting your intake.

RDA FOR THIAMIN	20% OF RDA	FOOD	CONTENT OF THIAMIN PER SERVING	TIMES EATEN PERWEEK
______	______	______	______	______
		______	______	______
		______	______	______
		______	______	______
		______	______	______
		______	______	______

RDA FOR RIBOFLAVIN	20% OF RDA	FOOD	CONTENT OF RIBOFLAVIN PER SERVING	TIMES EATEN PER WEEK
______	______	______	______	______
		______	______	______
		______	______	______
		______	______	______
		______	______	______
		______	______	______

RDA FOR NIACIN	20% OF RDA	FOOD	CONTENT OF NIACIN PER SERVING	TIMES EATEN PER WEEK
______	______	______	______	______
		______	______	______
		______	______	______
		______	______	______
		______	______	______
		______	______	______

This is an exercise to gain awareness of the nutrient content of your diet. It is not all inclusive. For example, pantothenic acid and biotin are not listed in the exercise. These vitamins are widely distributed in foods and are normally consumed in adequate amounts in the United States. The estimated safe and adequate daily dietary intakes for adults for pantothenic acid and biotin are 4 to 7 mg/day and 30 to 100 μg/day, respectively. Tables 13-6 and 13-8 reveal the widespread nature of these two vitamins. Eggs, meats, grain products, and legumes are all good sources of these vitamins. A diet that includes several daily servings from any or all of these groups likely supplies adequate amounts of these vitamins.

REFERENCES

1. Brown ML: Thiamin. In Brown ML, editor: *Present knowledge in nutrition,* ed 6, Washington, DC, 1990, International Life Sciences Institute.
2. Gubler CJ: Thiamin. In Machlin LJ, editor: *Handbook of vitamins,* ed 2, New York, 1991, Marcel Dekker.
3. Food and Nutrition Board, National Research Council: *Recommended dietary allowances,* ed 10, Washington, DC, 1989, National Academy Press.
4. Health and Welfare Canada: *Nutrition Recommendations,* The Report of the Scientific Review Committee, Ottawa, Canada, 1990, Canadian Government Publishing Centre.
5. *Dietary reference values for food energy and nutrients for the United Kingdom,* Report of the Panel on Dietary Reference Values of the Committee on Medical Aspects of Food Policy, Report on Health and Social Subjects No 4, London, 1991, Her Majesty's Stationery Office.
6. McCormick DB: Riboflavin. In Brown ML, editor: *Present knowledge of nutrition,* ed 6, Washington, DC, 1990, International Life Sciences Institute.
7. Cooper JM, Lopez R: Riboflavin. In Machlin LJ, editor: *Handbook of vitamins,* ed 2, New York, 1991, Marcel Dekker.
8. Winters LRT and others: Riboflavin requirements and exercise adaptation in older women, *Am J Clin Nutr* 56:526, 1992.
9. Boisuert WA, Gershoff S, Russell R: Riboflavin requirements of healthy elderly humans and its relationship to macronutrient composition of the diet, *J Nutr* 123:915, 1993.
10. United States Department of Agriculture: *Nationwide food consumption survey, continuing survey of food intakes by individuals,* Report Nos 85-3 and 85-4, Hyattsville, Md, 1986-1987, Human Nutrition Information Services, United States Department of Agriculture
11. McCormick DB: Vitamins. In Tietz NW, editor: *Textbook of clinical chemistry,* Philadelphia, 1986, WB Saunders.
12. Lopez R, Schwartz JV, Cooperman JM: Riboflavin deficiency in an adolescent population in New York City, *Am J Clin Nutr* 33:1283, 1980.
13. Jacob RA, Swendseid M: Niacin. In Brown ML, editor: *Present knowledge in nutrition,* ed 6, Washington, DC, 1990, International Life Sciences Institute.
14. Jacob RA and others: Biochemical markers for assessment of niacin status in young men: urinary and blood levels of niacin metabolites, *J Nutr* 119:591, 1989.
15. Block GA and others: Nutrient sources in the American diet: quantitative data from the National Health and Nutrition Examination Survey II, *Am J Epidemiol* 122:13, 1985.
16. Kleijnen J, Knipschild P: Niacin and vitamin B_6 in mental functioning: a review of controlled trials in humans, *Biol Psychiatry* 29:931, 1991.
17. Olson RE: Pantothenic acid. In Brown ML, editor: *Present knowledge in nutrition,* ed 6, Washington, DC, 1990, International Life Sciences Institute.
18. Fox HM: Pantothenic acid. In Machlin LJ, editor: *Handbook of vitamins,* ed 2, New York, 1991, Marcel Dekker.
19. Mock DM: Biotin. In Brown ML, editor: *Present knowledge in nutrition,* ed 6, Washington, DC, 1990, International Life Sciences Institute.
20. Bonjour JP: Biotin. In Machlin LJ, editor: *Handbook of vitamins,* ed 2, New York, 1991, Marcel Dekker.
21. Dakshinamurti R: Biotin. In Shils ME, Olson JA, Shike M, editors: *Modern nutrition in health and disease,* ed 8, Philadelphia, 1994, Lea & Febiger.
22. Fomon SJ, McCormick DB: B vitamins and choline. In Fomon SJ, editor: *Nutrition of normal infants,* St Louis, 1993, Mosby.
23. Marshall MW, Judd JT, Baker H: Effect of low and high fat diets varying in ratios of polyunsaturated to saturated fatty acids on biotin intakes and biotin in serum, red cells, and urine of adult men, *Nutr Res* 5:801, 1985.
24. Aukema HM, Holub BJ: Inositol. In Shils ME, Olson JA, Shike M, editors: *Modern nutrition in health and disease,* ed 8, Philadelphia, 1994, Lea & Febiger.
25. Zeisel SH and others: Choline, an essential nutrient for humans, *FASEB J* 5:2093, 1991.
26. Zeisel SH: Choline. In Shils ME, Olson JA, Shike M, editors: *Modern nutrition in health and disease,* ed 8, Philadelphia, 1994, Lea & Febiger.
27. Rebouche CJ: Carnitine function during the life cycle, *FASEB J* 6:3379, 1992.
28. Hayes KC: Taurine nutrition, *Nutr Res Rev* 1:99, 1988.
29. Sturman JA: Taurine in development, *J Nutr* 118:1169, 1988.
30. Hayes KC, Trautwein EA: Taurine. In Shils ME, Olson JA, Shike M, editors: *Modern nutrition in health and disease,* ed 8, Philadelphia, 1994, Lea & Febiger.
31. Smidt CR, Myers-Steinberg F, Rucker RB: Physiological importance of pyrroloquinoline quinone, *Proc Soc Exper Biol Med* 197:19, 1991.

~ ADDITIONAL READINGS ~

Beyer RE: An analysis of the role of coenzyme Q in free radical generation and as an antioxidant, *Biochem Cell Biol* 70:390, 1992.

Bieber LL: Carnitine, *Annu Rev Biochem* 57:261, 1988.

Blass JP: Thiamin and the Wernicke-Korsakoff syndrome. In Briggs MH, editor: *Vitamins in human biology and medicine,* Boca Raton, Fla, 1981, CRC Press.

Dong MH and others: Thiamin, riboflavin, and vitamin B_6 contents of selected foods as served, *JAMA* 76:156, 1980.

Dukshinanurti K, Chauhan J: Biotin, *Vitam Horm* 45:337, 1989.

Feller AG, Rudman D: Role of carnitine in human nutrition *J Nutr* 118:541, 1988.

Fry PC, Fox HM, Tao HG: Metabolic response to a pantothenic-deficient diet in humans, *J Nutr Sci Vitaminol (Tokyo)* 22:339, 1976.

Goldsmith GA: The B vitamins: thiamin, riboflavin, and niacin. In Beaton GM, McHenry EW, editors: *Nutrition, a comprehensive treatis,* vol 2, New York, 1964, Academic Press.

Haas RH: Thiamin and the brain, *Annu Rev Nutr* 8:483, 1988.

Henderson LM: Niacin, *Annu Rev Nutr* 3:289, 1983.

Hilker DM, Somogi JC: Antithiamins of plant origin: their chemical nature and mode of action, *Ann N Y Acad Sci* 378:137, 1982.

Holub BJ: Metabolism and function of myo-inositol and inositol phospholipids, *Annu Rev Nutr* 6:563, 1986.

Jarvis WT: Food faddism, cultism, and quackery, *Annu Rev Nutr* 3:35, 1983.

Lombardini JB: Taurine: retinal function, *Brain Res Rev* 16:151, 1991.

McCormick DB: Two interconnected B-vitamins: riboflavin and pyridonine, *Physio Rev* 69:1170, 1989.

McMahon K: Choline, an essential nutrient? *Nutr Today* 22:18, 1987.

Picone TA: Taurine update: metabolism and function, *Nutr Today* 22:16, 1987.

Plesofsky-Vig N, Brame R: Pantothenic acid and coenzyme A in cellular modification of proteins, *Annu Rev Nutr* 8:461, 1988.

Rana RS, Hokin LE: Role of phosphoinositides in transmembrane signaling, *Physiol Rev* 70:115, 1990.

Rebouche CJ, Paulson DJ: Carnitine metabolism and function in humans, *Annu Rev Nutr* 6:41, 1986.

Song WO and others: Effects of pantothenic acid status on the content of the vitamin in human milk, *Am J Clin Nutr* 40:317, 1984.

Wecker L: Neurochemical effects of choline supplementation, *Can J Physiol Pharmacol* 64:329, 1986.

Zeisel SH: Choline deficiency, *J Nutr Biochem* 1:332, 1990.

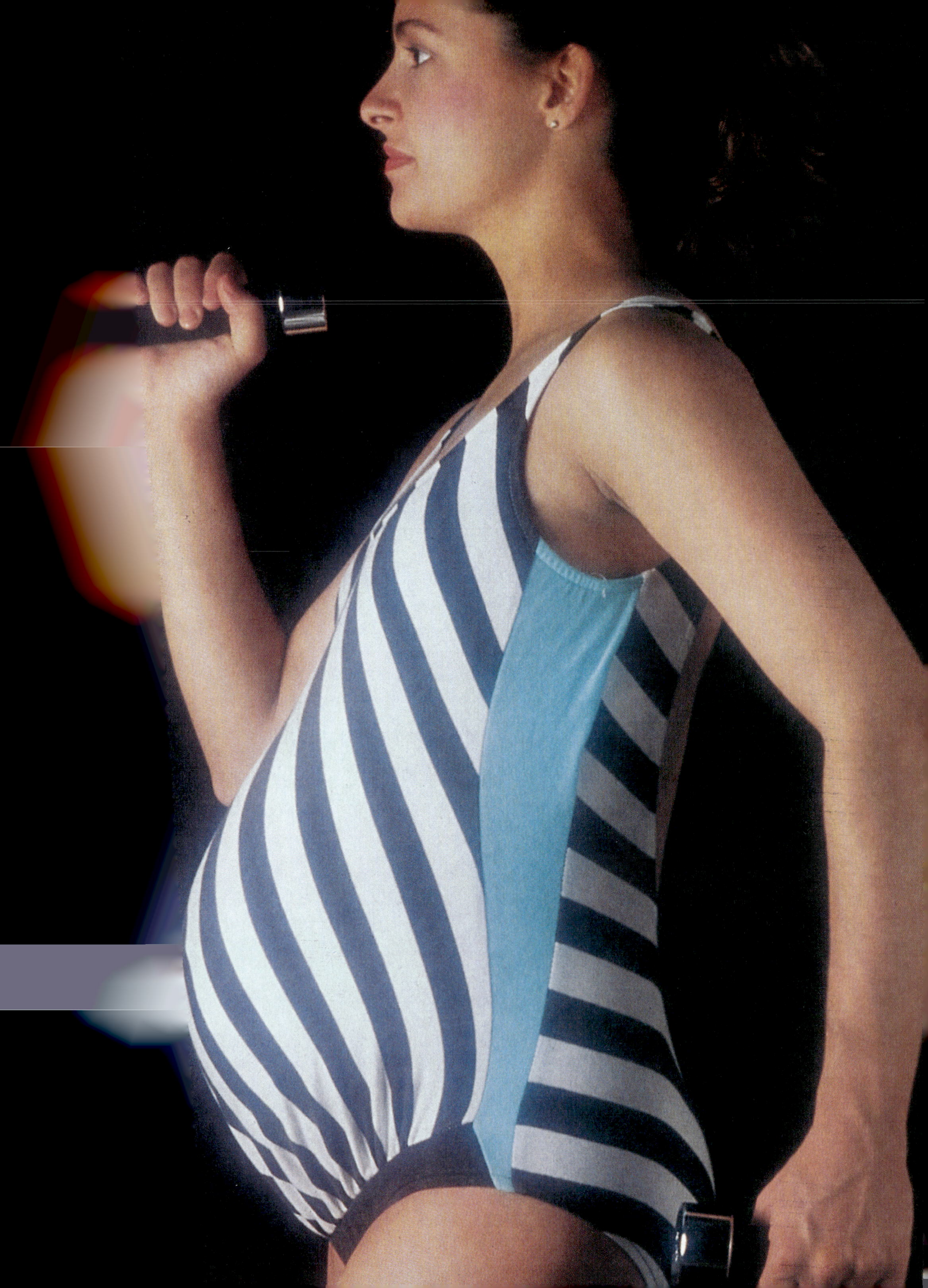

CHAPTER 14

NUTRITION IN PREGNANCY AND LACTATION

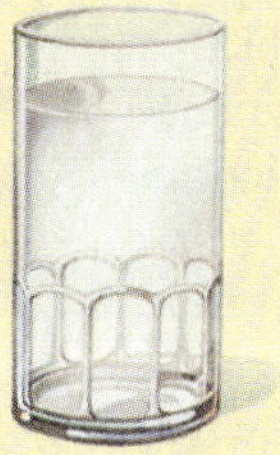

Nutrition before and during pregnancy and during lactation can have a significant effect on the long-term health of both infants and their mothers. The potential impact of nutrition is greater at this time than during any other stage of life. Infants who are well nourished in the womb have an increased chance of beginning their life in good physical and mental health. Infants who are undernourished in the womb are at risk of a variety of undesirable consequences, ranging from low–birth-weight to severe mental and physical retardation and death. The effect of undernutrition during pregnancy and lactation depends on the nutrient or nutrients involved and the stage at which undernutrition occurs. The nutritional status and health of both mother and child can be affected by the intake of such substances as alcohol, nicotine, and various drugs. Other factors involved in determining the success of pregnancy and lactation include the mother's age, the physical and emotional stresses to which she is subjected, and the presence of any infections or other diseases.

PREGNANCY

From a nutritional viewpoint, pregnancy is a vulnerable period, although it is a normal physiological process. The diet must meet the nutritional demands of the **embryo** or **fetus** developing in the **uterus**, in addition to those of the mother. This requires adequate nutrition both before and during pregnancy.

The importance of adequate nutrition for the fetus cannot be overemphasized. The future health of the developing child depends to a large extent on the nutritional foundations laid down during prenatal life. Nutritional deficits before birth can be partially compensated for by nutrition after birth, but the effects of inadequate fetal nutrition, especially in brain and nerve tissues, can never be completely reversed.

The effect of any nutritional deficiency during pregnancy depends on the stage of pregnancy in which it develops. Deficiencies in the early stages of pregnancy may cause spontaneous abortion. If the deficiencies occur when the major organs of the body are being formed, a variety of congenital abnormalities can result. Deficiency in the later stages of pregnancy may have little effect, apart from causing some retardation of growth.

It is difficult to isolate the precise effects of nutrition on reproduction. Maternal health is complex, being influenced by many factors in addition to diet, including genetic, environmental, social, and economic factors and any infections or other disease. These factors can also affect fetal development because the health of the fetus depends on the health of its mother. Also, the mother's nutrition before pregnancy is as important as her nutrition during pregnancy. Nutrition before and during pregnancy influences fetal growth and therefore the size and health of an infant at birth.

Fortunately, the nutritional needs of a pregnant woman are not the sum of the needs of the fetus plus the normal needs of a mature woman. A series of physiological adaptations within pregnant women improve their use of nutrients, through increased absorption, decreased excretion, or alterations in metabolism. Also, a woman who has been well nourished before pregnancy is equipped with reserves of several nutrients so that the needs of the fetus for these nutrients can be met without jeopardizing her health. The combined effect of physiological adaptations to pregnancy and adequate nutrition before pregnancy can allow a woman to bear a full-term, healthy infant without any extensive modification of her diet. It is recommended, however, that the mother's diet during pregnancy provide sufficient nutrients to avoid excessive depletion of her reserves and also to ensure that she is able to produce sufficient milk to nourish her infant after birth. It is also important to remember that the nutritional needs of pregnant teenagers are considerably higher than those of pregnant mature women.

FIGURE 14-1

Diagrammatic representation of a fetus and its link with the placenta via the umbilical cord.

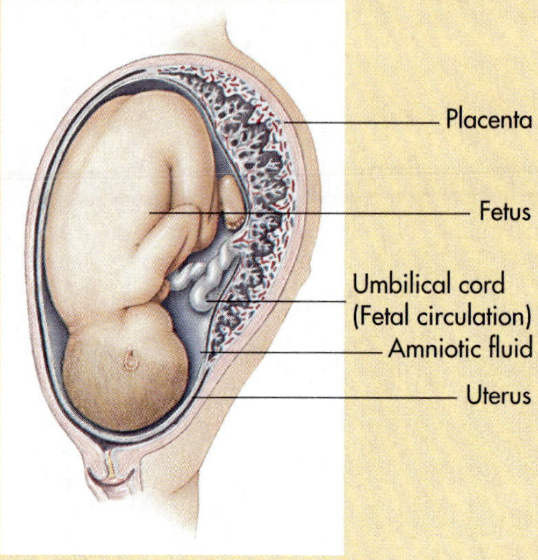

A developing fetus is completely dependent on its mother for all its nourishment. This nourishment is supplied primarily by the mother's blood, which comes into close contact with the fetal circulation in the **placenta**, allowing nutrients to be passed to the fetus via the **umbilical cord** (Figure 14-1 and boxed definitions). Because many nutrients (including most water-soluble vitamins) are transferred to the fetus against a concentration gradient, the nutrients are more concentrated in the fetal circulation than in the maternal circulation. In addition to allowing the delivery of nutrients to the fetus, the placenta also acts as an endocrine gland, synthesizing at least 10 hormones that control the metabolism of the fetus and, in some cases, the mother. During the latter part of **gestation** (pregnancy) some nutrients are available to the fetus from the **amniotic fluid,** which surrounds the infant as it develops.

In general, the nutrients supplied to a fetus come from three sources: directly from the mother's diet, from her stores of nutrients (primarily in the bones and liver), and from the synthesis of nutrients within the placenta. Adequate nutrition of the fetus while in the uterus (**intrauterine nutrition**) is especially important for the development of the infant's central nervous system and kidneys, which mature rapidly in the latter part of pregnancy.

The development of the placenta is clearly essential for the development of the fetus because the placenta controls the transfer of nutrients, hormones, and other substances (such as drugs) to the fetus. In chronically undernourished mothers the placenta is often smaller than normal, and the flow of blood through it is reduced.[1] This reduces the ability of the placenta to synthesize substances needed by the fetus, to transfer

Medical Terms Related to Pregnancy and Lactation

Amenorrhea: The absence of menstruation ("periods").
Colostrum: The first fluid secreted from the breast to nourish the infant before true milk is produced.
Conception: The fertilization of the female egg cell by the male sperm cell.
Congenital: Existing at or dating from birth.
Foremilk: Milk secreted at the beginning of one nursing period.
Gestation: The period from conception to delivery, i.e., the full course of pregnancy.
Hindmilk: Milk secreted at the end of one nursing period.
Multiparas: Women having their second or third (and so on) infant.
Neonatal: During the first 28 days of life.
Perinatal: At or close to the time of birth.
Pica: Practice of eating nonfood items, such as clay or dirt (also sometimes used to refer to the cravings for specific foods that can occur during pregnancy).
Placenta: Tissue embedded in the wall of the uterus in which the maternal and fetal circulations come into close contact. Materials that are transferred between the maternal and fetal circulations are said to "cross the placenta."
Postnatal: After birth.
Prenatal: Before birth.
Primiparas: Women having their first infant.
Trimester: A term applied to each of the successive 3-month periods of gestation. A pregnancy is divided into the first trimester, second trimester and third trimester.
Umbilical cord: The narrow tube connecting the placenta to the fetus. Maternal blood circulates through the placenta. Fetal blood circulates through the fetus and umbilical cord.

these substances and nutrients to the fetus, and to inhibit the transfer of potentially harmful substances into the fetus.

BIRTH SIZE

In the United States, approximately 7% of all infants born each year are classified as **low-birth-weight (LBW) infants,** weighing less that 5.5 lb (2500 g). More than two thirds of these infants are **premature,** defined as being born before completing 37 weeks of gestation. The other one third of LBW infants are born after a normal length of gestation (37 to 40 weeks) but exhibit **intrauterine growth retardation (IUGR)** resulting from malnutrition while growing in the uterus. LBW infants have a wide range of disorders, including neurodevelopmental problems, learning disorders, behavior problems, and increased infection rates. Compared with infants born weighing 5.5 lb or more, LBW infants are 30 times more likely to die during the **neonatal** period (the first 28 days of life) and twice as likely to be hospitalized in their first year of life.[2]

IUGR produces infants who are classified as **small for gestational age (SGA).** This is most likely to occur in infants who are born to women of low socioeconomic status and poor nutritional status; who are shorter and weigh less than their well-nourished counterparts when they conceive; who experience hypertension, viral infections, or other diseases; or who use drugs extensively before or during pregnancy. The undernourishment of an infant borne by a mother from this group may be caused by the poor nutritional status of the mother; poor blood supply to the fetus, causing reduced delivery of nutrients and oxygen; the inhibition of nutrient transfer between the maternal and fetal circulation; or hormonal changes.[3] The sequence of events leading to fetal growth retardation is shown in Figure 14-2.

FIGURE 14-2

Relationship between maternal and fetal malnutrition.

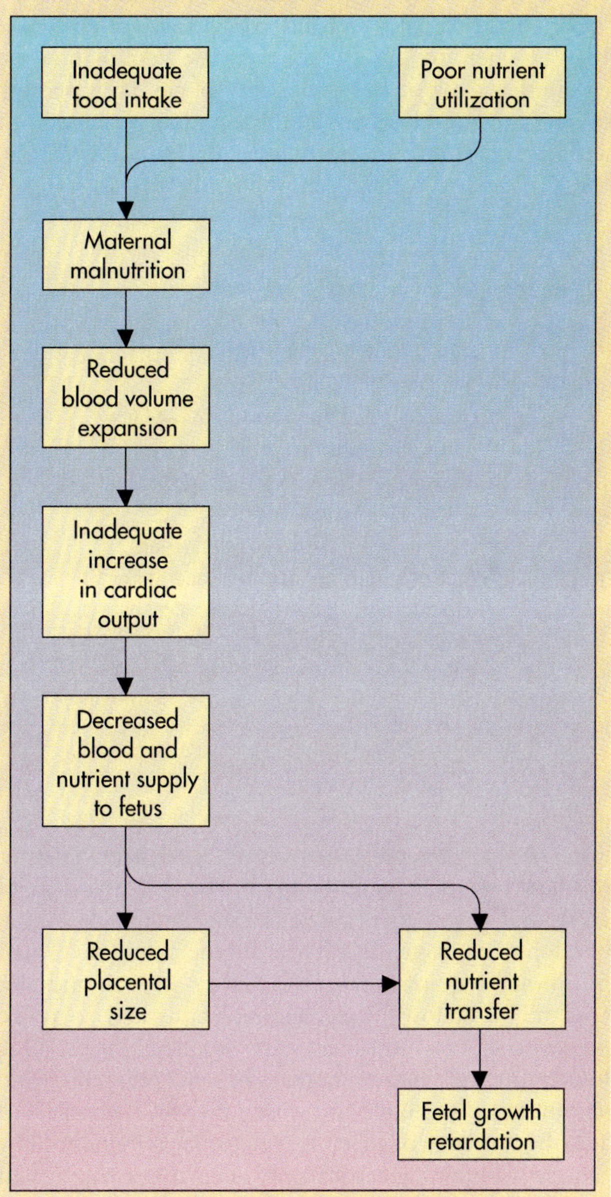

LBW caused by premature birth is most often associated with multiple births (for example, twins or triplets) or with mothers who gain too little weight (less than 16 lb, or 7 kg) or too much weight (more than 36 lb, or 16 kg) during pregnancy; smoke excessively (more than 11 cigarettes per day); or consume alcohol in excess (more than 1 oz of 100-proof alcohol per day). Because much of the development and maturation of the kidneys and lungs occurs in the later part of pregnancy, defects in these tissues are common in premature infants.

To reduce the chances of having a low–birth-weight (LBW) infant, pregnant women should do the following:

- Gain between 16 and 45 lb, depending on their weight before pregnancy.
- Smoke no more than 11 cigarettes per day and preferably none.
- Limit alcohol consumption to no more than one drink per day (with one drink equivalent to 1 oz of 100-proof alcohol).
- Eat a nutritious and varied diet, following the Food Guide Pyramid.

The half-million U.S. infants born each year to mothers under 18 years of age are at increased risk of LBW and impaired physical, social, and psychological development in general. Their mothers still have high nutritional requirements for their own growth and also tend to be of low socioeconomic status and so to be prone to poor nutritional status to begin with. One fourth of these teenage mothers become pregnant again within 1 year and one third within 2 years. Regardless of age, the outcome of a teenage pregnancy is influenced by the girl's physiological maturity. The closer the age of **menarche** (time of onset of periods) to the age of conception, the greater the nutritional demands on the mother and the risks of LBW and developmental abnormalities in their infants. Unfortunately, the infants born to teenage mothers are also at increased risk of physical abuse and neglect.

Various natural mechanisms can prevent malnourished women from carrying a potentially undernourished child to term. Only an estimated 60% of conceptions survive the first critical 4 weeks of gestation. Of these, another 10% fail to survive to 20 weeks. Intrauterine deaths after 20 weeks reduce the total proportion of conceptions that result in viable births to 50%. Also, approximately 1% of newborn infants suffer from perinatal handicaps that cause them to need special care. In the United States the mortality rate in the first year of life is 10 per 1000 live births, being highest among African-American and low-income women. Throughout the world, infant mortality ranges from as low as 5 per 1000 live births in Japan to as high as 20 per 1000 in many developing countries. There is general agreement that many infant deaths result from undernutrition and malnutrition before and during pregnancy and are therefore preventable.

PHYSIOLOGICAL ADJUSTMENTS

During pregnancy, many physiological adjustments influence the mother's need for nutrients and the efficiency with which her body uses nutrients. By the third month of pregnancy the total plasma volume of the blood rises to 1½ times normal in women having their first infant (**primiparas**) and to greater volumes in women who have already had at least one infant (**multiparas**). At the same time, the number of red cells in the blood increases by about 20%.[4] The expansion of blood volume is required to allow the circulation of blood through the placenta and allow it to carry nutrients and oxygen to the fetus and metabolic wastes away from the fetus.

The rate at which blood is filtered through the kidneys increases during pregnancy, allowing the body to excrete the additional metabolic wastes produced by the fetus and to get rid of other waste products that could harm the developing fetus. During pregnancy, water-soluble nutrients that are normally reabsorbed by the kidneys begin to be excreted in the urine in substantial amounts. This "renal squandering" of nutrients makes the mother's dietary needs for the nutrients greater than they would otherwise be.

To assist the circulation of the increased volume of blood, the capacity of the heart to pump fluid (the **cardiac output**) increases by one third during pregnancy. The amount of intercellular fluid—between the body's cells—also increases during pregnancy, and the total amount of water in the body (comprising both intracellular and extracellular fluid) increases by as much as 20% during pregnancy.

The increase in blood volume in pregnancy is more than twice as great as is the increase in the amounts of red cells, hemoglobin, plasma proteins, and many nutrients (Figure 14-3). This causes **hemodilution,** the dilution of the components of the blood. The fall in the concentration of nutrients in the blood caused by hemodilution in pregnancy can be misinterpreted as a sign of nutritional deficiency. To accurately assess the pregnant woman's nutritional status, standards different from those applied to nonpregnant women must be used. The total amount of a nutrient or other component of the blood may actually rise during pregnancy,

FIGURE 14-3

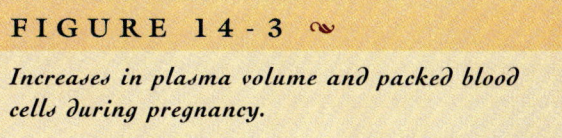

Increases in plasma volume and packed blood cells during pregnancy.

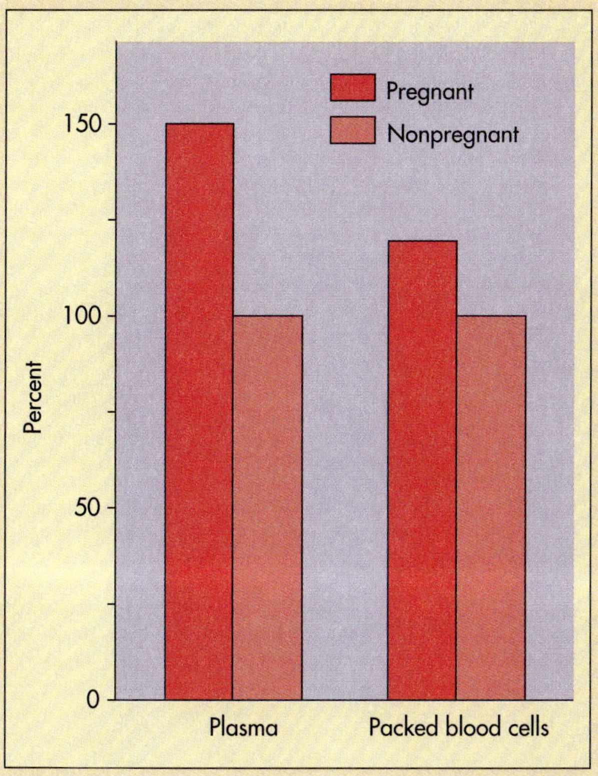

even though its concentration may fall. On the other hand, both the total amount and the plasma concentrations of cholesterol, phospholipids, free fatty acids, and fat-soluble vitamins (except vitamin A) normally increase during pregnancy.

It is common for gastric motility to decrease during pregnancy, thereby slowing the passage of food through the gastrointestinal tract and so enhancing the absorption of nutrients. Unfortunately, it may also cause nausea and constipation, and the constipation can cause considerable discomfort in the late stages of pregnancy. A decrease in the secretion of hydrochloric acid into the stomach also normally occurs, which theoretically should depress calcium and iron absorption. Other compensating factors, however, lead to increased absorption of calcium and iron in the last trimester of pregnancy.

Basal metabolic rate increases by 15% to 20% during pregnancy, reflecting the increased energy costs of pregnancy, principally because of the increased work done by the kidneys and heart.

The pregnant woman secretes over 30 hormones that serve to control and integrate all the physiological changes involved in pregnancy. Increased secretion of the hormones progesterone and estrogen and related placental hormones is particularly vital to ensure that pregnancy follows its normal course. Some of the hormonal secretions associated with pregnancy have nutritionally significant effects, in addition to the effects from the growth of the fetus. The following hormones have nutritional effects:

- Aldosterone (the salt-conserving hormone) and cortisone (secreted by the adrenal gland)
- Growth hormone, secreted by the pituitary gland
- Thyroid-stimulating hormone (TSH), which influences the regulation of metabolism by the thyroid gland
- The parathyroid hormone, which controls the metabolism of calcium, phosphorus, and magnesium

PHYSIOLOGICAL STAGES

Pregnancy can be divided into three main physiological stages—**implantation, organogenesis,** and **growth,** each with its own unique nutritional implications.

Implantation

Implantation is the name given to the first 2 weeks of gestation, when the fertilized ovum (or fertilized egg cell) becomes embedded in the wall of the uterus. Throughout this period the developing embryo is nourished by secretions of **uterine milk** from the uterine glands. The nutrients within uterine milk pass directly into the fertilized ovum and developing embryo. About one third of conceptions fail to survive through the implantation stage.

Organogenesis

The next 6 weeks of pregnancy are known as the period of organogenesis, or **embryogenesis,** or the **embryonic period.** During this stage the cells of the embryo begin to differentiate into distinct tissues and functional units that later become organs, such as the heart, lungs, and liver. The development of the skeleton also begins at this time. By the end of organogenesis, all of the major organs have begun to develop, although they mostly perform only minimal functions. During organogenesis the fetus obtains nourishment from the mother's blood and also from degenerating cells in the space between the embryo and the wall of the uterus.

Organogenesis is a particularly vulnerable time for the developing fetus, and the risk of problems from nutritional inadequacy is increased by the possibility that many mothers do not realize they are pregnant at this stage and may experience nausea, which depresses appetite and so limits the intake of nutrients. In such circumstances the previous nutritional history of the mother can be crucial, with a history of good nutrition being associated with significantly less risk to the fetus.

Folic Acid and Pregnancy

The link between supplemental folic acid and a reduced risk of neural tube defects (NTDs) has resulted in a number of governmental and professional organizations issuing statements and recommendations, including the following:

1991	The U.S. Centers for Disease Control recommended that women with a pregnancy previously affected by NTD should take supplements of 4 mg/day of folic acid when they plan to become pregnant again.*
1992	The U.S. Public Health Service recommended that all women capable of becoming pregnant should ingest 400 μg/day of folic acid (about two times the current RDA for nonpregnant, nonlactating women).†
1993	The American College of Obstetricians and Gynecologists recommended that women with a previous pregnancy affected by NTD should be offered treatment with 4 mg/day of folic acid starting 1 month before the time they plan to become pregnant and continuing through the first 3 months of pregnancy. Patients should be advised not to attempt these dosages (10 × RDA during pregnancy) by taking over-the-counter or prescription multivitamins with folic acid, because of the possible harmful levels of other vitamins (e.g., vitamin A)‡
1993	Health Protection Branch of Health and Welfare, Canada, recommended the following: (1) as early as possible when planning a pregnancy, women should consult their physician about folic acid supplements, (2) women with a previous NTD-affected pregnancy are at higher risk of another affected pregnancy, and they should consult their physician about folic acid supplements, and (3) all women of child bearing potential should follow Canada's *Food Guide to Healthy Eating* and take care to choose more foods higher in folate. Some good or excellent food sources of folate include dark green vegetables (e.g., broccoli, spinach, and peas), corn, dried peas, dried beans, lentils, and orange juice.§
1993	*United Kingdom Report of An Expert Advisory Group* recommended that all women with spina bifida or with a previous pregnancy affected by an NTD should be advised to take a supplement of 5 mg/day of folic acid if they wish to become pregnant or are at risk of pregnancy. All other women planning a pregnancy or who suspect they may be pregnant should take 0.4 mg/day as a medicinal or food supplement and should eat more folate-rich food. The expert advisory group also recommended that breads fortified with folic acid should be increased and that major educational programs should be undertaken.‖
1993	The American Academy of Pediatrics (AAP) endorsed the recommendations of the U.S. Centers for Disease Control and the U.S. Public Health Service. The AAP also recommended that the federal government of the United States devise and implement a program, such as food fortification, that will prevent folate-related NTD. The AAP further advised that surveillance with respect to effectiveness and/or adverse outcomes of implemented programs be initiated.¶

* U.S. Centers for Disease Control: *MMWR* 40:513, 1991.
† U.S. Centers for Disease Control: *MMWR* 41:1, 1992.
‡ American College of Obstetricians and Gynecologists Committee on Obstetrics: *Int J Gynecol Obstet* 42:75, 1993.
§ Health Protection Branch, Department of National Health and Welfare: *Can J Public Health* 84:208, 1993.
‖ Scottish Office Home and Health Department, Welsh Office and Department of Health and Social Services: *Report from an expert advisory group, Department of Health,* Letter from chief medical officers of the United Kingdom to Physicians, Nursing Officers, and Directors of Public Health, December 17, 1992.
¶ Committee on Genetics, American Academy of Pediatrics: *Pediatrics* 92:493, 1993.

Evidence from animal studies indicates that the presence of particular nutrients at specific times is crucial for the normal development of various tissues. The evidence suggests that there are **critical periods** of organogenesis, during which the absence of certain nutrients can cause specific congenital abnormalities. For example, riboflavin deficiency during a critical period has been associated with poor skeletal formation, pyridoxine and manganese deficiencies with neuromotor problems, and vitamin B_{12}, vitamin A, niacin, and folate deficiencies with defects in the central nervous system. It has been hard to confirm the role of nutritional deficiency in comparable effects in humans, but they do seem probable if deficiencies continue for long periods.

It has recently become clear that folate is important for the prevention of neural tube defects (NTD) (see Chapter 12), which are the most common congenital malformations in the United States.[4,5] Approximately 2500 to 3000 infants are born with NTD each year in the United States, out of a worldwide total of 300,000

TABLE 14-1

Sequence of developmental changes during pregnancy

STAGE	DEVELOPMENTAL CHANGE
WEEK	
3	Brain development begins
4	Heart functions
	Liver functions
5	Eyes and limbs develop
6	Teeth develop
8	Skeleton mineralization begins
MONTH	
3	Kidney functions
4	Lungs form
5	Fetus kicks and turns
6	Fetus swallows
7	Fetal nervous system controls breathing
8	Subcutaneous fat accumulates
9	Lungs function

FIGURE 14-4

Fetal growth curve.

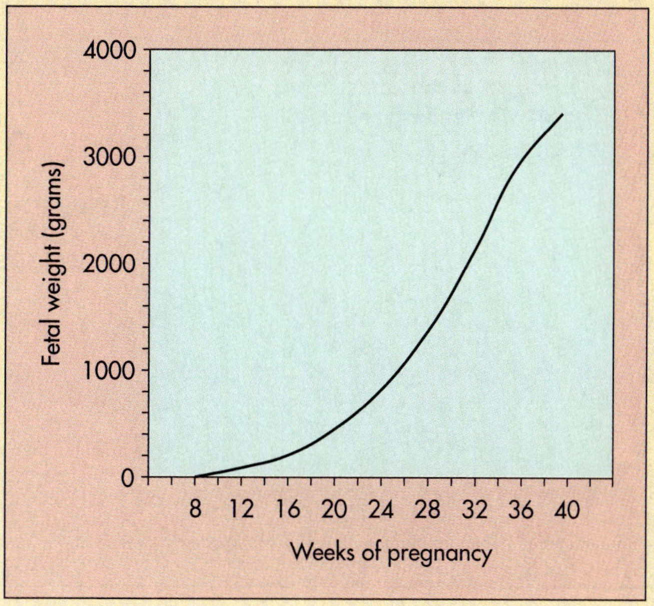

to 400,000 cases. The critical period for the formation of the neural tube is from day 17 to day 30 of pregnancy. The exact cause of NTD is unknown but is undoubtedly complex and involves both genetic and environmental factors. Recent research has demonstrated that ample folate intake can significantly reduce the risk of this form of fetal abnormality. As a result, authorities in several countries have issued statements on folate nutrition and the use of folate supplements before and during pregnancy (see box on p. 514).

When organogenesis is complete, the fetus weighs only about 6 g (0.2 oz) and is little more than 1 inch long. It does, however, have many of the structural and functional features of a newborn infant. The sequence of some key developmental changes during organogenesis is summarized in Table 14-1.

Growth

The remaining 7 months of pregnancy are known as the **growth period.** During this time the tissues and organs formed during organogenesis continue to grow and mature until they are able to sustain the infant's life when it leaves the womb. Most of the nutrients for growth are delivered through the placenta, although some are provided by the portions of amniotic fluid that the infant swallows during the latter part of pregnancy. A typical **fetal growth curve,** summarizing the course of the 500-fold increase in weight during the growth period, is shown in Figure 14-4.

Growth of the fetus occurs in three phases. During the first, known as **hyperplasia,** there is a rapid increase in the *number* of cells. The large numbers of cell divisions (cellular replication) involved require sufficient supplies of folate and vitamin B_{12}, which are both involved in the synthesis of nucleic acids, essential for cell division and cell growth. In the next phase, cellular replication continues with **hypertrophy,** when cells are *growing* in size. This requires sufficient supplies of amino acids and vitamin B_6. In the final phase of growth, hypertrophy or cellular growth predominates, whereas cellular division ceases.

The age at which a particular tissue reaches full maturity after birth varies from 1 year to several years. Nutritional deficiencies during the growth period in the womb and after birth tend to cause low weight and small size, rather than the more serious abnormalities associated with deficiencies at earlier times. Many tissues can function relatively normally with fewer or smaller cells than normal. Also, any depression of growth during a temporary period of undernutrition can be compensated for by increased growth when nutrition becomes adequate again.

The placenta The placenta develops early in pregnancy and begins to play its role in providing nourishment for the fetus. The placenta grows to weigh around 500 to 650 g (1.1 to 1.4 lb) at birth. Blood does not flow directly from the mother's circulation to the fetal circulation. The two independent circulatory systems do come into close enough contact, however, for nutrients to pass from the placenta to the fetus and for wastes to pass from the fetus to the placenta. Altogether, about 10

FIGURE 14-5

Pattern and components of weight gain during pregnancy.

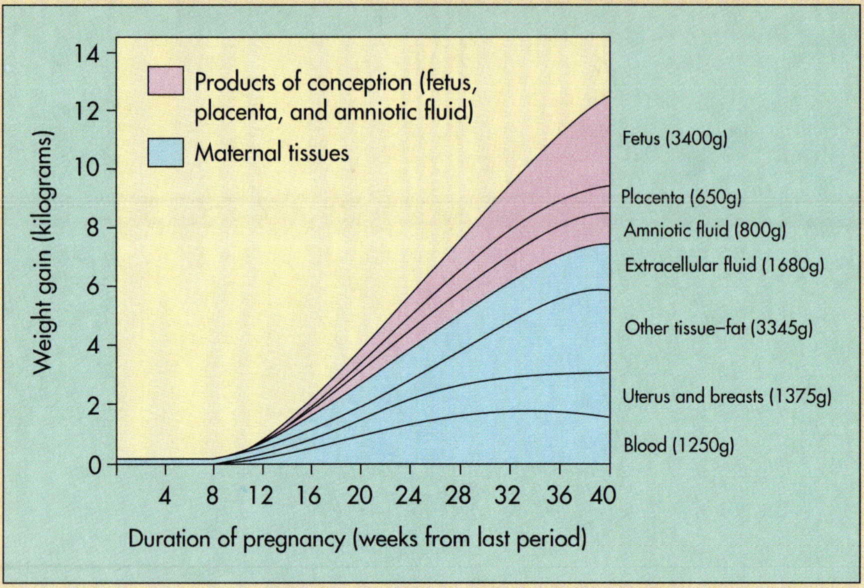

TABLE 14-2

Estimated fetal requirement for selected nutrients near term

NUTRIENT	DAILY REQUIREMENTS
Amino acids	2.2-2.5 g/kg
Calcium	86 mg/kg
Carbohydrate	11.2 g/kg
Energy	43.5 kcal/kg
As carbohydrate	80%
As fat	0%
As amino acids	20%
Fat	0.5 g/kg
Iron	0.9 mg/kg
Magnesium	1.4 mg/kg
Niacin	0.34 mg/kg
Riboflavin	0.02 mg/kg
Thiamin	0.01 mg/kg
Zinc	0.6 mg/kg

From Rosso P: *Nutrition and metabolism in pregnancy: mother and fetus,* New York, 1990, Oxford University Press.

to 11 square meters of surface area are available for the transfer of materials between the placental circulation and that of the fetus.

Free fatty acids and cholesterol can be transferred across the placenta by simple diffusion, carbohydrates (mainly glucose) cross by facilitated diffusion, and amino acids are transferred by active transport. Some proteins can cross the placenta into the fetus by a mechanism that is not well understood but is certainly highly selective. Most water-soluble vitamins are present in the fetal circulation at higher concentrations than in the maternal circulation and so presumably enter the fetus by active transport. Fat-soluble vitamins are present at lower concentrations in the fetus than in the mother and probably enter the fetus by passive diffusion. Both calcium and iron cross the placenta by active transport via mechanisms that are not well understood. Table 14-2 lists the estimated fetal requirement for selected nutrients at the end of pregnancy.

Components of weight gain during pregnancy As can be seen from Figure 14-4, the rate of fetal growth is slow during the first 2 months of pregnancy. By the twenty-fifth week of pregnancy the growth rate rises to about 6 g (0.2 oz)/day, then reaches 40 g (1.4 oz)/day by week 34. It then falls to around 13 g (0.4 oz)/day by the end of pregnancy. The average pattern of weight gain during pregnancy, broken into the individual components, is shown in Figure 14-5. The components of the weight gain during pregnancy can be divided into two general categories: the **products of conception** (the fetus, the amniotic fluid, and the placenta), and the increased amounts of **maternal tissues** (blood, extracellular fluid, uterus, breasts, and fat). The proportion of the total weight gain during pregnancy that can be attributed to each of these components is as follows:

- The fetus: 25% to 27%
- The placenta: 5%
- The amniotic fluid: 6%
- Expansion of blood volume: 10%
- Growth of uterus and breasts: 11%
- Increase in extracellular fluid: 13%
- Increase in maternal fat stores: 25% to 27%

TABLE 14-3

Fetal weight and maternal gains at different stages of pregnancy

AGE (WEEKS)	TOTAL FETAL WEIGHT (g[lb])	MATERNAL GAINS, INCLUDING FETUS (g[lb])
FIRST TRIMESTER		
10	5 (0.01)	650 (1.4)
SECOND TRIMESTER		
20	300 (0.7)	4000 (8.8)
THIRD TRIMESTER		
30	1500 (3.3)	8500 (18.7)
40	3400 (7.5)	12,500 (27.5)

FIGURE 14-6

Fetal weight as a percentage of maternal weight throughout the gestation of six mammalian species.

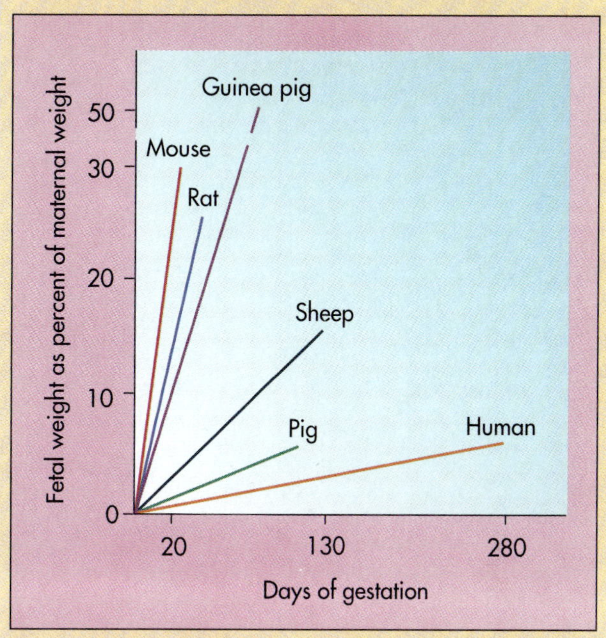

The weight gained during the first trimester (3 months) is almost entirely from growth of maternal tissues. During the second trimester, there are significant gains in both maternal and fetal tissue, and most of the weight gained in the third trimester is from fetal tissue. A women can gain, on average, between 0.335 and 0.45 kg (approximately ¾ to 1 lb)/week during the last half of the pregnancy. A typical weight-gain pattern for a woman in her first pregnancy is as follows:

0 to 10 weeks: 0.065 kg (0.14 lb)/week
10 to 20 weeks: 0.335 kg (0.74 lb)/week
20 to 30 weeks: 0.450 kg (1.0 lb)/week
30 to 40 weeks: 0.335 kg (0.74 lb)/week

Fetal weights at various stages of gestation and the corresponding increases in maternal weight are shown in Table 14-3.

The fact that a human fetus grows relatively slowly means that nutritional deficiencies must be present for a fairly long period to have a measurable effect on the development of the fetus. This contrasts with the situation in many animals used in nutritional investigations, in which a fetus develops quickly and large litters are commonplace (Figure 14-6). For this reason, experimental animals are more vulnerable to short-term nutritional deficiencies.

NUTRITIONAL NEEDS

Table 14-4 compares the recommended dietary allowances (RDAs) for pregnant and lactating women with those of adult, nonpregnant women. The nutritional needs of adolescent pregnant women are even greater than those shown. The percentage of increase in energy requirements is smaller than the percentage of increase in requirements for most nutrients. RDAs for both energy and niacin rise by just 14%, whereas those for other nutrients rise by between 16% and 100%.

For such nutrients as iron and vitamin A the RDA during pregnancy must be sufficient to build up stores within the fetus. Other such nutrients as vitamin D, vitamin C, and calcium are not stored by the fetus in significant amounts, so the RDA need only be sufficient to meet the needs for fetal growth.

Energy

Energy needs during pregnancy increase because of the additional energy required for the following:

- The growth and physical activity of the fetus (requiring 125 kcal/day by the end of pregnancy)
- The growth of the placenta
- The normal increase in maternal body size
- The additional work involved in carrying the weight of the fetus and extra maternal tissues
- The slow but steady rise in basal metabolic rate during pregnancy

On the other hand, any decrease in the mother's normal level of activity—resulting from taking more rest or stopping work, for example—causes some reduction in energy requirements. When all the changes in energy requirements are combined, a pregnant mother usually

TABLE 14-4

Recommended dietary allowances to meet needs of pregnancy and lactation: percentage of increase over those of nonpregnant women

	ADULT WOMEN (25-49 YEARS OF AGE)	PREGNANT WOMEN (THIRD TRIMESTER)	LACTATING MOTHERS*	PERCENTAGE OF INCREASE IN NEED OVER THAT OF NONPREGNANT WOMEN	
				PREGNANT	LACTATING
Energy (kcal)	2200	2500	2700	14	23
Protein (g)	50	60	65	20	30
Vitamin A (RE)	800	800	1300	0	33
Vitamin D (μg)	5	10	10	100	100
Vitamin E (TE, mg)	8	10	12	25	50
Vitamin C (mg)	60	70	95	16	58
Thiamin (mg)	1.1	1.5	1.6	35	45
Riboflavin (mg)	1.3	1.6	1.8	23	38
Niacin (NE, mg)	15	17	20	14	33
Vitamin B_6 (mg)	1.6	2.1	2.1	31	31
Folate (μg)†	(180)	400	(280)	†	†
Vitamin B_{12} (μg)	2	2.2	2.6	10	30
Calcium (mg)	800	1200	1200	50	50
Phosphorus (mg)	800	1200	1200	50	50
Iron (mg)‡	15	30	15	100	0
Zinc (mg)	12	15	19	25	58
Iodine (μg)	150	175	200	16	33
Selenium (μg)	55	65	75	20	36

NE, Niacin equivalent; *RE,* retinol equivalent; *TE,* tocopherol equivalent.

* During the first 6 months of lactation.

† Current recommendation from the U.S. Public Health Service is 400 μg/day for women of childbearing age (see box on p. 511).

‡ The increased iron requirement for pregnancy cannot be met by the usual American diet or from body stores; thus a supplement of 30 to 60 mg of elemental iron is recommended.

requires an additional 85,000 kcal over the 9 months of pregnancy. This is equivalent to an additional 300 kcal/day. If this increased energy need is not met, the mother may develop insufficient fat reserves to sustain a normal and successful period of lactation.

In addition to sustaining lactation, the fat that a mother accumulates during pregnancy acts as an energy reserve for any periods when her food intake is inadequate. If the level of ketones in the urine increases at any time during pregnancy, it suggests that the fat reserves are being depleted to meet the energy needs of the fetus and the mother and to spare protein for tissue growth.

The fetus accumulates no fat stores of its own during the first trimester of pregnancy and at 20 weeks contains only 0.5% fat (largely essential lipids in membranes and the nervous system). From 20 weeks onward, however, the percentage of fat in the fetus rises steadily to reach 16% by the end of pregnancy (Figure 14-7). Fat is synthesized in the fetus from glucose and from fatty acids (especially the essential fatty acids).

FIGURE 14-7

Change in percentage of fat content of the fetus during pregnancy.

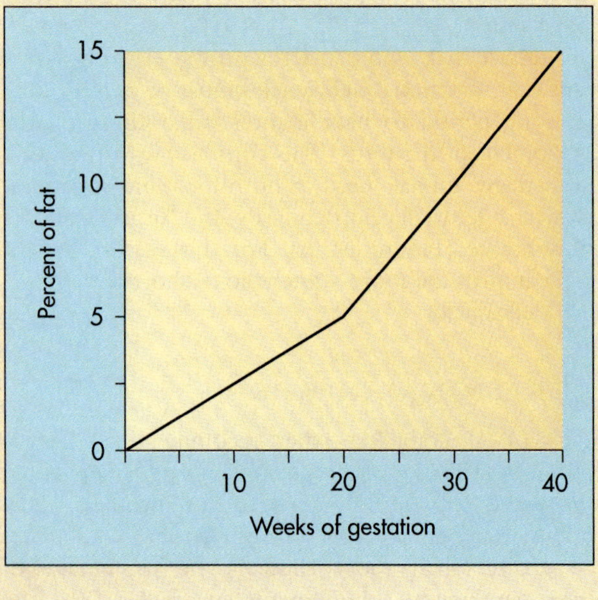

TABLE 14-5

Recommended total weight gain ranges for pregnant women, by prepregnancy body mass index (BMI)*

WEIGHT-FOR-HEIGHT CATEGORY	RECOMMENDED TOTAL GAIN	
	kg	lb
Low (BMI of <19.8)	12.5-18	28-40
Normal (BMI of 19.8-26.0)	11.5-16	25-35
High† (BMI of >26-29)	7-11.5	15-25

Young adolescent and African-American women should strive for gains at the upper end of the recommended range. Short women (<157 cm or 62 in) should strive for gains at the lower end of the range.

* BMI = Weight in kg/(height in m)^2.

† The recommended target weight gain for obese women (BMI of >29.0) is at least 6 kg (13 lb).

From National Academy of Sciences: *Nutrition during pregnancy: weight gain and nutrient supplements,* Washington, DC, 1990, National Academy Press.

Maternal Weight Gain

Recommendations on appropriate maternal weight gain have changed markedly over the past 60 years. In the early part of the century, unrestricted weight gain in pregnancy was widely encouraged, based on the logic that the mother was "eating for two." Various problems were eventually found to be associated with this advice, including difficulties of pregnancy and labor, **preeclampsia** (see p. 527), hypertension, and the birth of large infants prone to many health complications in early life. The next recommendation, popular in the 1940s and 1950s, was that energy intake should be restricted sufficiently to limit the total weight gain to between 10 and 15 lb (4 to 6 kg). This resulted in equally undesirable consequences, including IUGR and an increased risk of death during the first year of the infant's life. Current recommendations, calling for a weight gain of between 15 and 40 lb, are based on a better understanding of the physiology of pregnancy and the relationships between maternal size, weight gain, and fetal health.[6,7]

Recommended weight gains are highest for thin women and lowest for obese, overweight, and short women.[6] The Subcommittee on Nutritional Status and Weight Gain During Pregnancy of the U.S. National Academy of Sciences has recommended that all pregnant women have their body mass index (BMI) calculated when they first seek medical supervision. Their recommended weight gain during pregnancy is then based on their weight-for-height classification (Table 14-5). The recommended weight gain for a woman with normal prepregnancy BMI is 11.5 to 16 kg (25 to 35 lb). This is higher than the gain previously recommended by the National Academy of Sciences because of evidence that the higher value is associated with less risk of bearing an infant with IUGR. A higher weight gain range (12.5 to 18 kg [28 to 40 lb]) is recommended for women with low prepregnancy BMI, and a lower range (7 to 11.5 kg[15 to 25 lb]) is recommended for those with high prepregnancy BMI. Short women should aim for the lower end of whatever target range their BMI places them in, whereas African-American and very young women should strive to reach the upper end of their weight gain range. The recommended target weight gain range for women carrying twins is 16 to 20.5 kg (35 to 45 lb).

The rate of weight gain is as important as the total amount of weight gained. It is recommended that women of normal prepregnancy weight gain 0.4 kg (1 lb)/week in the second and third trimesters of pregnancy. Underweight women should try to gain 0.5 kg/week, whereas those who are overweight should limit their weight gain to 0.3 kg/week.

All of these recommendations are based on a large body of evidence suggesting that weight gain in pregnancy (especially during the second and third trimesters) is important for optimal growth of the fetus.

On average, each birth causes a woman's postpartum (after birth) weight to rise by 1 kg (2.2 lb) more than the normal weight gain with age.[6] The actual value for some women who gain excessive weight during pregnancy may be considerably greater than this average figure.

A weight-reducing program should never be undertaken during pregnancy, even by obese women. A reduction in energy intake to 50% of the recommended amount during the second and third trimesters of pregnancy causes a reduction in infant birth weight of about 330 g. If the energy restriction is limited to the third trimester of pregnancy, the birth weight is reduced by about 120 g.[8]

Protein

Recommendations for protein intake during pregnancy take into account the following factors:

- The estimated 925 g of protein (3.3 g/day) deposited during pregnancy in the fetal, placental, and maternal tissue
- An estimated twofold increase in nitrogen retention during pregnancy (indicated by nitrogen balance studies)
- Evidence suggesting that pregnant women with protein intakes higher than their estimated needs have more successful pregnancies
- Evidence linking low protein intakes with increased risks of problems during pregnancy

As a result, the U.S. RDAs for protein during pregnancy include an additional 10 g of protein per day, making a total RDA of 60 g. The World Health Organization (WHO), on the other hand, suggests only an additional 6 g of protein per day, which is an average of the estimated additional needs during the first, second, and third trimesters of pregnancy. In the United States most women consume more protein than the RDA during pregnancy (60 g/day), even when not pregnant.

Amino acids derived from ingested protein are transferred to the fetus to be used for the synthesis of fetal proteins. For the first 20 weeks of pregnancy, all amino acids needed for protein synthesis must be provided by the mother. After 20 weeks, the fetal liver becomes able to synthesize some of the nonessential amino acids for itself. About 20% of the amino acids transferred to the fetus are oxidized to provide energy, rather than being used for protein synthesis.

About half of the 1 kg of protein gained by a mother during pregnancy is in the fetal tissues. Most of the additional protein in maternal tissues is accumulated early in pregnancy, during the growth of the uterus, placenta, and mammary glands. If protein intake is restricted during pregnancy, the amount stored in the mother's body, rather than the amount transferred to the fetus, is reduced. However, the protein intake of the mother does influence the extent to which the infant achieves its potential birth length.

Severe protein restriction during pregnancy is associated with a decrease in the number of cells in a newborn infant's tissues. This is particularly serious in the brain, which can be irreversibly stunted by a prenatal protein deficiency. Other tissues that grow to a smaller proportion of their mature size during pregnancy are not as seriously affected. Protein and energy deficiencies during gestation can also result in poor use of food by the infant after birth.

Minerals

Calcium An infant's bones are poorly calcified at birth, but teeth begin to calcify at 5 months of gestation, and an appreciable amount of calcium is involved in fetal development. About 7 mg of calcium per day is required during the first trimester, rising to 110 mg/day in the second trimester and reaching 350 mg/day in the third trimester. Overall, the mother transfers about 30 g of calcium to her infant before birth. A well-nourished woman has more than 1000 g of stored calcium on which to draw, and the efficiency with which she absorbs calcium normally increases twofold during pregnancy. It is estimated that only 9 g of the 30 g of calcium provided to the fetus comes from the stores in the mother's bones. To minimize a pregnant woman's risk of developing osteoporosis in later life, her diet should contain reasonable amounts of calcium, no excessive amounts of phytic acid, and adequate vitamin D.

Iron Infants are born with high hemoglobin levels of 18 to 22 g/dl of blood and with a supply of iron stored in the liver sufficient to last for 3 to 6 months. To achieve these levels, the mother must transfer about 200 to 370 mg of iron to the fetus during gestation. In addition to the iron needed for transfer to the fetus, the pregnant woman requires additional iron for the formation of the placenta (30 to 170 mg), for the formation of the hemoglobin required by the expansion of blood volume (450 mg), and to compensate for the loss of blood during delivery (250 mg). Most of the iron used to make additional hemoglobin to cope with the expanded blood volume during pregnancy is eventually returned to the maternal stores. Once this is taken into account, the total requirement for iron over the course of pregnancy amounts to about 840 mg. In principle, the mother's iron stores could supply a total of up to 300 mg of iron during pregnancy, but unfortunately, many young women enter pregnancy with practically no reserves of iron. Each day, the diet or maternal stores must supply approximately 3 mg of iron.

The efficiency of iron absorption increases from 10% to 30% in the second half of pregnancy. To maintain maternal reserves and meet the needs of the fetus, the Food and Nutrition Board suggests that the RDA of 15 mg for nonpregnant women should be supplemented with an additional 15 mg of elemental iron during pregnancy. The National Academy of Sciences recommends supplements providing 30 mg of iron per day (beginning after 12 weeks of pregnancy) to prevent the depletion of maternal stores and the development of iron deficiency in the mother.[6] Iron deficiency in the mother does not lead to a deficiency in her infant but may increase the risk of LBW, premature delivery, or perinatal mortality.

Sodium The sodium required by the fetus, amniotic fluid, and the increase in maternal extracellular fluid during pregnancy increases the mother's requirement for sodium by 70 mg/day. As this increased need for sodium becomes accepted, obstetricians are abandoning the long-standing practice of advising pregnant women to restrict their sodium intake. The advice to restrict sodium intake was to help prevent hypertension induced by pregnancy, but sodium is apparently so important that if dietary intake is restricted, a variety of compensating hormonal and biochemical changes help conserve sodium in the mother's body.[9] When blood sodium levels first begin to fall, the kidneys produce more of the hormone renin, which initiates a series of responses that lead to increased conservation of sodium. If this mechanism fails or is insufficient, a deficiency of sodium develops and causes increased risk of eclampsia, premature delivery, and LBW. Because sodium intake in the United States is usually high (at 5 to 10 g/day), however, pregnant women are advised to continue their usual sodium intake, rather than either increasing or decreasing it.

Because diuretics cause increased loss of sodium, their use during pregnancy should be discouraged. The use of salt substitutes should also be discouraged because there is only limited information available about their effects on pregnant women.

Iodine Iodine deficiency before and during pregnancy can result in cretinism in the infant. There is also evidence that maternal iodine deficiencies that are not severe enough to cause cretinism can cause impaired motor and cognitive function in children.[10] Intakes of iodine that are sufficient to prevent goiter under normal circumstances frequently prove inadequate during pregnancy, leading to goiter in the mother (especially if she is adolescent). When the mother has goiter, the chances that the infant will develop goiter are increased tenfold. In Western countries the use of iodine-containing dough conditioners, colorings, and sterilizing materials in food processing is increasing, making the likelihood of iodine deficiency small. If a developing fetus is exposed to excessive amounts of iodine, this can also produce goiter, hypothyroidism, and damage to the hair.[11]

Zinc A total of 100 mg of zinc is estimated to accumulate within fetal and maternal tissues during pregnancy, at a rate that reaches 0.7 mg/day during the last trimester.[12] Assuming 25% absorption, approximately 3 mg of additional dietary zinc per day is required during the last trimester, in addition to the 12 mg RDA for nonpregnant and nonlactating women. The efficiency of zinc absorption is known to increase in pregnant rats, but it is unknown whether this also occurs in humans. Typical zinc intakes in pregnancy range between 9 and 14 mg/day, apart from those of vegetarians, whose intakes are lower.

Several cases of severe zinc deficiency in pregnancy are known to have resulted from inadequate treatment of **acrodermatitis enteropatica,** a hereditary impairment of zinc absorption. These cases were associated with a high incidence of obstetric complications and congenital malformations in the infants. It is unknown how common mild zinc deficiency is during pregnancy or what problems it may cause. Some reports have associated low plasma zinc levels in pregnancy with prolonged labor, pregnancy-induced hypertension, congenital malformations, and IUGR. Different studies in this area have produced inconsistent results, however, and most trials of zinc supplementation during pregnancy have had little or no impact on the course and outcome of the pregnancies.[6]

Giving pregnant women more than 60 mg of iron per day appears to interfere with the absorption of zinc and to depress plasma zinc levels. For this reason, large doses of supplemental iron should be avoided during pregnancy. If pregnant women take more than 30 mg of iron per day, they should also take supplemental zinc every day.

Other minerals Little work has been done to quantify the needs for other minerals during pregnancy. It seems reasonable to suppose that the adaptations of the body to pregnancy include increased efficiency of absorption and decreased excretion sufficient to cover some, if not all, of the additional mineral needs.

Low levels of copper, magnesium, and manganese have all been associated with defects in fetal development in animals. Excessively high levels of various minerals can also have adverse effects. The levels of minerals used to produce these adverse effects in animal studies far exceed the amounts found in normal diets, but such studies provide a warning of the dangers of excessive use of mineral supplements.

Fat-Soluble Vitamins

Although it is well established that adaptive mechanisms improve the body's use of minerals during pregnancy, there is no evidence of similar mechanisms for adapting to vitamin needs.

Vitamin A Animals consuming diets deficient in vitamin A are less likely to conceive and bear young, but little is known about the need for vitamin A during pregnancy. Excessive intakes of vitamin A during pregnancy can cause birth defects. Daily intakes as low as 7500 retinol equivalents (RE) during the first trimester have been shown to produce congenital abnormalities.

If the mother is adequately nourished and two thirds of her vitamin A intake is preformed vitamin A, her infant will be born with a reserve of vitamin A in the liver, even if the mother did not increase her vitamin A intake during pregnancy.

Vitamin D The need for vitamin D during pregnancy is estimated to be 10 μg (400 IU)/day, which is twice the RDA for the nonpregnant adult female. Both active forms of vitamin D readily cross the placenta to play an active role in the metabolism of calcium in the fetus. Because all milk, except buttermilk, is fortified with 400 IU/qt, mothers who consume enough milk to meet their calcium needs do not need an additional source of vitamin D. Excessive consumption of vitamin D during pregnancy should be avoided because of the possibility of inducing fetal hypercalcemia.

Vitamin E Vitamin E has been shown to promote normal reproduction and reduce the incidence of spontaneous abortion and stillbirth in animal studies, but so far no similar role in human reproduction has been firmly established. There is some evidence, however, that vitamin E may be of benefit to women who have experienced difficulty in conceiving or had repeated spontaneous abortions. Although the evidence supporting an important role for vitamin E in human pregnancy is not clear-cut, an additional 2 mg/day (bringing total intake to 10 mg/day) is recommended throughout pregnancy. This requirement appears to be met by a balanced diet, however, so there is little likelihood of a deficiency, unless the diet contains unusually high amounts of polyunsaturated fatty acids (PUFA). Because only small amounts of vitamin E cross the placenta, human infants have low tissue concentrations of this vitamin that persist for at least the first 6 years of life.

Vitamin K Vitamin K, which is necessary for the normal coagulation of blood, is involved in preventing **neonatal hemorrhaging** (bleeding soon after birth). For a time it became routine practice to give oral doses of menadione (synthetic vitamin K) to mothers in the last few weeks in pregnancy, and it was sometimes given by injection during labor. The inclusion of menadione in over-the-counter supplements for pregnancy is prohibited, but safe protection can be provided by the use of oral or injected natural vitamin K given either to the mother before birth or to the infant immediately after birth.

Water-Soluble Vitamins

Because there is little storage of water-soluble vitamins, pregnant women must rely on their daily intakes to meet all their needs. In general, the concentrations of the water-soluble vitamins in a pregnant woman's blood fall from their levels before pregnancy in part because of the increase in the mother's blood volume. However, the concentrations of these vitamins in the fetus tend to exceed those in the mother's blood by 50% to 100%.

> During pregnancy, water-soluble nutrients that are normally reabsorbed by the kidneys begin to be excreted in the urine in substantial amounts. This "renal squandering" of nutrients makes the mother's dietary needs for the nutrients greater than they would otherwise be.

Thiamin An additional intake of 0.4 mg of thiamin is recommended during pregnancy, making a total RDA of 1.5 mg/day. The relationship between thiamin needs and energy intake is believed to apply as normal during pregnancy. The urinary excretion of thiamin drops, however, indicating that more of the vitamin is being retained by the body. In some cases, supplementary thiamin can help relieve the nausea associated with pregnancy.

Riboflavin The increase in maternal body weight and the growth of the fetus and accessory tissues produce an increased need for riboflavin during pregnancy. An additional 0.3 mg/day is recommended, making a total of 1.6 mg/day. Riboflavin is present at higher levels in fetal blood than in maternal blood. Studies in animals have revealed that riboflavin deficiency interferes with the formation of cartilage, resulting in skeletal malformations, such as shortening of the long bones and fusion of the ribs.

Vitamin B_6 During pregnancy, vitamin B_6 is transferred to the fetus to maintain concentrations in fetal blood that are much higher than the concentrations in maternal blood. The RDA for pregnant women is set at 1.6 mg/day, which is 0.6 mg more than the RDA for nonpregnant adult women.

Pyridoxine has been used experimentally to help control the nausea and vomiting of pregnancy. It is unknown how this effect might be brought about, and it appears to be helpful only in some women. Pyridoxine levels of about one third of normal have been found in those with pregnancy-induced hypertension.

Women who have used oral contraceptives often enter pregnancy with low tissue levels of pyridoxine. There is no evidence that this affects the outcome of their pregnancy, but it can reduce the amount of pyridoxine in the mother's milk.

Folate As previously discussed, adequate folate nutrition before conception and in the early stages of pregnancy is required for the prevention of NTDs in infants. Later in pregnancy, folate is involved in promoting normal fetal growth and preventing macrocytic anemia of pregnancy. Adequate folate nutrition offers protection against other complications of pregnancy, including premature detachment of the placenta (**abruptio placentae**), hemorrhage, LBW, and fetal malformation.

It is logical to expect folate needs to increase during pregnancy because it is involved in the synthesis of deoxyribonucleic acid (DNA) and ribonucleic acid (RNA), which are required for cell division, growth, and the development of red blood cells. The RDA for folate during pregnancy is 400 μg/day. The U.S. Public Health Service and similar agencies in other developed countries have begun to recommend that all women capable of becoming pregnant should consume 400 μg of folate per day, rather than the RDA of 180 μg/day because many pregnancies are unplanned and folate is important in the earliest stage of pregnancy. Although it is possible to obtain the recommended amount of folate from a well-planned diet, a supplement of 300 μg can be used to ensure adequate intake.[6] Consuming sufficient folate is especially important for women who have had many pregnancies, who have suffered from chronic hemolytic anemia, or who are taking anticonvulsant drugs.

Once folate has been transferred into the fetus, it is converted to a form that cannot be returned to the mother. This ensures that fetal folate will not be depleted to meet the mother's needs at any later stage of the pregnancy.

TABLE 14-6

Comparison of dietary standards during pregnancy

	WHO/FAO*	UNITED STATES†	UNITED KINGDOM‡	CANADA§
Energy (kcal)	2485	2500	2510	2200
Protein (g)	56	60	49	75
Calcium (g)	1-1.2	1.2	1.25	1.3
Iron (mg)	‖	30	14.8	23
Vitamin A (μg RE)	600	800	700	800
Vitamin D (μg)	10	10	10	5
Thiamin (mg)	0.9	1.5	0.9	0.9
Riboflavin (mg)	1.4	1.6	1.4	1.3
Pyridoxine (mg)	No recommendation	2.2	1.2	No recommendation
Folate (μg)	470	400	300	385
Vitamin B_{12} (μg)	1.4	2.2	1.5	1.2
Vitamin C (mg)	50	70	50	40
Zinc (mg)	7.5	15	7	15

* From World Health Organization/Food and Agriculture Organization: *Diet, nutrition and the prevention of chronic diseases.* Report of a WHO study group Technical Report Series No 797, Geneva, Switzerland, 1990, World Health Organization.

† From Food and Nutrition Board, National Research Council: *Recommended dietary allowances,* ed 10, Washington, DC, 1989, National Academy Press.

‡ From *Dietary reference values for food, energy and nutrients for the United Kingdom,* Report of the Panel on Dietary Reference Values of the Committee on Medical Aspects of Food Policy, Report on Health and Social Subjects No 41, London, 1991, Her Majesty's Stationery Office.

§ From Health and Welfare Canada: *Nutrition recommendations,* The Report of the Scientific Review Committee, Ottawa, Canada, 1990, Supply and Services Canada.

‖ Recommended amount depends on iron status before pregnancy. The recommended intake for the nonreproducing adult woman is 2.5 mg of absorbed iron per day.

Strangely, there is a notable decrease in the efficiency of folate absorption and an increase in the rate of urinary excretion of folate during pregnancy.[12] This is probably an important factor in making folate deficiency a major cause for concern in pregnancy and making pregnancy the major cause of folate deficiency worldwide. There is evidence that iron deficiency can impose additional stress on folate metabolism, perhaps converting a subclinical folate deficiency into one with obvious clinical signs.

Vitamin B_{12} Vitamin B_{12} is absorbed more efficiently during pregnancy, and a large amount of the vitamin is transferred to the fetus. The level of vitamin B_{12} in fetal blood rises to twice the level in the maternal blood. The RDA for vitamin B_{12} during pregnancy is 4 μg/day.

Vitamin C The recommended allowance for vitamin C is increased by 10 mg during pregnancy. Vitamin C passes the placental barrier freely, and serum values of a fetus have been established as being two to four times those of the mother. There is some evidence that the placenta can synthesize vitamin C, which could account for higher levels in fetal tissues. Low maternal intakes of vitamin C are associated with the premature rupture of fetal membranes and increased neonatal death rates.

A comparison of the recommended dietary intakes during pregnancy, as suggested for different countries and shown in Table 14-6, makes it clear that, for some nutrients, such as calcium and riboflavin, there is fairly close agreement. For others, the differences are up to twofold, indicating that more data are needed.

Water Although we tend to rely on our sense of thirst to guide us to consume sufficient fluid, the pregnant woman must be encouraged to pay particular attention to her practices. It is recommended that she have at least 8 cups/day to ensure that her water intake is sufficient to facilitate digestion and absorption of nutrients, the elimination of metabolic waste through the kidneys, and lubrication of fecal material in the colon. The pregnant woman should choose fluids that contribute to overall nutrient needs.

ROLE OF NUTRITIONAL SUPPLEMENTS

Recommended dietary intakes during pregnancy call for increases over normal needs, ranging from 10% for vitamin B_{12} to 100% for iron and vitamin D. At the same time, it is suggested that energy intake be increased by only 300 kcal—approximately 14% to 15% (typical woman, 2000 to 2200 kcal)—above normal for most women. Therefore, to meet added needs for pregnancy and not exceed energy needs, it is absolutely essential to have foods of high nutrient density.

The selection of an adequate diet for pregnancy is relatively easy if we are concerned with an isolated day or two, but the pregnant woman must maintain a high level of nutritive intake for the normal gestation period of 280

TABLE 14-7

Recommended composition of multivitamin and mineral supplements for pregnant women

MINERAL	REQUIREMENT
Calcium	250 mg
Copper	2 mg
Folate	300 μg
Iron	30 mg
Vitamin B_6	2 mg
Vitamin C	50 mg
Vitamin D	5 μg
Zinc	15 mg

These are recommendations for supplements beginning in the second trimester. To promote absorption of these nutrients, the supplement should be taken between meals or at bedtime.

From Institute of Medicine, National Academy of Sciences: *Nutrition during pregnancy: weight gain and nutrient supplements,* Washington, DC, 1990, National Academy Press.

days. To do this, she must constantly be aware of her food choices. Taking this responsibility may result in extra pressure during a period that, for some women, is already characterized by some degree of emotional stress. To allow women a little more freedom in the selection of foods and an occasional indulgence in a favorite low-nutrient food, it is reasonable to suggest the use of a supplement that provides a balanced formula at protective levels. The recommended composition of a prenatal supplement for women who do not normally consume an adequate diet and those at nutritional risk is presented in Table 14-7.[6]

Iron supplements are recommended during pregnancy (30 mg/day),[6] and when hemoglobin levels drop below 10.5 to 11.0 g/dl, the recommended dose is increased to 60 to 120 mg/day.[6] The recommended dosage is decreased to 30 mg/day when hemoglobin concentration is in the recommended range. Ferrous fumarate, sulfate, and gluconate are most frequently recommended (Table 14-8). Because high levels of calcium or magnesium in supplements may interfere with the absorption of iron, the supplement should not contain excessive amounts of calcium and magnesium. Supplements that have therapeutic amounts of iron (more than 30 mg) should also contain zinc (15 mg) and copper (2 mg) because high levels of iron may interfere with the absorption or use of these trace minerals.

It is possible for some pregnant women to adapt their diets to provide a wide range of nutrients needed during the stress of pregnancy that nutritional supplementation is not necessary. This is especially true if they enter pregnancy in good nutritional health and do not suffer from nausea of pregnancy. However, supplements of iron, folate, and vitamin B_6 (for long-term users of oral contraceptives) are usually suggested. For

TABLE 14-8

Iron content of common supplements

		AMOUNT NEEDED TO PROVIDE	
	FE CONTENT	15 mg FE	30 mg FE
Ferrous fumarate	32%	47 mg	95 mg
Ferrous sulfate	20%	75 mg	150 mg
Ferrous gluconate	12%	125 mg	250 mg

complete vegetarians (those who consume no animal products), daily supplementation with 2 μg of vitamin B_{12} per day is recommended, with 400 IU or 10 μg of vitamin D per day and 600 mg of calcium per day.

DIETARY MODIFICATIONS

Selecting a diet to meet the nutritional needs of pregnancy is not particularly complicated, but it does require careful choice of foods. If the diet conforms to the guidance in the Food Guide Pyramid, it is necessary simply to choose the more nutrient-dense foods from each of the food groups. Women who have not followed the recommendations of the Food Guide Pyramid before pregnancy need to develop a substantially altered diet that follows the recommendations and is adequate in all nutrients. This is particularly important because their stores of some key nutrients may be at inadequate levels. Mothers who have experienced problems with earlier pregnancies—such as miscarriage, premature delivery, or LBW infants—should take particular care to select an appropriate diet during any subsequent pregnancy.

Nutrition is only one of many factors that determine the health of an infant, but it is one of the few significant factors over which the mother has complete control. Pregnancy is perhaps the best time to attempt nutrition education, because most mothers are motivated to "eat right" for the benefit of their developing child. There are many ways to select an adequate diet both during pregnancy and at other times, but the Daily Food Guide for Women, prepared by the California Department of Health, is one plan that is suitable for many different women in a variety of cultures (Table 14-9).

From the fifth to the fourteenth week of pregnancy, 50% to 70% of women experience some nausea and even vomiting because of hormonal changes within their bodies. The consumption of smaller and more frequent meals can help to reduce these problems for many women. This practice is also useful in the latter part of pregnancy, when large meals can cause discomfort because of the crowding of the abdomen by the presence of the fetus and accessory tissues.

Between the fourth and seventh months of pregnancy, many women experience an insatiable appetite.

TABLE 14-9

Daily food guide for women

FOOD GROUP	NONPREGNANT (11-24 YEARS)	NONPREGNANT (25-50 YEARS)	PREGNANT/LACTATING (11-50 YEARS)
Protein foods*	5	5	7
Milk products†	3	2	3
Bread, cereals, and grains‡	7	6	7
Whole grain	4	4	4
Enriched	3	2	3
Fruits and vegetables§			
Vitamin C–rich	1	1	1
Vitamin A–rich	1	1	1
Other	3	3	3
Unsaturated fats ‖	3	3	3

* Each serving from this group provides about 6 g of protein. In addition to protein, these foods are generally good sources of vitamin B_6, iron, and zinc. Animal sources of protein provide generous amounts of folate, magnesium, and fiber. A serving of an animal source of protein is 1 oz of cooked, boneless meat, and a serving of vegetable protein is ½ cup of cooked legumes, 2 Tbsp of peanut butter, ⅓ cup of nuts, or ¼ cup of seeds.

† Each serving from the milk group provides at least 250 mg of calcium. Fluid milk provides vitamin D. In addition, these foods are good sources of protein, riboflavin, and vitamins A, B_6, and B_{12}, and they supply some magnesium and zinc. A serving is 1 cup fluid milk, 6 to 8 oz of yogurt, or 1½ cup of ice cream.

‡ The bread, cereals, and grains group is divided into whole grain and enriched products. Whole grain products provide significantly more fiber, vitamin B_6, folate, magnesium, and zinc than do the enriched products. At least four of the minimum daily servings should be whole grain products. A serving is one slice of bread; ½ cup cooked cereal, rice, or pasta; ¾ cup of ready-to-eat cereal; or a small roll, muffin, or biscuit.

§ Fruits and vegetables are broken down into three groups: vitamin C–rich, vitamin A–rich, and others. Most are good sources of fiber and provide variable amounts of vitamins and minerals. A serving is 6 oz of juice, one average piece of whole fruit, ¼ of a melon, ½ cup of sliced or cooked fruit or vegetable, or 1 cup of raw leafy vegetables.

‖ These oils are good sources of vitamin E and the essential fatty acids. A serving is 1 tsp of vegetable oil or its approximate equivalent in kilocalories and fat (e.g., salad dressing).

Modified from Maternal and Child Health Branch: *Nutrition during pregnancy and the postpartum period,* Sacramento, 1990, California Department of Health Services.

During this period they can help control their food intake by eating a small meal just before the times when the hunger usually becomes most severe. It is important to try to maintain intake at a level that results in a steady weight gain of about 400 g/week (for women of normal prepregnancy weight) throughout the second and third trimesters. A diet that is relatively high in bulk and fluid may help in maintaining normal gastric motility at a time when there is a tendency toward constipation.

The selection of an appropriate diet during pregnancy is complicated because many women experience strong cravings and dislikes for certain foods. They often crave foods that they did not previously like and develop a strong dislike for foods they previously liked. In some cases the aroma or sight of a food (even a photograph) can evoke a strong reaction. The dislikes often develop for foods that are of no nutritional significance. If a dislike develops for nutritionally important foods, such as milk, the most reliable source of calcium, this can be of great concern. Similarly, most cravings cause few nutritional problems because they are for foods of nutritional value. If the craving is for energy-dense foods such as chocolate cake and ice cream, however, their consumption may restrict the intake of more nutritionally beneficial foods.

Some mothers develop the habit of **pica,** the eating of such nonfood items as dirt, paint chips, laundry starch, library paste, ice cubes, and clay. Nobody knows the physiological or psychological reasons for this, but it seems to occur most often in people who are deficient in iron. Some of the materials consumed, such as paint chips, may contain toxic substances (such as lead), whereas others (such as clay and starch) may contain ingredients that interfere with iron absorption.[13]

EFFECT OF NUTRITION ON OUTCOME OF PREGNANCY

The nutritional status of women when they conceive is considered to be as, if not more, important to the outcome of the pregnancy as is their diet during pregnancy. Nutritional status at conception is likely to reflect long-standing eating habits. Relatively few women are found to drastically alter these long-standing habits once they become pregnant.

The effect of the mother's diet before pregnancy is illustrated by data on infants born during periods of wartime starvation in the Netherlands and Russia.[14] The Netherlands study found that infants born during the period of starvation but conceived when their mothers' nutrition had been good were less likely to be stillborn, delivered prematurely, or have congenital malformation than infants both born and conceived during a period of starvation. This indicates the protective effect of a good diet before conception. Mothers whose infants were born during the siege of Leningrad in Russia and whose diets had been poor both before conception and throughout pregnancy produced twice the normal rate of stillbirths, a 41% incidence of premature delivery among live births, and a 31% increase in neonatal deaths among LBW infants. A reduced rate of conception was also found in these women.

Many studies have investigated the effects of nutrition during the course of pregnancy on the condition of the infant. Interpreting such studies is made difficult by the presence of a great many other variable factors, including age, number of previous pregnancies, interval between pregnancies, socioeconomic status, smoking and drinking habits, and the use of herbal teas, which may all have an influence on a pregnancy (see box). Some of the landmark studies are considered below.

One of the first studies to indicate a relationship between an infant's health and its mother's diet was performed by Burke and others.[15] This revealed that the chance of an infant's being born in a healthy condition was significantly greater when the mother's diet was rated as good or excellent than when it was rated as poor or very poor. Ebbs and his colleagues[16] then found a similar relationship, with Canadian mothers on good diets experiencing few complications during pregnancy and giving birth to infants who were more likely to survive the neonatal period than those born to mothers on poorer diets. Some time after these two studies, however, researchers at Vanderbilt University failed to demonstrate any relationship between the quality of maternal diet and the course and outcome of pregnancy.[17] They suggested that complications in some pregnancies might be causing a lowering in the quality of some mothers' diets, rather than preexisting poor diets causing the problems in pregnancy. None of the subjects in their study had a notably poor diet, however, and the subjects may have entered pregnancy with sufficiently good nutritional status to provide a buffer against the nutritional stress of pregnancy.

In 1959 a study in Britain by Thomson[18] did not detect any relationship between diet and the duration of gestation, fetal malformation, perinatal death, or failure of lactation. This study did, however, find a positive correlation between birth weight and maternal energy intake, although not when women of similar mean weight were compared. These conclusions were interpreted as indicating that abnormalities of reproduction were not caused by dietary deficiencies. They cannot, however, be used to suggest that dietary inadequacies are never responsible for abnormalities of pregnancy.

A widely publicized and highly controversial study in New York City that was published in 1982 assessed the effect on birth weight of dietary supplementation for women at high risk of reproductive complications.[19] The study failed to demonstrate any beneficial effect from daily consumption of a supplementary beverage providing 6 or 40 g of protein and 320 or 470 kcal of energy. However, a higher rate of premature births and neonatal deaths were found in the group receiving the supplement providing 40 g of protein and 470 kcal. This was possibly associated with a higher rate of intrauterine infection. The mothers taking the supplements gained more weight than did those who were not. The dietary supplement did overcome the adverse effects of smoking on the outcome of the pregnancies.

Factors that may Contribute to a Poor Course and Outcome of Pregnancy

- Being underweight or overweight before pregnancy
- Inadequate or excessive weight gain during pregnancy
- Anemia
- Inadequate expansion of plasma volume during pregnancy
- Previous pregnancy complications
- Adolescence
- A maternal age over 35 years
- A short interval between pregnancies
- High parity (large number of births)
- Existing medical complications (diabetes, hypertension, kidney disease, thyroid disease, etc.)
- Low socioeconomic status
- Substance abuse (alcohol, tobacco, recreational/street drugs, over-the-counter drugs, herbal remedies, excessive use of nutrient supplements, etc.)
- Pica
- Psychological problems
- Poor diet

Modified from Maternal and Child Health Branch: *Nutrition during pregnancy and the postpartum period,* Sacramento, 1990, California Department of Health Services.

The relationship between maternal nutrition, assessed on the basis of weight gain during pregnancy, and the outcome of pregnancy was evaluated in 1980 in a sample of 3581 U.S. women.[19] Maternal weight gain of 26 to 35 lb was found to be inversely correlated with the incidence of LBW deliveries and fetal mortality. In pregnant women gaining more than 35 lb, however, an increase in the incidence of LBW deliveries and fetal mortality was found. These results suggest that weight gain during pregnancy that is either below or above the optimal range can increase the chances of LBW at delivery and infant mortality. It was of particular concern that this study found that 23% of pregnant women in the United States (in 1980) gained less than 21 lb during pregnancy and 12% gained fewer than 16 lb. African-American women were 50% more likely than were white women to gain less than 21 lb, and 100% more likely to gain less than 16 lb. Overall, this study indicated that indiscriminate supplementation of pregnant women, who as a group were not chronically undernourished, had no effect on birth weight. A recent reanalysis of the data, however, found that supplementation of those women who were undernourished did have a positive effect on birth length and head circumference.[20]

An analysis by the Montreal Diet Dispensary of the use of dietary supplements in pregnancy found that mothers receiving supplements of milk, orange juice, and eggs, along with dietary counseling, gave birth to slightly larger infants. Supplements proved less effective, however, in women who had previously borne LBW infants.

An evaluation of the federally funded **Women, Infants and Children (WIC)** program investigated the impact of providing vouchers for food supplements (iron-fortified cereal, milk, cheese, eggs, and fruit) to women classified as nutritionally at risk and in low-income families. It detected an increase in birth weight of between 23 and 47 g and an increase in the head circumference of the infants. Participation in the WIC program was also found to significantly reduce fetal mortality.[21] A sample of Californians participating in the WIC program both during and for 5 to 7 months after their first pregnancy delivered second infants averaging 131 g heavier than those of participants in the program who only received supplementary foods for up to 2 months after the first pregnancy.[22]

These studies illustrate the varying signals that can come from studies in this area of nutrition in which a great many factors acting independently or interacting may be involved. Overall, however, a great many studies have demonstrated that good nutritional status before and during pregnancy significantly increases the chances of a normal pregnancy that produces a healthy infant.

NUTRITION-RELATED CONCERNS

Pregnancy-Induced Hypertension

Pregnancy-induced hypertension (PIH) is a condition that occurs most frequently in women who are underweight at conception, who fail to gain adequate weight in the early part of pregnancy, or who have a large and unexpected weight gain in the latter part of pregnancy. This condition used to be called **toxemia of pregnancy** and is also known as **preeclampsia**.

The high blood pressure from which PIH gets its name is frequently accompanied by proteinuria, generalized edema, headache, and blurred vision. If untreated, PIH can lead to **eclampsia** in which the mother suffers from convulsive seizures, thereby putting both mother and infant at considerable risk.

The treatment of PIH is different from that of hypertension that is unrelated to pregnancy. It primarily involves bed rest. Restriction of weight gain was previously recommended, but this is now considered unwise.

The cause of PIH is unknown, but it may involve nutritional factors. Because a variety of nutritional deficiencies have been reported in women with PIH, a nutritious diet before and during pregnancy may help prevent or minimize the severity of this condition.

Exercise

Many pregnant women continue to engage in active exercise programs throughout pregnancy, which can raise some concerns. In addition to having higher energy needs during pregnancy, women are also more susceptible to hypoglycemia and the loss of fluids during exercise. They are therefore advised to avoid exercising with an empty stomach and to drink fluids both before and during exercise. Strenuous exercise should be avoided because the diversion of blood to the exercising muscles can reduce the blood supply to the fetus by as much as 25%. There is also some danger that the rise in the mother's body temperature during strenuous exercise could cause an undesirable rise in fetal temperature and heart rate. Strenuous exercise has been associated with LBW infants in some studies, whereas moderate exercise has not.

Alcohol

In 1973 the publication of a research report describing **fetal alcohol syndrome (FAS),** caused by exposure of

Risk Factors for Pregnancy-Induced Hypertension

- Inadequate diet
- First pregnancy at less than 20 or more than 35 years of age
- Multiple gestation (i.e., twins, triplets, etc.)
- History of high blood pressure, kidney disease, or inadequate medical care
- Sudden weight gain
- Inadequate weight gain
- Excessive weight gain

Nutrition-Related Concerns in Pregnancy

- Pregnancy-induced hypertension
- Strenuous exercise
- Alcohol consumption
- Caffeine consumption
- Drug use
- Artificial sweetener consumption
- Nausea
- Edema
- Cigarette smoking
- Vegetarianism
- Maternal age greater than 35 years

Recommendations For Exercise During Pregnancy

- Moderate exercise is acceptable.
- Keep pulse rate below 140 beats per minute.
- Limit "workouts" to 15 minutes or less 3 times per week
- Do not exercise if any pregnancy-related health problems occur.
- Recommended activities are swimming, walking and bicycling on a stationary exercise bicycle.

the developing fetus to alcohol, raised considerable concern about the consumption of alcohol during pregnancy. Children born with FAS have characteristic facial malformations, are of low weight and height, have a smaller-than-normal head circumference, and exhibit mental and physical retardation. Before 1973 these symptoms had been found in children born to alcoholics, but the 1973 report detected it in children of "moderate" drinkers consuming around 1 to 2 oz of alcohol per day.

Further study led the Surgeon General to advise in 1981 that each pregnant woman should be told about the risk of alcohol consumption, counseled to avoid drinking, and urged to become aware of alcohol in food and drugs. There was little controversy about the risks of heavy drinking but considerable differences of professional opinion on the dangers of moderate drinking. A series of surveys were carried out to try to resolve these differences. The results, based on the responses of at least 65,000 women, confirmed the positive correlation between maternal alcohol consumption and the risk of fetal abnormality. Depending on the population group, the incidence of fetal abnormality attributable to alcohol varied between 1 in 300 and 1 in 2000 live births. Abnormalities were found in 30% to 40% of infants born to alcoholic mothers. Stillbirths were twice as prevalent in women who had consumed at least three drinks per day during pregnancy, and the incidence of spontaneous abortion in this group was three times that in those who had consumed one drink or less per day.

Results from animal studies suggest that individual drinking binges at a critical stage of pregnancy can also cause FAS, even if little alcohol is consumed throughout the pregnancy overall. Information about the effects of binge drinking on human pregnancy is limited, but it seems likely that it could have serious consequences for the developing fetus.

It is now clear that women of childbearing age should be advised that the only completely safe choice is not to consume alcohol during pregnancy. They should also be advised that the alcohol in beer and wine is just as damaging as the alcohol in spirits. The dose of alcohol taken is the only relevant factor, not its source. They should also be aware that some medicines contain alcohol and should be avoided during pregnancy. Although complete abstinence is the safest option, the American Council on Science and Health believes that a blanket recommendation of abstinence is unrealistic and unnecessary. They believe that 1 oz of alcohol per day (equivalent to two 12-oz glasses of beer or two 4-oz glasses of wine) is a safe upper limit. They also caution against binge drinking.

Caffeine

The evidence suggesting that caffeine consumption poses risks during pregnancy is much less convincing than the evidence against alcohol. Evidence against caffeine is based almost entirely on studies of rats, mice, and rabbits, which have shown that caffeine intakes as low as 80 mg/kg of body weight can cause irreversible effects on a developing fetus. Intakes of only 6 mg/kg could cause less serious and more reversible effects. The most frequently observed problems involve bone malformation causing deformed fingers and toes and cleft palate.

Because little is known about the differences in caffeine metabolism between species, it is difficult to determine the significance of these results for humans. If the effects on humans were directly comparable, the daily consumption of caffeine required to supply 80 mg of caffeine per kilogram to a woman weighing 110 to 132 lb (50 to 60 kg) would correspond to 25 to 35 cups of regular coffee, 75 to 100 cups of tea, or 50 12-oz cola drinks. Even if detectable effects were produced by the consumption of 6 mg/kg of caffeine, it seems unlikely that any problems could be caused by moderate consumption of coffee, tea, or cola drinks. A Finnish study compared 466 pairs of mothers of infants with and without deformities. It detected no difference in the incidence of deformity between mothers who consumed at least four cups of coffee per day and those who drank less.

Until definitive large-scale studies on humans are performed, the possibility of an association between caffeine consumption and birth defects cannot be ruled out. In the meantime the FDA urges pregnant women to be prudent in their use of caffeine and if possible to avoid it.

Drug Use

Only limited information is available on any adverse effects of prescription or over-the-counter drugs on the developing fetus. These drugs often affect the intake, absorption, and metabolism of nutrients and so may be a cause for concern. No drugs should be taken during pregnancy without adequate medical supervision. A pregnant woman's doctor assesses the balance of benefit and risk associated with the use of any drug. Herbal teas should also be avoided because many contain ingredients that could adversely affect fetal development.

Artificial Sweeteners

The use of saccharin is not recommended during pregnancy.[23] It is a weak carcinogen that crosses the placenta and becomes evenly distributed throughout the fetus, apart from its central nervous system. The use of aspartame should be restricted to less than the Accepted Daily Intake (ADI) of 50 mg/kg of body weight. For a 150-lb woman, this corresponds to approximately 17 cans of aspartame-sweetened soda per 24 hours.

Nausea

Severe nausea, or "morning sickness," during the early stages of pregnancy can have serious nutritional consequences in mothers entering pregnancy with low levels of nutrient stores. Eating smaller but more frequent meals and eating dry crackers before rising in the morning can help minimize this problem in many women. Some evidence indicates that some women find relief from nausea by drinking lemonade or by sniffing a lemon. Severe and continued nausea (**hyperemesis**) calls for hospitalization to control dehydration, electrolyte imbalances, or excessive weight loss.

Edema

Some edema occurs in most pregnancies, primarily in the extremities of the body and especially during the third trimester. Neither dietary modification nor salt restriction is appropriate to control edema of pregnancy because it is caused by hormonal, rather than dietary, factors.

Cigarette Smoking

Cigarette smoking has been shown to decrease infant birth weight and increase the risk of perinatal morbidity and mortality. The effects may be a result of the toxicity of carbon monoxide, nicotine, or other constituents of tobacco smoke; reduced blood flow to the uterus; or reduced food intake by the mother. Exposure to sidestream tobacco smoke also increases the risk.

Vegetarianism

Well-planned vegetarian diets containing a variety of plant foods, in addition to milk and eggs, are perfectly adequate to meet the nutrient needs of pregnant women. Less well-planned vegetarian diets may pose risks of inadequate intakes of iron, zinc, calcium, vitamin B_{12}, and high-quality protein. "New vegetarians," who avoid only some meats and animal foods, are at minimal risk of dietary inadequacy.

Age

Women who become pregnant when over 35 years of age have distinct nutritional needs, reflecting their longer medical history, the probably long-term use of oral contraceptives, and the possibility of a longer history of poor eating habits. Careful nutritional evaluation of these women can be used to provide guidance that may reduce the risk of nutritional inadequacies causing any complications of pregnancy.

LACTATION

Every mother must decide how to feed her infant for the first 3 to 6 months of life, with the choice in most cases being between breast-feeding and bottle-feeding using a formula based on cow's milk. For the few infants who are allergic to cow's milk, the choice is between breast-feeding and bottle-feeding using a formula that is not based on cow's milk. The decision to breast-feed can be changed at any time, but infants who are started on bottle-feeding can seldom be transferred to breast-feeding after the first few days of life.

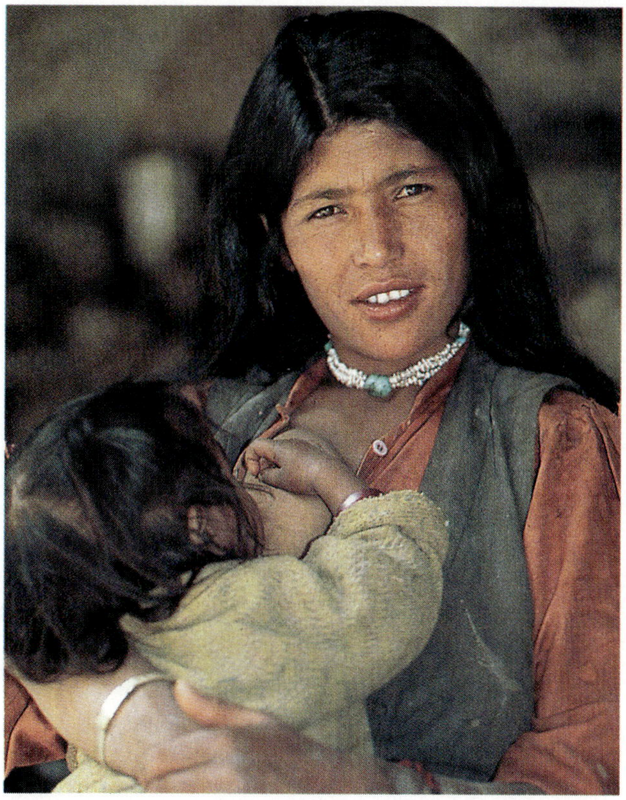

Breast-feeding has some well-documented nutritional, psychological, psychosocial, and social advantages over bottle-feeding, but bottle-feeding is a popular choice. In 1989, for example, only slightly more than 50% of U.S. mothers had chosen breast-feeding when discharged from the hospital. By 5 to 6 months after birth, only about 20% of U.S. infants were being breast-fed.[24] The decision between breast-feeding and bottle-feeding may have long-term consequences for both the child and the mother, as considered in more detail in Chapter 15. In addition to its nutritional advantages, breast-feeding is normally a satisfying emotional experience for the mother.

Current U.S. health objectives for the year 2000 aim to increase the proportion of infants who are breast-fed in the period immediately after delivery to at least 75% and to increase the proportion breast-fed for at least 5 to 6 months to 50%.[25] It is believed to be particularly important to encourage the feeding to the infant of the **colostrum,** the first fluid secreted by the mother before she begins to produce milk.

For many mothers, the decision of whether to choose breast- or bottle-feeding is a difficult emotional one, possibly influenced by the opinions of husbands, mothers, doctors, peers, and friends. For others, it may be a straightforward practical decision based on the need to return to work outside the home. Most women decide what method of feeding they favor very early, often in adolescence, long before they conceive. Few mothers have not decided on their preference by early pregnancy. Those who are not totally committed to their original decision, however, may be influenced in what path they eventually follow by the attitudes of nurses, doctors, and other medical personnel and by the practices in the hospital (such as rooming-in and provision for immediate physical contact with the infant).

Sometimes attempts to breast-feed are unsuccessful, forcing mothers to turn to bottle-feeding after a short time. The likelihood of successful breast-feeding depends on the general health and nutritional status of the mother and also on her attitude toward breast-feeding, her understanding of the process of lactation, and the support and encouragement she receives from medical personnel and her family.

Nutritional Needs of a Lactating Woman Relative to a Pregnant Woman

INCREASED	DECREASED	UNCHANGED
Energy	Iron	Calcium
Protein		Phosphorus
Vitamin A		Vitamin D
Thiamin		Vitamin B_6
Riboflavin		Folate
Niacin		
Vitamin E		
Vitamin C		
Manesium		
Selenium		
Zinc		
Iodine		

NUTRITIONAL NEEDS

The nutritive demands made on a mother by lactation are considerably greater than those made by pregnancy, although after the birth a mother may think she is no longer "eating for two." In the 4 months after birth, an infant doubles the birth weight that accumulated during 9 months of pregnancy. The milk secreted in 1 month represents more kilocalories than the total energy cost of a pregnancy. Fortunately, some of the energy and many of the nutrients stored during pregnancy are available to support milk production.

The recommended intakes of specific nutrients during lactation are summarized in Table 14-4. Most of these recommended intakes are based on our knowledge of the amount of milk produced during lactation, its nutritional content, and the amount of nutrient reserves held by the average mother. The RDAs during lactation are, however, based on even less quantitative data than are the RDAs during pregnancy. Nevertheless, it is fairly well established that the RDAs during lactation support the production of 750 ml of milk per day. This is the average amount of milk produced during lactation, although some studies have reported production of as much as 1000 to 1200 ml/day. Many mothers, especially in developing countries, are able to maintain a prolonged and satisfactory lactation period on diets that are well below the currently recommended standards. This is puzzling and suggests that it is necessary to reappraise the ability of lactating women to adapt to limited nutrient intakes.

Analysis of human milk reveals considerable variation in nutrient content not only among different women, but also in the same woman at different times. The amount of some nutrients can vary with the time of day, in addition to longer term variations. Also, the milk secreted first in any single nursing period (session on the breast), known as **foremilk,** often differs nutritionally from the **hindmilk** secreted at the end of that nursing period.

Table 14-10 lists nutrients whose abundance in milk may be affected by the mother's nutrient intake. It also identifies those nutrients that have been associated with recognizable deficiencies in breast-fed infants.

The Subcommittee on Nutrition During Lactation of the Committee on Nutritional Status During Pregnancy and Lactation of the U.S. National Academy of Sciences[24] reviewed the literature concerning the effects of maternal nutrition on the composition of human milk and reported its findings as follows:

- Even if the usual dietary intake of a macronutrient is less than that recommended in *Recommended Dietary Allowances*, there will be little or no effect on the total amount of that nutrient in the milk. However, the proportions of the different fatty acids in human milk vary with maternal dietary intake.
- The concentrations of major minerals (calcium, phosphorus, magnesium, sodium, and potassium) in human milk are not affected by the diet. Maternal intakes of selenium and iodine are positively related to their concentrations in human milk, but there is no convincing evidence that the concentrations of other trace elements in human milk are affected by maternal diet.
- The vitamin content of human milk is dependent upon the mother's current vitamin intake and her vitamin stores, but the strength of the relationships varies with the vitamin. Chronically low maternal intake of vitamins may result in milk that contains low amounts of these essential nutrients.
- The content of at least some nutrients in human milk may be maintained at a satisfactory level at the expense of maternal stores. This applies particularly to folate and calcium.

TABLE 14-10

Possible influences of maternal intake on the nutrient composition of human milk and nutrients for which clinical deficiency is recognizable in infants

NUTRIENT OR NUTRIENT CLASS	EFFECTS OF MATERNAL INTAKE ON MILK COMPOSITION*	RECOGNIZABLE NUTRITIONAL DEFICIENCY IN BREAST-FED INFANTS
Macronutrients		
Proteins	+	Unknown†
Lipids	+‡	Unknown
Lactose	o	Unknown
Minerals		
Calcium	o	Unknown
Phosphorus	o	Unknown
Magnesium	o	Unknown
Sodium	o	Unknown
Potassium	o	Unknown
Chlorine	o	Unknown
Iron	o	Yes§
Copper	o	Unknown
Zinc	+,o	Unknown
Manganese	+	Unknown
Selenium	+	Unknown
Iodine	+	Yes
Fluoride	+	Unknown
Vitamins		Yes
Vitamin C	+	Yes
Thiamin	+	Unknown
Riboflavin	+	Unknown
Niacin	+	Yes
Pantothenic acid	+	Yes
Vitamin B_6	+	Yes
Biotin	+	Yes
Folate	+	Yes
Vitamin B_{12}	+	Yes
Vitamin A	+	Yes
Vitamin D	+	Yes
Vitamin E	+	Yes
Vitamin K	+	Yes‖

* + denotes a positive effect of intake on nutrient content of milk. The magnitude of the effect varies widely among nutrients. *o* denotes no known effect of intake on nutrient content of milk.

† Evidence is not sufficiently conclusive to categorize as "no."

‡ Effect appears to be on type of fatty acids present but not on total content of triglycerides or cholesterol in the milk.

§ Deficiency is not related to maternal intake.

‖ Maternal intake is not the primary determinant of the infant's vitamin K status.

From Institute of Medicine/National Academy of Sciences: *Nutrition during lactation,* Washington, DC, 1991, National Academy Press.

- Increasing the mother's intake of a nutrient to levels above the RDA ordinarily does not result in unusually high levels of the nutrient in her milk; vitamins B_6, iodine, and selenium are exceptions. Studies have not been conducted to evaluate the possibility that high levels of nutrients in milk are toxic to the infant.
- Some studies suggest that poor maternal nutrition is associated with decreased concentrations of certain host-resistance factors in human milk, whereas other studies do not suggest this association.[24]

The nutritional composition of human milk is different from that of milk produced by other species or of infant formula. The specific properties of human milk that are unique are its physical structure and the type and concentration of macronutrients (proteins, fats, and carbohydrates), micronutrients (vitamins and minerals), enzymes, hormones, growth factors, host-resistance factors, immune-regulating substances, and antiinflammatory agents.

Energy

The additional energy required to sustain lactation is proportional to the amount of milk produced. The average 750 to 850 ml of milk secreted per day provides 67 kcal/100 ml, corresponding to 502 to 570 kcal/day overall. The energy efficiency of milk synthesis in the mother is about 90%, meaning that she requires an additional 550 to 625 kcal/day over nonlactating intakes to sustain her milk production. It is generally assumed that about 200 kcal/day can be obtained from the fat stored during pregnancy; so an additional intake of 355 to 425 kcal/day should be sufficient. However, in addition to the energy cost of producing milk, a lactating women may need more energy because of the increased physical activity involved in caring for her infant. Overall, the recommended energy intake (REI) during lactation is 500 kcal more than the woman's normal needs.

The recommended increase in energy intake during lactation is proportionately smaller than the recommended increase for many vitamins and minerals (Table 14-4). This means that the extra energy required by the lactating woman should come from foods of high nutrient density, such as nonfat milk, eggs, fruit, vegetables, and enriched or whole grain cereals.

Because the amount of extra energy required during lactation is almost twice the amount of extra energy required during pregnancy, it is appropriate for a nursing mother to add more food to her diet after the birth of her infant.

Protein

An additional 15 g of protein per day is recommended during lactation. This is readily available in typical North American diets, which usually contain significantly more protein than the recommended amounts.

Riboflavin

The mean riboflavin content of human milk is 0.04 mg/dl, although the specific amount varies with the mother's dietary intake of riboflavin. About 0.34 mg of riboflavin must be transferred to the milk of a lactating mother each day. Because only 75% of additional dietary riboflavin is used in milk production, the recommended riboflavin intake during lactation is 0.5 mg more than normal. Four glasses of milk per day should be sufficient to meet all riboflavin needs.

Vitamin C

Human milk contains approximately 5 to 6 mg of vitamin C per 100 ml. Increasing maternal intake of vitamin C from an originally low level produces a corresponding increase in the vitamin C content of the milk. The recommended vitamin C intake of 95 mg/day during lactation is readily obtained from two servings of citrus fruit or juice.

Vitamin B_6

The amount of vitamin B_6 in human milk is directly related to the mother's dietary intake, and it responds rapidly to changes in intake. Only 4% of the mother's intake is actually transferred to her milk, which contains an average of 90 to 100 μg of vitamin B_6 per 100 ml.

Mothers who have used oral contraceptives for long periods are reported to have lower-than-normal levels of vitamin B_6 in their milk. This is presumably related to the fact that the estrogen hormones in oral contraceptives increase vitamin B_6 requirements. Because modern oral contraceptives contain less estrogen than did earlier formulations, their effect on vitamin B_6 use and the vitamin B_6 content of milk should be less.

Folate

The high incidence of megaloblastic anemia caused by folate deficiency in lactating women suggests that lactation drains maternal reserves of folate. This problem is complicated by the fact that folate deficiency is the most common nutritional problem during pregnancy, and many women may enter lactation with practically no folate reserves. Recent analyses indicate that the folate content of human milk is approximately 100 μg/100 ml. This is twice the value that was used by the RDA committee to estimate folate requirements during lactation.[26]

Vitamin B_{12}

The concentration of vitamin B_{12} in the milk of women on a mixed diet varies from 0.3 to 3.2 μg/L. The concentration in the milk of strict vegetarians is low, at 0.05 to 0.075 μg/L.

Vitamin A

Most infants have significant reserves of vitamin A in the liver, but their mothers' milk provides them with additional vitamin A and related carotenoids. A maternal intake of 6500 IU (1300 RE), which is easily achieved by regular consumption of green and yellow fruits and vegetables, produces milk with 60 to 70 RE (200 to 233 IU)/100 ml. This is sufficient to meet all the needs of the infant.

Vitamin D

Vitamin D is needed to protect the infant against rickets. Relatively little of this fat-soluble vitamin is transferred to the mother's milk, which contains 0.05 to 0.15 μg (2 to 6 IU)/dl. This means that infants are dependent on the synthesis of vitamin D in their skin on exposure to sunlight or perhaps on a dietary supplement of vitamin D. A daily intake of 400 IU of vitamin D, the amount in 1 qt of fortified milk, is considered adequate for lactating women.

Vitamin K

Although the amount of vitamin K in human milk is insufficient to meet the needs of the infant, it can be increased by adding vitamin K to the mother's diet. It is also significant that supplemental vitamin K taken by the mother has a small impact on the amount of vitamin K in her milk until 48 hours after the supplement was taken.

Vitamin K is required to protect a newborn infant from hemorrhage in its first few days of life, and even the

Some of the Hormones Involved in the Regulation of Lactation

HORMONE	SOURCE	FUNCTION
Estrogen	Ovary and placenta	Stimulates breast development during pregnancy
Progesterone	Ovary and placenta	Stimulates breast development during pregnancy
Prolactin	Anterior pituitary gland	Stimulates milk production
Oxytocin	Posterior pituitary gland	Stimulates the let-down reflex

FIGURE 14-8

Hormonal control of lactation.

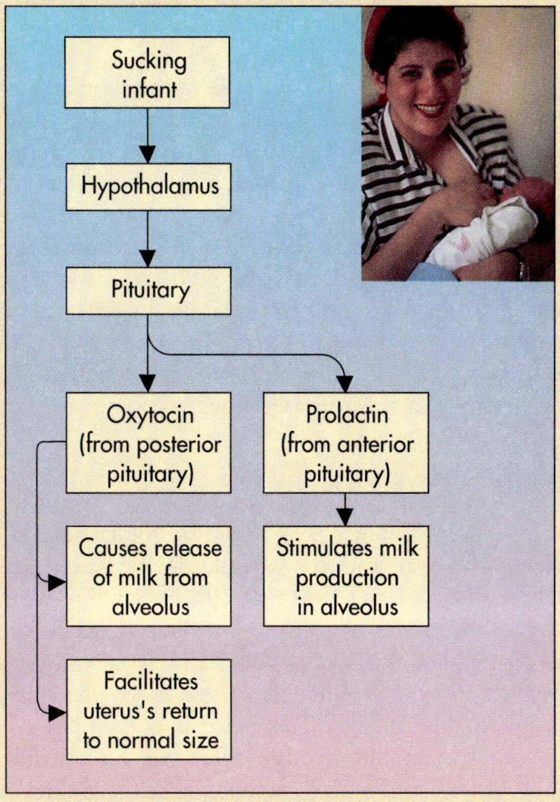

milk produced by a mother who has consumed large amounts of vitamin K may not offer sufficient protection. For this reason, breast-fed infants are given a supplement of natural vitamin K, either orally or by injection, immediately after birth.

CONTAMINANTS OF HUMAN MILK

The extent to which drugs, pesticide and herbicide residues, and other contaminants are transferred to a mother's milk and their effects on the infant are not well understood. When DDT (which can be stored in body fat) was in general use, there was concern that it might reach dangerously high levels in human milk during a first lactation. Oral contraceptives cause decreased milk production, and the use of sedatives decreases the strength of the infant's suckling reflex.

It appears that variable amounts of almost all drugs taken by a mother appear in her milk, with variable and largely unknown effects on her infant. It is best for a mother to avoid all drugs while breast-feeding, and they should certainly be taken only with the advice of a physician.

Alcohol is found in human milk in proportion to the amount consumed by the mother. The small amount associated with an occasional moderate drink has a small sedative effect on the infant and is probably relatively harmless. More frequent use of alcohol should be avoided.

DIETARY SUPPLEMENTS

In view of the considerable increase in nutrient requirements during lactation, it is probably advisable for the lactating mother to continue to take the supplements used during pregnancy. Only well-balanced supplements are appropriate, however, not those which contain beneficial amounts of selected nutrients and insignificant amounts of others. Any use of supplements should not detract from the fundamental importance of a well-chosen mixed diet. In particular, a well-chosen diet can provide the required fiber, energy, high-quality protein, and trace elements that are not supplied by most supplements.

STIMULATION OF LACTATION

The regulation of lactation is under the control of many hormones, including estrogen, progesterone, prolactin, and oxytocin (see box). Estrogen and progesterone levels that are maintained at high levels during pregnancy fall dramatically after the delivery of the infant, events associated with the establishment of lactation. The flow of milk is initiated when an infant begins to suck at the breast. A vigorous sucking action stimulates the pituitary gland to produce the hormones **prolactin** and **oxytocin** (Figure 14-8). Prolactin is released from the anterior pituitary gland and stimulates the production or secretion of milk by the **alveoli** cells of the mammary gland within the breast. Oxytocin is released from the posterior pituitary gland and stimulates the contraction of muscle cells surrounding the alveoli to cause the release of the milk (this is known as **milk ejection** or the **let-down reflex**). Oxytocin also acts on the walls of the uterus, causing strong contractions that help it to return to its normal size.

Almost every culture has its own medicinal or food

galactogogues, which are substances believed to stimulate lactation. These include garlic, cottonseed, candy, large quantities of milk, and small quantities of beer. Whether any are actually effective in stimulating lactation is uncertain.

The relationship between a lactating woman's fluid intake and the volume of milk secreted has not been fully investigated. It is known, however, that the volume of milk produced remains constant, even when fluid intake is low. This puts the lactating woman at increased risk of dehydration if her fluid intake is low. On the other hand, drinking more fluid than is required to satisfy natural thirst may decrease milk production by affecting the secretion of the pituitary hormones that regulate milk production. Overall, liberal—but not excessive—fluid intake is advisable during lactation.

FOOD AVOIDANCE

Many lactating women avoid specific foods because of widespread beliefs that they should not be eaten during lactation. One study found that 59% of lactating women avoid cabbage, beans, garlic, and onions; 52% avoid chocolate; 21% avoid alcohol; and 18% avoid carbonated beverages, on the grounds that these foods produce gas or colic in their infants. This belief is not supported by any sound data, but because there are no nutritional disadvantages and some advantages in avoiding the foods involved, the practice should cause no concern. Another study found that the consumption of milk by mothers of certain sensitive infants could produce colic in the infants. The avoidance of milk and other dairy products by lactating women is a cause of concern because of the important role of milk in providing calcium and vitamin D. If milk and other dairy products are avoided, sufficient calcium and vitamin D must be supplied from other sources, most feasibly from supplements.

SUCCESS AND DURATION OF LACTATION

Attempts to breast-feed are not always successful, forcing mothers to turn to formula feeding after a short time. Many attempts have been made to determine the factors influencing the success of lactation. Some evidence suggests that the output of milk during lactation is directly proportional to the mother's metabolic body size (body weight in kilograms raised to the power of ¾). There is also evidence of a strong positive correlation between the rise in temperature of the mammary skin caused by nursing a child and the amount of milk secreted. Other studies have shown that the course of lactation is established by the end of the first week, when the daily output of milk should reach 500 ml if the lactation is to prove successful. In addition, there is little doubt that a positive attitude in the mother and support from family and friends can contribute significantly to the success of breast-feeding.

Women who were severely malnourished in childhood may have suffered impaired development of secondary sexual characteristics, resulting in inadequate mammary tissue and consequent difficulties in breast-feeding. Nevertheless, a great many undernourished women succeed in breast-feeding as evidenced in the developing countries of the world.

The length of the breast-feeding period depends on many different factors. Mothers in higher socioeconomic and educational groups feed their infants more frequently and for longer periods. At present, only one infant in five is breast-fed for 6 months or more in the United States. In many cultures breast-feeding normally continues for 2 to 3 years, with milk being the only (sometimes inadequate) source of food for a year or more. In other cultures, breast milk may be supplemented with other foods as early as 3 or 4 weeks after birth. Such early supplementation with food may cause less vigorous sucking, which in turn causes a reduction in milk output and usually early weaning. Mothers in this group tend to experience an earlier return to a regular pattern of ovulation, causing subsequent pregnancies to occur sooner.

Breast-feeding has a contraceptive effect, because when sucking is strong and prolonged, the hormonal effects it induces delay both ovulation and the return of a regular menstrual cycle. In at least 50% of women, the first menstrual cycle after birth does not include the production of an egg cell (or ovum). The risk of pregnancy during the absence of menstruation (**amenorrhea**) caused by lactation is initially 5% but rises with each menstrual cycle.

ISSUES AND OPINIONS

The Nutrition of Pregnant Adolescents

Approximately 10% of American females between 15 and 19 years of age become pregnant each year, although around half of these pregnancies are terminated. The pregnancies that are continued to term produce a high proportion of premature infants of low birth weight who are at increased risk of dying at birth or requiring intensive care. Infants who are born to adolescent mothers and survive the initial period after birth are at almost twice the risk of physical problems or death as are infants born to older women.

Many factors underlie the increased vulnerability of infants born to adolescent mothers. One key factor is the low socioeconomic status of many pregnant adolescents, which puts the mothers at risk for poor nutritional status before pregnancy and deteriorating nutritional status throughout pregnancy. This key factor operates together with the fact that adolescents are in any case going through a nutritionally critical period of their lives (even without the added stress of pregnancy), and the relatively poor level of nutritional knowledge among adolescents in general.

In light of the special nutritional needs of pregnant adolescents, the American Dietetic Association (ADA) has published specific recommendations for their nutritional care.* In particular, the ADA recommends that all pregnant adolescents should have access to professional nutritional care via programs specifically targeted at them. The ADA has made three main recommendations concerning the services these programs should provide:

- The programs should be targeted toward the unique biological, psychosocial, developmental, and economic factors that affect the nutritional needs of pregnant adolescents.
- The programs should be funded in such a way to ensure that financial and social barriers do not prevent pregnant adolescents from receiving nutritional care from the earliest days of pregnancy and continuously during and after pregnancy.
- The programs should include the provision of supplemental food and other assistance required to optimize the nutritional status of all the adolescents participating in the programs.

Such programs will be expensive, but large sums of public money are already spent on *reacting to* the effects of poor nutrition on pregnant adolescents and their children. Therefore, it would be better to spend more money on preventing the problems in the first place. Many of the existing costs to the community of adolescent pregnancy result from the higher proportion of infants born to adolescent mothers who require intensive hospital care. Because many of the mothers are teenagers from poor socioeconomic backgrounds, the costs of their medical care are eventually paid by the community through medical assistance programs. In addition, about 40% of adolescent mothers have a second child while still teenagers, despite the existence of programs designed to encourage them to wait until they are older.

The major existing program to provide nutritional support to pregnant adolescents is the Special Supplemental Food Program for Woman, Infants, and Children. The impact of this program (and the importance of building on it) is demonstrated by the finding that adolescents who do not enroll or enroll late in pregnancy are less likely to gain sufficient weight during their pregnancy than are those who enroll at an early stage of pregnancy.

* Rees JM, Worthington-Roberts B: *J Am Diet Assoc* 94:449, 1994.

BY NOW YOU SHOULD KNOW

- The health of an infant is influenced by the nutritional status of the mother before and during pregnancy.
- The nutritional needs of the pregnant woman are greater than her normal needs but less than the sum of the needs of a nonpregnant woman and the fetus.
- Low–birth-weight (LBW) infants are at greater risk of illness within the first year of their lives than are infants that weigh over 5.5 lb at birth.
- A variety of physiological adaptations make pregnant women more efficient at absorbing and using nutrients than nonpregnant women.
- At the time of conception, a woman's folate status is one of many factors that determine the risk of her infant's developing neural tube defects.
- In the first 3 months of pregnancy the fetus grows to a weight of only about 1 oz, but this is the crucial period of cell differentiation. The quality of the mother's diet and the extent of her nutrient reserves have a major influence on the development of the fetus at this stage.
- Because the increase in energy requirements during pregnancy is proportionately less than the increase in the requirements for other nutrients, the mother must choose foods of high nutrient density.
- The need during pregnancy for all nutrients, except iron, can be readily met by the diet. Pregnant women are advised to use a supplement to ensure an adequate intake of iron and possibly to balance amounts of other vitamins and minerals provided by diet.
- Total weight gain during pregnancy should be between 25 to 35 lb for women of normal prepregnancy weight, between 28 and 40 lb for underweight women, and between 15 and 25 lb for overweight women.
- Use of alcohol and caffeine should be kept to a minimum during pregnancy.
- Over 50% of American women choose to breastfeed their infants because of the nutritional, immunological, and psychological benefits.
- Current Health Objectives for the United States call for 75% of infants to be breast-fed at the time of discharge from hospital and 50% at 6 months of age by the year 2000.
- The nutritional needs of lactating women for most nutrients are higher than they are for pregnant women. However, the needs for protein and iron are less during lactation than during pregnancy.
- Because of the high nutritional demands on the lactating woman, she is encouraged to continue taking a prenatal vitamin/mineral supplement throughout lactation.

STUDY QUESTIONS

1. Define the following terms: *placenta, amniotic fluid, intrauterine growth retardation, uterine milk, implantation, organogenesis, fetus, pregnancy-induced hypertension, eclampsia, macrocytic anemia, colostrum,* and *lactation.*
2. What are the particular nutritional needs of the pregnant woman during each trimester of pregnancy and during lactation after she has given birth?
3. How does the fertilized ovum develop into a viable infant?
4. How do the amount and pattern of weight gain influence the outcome of pregnancy?
5. List the reasons why a woman should not gain too little or too much weight during pregnancy.
6. Describe the way in which the fetus receives nourishment during gestation.
7. If a pregnant woman is complaining of constipation, what dietary recommendations would you make?
8. What precautions should a pregnant woman take to guard against osteomalacia?

CRITICAL ANALYSIS

1. Your friend just learned from her physician that she is 1 month pregnant. The RDA for pregnancy includes an additional 10 g of protein per day (50 to 60 g/day) and an additional 300 kcal/day. How would you incorporate these additions into your friend's diet?

   One of the easier ways is to use the exchange system in determining the protein and energy values of foods. Although the true protein and energy content of a given food may vary somewhat from the values stated for its exchange group, the exchange group values are close enough to use to modify diets. Most dietitians use only the low fat exchange groups for meats and meat substitutes and dairy products, unless the expectant mother is underweight. Below are the remaining exchange groups, the protein and calorie values for each group, and a few foods from each group. Use these group values and the example foods to create a combination of foods that supply 10 g of protein and 300 kcal. You can design one or two snacks or small meals with your combination. You may also choose foods from the full listings of the exchange groups which are found in Appendix H.

EXCHANGE GROUP	PROTEIN (g)	Kcal	EXAMPLE FOODS
Skim milk	8	90	Skim or nonfat milk, 1 cup Nonfat yogurt (plain), 1 cup
Low fat milk	8	120	Low-fat milk, 1 cup Low-fat yogurt (plain), 1 cup
Lean meats	7	55	1 egg white Egg substitutes with less than 55 kcal / ¼ cup Canadian bacon, 1 oz Low-fat (95% fat-free) deli meats (ham, chicken, turkey), 1 oz Lean beef or pork, 1 oz Chicken breast meat, 1 oz Fish, any, fresh, 1 oz Cottage cheese, ¼ cup
Medium fat meats	7	75	Ground beef, beef roasts, beef steaks, 1 oz Most pork products, 1 oz Tuna, canned in oil, drained, 1 oz Cheese: diet cheeses, Mozzarella, 1 oz; Ricotta, ¼ cup 1 whole egg Tofu, 2 ½″ × 2 ¾″ × 1″
Fruits	0	60	1 apple (2″ diameter) ½ banana, 9″ long ½ grapefruit, medium 1 orange (2 ½ inches diameter) ½ large or 1 small pear 1 ¼ cup strawberries, whole
Vegetables	2	25	1 cup raw or ½ cup cooked (asparagus, green beans, broccoli, carrots, cooked cabbage, cauliflower, green peppers, cooked mushrooms, onions, tomatoes, zucchini)
Starches/breads	3	80	¾ cup ready-to-eat unsweetened cereal ½ cup cooked cereal ¼ cup baked beans ⅓ cup cooked beans or peas (kidney, white, split, black-eyed)
Fats	0	45	Butter or margarine, 1 tsp Mayonnaise, 1 tsp Oil, any, 1 tsp Reduced calorie butter, margarine, mayonnaise, 1 Tbsp Reduced calorie salad dressing, 2 Tbsp Salad dressing, 1 Tbsp

FOOD	AMOUNT	PROTEIN (g)	KCAL

Although it is not difficult to select some foods that just meet the increased RDAs for protein and energy, you may have found that the result is a list of foods that do not sound like a meal or snack that anyone would be interested in eating. For this reason, and because exceeding the increased RDA for protein by a few grams is not normally harmful, you can design such meals or snacks with foods that supply more than 10 g of protein. For instance, a sandwich made with 1 oz of lean meat and two pieces of bread would supply 13 g of protein and 215 kcal. To accommodate your friend's preferences, you might allow an additional ounce of lean meat. The sandwich now supplies 20 g of protein and 270 kcal. One teaspoon of mayonnaise brings the kcals to 315. This diet now meets the increased RDAs. The sandwich supplies 10 g of protein more than recommended, but this is not normally cause for concern (it would be cause for concern if the expectant mother had been prescribed a protein restricted diet; in that case, you would try to just meet the mother's protein needs, as prescribed by a physician).

Another strategy is to use combination foods. Below are some popular combination foods and the number of exchanges they represent. Calculate the total grams of protein and the calories supplied by each food using the grams of protein and calorie values for each exchange group.

FOOD	AMOUNT	EXCHANGES	PROTEIN (g)	Kcal
Casserole, homemade	1 cup	2 starch/bread, 2 medium-fat meat, 1 fat	________	________
Cheese pizza, thin crust	¼ of 15-oz or ¼ of 10-inch pizza	2 starch/bread, 1 medium-fat meat, 1 fat	________	________
Chili with beans, canned	1 cup	2 starch/bread, 2 medium-fat meat, 2 fat	________	________
Macaroni and cheese	1 cup	2 starch/bread, 1 medium-fat meat, 2 fat	________	________

REFERENCES

1. Rosso P: Placental growth, development and function in relation to maternal malnutrition, *Fed Proc* 39:250, 1980.

2. Institute of Medicine, National Academy of Sciences: *Preventing low birthweight,* Washington, DC, 1985, National Academy Press.

3. Rosso P: Nutrition and maternal fetal exchange, *Am J Clin Nutr* 34:744, 1981.

4. Medical Research Council Vitamin Study Research Group: Prevention of neural tube defects: results of the Medical Council Vitamin Study, *Lancet* 338:131, 1991.

5. Czeizel AE, Dudas I: Prevention of the first occurrence of neural tube defects by periconceptual vitamin supplementation, *N Engl J Med* 327:1832, 1992.

6. Institute of Medicine, National Academy of Sciences: *Nutrition during pregnancy: weight gain and nutrient supplements,* Washington, DC, 1990, National Academy Press.

7. Shepard MJ, Hellenbrand KG, Bracken MB: Proportional weight gain and complications of pregnancy, labor, and delivery in healthy women of normal prepregnancy weight, *Am J Obstet Gynecol* 155:947, 1986.

8. McGanity WJ, Dawson EB, Fogelman A: Nutrition in pregnancy and lactation. In Shils ME, Olson JA, Shike M, editors: *Modern nutrition in health and disease,* ed 8, Philadelphia, 1994, Lea & Febiger.

9. Pike RL, Smiciklas HA: A reappraisal of sodium restriction during pregnancy, *Int J Gynecol Obstet* 10:1, 1972.

10. Pharoah POD, Hornabrook RW: Endemic creatinism of recent onset in New Guinea, *Lancet* 2:1038, 1974.

11. Pennington JA: A review of iodine toxicity reports, *J Am Diet Assoc* 90:1571, 1990.

12. McPartlin JA and others: Accelerated folate breakdown in pregnancy, *Lancet* 341:148, 1993.

13. Committee on Nutrition of the Mother and Preschool Child, Food and Nutrition Board, Commission on Life Sciences, National Research Council: *Alternative dietary practices and nutritional abuses in pregnancy,* Washington, DC, 1982, National Academy Press.

14. Stein Z and others: *Famine and human development,* New York, 1975, Oxford University Press.

15. Burke BS and others: Nutrition studies during pregnancy vs. relation of maternal nutrition to condition of infant at birth: study of siblings, *J Nutr* 38:453, 1949.

16. Ebbs JF, Tisdall FF, Scott WA: Influence of prenatal diet on mother and child, *J Nutr* 22:515, 1941.

17. McGanity WJ and others: The Vanderbilt Cooperative study of maternal and infant nutrition. Vol. 7. Some nutritional implications, *J Am Diet Assoc* 31:582, 1955.

18. Thomson AM: Diet in pregnancy. Vol 3. Diet in relation to the course and outcome of pregnancy, *Br J Nutr* 13:509, 1959.

19. Rush D, Stern Z, Susser M: *Diet in pregnancy: a randomized controlled trial of nutritional supplements,* New York, 1980, Liss.

20. Rosso P: *Nutrition and metabolism in pregnancy: mother and fetus,* New York, 1990, Oxford University Press.

21. Rush D and others: Historical study of pregnancy outcomes, *Am J Clin Nutr* 48:412, 1988.

22. Caan B and others: Benefits associated with WIC supplemental feeding during the interpregnancy interval, *Am J Clin Nutr* 45:29, 1987.

23. Pitkin RM and others: Placental transmission and fetal distribution of saccharin, *Am J Obstet Gynecol* 111:280, 1971.

24. Institute of Medicine, National Academy of Sciences: *Nutrition during lactation,* Washington, DC, 1991, National Academy Press.

25. Department of Health and Human Services: *Healthy people 2000: national health promotion and disease prevention objectives,* Washington, DC, 1990, Office of the Assistant Secretary of Health.

26. O'Connor DL, Tamura T, Picciano MF: Presence of pteroylpolyglutamates in human milk, *Am J Clin Nutr* 53:930, 1991.

~ ADDITIONAL READINGS ~

Abrams B, Parker J: Overweight and pregnancy complications, *Int J Obesity* 12:293, 1988.

Behrman RE: Preventing low birth weight: a pediatric perspective, *J Pediatr* 107:842, 1985.

Bennett PN, editor: *Drugs and human lactation,* New York, 1988, Elsevier.

Committee on Drugs, American Academy of Pediatrics: Transfer of drugs and other chemicals into human breast milk, *Pediatrics* 84:924, 1989.

Kuller JM: Effects on the fetus and newborn of medications commonly used during pregnancy, *J Perinat Neonat Nurs* 3:73, 1990.

Lawrence RE: *Breastfeeding: a guide for the medical profession,* ed 4, St Louis, 1994, Mosby.

Neifert MR, Seacat JM: Contemporary breastfeeding management, *Clin Perinatol* 12:319, 1985.

Neville MC, Neifert MR, editors: *Lactation: physiology, nutrition, and breastfeeding,* New York, 1983, Plenum Press.

Sayetta RB: Pica: an overview, *Am Fam Physician* 33:181, 1986.

Stewart DE and others: Anorexia nervosa, bulimia, and pregnancy, *Am J Obstet Gynecol* 157:1194, 1987.

Weiner L, Rosett HL: Pregnancy and alcohol, *Clin Nutr* 4:10, 1985.

Weisburg E: Smoking and reproductive health, *Clin Reprod Fertil* 3:175, 1985.

Worthington-Roberts B: Nutrition support of successful reproduction, *J Nutr Educ* 19:1, 1987.

Worthington-Roberts B, Williams SR: *Nutrition in pregnancy and lactation,* ed 5, St Louis, 1993, Mosby.

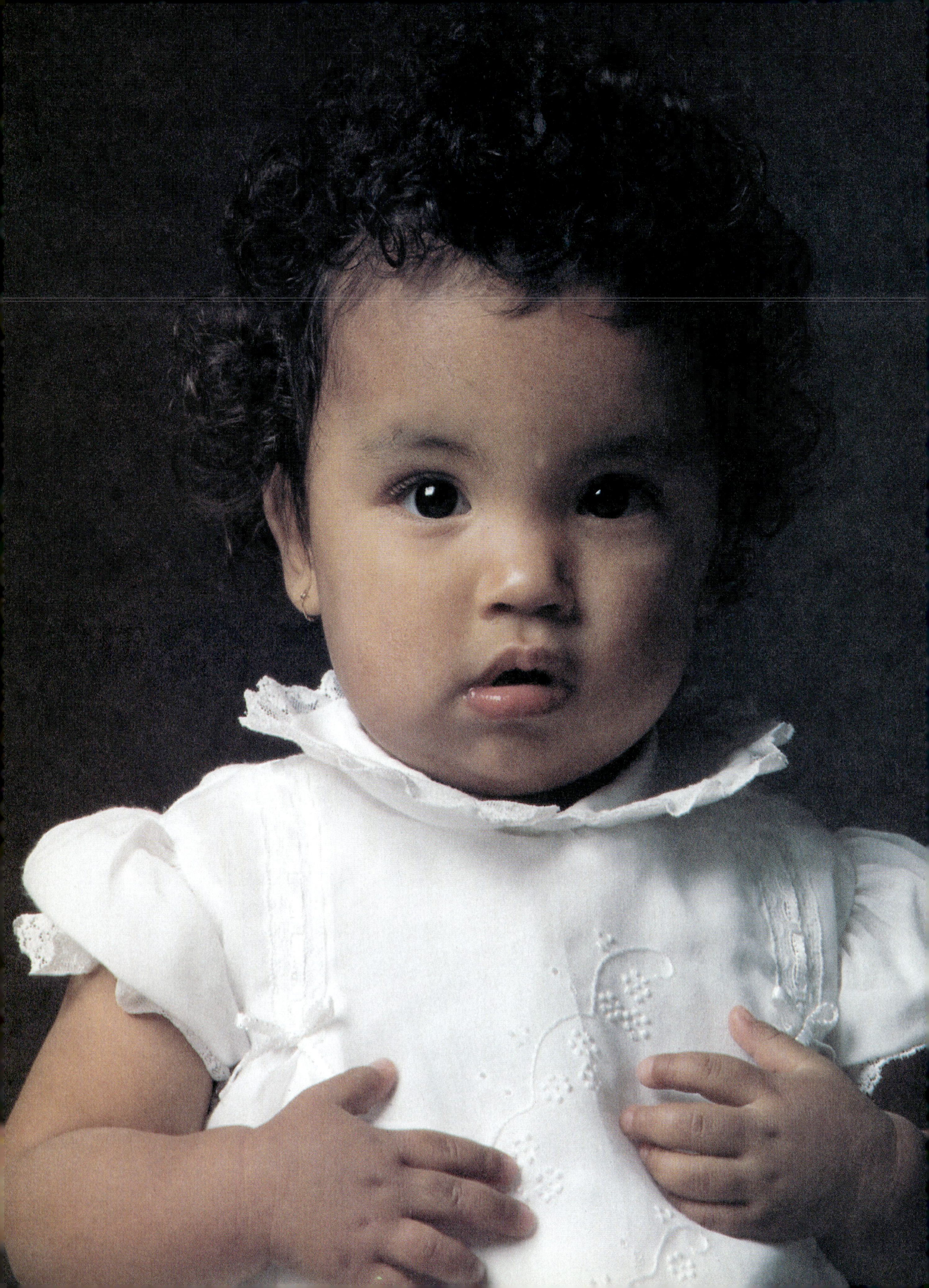

CHAPTER 15

INFANT NUTRITION

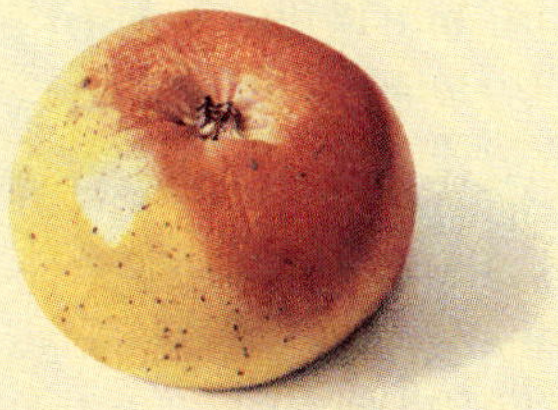

An infant's nutrition during the first year of life is critically important for his or her development and health throughout life. Because parents and other caretakers make all the food choices for an infant during this vital period, it is important that they receive adequate nutritional advice for the infant. Fortunately, infants are amazingly resilient and thrive on many different feeding patterns. However, nutritionists can now give detailed advice about the optimal diet during infancy, including the best methods of introducing an infant to foods available from the family table. Nutritionists are also continuing to increase their understanding of the role of nutrition in infancy and the influence of early nutrition on health throughout life.

The quality of nutrition an infant receives in its first year affects its health for the rest of its life. This is largely because the growth, development, and maturation of body tissues occur more rapidly in the first year of life than at any other time, except in the womb. The adequately nourished infant is more likely to achieve normal physical and mental development. Inadequate infant nourishment brings risks of stunted growth and a range of biochemical changes that impair development.

The impact of any nutritional deficiency on an infant's health depends on when the deficiency occurs and how long it lasts. Many problems can be prevented if the deficiency is corrected reasonably soon, but if the deficiency persists for too long, permanent damage can result. The chances of permanent damage are highest during specific critical periods, which vary, depending on the tissues and nutrients concerned. The critical period for brain growth, for example, spans the first 2 years of life, demanding adequate supplies of protein and essential fatty acids. Tooth development, on the other hand, occurs largely throughout the first 6 years of life and demands adequate calcium, phosphorus, and vitamins A, D, and C.

The success of nutrition during infancy depends on the choice of early feeding methods, the correct use of nutrient supplements, the pattern and timing of the introduction of solid foods, and careful monitoring of growth, nutritional status, and any diseases. Each of these factors is influenced by a complex combination of social, environmental, economic, and behavioral variables, in addition to basic nutritional considerations.

There are many gaps in our knowledge of the route to optimal nutrition, sometimes causing nutritionists and pediatricians to make seemingly contradictory recommendations. The more we learn, however, the more the various kinds of health professionals agree on the appropriate strategy for infant feeding. Fortunately, infants seem able to thrive on a wide variety of feeding patterns. In years to come, we may learn much more about the differing long-term consequences of different feeding patterns, which at present most seem to produce healthy infants and children. Any such consequences, however, are likely to be subtle and difficult to identify from short-term studies.

The period of infant feeding can be regarded as consisting of three overlapping phases:

- The **nursing phase,** when human milk or an appropriate formula is the sole source of nutrients
- The **transitional phase,** when other specially prepared foods are introduced to complement human milk or formula
- The **modified adult phase,** when the majority of the infant's nutrients are provided by selected foods available from the family's normal diet

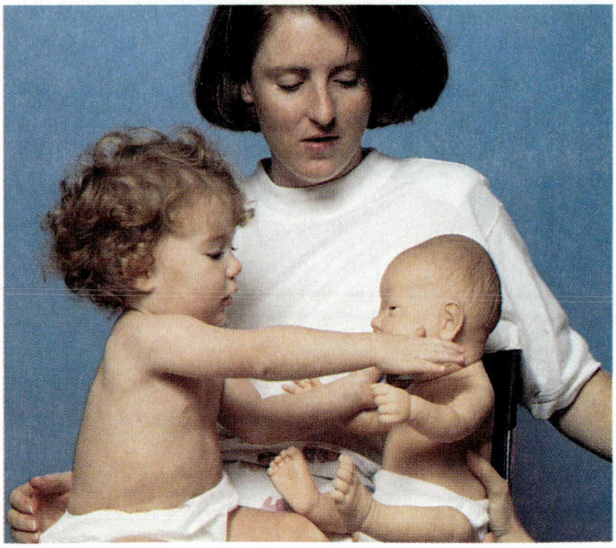

A full-term infant's weight should double in 4 to 6 months and should triple in 1 year.

One simple way to judge the nutritional adequacy of an infant's diet is to monitor the infant's rate of growth. The weight of a full-term infant should rise to double its birth weight in 4 to 6 months and to triple its birth weight in 1 year. This is certainly not the only measure of successful infant nutrition, but it is a simple and reasonably reliable one.

BREAST-FEEDING

At the turn of the century almost all U.S. infants were breast-fed. By 1946 the proportion being breast-fed had fallen to 65%, and then continued to decline to 37% in 1956. By 1971 only about 25% of infants were being breast-fed at the time of discharge from hospital. The trend was then reversed, rising to 58% by 1984 and then declining again slightly to 53% by 1989, where it has remained through 1992(Figure 15-1).

Studies show that the women most likely to breast-feed are older, more educated, and from higher socioeconomic groups than women who opt for formula feeding. Those choosing breast-feeding are also the most likely to be concerned about environmental influences on health, to feel "natural is best," and to be nonsmokers.[1] Other studies find that women report feeding their children in the way that they themselves were fed when young. Current data indicate that 19% of U.S. infants are breast-fed until 6 months of age, compared with 7% in 1971. Overall, it appears that more women are choosing to breast-feed and are breast-feeding for longer than was the case 25 years ago.

Changes in the pattern of feeding that are first adopted by better-educated women are frequently followed several years later by less-educated women and

FIGURE 15-1

Changes in the incidence of breast-feeding at hospital discharge in the United States (1946-1989).

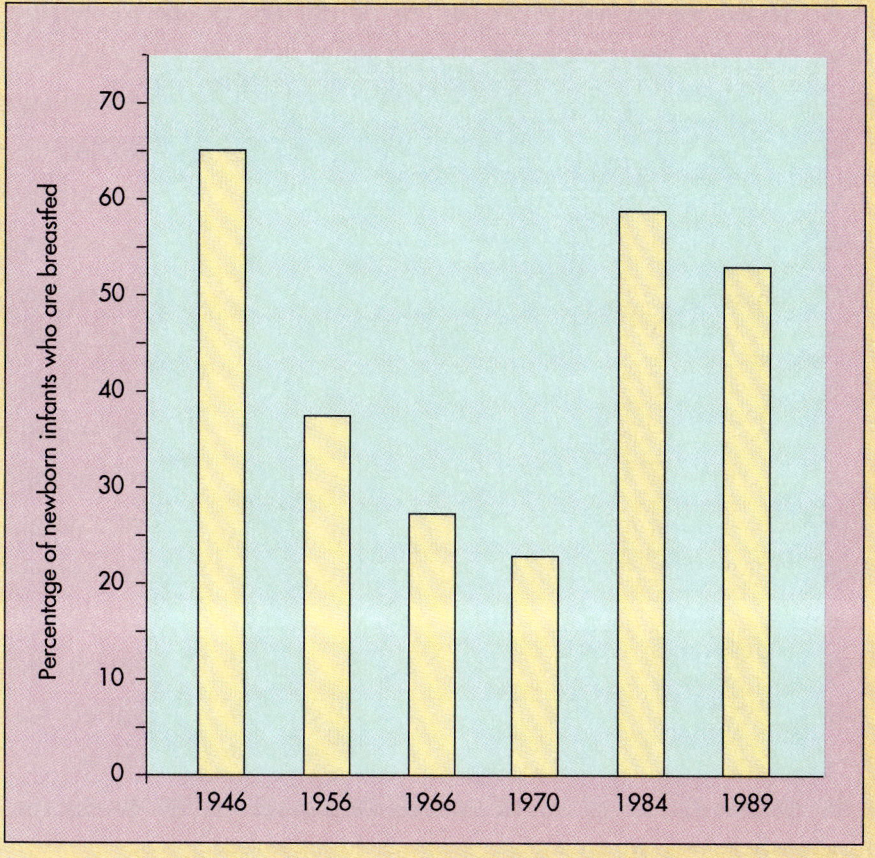

those of lower socioeconomic status. The current trend toward breast-feeding is being reinforced by the recommendation from health professionals that human milk (or modified cow's milk formula, if breast-feeding is impossible) should be the *sole* source of nutrition in the first 4 to 6 months of life and the *major* source for the first year.

The decision to breast-feed is influenced by consideration of the health benefits for the baby, the fact that it fosters a close relationship between mother and baby, and the belief that it is the "natural" thing to do. One study has found that over 50% of mothers choose their preferred method of infant feeding before pregnancy, 86% by the end of the first trimester, and all by the last trimester.[2] This indicates the wisdom of directing education programs at girls early in their schooling, rather than waiting for them to receive information from a physician at a time when it may have little influence on their choice.

The lower incidence of breast-feeding in developed countries, as compared with developing countries, has been largely attributed to the availability of alternative feeding methods and the large numbers of women working outside of the home in developed countries. In developing countries, alternatives to breast-feeding are too costly for most families, the water supply may be contaminated, refrigeration may not be available, and knowledge of how to prepare and handle infant formula may be limited. If a child in a developing country is to survive the neonatal period, breast-feeding is almost essential.

Failure of women to breast-feed results in the loss of one of a country's best natural resources—human milk. In developing countries, formula feeding is usually a rare alternative used by affluent families or to save lives. In developed countries women are more free to weigh the advantages and disadvantages of breast-feeding in their own individual situation, before choosing their method of infant feeding.

There is almost complete agreement that breast-feeding is nutritionally superior to formula feeding for practically all infants. It is nevertheless important that women are not forced into breast-feeding, because reasonable alternatives are available. Women should be made aware that breast-feeding is regarded as the ideal infant feeding method but should not be made to feel guilty if they choose not to breast-feed.

FIGURE 15-2

Differences in the composition of human milk and cow's milk.

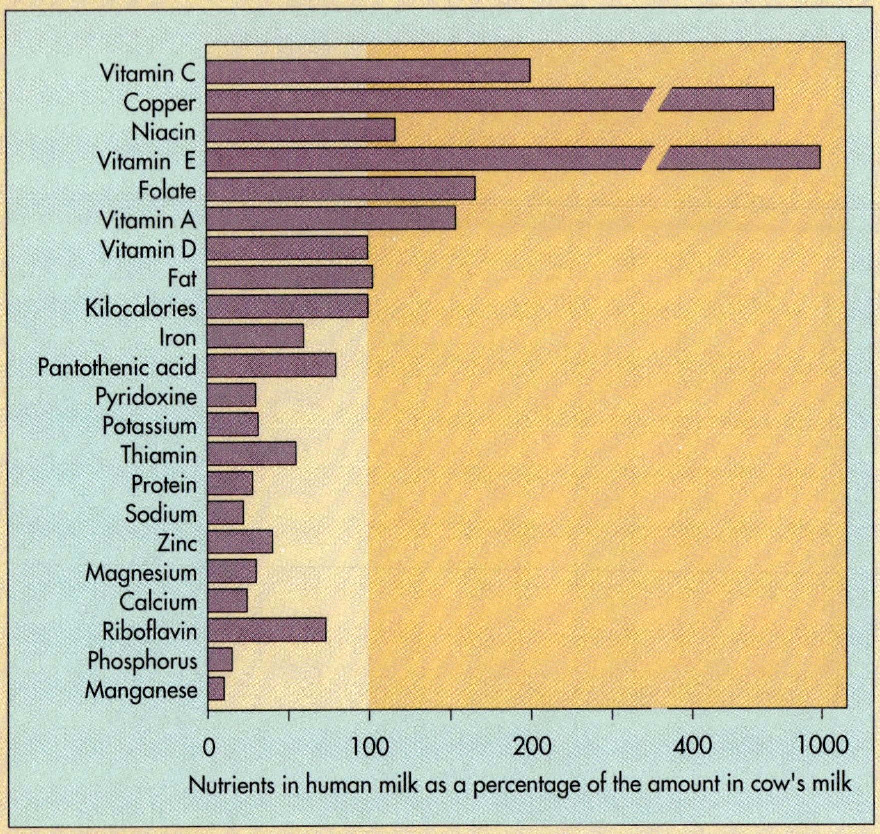

CONSIDERATIONS FAVORING BREAST-FEEDING

NUTRITIONAL FACTORS

It is generally believed that the milk of each species provides the most suitable nutrient mixture to sustain the growth of its offspring, and therefore human milk is the best food for newborn humans. If cow's milk must be used to feed human infants, its nutrient composition should be modified to approximately match the composition of human milk. Some key differences between the nutrient composition of human milk and cow's milk are presented in Figure 15-2 and Table 15-1. These indicate that human milk contains more of some nutrients than does cow's milk and less of others, whereas some nutrients are present in both types of milk in roughly similar amounts. It is also relevant that the milk of any one species contains some nutrients in whatever form is best suited to the digestive capacities of their own offspring. The fact that human milk contains less of some nutrients, such as protein and calcium, than does cow's milk is believed to reflect differences in the nutrient needs for growth between the two species. A calf must double its weight in 2 months, whereas a human infant doubles its weight in 4 months.

ENERGY

The energy contents of human and cow's milk are similar (at about 64 kcal/100 ml), as are their total fat contents (at between 3.7% and 3.9%). Fat provides 51% of the energy available from human milk, carbohydrate provides 43%, and protein 6%. The corresponding figures for cow's milk are 50% from fat, 30% from carbohydrate, and 20% from protein. For infant formula, the energy is provided in the ratio of 48% from fat, 43% from carbohydrate, and 9% from protein (Figure 15-3).

During gestation, a fetus derives most of its energy from glucose. In the first 24 hours after birth, it converts all of the glycogen stored in its liver to glucose for use as an energy source. It then relies on a mixture of glucose and fatty acids derived from both its diet and body fat stores. More than 97% of the fat in human milk and infant formula is present in the form of triglycerides. Free fatty acids can be released from the triglycerides by a lipase enzyme present in human milk. Fatty acids are the preferred source of energy throughout the suckling period. The switch from reliance on glucose to reliance on fatty acids as an energy source calls for a source of carnitine needed for fatty acid transport into the mitochondria. Newborns cannot synthesize the carnitine they need and so must obtain it from either human milk or

TABLE 15-1

Composition of mature human milk, cow's milk, and cow's milk–based formula per 100 ml

NUTRIENT	MATURE HUMAN MILK*	COW'S MILK	COW'S MILK–BASED FORMULA
Energy (kcal)	64	64	67
Fat (g)	3.7	3.6	3.6-3.8
Lactose (g)	7.2	4.8	6.9-7.2
Protein (g)	0.9	3.2	1.4
Casein (g)	0.25	2.6	†
Lactalbumin (g)	0.26	0.1	†
Calcium (mg)	30	115	42-49
Phosphorus (mg)	15	91	28-38
Zinc (mg)	0.16	0.4	0.5
Iron (mg)	0.03	0.05	1.2‡
Vitamins			
A (RE)	77	30-70	60
Carotene (RE)	8.5		
D (IU)	5	5	40-43
E (mg)	0.4	0.04	2
C (mg)	6	3	9.5-21
K (μg)	0.16	0.1-0.4	5.5-5.8
Folate (μg)	10	6.0	5-10.6
Niacin (mg)	0.20	0.166	0.5-0.85
Pantothenic acid (mg)	0.26	0.32	0.21-0.32
Pyridoxine (μg)	20	55.4	40
Riboflavin (μg)	58	91.4	100
Thiamin (μg)	20.8	38.8	50-70
Sodium (mg)	12	52	15-18
Potassium (mg)	45	140	56-73
Chloride (mg)	39	97	38-43
Magnesium (mg)	3	9.6	4.1-5.3
Copper (μg)	24	3	6-9.5
Iodine (μg)	11-27	20-50	3.4-10
Manganese (μg)	0.4	4	1.2-1.5
Selenium (μg)	1.5	0-10	0.5-2

RE, Retinol equivalent; *IU*, international unit.
* Mature human milk is that produced after 1 month of lactation.
† Percentages of casein and whey proteins vary with type (casein-predominant formulas and whey-predominant formulas).
‡ Also available with 0.1 mg/100 ml.

From Fomon SJ: *Infant nutrition,* St Louis, 1993, Mosby.

formula. Carnitine is now added to milk-free formulas marketed in the United States. Infants fed carnitine-free formulas have been found to have low plasma carnitine levels and high plasma free fatty acid levels, both suggesting an impaired use of fat as an energy source.[3]

CARBOHYDRATE

The main sugar in milk is the disaccharide lactose, which is present at a higher concentration in human milk than in cow's milk. Several factors make lactose a suitable form of carbohydrate for infant nutrition: it facilitates the absorption of calcium, zinc, iron, and manganese,[4] and it is the only source of the monosaccharide galactose. Galactose is essential for the formation of the myelin sheath surrounding many nerves and therefore is essential for the normal development of the nervous system.

Lactose is the carbohydrate added to all milk-based commercially prepared formulas. Its low solubility makes it unsuitable for use in formula prepared at home. Soy-based formulas use sucrose as the added carbohydrate, which cannot act as a source of galactose and promotes the growth of bacteria that can cause gastrointestinal distress.

Human milk contains an amylase enzyme that allows a breast-fed infant to digest starch from other foods at a stage in life when little or no pancreatic amylase is produced.[5]

PROTEIN

Human milk contains only one fourth as much protein as does cow's milk. Both forms of milk contain **whey proteins** and **casein proteins,** but the whey proteins predominate in human milk, whereas the casein proteins predominate in cow's milk (Figure 15-4 and Table 15-2). The whey proteins that predominate in human milk have an amino acid pattern that closely matches the

FIGURE 15-3

Comparison of the percentage of total energy provided by fat, carbohydrate, and protein in human milk, cow's milk, and infant formula.

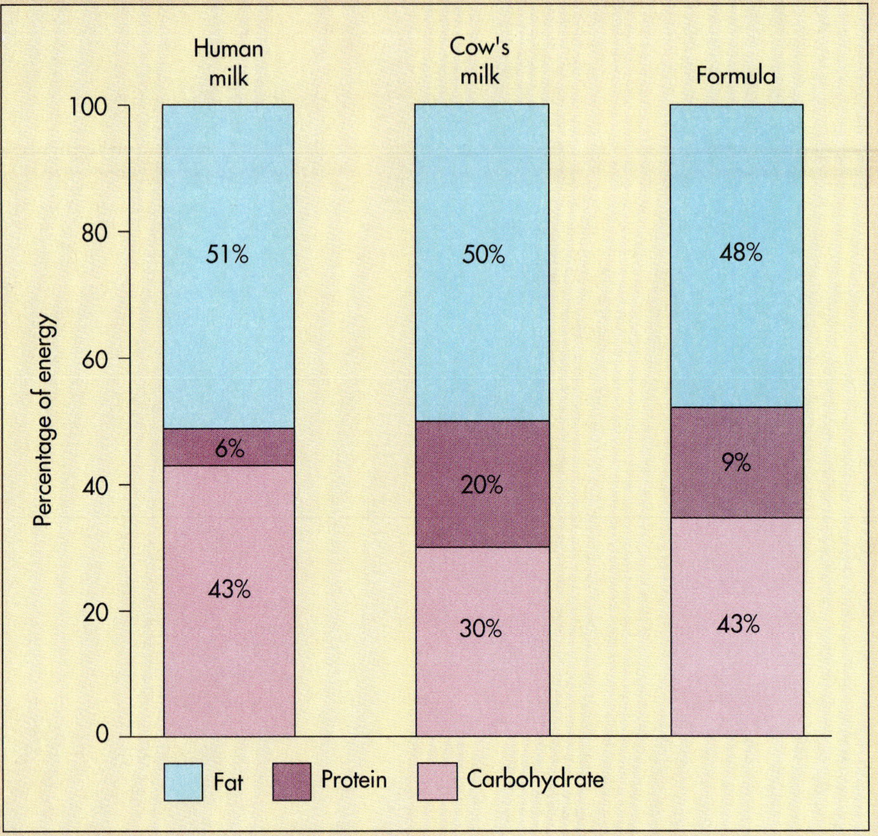

TABLE 15-2

Protein composition of human milk and cow's milk

	HUMAN MILK (g/100 ml)	COW'S MILK (g/100 ml)
Total proteins	0.95	3.3
Caseins	0.25	2.6
Whey proteins	0.70	0.67
α-lactalbumin	0.26 (37)*	0.12 (18)
β-lactoglobulin	—	0.30 (45)
Lactoferrin	0.17 (24)	trace
Serum albumin	0.05 (7)	0.03 (4)
Lysozyme	0.05 (7)	trace
Immunoglobulins	0.105 (15)	0.066 (10)
Other	0.07 (10)	0.15 (23)
Total nonprotein nitrogen	0.5 [26]†	0.28 [5]

* Numbers in parentheses indicate percentages of whey proteins.
† Number in brackets indicates nonprotein nitrogen as a percentage of total nitrogen.

From Hambreaus L: *Nutr Abstr Rev Rev Clin Nutr* 54:219, 1984.

amino acid pattern of body proteins in general. The whey proteins also provide more of the essential amino acids than do the casein proteins. When casein proteins enter the stomach, the enzyme rennin causes them to form a hard curd. Whey proteins, on the other hand, form a soft, flocculent curd that is more rapidly digested and absorbed by an infant. Human milk also contains protein-splitting enzymes (proteases) that break proteins into small peptides that are more readily degraded by an infant's digestive enzymes. These enzymes in cow's milk and formula are destroyed by the heat of pasteurization.

Another significant difference between human milk and cow's milk is the higher cysteine/methionine ratio of human milk. This is important because the liver and kidney of an immature human infant may lack the enzyme necessary to convert methionine to cysteine, which is a conditionally essential amino acid during infancy. Human milk also has a lower proportion of the amino acid phenylalanine than does cow's milk. This difference is important in infants with phenylketonuria (PKU), who can use and tolerate only a small amount of phenylalanine.[6] PKU is a genetic defect of phenylalanine metabolism in which a deficiency of the enzyme pheny-

FIGURE 15-4

Comparison of the amounts of the different types of protein in human milk and cow's milk.

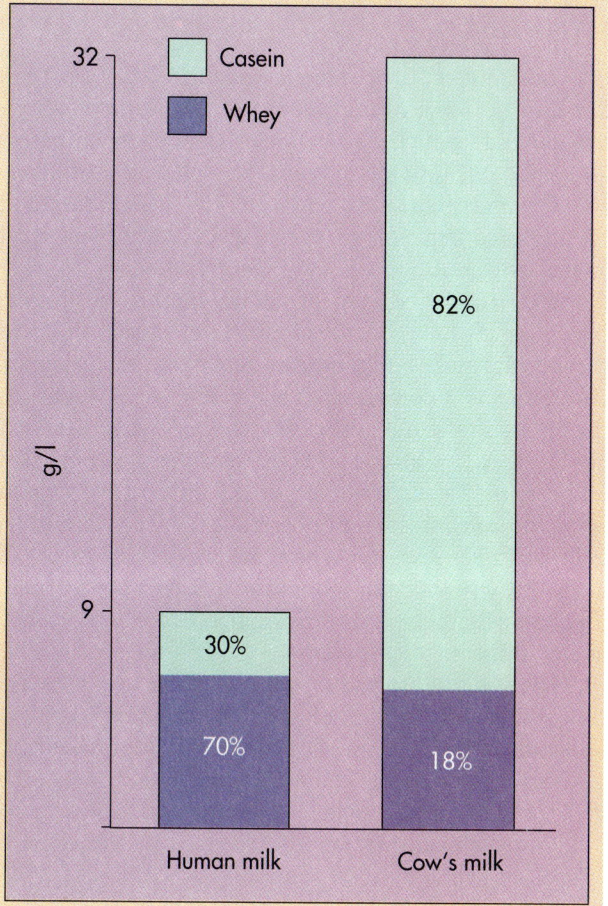

Benefits of Human Milk Over Cow's Milk

PROTEIN

- More whey proteins
- Less casein
- Higher cysteine-to-methionine ratio
- Less phenylalanine
- More taurine
- More peptidase

LIPIDS

- Less saturated fatty acids
- More medium-chain fatty acids
- Less short-chain fatty acids
- More lipase enzyme
- More digestible
- Palmitic acid on position two of triglycerides
- More linoleic acid
- Higher polyunsaturated/saturated fatty acid ratio
- More fat in hindmilk
- More cholesterol

MINERALS

- Less calcium
- Less sodium
- Higher calcium/phosphorus ratio
- Iron and zinc in more available form
- Higher copper to zinc ratio

lalanine hydrolase decreases the conversion of phenylalanine to tyrosine. If infants with PKU consume too much phenylalanine, the accumulation of abnormal metabolites of this amino acid can cause brain damage.

The sulfur-containing amino acid **taurine** has recently been identified as a possible dietary essential for infants because of its role in the development of the central nervous system. Human milk produced by mothers who consume a mixed (omniverous) diet contains sufficient taurine, but it is present only at low levels in the milk of vegans and in cow's milk. Taurine is added to most infant formulas at a level of 40 to 45 mg/L.

Of the nitrogen in human milk, 26% is nonprotein nitrogen, compared with 5% in cow's milk, but the nutritional significance of this difference is unclear.

LIPID

The lipid (or "fat") in human milk is almost all in the form of triglycerides, and it differs in several respects from the lipid in cow's milk. The fatty acids in human milk are less saturated than those of cow's milk, are largely of medium-chain length (10 to 14 carbon atoms), and are used more effectively than are the fatty acids in cow's milk. About 90% of human milk fat is digested, compared with 60% of butterfat. This difference is partly a result of the activity of a fat-splitting enzyme (a bile-salt–stimulated lipase) in human milk.

The palmitic acid in human milk is found on the central (position two) carbon of triglycerides, whereas in other milks, it is attached to the outer carbons (positions one and three). An enzyme in human milk splits off the fatty acids at positions one and three of a triglyceride, releasing monoglyceride carrying palmitic acid on position two. This monoglyceride is absorbed intact, with the result that there is little free palmitic acid in the intestine of a breast-fed infant. This is a desirable situation because free palmitic acid can interfere with calcium absorption.

The total lipid content of human milk varies between 2% and 10%, but it is not influenced by the mother's diet. The pattern of fatty acids in human milk, however, does reflect the fatty acid composition of the mother's diet. Human milk contains a high proportion of the essential fatty acids linoleic and α-linolenic acid. These account for 14% to 25% and 1% to 1.5%, respectively, of the fatty acids in human milk and allow human milk to protect an infant against a deficiency of essential fatty acids.

Alpha-linolenic acid is converted to eicosapentanoic acid (EPA) and docosahexaenoic acid (DHA). These long-chain fatty acids are important for maintaining the membrane fluidity needed for the initiation and propagation of nerve impulses. Infants have only a limited ability to convert α-linolenic acid to EPA and DHA, but they are both present in human milk. In cow's milk and infant formula, on the other hand, EPA and DHA are either absent or present at low levels.

The cholesterol provided by human milk is important because it is needed to assist the development of the infant's nervous system. It is also desirable that an infant be exposed to dietary cholesterol early in life to allow its body to become able to adjust the rate of cholesterol synthesis in the liver. By changing the rate of synthesis in harmony with changes in the dietary availability of cholesterol, the body is able to maintain sufficient supplies of cholesterol while at the same time protect against excess production when dietary cholesterol levels are high. The cholesterol content of human milk is not affected by variations in the mother's cholesterol intake. Infant formulas do not contain any cholesterol.

VITAMINS

The vitamin content of human milk generally reflects the vitamin intake and nutritional status of the mother. This means that a good supply of vitamins to the breast-fed infant can be maintained by supplementing the mother's diet with extra vitamins, if necessary. If the mother's vitamin supply and nutritional status are already high, additional supplementation only raises the vitamin content of her milk up to a natural plateau, after which the mother excretes additional vitamins, rather than passing them on to her infant.

One exception to the general rule that the vitamin content of milk reflects maternal intake and nutritional status is folate. The folate content of human milk remains relatively stable, unless the mother's diet has been poor. The absorption of folate by an infant is enhanced by another factor in human milk, possibly a folate-binding protein.

Human milk may be low in vitamin K, and all infants should receive a vitamin K supplement soon after birth. Infant formulas are supplemented with vitamin K to a concentration that is 10 to 20 times greater than that of human milk.

The heat-labile vitamins within human milk—thiamin, vitamin C, and vitamin B_6—are almost completely available to the infant. The higher amounts of these vitamins originally present in cow's milk may be substantially reduced by the heat used in pasteurization of milk and the oversterilization of formula.

Mothers who follow strict vegetarian diets, have deeply pigmented skin, or do not have adequate exposure to sunlight may have critically low vitamin D levels and may produce milk with insufficient vitamin D to prevent rickets in their infants.

MINERALS

For most minerals the mineral content of the mother's diet and her level of mineral stores have little effect on the mineral content of her milk. This has been established for calcium, magnesium, phosphorus, iron, copper, sodium, potassium, and chloride. The iodine and selenium content of milk *is* influenced by maternal intake, however.

The calcium content of human milk is one fourth that of cow's milk, but this lower level is well suited to the calcium needs of the growing infant. Human milk also contains a considerably lower level of phosphorus than does cow's milk, providing only one sixth as much per liter or per 100 kcal and one third as much per gram of protein. Taken together, these differences yield a favorable calcium/phosphorus ratio of 2:1 in human milk but a significantly lower ratio of 1.25:1 in cow's milk. The low calcium/phosphorus ratio in cow's milk may contribute to the development of hypocalcemic tetany in formula-fed infants.

The sodium content of human milk is low, which is compatible with the limited ability of an infant's kidneys to handle excess sodium. The sodium content of human colostrum is 600 mg/L but declines to 180 mg/L of milk by the time the infant is 1 month old. The level of sodium in human milk is not influenced by the amount of sodium in the mother's diet.

TRACE MINERALS

As knowledge increases about the role of trace minerals in human health, the trace mineral content of human milk is being used as a standard to estimate an infant's needs for these minerals. The information gained is also being used as a guide to the appropriate trace mineral content of infant formula. This guidance is important because certain processes used to modify cow's milk for use in infant formulas may remove some of the trace minerals from the cow's milk. Caregivers who use distilled water to prepare formula, because of worries about contaminants in tap water, may further reduce the trace mineral content of their infant's diet.

The iron content of human milk is low (0.3 mg/L), but the iron in human milk has a higher bioavailability (50%) than any other dietary source of iron. This may partially be because of the presence of the iron-containing protein **lactoferrin** in human milk. The high bioavailability of the iron in human milk and the fact that most infants are born with a 3- to 6-month reserve of iron mean that normal, adequately nourished breast-fed infants do not need another source of iron until they are 4 to 6 months old. Additional iron may be needed by breast-fed infants if they suffer significant blood loss or have an unusually high rate of growth.

Iron-deficiency anemia remains a risk to some infants, however, especially those fed formula with iron in a less bioavailable form. There is some evidence that before the traditional symptoms of iron-deficiency anemia develop, affected infants may show behavioral changes, such as tension, decreased responsiveness to stimuli, and lethargy. For these reasons many health professionals recommend the use of an iron-fortified formula starting at birth to prevent the development of iron deficiency later in infancy.

Human milk is known to contain a substance that enhances the absorption of zinc. It has also been suggested that the high copper/zinc ratio of 1:5 in human milk (compared with 1:15 in cow's milk) is associated with decreased cholesterol synthesis.

There is no evidence of copper deficiency in exclusively breast-fed infants.

IMMUNOLOGICAL FACTORS

Both colostrum and mature human milk contain **host-resistance factors,** which confer some immunity from infection to the breast-fed infant. The greatest concentration of these factors is found in colostrum, but significant amounts are found in mature milk. They include the enzymes **lysozyme** and **lactoperoxidase, lymphocytes, macrophages, *Lactobacillus bifidus* factor, lactoferrin, immunoglobulins,** and **interferon.**[7,8] All of these factors bestow what is called **passive immunity** to the breast-fed infant, meaning that they provide a form of immunity that does not require the activation of the infant's own immune defenses. Several of these factors are discussed below.

The enzyme lysozyme attacks and digests the cell walls of bacteria after the bacteria have been inactivated by peroxides and vitamin C present in both human milk and infant saliva. The lactoperoxidase enzyme acts by killing *Streptococcus* bacteria. Lymphocytes are the white blood cells responsible for mediating most aspects of the immune system, with its ability to attack a wide range of infectious microorganisms. The macrophages engulf and digest microorganisms by phagocytosis. They also synthesize and release lysozyme, lactoferrin, and "complement" proteins (a series of proteins that assist in the destruction of infectious microorganisms and infected cells).

Lactobacillus bifidus factor is a nitrogen-containing carbohydrate that encourages the growth of the bacterium *L. bifidus.* This bacterium converts lactose into acetic acid or lactic acid, thereby inhibiting the growth of pathogenic (disease-causing) microorganisms. The bacterium also competes with undesirable *Escherichia coli* bacteria and so inhibits their growth.

Lactoferrin is an iron-containing protein that inhibits the growth of *Staphylococcus* and *E. coli* bacteria by binding to the iron they need for growth. If an excess of iron is present in the diet, however, the lactoferrin may become saturated, thus allowing some of the additional iron to assist the growth of infectious microorganisms. This means that infants whose diets contain supplementary iron may be at increased risk of certain infections.

Immunoglobulins are the defensive proteins that include all types of antibodies. One class is known as **secretory IgA** and plays a major role in defending an infant against viruses, bacteria, and other pathogens and harmful food components in the first few days of life. It acts within the gastrointestinal tract and is especially effective against pathogens to which the mother has been exposed, such as polio virus, *Streptococcus,* and *Pneumococcus.* Human milk also contains **IgG** and **IgM** immunoglobulins but at a much lower level than that of IgA. It is interesting that the infant makes relatively low levels of its own IgA immunoglobulins and high levels of its own IgG and IgM immunoglobulins during the first year of life. This is an example of the functional development of the infant working in harmony with the composition of the milk it receives from its mother. Although immunoglobulins are proteins, they are relatively resistant to digestion in the infant's gastrointestinal tract and can survive the high acidity (low pH level) of the stomach.

Interferon is a small protein that plays a major role in defending the body against viral infection. It is produced by lymphocytes. In addition, some of the fatty acids and monoglycerides in human milk are able to penetrate the membranes of bacteria and some viruses to destroy them.

The passive immunity delivered to breast-fed infants via colostrum and milk can protect infants reared in conditions of poor sanitation against many life-threatening diseases. Even breast-fed infants raised in good environments have fewer respiratory and intestinal infections than do their formula-fed counterparts. It is also becoming clear that breast-feeding can bestow significant protection against illnesses later in life, by mechanisms that are not well understood (Table 15-3). Both retrospective and prospective epidemiological studies have found that breast-feeding is associated with protection against the development later in life of insulin-dependent diabetes mellitus, lymphoma, celiac disease, and Crohn's disease.[9]

PSYCHOLOGICAL FACTORS

The psychological advantages of breast-feeding are widely discussed but have proved difficult to document. Women who are allowed close physical contact with their infants in the delivery room immediately after birth are more likely to breast-feed successfully than are mothers who are initially separated from their infants for at least 8 hours.[10]

It is generally agreed that an infant derives a sense of security and belonging from the warmth of the mother's

TABLE 15-3

*Relative risk for developing selected illnesses throughout life for formula-fed, as compared with human milk-fed, infants**

ILLNESS	NEONATES (0-1 MONTH)	INFANTS (1 MONTH-1 YEAR)	CHILDHOOD/ ADOLESCENCE (>1-16 YEARS)	YOUNG ADULTS (>16 YEARS)
Necrotizing enterocolitis	2.8			
Diarrhea	14			
Septicemia	3.2	4-10		
Meningitis	3.2	4-16	3	
Atopic eczema		2.8		
Respiratory illness		2.3-5		
Otitis media		8.6	3.3-4.3	
Sudden infant death syndrome		3.5-7.7		
Colitis			2.7	1.8
Crohn's disease			2.1	1.7
Cancer (all types)			1.8	
Lymphoma			6.0	
Brain cancer			1.8	
Soft tissue sarcoma			1.6	

* The relative risk for breast-fed infants is 1.

From Ellis L, Picciano MF: *Nutr Today* 27:6, 1992.

body and from being held, rather than from the breast-feeding process as such. One classic study with monkeys showed that those fed from a bottle and being held by a warm surrogate mother were as well-adjusted as those nursed by their real mother. Research with dogs and ducks has identified a critical period during the first few days of life, when imprinting (or learning) occurs, which proves remarkably resistant to later modification.

The effect of the mother's presence on her child during the earliest days of life may well have long-term benefits for the child's later development. So far, however, psychologists have been unable to identify consistent differences in personality between breast-fed and formula-fed infants.

Breast-feeding certainly increases a mother's feeling of competence in dealing with her child. It increases the mother's belief that she is developing a unique relationship with her child and is fulfilling her natural maternal role. It is possible that breast-feeding bestows greater psychological advantages on the mother than on her infant.[11]

FERTILITY FACTORS

Breast-feeding has long been recognized as an important, although far from foolproof, factor in birth control. It appears that as long as a child is sucking vigorously at the breast each day, the mother's ovulation cycle is unlikely to return to a normal fertility pattern. This is probably because sucking stimulates the secretion of prolactin from the pituitary gland and suppresses the release of gonadotrophin-releasing hormone from the hypothalamus. Gonadotrophin-releasing hormone is necessary for the release of leutenizing hormone from the pituitary gland, which in turn is necessary for the maturation of the follicles in the ovary, which leads to ovulation. No direct role for prolactin in modifying fertility is yet known.[12]

In general, mothers whose infants are solely breast-fed and nurse regularly do not begin to ovulate again until 12 months after delivery. If solid foods are introduced early, in addition to breast-feeding, an earlier return to ovulation, menstruation, and fertility occurs. This reflects the decreased frequency, intensity, and duration of the nursing sessions because a considerable proportion of the infant's nutritional needs is satisfied by the solid food the infant receives. Mothers of formula-fed infants begin to ovulate and menstruate regularly within 3 to 6 months after birth.

OTHER FACTORS

Scientists are continually identifying additional ways in which breast-feeding offers unique benefits to both infants and their mothers. There is some evidence that breast-feeding protects against the development of obesity.[13] The risk of breast cancer is lower among women who have breast-fed a child than among those who have not. Breast-feeding also promotes the contractions of the uterus that quickly return it to its normal size after birth. Human milk contains a wide range of hormones and other biologically active substances, in addition to

Hormones and Hormonelike Substances in Human Milk

PITUITARY HORMONES	**STEROIDS**
Prolactin	Estradiol
Growth hormone	Estriol
Thyroid-stimulating hormone	Progesterone
Follicle-stimulating hormone	Testosterone
Luteinizing hormone	17-Ketosteroids
Adrenocorticotropin	Corticosterone
Oxytocin	Vitamin D
Neurotensin	
BRAIN-GUT PEPTIDES	**NONSTEROIDS**
Thyrotropin-releasing hormone	Thyroxin
Growth hormone–releasing hormone	Tri-iodothyroxin
Vasoactive intestinal peptide	Prostaglandins
Bombesin	(E2 and F2α)
Luteinizing hormone–releasing hormone	c AMP
Cholecystokinin	cGMP
Gastrin	Melatonin
Gastric inhibitory peptide	
GROWTH FACTORS	
Epidermal growth factor	
Insulin-like growth factors (I and II)	
Neural growth factor	

From Ellis L, Picciano MF: *Nutr Today* 27:6, 1992.

the specific substances discussed previously (see box). The function of many of these substances is not fully known, although animal studies suggest that they either assist in the synthesis and secretion of milk or play a role in the regulation of infant development.[14]

Overall, the advantages of breast-feeding are so compelling that an official *U.S. health objective for the nation for the year 2000* is to "increase to at least 75% the proportion of mothers who breast-feed their babies in the early postpartum period and to at least 50% the proportion who continue breast-feeding until their babies are 5 to 6 months old," from the 1988 baseline of 54% and 21%, respectively.[15]

CONTRAINDICATIONS

Because up to 50% of mothers choose not to breast-feed their infants, they obviously believe that alternative methods either offer them advantages or are equally satisfactory or that breast-feeding has disadvantages in their situation. Among the factors considered to be disadvantageous are the constant fatigue experienced by many breast-feeding mothers, the lack of freedom to return to work or a normal social life, the possibility of breast infection, and the mother's desire to quickly restore her figure to normal. Many mothers also worry about being unable to secrete sufficient milk.

Some mothers abandon attempts at breast-feeding early because they do not appreciate that proper lactation may be delayed until 3 to 5 days after birth and that the appearance of colostrum is naturally different from that of true milk. This difference in appearance can make some mothers feel that their milk "has turned to water." Some mothers may also be unprepared for some degree of physical discomfort because of the engorgement of the breasts when their milk first "comes in." Economic pressures on hospitals and the cost-containment policies of health insurance companies mean that many mothers are routinely discharged from the hospital 24 hours after delivery with no instruction or support to help them begin breast-feeding and no opportunity to establish satisfactory lactation practices before leaving the hospital or birthing facility.

CONTAMINANTS

Some mothers are deterred from breast-feeding by concerns about environmental contaminants being passed on to their infants within their milk. In areas of high insecticide use, some insecticides can be present in human milk. Dichlorodiphenyltrichloroethane (DDT), polychlorinated biphenyls (PCBs), hexachlorobenzene, dieldrin, and heptachlor epoxide have all been found in human milk in areas where these chemicals are widely used. The insecticide levels in human milk tend to be higher than those in cow's milk because humans are at the top of the food chain, with concentration of the insecticides possible at each level on the way up the food chain. One study investigated 858 children from birth to 5 years whose mothers' milk was known to contain PCBs and a metabolite of DDT (dichlorodiphenyl ethane, [DDE]). This study found no evidence of changes in the infants' growth rates, general health, or number of physician visits because of illness.[9] Because these children are still being studied, updates on their progress can be expected. In general, concern about contamination of human milk with DDT, PCBs, and other environmental contaminants is subsiding because of stricter control over the use of the chemicals involved. It is also relevant that heavy metals such as lead, mercury, arsenic, and cadmium are found in higher concentrations in certain water supplies, cow's milk, and reconstituted formulas than in human milk.[9]

Other possible contaminants are drugs taken by the mother. Nicotine, caffeine, and amphetamines should not be taken by a nursing mother. Nicotine may reduce the volume of milk produced. Caffeine and amphetamines can be passed on via milk to cause irritability and poor sleeping patterns in infants. Tranquilizers are also a cause for concern. They can cause a child to suck less vigorously, which in turn leads to a reduction in the volume of milk produced. Some less commonly used drugs that are also incompatible with breast-feeding are anticancer drugs, radioactive pharmaceuticals, lithium, lactation suppressants, certain antithyroid drugs, and anticoagulants. More detailed information can be obtained from the report of the Committee on Drugs of the American Academy of Pediatrics.[16]

ILLNESS OF MOTHER

If a mother is acutely or chronically ill, it may not be feasible for her to breast-feed her infant. However, mothers who suffer from short-term infections such as the breast infection, mastitis, may be able to continue breast-feeding until the infection responds to treatment. If they must refrain from breast-feeding for a short time, they may be able to maintain lactation by regular use of a breast pump until nursing can be resumed.

The disease of greatest concern nowadays is acquired immunodeficiency syndrome (AIDS), caused by infection with human immunodeficiency virus (HIV). Available data indicate that HIV infection is transmitted to infants via the placenta from about 30% to 40% of infected mothers. An additional 18% of infected mothers may pass the virus to their infants via their milk. Infants who have been infected with HIV by their mothers cannot be identified immediately because the infection is detected by testing for the presence of anti-HIV antibodies, and all infants born to infected mothers receive some of these antibodies from their mother by passive immunity. In the United States, where the success of formula feeding is ensured, mothers infected with HIV should not breast-feed their infants because the risk of transmitting the virus in their milk is too high. In the developing world, more than 50% of infants who are not breast-fed die within 1 year of birth. Mothers with HIV infection in these countries should be encouraged to breast-feed their infants because the risk of transmitting the virus via their milk is only 18%. Laboratory investigations have shown that a protein in human milk that has not yet been fully characterized suppresses the multiplication of HIV. This protein is not found in cow's milk.

Another virus that can be transmitted via milk is human T-cell lymphotropic virus type I (HTLV-I), which causes a form of leukemia known as *adult T-cell leukemia*. This virus is currently spreading rapidly throughout the Far East. Although HTLV-I is not yet widely prevalent in the Western world, it is possible that it may develop into a significant public health problem in the future. In the meantime, mothers known to be infected with HTLV-I should not breast-feed their infants.

ECONOMIC FACTORS

The cost to a mother of the additional food needed to sustain milk production may be higher or lower than the cost of formula feeding, depending on the type of diet she follows and her choice of formula type (Table 15-4). It is certainly feasible for her to consume an adequate diet to sustain breast-feeding at less additional cost than is required for formula feeding. The figures quoted in Table 15-4 for the cost of formula feeding do not include the cost of the equipment needed. Overall, shortage of money alone should not be a factor deterring mothers from breast-feeding. The need for mothers from poor families to go out to work, however, may be a significant factor influencing a decision to use formula feeding.

TABLE 15-4

Relative costs (in U.S. dollars) per week of breast-feeding and bottle-feeding (based on 750 ml/day)

FEEDING METHOD	COST ($)
BREAST-FEEDING	
Thrifty food plan	3.15
Liberal food plan	5.74
BOTTLE-FEEDING	
Whole fluid milk and sugar	2.85
Evaporated milk and sugar	2.46
Concentrated liquid formula (13 oz)	7.00
Powdered formula (1-lb can)	8.84
Ready-to-use formula	
Large can (32 oz)	10.65
Serving-size bottle (8 oz)	15.75

SOCIAL FACTORS

For many mothers the freedom to return to a normal social and working life is the dominant factor influencing their decision to use formula feeding. Even mothers who have had a satisfying and successful experience of breast-feeding consider the loss of freedom and restriction on their social life to be the major disadvantage of breast-feeding. Most mothers who breast-feed, however, find that they can occasionally use formula feeding when social events demand it, without any problems for either themselves or their infant. The mother may experience some discomfort because of the engorgement of her breasts when her infant does not feed on a normal schedule, but use of a breast pump can easily resolve this problem.

As women form an increasing proportion of the workforce, many employers are making efforts to meet the needs of women who breast-feed their infants. These include offering flex-time work schedules, on-site infant day-care centers, and nursing rooms for mothers to feed their infants or remove milk using a breast pump and refrigerate it for later use. Such measures mean that increasing numbers of mothers can combine an early return to work with successful breast-feeding.

FORMULA-FEEDING (BOTTLE-FEEDING)

The availability and success of infant formulas lead many mothers to prefer them to breast milk for the sustenance of their infants. Most of the formulas available in the United States are based on cow's milk, although alternatives based on soy protein and protein hydrolysates are also available. The formulas all contain added carbohydrate (lactose or sucrose), fats (a mixture of vegetable oils), minerals, and vitamins. The Committee on Nutrition of the American Academy of Pediatrics recommended levels of nutrients to be present in formulas (Table 15-5). These recommendations were adopted as law in the Infant Formula Act of 1980 (revised in 1986). This act establishes a minimal standard for 29 nutrients and a maximal allowable limit for 9 of these nutrients. The act also requires the quantities of each nutrient present to be listed on the label. Some nutrients are added to formula in a higher concentration than found in human milk to compensate for the lower bioavailability of the nutrients when they are present in formula.[17]

Formula is usually warmed to body temperature before feeding, although unwarmed formula is well tolerated by 50% of young infants and 75% of older infants. Giving the formula without warming has no adverse effect on the growth rate of infants. Feeding ice-cold formula, however, lowers the temperature of the infant's stomach contents for at least an hour and slows digestion by decreasing the activity of the digestive enzymes.

The practice of offering infants a bottle at bedtime and allowing them to fall asleep with the bottle in their mouth is a cause of **nursing bottle syndrome.** This is associated with a high incidence of tooth decay caused by the presence of the sugar-containing fluid (whether formula or fruit juice) close to the teeth. In addition to not leaving an infant with a bottle in its mouth, it is recommended that fruit juices be fed only by cup.

USE OF COW'S MILK IN INFANCY

In the first year of life, infants should not be fed whole cow's milk, skim milk, 1% to 2% fat milk, or evaporated milk.[18] These milks are considerably less expensive than formula preparations but have many nutritional disadvantages. They should not be used until the infant reaches 1 year of age, when at least two thirds of an infant's energy needs are being met by other foods. Infants fed cow's milk can develop iron deficiency because of the low level of iron in cow's milk. In addition, the high sodium and protein content of cow's milk increases the solute load on an infant's kidneys and brings a risk of dehydration as urine volume increases. The limited amounts of vitamin C, essential fatty acids, bioavailable zinc, and perhaps other trace minerals may be insufficient to prevent deficiency of these nutrients.

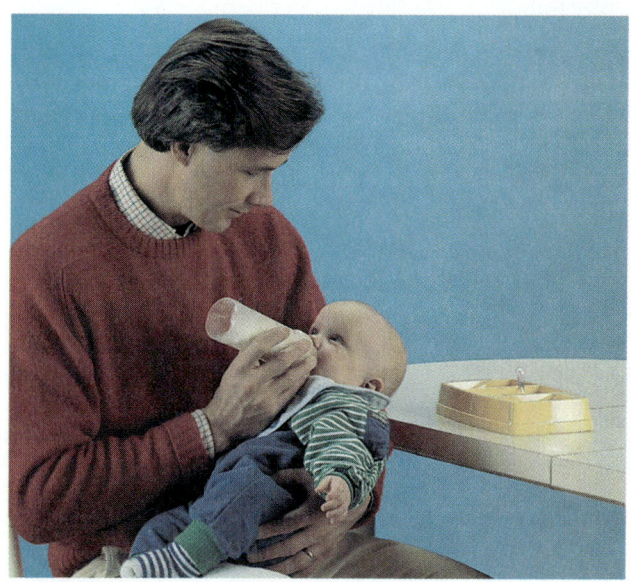

The use of skim milk can cause an infant to consume too much protein if the infant consumes enough milk to meet energy needs or, because of skim milk's low energy density, to consume an insufficient amount of milk to meet the infant's energy needs. Unmodified cow's milk also carries a greater risk of inducing milk allergy than do modified formulas.

> Feeding infants whole unmodified cow's milk may cause the following:
> - Low vitamin C intakes
> - Iron deficiency
> - Increased renal solute load
> - Allergies
> - Essential fatty acid deficiencies

ADEQUACY OF A MILK DIET

The recommended levels of nutrient supplementation in infant's diets are shown in Table 15-6.

The small amount of iron in human milk is well used, with up to 50% being absorbed. For infants older than 6 months, however, human milk cannot provide sufficient iron to maintain iron stores because iron absorption from human milk decreases when other foods are fed. When weaned onto iron-fortified cereals, infants should be given an iron supplement or some iron-fortified formula. Formula-fed infants should be given an iron-fortified formula throughout the first year of life to prevent the development of iron deficiency.

TABLE 15-5

Recommended nutrient levels of infant formulas per 100 kcal

NUTRIENT	RANGE	
	LOWEST ADEQUATE	NOT TO EXCEED[a]
Protein (g)	1.8[b]	4.5[b]
Fat (g)	3.3 (30% of cal)	6 (54% of cal)
Including essential fatty acid (linoleate) (mg)	300 (2.7% of cal)	
Vitamins		
A (IU)	250 (75 μg)[c]	750 (225 μg)[c]
D (IU)	40 (1 μg)[d]	100 (2.5 μg)[d]
K (μg)[e]	4	—
E (IU)	0.7 (0.5 mg),[f] at least 0.71U (0.5 mg)/g linoleic acid	—
C (ascorbic acid) (mg)	8	—
B_1 (thiamin) (μg)	40	—
B_2 (riboflavin) (μg)	60	—
B_6 (pyridoxine) (μg)	35 (15 μg/g of protein)	—
B_{12} (μg)	0.15	—
Niacin (μg)	250 (or 0.8 mg niacin equivalents)	—
Folic acid (μg)	4	—
Panthotenic acid (μg)	300	—
Biotin (μg)	1.4[g]	—
Choline (mg)	7[g]	—
Inositol (mg)	4[g]	—
Minerals[h]		
Calcium (mg)	60[i]	—
Phosphorus (mg)	30[i]	—
Magnesium (mg)	6	—
Iron (mg)	0.15	2.5[j]
Iodine (μg)	5	25
Zinc (mg)	0.5	—
Copper (μg)	60	—
Manganese (μg)	5	—
Sodium (mg)	20 (5.8 mEq)	60 (17.5 mEq)
Potassium (mg)	80 (13.7 mEq)	200 (34.3 mEq)
Chloride (mg)	55 (10.4 mEq)	150 (28.3 mEq)
Selenium (μg)[k]	3	—

[a] Where no upper limit is given, toxicity is not well defined; massive excesses may have adverse consequences.
[b] At least nutritionally equivalent to casein quality recommended as outlined in *Pediatrics* 57:278, 1978.
[c] Retinol equivalents.
[d] Cholecalciferol.
[e] Any vitamin K added shall be in the form of phylloquinone.
[f] d-Alpha tocopherol equivalents.
[g] Average present in milk-based formulas; should be included in this amount in other formulas.
[h] Formula should be made with water low in fluoride and in any case contain less than 45 μg/100 kcal. For explanation, see *Pediatrics,* 77:758, 1988.
[i] Calcium-to-phosphorus ratio should be no less than 1.1 nor more than 2.
[j] Prudence indicates that there should be an upper limit on iron. If formula is labeled "infant formula with iron," it must contain not less than 1 mg/100 kcal.
[k] Selenium is not included in 1987 recommendations. The level that causes toxicity is very narrow.

From Barness L, editor: *Pediatric nutrition handbook,* ed 3, Elk Grove Village, Ill, 1993, American Academy of Pediatrics.

The amount of vitamin D in human milk depends to some extent on the mother's diet, and even under ideal conditions it is not a dependable source of all the vitamin D needed by an infant. An infant who is regularly exposed to the ultraviolet rays of the sun manufactures sufficient vitamin D to overcome any dietary deficit. If breast-fed infants are not exposed to regular sunshine, they should be given a daily supplement of 10 μg (400 international units [IU]) of vitamin D, preferably beginning by the fifth day of life. Cod liver oil was once a popular source of vitamin D, but it has now been largely replaced by water-miscible preparations. The new prepa-

TABLE 15-6

Recommended supplementation of infant diets

TYPE OF FEEDING	VITAMIN K	VITAMIN D	FLUORIDE	IRON
Human milk	Single intramuscular dose of 0.5 to 1 mg or oral dose of 1 to 2 mg	10 μg/day	0.25 mg/day	1 mg/kg/day*
Formula	Single intramuscular dose of 0.5 to 1 mg or oral dose of 1 to 2 mg	—	0.25 mg/day†	—

* If an iron-fortified cereal is not used after 6 months of age.
† If fluoride content of water is less than 0.3 parts per million.

rations do not place the infant at risk of developing lipoid pneumonia because of the aspiration of oily particles of cod liver oil into the lungs. Vitamin D supplementation is not required for infants fed prepared formulas and is probably undesirable as is the use of other vitamin D-fortified foods because of the risk of toxicity from consumption of too much vitamin D.

Except for infants fed a formula prepared with fluoridated water, all infants should be given a fluoride supplement of 0.25 mg/day in the first year of life. This is recommended so that infants develop resistance to tooth decay. Such supplements are available only with a prescription because of the dangers associated with excess fluoride consumption.

All infants should receive 0.5 to 1.0 mg of vitamin K by injection, or 1 to 2 mg orally, once shortly after birth. Infants fed human milk maintain lower plasma levels of vitamin K than do formula-fed infants largely because formula is typically supplemented with the vitamin to a relatively high level of 5 μg/100ml. The minimal level of supplementary vitamin K in formula was set at 4 μg/100 ml at a time when the level of vitamin K in human milk was believed to be 1.5 μg/100 ml, 10 times the currently expected value.

NUTRITIVE NEEDS OF INFANTS

Precise information on the nutritive needs of infants is available for only a few nutrients. Levels of intake that appear to support the growth of healthy infants are used as guidance when setting recommended dietary allowances (RDAs) (Table 15-7).

ENERGY

An average daily energy intake of 49 kcal/lb or 108 kcal/kg has traditionally been considered adequate to meet an infant's needs during the first 6 months of life. Research findings, however, indicate that the level of energy required falls to about 71 kcal/kg/day by the fourth month. Of the energy intake, 50% is used to meet basal energy needs, 25% for activity, and 25% to cover the energy needs for growth (which averages 15 to 35 g/day). Infants have a surface area/weight ratio twice as great as that of adults, and so they lose proportionately more energy as heat.

Human milk or infant formula provides all of the energy needed by a newborn infant. Milk or formula is the recommended sole source of energy for the first 6 months, but in practice, most infants receive 15% of their energy from supplemental foods by the age of 4 months.[20]

Excessive energy intake leading to rapid weight gain is as undesirable in infants as it is in adults. It is important for parents to realize that maximal growth is not the same as optimal growth: infants can be made to grow faster than is best for them by overfeeding. Attempts to prove any link between weight in infancy and obesity in childhood, adolescence, and adulthood have been far from conclusive.

PROTEIN

The need for protein during infancy is relatively high because of the rapid growth of the skeleton, muscles, and other tissues. A daily intake of 2.2 g of high biological value protein per kilogram of body weight is sufficient for normal growth, provided that energy intake is also adequate. At 3 weeks of age, 60% to 75% of dietary protein is used for growth and the rest is used for maintenance of existing tissues. By 4 months of age, 45% is used for growth and 55% for maintenance. By 5 months, total protein needs have dropped to 1.4 g/kg/day.

If protein of lower biological value is used, the amounts required increase accordingly. Infants should only be given proteins with a biological value of 70% to 85%, such as milk, meat, and eggs. In general, a protein intake that provides 6.5% to 8% of total dietary energy meets an infant's protein requirement. There is no evidence of any advantages from protein intakes that are above that level.

Surplus dietary protein must be deaminated in the liver, leading to excretion of its nitrogen as urea and use

TABLE 15-7

Recommended dietary allowances (United States*) and recommended nutrient intakes (Canada†) for infants

NUTRIENT	RDAs and RNIs FOR AGE (0-0.5 MONTH)		RDAs and RNIs FOR AGE (0.5-1 MONTH)	
	UNITED STATES	CANADA	UNITED STATES	CANADA
Kcal	650	600	850	900
Protein (g)	13	12	14	12
Calcium (mg)	400	250	600	400
Magnesium (mg)	40	20	60	32
Iron (mg)	6	0.3	10	7
Iodine (μg)	40	30	50	40
Zinc (mg)	5	2	5	3
Selenium (μg)	10	—	15	—
Vitamin A (μg RE)	375	400	375	400
Vitamin D (μg)	7.5	10	10	10
Vitamin E (mg α TE)	3	3	4	3
Vitamin C (mg)	30	20	35	20
Folate (μg)	25	50	35	50
Niacin (mg NE)	5	4	6	7
Riboflavin (mg)	0.4	0.3	0.5	0.5
Thiamin (mg)	0.3	0.3	0.4	0.4
Pyridoxine (mg)	0.3	—	0.6	—
Vitamin B_{12} (μg)	0.3	0.3	0.5	0.3
PROVISIONAL ALLOWANCES				
Chromium (μg)	10-40	—	20-60	—
Molybdenum (μg)	15-30	—	20-40	—
Manganese (mg)	0.3-0.6	—	0.6-1	—
Copper (mg)	0.4-0.6	—	0.6-0.7	—
Fluoride (mg)	0.1-0.5	—	0.2-1	—

RE, Retinol equivalent; *TE,* tocopherol equivalent; NE, niacin equivalent.

* From National Research Council: *Recommended dietary allowances,* ed 10, Washington, DC, 1989, National Academy Press.

† From Health and Welfare Canada: *Recommended nutrient intakes,* Ottawa, Canada, 1990, Supply and Service Canada.

of the remainder as an energy source. Because infants have a limited ability to concentrate waste metabolites, such as urea, sufficient water must be available for them to excrete the urea derived from excess protein. If enough water is not available, urea accumulates in the blood, causing protein edema. Consumption of excess protein can also lead to undesirable growth of the liver (hypertrophy) because of its need to produce the deaminase enzymes required for protein metabolism. All of these considerations mean that an infant's protein intake should not exceed 6 g/kg of body weight (four times the recommended intake).

The higher rate of infection found in infants fed cow's milk may be caused by mechanisms that normally produce antibodies being diverted to deal with excess milk proteins. Infants fed unmodified whole cow's milk, which contains twice the protein of human milk, can develop hypochromic microcytic anemia. This is caused by gastric bleeding, leading to loss of blood in the feces, apparently from an allergic response to the undiluted cow's milk protein.

The amino acid requirements of infants are proportionately higher than those of adults. In addition to the eight amino acids needed by adults, histidine is an essential amino acid for infants, although adequately met by either human milk or formula.

One study of the diets of 637 infants found that from the age of 6 months, their diets provided 12% more protein than the RDA. The level of excess increased until the infants were consuming more than twice the RDA by the age of 12 months.[20] Cow's milk and food from the family table provided 50% of the protein at 8 months and 80% at 12 months.

WATER-SOLUBLE VITAMINS

Human milk usually provides the infant's requirements for the water-soluble vitamins if the mother's diet is adequate. In many cases the RDA is set well above the level achievable with human milk feeding to account for differences in bioavailability and possible losses from processing.

The recommended amount of **thiamin** was estimated from the mean thiamin concentration of human milk, plus some additional safety margin, at 0.3 mg/L, or 0.4 mg/100 kcal. Studies of the thiamin content of human milk also suggest that the minimal daily requirement is 0.17 mg/day. The recommended intakes of 0.3 mg/day during the first 6 months of life and 0.4 mg/day in the second 6 months are well above the estimated requirements.

The recommended daily intake of 5 to 6 mg **niacin** equivalents (NEs) cannot be met by human milk, which provides 0.15 mg of niacin and 21 mg of tryptophan per 100 ml. This is equivalent to 3.7 NE/750 ml of milk, or 7 NE/1000 kcal. There is no evidence that breast-fed infants require supplemental niacin.

The RDAs for infants are set so that a progressively increasing amount of **pyridoxine** is given to an infant during the first year of life. Infants fed diets very low in pyridoxine can develop seizures. The amount in human milk reflects the mother's intake and increases quickly when the mother takes a supplement. Milk from mothers who use oral contraceptives for more than 30 months before pregnancy may have marginal levels of pyridoxine. Infant formulas contain sufficient pyridoxine to satisfy an infant's needs, at a level of 0.115 mg of pyridoxine per gram of protein, or 0.04 mg/100 kcal.

An infant probably needs 3.5 μg of folate per kg of body weight. Human milk and infant formulas provide considerably more folate than this.[21]

The daily intake of **vitamin B_{12}** from human milk is about 0.35 to 0.40 μg, whereas the RDA during the first 6 months of life is 0.3 μg. Because reserves build up during fetal life, there is little likelihood of vitamin B_{12} deficiency in breast-fed infants, unless the mother is a vegan. There have been many claims that vitamin B_{12} is a growth stimulant for infants. The American Academy of Pediatrics surveyed 13 studies of the effect of oral or intramuscular vitamin B_{12} on 546 "normal children." Only two of the studies—involving 69 children—reported a significant and stimulating growth effect, and all the children showing enhanced growth were underweight at the beginning of the study.

The RDA for **vitamin C** in infancy is 30 to 35 mg/day. Breast-fed infants usually receive adequate amounts, and formula has additional vitamin C to counteract the losses during pasteurization.

FAT-SOLUBLE VITAMINS

An infant is normally born with reserves of **vitamin A** stored in its liver, to an extent determined by the vitamin A status of the mother. The RDA for vitamin A in infancy is 375 μg retinol equivalents (REs), which is less than the amount normally supplied by a daily intake of 750 ml of human milk. Vitamin A toxicity becomes a problem when intakes rise to between 25,000 and 50,000 RE/day and are maintained for about 30 days. The main effects of vitamin A toxicity in an infant are a buildup of intracranial pressure and hydrocephalus.

Vitamin D is crucial in infancy to sustain the rapid calcification of bones and teeth. One hundred IU/day prevents rickets, 300 IU/day cures rickets, and 400 IU(10 μg)/day promotes good calcium absorption and skeletal growth. Because human milk contains only 50 IU/L, a vitamin D supplement of 400 IU/day is recommended during the first week of life. Supplementation with vitamin D is not required for formula-fed infants. There are no known advantages of vitamin D intakes in excess of 400 IU/day, and intakes greater than 1800 IU/day may actually cause a decrease in calcium absorption. There is also evidence that sensitive infants consuming from 1000 to 3000 IU/day may exhibit hypercalcemia, decreased appetite, and retarded growth.

Because little **vitamin E** crosses the placenta, infants are born with low tissue concentrations of this vitamin. An intake of 3 to 4 mg tocopherol equivalents (TE) of vitamin E is advisable during the first year of life. Both human milk and formula supply the required amount of vitamin E. Premature infants have lower stores of vitamin E and a reduced ability to absorb it. They can develop anemia because of the rupture of red blood cell membranes caused by the lack of the antioxidant protection afforded by vitamin E. Diets high in polyunsaturated fatty acids (PUFAs) make this situation worse.

MINERALS

Considerable amounts of **calcium** are needed to sustain the rapid rate of calcification of bone tissue and teeth during infancy. Milk contains sufficient calcium to meet the infant's needs, but sufficient vitamin D must also be available to allow the efficient absorption of calcium from milk. The RDAs for calcium during infancy, of 400 to 600 mg/day, are intended only for formula-fed infants, who absorb only one third to half of the calcium they consume. The calcium/phosphorus ratio of 1.2:1 in cow's milk (compared with 2:1 in human milk) is too low for the newborn infant. However, a calcium/phosphorus ratio of anywhere between 1:1 and 2:1 is recommended for formulas.

Full-term infants normally have sufficient reserves of **iron** to meet their needs for the first 3 months of life. Premature infants, however, have received less iron from their mother while in the womb and so need to be provided with iron early in life. Twins also have lower-than-normal reserves of iron because the mother's supply has been shared between them. Human milk provides adequate iron for breast-fed infants. Many pediatric nutritionists now recommend that formula-fed infants should be given formula fortified with ferrous sulfate (at 12 mg/L) throughout the first year of life. Only 4% of such supplemental dietary iron is absorbed, but this is sufficient to prevent development of iron deficiency. The dietary allowances for iron are for infants who are not breast-fed and are based on an average dietary need of 1 mg/kg/day. The total recommended intakes of between 6 and 10 mg/day can be provided by iron-fortified formulas and iron-enriched infant cereals, containing 12 mg of iron per ounce.

Studies have shown that most infants are in negative **zinc** balance during the first weeks and possibly months of life. This has focused attention on the importance of zinc in early feeding, especially because the mineral is known to be required for normal growth and the development of the brain. Colostrum is rich in zinc (at 4 mg/L), but the level in mature milk declines to 1.2 mg/L at 6 months and to 0.5 mg/L by 1 year. Zinc in human milk is more bioavailable than is the zinc in cow's milk. All commercial formulas sold in the United States currently contain 5 to 6 mg of zinc/L. The RDA for zinc in infancy is 5 mg/day, although this appears to be unnecessarily high.

Past concerns over the amount of **iodine** available to infants have been alleviated by an increase in the amount available from milk because of increases in the amounts available in mothers' diets. Soy-based infant formulas may be supplemented with iodine to counteract the effect of goitrogens in soy products. The RDA for iodine in infancy is 40 to 50 μg/day.

Fluoride is an important component of an infant's diet because of its role in the development of teeth that are resistant to decay. Because relatively little fluoride crosses the placenta from mother to infant, it is important that infants receive up to 1 mg/day throughout their first year. Human milk contains relatively little fluoride. Formula prepared with fluoridated water has been found to contain as much as 0.9 mg of fluoride per liter. When a variety of baby foods are added to the diet, infants generally receive around 1.2 mg of fluoride per day. A fluoride supplement providing 0.25 mg/day should be provided (with a prescription) for infants whose fluoride intake is likely to be marginal.

Estimates of the requirements for other trace minerals during infancy are based largely on analysis of the amounts in human milk. Because these values vary widely, both among different mothers and within the same mother at different times, recommendations quote a range of values. The best current estimates of recommended intakes are shown in Table 15-7.

WATER OR FLUID

The greater surface area/weight ratio of infants relative to adults causes them to lose water and heat at almost twice the rate of adults. This makes it vital to ensure that an infant consumes sufficient water. Most breast-fed and formula-fed infants receive adequate water in their milk or formula. When solid foods are introduced, they must be accompanied by sufficient water to satisfy the baby's thirst.

An infant fed on human milk requires 20 ml of water per kilogram of body weight to allow the kidneys to handle the excretion of soluble wastes. If cow's milk formula is used, 61 ml/kg is required. If undiluted cow's milk is fed to infants, they require 87 ml of water per kg of body weight. For an infant living at normal room temperature (70° F or 21° C), any one of these sources of milk contains sufficient water. At 93° F (34° C), more water is lost through the skin and the cow's milk does not provide enough water to meet the infant's needs. Even when formula feeding is used, a child should be offered additional water when the environmental temperature is high. It is not only unnecessary to offer additional water to breast-fed infants, but also it is discouraged in areas of the world where water contamination is likely.

Thirsty infants act like hungry infants; so parents sometimes offer food when infants really need water. If they eat the food, their need for water increases, making the thirst more severe. Parents should be aware of the importance of offering fluids to their infants in such situations.

EFFECTS OF DRUGS

The need for many nutrients in infancy may be increased by the use of drugs. There is considerable evidence that anticonvulsant drugs increase the need for both vitamin D and folate. Antibiotics influence the availability of several nutrients, such as vitamin B_{12} and vitamin K.

INTRODUCTION TO SOLID FOODS

At the turn of the century, pediatricians were recommending that the milk diet of an infant not be supplemented with food, such as meat or cereal, until the infant was 1 year old. In 1917 Emmett Holt suggested that a meat broth could safely be introduced at 8 or 9 months of age. By 1956 opinion had swung dramatically to the point where some pediatricians recommended that at 2 or 3 weeks of age infants should be consuming solid foods as part of a three-meals-per-day diet.

Current Recommendations for the Optimal Feeding of Infants

- Use only breast-feeding for the first 4 to 6 months.
- Begin to introduce some solid foods by 6 months.
- Make the transition to foods from the family table gradually and at whatever pace suits the infant.

The trend toward earlier introduction of solid foods was not supported by any nutritional or physiological evidence in its favor. It prompted The American Academy of Pediatrics to undertake a survey to try to determine the bases of pediatricians' recommendations.

This survey confirmed that most pediatricians were recommending the use of cereal by 3 to 6 weeks of age, developing into a full diet of meat, eggs, fruit, vegetables, and cereals by the time an infant was 4 to 5 months old. These recommendations had developed in response to the wishes of parents to follow this supposedly "progressive" procedure and were not based on any evidence that infants needed solid foods so early in life.

The pendulum of opinion has now swung back to the current recommendation that milk should be the sole source of nourishment in the first 4 to 6 months of life and the main source for the rest of the first year.[22] Although this recommendation is almost universally accepted by nutrition professionals, several surveys of infant feeding practices show that a significant number of mothers introduce solid foods earlier than recommended. In 1988, for example, 35% of infants were introduced to solid foods by 2 months and 53% by 3 months.

Solid food added to an infant's diet is called **beikost** (a German word meaning foods, other than milk, fed to infants). If it is not introduced until after 6 months of age, the sequence in which different foods are introduced is not particularly important. If introduced earlier, however, the foods used and the sequence in which they are introduced should reflect an infant's nutritional needs, physiological readiness to use the foods, and physical ability to handle them. These three factors are considered in more detail below.

NUTRITIONAL NEEDS

All of the nutrients required by an infant in its first 4 to 6 months of life can be provided by a milk diet supplemented with iron, fluoride, and vitamin D. The supplements can be taken on their own or added to milk or formula; so there is no nutritional need to introduce solid foods before 4 to 6 months of age. The major objection to introducing solid foods earlier than this is the possibility of overfeeding and the potential that the infant will develop allergies.

By the time an infant reaches 6 months of age, a milk diet alone cannot provide sufficient energy or protein for a growing infant. This is the stage at which infant cereal is usually added to the diet. It should be mixed with milk to a consistency that allows it to be swallowed, but not sucked, from the spoon. Several types of cereal grain—such as rice, wheat, and oats—should be introduced individually 1 week at a time. This allows sufficient time for any potential allergy to be identified.

A few weeks after the introduction of cereals, various strained fruits can be given, again one at a time over several weeks. It is nutritionally unnecessary to add sugar to fruit, although some commercial infant fruit products contain small amounts of sugar to compensate for natural variations in the sweetness of fruit used in different batches. Bananas that are fully ripened so that the starch has changed to sugar are an acceptable fruit for infants at this stage. Vegetables can be introduced after fruits, again one at a time. By 9 months of age, infant cereals should provide 8% to 10% of an infant's energy intake, whereas other solid baby foods should provide 30% to 40%.[20]

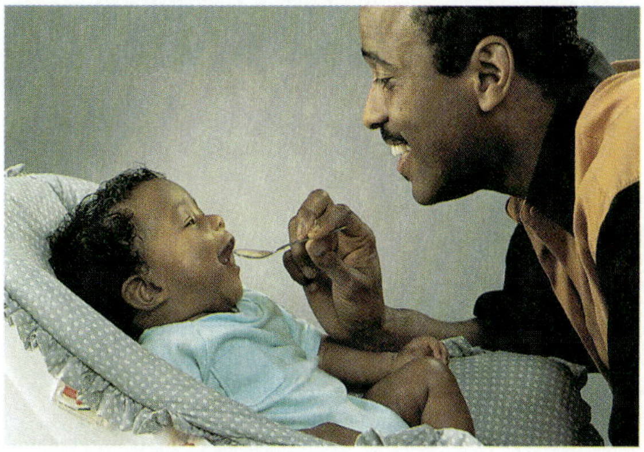

The introduction of solid foods to an infant who is ready can be a pleasant experience for the parent and the child.

Egg, meat, and cottage cheese are considered suitable foods to help provide sufficient protein for the infant being introduced to solid foods. Egg is **allergenic** to some infants and should not be given to infants from families with a history of food allergy.

As solid foods are introduced, it is desirable to keep the proportion of kilocalories provided by protein at 7% to 16%; from fat, at 35% to 45%; and from carbohydrate, at 29% to 58%. These proportions are close to the proportions found in human milk. The percentages of kilocalories provided by the protein, fat, and carbohydrate in selected infant foods are shown in Table 15-8.

PHYSICAL DEVELOPMENT

Infants are born with rooting, sucking, and extrusion reflexes, which equip them to live on a diet of milk. These reflexes are replaced with the ability to swallow semisolid foods, as the infant matures. Infants vary in the rate at which their physical development equips them to cope with semisolid and solid foods. At birth, the lower jaw is poorly developed and fat pads in the cheeks help to give the mouth the shape needed for sucking. As the infant matures, the contour of the jaw changes and the fat pads disappear. This allows the infant to swallow, rather than to simply suck.

The ability to swallow usually develops between 3 and 5 months of age. Before that time the extrusion reflex causes the infant to push out food or other objects placed at the front of the tongue. This must be replaced by the swallowing reflex, in which food placed at the front of the tongue is rolled into a ball and pushed to the top of the esophagus. Any solid or semisolid food given before the age of 3 to 5 months must either be placed far

TABLE 15-8

Energy density and distribution of energy-yielding nutrients in infant foods

	Kcal/100 g	PROTEIN (%)	FAT (%)	CARBOHYDRATE (%)
Egg yolk	192	21	76	3
Meats	106	53	46	1
Fruits	85	2	2	96
Soups and dinners	58	16	28	56
Vegetables	45	14	6	80
Human milk	67	6	56	38
Nonfat milk	35	40	3	57
Whole milk	67	22	48	30

back in the mouth or must be sufficiently fluid for the infant to suck it.

In most infants the first teeth erupt at about 5 to 6 months of age. It is important that an infant be given an opportunity to learn to chew at this time. Dry toast can be used to stimulate chewing. Hard materials, such as crisp bacon and certain flint-like commercial biscuits, should be avoided because they can irritate the throat. Several cases of choking have been reported involving infants fed hot dogs, nuts, grapes, and raw carrots. All such foods should be avoided.

An infant's physical readiness for solid food depends on the following:

- The ability to chew
- The ability to swallow
- The eruption of teeth

An infant is physiologically ready for solid foods when the following occur:

- Saliva is produced.
- Enzymes for the digestion of starch and unemulsified fat are produced.
- The kidneys mature to be able to handle the increased solute load produced by solid food.
- Gastric acidity increases toward adult levels.

PHYSIOLOGICAL DEVELOPMENT

The ability of an infant to handle foods other than milk also depends on its physiological development. To digest and use solid food effectively, an infant must be producing sufficient saliva to moisten the food and sufficient digestive enzymes to digest the food, its stomach must be able to produce sufficient acid, and its kidneys must be mature enough to handle the increased solute load generated by solid food.

An infant produces little saliva immediately after birth but may produce enough to cause drooling by the age of 2 to 3 months. Because the enzymes in saliva are involved only in the digestion of starches, they are unnecessary for infants receiving milk alone. Proteolytic enzymes are present in the stomach and the intestine from birth in sufficient quantities to digest milk protein within a soft, flocculent, and dilute curd. The levels of these enzymes steadily increase until they are able to digest most proteins by the time the infant is 4 to 6 months old.

The interior of an infant's stomach is not as acidic as that of an adult stomach. This initial "low gastric acidity" means that nitrates in food are more readily converted into nitrites, which in turn react with amines in the intestines to produce nitrosamines. Because nitrosamines are potential carcinogens, it is important to prevent overconsumption of nitrates by infants. Vegetables that are rich in nitrates and so should be avoided in early infancy (less than 6 months of age) include beets, spinach, turnips, collard greens, and broccoli. Another problem associated with nitrates is the ability of the nitrites they generate to be absorbed and to convert hemoglobin to methemoglobin, which has a reduced capacity to carry oxygen.

The kidneys of full-term infants are not fully mature. The glomeruli within the kidneys can filter fluid from the blood efficiently, but the tubules of the kidneys cannot reabsorb water and some solutes efficiently. This situation lasts for only the first 6 to 8 weeks of life and means that high-protein and high-sodium diets should be avoided during that time. This is particularly important for infants who have excessive fluid loss, such as those living in hot climates, suffering from diarrhea, or eating foods of high-energy density.

OTHER CONSIDERATIONS

The major argument used in favor of giving solid food in the first few months of life is that the infant becomes accustomed to a wide variety of flavors and textures of food and will continue to accept varied foods later in life. Beal,[22] however, found that there was little relationship between the age at which a child was first offered solid foods and the age at which the food was accepted. She reported a period of difficulty in the mother-child relationship, when mothers try to give solids and semisolids to infants who are not ready for them. She believed that the feeding of semisolids between the ninth and twelfth weeks increased the incidence of feeding problems and food dislikes in the infant.

Some parents believe that the introduction of solid food makes it more likely that their infant will sleep through the night.[23] There is no experimental evidence to support this belief.[24]

Although the findings are inconsistent, many studies report an increased incidence of food allergy among infants introduced to a variety of foods at an early age. This possibility is particularly important to infants in families with a history of food allergy. Allergists suggest that such infants should be introduced to solid foods at a later date than are other infants and should be given such foods as vegetables, fruits, and rice cereal, which are not strong allergens. Throughout the first year of life it is also advisable not to feed major allergens such as cow's milk, soy, and peanuts to infants at risk of food allergy.[25]

Solid foods should be added to an infant's diet in the following order:

- Cereal
  - Rice
  - Oats
  - Barley
- Fruit
- Vegetables (avoiding nitrate-containing vegetables)
- Eggs
- Meat

Young infants have low levels of many cellular enzymes, in addition to having low levels of many digestive enzymes. Phenylalanine hydroxylase, required for the metabolism of phenylalanine, is one well-known case in point. A diet high in protein may tax the infant's ability to use all the phenylalanine released by the digestion of the protein.

Concern over the use of food additives in infant foods has focused on the use of salt (sodium chloride), monosodium glutamate, sugar, and modified starch. All of these have been added to many commercially prepared infant foods, although mainly to make them more suited to the taste of the mothers using them rather than to adapt them to the likely taste preferences of infants. Infants have been found to eat the same amount of a food, regardless of whether salt is added to it.[26] The FDA has ruled that the level of salt in infant foods should not exceed 0.25%, in contrast with the 1% often found before this ruling. Many manufacturers have since stopped adding salt to infant foods and advise parents not to season the food according to their own taste. The main concern about the use of salt is that the immature kidneys of infants cannot excrete excess electrolytes efficiently.

Concern about the use of monosodium glutamate in infant foods is based on reports that mice fed large quantities of this flavor enhancer develop brain tumors. There is no evidence that the smaller amounts used in infant foods pose any threat to the infants, but food manufacturers have now voluntarily stopped using it.

The addition of sugar to infant foods is criticized by people who believe it may contribute to the development of a "sweet tooth." Many fruits that are labeled as containing sugar may only contain the natural sugar of the fruit or sugar added to return the sugar content to its natural level. Honey is often used to sweeten homemade infant foods, but it should not be given to infants younger than 1 year old. Some honey contains spores of *Clostridium botulinum,* which are resistant to heat and are not inactivated by the low acidity of the infant stomach. If these spores germinate in the gastrointestinal tract, they can cause botulism, which is often fatal.

The modified starches used in baby foods are primarily corn, potato, wheat, or cassava starches, which have been chemically treated to make them more suitable for infant food. The treatment makes the starches more stable and more efficient thickeners of the food to which they are added. The small amounts of modified starches added to infant foods have been found to be easily digested and safe constituents of an infant's diet.[27]

EFFECTS OF EARLY FEEDING ON LATER DEVELOPMENT

There is considerable interest about possible effects of early feeding practices on later development, but it is difficult to obtain reliable information in this area. Most concern has been focused on the possibility that some infant feeding practices may predispose a child to degenerative diseases later in life.

One major issue has been whether an increase in the number of fat cells caused by overfeeding in infancy can contribute to obesity throughout life. Studies have not found strong evidence to support this idea (see Issues and Opinions Box, Chapter 6).

There is also popular concern that saturated fat and cholesterol consumed in infancy may increase the risk of atherosclerosis later in life. Cholesterol must not be eliminated from the diets of infants and children because of its essential role in metabolism. Nor is it appropriate to restrict the fat intake of children under 2 years of age because this might leave them deficient in the energy needed for growth. If polyunsaturated fats are substituted for saturated fats in an infant's diet, the amount of vitamin E must be increased to give sufficient antioxidant protection.

Giving infants large amounts of salt before their kidneys can efficiently excrete excess sodium may increase the risk of high blood pressure in adulthood.

In any cases in which an infant's diet can increase the risk of disease later in life, the dangers are greatest for infants from families with a history of the diseases concerned.

ADEQUACY OF INFANTS' DIETS

Most recent surveys indicate that most American infants consume at least the RDA amounts of most nutrients.[19,20] A larger number of infants, however, are fed whole or skim cow's milk, rather than human milk or infant formula.[28] These infants receive three times the RDA for protein and one and a half times the maximal "safe" amount of sodium, but only two thirds of the RDA for iron and half the recommended intake of linoleic acid. The consequences of these practices are unknown.

The adequacy of infants' diets is best assessed by analyzing the rate and pattern of their growth. To help assess growth, the National Center for Health Statistics has developed **growth charts** that display the expected patterns at percentiles from 5 to 95 (Figures 15-5 and 15-6).

Failure to thrive in infants is primarily a result of inadequate food intake. This may be caused by illness, a failure to absorb food efficiently, or social factors such as poverty, neglect, or vegetarianism.

Concern over the possibility that some infants are nutritionally disadvantaged from birth led to the implementation of the Women, Infants and Children program (WIC). As discussed in Chapter 14, this helps to provide food for pregnant and lactating women and their infants and children under 5. To be eligible for participation, the women, infants, and children must be from families with an income at or near the poverty level and must show some evidence of nutritional risk. There were approximately 4.9 million participants per month in this U.S. federally assisted program in 1992. Funding has risen from $20 million in 1974 to over $2.5 billion in 1992, yet it is estimated that only 60% of those eligible are enrolled in the program. The U.S. government's General Accounting Office estimated that each dollar invested in WIC saves $2.89 in health care within the first year of life and $3.50 over 18 years.[28]

FIGURE 15-5

Weight and height for age chart for girls from birth to 36 months.

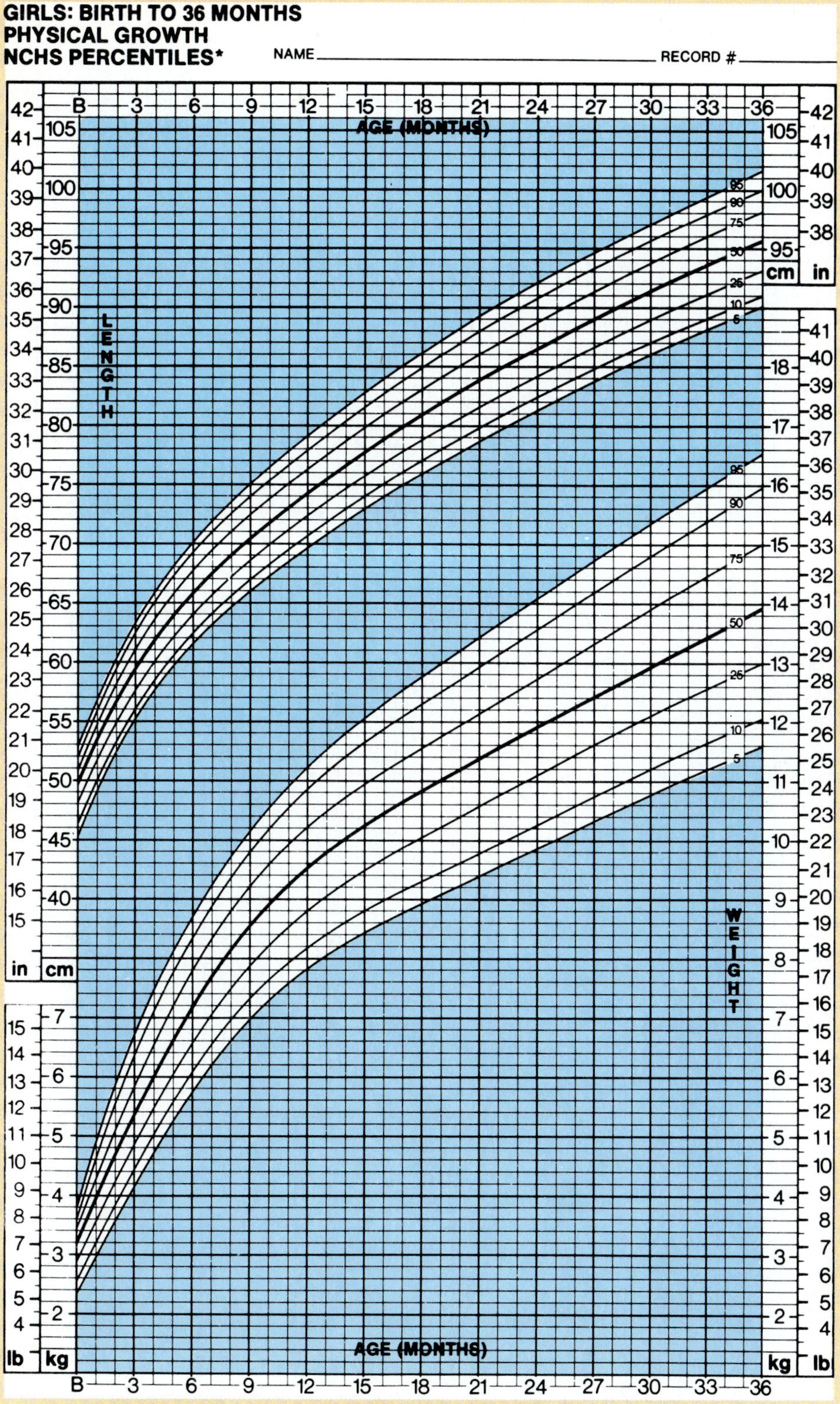

FIGURE 15-6

Weight and height for age chart for boys from birth to 36 months.

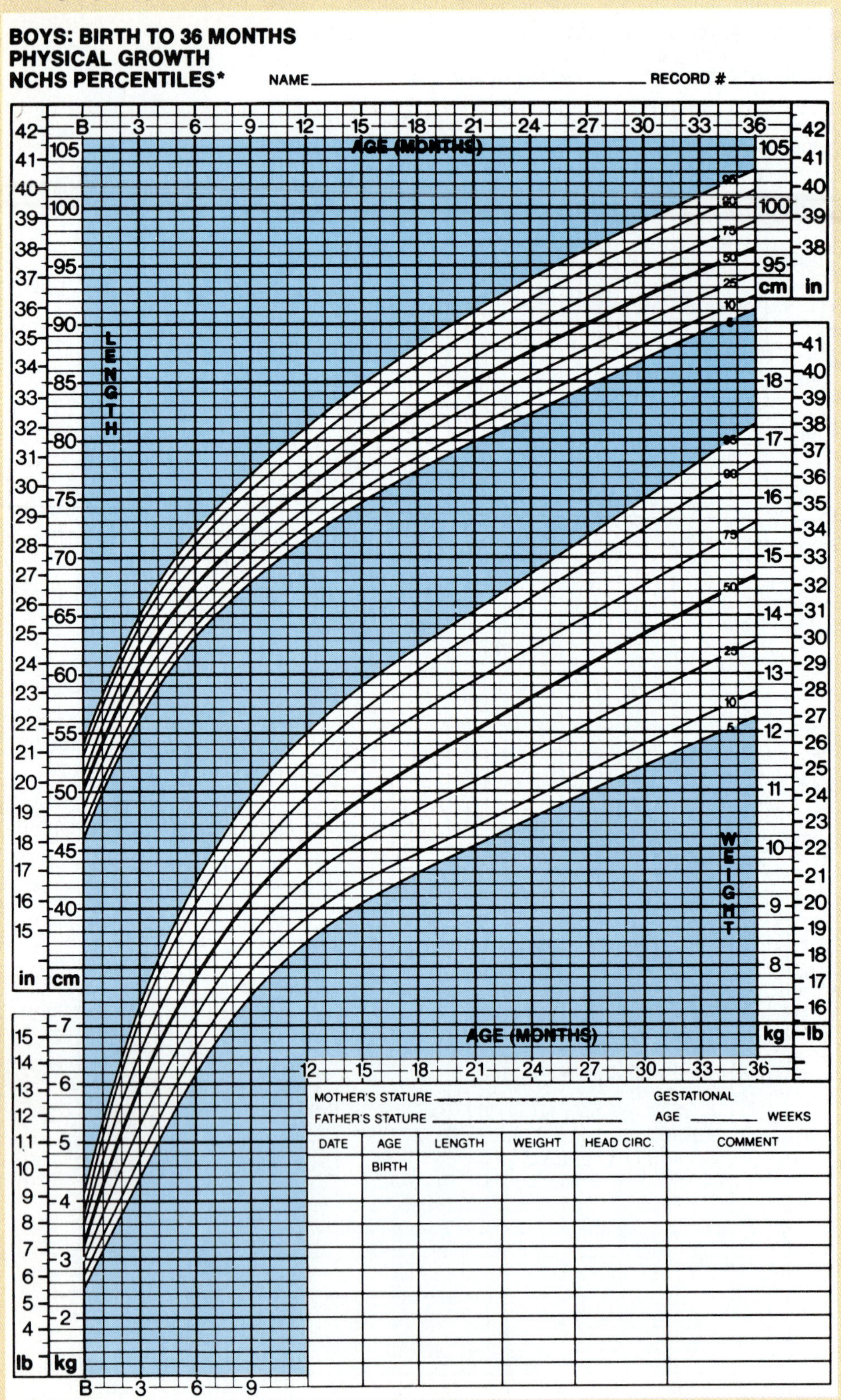

ISSUES AND OPINIONS

Is It Safe for Lactating Mothers To Restrict Their Energy Intake?

Women who have just given birth are often anxious to lose the excess weight put on during pregnancy and to recover their prepregnancy figure. In addition to the effects of weight gain on their appearance, some women who have put on weight during pregnancy may be concerned about the medical risks associated with weight gain. Breast-feeding may itself help many women to regain their prepregnancy figure, because the body must meet the energy costs of lactation in addition to the mother's normal energy needs. Nevertheless, many lactating women feel the need to make additional efforts to lose weight, and many adopt energy-restricted diets to achieve the weight loss they desire.* Some concern has been expressed about the practice of dieting by lactating women because their bodies must cope with the additional nutritional demands of lactation, and they may also need to replenish nutrient stores that have become depleted during pregnancy.

A recent study investigated the effects of dieting on 22 apparently healthy and well-nourished breast-feeding mothers.† The women voluntarily restricted their energy intake to 25% less than their predicted energy needs for 10 weeks. This regimen was designed to produce weight loss at a rate of about 1 pound per week. The women's average kilocalorie intake before dieting of 2300 kcal/day was reduced to an average of 1765 kcal/day for the 10 weeks of the study.

By the end of the study period, the participants had actually lost an average of 10.6 pounds. Their waist and hip circumferences were reduced, as were the sums of three separate skinfold thickness measurements (in the triceps, suprailiac, and abdominal regions). Despite this substantial loss of weight, the women's average daily milk production remained within the normal desirable range. At the start of the study, milk production averaged 759 ml/day; by the end of the study it averaged 802 ml/day. The women also consumed nutritionally adequate diets throughout the study, with only iron and thiamin intakes falling slightly below the RDA levels for lactating women.

The results of this study suggest that it is perfectly safe for a healthy lactating woman to lose excess weight at a rate of about 1 pound (0.45 kg)/week, without compromising her ability to breast-feed her infant. Throughout the study period, however, the women received counseling, monitoring, and encouragement from health care professionals. All lactating women who diet to lose weight should receive similar counseling and monitoring by a physician or registered dietitian.

* Strode MA, Dewey KG, Lonnerdal B: *Acta Paediatr Scand* 75:222, 1986.

† Dusdieker LB, Hemingway DL, Stumbo PJ: *Am J Clin Nutr* 59:833, 1994.

BY NOW YOU SHOULD KNOW

- Infant feeding can be divided into three chronological phases: the nursing phase, the transitional feeding phase, and the modified adult diet phase.
- There are many ways to adequately feed an infant, but breast-feeding is the preferred method for practically all infants. Breast-feeding may not, however, be the preferable form of feeding for many parents.
- The choice of infant feeding method is made on the basis of nutritional, immunological, psychological, economic, and social considerations.
- Colostrum is secreted from a mother's breast in the first few days after birth. It contains high concentrations of immune factors that protect the infant against infection.
- Infant formulas are most often made from cow's milk that is modified to resemble the nutrient composition of human milk. Some formulas are based on soy protein or protein hydrolysates. Formulas do not contain the immunological factors present in human milk.
- A U.S. national health objective for the year 2000 is to have 75% of all babies breast-fed when discharged from the hospital and 50% still breast-fed at 6 months.
- Breast-fed infants need supplemental amounts of vitamin D, fluoride, and (after 6 months) iron.
- Infants fed iron-fortified formulas made with fluoridated water do not need any additional supplementation.
- Formula-fed infants are at greater risk of developing certain illnesses throughout their lives than are infants who are breast-fed.
- Allowing an infant to fall asleep with a bottle in his or her mouth containing formula, milk, or juice increases the risk of tooth decay (nursing bottle syndrome).
- Infants should be introduced to solid foods between 4 and 6 months of age.
- Solid foods should be introduced gradually and individually, allowing monitoring for allergic reactions.
- The growth pattern of infants is the best indication of an adequate diet.
- An infant normally doubles in weight within 4 months of birth and triples in weight within 12 months.

~ STUDY QUESTIONS ~

1. Define the following terms: *colostrum, beikost, immunoglobulin, lactalbumin, lactoferrin,* and *bifidus factor.* What is the significance of each in infant feeding?
2. What supplements should be given to an infant, and when and why should they be given?
3. List the various ways in which a breast-fed infant receives additional protection against infection.
4. What are the nutritional and psychological advantages of breast-feeding?
5. What are the economic factors involved in the choice between breast-feeding and formula-feeding?
6. How is formula made nutritionally adequate for the feeding of an infant?
7. Explain how growth charts, such as those shown in Figures 15-5 and 15-6, are used to assess the development of a child.

~ CRITICAL ANALYSIS ~

1. Although an infant's height and weight recorded on a growth chart, are the criteria most often used to assess nutritional adequacy, this method can only assess dietary adequacy over a period of weeks or months. When there is concern about whether a breast-fed infant is receiving an adequate supply of milk, the most practical method to measure this is to weigh the infant on an infant scale (which is able to weigh in the range of 0 to 20 kg much more accurately than an adult scale) before and after a feeding. If the mother and infant can be made comfortable, this method can estimate the amount of milk the infant receives and thus the nutrients supplied. The increase in weight after feeding must result from milk intake. Assume that 1 ml of milk, like 1 ml of water, weighs 1 g. If an infant weighs 50 g more after breastfeeding, he or she consumed 50 ml of milk (approximately). The energy and protein content of 100 ml of milk are listed in Table 15-1. If an infant consumed 50 ml of milk and the energy content of 100 ml is 64 kcal, the infant consumed 32 kcal.
   a. Anna M. tells you she is concerned that her 1-month-old infant is not getting enough nourishment from breast milk alone. The infant's weight before feeding is 3900 g (3.9 kg) and 3980 g after feeding. Calculate the calories and protein from this feeding: _______kcal and _______g of protein
   b. Anna M. indicates that her infant usually nurses 8 times per day. Calculate the infant's daily energy and protein intake: _________kcal and ______g of protein
   c. Data cited in the chapter indicate that 108 kcal/kg has been considered adequate for infants during the first 6 months. The energy required falls to about 71 kcal/kg/day after 4 months of age. Is Anna M.'s infant receiving approximately 108 kcal/kg/day? Similarly, 2.2 g/kg/day of high quality protein are recommended during the first 5 months. Has Anna M.'s infant achieved this level of protein intake?

REFERENCES

1. Ryan AS, Martinez GA: Breast-feeding and the working mother: a profile, *Pediatrics* 83:524, 1991.
2. Sarett HP, Bain KR, O'Leary JC: Decisions on breast-feeding or formula feeding and trends in infant-feeding practices, *Am J Dis Child* 137:719, 1983.
3. Rebouche CJ: Carnitine metabolism and human nutrition, *J Appl Nutr* 40:99, 1988.
4. Ziegler EE, Fomon SJ: Lactose enhances mineral absorption in infancy, *J Pediatr Gastroenterol Nutr* 2:288, 1983.
5. Lindberg T, Skude G: Amylase in human milk, *Pediatrics* 70:235, 1982.
6. Greve LC and others: Breast-feeding in the management of the newborn with phenylketonuria: a practical approach to dietary therapy, *JAMA* 94:305, 1994.
7. Goldman AS, Goldblum RM: Immunologic systems in human milk: characteristics and effects. In Lebenthal E, editor: *Textbook of gastroenterology and nutrition in early infancy,* ed 2, New York, 1989, Raven Press.
8. Goldman AS, Goldblum RM: Human milk: immunologic-nutritional relationships, *Ann N Y Acad Sci* 587:236, 1990.
9. Institute of Medicine/National Academy of Sciences: *Nutrition during lactation,* Washington, DC, 1991, National Academy Press.
10. Sosa R and others: The effect of early mother-infant contact on breast-feeding, infection and growth. In *Breast-feeding and the mother,* Ciba Foundation Symposium 45, Amsterdam, 1976, Elsevier.
11. Virden SF: The relationship between infant feeding method and maternal role adjustment, *J Nurse Midwifery* 33:31, 1988.
12. McNeilly AS, Glasier A, Howie PW: Endocrine control of lactational infertility. In Dobbing J, editor: *Maternal nutrition and lactational infertility,* New York, 1985, Raven Press.
13. Kramer MS: Do breast-feeding and delayed introduction of solid foods protect against subsequent obesity? *J Pediatr* 98:883, 1981.
14. Ellis LA, Picciano MF: Milk-borne hormones: regulators of development in neonate, *Nutr Today* 27:6, 1992.
15. U.S. Department of Health and Human Services: *Healthy people 2000: national health promotion and disease prevention objectives,* Washington, DC, 1991, Public Health Service.
16. Committee on Drugs/American Academy of Pediatrics: Transfer of drugs and other chemicals into human milk, *Pediatrics* 84:924, 1989.
17. Barness L, editor: *Pediatric nutrition handbook,* ed 3, Elk Grove Village, Ill, 1993, American Academy of Pediatrics.
18. Committee on Nutrition/American Academy of Pediatrics: The use of whole cow's milk in infancy, *Pediatrics* 89:1105, 1992.
19. Purvis GA, Bartholmey SJ: Infant feeding practices: commercially prepared baby foods. In Tsang RC, Nichols BL, editors: *Nutrition during infancy,* St Louis, 1988, Mosby.
20. Smith AM, Picciano MF, Deering RH: Folate intake and blood concentrations of term infants, *Am J Clin Nutr* 41:590, 1985.
21. Committee on Nutrition/American Academy of Pediatrics: On the feeding of supplemental foods to infants, *Pediatrics* 65:1178, 1980.
22. Beal VA: On the acceptance of solid foods and other food patterns of infants and children, *Pediatrics* 20:448, 1957.
23. Macknin ML, Medendorp SV, Maier WC: Infant sleep and bedtime cereal, *Am J Dis Child* 143:1066, 1989.
24. Fomon SJ: *Infant nutrition,* St Louis, 1993, Mosby.
25. Fomon SJ, Thomas LN, Filer LJ Jr: Acceptance of unsalted strained foods by normal infants, *J Pediatr* 76:242, 1970.
26. Filer LJ Jr: Modified food starch—an update, *J Am Diet Assoc* 88:342, 1988.
27. Martinez GA, Ryan AS, Malec DJ: Nutrient intakes of American infants and children fed cow's milk or infant formula, *Am J Dis Child* 139:1010, 1985.
28. Splett PL: Federal food assistance programs: a step to food security for many, *Nutr Today* 29:6, 1994.

~ ADDITIONAL READINGS ~

Adair LS, Popkin BM, Guilkey DK: The duration of breast-feeding: how is it affected by biological, sociodemographic, health sector, and food industry factors? *Demography* 30:63, 1993.

American Dietetic Association: Position on promotion and support of breast feeding, *J Am Diet Assoc* 93:467, 1993.

Atkinson SA, Hanson LA, Chandra RK: *Human lactation,* vol 4, *Breast-feeding, nutrition, infection, and infant growth in developed and emerging countries,* Newfoundland, Canada, 1990, ARTS Biomedical.

Barness LA, Gilbert-Barness EF: What lies ahead in infant nutrition, *Semin Perinatol* 13:112, 1989.

Curtis DM: Infant nutrition supplementation, *J Pediatr* 117:S110, 1990.

Dewey KG and others: Adequacy of energy intake among breast-fed infants in the DARLING study: relationships to growth velocity, morbidity, and activity levels, Davis area research on lactation, infant nutrition and growth, *J Pediatr* 119:538, 1991.

Dewey KG and others: Maternal versus infant factors related to breast milk intake and residual milk volume: the DARLING study, *Pediatrics* 87:829, 1991.

Dewey KG and others: Growth of breast-fed and formula-fed infants from 0 to 18 months: the DARLING study, *Pediatrics* 89:1035, 1992.

Edelman R: Infant nutrition and immunity, *Ann N Y Acad Sci* 587:232, 1990.

Goldman AS, Atkinson SA, Hanson LA: *Human lactation,* vol 3, *The effect of human milk on the recipient infant,* New York, 1987, Plenum Press.

Grummer-Strawn LM: Does prolonged breast-feeding impair child growth? a critical review, *Pediatrics* 91:766, 1993.

Hamosh M: Human milk composition and function in the infant, *Semin Pediatr Gastroenterol Nutr* 3:4, 1992.

Hamosh M, Goldman AS: *Human lactation,* vol 2, *Maternal and environmental factors,* New York, 1986, Plenum Press.

Heird WC: Advances in infant nutrition over the past quarter century, *J Am Coll Nutr* 8:22S, 1989.

Jensen RG, Neville MC: *Human lactation,* vol 1, *Maternal and environmental factors,* New York, 1985, Plenum Press.

Lawrence RA: The pediatrician's role in infant feeding decision-making, *Pediatr Rev* 14:265, 1993.

Lucas A: Does early diet program future outcome? *Acta Paediatr Scand Suppl* 365:58, 1990.

Mastecky J, Blair C, Ogra, PL: Immunology of milk and the neonate, New York, 1991, Plenum Press.

Mathew OP: Science of bottle feeding, *J Pediatr* 119:511, 1991.

Menella JA, Beauchamp GK: Early flavor experiences: when do they start? *Nutr Today* 29:15, 1994.

Milner JA: Trace minerals in the nutrition of children, *J Pediatr* 117:S147, 1990.

Picciano MF, Lonnerdal B: *Human lactation,* vol 5, *Mechanisms regulating lactation and infant nutrient utilization,* New York, 1992, Wiley-Liss.

Pipes PL, Trahms CA: Nutrition in infancy and childhood, ed 5, St Louis, 1993, Mosby.

Rogan WJ and others: Should the presence of carcinogens in breast milk discourage breast feeding? *Regul Toxicol Pharmacol* 13:228, 1991.

Savilahti E, Kuitunen M: Allergenicity of cow milk proteins, *J Pediatr* 121:S12, 1992.

Walker-Smith JA: Cow milk–sensitive enteropathy: predisposing factors and treatment, *J Pediatr* 121:S111, 1992.

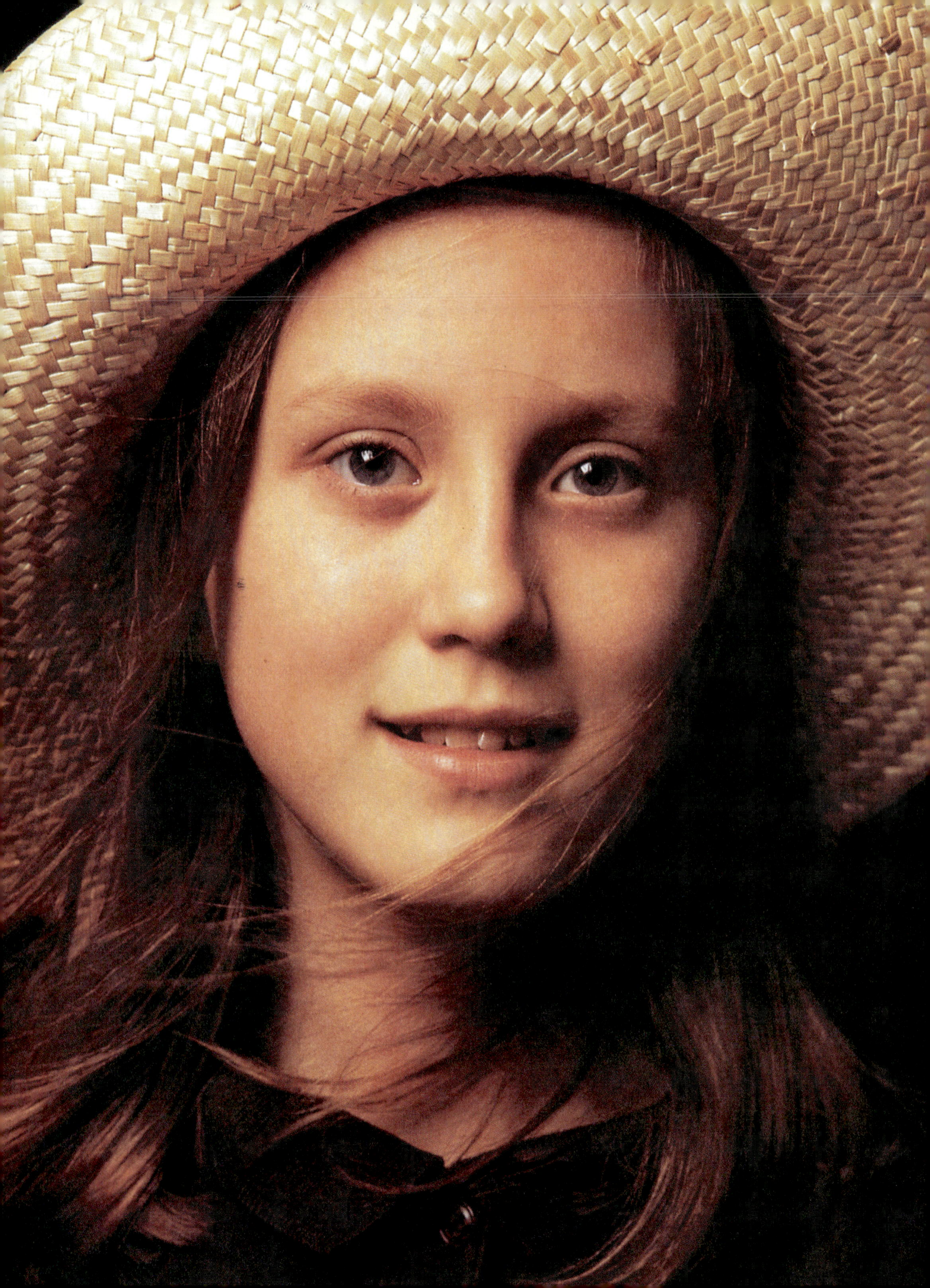

CHAPTER 16

NUTRITION FROM CHILDHOOD THROUGH ADOLESCENCE

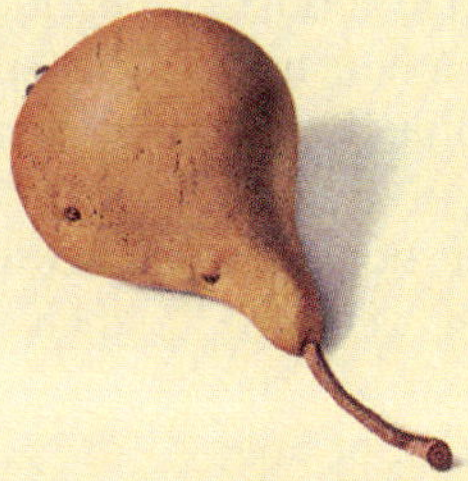

Relatively little research has been done on the nutritional needs and problems of people from 2 to 16 years of age largely because few nutritional problems appear during this period. Although this is a crucial period of growth, children and adolescents are amazingly resilient in the face of short-term nutrient deficiencies. There is little information on which to judge the long-term consequences of specific eating patterns during childhood and adolescence but every reason to believe they are significant. Nutrient adequacy during childhood and adolescence definitely offers some protection against the degenerative diseases associated with aging.

By the time a child is 1 year old, the digestive system, liver, and kidneys are able to cope with a wide variety of foods available from the family table. The reduction in the rate of growth and the increased capacity of the stomach mean that the frequent feeding in infancy can be replaced by less frequent, larger meals. Sometime between the ages of 6 months and 1 year most infants make the gradual changeover from a milk-based diet to one that closely resembles the diet they consume throughout childhood, adolescence, and adulthood.

CHILDHOOD

The overall relative rate of growth in childhood is less than it is during infancy. A typical infant may triple in weight during its first year and then only double in weight during the rest of the preschool period. Growth does continue throughout childhood, however, and must be sustained by an adequate supply of nutrients. Children tend to grow in spurts, and so the nutrients available in their diet at all times should be able to meet the demand for nutrients during growth spurts.

The dietary standards for children proposed by the Food and Nutrition Board represent the intakes believed to promote optimal health in practically all children in each age-group. In times of rapid growth, these standards are probably realistic estimates of the amount of nutrients required. In other times, they probably provide a substantial excess of most nutrients. Firm experimental evidence to back up the dietary standards is available for a few nutrients. For others, the standards are calculated from knowledge about the rate of growth the nutrients must sustain. Some other standards are based on extrapolation from information on adult needs. The remaining standards simply reflect the level of the nutrients that are known to be consumed by apparently healthy children.

Figure 16-1 illustrates some of the changing nutritional needs during childhood and adolescence relative to the needs of children aged between 1 and 3 years. The rate at which the need for different nutrients increases varies from one nutrient to another. Fortunately, however, the increase in the need for kilocalories is often at least as great as the increase in the need for a specific nutrient. This tends to ensure that a person consuming adequate energy also consumes adequate nutrients, provided that he or she consumes a mixed and reasonably appropriate diet.

The increase in energy needs with age reflects increases in the energy needed by basal metabolism, increased activity, and increased growth of muscle and adipose tissue. Recommended Energy Intakes (REIs) make no distinction between boys and girls until age 11. Several studies, however, indicate that boys as young as 6 have greater energy needs than do girls and that the boys eat more to meet their greater needs.

Many water-soluble vitamins are involved in energy metabolism, including thiamin, riboflavin, niacin, and pantothenic acid. Accordingly, the needs for many water-soluble vitamins increase in proportion to total energy needs. Pyridoxine is required in greater amounts during periods of rapid tissue growth, reflecting this vitamin's role in the use of dietary protein and the synthesis of new tissue protein. The increase in muscle mass during growth requires that a positive nitrogen balance be maintained. This is usually ensured by daily consumption of 1.5 to 2 g of protein per kilogram of body weight. Nutrients involved in blood formation are also important during growth because the vascular system must grow to bring blood to all new cells. This increase in the vascular system demands adequate supplies of iron, protein, folate, and pyridoxine. Bone growth creates a need for calcium, phosphorus, fluoride, and vitamin D. The body's need for vitamins A and C is also believed to increase during growth because of the involvement of vitamin A in bone growth and maintaining epithelial cells and the involvement of vitamin C in the synthesis of collagen.

Nutrition is not the only factor determining the rate of growth. Many other environmental factors influence

NUTRIENTS NEEDED FOR ENERGY METABOLSIM:

Thiamin
Riboflavin
Niacin
Pantothenic acid

NUTRIENTS NEEDED FOR MUSCLE GROWTH

Protein
Pyridoxine
Potassium
Folate
Vitamin B_{12}
Zinc

NUTRIENTS NEEDED FOR BLOOD FORMATION

Protein
Iron
Pyridoxine
Folate
Vitamin B_{12}
Vitamin C
Copper

NUTRIENTS NEEDED FOR BONE FORMATION

Calcium
Phosphorus
Vitamin A
Vitamin D
Vitamin C
Protein
Manganese

FIGURE 16-1

Changes in recommended nutrient intakes from the ages of 4 to 18 years, relative to recommended intakes for the 1-to 3-year-old child.

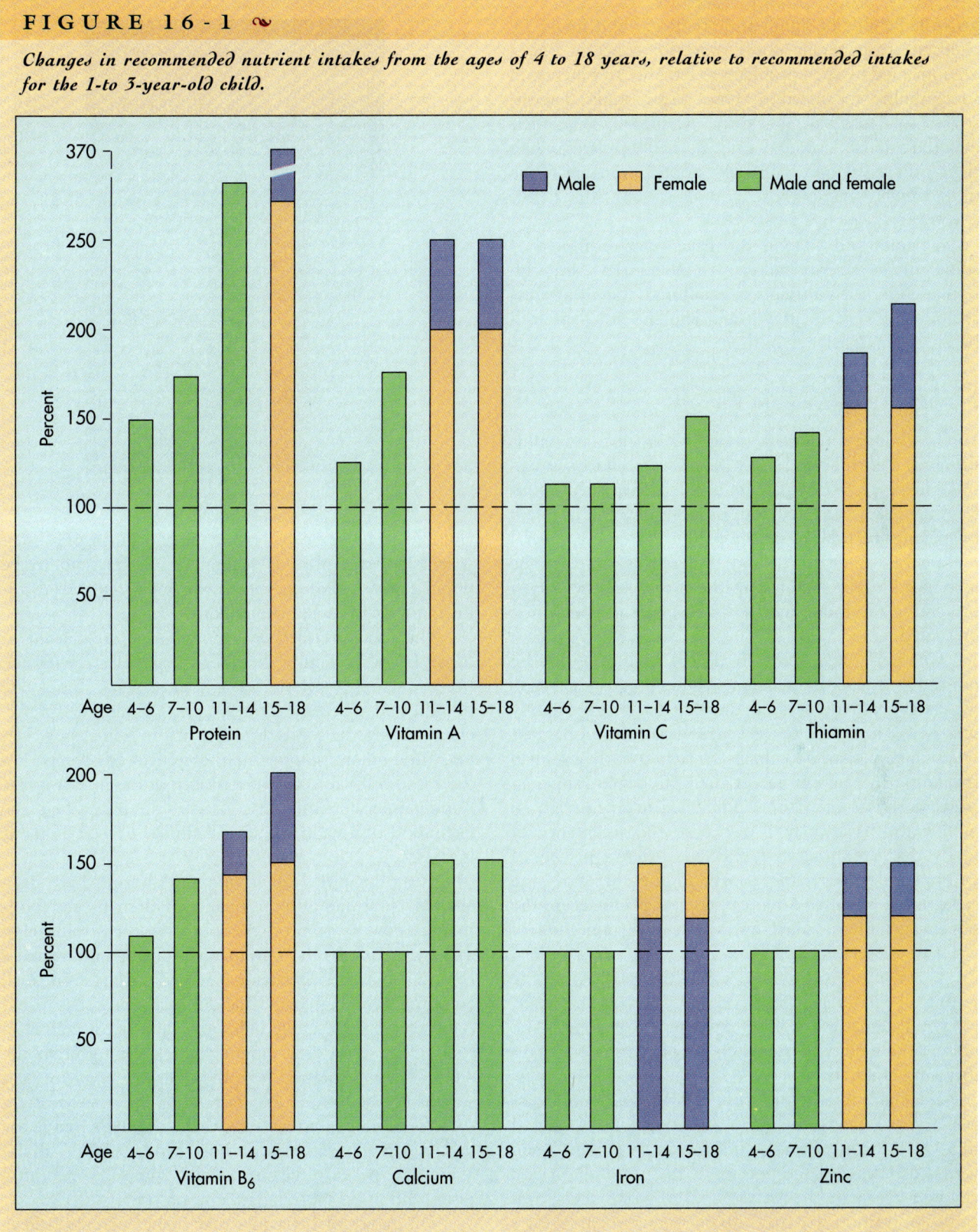

what proportion of a person's genetically determined maximal size is actually attained. These other factors include the standard of medical care and sanitation the growing child enjoys and his or her participation in regular exercise.

Children's appetites appear to automatically adjust to their changing needs for nutrients. Many parents become concerned if their child goes through a period of seeming to eat very little, but such periods usually give way to more hearty eating just as the child has a spurt of growth. Periods of significantly reduced food intake by children are generally not a cause for concern, unless accompanied by such problems as lethargy and increased susceptibility to infection. One classic study demonstrated that many parents worry needlessly about their children's diets. It found that mothers tended to rate their children's food habits as "poor," even when the diets actually met all the criteria for nutritional adequacy.[1]

Thiamin and vitamin B_{12} have been promoted as stimulants to appetite and growth in children. Although both are essential nutrients in childhood, these nutrients are of value only if growth and appetite are depressed because of a deficiency of them.

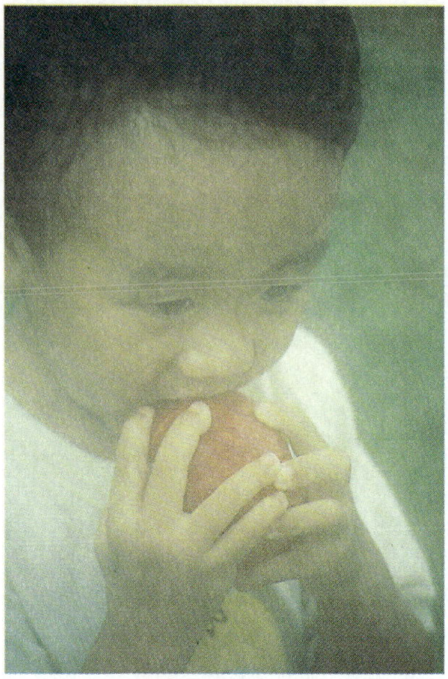

FOOD PREFERENCES

Young children generally prefer foods that are mild-flavored, colorful, soft, moist, lukewarm, and served in small helpings. When parents become concerned about food being rejected, they can often resolve the problem by making the food more compatible with these general preferences. Children's food preferences can also be influenced by the time of day, the attitude of the person presenting the food, and the atmosphere in which it is presented.[2]

Children often react to flavors that may not be noticed by adults. For example, children may reject milk with a slight taint or food that has been only slightly scorched. They often refuse vegetables of the cabbage or onion family that have been cooked quickly in small amounts of water but accept them if cooked longer in larger amounts of water. Adding a sauce or cream to modify the flavor may also lead to the acceptance of foods that are otherwise rejected. After a period of getting used to vegetables cooked for long times in large amounts of water, children can then begin to accept the same vegetables cooked quickly in small amounts of water to conserve nutrients.[3,4]

Color provided by the food, the plate, and the setting all encourage children to eat. It is best, however, to avoid unnatural colors and shapes of food. The presence of inedible material on the plate poses a danger to young children.

It is more satisfactory from a psychological point of view to offer young children a small portion of food and then have them return for more than to present them with a dauntingly large portion at the outset. Allowing children to serve themselves and so make their own choice of portion size may also encourage them to eat a food or a meal.

Vegetables are generally unpopular with children, relative to other foods, but raw vegetables are much more popular among children than are cooked vegetables. The tendency of children to dislike vegetables may be because of the way they are cooked, or the children may react to subtle clues concerning their parents' own dislike of vegetables. Fruits tend to be popular with children, with meat, milk, and bread following fruit in preference rankings.

The food preferences of youngsters are related to those of other family members, especially the father, because family preferences influence what foods are bought and when they are bought.[5] Children's preferences among the foods available in the home, however, bear little relationship to the preferences of parents. If a food is liked or rejected by a sibling or other peer in the home, especially one in a leadership role, then the likelihood of a child showing a similar like or dislike is increased.[2]

The principles of behavior modification have been applied to attempts to persuade children to eat foods that are new to them often enough for them to develop a liking for the foods. This involves giving an immediate reward for desired behavior (such as tasting even small amounts of vegetables), while doing nothing that would reinforce an undesirable behavior (such as the refusal of food). The rewards given must be meaningful to the child, clearly associated with the desirable behavior, and should not be food (e.g., candy).[6] As the desired eating pattern develops, the reward can be given less frequently and eventually withdrawn. For some children, praise alone may prove sufficient reward, whereas others may respond only to more tangible nonfood rewards.

The range of behaviors that makes parents believe their child has an eating problem includes frequent refusal to eat, dawdling, spitting out food, and playing with food (which is in fact a normal part of a child's exploration of its environment). Parents respond with a variety of strategies, including reasoning with the children, coaxing them, threatening them, punishing them,

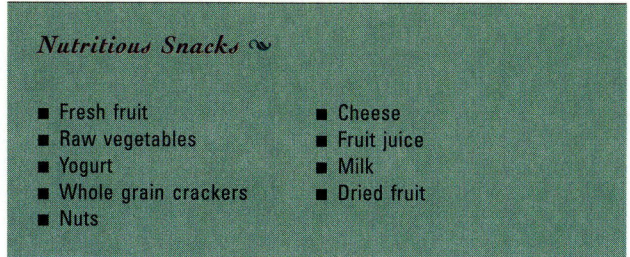

Nutritious Snacks

- Fresh fruit
- Raw vegetables
- Yogurt
- Whole grain crackers
- Nuts
- Cheese
- Fruit juice
- Milk
- Dried fruit

denying them some privilege, or offering rewards. Child psychologists have long debated the effectiveness of the various methods. They agree, however, that the most significant problems arise when children learn to use food to manipulate their parents or other caretakers.[7]

It is important to remember that children are just as individual in their preferences as are adults. Just because a child's preferences and habits do not fit in with broad generalizations of expected or desired behavior does not necessarily mean that they are a cause for concern.

MEAL PATTERNS

Children between the ages of 1 and 5 years generally eat more than three times a day; they normally eat between five and seven times a day. It has been found that the frequency of eating is not related to nutrient intake, except for children who eat fewer than four times per day or more than six times per day.[8]

SNACKS

During periods of high nutritive needs, such as growth spurts, snacks are almost essential. Small children may be unable to take in sufficient food from main meals to meet their nutrient needs because of the small capacity of their stomachs. On the other hand, if energy-dense snacks are consumed too close to mealtimes, they may significantly reduce the amount of food eaten at mealtimes.

There is evidence that a considerable proportion of children's snacks are eaten while watching television. These snacks, superimposed on a sedentary lifestyle, are a significant factor increasing a child's risk of obesity. It has been found that the prevalence of childhood obesity is directly related to the amount of time spent watching television.[9] On the other hand, some research has shown that the use of smaller, more frequent snack-type meals results in the formation of less adipose tissue and better nutrient use in children. It is important to remember that excess consumption of any food, regardless of how nutritious it is, leads to reduced consumption of other foods that may be needed to provide a balanced nutrient intake overall. Therefore, overdependence on any one type of food can lead to nutritional imbalances.[10]

Although the amount of food eaten as meals and snacks can vary widely from day to day, most children appear to regulate their energy intake over each 24-hour period to match their energy needs.[11] The adults who purchase food for children must take the responsibility of ensuring that the snacks contribute to the nutritional adequacy of the children's diets.

A United States Department of Agriculture (USDA) survey in 1985 and 1986 found that 76% to 83% of children had at least one snack per day. The snack or snacks provided about 20% of the daily calories and over 15% of the daily intake of fiber, vitamins C and E, riboflavin, calcium, phosphorus, magnesium, copper, and potassium. This indicates that the snacks were relatively nutritious, although they contained a somewhat higher proportion of the needs for energy than that for specific nutrients. The adequacy of the children's nutrient and energy intake overall was found to increase in line with the number of snacks consumed. This indicates that the snacks tended to be of acceptable nutrient density and were not primarily composed of refined carbohydrates, including sugar. Because eating patterns involving frequent snacks are becoming more common, nutritionists should promote attitudes that lead to selection of nutritionally beneficial snacks.

FOOD JAGS

Young children sometimes go on "food jags," when they accept only a limited variety of foods. In many cases, the foods accepted during food jags can form a nutritionally adequate but monotonous or unconventional diet. Such food jag periods should be little cause for concern, unless the foods provide excess amounts of fats, sugar, or salt. Food jags seldom persist for long, and there is no evidence that they lead to restrictive food preferences in adulthood. In general, however, the nutritive quality of the diet at all stages of life is directly related to the number of different types of food eaten each day. This emphasizes the importance of encouraging children to eat a wide variety of foods without becoming overconcerned by occasional short-term food jags. Although children can instinctively adjust their energy intake to an appropriate level, they cannot automatically choose foods that provide all the nutrients they require.[12] This again emphasizes the importance of introducing a wide variety of foods to children in their early habit-forming years and the important role of parents or caregivers in ensuring that only appropriate foods are available from which the child may select.

THE ADEQUACY OF DIETS

The 1985 and 1986 USDA surveys of children aged 1 to 5 years found that the average intake of all nutrients exceeded the recommended dietary allowances (RDAs), with the exception of iron and zinc for 1- to 3-year-olds and vitamin E and zinc for 4- and 5-year-olds.[13]

Children raised on a strict vegetarian diet (vegan) are at increased risk of growth retardation, rickets, and anemia. Their diets may contain relatively low amounts of available iron, protein, zinc, vitamin D, folate, vitamin B_{12}, and calcium. Because children have smaller stomachs than do adults, it is difficult for them to eat enough of the high-fiber foods in a vegetarian diet to meet their energy needs. Once any fetal reserves of vitamin B_{12} have been depleted, hardly any of this vitamin will be present in a strict vegan diet. Alarmingly low amounts of calcium and vitamin D are provided by a vegan diet, predisposing vegan children to rickets. The total iron intake of vegetarians can be relatively high, but this iron is of limited bioavailability because it contains no heme iron. The high fiber content of a vegetarian diet also limits the bioavailability of iron, zinc, calcium, and possibly other minerals. Growth statistics clearly indicate that vegan children are more likely to fall into the lower percentiles of height and weight.

Similarly, data from the National Health and Nutrition Examination Survey (NHANES) III show that mean energy intakes for 1-to 2-year-old children were approximately 1200 kcal/day and for 3-to 5-year-old children were 1500 kcal/day. Children for whom dietary data were analyzed met or exceeded the RDA for all nutrients except zinc and vitamin E. Children of ages 1 to 2 years met over 95% but not 100% of their RDAs. The NHANES II survey found no biochemical or clinical evidence of frank nutrient deficiency conditions in children, apart from impaired iron status in 9% of children aged 1 to 2 and in 5% of children aged 3 to 10. The preliminary analysis of NHANES III data indicates a decline to 3% in the prevalence of iron-deficiency anemia among preschool children.[14]

Figure 16-2 summarizes the mean total food energy intake (TFEI) and mean percentage of TFEI obtained from total dietary fat and from saturated fat for children aged 1 to 15 years as surveyed by NHANES III.[15] A recent survey of Canadian children found percentages of total energy derived from fat and saturated fat of 35% and 13%, respectively, which are similar to the findings for American children.[16]

The NHANES III survey was conducted from October 1988 to October 1991. It found that mean percentages of children's TFEI derived from fat and saturated fat had *decreased* since the NHANES II survey of 1976 to 1980.[17] This is in line with the general trend, found in many different surveys, toward diets in which fats provide a lower proportion of total energy. The American Academy of Pediatrics recommends that the proportions of fat and cholesterol in children's diets gradually decline throughout childhood, toward the proportions recommended for adults. The official "dietary goal" for children older than 2 years of age is that only 30% of total energy should come from dietary fat and 10% from saturated fat.[18] The Academy of Pediatrics warns, however, that attempting to provide less than 30% of a child's energy from fat might lead to inappropriate use of more restricted diets. These low-fat diets might lead to growth failure and stunting. To avoid these dangers, the foods used to replace energy previously derived from fat need to be chosen carefully if nutrient adequacy is to be maintained.[19]

EVALUATION OF NUTRITIONAL STATUS

The pattern of a child's growth is an easily measured indicator of his or her nutritional status. The National Center for Health Statistics published standard growth curves in 1979, based on cross sectional data on the U.S. population. The most useful of these curves indicate either expected height for age or expected weight for height. The height-for-age curves can be used to detect abnormal shortness or tallness for age, and the weight-for-height curves can indicate abnormal thinness or fatness. Weight-for-age curves also exist but are of little use when considered without taking height into account. A range of growth curves for children can be seen in Figures 16-3 through 16-6. Growth curves for children from birth to 3 years of age are shown in Figures 15-5 to 15-8.

The growth of a particular child can be compared with the typical growth of other children of the same age or height by plotting the child's individual data on the appropriate growth curve. Any child who falls below the fifth percentile, meaning that only 5% or less of those of the same age shows as little growth as the child, should be screened to determine whether nutritional or other environmental factors might be causing retarded growth. It is also important to compare each measurement with the previous ones to determine whether the relative rate of growth is changing, indicating improvement or deterioration in nutritional status. A trend toward the upper percentiles of weight for height is a sign that energy intake should be restricted or energy expenditure increased to avoid the onset of obesity. Individual growth curves are used as a straightforward way of monitoring children's growth in many schools in Western countries.

FIGURE 16-2

Mean daily Total Food Energy Intake (TFEI) and mean percentages of TFEI from total dietary fat and saturated fat for children.

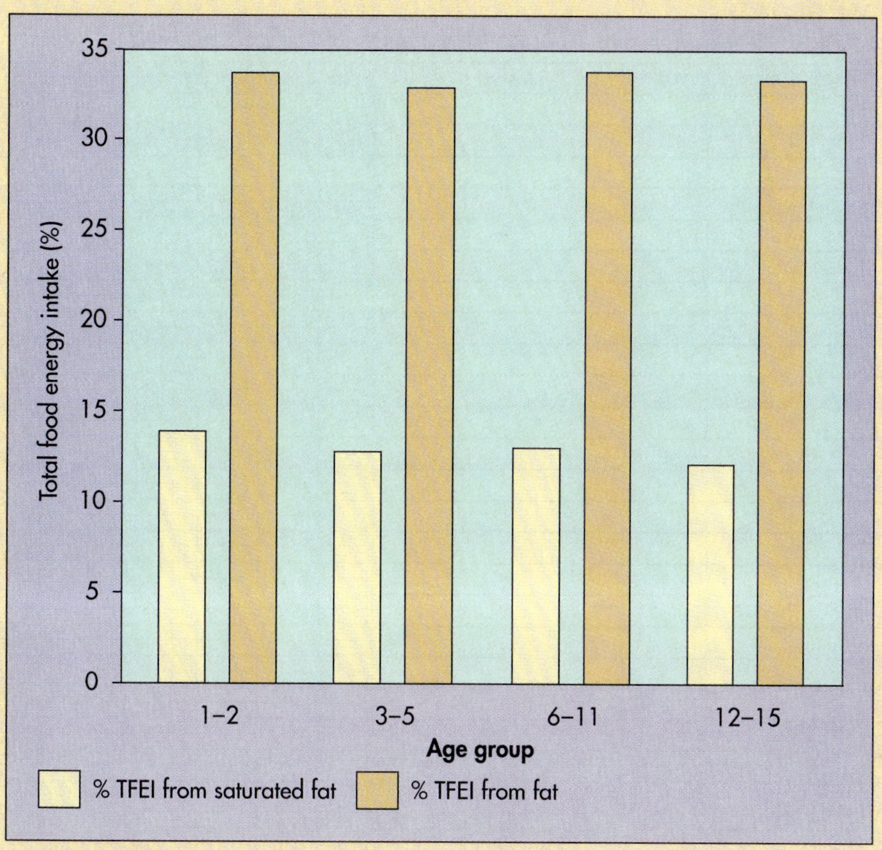

Actual weight gain in relation to expected weight gain, according to standard weight tables, has been proposed as a reliable quantitative measure of the adequacy of growth. The rate of gain is considered unacceptable if it is less than half the expected rate. Because factors that accelerate or retard growth affect weight before they affect height, weight-for-height measurements give a good indication of recent nutritional status, whereas height-for-age measurements are more indicative of long-term nutritional status.

NUTRITION-RELATED PROBLEMS

Severe malnutrition of children seldom occurs in the United States and Canada. This is because of the universal availability of medical care, nutrition intervention programs, and improved methods for detecting nutritional problems before they develop into full-fledged deficiency syndromes. Pellagra and beriberi are now virtually unknown in North America, and only occasional cases of scurvy and rickets arise. However, surveys conducted by the Centers for Disease Control have found significant nutrition-related growth retardation and iron deficiency among children aged 5 years and younger from low-income families. Current U.S. national health objectives for the year 2000 aim to reduce the prevalence of growth retardation among low-income groups to less than 10% (from a 1987 baseline of 11%) and to reduce iron deficiency to an incidence of 3% among children aged 1 to 2 years (from a 1987 baseline of 9%) and to 3% for children aged 3 to 4 years (from a 1987 baseline of 4%).[20] The most common manifestations of poor nutrition in North American children are growth retardation, anemia, obesity, and poor dental health.

Anemia

Anemia, primarily caused by a lack of dietary iron, is most commonly found in children from the lower socioeconomic groups. Of children in these groups, 10% to 21% have hemoglobin levels of less than 10 g/dl of blood, indicative of iron deficiency. In addition to its consequences on physical and physiological functions, as discussed in Chapter 10, there is growing evidence of an adverse effect on behavioral and cognitive performance. The lack of dietary iron can result from parents' lack of knowledge about dietary sources of iron and the importance of iron in good nutrition, from the restric-

Text continued on p. 584.

FIGURE 16-3

Weight for height for prepubertal boys, 2 to 11½ years of age.

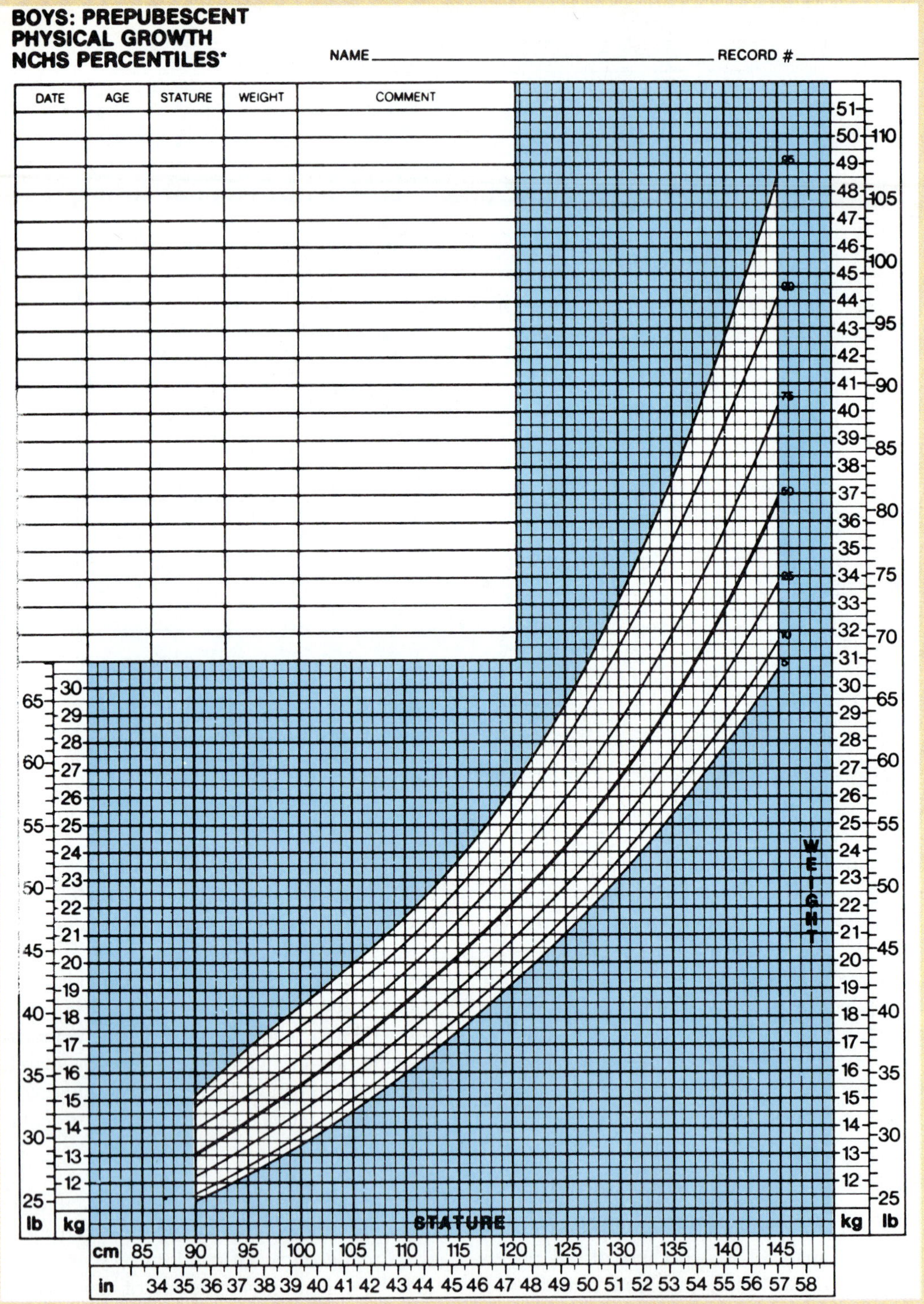

FIGURE 16-4

Weight for height for prepubertal girls, 2 to 10 years of age.

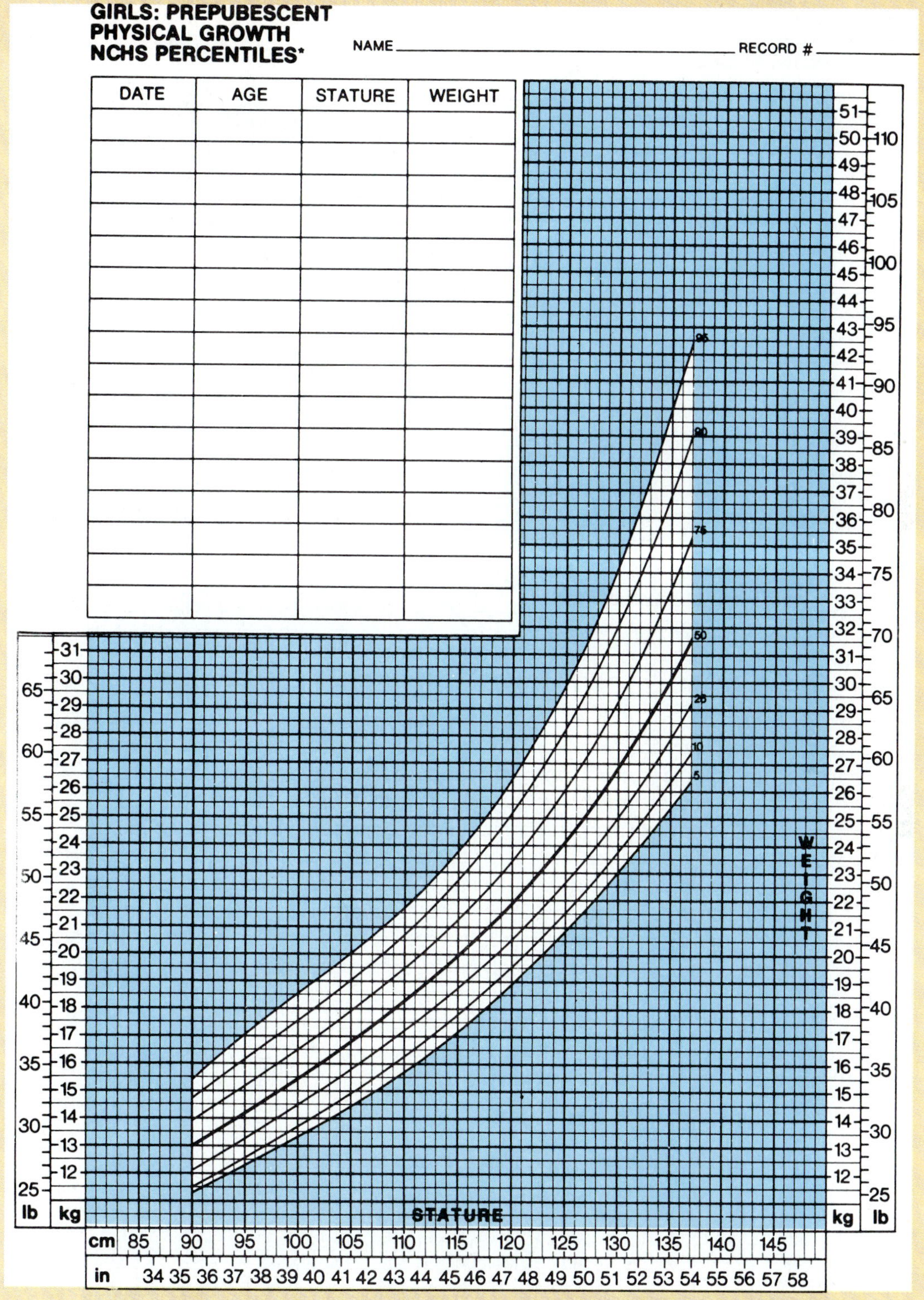

FIGURE 16-5

Height and weight for age for boys from 2 to 18 years of age.

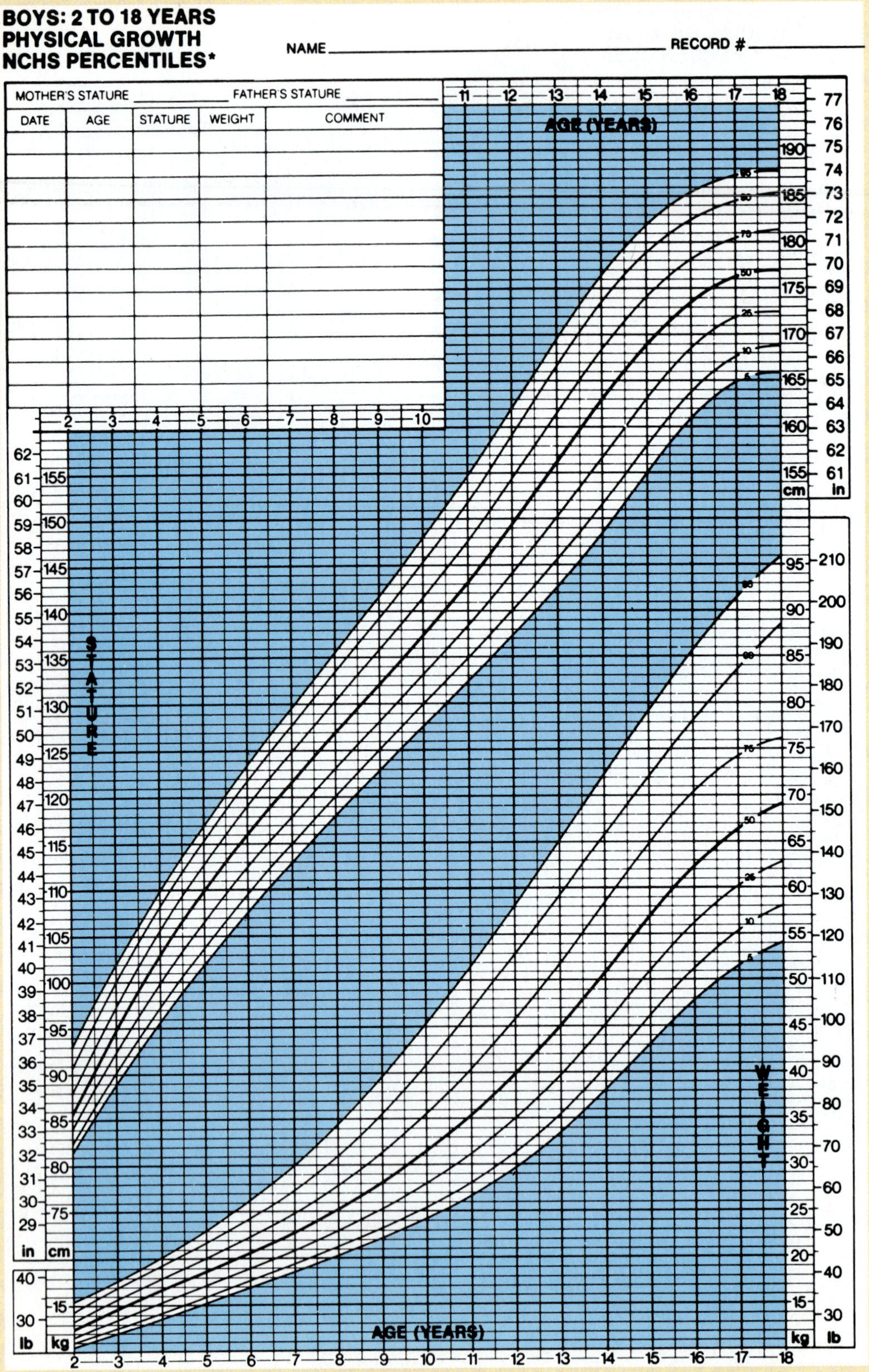

FIGURE 16-6

Height and weight for age for girls from 2 to 18 years of age.

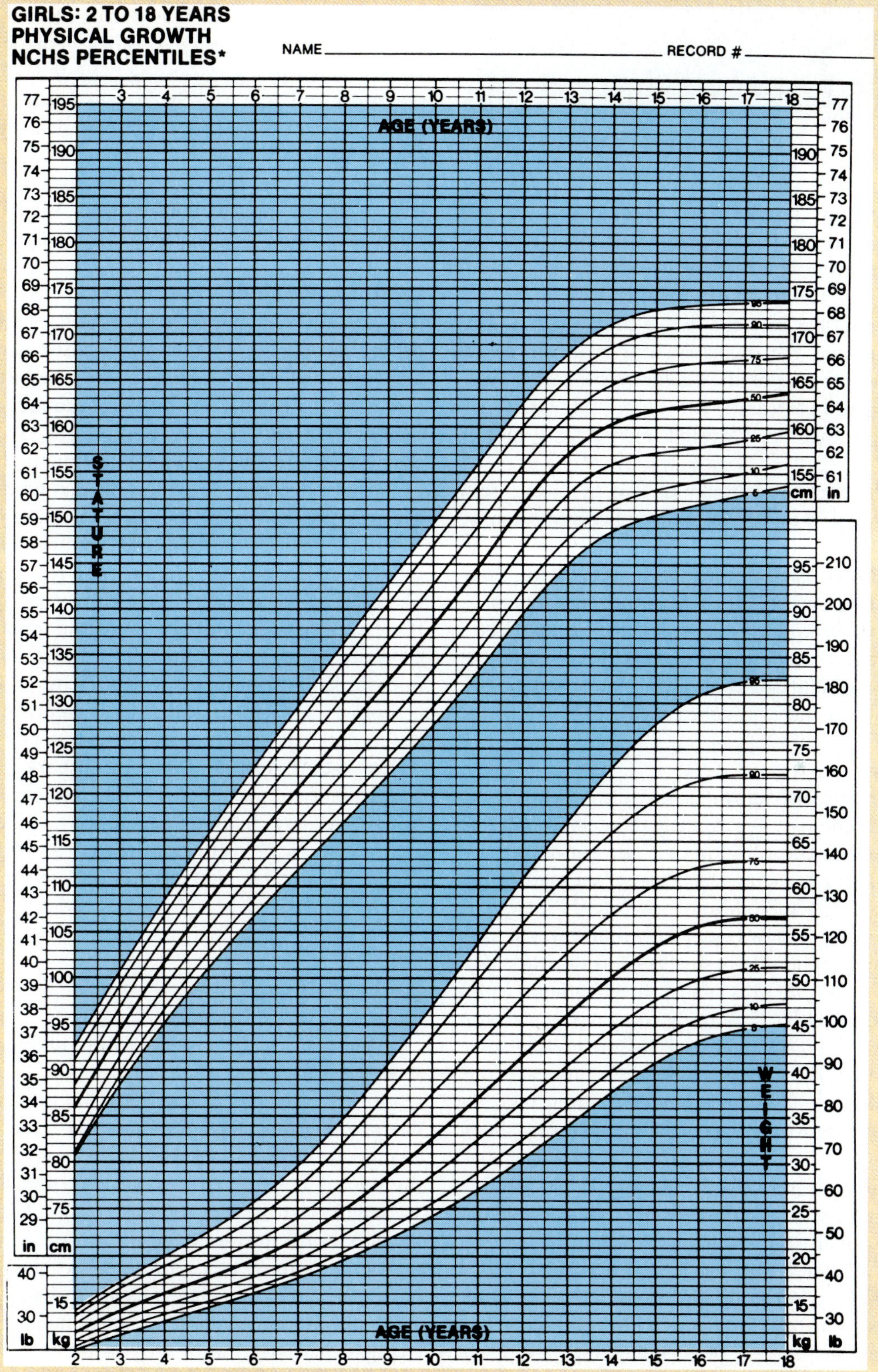

The Main Nutrition-Related Problems in Children

- Growth retardation
- Anemia
- Obesity
- Poor dental health

tive effect of poverty on the amount and variety of foods purchased, or from the difficulty of providing adequate dietary iron, even in favorable circumstances. In some children, infestation with intestinal parasites can worsen the problem. A few instances of anemia have been recorded as resulting from the use of cow's milk, which is low in iron, and the exclusion of a wide variety of foods after the first year of life. Children with anemia are usually lethargic, easily tired, and highly susceptible to infections, and they may exhibit mental and motor impairments.

Childhood anemia is usually treated by giving iron salts that provide 30 to 100 mg of iron per day, often in conjunction with vitamin C to enhance its absorption, until hemoglobin levels return to normal. The child should then adopt a diet that is high in iron-containing foods, such as meat, green leafy vegetables, and iron-fortified cereals. Nutrition health objectives for the nation for the year 2000 call for reducing the prevalence of childhood anemia and iron deficiency by 50%.

Obesity

Childhood obesity, also known as juvenile-onset obesity, is currently on the rise, is extremely difficult to correct, and often persists into adulthood. The prevalence of obesity in children is increasing. Current estimates suggest that about 27% of children aged 6 to 11 years are obese. Many parents unwittingly contribute to the development of childhood obesity by introducing solid foods before 4 to 6 months of age, by equating weight gain with good health, or by using food as a reward for good behavior. Even subtle factors, such as how much a parent talks to a child at mealtime, can influence the amount of food a child eats. Thinner children tend to talk with their parents more at mealtimes, causing them to eat less.

Any tendency toward obesity is worsened by inactivity. Too many pale and flabby American children spend their summers in air-conditioned houses, immobilized in front of the television and drinking beverages of low-nutrient density. Encouraging exercise is one of the most effective ways to help children stay within an acceptable weight range. Encouraging obese children to adopt an activity pattern of regular exercise and an eating pattern that allows them to "grow into their weight" proves more successful than trying to achieve any actual weight loss. Success in treating childhood obesity requires a persistent effort and must be backed up by appropriate nutritional guidance for the parents.

Obese children are subject to considerable psychosocial disadvantages, such as ridicule, teasing, and being excluded from games and other activities. This can worsen their obesity by causing them to lead increasingly sedentary and solitary lives in which they use food as a source of comfort. Obese children usually have poor self-images and experience feelings of rejection and inferiority. At the other side of the growth continuum is the 8% of low-income children who suffer from growth retardation, down from a baseline of 11%.

Dental Health

A child's diet influences dental health by affecting both tooth formation and the oral environment to which teeth are subjected. Vitamin A is required for the formation of tooth enamel, vitamin C is required to form the dentin layer, and calcium, phosphorus, and vitamin D are necessary for the calcification of teeth. The availability of fluoride during calcification also greatly decreases the susceptibility of teeth to decay.

Once a tooth has erupted, the major dietary factor influencing decay is the presence of a fermentable carbohydrate able to adhere to the tooth surface. The stickier the carbohydrates in the diet and the longer a tooth is exposed to sugar, the greater is the risk of caries as microorganisms normally present in the mouth ferment carbohydrate to form acid. The presence of fluoride in the mouth (provided mainly by water) is the major dietary factor able to protect against tooth decay. The susceptibility to tooth decay is also influenced by genetic factors, but few children are endowed with either caries-resistant teeth or teeth that cannot be protected from decay by a suitable diet and appropriate use of fluoride.

ADOLESCENCE

The period of transition from childhood to adulthood, known as *adolescence,* is a relatively short stage of life that is accompanied by dramatic physical, biochemical, and emotional changes. One of the main changes is the onset of **puberty,** the period during which the reproductive organs become functionally active and secondary sexual characteristics appear. Adolescence influences both nutritional needs and the absorption and use of nutrients. It is accompanied by rapid enlargement of organs and tissues. The hormonal changes that mediate puberty also cause more general physiological changes that affect nutritional needs.

The time of onset of rapid growth and puberty in adolescence depends more on a person's weight and possibly body composition than on his or her age. This suggests that nutritional status may play an important role in determining a person's state of physiological maturity. The critical weight required before puberty begins is believed to be approximately 66 lb (30 kg). This weight corresponds to a critical body composition of 10% of body weight as fat. Passing these weight and body composition landmarks leads to a height growth spurt that begins shortly after 10 years of age and peaks at 12 in girls and between 12 and 14 in boys. A weight growth spurt begins about 6 months later than does the height growth spurt in both boys and girls. The period of rapid growth lasts for 2½ to 3 years. So the period of greatest nutritional need is between the ages of 12 and 15 for boys and 10 and 13 for girls.

The onset of girls' menstrual periods, known as **menarche**, occurs after the period of rapid weight gain, when a weight of around 103 lb (47 kg) is reached and fat stores have doubled to about 20% of body weight. It was once widely believed that menarche could not occur until body fat accounted for at least 17% of weight and that ovulation would stop whenever body fat levels fell below this critical point. This belief has been challenged in recent years, but a body composition in which 22% of weight is from fat does seem to be required to maintain regular ovulation.

The sexual development of boys coincides with the beginning of the growth spurt. In both males and females, proper sexual development throughout puberty depends on adequate zinc status.

Growth rates and hence nutrient needs vary widely among adolescents. This has led to the suggestion that a sexual maturity rating (SMR), based on the appearance of secondary sexual characteristics, is more meaningful than age as an indicator of nutritional needs.

Both males and females reach their adult stature by 20 years of age, but their bone mass continues to increase until the ages of 30 to 35. The percentage of adipose tissue (fat) in mature women is about twice that of men, and the percentage of lean tissue in women is about two thirds of the percentage found in men.

As children mature into adolescents, their lifestyle changes dramatically, with equally dramatic changes in their eating habits. They become more independent and mobile, eating more meals and snacks out of the home. They also share more food with their peers, learn new food preferences, and discard old eating habits. There are currently 39 million Americans (17% of the U.S. population) between 10 and 19 years of age, an age when dietary patterns and attitudes are formed. They are a prime target for nutrition education and for marketing strategies designed to establish brand loyalties at an early age. The RDAs for adolescents are shown in Table 16-1.

SPECIFIC NUTRITIONAL NEEDS

Data from dietary surveys indicate that energy intakes peak between 12 and 13 years of age for girls and at age 16 for boys. For most adolescents, "eating to appetite" (that is, eating until feeling satisfied) serves as a reasonably effective way of achieving sufficient energy intake while avoiding excessive intake.

Protein intakes of 89 g and 111 g for boys and 62 g and 67 g for girls 12 to 15 years of age and 16 to 19 years of age, respectively, account for 13% to 14% of total energy intake (NHANES III, 1989-1991). This usually corresponds to more than the 1 g of protein per kilogram of body weight required to meet protein needs for growth and maintenance. Protein becomes a limiting factor in growth, only if energy intake is so restricted that dietary protein must be used as an energy source. During adolescence the lean body mass of males increases by an average of 35 kg, whereas the corresponding figure in females is 19 kg.

The minerals most likely to be available in less-than-adequate amounts during adolescence are calcium, iron, and zinc because the need for these minerals increases significantly during periods of rapid growth. In the NHANES III study, mean intakes for girls provided approximately 63% of the RDAs for zinc, 66% for calcium, and 80% for iron, whereas intakes for boys provided at least 95% for all of these minerals. Although some experts recommend calcium intakes of 1200 mg/day, at least 900 mg/day is required during periods of growth in adolescence. This allows retention of at least 300 mg of calcium per day. The considerable expansion of blood volume during growth causes a need for iron to sustain hemoglobin production. Iron is also required to form the myoglobin within new muscle tissue. Boys need more iron than do girls to sustain growth alone, but this difference is more than offset by the extra iron girls need to replace losses during menstruation. The RDA for girls is set at 15 mg/day, whereas the figure for boys is 12 mg/day. Adolescents must consume between 12 and 15 mg of zinc per day to ensure that at least 0.4 mg/day is retained within the body. Zinc intakes can easily fall below the recommended levels, especially in girls. The zinc/protein ratio of food averages 1.5 mg of zinc per 10 g of protein, suggesting that adequate zinc is provided only by diets containing at least 100 g of protein. At least half of the salt used by adolescents should be iodized to protect against the risk of goiter caused by iodine deficiency.

There is some concern that peer pressure and the forceful marketing of soft drinks may cause some adolescents to consume insufficient milk. The use of milk is important in maintaining a calcium intake required for healthy bones. Even more concern has been caused by the finding of considerably reduced bone mass in adolescent female runners and gymnasts who have amenorrhea (cessation of menstrual periods). Any restriction of bone mass during adolescence may significantly increase the risk of osteoporosis in later life. Girls, especially those who are athletes, should be encouraged to maintain an

TABLE 16-1

Recommended dietary allowances of nutrients for adolescent males and females and pregnant adolescents

	MALES		FEMALES		PREGNANT FEMALES	
	11-14 YEARS	15-18 YEARS	11-14 YEARS	15-18 YEARS	11-14 YEARS	15-18 YEARS
Weight (kg)	45	66	46	55	46	55
Energy (kcal)	2500	3000	2200	2200	2500	2500
Protein (g)	45	59	46	44	56	54
Vitamin A (μg RE)	1000	1000	800	800	800	800
Vitamin A (IU)	5000	5000	4000	4000	4000	4000
Vitamin D (μg)	10	10	10	10	10	10
Vitamin D (IU)	400	400	400	400	400	400
Vitamin E (mg α-TE)	10	10	8	8	10	10
Vitamin C (mg)	50	60	50	60	70	70
Folate (μg)*	150	200	150	180	400	400
Niacin (mg)	17	20	15	15	17	17
Riboflavin (mg)	1.5	1.8	1.3	1.3	1.6	1.6
Thiamin (mg)	1.3	1.5	1.1	1.1	1.5	1.5
Vitamin B_6 (mg)	1.7	2	1.4	1.5	2.2	2.2
Vitamin B_{12} (μg)	2	2	2	2.1	2.2	2.2
Calcium (mg)	1200	1200	1200	1200	1200	1200
Phosphorus (mg)	1200	1200	1200	1200	1200	1200
Iodine (μg)	150	150	150	150	175	175
Iron (mg)	12	12	15	15	30	30
Magnesium (mg)	270	400	280	300	320	320
Zinc (mg)	15	15	12	12	15	15
Selenium (μg)	40	50	45	50	65	65

RE, Retinol equivalent; *IU,* International unit; *α-TE,* alpha-tocopherol equivalent.

* Current recommendation by the Centers for Disease Control is 400 μg/day for all women of childbearing potential.

Based on National Academy of Sciences, *Recommended dietary allowances,* ed 10, Washington, DC, 1989, National Academy Press.

adequate intake of dairy products to provide the calcium needs. They should be strongly discouraged from using soft drinks in place of milk.

The need for the vitamins thiamin, riboflavin, and niacin—involved in energy metabolism—increases in proportion to increased energy intake. Folate and vitamin B_{12}, essential for DNA and RNA synthesis, are also needed in greater amounts during periods of rapid growth. Growth also depends on increased amino acid metabolism, particularly the transamination reactions involved in synthesizing nonessential amino acids, and therefore the need for vitamin B_6 increases in line with increased growth. During adolescence there is an increase in lean body mass of 35% in males and 19% in females. Vitamin D is required for the proper growth of the skeleton, and vitamins A, C, and E are required for the formation and proper functioning of new cells. Although mean intakes, as reported in NHANES III, of all vitamins for boys and of all but vitamins A and E for 12- to 15-year-old girls met the appropriate RDAs, the vitamins most likely to be present in inadequate amounts during adolescence for many are vitamins A, B_6, C, and folate. These inadequacies could be alleviated by recommended intakes of at least five servings of fruits and vegetables.

CONCERNS ABOUT ADOLESCENTS' DIETS

Dietary inadequacy is more common among adolescent girls than in any other segment of the population. The significance of this statistic is increased by the fact that adolescence is a time when adequate nutrition is particularly vital, and inadequate nutrition can lead to health problems that persist throughout life. Poor nutrition during adolescence can be caused by a wide variety of factors, including emotional instability, inappropriate desires to be thin, and general instability in lifestyle and social circumstances.

Special concern is focused on nutritional inadequacy in female adolescents because they may become pregnant and need to cope with the additional nutritional, physical, and emotional demands of pregnancy, childbirth, and lactation. One out of four North American mothers bearing a first child is less than 20 years old. Six percent of all deaths among 18- to 19-year-old girls result from complications of pregnancy. Poor nutritional intake in the years before pregnancy can leave a woman much more vulnerable to problems during pregnancy and cause her infant to be at greater risk of health problems at and after birth. Poor nutrition undoubtedly

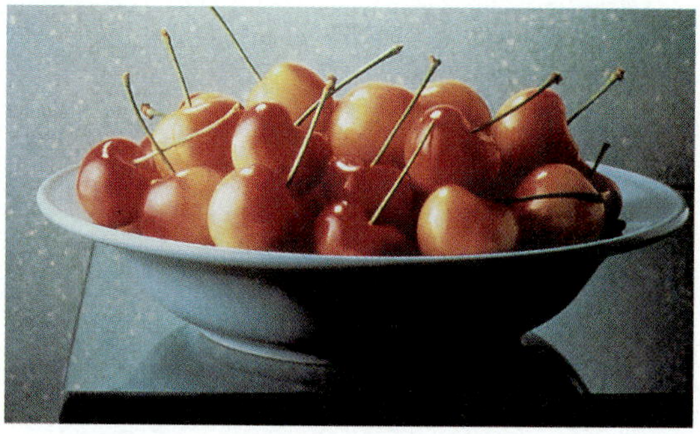

Snacks can play an important role in nutrition.

contributes to the facts that, compared with older women, teenagers have more stillbirths and premature deliveries, have a higher mortality rate, and give birth to children more likely to have congenital defects and insufficient nutrient reserves for the first few months of life. The shorter the period between menarche and conception, the greater the obstetrical risk to the mother. The concern of nutritionists over the diets of adolescents has prompted a concerted effort to educate and cooperate with this group to try to improve its nutritional status.

Factors Influencing Eating Habits

A few studies have focused on the factors that influence adolescents' eating habits. These studies show that young girls who were concerned about their health, were emotionally stable, conformed to social expectations, and came from homes with good family relationships made the most appropriate food choices. The studies found that girls who were motivated by considerations of group status, sociability, independence from parental control, or the enjoyment of eating made significantly less appropriate food choices. Parental criticism of their eating habits led girls to skip meals more frequently. Lunch was the meal skipped most commonly, followed by breakfast.

Adolescents were found to eat better meals in winter than in summer because their winter schedules were more regimented. The likelihood that an adolescent's meals were nutritionally inadequate was found to increase with the proportion of meals eaten away from home. This is especially true when lunch money is used to buy lunches outside the school and probably reflects conformity to the habits of peer groups. The trend toward shorter lunch periods in high schools and restrictions on leaving school property may discourage some inappropriate eating at lunchtime.

The following specific practices and beliefs commonly caused nutritional problems in the adolescents surveyed:

- The skipping of one or more meals each day
- Inappropriate choices of snack foods
- Lack of supervision in food choices made away from home
- Fear of obesity, especially among girls
- Concern that certain foods would aggravate acne
- Lack of time to consume regular meals
- Lack of companionship while consuming meals
- Drinking no milk (perhaps as a rebellion against parental influence)
- Beginning to consume alcohol

BREAKFAST

Many adolescents skip breakfast, but a good breakfast should be included in all diets. The supply of readily usable carbohydrate in most breakfasts causes a rapid increase in blood glucose levels and a related decrease in reaction time in responding to environmental stimuli. A good breakfast improves physical performance and reduces susceptibility to accidents. Although a person's immediate recall is better if he or she skips breakfast, problem-solving ability is reduced. A good breakfast generally provides a range of important nutrients, particularly vitamin C, calcium, and riboflavin.

There are many reasons for adolescents (and others) skipping breakfast, including lack of time, lack of appetite, and fear of becoming fat. The tendency of a person to eat breakfast is also influenced by the availability of someone to prepare it and someone with whom to eat it and by the availability of suitable food and the acceptance of the breakfast-eating habit within a person's peer group.

A "good" breakfast need not consist of the conventional fruit, cereal, toast, and beverage mixture. It can be any combination of foods providing at least 300 kcal of energy and sufficient protein and fat to induce a feeling of satiety until the next meal. The best breakfasts contribute a variety of nutrients to the daily diet, with riboflavin, calcium, and vitamin C intakes found to be higher among those who ate breakfast than among those who did not.

The National Evaluation of School Nutrition programs have demonstrated that the School Breakfast Program has significantly increased the likelihood that children will eat breakfast. This program, which is available to schools enrolling children who are from low-income families or who must travel long distances to school, is offered by 33% of American schools. The four million children participating in the program each day have been found to consume significantly more nutrients than do nonparticipants. Low-income participants have shown significant academic improvement. In schools where breakfast is not offered, it is estimated that a total of three million children skip breakfast each day.[21]

TABLE 16-2

School lunch pattern—National School Lunch Program

COMPONENTS		MINIMUM QUANTITIES: GROUP I: AGE 1-2 YEARS; PRESCHOOL	MINIMUM QUANTITIES: GROUP II: AGE 3-4 YEARS; PRESCHOOL	MINIMUM QUANTITIES: GROUP III: AGE 5-8 YEARS; GR. K-3	MINIMUM QUANTITIES: GROUP IV: AGE 9 YEARS AND OLDER; GR. 4-12	RECOMMENDED QUANTITIES*: GROUP V: AGE 12 YEARS AND OLDER; GR. 7-12
Milk	Whole and unflavored lowfat milk must be offered†	¾ cup (6 fl oz)	¾ cup (6 fl oz)	½ pt (8 fl oz)	½ pt (8 fl oz)	½ pt (8 fl oz)
Meat or meat alternate (quantity of the edible portion as served)	Lean meat, poultry, or fish	1 oz	1½ oz	1½ oz	2 oz	3 oz
	Cheese	1 oz	1½ oz	1½ oz	2 oz	3 oz
	Large egg	½	¾	¾	1	1½
	Cooked dry beans or peas	¼ cup	⅜ cup	⅜ cup	½ cup	¾ cup
	Peanut butter or an equivalent quantity of any combination of above	2 Tbsp	3 Tbsp	3 Tbsp	4 Tbsp	6 Tbsp
Vegetable or fruit	2 or more servings of vegetable or fruit or both to total ½-¾ cup	½ cup	½ cup	½ cup	¾ cup	¾ cup
Bread or bread alternate (servings per week)	Must be enriched or whole grain—at least ½ serving‡ for group I or 1 serving‡ for groups II-V must be served daily	5	8	8	8	10

* The minimal portion sizes for these children are the portion sizes for group IV.

† This requirement does not prohibit offering other milk, such as flavored milk or skim milk, along with the above.

‡ Serving, 1 slice of bread; $\frac{1}{2}$ cup of cooked rice, macaroni, noodles, other pasta products, other cereal products, such as bulgur and corn grits; 1 biscuit, roll, muffin, or similiar products; or any combination of these.

From Food and Nutrition Service, U.S. Department of Agriculture: *Meal pattern requirements and offer versus serve manual*, FNS-265, Washington, DC, 1990, U.S. Government Printing Office.

SCHOOL LUNCH

The National School Lunch Program can be considered an important factor in the nutrient intake of school children. From its inception in 1946, the School Lunch Act in the United States required that a type A lunch provide a third or more of the daily nutrient intake of the 10- to 12-year-old child, with adjustments made for younger and older children. To encourage the preparation of nutritious lunches, the USDA provided subsidies in the form of technical advice, surplus agricultural commodities, or foods purchased by the government as part of the price support programs, as well as a cash subsidy. To qualify for reimbursement, a school must offer as a plate lunch a meal containing specific food components (as indicated in Table 16-2).

Almost all primary and secondary public schools in the United States offer school lunches to students. Nearly half of the lunches are provided free or at a reduced price to children from low-income families. In the 1992 fiscal year, 42.7 million school students (58% of all students) participated in the school lunch program. The required federal funding totaled $3.8 billion, distributed among 92,300 schools.

The School Lunch Program has been modified in recent years to allow more choice to the students and to reduce food waste. The current regulations require all schools to *offer all five components of the meal* and to *serve at least three* to the child. A la carte lines, salad bars, and "hamburger basket" options are also included to appeal to the preferences of students in secondary schools but do not qualify for reimbursement.

In addition to providing nutrients, the School Lunch Program is designed to reduce the fat and sodium contents of the foods consumed. In general, it is intended to bring school meals in line with the USDA and the Department of Health and Human Services (DHHS) Dietary Guidelines for Americans and to assist in achieving the Healthy People 2000 National Health Promotion and Disease Prevention Objectives. In some states special training and support is provided for school food service personnel to assist in the transition to more healthful school lunches.

Evaluation of the School Lunch Program has shown that participants have an overall higher quality diet than do nonparticipants. Participants have also been found to have higher weights for their age than do nonparticipants. One recent study found that low-income participants consumed more protein, calcium, riboflavin, phosphorus, vitamin A, and vitamin B_6 than did nonparticipants of similar income but less magnesium and vitamin C.

In October of 1994 the USDA passed a regulation that the School Lunch Program must conform with current dietary guidelines. These regulations introduce a system called *Nu Menu,* which retains the present nutrient but not the specific food standards and expands the requirement to quantify the fat component. By 1996, on a weekly average (not on a daily average or for specific foods), meals must provide less than 30% of total energy from fat and less than 10% from saturated fat.

The School Lunch Program is supplemented by the Special Milk Program, which provides half a pint of milk to certain schools and childcare centers. A number of other innovative nutrition intervention programs, such as the summer food program, are being investigated as possible ways to improve the nutrition of school children, especially those from economically deprived groups.

FAST FOODS

Many parents and health professionals are concerned about the tendency of adolescents to obtain meals from fast-food establishments. Research, however, suggests that most adolescents obtain only a small proportion of their food from these establishments, and even if there is a problem associated with fast food, it is over-rated.

The main objections to fast food have been the limited selection available and the belief that the foods are high in both fat and salt. Criticisms that fast food did not provide sufficient amounts of vitamins A and C and fiber and did provide too much salt and fat have led many establishments to add salads, raw vegetables, or coleslaw, low-fat milk, and reduced-fat dressing to their menus. The nutritional image of fast-food outlets is also considerably enhanced by the availability of milk and fruit juice as an alternative to soft drinks and coffee.

The information in Table 16-3 shows that most of the foods traditionally available in fast-food outlets actually have considerable nutritional merit, even when assessed on a nutrient-density basis. A complete analysis of foods provided in fast-food establishments is included in Appendix E. Many fast-food chains now provide nutrient information on all menu items at the point of purchase. This is a commendable practice that might well be copied by more expensive restaurants, whose customers may be nutritionally vulnerable adults.

SNACKS

Until recently, nutritionists tended to emphasize the importance of three "good" meals per day and to ignore the possibility that snacks could provide anything other than foods of low-nutrient density. It is now recognized, however, that smaller, more frequent meals may have many physiological and nutritional advantages. Nutritionists also recognize that "snacking" is a way of life with many teenagers and are focusing their attention on ways to improve the nutritional quality of snacks. Studies have shown that the nutritional quality of most diets actually increases as the number of snacks taken increases.

Surveys indicate that snacks are eaten by more than 75% of adolescents, providing between one fourth and one third of their energy intake. The extent to which snacks contribute to the intake of specific nutrients obviously depends on which snacks are taken. Contrary to popular belief, there are few foods that are used more regularly as snacks than for meals. The few that do fall into that category include ice cream and candy but not salty snacks or soft drinks, which are more frequently reported to be consumed as part of a meal than as snacks. About one fourth of all teenagers use milk and fruits as snacks more frequently that they use traditional snack foods. Overall, the most commonly reported snack foods are cakes, cookies, milk, soft drinks, salty snack food, frozen desserts, and fruit.

Once adults have accepted that snacking can be an acceptable part of the daily diet, they can do much to ensure that the snacks taken by adolescents make a significant contribution to good nutrition. They can make nutritious snacks such as fruits, nuts, cheese, and milk readily available for adolescents in their care. Making nutritious snacks available, alongside other less nutritious ones, may prove a more successful way of improving an adolescent's nutritional status than banning certain snacks or trying to discourage snacking.

Snacking should be encouraged as an integral part of a mixed diet. It need only be questioned and discouraged if it contributes to overeating. Excessive snacking only during the evening hours in what is known as "night-eating syndrome" has been implicated as a cause of obesity.

TABLE 16-3

Index of nutrient quality (INQ)* of menu items offered by a fast-food restaurant

MENU ITEM†	PROTEIN	VITAMIN A	VITAMIN C	THIAMIN	RIBOFLAVIN	NIACIN	CALCIUM	IRON	NUTRITIOUS?‡
Regular hamburger	2	0.4	0.3	1.5	1.1	2.2	0.5	1.4	Yes
Regular cheeseburger	2	0.5	0.2	1.2	1.3	2	1.1	1.1	Yes
Large hamburger	2	0.2	0.2	1.0	1.3	2.6	0.4	1.5	Yes
Large cheeseburger	2.4	0.6	0.2	1	1.5	3.2	1.1	1	Yes
Double patty hamburger	1.9	0.3	0.2	1	0.9	1.7	0.7	1	Yes
Fish sandwich	1.6	0.2	0.4	1	0.9	1.1	0.6	0.5	No
Apple pie	0.3	0.1	0.3	0.1	0.1	0.5	0.1	0.3	No
Cookies	0.6	0.1	0.2	1.4	1	0.3	0.1	0.6	No
Chocolate shake	1.2	0.4	0.03	0.5	3.1	0.2	2	0.3	Yes
Egg on English muffin	2.1	0.5	0.2	1.5	2.2	1.3	1.2	1.1	Yes
Hot cakes	0.7	0.2	0.2	1	1.2	0.9	0.7	0.6	No
Scrambled eggs	2.9	1.4	0.2	0.6	4.8	0.3	0.7	1.7	Yes
Pork sausage	1.9	0.1	0.1	1.8	0.9	3.5	0.2	0.6	No
English muffin, buttered	1.2	0.3	0.1	1.7	1	3.8	1	1	Yes
French fries	0.6	0.1	1.9	1	0.2	1.5	0.1	0.3	No

* Percentage of nutrient requirement supplied by each item as purchased, divided by percentage of energy requirement supplied by each item, as purchased. The nutrient requirements were set as the U.S. Recommended Daily Allowance for each nutrient except protein, in which case the requirement was set as 55 g daily. The energy requirement was set as 2200 kcal daily.

† Nutrient compositions on menu items determined by Wisconsin Alumni Research Foundation Institute, Inc, Madison, Wis, 1975.

‡ Based on standard of four nutrients with INQ >1 or two nutrients with INQ >2. Other foods may qualify, if additional nutrients are considered.

From Shannon BM, Parks SC: *J Am Diet Assoc* 76:242, 1980.

OBESITY

Between 30% and 35% of American teenagers are overweight, and statistics suggest that 80% of those teenagers will remain overweight as adults. Between 3% and 20% of American teenagers are obese. Many teenagers, especially girls, believe they are fat or are fearful of becoming fat, striving to attain an unrealistic or unhealthy body size comparable to those of fashion models. Many of these teenage girls embark on self-directed weight-reduction programs that can be hazardous to health. Such inappropriate dieting by teenagers, who have high nutrient needs, is one of the major nutritional concerns in America. It may be particularly damaging if weight-reduction programs are followed intermittently, causing periods of rapid weight loss that are followed by periods of rapid weight gain.

A frequent cause of overweight and obesity in teenagers is an inappropriately low level of activity, rather than excessive food intake. The prevalence of obesity increases by about 2% for every hour per day of inactivity associated with watching television. Recent evidence suggests that the metabolic rate while watching television falls significantly lower than the rate when resting in other ways.[22]

Obese youngsters have been found to have significantly lower serum iron levels than nonobese youngsters, yet accompanied by normal hemoglobin levels. This could be a result of low levels of myoglobin and other iron-containing pigments in muscles, which may cause an unconscious reduction in activity because of the reduced availability of oxygen to the muscle cells.

Because the activity patterns developed during late adolescence often prevail throughout adulthood, this is an opportune time to initiate a healthful, active life-style that helps maintain good weight throughout life. It is also important to learn early in life the importance of responding to satiety signals, allowing food intake to match the prevailing need.

ALCOHOL

Although in most states the legal drinking age is 21, 80% of 12- to 17-year-olds report having at least one alcoholic drink a month and 3% have one per day. It is estimated that 39% of adolescents are moderate drinkers and 28% are "problem" drinkers. This suggests that alcohol consumption by adolescents is both a nutritional and a social problem. Because people generally underreport their alcohol intake, the problem is probably more prevalent and serious than these statistics suggest. Research shows that teenagers under the influence of alcohol are more likely to have casual sex, thereby putting themselves at a greater risk of an unintentional pregnancy or contracting the human immunodeficiency virus (HIV), both of which are health problems with nutritional implications.

"Hard" liquor contributes only energy to the diet. Beer contributes some thiamin and niacin, but this cannot justify its use as part of a well-chosen diet. Alcohol adversely affects the absorption of both zinc and folate, two nutrients that are required for normal growth. The effect of alcohol consumption during pregnancy is discussed in Chapter 14.

SPECIAL CONCERNS RELATING TO ADOLESCENT GIRLS

Use of Oral Contraceptives

Oral contraceptives are widely used by adolescent girls and are associated with some undesirable nutritional consequences. The most common effects are a decrease in serum and red blood cell folate levels and an associated increase in megaloblastic anemia. Taking folate supplements to protect against this problem poses other problems because folate supplements, especially if taken together with iron supplements, cause a reduction in serum zinc levels. This in turn may adversely affect skeletal and muscle growth, sexual development, wound healing, and immune function. The long-term use of oral contraceptives before pregnancy is associated with a reduction in the vitamin B_6 content of human milk to levels incapable of meeting an infant's needs.

On the positive side, oral contraceptive use may decrease an adolescent girl's need for iron by reducing blood losses during menstruation and increasing iron absorption. The estrogen content of oral contraceptives may also lead to an enhanced conversion of carotene to vitamin A, raised serum copper levels, and enhanced calcium absorption.

Premenstrual Syndrome

Premenstrual syndrome (PMS) is the name given to a group of psychological and physical symptoms that recur each month in some women, some time between ovulation and the beginning of menstruation. The symptoms include tension, depression, fatigue, aggression, crying spells, headaches, abdominal bloating, breast tenderness, abnormal thirst, and food cravings. Almost any combination of these symptoms can occur in individual women. Proposed physiological causes of PMS include hormonal imbalance, water retention, hypoglycemia, and prostaglandin deficiency. PMS is a condition distinct from the **dysmenorrhea** (cramps, headache, nausea, and diarrhea) associated with menstrual flow. In fact, the two conditions seldom, if ever, occur in the same woman.

Many nutritional therapies have been proposed for PMS, but none has proved more than minimally successful. The suggested therapies include supplements or megadoses of vitamin B_6, essential fatty acids, magnesium, zinc, vitamin C, and vitamin E and the avoidance of caffeine, alcohol, and salt. At present there is no effective nutritional or psychological treatment for PMS.

Lactation

Although adolescent girls may be encouraged to breastfeed for their infant's benefit, there is concern about the impact of lactation on the bone mineral status of the adolescent mother. Studies have found a significant decrease in bone mineral after 2 to 16 weeks of lactation, accompanied by low dietary intakes of calcium and phosphorus. It is questionable whether it is acceptable for an adolescent mother to meet the nutritional demands of lactation superimposed on those of adolescent growth.

Predisposition to Osteoporosis

A young woman's diet during adolescence can have a considerable influence on her risk of osteoporosis in later life. Excessive exercise, a high fiber intake, and a low fat intake reduce circulating estrogen levels, leading to decreased bone mass. The peak bone mass, attained between the ages of 20 and 35, is one of the main factors determining a woman's risk of osteoporosis after menopause. This is one more reason for encouraging adolescent girls to eat an appropriate diet and exercise sufficiently but not to excess.

Anorexia Nervosa and Bulimia

Anorexia nervosa is best described as a state of emaciation brought about by voluntary starvation. It occurs primarily in adolescent girls, most commonly from middle- and upper-class families. Unless recognized in its early stages, anorexia nervosa is difficult to treat because the patient refuses to eat. Instead of being lethargic and apathetic, as might be expected in undernutrition, those with anorexia have a compulsion to be active. Most cases of anorexia nervosa have a psychological basis.

Anorectic adolescents usually experience amenorrhea and sometimes fatal electrolyte imbalances. They deny that they are emaciated, in spite of a skeleton-like appearance, and relentlessly continue to pursue thinness through starvation and exercise. Successful treatment depends on resolving the underlying psychological problems, correcting disturbed family interactions, and restoring normal food intake. This almost always requires psychiatric and nutritional care and, in severe cases, hospitalization.

A related phenomenon known as "gorge and purge" or bulimia occurs among adolescents (mainly girls) from similar backgrounds to those of adolescents susceptible to anorexia nervosa. Bulimic individuals consume enormous quantities of food and then immediately induce vomiting or take laxatives to purge themselves of the food and its nutrients. Bulimia is also primarily a psychological condition. Unlike anorexia, it carries a high economic cost in addition to its nutritional and psychological costs because large quantities of food are bought to meet the compulsion to gorge. Some of the warning signs and personal characteristics that distin-

TABLE 16-4

Warning signs and personal characteristics that distinguish persons with anorexia nervosa and bulimia

ANOREXIA NERVOSA	BULIMIA
Turns away from food to cope	Turns to food to cope
Introverted	Extroverted
Avoids intimacy	Seeks intimacy
Negates feminine role	Aspires to feminine role
Maintains rigid control—perfectionist	Loses control—steals, uses drugs, promiscuous
Distorted body image	Infrequent body distortions
Denies illness	Recognizes illness
Significant and abnormal weight loss of 25% or more, with no known medical illness accounting for the loss	Within 10 to 15 lb of normal body weight
Intense fear of gaining weight	Exhibits concern about weight and makes attempts to control weight by diet, vomiting, or laxative and diuretic abuse
Reduction in food intake, denial of hunger, and decrease in consumption of fat-containing foods	Eating pattern may alternate between binges and fasts
Amenorrhea in women	Most are secretive about binges and vomiting
Prolonged exercising, despite fatigue and weakness	During a binge, consumes food that has a high caloric content
Peculiar patterns of handling food	Depressive moods may occur
Some exhibit bulimic episodes of binge eating, followed by vomiting or laxative abuse	Death resulting from hypokalemia (low blood potassium level) and suicide
Symptoms of electrolyte imbalance, anemia, and endocrine and immune dysfunction	
Death resulting from starvation, hypothermia, or cardiac failure	

FIGURE 16-7

Possible signs and symptoms accompanying weight loss in eating disorders.

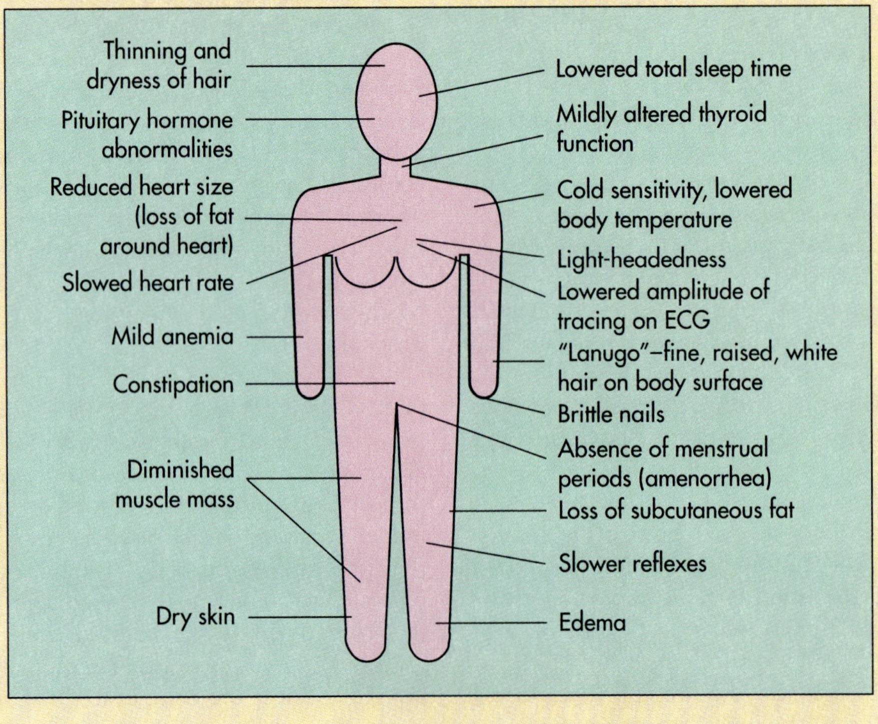

guish anorexia from bulimia are shown in Table 16-4 and Figure 16-7.

IMPROVING NUTRITIONAL HABITS

It has been well documented that knowledge about the requirements for good nutrition does not necessarily lead to the adoption of appropriate nutritional habits. *Motivation* appears to be the key to the application of nutritionally sound eating patterns. The most effective motivation in adolescence is the desire for vitality, good looks, and popularity. Concern about the likely long-term effects of eating habits on health has little impact on adolescents. Group sessions appear to be one of the most effective ways of getting adolescents to accept the need for healthful eating patterns and of motivating them to adopt these patterns. A positive approach that emphasizes the advantages of good eating habits proves more successful than does the negative approach of emphasizing the disadvantages of poor nutrition. Therefore it is important to start from the base of a person's existing food habits, reinforce the existing good aspects of their diet, and try to gradually replace the poor habits with new and more appropriate ones. It is also important for people to recognize that a good diet will not just happen, but it must be properly planned.

ISSUES AND OPINIONS

Drinking Too Much Juice Can Cause Malnutrition in Early Childhood

Fruit juices are popular with children of all ages. Children like them because they are sweet, and parents offer them because they consider them to be healthful and nutritious. Surveys in the United States report that almost 90% of infants consume fruit juices by 12 months of age. Children under 5 years of age consume more juice than those in any other age-group, averaging an annual 9 gallons per child. Apple juice accounts for approximately half of the juice consumed by young children.

Malabsorption of fructose and sorbitol present in apple juice has been associated with chronic nonspecific diarrhea of childhood (CNSD), which affects children aged 1 to 4 years. This association was described in a recent review article,* and the American Academy of Pediatrics issued a statement† advising pediatricians to obtain information regarding sorbitol-containing juice consumption in children who have diarrhea, abdominal pain, or bloating. However, CNSD is not usually associated with failure to thrive (FTT), unless restrictive diets are used to control the diarrhea.

Overconsumption of juice may also create dietary imbalances and/or nutrient deficiencies, whether or not their consumption causes carbohydrate malabsorption or diarrhea. This is particularly true if the juice is used exclusively as a beverage, thus eliminating milk consumption.

A recent study‡ reported the cases of eight toddlers, aged 14 to 27 months, who were not growing because a disproportionate amount of their energy was derived from fruit juices, principally apple juice. Factors attributable to both parents and children were responsible for the excessive juice consumption. Many of the children were described as picky eaters, and their parents or caregivers felt they had little control over the toddler's food or beverage selections. In these cases, they tended to give apple juice, which was well received, to minimize feeding struggles.

It is not known whether the excessive juice consumption simply replaced foods of higher energy and nutrient density, leading to inadequate dietary intakes, or whether carbohydrate malabsorption also contributed to the poor weight gain of these patients.

The diets of five toddlers contained inadequate iron and zinc. Three children showed biochemical evidence of iron deficiency, but none had low serum zinc levels. Because iron and zinc deficiencies may affect appetite, it is possible that iron deficiency contributed to the poor appetite and behavioral feeding difficulties of some patients.

These experiences with fruit juices emphasize that appropriate nutrition for children requires a balanced intake of a variety of foods. Any single food consumed in excess, even if it is perceived as being healthful and nutritious and recognized as desirable in moderation, can result in dietary imbalances and affect the weight gain and subsequent growth and development of children.

* Lifshitz F and others: *J Pediatr* 89:825, 1992.

† American Academy of Pediatrics, Committee on Nutrition: *AAP News* 7:11, 1991.

‡ Smith MM, Lifshitz F: *Pediatrics* 93:438, 1994.

~ BY NOW YOU SHOULD KNOW ~

- Requirements for various nutrients are higher during the period of growth than at any other time throughout life. The rate of increase in nutrient needs with age depends on the nutrients concerned and is determined by which tissues are undergoing most growth at any one time.
- Snacks can make a major contribution to the energy and nutrients supplied by the diet during childhood and adolescence.
- Iron, folate, calcium, and zinc are the nutrients most likely to be inadequately supplied by the diets of young children.
- Growth curves are used to monitor how a child is developing, in comparison with other children.
- The most common nutrition-related problems during childhood are growth retardation, anemia, obesity, and dental caries.
- Nutritional concerns during adolescence focus on eating disorders and inappropriate food patterns, including skipping meals, snacking habits, fad dieting, and the use of alcohol and drugs. Additional concerns about adolescent females focus on premenstrual syndrome, pregnancy, lactation, and the use of oral contraceptives.
- Food habits formed during adolescence can influence health throughout adulthood and can set the pattern of food habits that will be followed throughout life.
- The National School Lunch Program, the Special Milk Program, and the Breakfast Program have all been important in improving the nutrient intake of American schoolchildren.

STUDY QUESTIONS

1. List the nutrients that influence normal tooth function, and explain the role of each nutrient.
2. In an interview with a child about his or her food consumption patterns you find that the child skips breakfast. What are the nutritional and physical implications of skipping breakfast?
3. A child is in the 80th percentile for height on the growth curve. Explain what this means.
4. You have a friend whose child has been on a food jag for about 3 weeks, eating only hot dogs on buns and soda. What do you advise your friend to do?
5. How would you expect a child with iron-deficiency anemia to behave? Would you expect the child to look any different from adequately nourished children?
6. Explain the differences and similarities between anorexia nervosa and bulimia.
7. Why are there more nutritional concerns about girls during adolescence than about boys?

CRITICAL ANALYSIS

1. Assessing the adequacy of a young child's diet can be a challenge. One way to do this is to compare the child's intake with the recommended number of servings from each food group. Consider the case of John, a 12-month-old male. He weighs 18.75 lb and is 28 inches in length. By plotting these measurements on the appropriate growth charts, you discover that he is near the fifth percentile of weight for age (i.e., approximately 95% of males at this age weigh more than John) and at or below the fifth percentile of height for age. This indicates that John is small for his age. His mother has asked you for a dietary assessment to rule out dietary inadequacy as the problem. His intake for the previous day, as recalled by his mother, is listed in the next column:

½ cup milk
¼ cup ready-to-eat cereal
½ slice toast with 1 tsp margarine and 1 tsp jelly
½ cup orange juice
½ medium apple (about 4 Tbsp)
6 saltine crackers
1 oz cheese
2 baby carrots (about 1 Tbsp)
1 oz chicken
½ cup rice
1 cup juice

Compare John's intake (fill in the spaces) with the following recommended servings. What recommendations would you make?

FOOD GROUP	SERVING SIZE	RECOMMENDED SERVINGS PER DAY	NUMBER OF JOHN'S SERVINGS
Milk/dairy	½ cup	4-5	________
Meats/meat substitutes	1 oz or 2-4 Tbsp	1	________
Vegetables and fruits		4-5	
Vegetables			________
Cooked, raw	1-2 Tbsp		
Fruits			
Canned, raw	2-4 Tbsp		
Juice	2-4 oz		
Grains and grain products	½ slice	3	________

REFERENCES

1. Beal VA: On the acceptance of solid foods and other food patterns of infants and children, *Pediatrics* 20:448, 1957.
2. Birch LL: The acquisition of food acceptance patterns in children. In Boakes R, Papplewell D, Burton M, editors: *Eating habits,* Chichester, England, 1986, Wiley.
3. Ashbrook S, Doyle M: Infants' acceptance of strong and mild flavored vegetables, *J Nutr Educ* 17:5, 1985.
4. Breckenridge M: Food patterns of five to twelve year old children, *J Am Diet Assoc* 35:704, 1959.
5. Bryan MS, Lowenberg ME: The father's influence on young children's food preferences, *J Am Diet Assoc* 34:30, 1958.
6. Ireton CL, Guthrie HA: Modification of vegetable-eating behavior in preschool children, *J Nutr Educ* 4:100, 1972.
7. Birch LL, Marlin DW, Rotter J: Eating as the "means" activity in a contingency: effects on young children's food preferences, *Child Dev* 55:431, 1984.
8. Eppright ES and others: The North Central Regional Study of diets of preschool children, *J Home Econ* 62:407, 1970.
9. Dietz WH, Gortmaker SL: Do we fatten our children at the television set? obesity and television viewing in children and adolescents, *Pediatrics* 75:807, 1985.
10. Smith MM, Lifshitz F: Excessive fruit juice consumption as a contributing factor in nonorganic failure to thrive, *Pediatrics* 93:438, 1994.
11. Birch LL and others: The variability of young children's energy intake, *New Engl J Med* 324:232, 1991.
12. Story M, Brown JE: Do young children instinctively know what to eat? the studies of Clara Davis revisited, *N Engl J Med* 316:103, 1987.
13. Nationwide Food Consumption Survey—continuing survey of food intake by individuals, 1986, *Nutr Today,* p. 36, Sept/Oct 1987.
14. Institute of Medicine: *Iron deficiency anemia: recommended guidelines for the prevention, detection, and management among U.S. children and women of childbearing age,* Washington, DC, 1993, National Academy of Sciences.
15. Daily dietary fat and total food-energy intakes—Third National Health and Nutrition Examination Survey, phase I, 1988-91, *Morbid Mortal Weekly Rep* 43:116, 1994.
16. Gibson RS, MacDonald CA, Smit Vanderkooy PD: Dietary fat patterns of some Canadian preschool children in relation to indices of growth, iron, zinc, and dietary status, *J Can Diet Assoc* 54:33, 1993.
17. Life Sciences Research Office, Federation of American Societies for Experimental Biology Nutritional Monitoring in the U.S.: *An update report on nutrition monitoring,* U.S. Public Health Service Pub No 89-1255, Washington, DC, 1989, U.S. Department of Health and Human Services.
18. American Academy of Pediatrics/Committee on Nutrition: Statement on cholesterol, *Pediatrics* 90:469, 1992.
19. Lifshitz F: Growth failure, a complication of dietary treatment of hypercholesterolemia, *Am J Dis Child* 143:537, 1989.
20. U.S. Department of Health and Human Services: *Healthy people 2000: national health promotion and disease prevention objectives,* Washington, DC, 1991, Public Health Service.
21. Hanes S, Vermeersch J, Gale S: The national evaluation of school nutrition programs: program impact on dietary intake, *Am J Clin Nutr* 40:390, 1984.
22. Klesges RC, Shelton ML, Klesges LM: Effect of television on metabolic rate: potential implications for childhood obesity, *Pediatrics* 91:281, 1993.

ADDITIONAL READINGS

American Dietetic Association: Position paper on vegetarian approach to eating, *J Am Diet Assoc* 88:351, 1988.

American Dietetic Association: Position paper on nutrition intervention in the treatment of anorexia nervosa, bulimia nervosa and binge eating, *J Am Diet Assoc* 94:902, 1994.

Birch LL and others: Children's lunch intake: effects of midmorning snacks varying in energy density and fat content, *Appetite* 20:83, 1993.

Casey R, Rozin P: Changing children's food preferences: parent opinions, *Appetite* 12:171, 1989.

Dietz W: Factors associated with childhood obesity, *Nutrition* 7:290, 1991.

Dwyer JT: Nutritional consequences of vegetarianism, *Annu Rev Nutr* 11:61, 1991.

Fast-food fare. Consumer guidelines, *New Engl J Med* 321:752, 1989.

Gazzaniga JM, Burns TL: Relationship between diet composition and body fatness, with adjustment for resting energy expenditure and physical activity, in preadolescent children, *Am J Clin Nutr* 58:21, 1993.

Koff E, Rierdan J: Perceptions of weight and attitudes toward eating in early adolescent girls, *J Adolesc Health* 12:307, 1991.

Kreipe RE, Churchill BH, Strauss J: Long-term outcome of adolescents with anorexia nervosa, *Am J Dis Child* 143:1322, 1989.

Lask B and others: Zinc deficiency and childhood-onset anorexia nervosa, *J Clin Psychiatry* 54(2):63, 1993.

Lechky O: If children are developing poorly, ask what they had for breakfast, *Can Med Assoc J* 143:210, 1990.

Lifshitz F: Children on adult diets: is it harmful? Is it healthful? *J Am Coll Nutr* 11(Suppl):84S, 1992.

Nicklas TA and others: Breakfast consumption affects adequacy of total daily intake in children, *J Am Diet Assoc* 93:886, 1993.

Pipes PL, Trahms CM: Nutrition in infancy and childhood, ed 5, St Louis, 1993, Mosby.

Sanders TAB, Reddy S: Vegetarian diets and children, *Am J Clin Nutr* 59 (suppl): 1176S, 1994.

Shea S and others: Variability and self-regulation of energy intake in young children in their everyday environment, *Pediatrics* 90:542, 1992.

Snyder MP, Story M, Trenkner LL: Reducing fat and sodium in school lunch programs: the LUNCHPOWER intervention study, *J Am Diet Assoc* 92:1087, 1992.

Splett P: Federal food assistance programs: a step to food security, *Nutr Today* 29(2):6, 1994.

Steiger H, Puentes-Neuman G, Leung FY: Personality and family features of adolescent girls with eating symptoms: evidence for restricter/binger differences in a nonclinical population, *Addict Behav* 16:303, 1991.

Swadi H: Alcohol abuse in adolescence: an update, *Arch Dis Child* 68:341, 1993.

Thornton LP, DeBlassie RR: Treating bulimia, *Adolescence* 24:631, 1989.

Woodhead JC and others: Gender-related differences in iron absorption by preadolescent children, *Pediatr Res* 29:435, 1991.

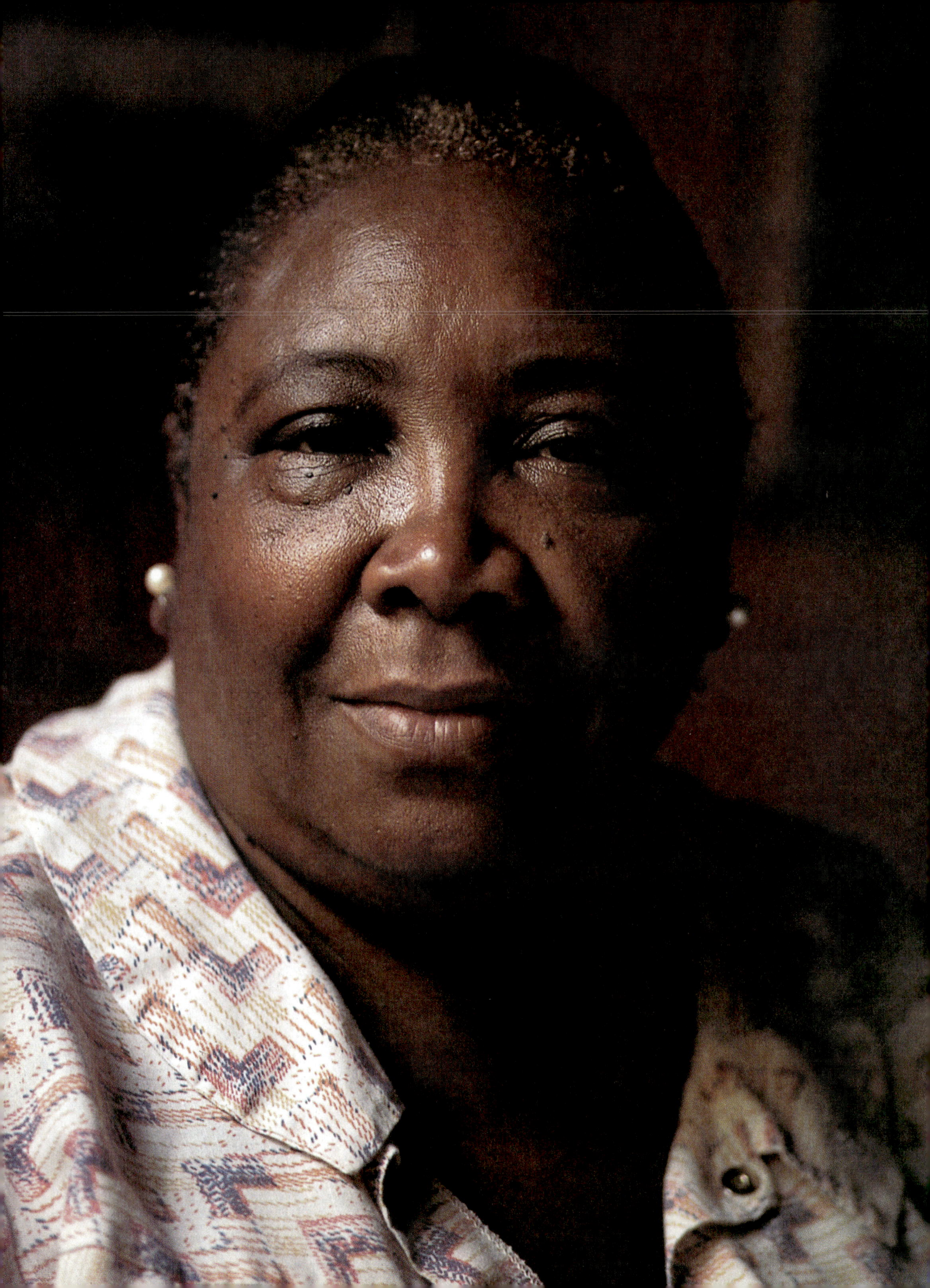

CHAPTER 17

NUTRITION IN THE LATER YEARS

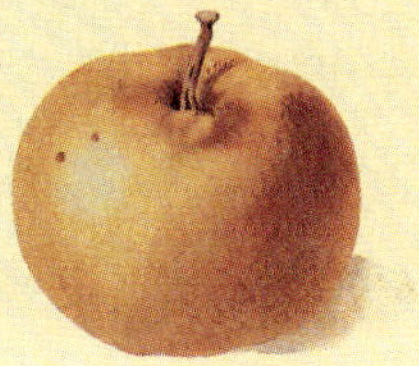

The increasing number of people who survive to enjoy their renaissance years has caused increasing interest in the nutritional needs of elderly persons. These needs are influenced by the physical condition and activity of elderly people and by each person's nutritional history. Many social, environmental, psychological, and physiological factors also play a role in determining nutritional needs in the later years. Many social programs have been developed to help senior citizens receive adequate nutrition and to enjoy good health.

Aging is an unavoidable part of life, although most of us would like to delay its onset and slow its progress. Many scientists, laypersons, and charlatans continue humanity's perpetual search for the "Fountain of Youth": some chemical or some way of life that bestows good health and great longevity on its users or adherents. Needless to say, immortality remains elusive, yet people are living longer and healthier lives for many reasons. One of the most significant reasons is the improved nutrition of the modern Western population, compared with its predecessors.

The branch of medicine dedicated to the care of the aging is known as **geriatrics**. **Gerontology** is a wider discipline concerned with the psychological, sociological, economic, physiological, and medical aspects of aging. The physiological and medical aspects of aging alone are sometimes referred to as **biogerontology.** There has been a surge of activity in geriatrics, gerontology, and biogerontology in recent years.

In 1900, three million people in the United States (4% of the population) were over 65 years of age. In 1987 the U.S. Bureau of Census reported that about 12% of the U.S. population was 65 years of age or older, amounting to about 30 million people.[1] By the year 2030 there will be more than 65 million Americans aged 65 and over, accounting for 21% of the population. There will be an even greater increase in the proportion of elderly people over 70 years of age, and those over 85 years of age will be the most rapidly growing segment of the population.

National goals and objectives for older Americans were recently set out in *Healthy People 2000: National Health Promotion and Disease Prevention Objectives.*[2] The main goal is to prevent older Americans from becoming disabled and to help those who are already disabled to avoid further disability. In general, the aim is to preserve as much physical and mental function as possible and thus increase the span of "healthy life." A healthy life is defined as one in which functional independence is maintained. At present, 65-year-old Americans can expect, on average, to live for an additional 16.4 years and be functionally independent for about 12 of these years. By the year 2000 the national goal is to increase "active" or "functional" life expectancy at 65 to at least 14 years for men and 16 years for women.

Table 17-1 indicates that life expectancy at birth is still increasing slowly and is substantially greater for women than for men. As life expectancy has risen, so the major causes of death have changed. Most significantly, infectious diseases have been replaced by degenerative diseases as the major causes of death (Table 17-2). A person's susceptibility to the three leading causes of death—heart disease, cancer, and stroke—is affected by his or her diet. Therefore nutrition has a vital role to play in prolonging a healthy life.

TABLE 17-1

Life expectancy determined at year of birth

YEAR OF BIRTH	LIFE EXPECTANCY (YEARS)
1850	40
1900	47
1940	63
1950	68
1960	70
1970	70
1980	73 (men, 69; women, 77)
1990	74.5 (men, 72.1; women, 79)
1991	75.7 (men 72.2; women 79.1)

TABLE 17-2

Leading causes of death in the United States

CAUSE	DEATHS (%)
1900*	
Pneumonia	12
Tuberculosis	11
Diarrhea	8
Heart diseases	8
Stroke	6
1987†	
Heart diseases	36
Cancers	22
Stroke	7
Accidents	4
Lung diseases	4

* From National Center for Health Statistics *Monthly Vital Statistics Report* 37(1), April 1, 1968.

† *The Surgeon General's Report on Nutrition and Health,* U.S. Public Health Services, Pub No 88-50210, Washington, DC, 1988, U.S. Government Printing Office.

The U.S. commitment to the study of nutrition and aging is evident from the establishment of the United States Department of Agriculture (USDA) Center on Aging at Tufts University in 1982. The Center on Aging is the site of the most advanced research in the world on human nutrition and aging, with scientists examining the function and nutritional consequences of the many organ systems that change during maturation. Housed in a 15-story building that is a combination of laboratories, offices, and modern hotel-type accommodations, the center has the capacity to conduct research at all levels—from molecular biology, to animal and human studies, to population studies. For the first time, senior citizens are participating in research that will affect their generation and provide preventive dietary guidance for future generations (Figure 17-1).

FIGURE 17-1

Dr. Robert Russell, Director of Human Studies (left), and Dr. Irwin Rosenberg, Center Director (right), of the United States Department of Agriculture Human Nutrition Research Center on Aging at Tufts University, prepare a research volunteer for insertion of a gastric tube used to measure acidity of the stomach and intestine. A student observes.

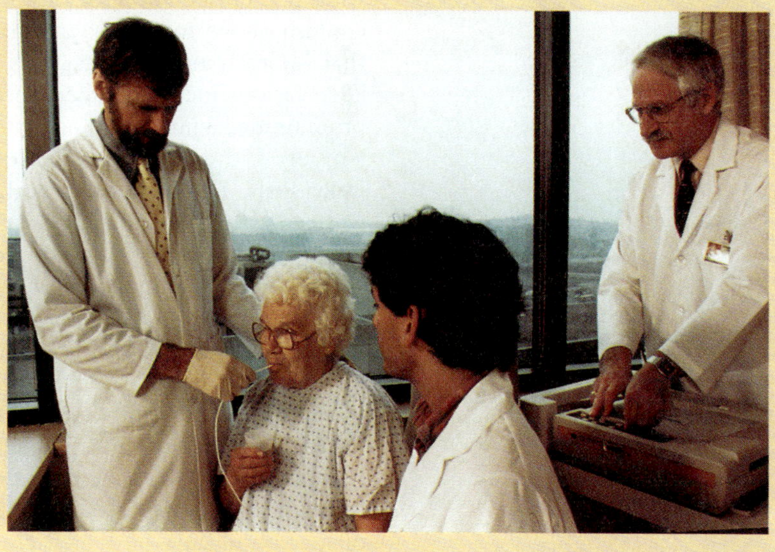

THE AGING PROCESS

Aging is influenced by both genetic and environmental factors. Genetic factors are believed to determine the maximal age an individual can attain, whereas environmental factors determine how close he or she gets to achieving that maximal age and how healthy and active he or she remains throughout aging. Many different theories of aging attempt to lay more detail on the foundation of these broad generalizations.

The various theories of aging fall into two broad categories. According to **systemic** theories, aging must be understood from the viewpoint of whole organisms or at least intact body systems. **Cellular** theories, on the other hand, focus on changes taking place within individual cells.

Selected Theories of Aging

SYSTEMIC	CELLULAR
Rate of living	Program theories
Cerebral clock	Suicide protein
Homeostases failure	Gene depletion
Endocrine malfunction	Codon restriction
Immune system malfunction	Error theories
	Error catastrophe
	Altered protein degradation
	Free radical damage
	Somatic mutation
	DNA repair
	Cross-linking

From Dice JF: *World Rev Nutr Diet* 63:175, 1990.

Some of the most accepted systemic theories can be summarized as follows:

- The **rate of living theory** suggests that the rate of aging is closely related to a person's basal metabolic rate (BMR). According to this theory, the higher the BMR, the shorter the life span, and vice versa. It is suggested that this effect might be mediated by the accumulation of some deleterious products of metabolism or by the steady depletion of some vital substance as a result of metabolism.
- The **cerebral clock theory** suggests that the brain somehow monitors the rate of metabolism and controls the rate of aging accordingly. Thus some kind of cerebral "clock" is forming a link between the "rate of living" and the rate of aging.
- The **homeostasis failure theory** suggests that the underlying cause of aging is a failure of the many complex networks of homeostasis, which normally keep the body stable and able to respond to change in an appropriate way. As homeostatic control deteriorates, so the ability of the body to behave as an integrated whole deteriorates, leading to some ultimate catastrophe that causes death.

TABLE 17-3

Neurological and behavioral effects of vitamin deficiencies

VITAMIN	MANIFESTATIONS OR SYMPTOMS
Thiamin (B_1)	Beriberi, Wernicke-Korsakoff's psychosis
Niacin	Pellagra, dementia
Pantothenic acid	Myelin degeneration
Pyridoxine (B_6)	Peripheral neuropathy, convulsions
Folate	Irritability, depression
Cobalamin (B_{12})	Peripheral neuropathy, subacute combined system degeneration, dementia
Vitamin E	Spinocerebellar degeneration, peripheral axonopathy

From Rosenberg IH: Nutrition and aging. In Hazzard WR and others: *Principles of geriatric medicine and gerontology, ed 3, New York, 1994, McGraw-Hill Professions Division.*

- The **endocrine malfunction theory** proposes that some malfunction of hormonal control is the key to aging.
- The **immune system malfunction theory** suggests that a steady deterioration of the immune system leads to the slow deterioration of the body that is called aging.

Researchers who prefer cellular theories of aging concentrate their attention on single cells under laboratory conditions and then attempt to apply their findings to the cells of the intact body. For example, a human connective tissue cell (fibroblast) grown in the laboratory is able to multiply through no more than about 50 to 60 cell divisions. After that time, the resulting cells are unable to multiply further under the conditions of the culture. When examined, the cells are found to have many of the biochemical and structural characteristics of cells in aged tissues taken from intact bodies. If fibroblasts are taken from people of different ages and then cultured, the number of cell divisions they can pass through in culture is inversely related to the age of the person from whom the cells are derived. In other words, cells from older people appear to have less capacity to survive and grow in culture than do cells from younger people. Such results as these encourage many researchers to believe that examining the biochemical characteristics of individual cells might reveal the secrets of aging.

The various specific cellular theories of aging are often divided into **programmed aging theories** and **error theories** (see Table 17-3), although the two categories do overlap. Programmed aging theories suggest that cells are somehow genetically programmed to age and die at a specific time. They have developed from knowledge that programmed cell death definitely occurs during early development. One major problem with programmed aging theories is that they require aging to have been naturally selected during the course of evolution.[3] There is a vigorous and continuing debate about whether and how natural selection, normally associated with the preservation of advantageous characteristics, could have led to the programming of an aging process that is clearly not advantageous to the individuals who age. Various ideas have been proposed to explain how programmed aging could have arisen during evolution as a result of advantages it confers on species rather than on individuals. The merits and weaknesses of these theories will be debated for a long time to come.

Error theories of aging propose that aging is caused by the steady accumulation of aberrant macromolecules because of errors in the normal operations of the cell. The effect of one error makes further errors more likely, leading to a "cascade" of errors that result in eventual catastrophe. Different error theories propose different sources of the errors and different target molecules that accumulate the errors. Proteins, DNA molecules, RNA molecules, carbohydrates, and lipids are the main types of macromolecules in which crucial errors might accumulate. Free radicals, chemical cross-linking agents, and chemical mutagens (able to cause mutations in DNA) are the main types of chemical agents proposed as causes of the errors.

Most of the theories of aging are currently under active investigation. It is hoped that this continuing research will narrow the list of possibilities and perhaps focus attention on the specific ways in which diet might affect the aging process.

NUTRITIONAL DEPRIVATION AND AGING

An interesting series of experiments has shown that restricting the energy available from the diet can increase the life span of rats, hamsters, mice, cattle, fruitflies, and worms by as much as 70%.[4] The life span of such animals can also be extended by periods of excess energy consumption interspersed by periods of starvation or by feeding a diet with sufficient energy but insufficient protein.

The extension of life achieved in these experiments is apparently not caused by any reduction in metabolic rate, retardation of growth, or delay in maturation. A variety of biochemical and physiological changes have been observed in the animals concerned, but their significance is unclear. It is also unknown whether similar dietary restriction extends the human life span.[5] Even if the methods are applicable to humans, it is questionable whether many people would wish to adopt them given the rigid dietary control involved. Many people might choose a slightly shorter life of higher quality in preference to a longer life of significantly reduced quality.

THE ROLE OF GENETICS

Scientists have identified specific genes in simple organisms, such as the nematode or round worm *Caenorhabditis elegans,* which can either accelerate or slow the aging process.[6] The further analysis of these genes offers one of the most promising avenues toward better understanding of the role of genetics in aging.

Studies with identical and nonidentical twins have revealed some information about the role of genetics in human aging. Identical twins have the same complement of genes because they are derived from the same fertilized egg cell (**zygote**), which splits after fertilization to yield two genetically identical fetuses. Such twins are known as **monozygotic twins** (derived from one zygote). Nonidentical twins are derived from different egg cells, which happened to be released and fertilized within their mother at the same time. These **dizygotic twins** (derived from two different zygotes) each contain a different complement of genes. Studies have found that the life spans of pairs of monozygotic twins are more similar than are the life spans of pairs of dizygotic twins. This is strong evidence suggesting that a person's genetic make-up does play a significant role in influencing his or her likely life span. It is difficult to get detailed information on the role of genetics in human aging, however, because it is impossible and unethical to control the many environmental factors that may also influence aging, to distinguish environmental effects from genetic ones.

Some possible clues come from a variety of inherited diseases that appear to produce premature aging in humans. Two examples of such diseases are progeria (Hutchinson-Gilford syndrome) and Werner's syndrome. Each of these syndromes is apparently caused by a single gene. In the case of Hutchinson-Gilford syndrome, the presence of an autosomal dominant gene results in premature balding, wrinkling, age-pigment spotting of the skin, and death from heart failure by about 12 years of age. Werner's syndrome is associated with similar symptoms in early adulthood, leading to death from atherosclerosis by about age 40, and is caused by an autosomal recessive gene.

Taken all together, current evidence suggests that between 70 and 240 different genes may affect human aging. Researchers can be expected to steadily identify these genes, work out their functions, and thus gain increasing knowledge on the extent to which our genes influence how long we will live and from what we will die.

The entire collection of genetic material in the nucleus of each cell of the human body is called the *genome.* The typical human genome consists of the deoxyribonucleic acid (DNA) within 23 pairs of chromosomes (so there are 46 individual chromosomes). One member of each pair of chromosomes is derived from each parent. It is estimated that humans have 100,000 or more genes, and about 2000 have been identified. The pair of chromosomes in the human genome that determine sex is called the sex chromosomes (known as *X* and *Y*). The other 44 chromosomes in the human genome are called autosomes. Genes that produce effects even if only one copy of them is present are called *dominant genes* (for example, the gene responsible for producing brown eyes). Genes that produce an effect only when there are two copies of them present are called *recessive genes* (for example, the gene responsible for blue eyes). Thus an autosomal dominant gene is one present on an autosome that will definitely have effects in the individual. An autosomal recessive gene, on the other hand, must be present on both members of a pair of chromosomes to have an effect in the individual.

NUTRITION AND AGING

The study of nutrition and aging is complicated by the fact that people's nutritional needs grow more complex as they age for both physiological and social reasons. Different elderly people have different and long histories, including many variables that can affect their nutritional needs. They have had different illnesses, been exposed to different physical and emotional traumas, and followed different diets. The differing effects of these historical factors are superimposed on the normal genetic variation among different people. Wide variations in the ability of elderly people to digest, absorb, and use specific nutrients also complicate attempts to generalize about their nutritional needs.

Research in this area is further complicated by the fact that it is hardly feasible to study individual people throughout 50 or 60 years of life, in contrast with the relative ease—for example—of monitoring individual infants throughout their first year. This has forced scientists investigating the links between nutrition and aging to rely largely on data from "cross-sectional" studies, in which many different people of different ages are exam-

FIGURE 17-2

Physiological changes with age.

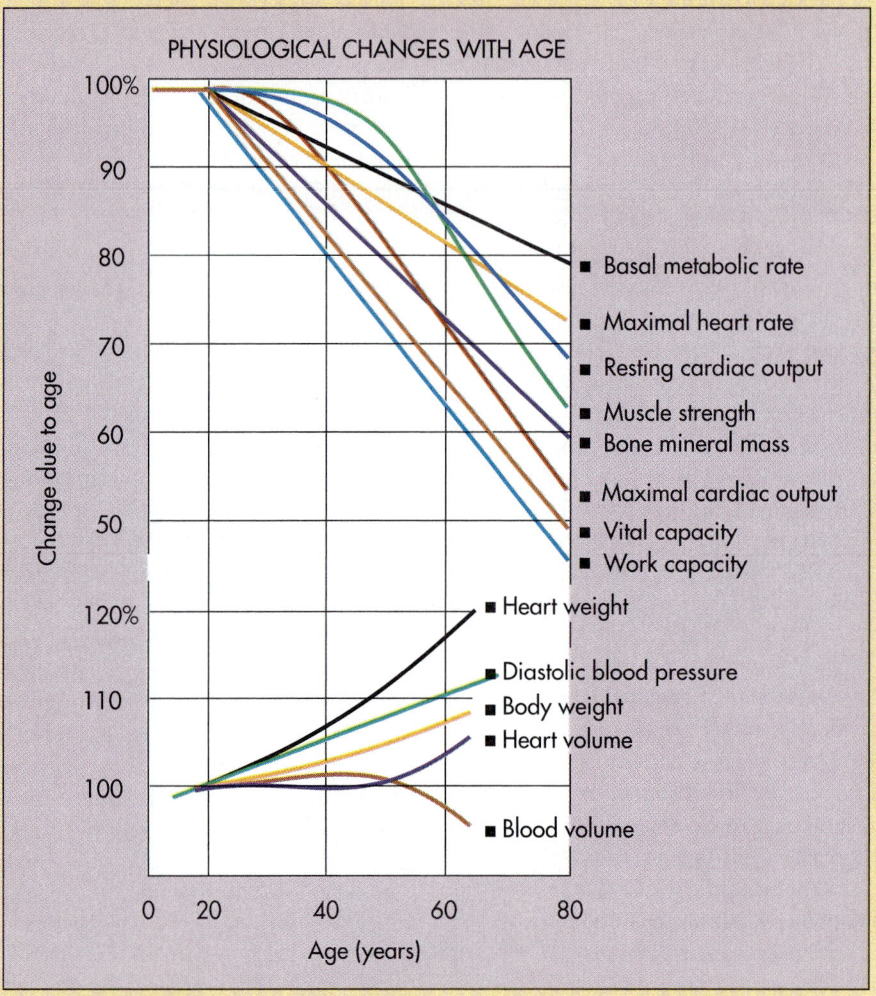

ined. However, a few "longitudinal" studies, which monitor specific individuals over long periods, are now either complete or underway. These studies should provide much useful information on the biochemical and physiological changes associated with aging. They may help to explain why chronological age (age in years) is not an accurate predictor of physiological age (the stage of physiological aging of the body).

In considering the role of nutrition in aging, we are concerned with not only how nutrition affects the aging process, but also how aging affects the need for nutrients.

PHYSIOLOGICAL CHANGES WITH AGE

Some of the main physiological changes that accompany aging are summarized in Figure 17-2. The specific values used in Figure 17-2 are for men, and although similar general trends are expected for women, comparable data for women are not available. The changes involved are inevitable consequences of aging, although the rate at which they occur can be modified by nutrition and physical exercise. Some of the physiological changes associated with aging have a direct influence on the aging person's nutrient needs. Details of some such changes are given in the box on p. 607.

Loss of Lean Mass

The decline in muscle mass between the ages of 45 and 78 is illustrated in Figure 17-3.[7] For people living beyond the age of 78, the rate of muscle loss accelerates. One direct consequence of the loss of lean mass with aging is a reduction of basal energy needs by about 100 kcal per decade. This, coupled with reduced energy needs for activity, can result in total energy needs that may be satisfied by a total food intake containing insufficient micronutrients (particularly vitamin D, magnesium, calcium, and zinc).

Age-Related Changes in Physiological Function That Influence Nutrient Needs

- Energy requirements decline as the muscle mass of the aging person decreases; fewer calories are used in physical activity.
- Peripheral tissues of older persons take up fat-soluble vitamins at slower rates; thus vitamin A intake in elderly people results in higher circulating levels of vitamin A.
- There is a decline in immune function with age that may be responsible in part for the increased susceptibility to conditions such as infection and malignancy. At the same time, there is evidence that increased vitamin and mineral intake, including zinc, may counteract this age-related change.
- While the efficiency of nutrient absorption is relatively well maintained during aging, intestinal absorption of calcium declines.
- Skin synthesis of vitamin D diminishes.
- Metabolic use of vitamin B_6 in older subjects is less efficient.
- One third of individuals over age 70 lose entirely or have a significantly diminished capacity to secrete stomach acid. The effect of lower stomach acid on the absorption of vitamin B_{12}, calcium, iron, folic acid, and possibly zinc appears to explain some of the increased tendency for depletion of some of those micronutrients with age and the possible need for increased intake by diet or the use of supplements.
- The senses of both smell and taste decline with age.

From Rosenberg IH: Nutrition and aging. In Hazzard WR: *Principles of gerontology,* ed 3, New York, 1994, McGraw-Hill Professions Division.

Frontera and coworkers[7] found that declining muscle mass was the major factor in the decline in muscle strength with age. Therefore attempts to maintain muscle strength during aging should focus on steps that minimize the loss of muscle mass. One of the most effective measures to achieve this aim is engaging in regular exercise. People should ideally exercise regularly throughout life, but muscle size and strength can be increased even in frail and institutionalized women up to age 100 who take up exercise.[8] Any increase in muscle size achieved in aging people decreases the possibility of micronutrient deficiencies by increasing their energy intake.

Falling Bone Mass

The decline in bone mass that accompanies aging brings an increased risk of osteoporosis. One important factor involved in the decline in bone mass is the decreased synthesis of vitamin D in the skin of elderly people. This decrease is a result of both reduced efficiency of vitamin D synthesis and decreased exposure to sunlight.[9] Vitamin D intake also usually declines with age, making this vitamin a key target for efforts to slow the decline in bone mass with age. Giving elderly persons vitamin D supplements has been shown to have a significant beneficial effect on bone mineral status. Calcium supplementation is also found to produce clear benefits in people whose calcium intake would otherwise be less than 400 mg/day.

FIGURE 17-3

The decline in muscle mass with age.

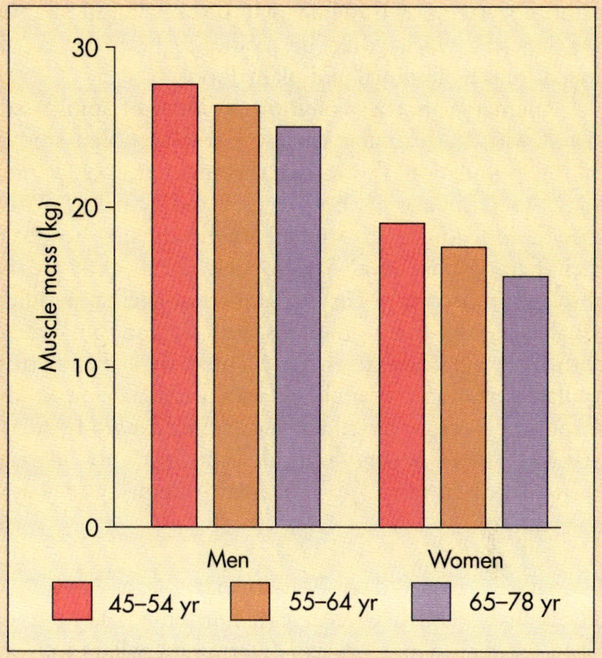

Postmenopausal women are at the greatest risk of osteoporosis, although it also affects a smaller proportion of men. For a more detailed discussion of this condition, see Chapter 9.

Vascular Changes

Cardiovascular disease is one of the major causes of death and illness in elderly persons. The risk of cardiovascular disease has been clearly shown to be influenced by nutritional factors, particularly the consumption of dietary fat (see Chapter 4). Some degree of atherosclerosis is an inevitable consequence of aging, but the extent to which an aging person is at risk of cardiovascular disease is strongly influenced by his or her lifelong dietary history, superimposed on genetic factors.

One recently discovered additional factor is the circulating level of the nonprotein amino acid homocysteine. High levels of plasma homocysteine are known to cause premature vascular disease and mental retardation in individuals carrying a specific genetic defect. In normal individuals, however, homocysteine levels have been found to increase with aging.[10] This observation suggests that homocysteine may be involved in the vascular changes that lead to cardiovascular disease in elderly persons. Several vitamins are involved in regulating homocysteine metabolism, including folate, vitamin B_6, and vitamin B_{12}. Giving elderly men and postmenopausal women folate or vitamin B_{12} supplements has been shown to reduce homocysteine levels. This suggests that at least part of the explanation for the increase in homocysteine with aging may be subclinical vitamin deficiencies, which could be readily reversed by a balanced intake of animal and plant foods.

Anemia is another common problem of aging associated with the vascular system. Cross-sectional studies of the population show that the incidence of anemia increases with age in both males and females. When specific individuals are studied longitudinally, however, their hemoglobin levels do not fall significantly in the absence of disease.[11] This suggests that anemia in aging usually accompanies other diseases. It can be treated with iron supplements and prevented by a diet rich in available iron and vitamin C (which enhances iron absorption). Because megaloblastic anemia caused by folate deficiency often occurs alongside iron-deficiency anemia, particular attention to dietary folate adequacy may also be required.

Changes in Brain Function

The brain is sensitive to changes in nutrient intake, and the brain also plays a major role in determining what foods are eaten and in what amounts. The brain requires a continual supply of glucose in appropriate amounts. Either too much glucose in the blood (hyperglycemia) or too little (hypoglycemia) can quickly cause the brain to slip into coma. The brain also requires many vitamins and minerals, particularly the seven vitamins listed in Table 17-3.

Recent studies have found that aging is associated with declining levels of vitamin B_6, vitamin B_{12}, and folate. It seems possible that some of the impairments of brain function, including memory loss and reduced cognitive ability, may be caused by mild deficiencies of these and other vitamins.[12] Healthy elderly people with low blood levels of a variety of vitamins achieve lower scores in memory and nonverbal abstract thinking tests than do those with higher vitamin levels.

Failing Vision

The impairment of vision that can accompany aging is often the greatest single factor reducing an elderly person's quality of life. Just under 50% of Americans aged 75 through 85 have suffered significant loss of vision from cataracts,[13] but in most cases this is readily corrected by surgery. A significant body of evidence now suggests that the onset of cataracts can be prevented or at least delayed by appropriate nutritional and behavioral modification.[13] Vitamin C, vitamin E, and β-carotene have all been shown to provide some protection against cataract formation, presumably from their ability to prevent oxidative damage. The most significant behavioral changes that can reduce the risk of cataracts are the avoidance of smoking (or other people's smoke) and avoidance of excessively bright light.

Evidence also suggests that antioxidant nutrients such as vitamin C, vitamin E, and β-carotene can offer some protection against macular degeneration, which is the most common cause of blindness in elderly persons. This condition is believed to result from oxidative damage to the photoreceptors of the retina. It affects almost one third of Americans over 65, and its incidence increases with age. The role of antioxidant nutrients in protecting against macular degeneration is not yet firmly established. The possible protective effects of these nutrients, however, are an additional reason for ensuring that elderly people consume sufficient yellow, orange, or dark green fruits and vegetables, or receive antioxidant nutrient supplementation at a comparable level, if sufficient dietary intake cannot be maintained.

Declining Immunity

The mass of immune tissue declines throughout life, leading to a steady decline in immune function.[14] This decline is almost certainly related to the increase in susceptibility to infection and some cancers that accompanies aging. The immune system is known to require a wide variety of nutrients and to be sensitive to changes in both macronutrient and micronutrient status. Therefore adequate nutrition and appropriate nutritional intervention can play a big part in maintaining a person's immune defenses at their maximal possible level. This role of good nutrition in immune function applies to people of all ages, but is especially important for aged persons,[15] when some decline in immune function is inevitable.

Obesity

Many people put on weight as they age, for many different reasons, including declining metabolic rate, reduced levels of exercise, and increased wealth and the concomitant opportunity to consume rich food. As part of this trend, obesity becomes a problem for significant numbers of people as they age. Elderly women are two to three times more likely to be obese as are elderly men. Obesity in elderly people is associated with an increased incidence of diabetes.

The most prevalent nutrition-related problems in elderly persons are the following:

- Obesity
- Undernutrition
- Osteoporosis
- Diabetes
- Cardiovascular disease

The incidence of obesity in both men and women over 80 years of age is less than in men and women aged between 60 and 80, which may reflect the high mortality rate among obese people when they are 60 to 80 years of age.

Weight Loss

Although many aging people become overweight or obese, many encounter the opposite problem of unintentional and undesirable weight loss. This may be a result of psychological factors, a generalized deterioration in physical condition, or the presence of some disease.[16] The lost weight generally includes both lean body tissue and body fat.

SOCIAL FACTORS AFFECTING NUTRITION OF ELDERLY PERSONS

Three main social factors affect the nutrition of elderly people: their long-standing food habits, economic considerations, and susceptibility to nutrition misinformation.

Long-Standing Food Habits

The food patterns and preferences of elderly people are largely the result of their long-standing food habits. These food habits reflect each person's ethnic, social, and economic background and the availability of foods at the time when the habits were established. People of 70 or 80 years of age tend to have food habits that were established 50 or 60 years ago, when the food distribution system in America was much simpler and more restricted than it is now. These people may still regard fruits and vegetables as seasonal items that should be bought only at certain times of the year. Therefore even though the fruits and vegetables are available all year, elderly persons may buy them only at the times they consider them to be "in season." This attitude may be one of the main causes of vitamin A, vitamin C, and folate inadequacies in elderly persons, although the relatively high cost of some good food sources may also be a factor.

Foods that are associated with pleasant experiences early in life may be strongly preferred when an elderly person is ill, under stress, or lonely. Many old people, for example, crave for such foods as bread and milk, brown sugar on toast, or homemade ice cream because they associate the foods with happy memories and find that eating them creates a sense of security and well-being. The psychological and social meanings of such foods can be an important part in helping an elderly person recover from illness or adjust to changed circumstances.

Elderly people often hold rigid long-established beliefs about the specific nutritional merits of some foods and adverse effects of others. Common beliefs among elderly persons are that eating fish causes worms, that some fruits should not be eaten with milk, that cheese causes constipation, and that milk is suitable only for infants. Such ideas can have a major effect on an elderly person's diet and must be taken into account when delivering nutritional education to elderly people.

Because an elderly person's eating habits are deeply ingrained and have many social and psychological implications, attempts to change his or her diet should be made with great sensitivity to each individual's feelings. Major modifications may often be unwise or unnecessary. Where modification is required, it should be introduced gradually, under nonstressful circumstances, and with as much attention to individual preferences as possible. Some medical and metabolic problems such as ulcers, diabetes, hypertension, or allergies require rapid modification of an elderly person's eating habits. In such cases the sympathetic help of a counselor can be invaluable in making the transition.

Economic Considerations

Economic pressures play an important role in determining the food choices of many elderly people. Many of them are living on fixed incomes that were set when salaries and living costs were much lower. This forces many elderly people to buy only the cheapest foods that provide sufficient bulk and energy to satisfy their hunger. The foods chosen are often largely carbohydrate, such as bread and cereals, with a limited content of protein, vitamins, and minerals. More dependable and varied sources of nutrients such as meat, milk, and fresh fruits and vegetables are too expensive for many elderly people to purchase regularly. Another factor favoring the purchase of carbohydrate-rich foods is that many are easily stored, allowing use of small amounts.

The disappearance of many local grocery stores and their replacement by large supermarkets in suburban shopping plazas has also caused problems for elderly persons. Although the large stores offer a wide variety of foods at relatively low prices, it is difficult or expensive (or both) and sometimes impossible to reach them. Once inside such stores, many elderly people become overwhelmed and confused by the wide choice available. They often choose instead to shop in smaller delicatessens or service stores where prices are higher but where they may feel more welcomed and more secure.

Nutrition Misinformation

Many old people are haunted by the fear that they may become ill and unable to look after themselves or bear the cost of medical care. This makes them easy prey for the promoters of "health foods" and food supplements, who may promise good health, "eternal youth," increased vitality, and protection from the degenerative diseases of aging. It is sadly all too common for door-to-door salespeople to persuade elderly people to part with a significant proportion of their income in return for worthless and overpriced products. The ruling that any such contract can be voided within 1 to 3 days offers some protection to people who enter into agreements they later regret or are advised against. It is of even greater concern that many old people may rely on false panaceas offered by salespeople, rather than seeking the medical help that they need. This can cause an initially easily treatable condition to deteriorate into one that is much more difficult and expensive to treat.

PSYCHOLOGICAL FACTORS AFFECTING NUTRITION OF ELDERLY PERSONS

The main psychological factors affecting the nutrition of elderly people are living alone, depression, and anxiety.

Living Alone

Old people who preserve their independence by living alone may find that this leads to altered eating patterns. The lack of motivation to cook meals can lead to skipping meals or the frequent use of snack meals at irregular times. This often leads to a poorly balanced diet. Inexpensive living quarters may also lack adequate cooking and refrigeration facilities. Many older people follow an erratic eating pattern, including days of just nibbling, days of overeating, and days in which almost nothing is eaten. It has been found, not surprisingly, that many older people gain more pleasure from eating when they eat in company, rather than on their own.

Depression

Depression is a common accompaniment to aging, and it can have a major influence on food intake. Sometimes depression may cause overeating, whereas at other times or in other people it can lead to undereating. Overeating results from the use of food as a comforting experience that can relieve boredom. It can lead to overweight and obesity, which can in turn increase the risk of many of the degenerative diseases associated with aging. Undereating can obviously lead to undernutrition, which can also increase susceptibility to illness—for example, by reducing the effectiveness of the immune system. Depression in elderly persons can often be quickly alleviated if it causes family and friends to take more interest in the old person and socialize with him or her more frequently.

Anxiety

Anxiety and emotional stress can lead to changes in eating patterns, in addition to changes in the efficiency with which the body uses nutrients. People who are anxious or concerned frequently report a loss of appetite. Physiological effects of anxiety include decreased secretion of digestive juices, leading to a reduction in the efficiency of nutrient absorption from food.

THE INFLUENCE OF DRUGS

Elderly people in developed countries are often heavy users of both over-the-counter and prescription drugs. These drugs may affect the intake of nutrients in a variety of ways. Some drugs alter the sensation of taste and the perception of smell in ways that modify the user's appetite and food preferences. Many drugs have physiological effects on the gastrointestinal tract that can alter the absorption and use of nutrients. Such drugs can alter the pH level of the gastrointestinal environment, modify the secretion of digestive juices, bind to certain nutrients and thus inhibit their absorption, change the level of motility of the gastrointestinal tract, or alter its bacterial population. The metabolism of absorbed nutrients can be affected by drugs that change the amounts or activities of specific enzymes. Drugs can also increase the need for specific nutrients or alter the extent to which some nutrients are excreted from the body.

Some drugs known to cause an increased need for various nutrients are listed in Tables 17-4 and 17-5. High doses of some nutrients supplied by supplements can interfere with the action of some drugs. Folate and vitamin B_6, for example, can interfere with the action of anticonvulsants. Interventions designed to compensate for the effects of drug use on nutrition by administering high doses of supplementary nutrients should be supervised by a physician.

The rate of drug metabolism and detoxification by the liver is slower in elderly persons than in the young and middle-aged persons. This causes drugs to remain in the body longer and to exert their effects more slowly.

NUTRIENT NEEDS OF ELDERLY PERSONS

Information on the specific nutrient needs of people over 40 years old is scarce. The information available is largely based on studies of the intakes of apparently healthy people, rather than on experimental studies designed to quantify needs. Energy and the nutrients involved in energy metabolism are known to be required by elderly persons in significantly lower amounts than required by young adults. Until more definitive information is available, it is suggested that the intakes for most nutrients remain constant throughout adult life.

The current recommended dietary allowances (RDAs) and recommended nutrient intakes (RNIs) for men and women over 51 are shown in Table 17-6.[18] Careful analysis of the data reveals that foods of a high nutrient density are needed to provide the recommended amount of nutrients in a diet that meets the reduced energy needs of older people. Therefore people over 51 years of age have reduced opportunity to indulge in foods of low nutrient density—such as alco-

TABLE 17-4

Drug-nutrient interactions possible with some prescription drugs commonly used by the elderly

TYPE OF DRUG	MECHANISM/RISK OF INTERFERENCE	NUTRITIONAL CONSIDERATIONS
ANTIARRHYTHMIC DRUG		
Quinidine	Vitamin K deficiency if given with anticoagulants.	With high intake of fruit, juices: quinidine toxicity.
ANTICOAGULANT		
Warfarin	Antagonism of anticoagulant effects by vitamin K.	Large amounts of vitamin K–containing foods (cabbage, green peas, turnip greens, broccoli) should be avoided.
ANTICONVULSANTS		
Phenytoin	Impaired nutrient metabolism and utilization: folate deficiency. Increases activation of 25-OH-vitamin D: osteomalacia (long-term use).	Should be taken with food or immediately after meals to minimize gastric irritation. Folic acid supplement may be prescribed (limit 1 mg/day).
Primidone	Impaired nutrient metabolism and utilization: folate deficiency; neurologic complications. May interfere with bone mineralization via interruption of vitamin K–dependent bone proteins.	Supplementation with vitamin K may be considered.
ANTIDEPRESSANTS		
Imipramine	Possible inducement of riboflavin deficiency; interferes with assessment of riboflavin status. Acidifies urine. Causes gastric discomfort; constipation.	Should be administered with or immediately after food to reduce gastric irritation. May require increase in dietary fiber and fluid to overcome drug-induced constipation.
Phenelzine	Monoamine oxidase antidepressant: concomitant intake of tyramine foods can precipitate sudden hypertensive crisis. Can cause gastrointestinal distress, dry mouth, and appetite changes.	Foods and beverages high in tyramine and other pressor amines should be avoided. Body weight should be checked, and any unusual changes reported. Sugarless candy or gum may help stimulate salivary flow.
ANTIGOUT DRUG		
Colchicine	Damage to intestinal mucosa: decreased absorption of vitamin B_{12}, carotene, fat, cholesterol, lactose, D-xylose. Long-term administration leads to megaloblastic anemia.	To reduce gastric irritation, should be taken with water immediately before or after meals. Encourage adequate fluid intake.
ANTIHYPERTENSIVE DRUG		
Hydralazine	Administration with food: increased drug bioavailability. Vitamin B_6 deficiency: risk vitamin B_6 deficiency, causing neuritis.	Medication should be taken with food. Diet restricted in kilocalories and sodium may be warranted. Supplementation with vitamin B_6 may be considered.

Continued.

holic beverages and foods rich in sugar and fat—if they are to be adequately nourished by their diet without the assistance of vitamin and mineral supplements.

ENERGY

Aging is accompanied by a decrease in energy needs because of decreasing activity and a steady decline in metabolic rate. Differences in different people's energy requirements tend to become more pronounced with age.

The RDAs for energy for people over 51 years of age amount to 2300 kcal for the average 77-kg man and 1900 kcal for the average 65-kg woman. The Food and Agricultural Organization/World Health Organization (FAO/WHO) recommends a decrease in energy intake of 5% per decade between the ages of 39 and 59, then 10% from 60 to 69, and a further 10% for people older

TABLE 17-4

Drug-nutrient interactions possible with some prescription drugs commonly used by the elderly (continued)

TYPE OF DRUG	MECHANISM/RISK OF INTERFERENCE	NUTRITIONAL CONSIDERATIONS
ANTIINFECTIVE DRUGS		
Isoniazid	Altered nutrient excretion and vitamin B_6 antagonist: vitamin B_6 deficiency; pellagra secondary to vitamin B_6 deficiency. Interferes with vitamin D metabolism: risk of osteomalacia. Administration with food: decreased drug absorption.	Supplementation with vitamin B_6, niacin, and vitamin D may be considered. Risk of osteomalacia is greatest in homebound or institutionalized elderly who do not drink milk. Should be taken on an empty stomach with water.
Sulfadiazine (a sulfonamide)	Impaired folacin absorption. Anorexia. Administration with food alters GI motility and transit time: decreased drug absorption rate.	Foods rich in folacin should be encouraged. Supplementation with folic acid may be considered. To minimize gastric irritation, drug should be taken with food or water or after meals. Adequate fluid intake should be encouraged.
Tetracycline	Impaired nutrient metabolism and utilization. Interferes with vitamin K intestinal synthesis. Milk, dairy products, and iron supplements decrease drug absorption.	Supplementation with riboflavin, ascorbic acid, and calcium may be considered. Should be taken on an empty stomach with water. No milk, dairy products, or iron-containing foods should be taken within 3 hours of drug administration. Adequate fluids should be encouraged.
ANTIINFLAMMATORY DRUG		
Penicillamine	Appetite suppression: weight loss.	Supplementation with multivitamin and mineral pill may be advised, because the drug can increase need for vitamin B_6 and zinc. Should not be administered with iron or other mineral supplements. Should be taken 1 hour before or 3 hours after meals. Adequate fluid intake is necessary.
ANTIPARKINSON DRUG		
Levodopa	Vitamin B_6 causes accelerated conversion of levodopa to dopamine: decreased dopamine penetration of blood-brain barrier.	Intake of vitamin B_6 in diet and supplements should be restricted. Foods high in amino acids should be limited.
CARDIAC STIMULANT		
Digoxin	Anorexia and nausea: weight loss. Low potassium intake: digoxin toxicity. Bran cereal: slows drug absorption.	Well-balanced meals and adequate potassium intake should be encouraged. High-sodium foods should be avoided. Bran should be avoided in the meal that accompanies or follows drug administration.

than 70. In general, however, the correct energy intake is the intake that either maintains desirable weight for height or adjusts weight for height to the desirable level.

Studies on the nutritive intakes of older people consistently reveal low intakes. This may result from attempts to lose weight, the inability to buy or eat sufficient food, or failure to eat regular meals or—alternatively—may reflect an inability to remember and accurately report what is eaten. If the reported diets have indeed been accurate, they will fail to provide sufficient amounts of many nutrients (particularly calcium, iron, and several vitamins), in addition to supplying insufficient energy. Although such diets may seem to contain sufficient protein, the diversion of protein for use as an energy source may leave insufficient protein for the maintenance of body tissues. Diets providing less than 1800 kcal/day have been shown experimentally to result in negative nitrogen balance. The National Health and Nutrition Examination Survey (NHANES) III survey in 1988-1991 found a progressive decline in energy intake by elderly persons from an average of 2110 and 1578 kcal/day for men and women ages 60 to 69, respectively,

TABLE 17-4

Drug-nutrient interactions possible with some prescription drugs commonly used by the elderly (continued)

TYPE OF DRUG	MECHANISM/RISK OF INTERFERENCE	NUTRITIONAL CONSIDERATIONS
DIURETICS		
Furosemide	Enhances excretion of sodium, chloride, potassium, magnesium, calcium, and water.	High-sodium foods should be restricted. Foods rich in potassium, calcium, and magnesium should be encouraged.
Spironolactone	Enhances excretion of sodium, chloride, and water. Reduces excretion of potassium.	Potassium supplements should not be used, nor should a salt substitute.
Thiazides	Enhance excretion of sodium, potassium, magnesium, and water.	High-sodium foods should be restricted. Foods rich in potassium and magnesium should be encouraged.
LIPID-LOWERING DRUG		
Cholestyramine	Interferes with bile acid activity: vitamins A, D, E, K, and folate deficiencies.	Supplementation is recommended with vitamins A, D, K (if hypoprothrombinemia occurs) and folate (for those with reduced levels of serum or red blood cell folate). Low-cholesterol diet is indicated. A high-bulk diet and increased fluid intake should be encouraged as tolerated.
TRANQUILIZER		
Chlorpromazine	Increases appetite. Possible inducement of riboflavin deficiency; interferes with assessment of riboflavin status. May result in constipation, fecal impaction; sore mouth and gums.	May require increase in dietary fiber and fluid to overcome drug-induced constipation. Sore mouth may be relieved by rinsing mouth or taking frequent sips of water. Sugarless candy or gum may also help stimulate salivary flow.

From Schlenker ED: *Nutrition in aging,* St Louis, 1993, Mosby.

to 1887 and 1435 kcal/day for those aged 70 to 79, to 1776 and 1329 kcal/day for those aged more than 80.[19] Associated protein intakes were 84g, 74g, and 96g for men and 64g, 58g, and 52g for women in the respective age groups.

The fact that many elderly people consume insufficient kilocalories may explain much of the fatigue, lassitude, and lack of interest in life often found in elderly persons. Increased activity could be expected to stimulate the appetite and so provide elderly people with both the energy and other nutrients needed to prevent fatigue, lethargy, and depression. This possibility emphasizes the importance of trying to keep elderly people as active as possible.

PROTEIN

The total amount of protein synthesized each day declines only slightly with age, although muscle protein turnover drops from 30% of total protein turnover to 20%. The RDAs suggest that a total protein intake of 0.8 g/kg of body weight per day should be maintained throughout adulthood. Evidence exists, however, suggesting that more than this recommended amount of protein is required to maintain nitrogen balance.[11] Protein intakes in elderly persons usually account for 12% of total energy intakes. These intakes are greater than the RDAs for protein, and most elderly people who are free of debilitating disease or disability do not appear to be at risk of protein deficiency.

MINERALS

Most concern about the mineral supply in the diets of elderly persons is focused on calcium and zinc. It is possible, but not proven, that older people have an increased need for dietary calcium. This is particularly likely in women because of their susceptibility to osteoporosis. The efficiency of calcium absorption certainly declines with age, accompanied by increased excretion of calcium and the loss of bone mass. There is evidence, however, that increasing the calcium intake of postmenopausal women is of little value, unless accompanied by adequate vitamin D and the administration of estrogen. Dietary surveys of elderly persons often find calcium intakes of less than two thirds of the RDA.[20] It is probably more important to increase calcium intake to the current standards than to raise the standards.

TABLE 17-5

Nutritional considerations with over-the-counter drugs commonly used by the elderly

CLASSIFICATION/DRUG	EXAMPLES	NUTRITIONAL CONSIDERATIONS
ANALGESICS		
Aspirin	Bayer, Bufferin, Excedrin	Chronic ingestion may be associated with depressed plasma ascorbic acid and folate levels; supplemental therapy may be indicated. May cause iron-deficiency anemia as a result of gastrointestinal (GI) blood loss.
Acetaminophen	Datril, Tylenol	Coadministration with a high-carbohydrate meal may significantly retard absorption. Individuals with poor nutrition or who have ingested alcohol over prolonged periods are prone to liver disease, and drug may cause anorexia, nausea, vomiting, dyspepsia, constipation, or diarrhea. May increase urinary loss of ascorbic acid.
ANTACIDS		
Aluminum hydroxide	Amphojel	Large doses for prolonged periods along with a diet low in phosphorus and protein can result in phosphorus-deficiency syndrome—the elderly person in poor nutritional status is at high risk. Vitamin A and thiamin deficiencies can occur as a result of reduced absorption. Constipation occurs commonly, and intestinal obstruction has been reported.
Magnesium hydroxide	Milk of Magnesia	Excessive dosage can cause nausea, abdominal cramps, diarrhea, alkalinization of urine, and dehydration. Magnesium toxicity can develop in those with kidney failure.
ANTIDIARRHEAL DRUGS	Lomotil, Kaopectate	May cause nausea, vomiting, abdominal discomfort, constipation, and fecal impaction. Caffeine beverages and alcohol should be avoided, since both increase peristalsis. Prolonged use may interfere with intestinal absorption of nutrients and promote constipation.
ANTIEMETICS	Dramamine, Bonine	May cause dry mouth, nose, and throat; epigastric distress; and constipation.
ANTIHISTAMINES	Benedryl, Chlor-Trimeton	GI side effects may be lessened by administration of drug with meals or milk. Dry mouth may be relieved by sugarless candy or gum or rinses with water. Elderly people are especially likely to experience dizziness, sedation, and hypotension.
COLD PREPARATIONS	Robitussin	Fluid intake should be increased to 2 to 3 L daily to help thin and mobilize respiratory secretions, but the elderly should be monitored closely to avoid fluid overload.
LAXATIVES		
Bulk-forming	Metamucil, Mitrolan	Adequate fluid intake must be maintained; fecal impaction can occur if fluid intake by mouth is insufficient. Can decrease appetite through abdominal fullness. Products contain varying amounts of sugar and salt. Electrolyte imbalance is possible with chronic use.
Fecal softeners	Colace	Adequate fluid intake must be maintained.
Stimulants	Bisacolax, Correctol, Dulcolax, Ex-Lax	Abuse can cause electrolyte imbalance, including potassium depletion; malabsorption, with weight loss, can also occur. Frequent use may result in laxative dependence.

From Schlenker ED: *Nutrition in aging,* St Louis, 1993, Mosby.

TABLE 17-6

Recommended dietary allowances (United States) and recommended nutrient intakes (Canada) for people over 51 years of age

	MALE		FEMALE	
	UNITED STATES	CANADA	UNITED STATES	CANADA
Protein (g)	63	60-57	50	47
Calcium (mg)	800	800	800	800
Phosphorus (mg)	800	1000	800	1000
Magnesium (mg)	350	250-230	280	210
Iron (mg)	10	9	10	8
Zinc (mg)	15	12	12	9
Iodine (μg)	150	160	150	160
Selenium (μg)	70	—	55	—
Vitamin A (RE)	1000	1000	800	800
Vitamin D (μg)	5	5	5	5
Vitamin E (mg)	10	7-6	8	6-5
Ascorbic acid (mg)	60	40	60	30
Thiamin (mg)	1.2	0.9-0.8	1.0	0.8
Riboflavin (mg)	1.4	1.3-1	1.2	1
Niacin (mg)	15	16-14	13	14
Pyridoxine (mg)	2.0	—	1.6	—
Folate (μg)	200	220-205	180	190
Vitamin B_{12} (μg)	3.0	2	2.0	2

RE, Retinol equivalent.

Many elderly patients are reported to have marginal zinc stores. This can be a result of intakes that are generally below the RDA, sometimes from decreased meat intakes, medical conditions that impair zinc status, or the use of drugs that either reduce zinc absorption or increase zinc excretion. Supplements to improve zinc status should be used with caution, however, because excessive zinc intake can cause gastrointestinal irritation, copper deficiency, anemia, hypercholesterolemia, and impaired immune function.

There is no evidence to suggest that the RDAs for any other minerals are inadequate. Where mineral deficiency is suspected, each case should be evaluated to determine the appropriate degree of dietary modification or nutrient supplementation.

VITAMINS

The link between vitamins and aging has been the focus of a considerable amount of recent research.[21] Inadequate dietary intake of vitamins appears to cause a considerable amount of vitamin malnutrition in elderly persons. There is also strong evidence that the aging process itself affects the requirements for some vitamins. The available information suggests that the current RDAs for elderly persons for vitamin D, riboflavin, vitamin B_6, and vitamin B_{12} are too low. On the other hand, the RDA for vitamin A appears to be too high. The present RDAs for thiamin, vitamin C, and folate are believed to be about right.

OTHER NUTRIENTS

There is little specific information available about older people's requirements for other nutrients. For most nutrients, the decline in the efficiency of absorption that accompanies aging appears to be counterbalanced by a declining need for the nutrients.

Elderly persons are vulnerable to both dehydration and fluid retention because of the consumption of too little or too much water, respectively. One milliliter of water per kilocalorie consumed should be adequate. Older people often lose their ability to automatically adjust their fluid intake to meet their needs and often need to be encouraged to drink sufficient fluids. Some elderly people voluntarily restrict fluid intake because they are either incontinent or disabled and have problems gaining access to toilet facilities. The readily observable symptoms of dehydration are dry lips and skin, decreased excretion of urine, confusion, and raised body temperature. People who care for elderly persons should be alerted to these symptoms and be ready to encourage increased fluid consumption if required.[22] Retention of too much fluid by elderly persons is usually caused by physiological changes that reduce the capacity to excrete fluid.

TABLE 17-7

Dietary intakes of respondents 65 years of age and older in NHANES I (1971-74), NHANES III (1989-1991), NFCS (1977-1978), NFCS (1987-1988), the RLEDS (1990)

	NHANES I		NHANES III		NFCS (1977-1988)*		NFCS (1987-88)*		RLEDS (1990)†	
NUTRIENT	**MEN**	**WOMEN**	**MEN**	**WOMEN**	**MEN**	**WOMEN**	**MEN**	**WOMEN**	**MEN**	**WOMEN**
Protein (g)	72	53	79	61	84	60	74-81	58-61	74-77	54-62
Calcium (mg)	602	495	842	672	729	566	762-745	542-579	714-717	564-627
Magnesium (mg)			314	250	287	227	265-276	213-220	272-289	220-262
Iron (mg)	12.1	9.2	16.4	12.9	14.5	10.6	14-15	11-12	14-15	12-14
Thiamin (mg)	1.24	0.96	1.8	1.4	1.37	1.07	1.5-1.6	1.2	1.5-1.6	1.2-1.3
Riboflavin (mg)	1.77	1.3	2.1	1.7	1.78	1.41	1.9-2.0	1.5	1.8-1.9	1.4-1.6
Vitamin C (mg)	88	90	106	105	91	87	103-106	94	100-105	100-103
Vitamin B_6 (mg)			2.0	1.6	1.58	1.24	1.7-1.8	1.4	1.8-1.9	1.4-1.6
Vitamin B_{12} (µg)			5.7	3.9	5.9	4.4	6-8	4-5	4-7	4-7
Vitamin A (IU)			8205	7650	7164	6458	7792-8236	6920-6742	3573-3783	4139-4109

NHANES, National Health and Nutrition Examination Survey. Underlined values fall below recommended levels.

* National Food Consumption Survey (NFCS) 1987-1988 values are for individuals 60 to 60 years of age and older.

† Ross Laboratory Elderly Dietary Survey (RLEDS) 1990 values are for individuals 65 to 74 years of age and older.

ADEQUACY OF DIETS OF THE ELDERLY

Some findings of the major surveys assessing the dietary intake of elderly persons in the United States are summarized in Table 17-7. The data indicate that many elderly persons consume less than the recommended amounts of calcium, magnesium, phosphorus, and vitamin B_6. The Ross Laboratory Elderly Dietary Survey (RLEDS) also found that 20% to 28% of noninstitutionalized elderly people consumed less than two thirds of the RDA for folate, and 42% to 60% consumed less than two thirds of the RDA for zinc. Several other studies, however, suggest that this slight downward trend in nutrient intakes gives way to a much more pronounced downward trend from the age of 75 onward. Some other studies have found a higher mortality rate among elderly people consuming less than 40% of the RDAs of one or more nutrients. Comparison of data from elderly people and younger people in the NHANES and Nationwide Food Consumption Survey (NFCS) surveys suggests that only a slight decline in nutrient adequacy accompanies aging. Preliminary analyses of NHANES III data indicate that total food energy intake from total dietary fat (33.9%) and from total saturated fat (11.9%) has decreased in all age-groups, including individuals aged 60 years or greater. Mean serum cholesterol values also decreased from NHANES II to NHANES III. NHANES III dietary intake data showed that men aged 60 to 90 years received the RDA for iron, calcium and phosphorus but about 85% of the RDA for magnesium, whereas women in this age group had over 80% of the RDA for calcium and magnesium and recommended intakes of other minerals. Similarly, NHANES III data showed average intakes of people over 60 years old meeting the RDA for all vitamins except for slightly marginal intakes of vitamin E.

The nutrients most likely to be present in inadequate amounts in the diets of elderly persons are the following:

- Vitamin D
- Vitamin E
- Thiamin
- Riboflavin
- Folic acid
- Calcium
- Zinc

ASSESSING NUTRITIONAL STATUS OF ELDERLY PERSONS

Attempts to evaluate the nutritional status of elderly persons by biochemical analysis of blood and urine have been confined almost entirely to NHANES surveys and the Ten-State Nutrition Study. The Ten-State Nutrition Study (1976-1980) found low blood or urine levels of two or more nutrients in less than 8% of white people over the age of 60 but in 25% of African-American and Hispanic people over 60. More than 60%

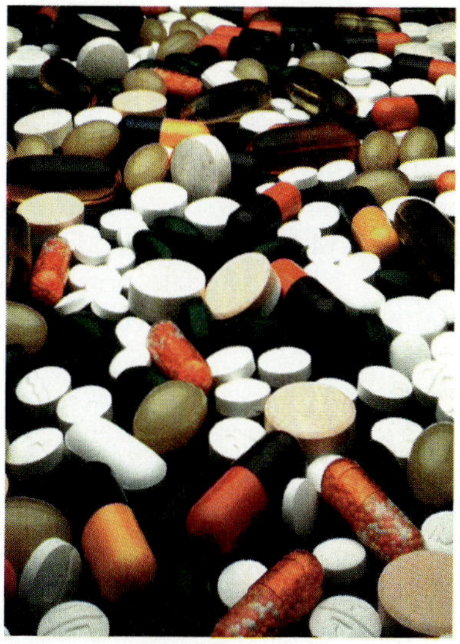

Approximately 40% of elderly people take dietary supplements.

of African-Americans and 50% of Hispanics had satisfactory levels of all nutrients for which they were tested. The NHANES I and II studies found that 29% of African-Americans over the age of 60 had low hemoglobin levels.

A survey of the nutritional status of elderly Canadians found low serum folate levels to be the most prevalent nutritional problem. Low folate levels were found in 60% of the men and 61% of the women aged over 65. About 30% of the elderly men and 12% of the elderly women surveyed had low urinary thiamin values.

Other, less comprehensive surveys have found that 70% of a group of elderly people had delayed prothrombin times, indicating a deficiency of vitamin K. This was associated with liver disease or the use of salicylates (aspirin) or antibiotics.

In 1991 a Nutritional Screening Initiative was set up in the United States to identify nutritional problems in elderly persons and improve the delivery of nutrition services to those at greatest risk. This initiative has been widely supported by health professionals. It should lead to improved diagnosis and treatment of nutrition-related problems in elderly persons.[23]

DIETARY SUPPLEMENTS FOR ELDERLY PERSONS

Many elderly people make use of dietary supplements in an attempt to improve their nutritional status. One study found that around 40% of the people surveyed who were aged 65 or older were using supplements. In Canada 34% of older men and 46% of older women used supplements, as did 35% of elderly persons in California.

Few of the supplements used by the elderly people surveyed were taken with the recommendation of physicians. It was also found that few of the supplement preparations contained nutrients in quantities that correlated with the people's actual nutrient needs. Some people used products that met some but not all of their nutrient needs, others consumed supplements that provided nutrients they were already receiving in adequate amounts, and some used supplements that provided all the nutrients that were inadequately supplied by their diets. Few of the people who were consuming insufficient dietary calcium were taking calcium supplements. About half of the elderly people surveyed had nutritionally adequate diets and no need of supplementation.

INTERVENTION PROGRAMS

Concern about the nutritional adequacy of elderly people's diets has led to the establishment of several nutrition intervention programs aimed at this group. These programs include the Home-Delivered Meals (Meals-on-Wheels) Program and The Congregate Dining Program.

The Home-Delivered Meals Program is designed for homebound elderly people who have inadequate cooking facilities or are unable to shop for and prepare food. A hot meal is delivered to the elderly person's home on 3 to 7 days each week. In some cases the hot meal is also accompanied by food to be refrigerated for the evening meal and possibly also food for the next day's breakfast.

The Congregate Dining Program was created in 1965 and was the first U.S. federal nutrition program specifically targeted to elderly persons. It is designed to meet both social and nutritional needs of elderly persons. Participants are transported to a centrally located "diners' club" where they receive an appetizing and nutritionally adequate meal in a pleasant social atmosphere with the company of others. They can also participate in a variety of recreational, social, and educational experiences.

Both the Home-Delivered Meals and the Congregate Dining Programs are designed to meet the nutritional needs of elderly people, regardless of their income. Those who can pay the full cost of their meals do so, and others receive their meals at reduced cost or no cost, depending on their economic circumstances. Food stamps can be used to pay for the meals.

Approximately 929,000 meals are served each day to older Americans who participate in these programs: 60% at Congregate Dining sites and 40% through Home-Delivered Meals. The USDA support for the nutrition programs of elderly persons was almost $143 million in 1993.

NUTRITION EDUCATION

Nutrition education is offered to participants in the Congregate Meals Program and can also be delivered to elderly persons in various other settings. A variety of approaches has been assessed, but one of the most successful involves the use of "peer educators." This involves training selected participants in the program to qualify them to provide information to other participants. This ensures that the front-line educators are readily accepted by the other participants because they are in the same peer group. Those selected to be educators regard it as an honor and tend to be highly motivated. They prove to be effective leaders who are able to devote a significant amount of time to their nutrition education tasks. Much of the actual educational information they deliver is focused on food purchasing choices. Other topics include the relationship between nutrition and health, food additives, the information available on labels, the selection and preparation of small amounts of food, and economic aspects of nutrition.

ISSUES AND OPINIONS

Enhancing The Golden Years Through Research

by the United States Department Of Agriculture Human Nutrition Research Center on Aging at Tufts University

The mission of the research program at The United States Department of Agriculture (USDA) Human Nutrition Center on Aging at Tufts University in Boston is to determine why some people age well, whereas others must deal with health conditions that interfere with the full enjoyment of life.

Nutrition scientists agree that how and what an individual eats have a considerable effect on the length and quality of life. Poor nutritional practices are believed to underlie and possibly contribute to diseases such as diabetes, cardiovascular disease, osteoporosis, and certain types of cancer. Consequently, scientists at the Human Nutrition Center on Aging are investigating how diet and other modifiable lifestyle factors can delay or prevent the onset of many degenerative conditions associated with aging.

Senior citizens are active participants in the research program at Tufts University on various aspects of aging. Approximately 2000 people are evaluated each year for admission to studies that will undoubtedly affect the next generation of senior citizens. Some of the most recent findings from the Center on Aging on the relationships between nutrition and aging include the following:

- Vitamin C intake is positively related to high blood levels of high-density lipoprotein, which are in turn associated with reduced risk of cardiovascular disease.
- A hormonal form of vitamin D can influence the aging of the skin and affect skin diseases such as psoriasis.
- The ability of the skin to synthesize vitamin D in sunlight dramatically decreases with age, causing a corresponding increase in the dietary requirement for this vitamin.
- The decreased ability to produce stomach acid found in about 20% of the elderly population interferes with the absorption of several vitamins and minerals.
- Elderly women who ingest low levels of calcium lose mineral from the spine at a significantly greater rate than women whose intakes exceed the Recommended Dietary Allowance (RDA).
- Calcium supplements taken with a meal decrease iron absorption from that meal.
- Under experimental conditions, vitamin E plays an important role in the immune system and may act to reverse age-related declines in immune responses.
- Vitamin B_6 requirements are increased in the elderly, whereas vitamin A requirements may be reduced in this age-group.

These findings, and those from other research centers around the world, are being incorporated into nutrition and health policies and dietary recommendations intended to enhance the quality of life among our maturing and aging citizens and to reduce health care costs. Many of the findings of current research on nutrition and aging affect the present generation of senior citizens. They also provide the basis for the development of more effective preventive measures for the next generation.

BY NOW YOU SHOULD KNOW

- Since 1900, the proportion of Americans living beyond the age of 65 has increased.
- Elderly people are such a heterogeneous group that it is difficult to generalize about their nutritional needs.
- Aging occurs at different rates in different people, even under similar environmental conditions.
- There are many theories about the biochemical and physiological bases of aging.
- Nutrient intake, nutrient use, and nutrient needs are determined by a variety of physical, physiological, psychological, and social factors.
- For almost all nutrients, the decline in the amounts required by the body is counteracted by a reduced efficiency of absorption and metabolism, meaning that dietary requirements change little during adulthood.
- Elderly persons are vulnerable to many nutrition-related problems, including cardiovascular diseases, osteoporosis, impaired immunity, drug-induced malnutrition, and impaired cognitive function.
- The RDAs for elderly persons are largely extrapolated from the RDAs for younger adults.
- The use of vitamin and mineral supplements is widespread among the elderly population, although they often do not correct nutritional deficits.
- Federally-funded programs, such as Meals-on-Wheels and the Congregate Meals Program, are designed to help elderly persons maintain their independence while obtaining good nutrition and social stimulation.
- The Congregate Meals Program requires all participants to be offered nutrition education. Peer education has proved a successful method of delivering this education.

STUDY QUESTIONS

1. Define the terms *geriatrics, gerontology,* and *biogerontology.*
2. Why are the RDAs similar for people under and over 50 years of age?
3. Why is there more concern about the effect of drugs on the nutrient needs of elderly persons than on the nutrient needs of young persons?
4. Describe the major nutrition-related problems of elderly persons.
5. Explain why it is important to monitor the amount of water in an elderly person's diet.

CRITICAL ANALYSIS

1. The data from several dietary intake surveys (Table 17-7) indicate that the mean intakes of Americans who are 51 years of age or older are meeting most of the current RDAs. However, data not shown but discussed in the text also indicate that sizable percentages of this population have intakes of particular nutrients, such as vitamin C and folic acid, that do not meet current RDAs. Many factors may be involved, including decreased appetite, a habit of consuming fresh fruits and vegetables only during the traditional growing season, limited economic resources or ability to travel, or limited knowledge of the nutrient content of foods. Faced with this situation, part of a nutritionist's job is to identify some food sources of these nutrients.

   Listed below are some of the nutrients most commonly associated with low intakes in older Americans.

   a. For each nutrient, fill in the RDA for an adult male or female 51+ years of age and identify two or three foods that are good to excellent sources of each nutrient. There are a number of ways to classify foods as good to excellent sources of a nutrient; use the following (somewhat arbitrary) criteria: a good food source supplies at least 10% of the RDA for a given nutrient, whereas an excellent source supplies 25% or more of the RDA for that nutrient.
   b. Try to identify one or two foods that are a good to excellent sources of two or more of the nutrients (for example, identify a food that is an excellent source of vitamin C and a good source of folic acid).
   c. How much will it cost to buy these foods? Look up the cost of each food by looking in the newspaper (grocery store advertisements frequently run in Sunday editions and also at least once during the week, often in a special food section), checking store flyers that come in the mail, or observing on your next shopping trip. Remember to calculate the cost of one serving. Thus if the price of the item is $1.00 for a pound, but the normal serving size is ¼ lb, the cost of 1 serving is $0.25. Although there is often some loss or waste of food during preparation, which can affect the cost, we will settle for an estimate of the cost for now. At current prices, how much would it cost to add one serving of the cheapest food source of each nutrient for 1 day? Can the cost be decreased if a food is a good to excellent source of more than one of the nutrients? An increase of $1.00 per day may seem like a small increase but will be beyond the means of at least some people. On the other hand, by including some of the foods you listed, other foods that are less nutrient dense may be dropped from the shopping list; so the food bill may not increase by as much as the per serving costs may indicate.

NUTRIENT	FOOD SOURCES	RDA	AMOUNT OF NUTRIENT PER SERVING	COST PER SERVING
Vitamin C	1.			
	2.			
Folic acid	1.			
	2.			
Iron	1.			
	2.			
Vitamin B_6	1.			
	2.			

REFERENCES

1. U.S. Bureau of the Census: *Projections of the population of the United States, by age, sex, and race: 1988 to 2080,* Current Population Report Series P-25, No 1018, Washington, DC, 1991, U.S. Government Printing Office.
2. U.S. Department of Health and Human Services: *Healthy people 2000: national health promotion and disease prevention objectives,* DHHS Pub No (PHS) 91-50213, Washington, DC, 1990, U.S. Government Printing Office.
3. Hayflick L: Origins of longevity. In Warner HR and others, editors: *Modern biological theories of aging,* New York, 1987, Raven Press.
4. Dice JF: Nutrition, genetics and aging. In Simopoulos AP, Childs B, editors: Genetic variation and nutrition, *World Rev Nutr Diet* 63:175, 1990.

5. Widdowson EM: Physiological processes of aging: are there special nutritional requirements for elderly people? Do McCay's findings apply to humans, *Am J Clin Nutr* 55:1246S, 1992.

6. Johnson TE: Developmentally programmed aging: future directions. In Warner HR and others, editors: *Modern biological theories of aging,* New York, 1987, Raven Press.

7. Frontera WR and others: A cross-sectional study of muscle strength and mass in 45- to 78-year-old men and women, *J Appl Physiol* 71:644, 1991.

8. Fiatarone MA and others: High intensity strength training in nonagenerians: effect on skeletal muscle, *Clin Res* 37:330A, 1989.

9. Dawson-Hughes B and others: A controlled trial of the effect of calcium supplementation on bone density in postmenopausal women, *N Engl J Med* 323:878, 1990.

10. Rosenberg IH: Nutrition and aging. In Hazzard WR and others: *Principles of gerontology,* ed 3, New York, 1994, McGraw-Hill Professions Division.

11. Baldwin JG: True anemia: incidence and significance in the elderly, *Geriatrics* 44:33, 1989.

12. Rosenberg IH, Miller JW: Nutritional factors in physical and cognitive function of the elderly, *Am J Clin Nutr* 55:1237S, 1992.

13. Taylor A: Role of nutrients in delaying cataracts, *Ann N Y Acad Sci* 669:111, 1992.

14. Thomas ML, Weigle WO: The cellular and subcellular basis of immunosenescence, *Adv Immunol* 46:221, 1989.

15. Chandra RK: Nutritional regulation of immunity and risk of illness in old age, *Immunology* 67:141, 1989.

16. Fischer J, Johnson MA: Low body weight and weight loss in the aged, *J Am Diet Assoc* 90:1697, 1990.

17. Ryan AS and others: Dietary patterns of older adults in the United States: NHANES II 1976-1980, *Am J Hum Biol* 1:321, 1989.

18. Food and Nutrition Board/Institute of Medicine: *Recommended Dietary Allowances,* ed 10, Washington, DC, 1989, National Academy Press.

19. Lenfant C: Daily dietary fat and total food-energy intakes—Third National Health and Nutrition Examination Survey, Phase I, 1988-1991, *Morb Mortal Weekly Rep* 43:116, 1994.

20. Ryan AS, Craig LD, Finn SC: Nutrient intakes and dietary patterns of older Americans: a national study, *J Gerontol* 47:M145, 1992.

21. Russell RM, Sutter PM: Vitamin requirements of elderly people: an update, *Am J Clin Nutr* 58:4, 1993.

22. Rolls BJ, Phillips PA: Aging and disturbances of thirst and fluid balance, *Nutr Rev* 48:137, 1990.

23. Dwyer JT: *Screening older Americans' nutritional health: current practices and future possibilities,* Washington, DC, 1991, Nutrition Screening Initiative.

~ ADDITIONAL READINGS ~

Ahmed FE: Effect of nutrition on the health of the elderly, *J Am Diet Assoc* 92:1102, 1992.

Blumberg JB: Changing nutrient requirements in older adults, *Nutr Today* 27:15, 1992.

Blumberg JB, Suter P: Pharmacology, nutrition, and the elderly: interactions and implications. In Chernoff R, editor: *Geriatric nutrition,* Rockville, MD, 1991, Aspen.

Chandra RK: Nutrition and immunity in the elderly, *Nutr Rev* 50:367, 1992.

Dwyer JT: The nutritional screening initiative: strategies to detect and prevent malnutrition in the elderly, *Nutr Today* 29:18, 1994.

Dwyer JT, Coletti J, Campbell D: Maximizing nutrition in the second fifty years, *Clin Appl Nutr* 1:19, 1991.

Evans WJ: Exercise, nutrition, and aging, *J Nutr* 122:796, 1992.

Evans WJ, Rosenberg IH, Thompson J: *Biomarkers—the 10 determinants of aging you can control,* New York, 1991, Simon & Schuster.

Fiatarone MA: Exercise. In Morley JE, Koreman SG, editors: *Endocrinology and metabolism in the elderly,* Boston, 1992, Blackwell Scientific Publications.

Hartz SC, Russell RM, Rosenberg IH, editors: *Nutrition in the elderly: the Boston Nutritional Status Survey,* London, 1992, Smith-Gordon and Company.

Hosoda S: The gastrointestinal tract and nutrition in the aging process: an overview, *Nutr Rev* 50:372, 1992.

Kiebzak GM: Age-related bone changes, *Exper Gerontol* 26:171, 1991.

Lakatta EG: Interaction between nutrition and aging: a summary of effects on the cardiovascular system, *Nutr Rev* 50:419, 1992.

Meydani M: Protective role of dietary vitamin E on oxidative stress in aging, *AgE* 15:89, 1992.

Poehlman ET: Energy expenditure and requirements in aging humans, *J Nutr* 122:2057, 1992.

Rolls BJ: Appetite, hunger, and satiety in the elderly, *Crit Rev Food Sci Nutr* 33:39, 1993.

Russell RM: Changes in gastrointestinal function attributed to aging, *Am J Clin Nutr* 55:1203S, 1992.

Russell RM: Vitamin requirements in old age, *Age Nutr* 3:20, 1992.

Sawada T: The influence of aging and nutrition on the occurrence of cerebrovascular diseases, *Nutr Rev* 50:413, 1992.

Schiffman SS: Perception of taste and smell in elderly persons, *Crit Rev Food Sci Nutr* 33:17, 1993.

Toner HM, Morris JD: A social-psychological perspective of dietary quality in later adulthood, *J Nutr Elderly* 11:35, 1992.

Wood RJ: Mineral needs of the elderly: developing a research agenda for the 1990s, *Age* 40:120, 1991.

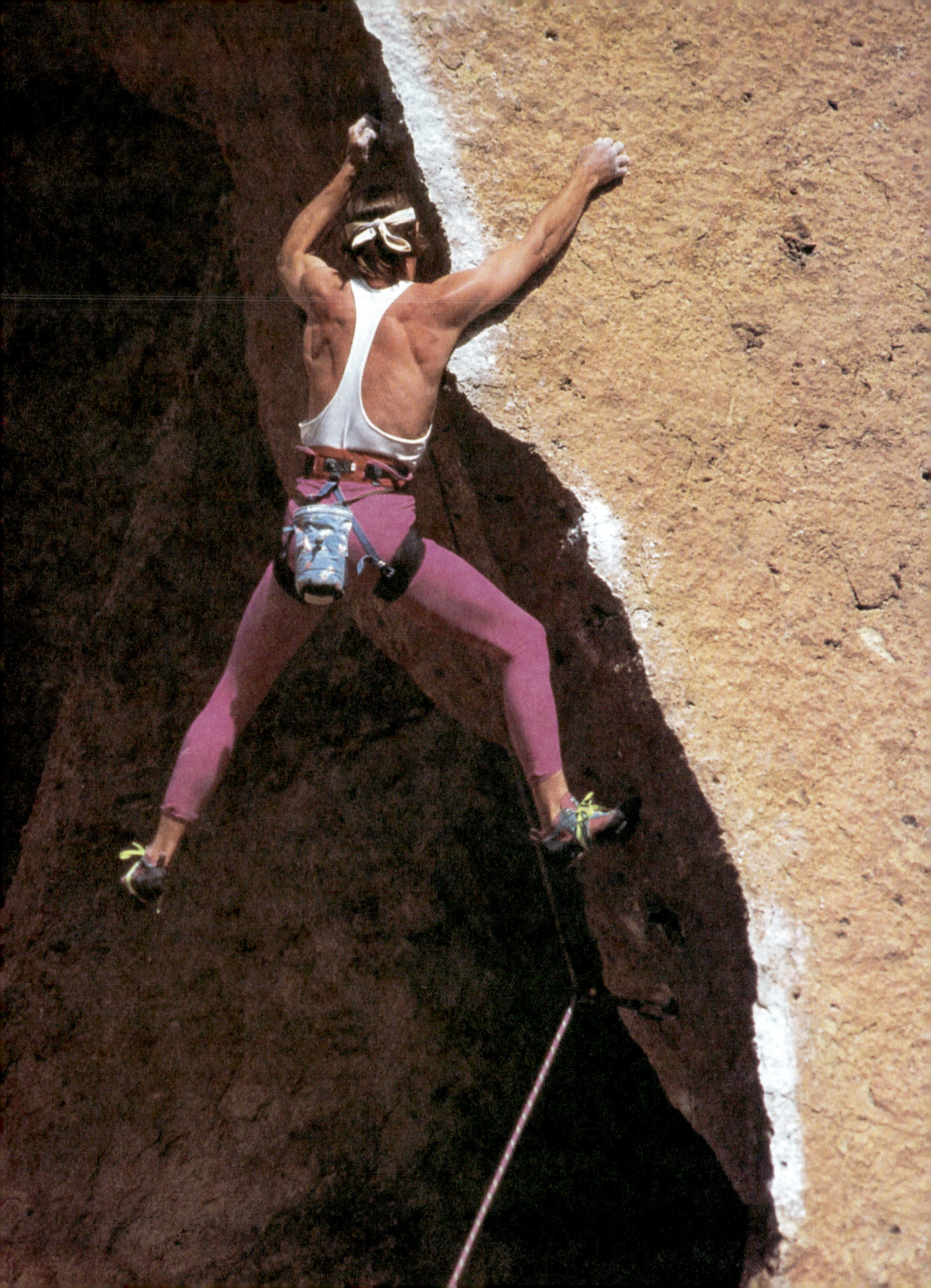

CHAPTER 18

NUTRITION AND PHYSICAL FITNESS

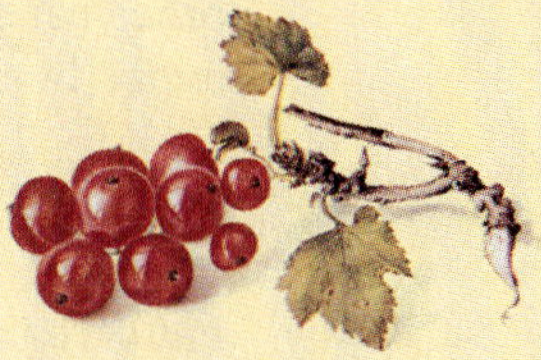

It is not difficult to convince athletes and other people concerned with physical fitness that good nutrition is important for fitness and good athletic performance. It is much more difficult to convince them that the nutritional requirements of athletes are similar to the requirements of less active people. In general, athletes need more energy and more water than nonathletic people but only slightly increased amounts of protein, minerals, and vitamins. Optimal athletic performance is influenced more by a lifetime of good nutritional habits than by the use or avoidance of particular foods. There is no magic food or combination of foods that compensates for lack of ability and lack of training. Good nutrition, however, may make a sufficient difference to provide the "competitive edge." For people concerned with general good health rather than athletic success, attention to both diet and exercise provides a good basis for fitness. This chapter provides guidance and reassurance that should assist the person interested in fitness and nutrition.

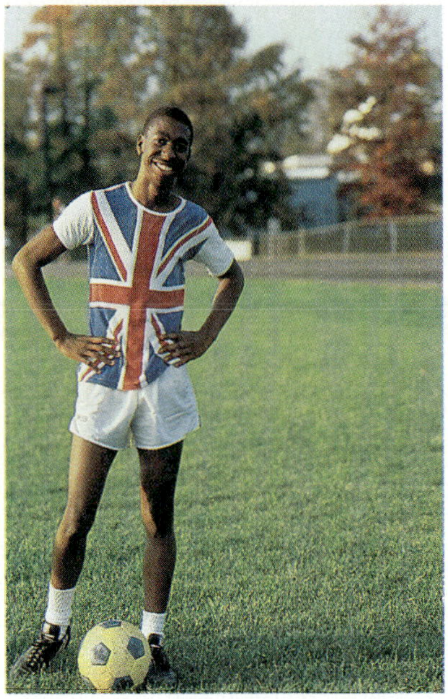

Athletes have been experimenting for centuries in the hope of finding the perfect diet to ensure optimal performance during competition. Only since 1960, however, has there been much systematic research to try to identify the best dietary practices for athletes.

Good nutritional practice for athletes is not substantially different from the nutritional practice that should be recommended to everyone. For all people the first rule of good nutrition is to eat a variety of foods in amounts that maintain a healthy body weight. The foods should be chosen to provide protein, minerals, and vitamins in the amounts suggested by the recommended dietary allowances (RDAs) for the appropriate age-group. Energy should be provided by carbohydrate, lipid, and protein in the following proportions: 60% to 70% from carbohydrate; 25% to 30% from lipid, and 12% to 15% from protein. People who exercise regularly need some vitamins, such as thiamin, riboflavin, and niacin, in slightly greater amounts than more sedentary people need. The increased need for these vitamins is in direct proportion to the increased energy need caused by the increased activity and is likely to be met by the increased food intake. People who exercise strenuously in warm, humid climates should be especially careful to consume sufficient water.

WATER

Water probably has a greater effect on athletic performance than any other nutrient.[1] It is the only nutrient lost during strenuous exercise in amounts several times greater than amounts lost by people who are not exercising. These losses are largely caused by the secretion of water within sweat as part of the body's temperature regulatory system. If the water lost via sweat is not replaced, blood volume falls and body temperature rises, causing loss of coordination and confusion. To replace the lost water, extra fluids must be consumed. Although a small amount of additional water is produced by the increased metabolism that provides the energy to sustain exercise, this amount is insignificant compared to the amount of water lost. Most people obtain around two thirds of their water intake from drinking fluids and between 20% and 40% from solid foods. Athletes, on the other hand, must obtain as much as 90% of their water intake by drinking fluids.

DEHYDRATION AND WATER NEEDS

Fluid replacement to avoid dehydration is an essential nutritional accompaniment to exercise. It is particularly critical for endurance athletes, such as marathon runners. A marathon runner can easily lose a quart of water per hour. As body fluids are lost, the sensation of thirst normally increases, causing people to automatically drink sufficient water and other beverages to compensate for the losses. During the rapid water loss experienced by athletes, however, the thirst sensation may not develop quickly enough to stimulate sufficient fluid intake to prevent dehydration. The fact that athletes are preoccupied by the intensity of competition can also cause them to ignore their developing need for water. It is important, therefore, for athletes to make a conscious effort to consume adequate fluids before, after, and possibly during competition. One simple guide is that they should consume sufficient fluid after competition to return to their precompetition weight.

The loss of as little as 2% of body water can cause a significant deterioration in athletic performance. A 70-kg man can easily lose this proportion of body water in 1 hour by producing 1.5 quarts of sweat. Significantly greater losses can occur during persistent strenuous exercise, such as marathon running. In addition to impairing athletic performance, such unreplaced water losses can cause lethargy, nausea, severe heat exhaustion, and heat stroke.

Sweat contains a lower concentration of dissolved electrolytes than does plasma (see box), but substantial amounts of electrolytes are lost from the body within sweat. Continuous exercise for several hours can cause sufficient sodium losses to cause **hyponatremia.** This is a serious and potentially fatal condition but one that is readily preventable by consuming sufficient sodium-containing beverages (Table 18-1).

Prolonged exercise can also cause hypoglycemia and glycogen depletion, both of which contribute to the sensation of fatigue. Consuming carbohydrate during exercise improves performance by providing additional

TABLE 18-1

Carbohydrate and electrolyte content of sports drinks, soft drinks, fruit juices, and water

BEVERAGE	CARBOHYDRATE (g/L)	Na(mEq/L)	K(mEq/L)
Gatorade	60	21	3
Isostar	73	24	4
Dioralyte	16	60	20
Coca Cola	107	2	0
Sprite	102	5	0
Cranberry juice	150	2	7
Orange juice	118	0.5	58
Water	0	trace	trace

Modified from Gisolfi CV, Duchman SM: *Med Sci Sports Exerc* 24:79, 1992.

supplies of energy.[2] The three most beneficial components of any fluids consumed during exercise are water, electrolytes, and carbohydrate. The carbohydrate, sodium, and potassium contents of various sports drinks, soft drinks, fruit juices, and water are listed in Table 18-1. Choosing a beverage that suits the taste of the person who drinks it obviously encourages the consumption of sufficient fluid. Consuming beverages containing carbohydrates and electrolytes after exercise has been shown to accelerate the return of blood volume and muscle glycogen levels to normal.[3]

Each person's needs for fluids, carbohydrate, and electrolytes vary, but, in general, a combination of both water and a sports drink or soft drink is recommended. For events lasting less than 1 hour, 300 to 500 ml of a beverage containing 60 to 100 g of carbohydrate per liter is recommended along with between 500 and 1000 ml of water. For events lasting between 1 and 3 hours, 300 to 500 ml of water is recommended before the event, followed by 800 to 1600 ml/hr of a cool beverage containing 60 to 80 g of carbohydrate per liter and 10 to 20 mEq of sodium per liter. For events lasting more than 3 hours, 300 to 500 ml of water is recommended before the event, followed by 500 to 1000 ml/hour of a cool beverage containing 60 to 80 g of carbohydrate per liter and 20 to 30 mEq of sodium per liter.[1] For a discussion of milliequivalents see box, top right.

If problems of dehydration and overheating do arise, they are best treated by cooling the body as fast as possible (in a shower or bath or by rubbing with ice cubes) and drinking cold water. In severe cases, intravenous rehydration by medical personnel is used.

The two groups of athletes most vulnerable to dehydration are marathon runners and wrestlers. Marathon runners can lose 8 to 13 pounds of fluid during a race, which must be replaced during the race to prevent severe cardiovascular problems caused by the reduction in blood volume. Wrestlers have problems with dehydration because they sometimes purposely dehydrate themselves to qualify for competition in the lowest possible weight class. The use of diuretics, hot showers, whirlpools, and sweatboxes is prohibited in competition, but the use of laxatives, intense sweat-producing exercise, and food and fluid restriction is not. Such methods, however, can impair the wrestler's competitive performance, even if partial rehydration occurs between the weigh-in and competition. The large fluctuations in body weight are bound to stress the body and almost certainly reduce the wrestler's ability to perform at his best. It is difficult, however, to convince a young man eager to win that his chances are greater at the bottom end of his natural weight class than at the top end of the lower weight class.

Electrolyte Concentration of Plasma and Sweat

	SODIUM (mEq/L)	Cl	K
Plasma	140	101	4
Sweat	40–60	30–50	3–4

1 mEq of Na = 23 mg, 1 mEq of Cl = 35 mg, and 1 mEq of K = 39 mg.

ENERGY

As discussed in Chapter 6, the energy cost of an activity is determined by the type of activity, the duration of the activity, and the weight of the person performing the activity. Obviously, the more strenuous the activity, the longer it is performed, and the heavier the person performing it, the higher is the energy cost. For a 125-pound (58-kg) person, typical energy costs of various activities are as follows:

- 176 kcal/hour for walking slowly
- 241 kcal/hour for swimming the crawl
- 495 kcal/hour for playing in a vigorous game of basketball
- 777 kcal/hour for running at 9 miles/hour

Comparable figures for a 205-pound person are 266, 392, 807, and 1269 kcal/hr, respectively. An impression of the wide variation in the energy costs of different exercises can be gained from Figure 18-1.

People participating in athletic training usually require between 3000 and 5000 kcal/day, but requirements may be at least twice as high. A swimmer training for 5 hours/day, for example, can easily require as much

FIGURE 18-1

Energy costs of various kinds of exercise.

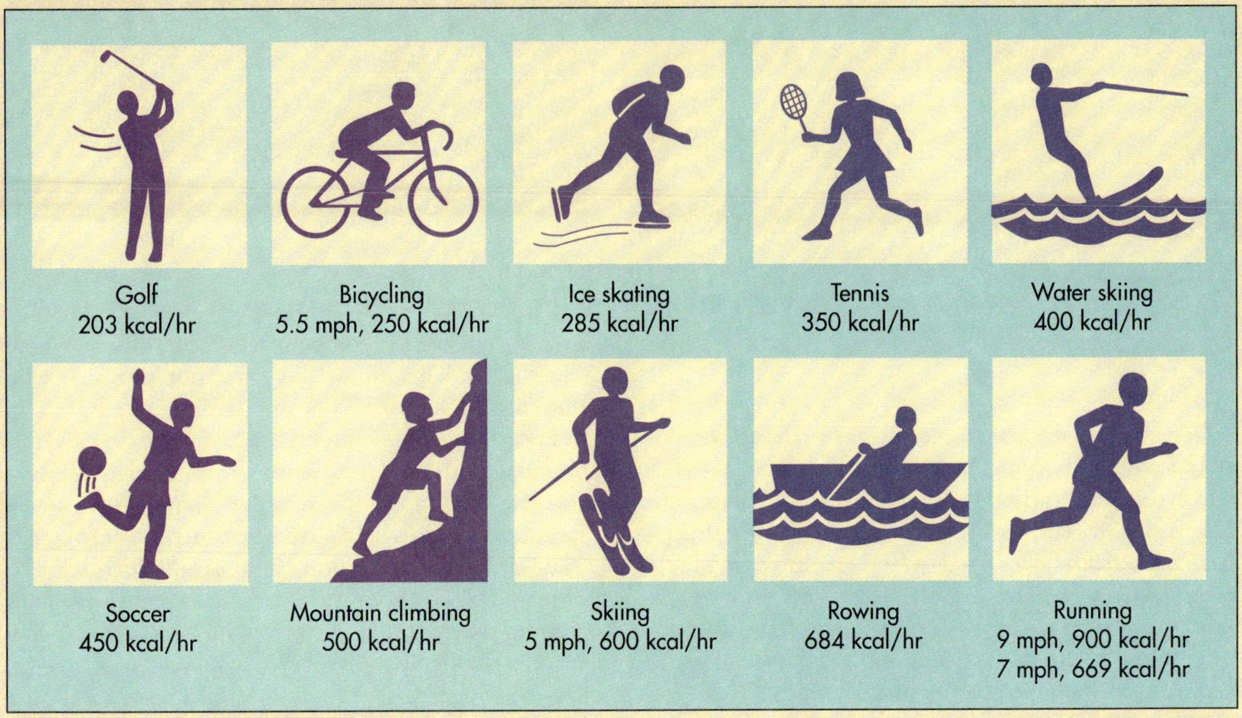
Golf
203 kcal/hr
Bicycling
5.5 mph, 250 kcal/hr
Ice skating
285 kcal/hr
Tennis
350 kcal/hr
Water skiing
400 kcal/hr
Soccer
450 kcal/hr
Mountain climbing
500 kcal/hr
Skiing
5 mph, 600 kcal/hr
Rowing
684 kcal/hr
Running
9 mph, 900 kcal/hr
7 mph, 669 kcal/hr

Aerobic and Anaerobic Exercise

During exercise of low or moderate intensity, such as jogging or distance swimming, the blood supply can deliver sufficient oxygen to muscles to allow the complete oxidation of glucose into carbon dioxide and water. Under these **aerobic** conditions the maximum amount of energy can be released from each glucose molecule.

During intense exercise, such as sprint running or swimming, oxygen is used up so quickly that **anaerobic** conditions can develop in the muscles. In these conditions the pyruvic acid derived from glucose by glycolysis is converted into lactic acid, instead of being passed into the mitochondria for oxidation. This allows release of only a small proportion of the energy available from each glucose molecule. The lactic acid accumulates in the muscles, causing a tingling sensation and then stiffness and pain.

Athletes performing aerobic exercise can continue indefinitely. Those performing anaerobic exercise can do so only for short periods before muscle pain and stiffness force them to rest and let their muscles become reoxygenated and recover.

as 7000 kcal/day. Athletes can usually rely on their natural appetite and satiety signals to regulate their food intake. As always, however, the appropriate total energy intake is whatever level maintains desirable and healthy weight.

SOURCES OF ENERGY

All of the energy required by the body must be released from the metabolism of carbohydrates, fats, protein, or alcohol. Alcohol should not be used as a source of energy before or during exercise because it promotes dehydration, hampers coordination, and generally impairs performance. Obtaining more than 12% to 15% of energy from protein is unnecessarily expensive, both metabolically and financially. Many people incorrectly believe that because muscle is mainly protein and muscle powers exercise, large amounts of protein must be eaten to meet the energy costs of exercise. In reality, muscles derive most of their energy from the metabolism of carbohydrate. Carbohydrate is provided initially by glucose already in the blood and then from glucose derived from the breakdown of glycogen in muscles and the liver. When these supplies of energy decline, reserves of body fat can be mobilized. Most athletes carry less body fat than other people, but they usually contain at least 15 pounds of fat reserves, which is capable of providing 50,000 kcal of energy. Only a small portion of this storage fat is actually used, however, even during an endurance event. Protein is only used as a major source of energy if insufficient energy is available from carbohydrate and fat. The relative use made of blood glucose, glycogen, and fat as energy sources during exercise is depicted in Figure 18-2.

FIGURE 18-2

The relative use made of energy sources in the body as exercise continues.

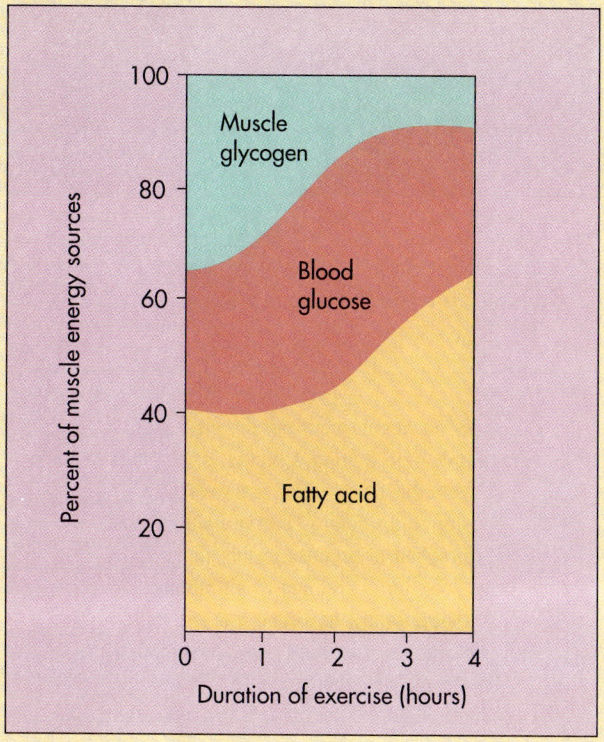

Classic Carbohydrate Loading Regimen*

Days 1-3	Regular exercise Moderate (350 g) carbohydrate diet
Days 4-5	Decreasing exercise High (550 g) complex carbohydrate diet
Day 6	Physical rest High (550 g) or 60% to 65% calories complex carbohydrate diet
Day 7	Day of event Usual diet

* No longer recommended (see text).

As an athlete becomes used to exercise by training, the ability to use fat as an energy source increases by as much as 50%. This allows the more limited supplies of carbohydrate to last longer.

Although the use of protein as an energy source is minor compared with the use made of carbohydrate and fat, recent research indicates that endurance exercise does increase the protein needs of athletes. In most cases, participation in endurance exercise increases the athlete's need for protein to between 150% and 175% of the RDA. In rare cases the need for protein may be as much as 200% of the RDA. The RDA for protein is 0.8 g/kg of body weight. Thus endurance athletes' protein needs may rise to between 1.2 and 1.6 g/kg/day. Athletes participating in events requiring strength rather than endurance usually experience only a slight increase in protein need to about 0.9 g/kg/day, or 112% of the RDA.[4] There is no evidence that eating more protein than the amounts listed here can increase metabolic efficiency or lead to enhanced strength or endurance. One drawback of excess protein consumption by athletes is that it increases the need for water because of the increased amount of urine that must be produced to excrete nitrogen as urea. A diet providing 12% to 15% of its total energy as protein should meet the protein needs of most athletes, unless the diet provides insufficient energy overall.

CARBOHYDRATE LOADING

After athletes have engaged in continuous strenuous exercise for a long time, they often experience what is known as "hitting the wall," at which point they find it difficult to keep going. This point corresponds to the time when the reserves of the carbohydrate glycogen in the muscles have been used up. It seems reasonable to suppose that athletes might be able to compete more effectively and longer if their glycogen reserves could be built up beforehand. This is the aim of a dietary and exercise regimen known as **carbohydrate loading.** The original, or "classic," carbohydrate loading regimen involved 3 days on a low carbohydrate diet accompanied by strenuous exercise, followed by 4 days on a high carbohydrate diet with minimum exercise (see box).

This program proved to have several undesirable side effects, namely depression, lethargy, loss of muscle tissue, stiffness, cramps, weight gain, and early fatigue. Most sports physiologists now recommend a simpler version of carbohydrate loading that involves consuming larger-than-usual amounts of complex carbohydrates, such as breads and pasta, during the 2 to 3 days before an event. Only a small benefit, if any, however, can be expected from the use of either method of carbohydrate loading.[5]

AMINO ACID AND PROTEIN SUPPLEMENTS

The widely promoted practice of supplementing the diets of athletes with individual amino acids or mixtures of amino acids in the form of protein hydrolysates is of no value. In fact, it may contribute to undesirable imbalances in the amino acid content of the diet.

Many athletes use amino acid or protein supplements (or both) to try to increase muscle mass. This approach is described as "muscle building" or "bulking up," but increased muscle mass can only be achieved by long-term training, not by the use of dietary "quick fixes." Without a training program, extra dietary protein is converted to storage fat, with the additional nitrogen being excreted as urea. Because most diets in the United States already contain considerably more than the recommended amounts of protein, there is no reason to promote or use protein supplements.

Nutritional Knowledge of Athletes and Coaches

Several studies have indicated that athletes and coaches have many misconceptions about the role of diet in athletic performance[7,8] In many cases, however, the level of knowledge is considerably better than the actual practices adopted suggest. This fact is especially true of girls, who often follow practices they know to be inadvisable. In general, male athletes eat considerably better diets than do female athletes.

VITAMIN AND MINERAL SUPPLEMENTS

The belief that "if a little is good, then more must be better" seems to lie behind many of the claims that vitamin and mineral supplements can enhance athletic performance. Although athletes do have increased needs for the nutrients involved in energy metabolism because of their increased energy needs, most mixed and reasonably well-chosen diets, especially the high-energy diets of physically active people, provide more than enough of all such nutrients.

Studies on the effects of high doses of vitamin C or vitamin E found a beneficial effect on performance only in people who were deficient in these vitamins to begin with. There is absolutely no evidence that megadoses of vitamins can improve athletic performance. There is, however, considerable reason to be concerned about the adverse effects of vitamin supplements that provide vitamins at hundreds of times the amount needed for normal metabolism.

There is a similar lack of evidence to suggest that large intakes of minerals can improve performance and considerable evidence that high mineral intakes can be harmful. The effects of iron and calcium supplements have received most attention. Endurance athletes tend to have a higher incidence of iron depletion, which may impair their performance.[6] This form of iron depletion, known as *sports anemia*, has been attributed to the loss of iron in sweat, the loss of blood as a result of bleeding into the gastrointestinal tract, or the breakdown of red blood cells as a result of the repeated impact of the feet on the ground. Iron supplements can be beneficial in people with evidence of this or any other form of iron deficiency. However, no benefit has been attributed to the consumption of excess iron, and iron supplements should be used only after consultation with a physician. African Americans, 20% of whom suffer from a genetic predisposition for iron overload, should have their iron status assessed before supplementing their diet. Calcium supplements may be beneficial for the promotion of increased bone mass in amenhorreic women taking exercise, especially those suffering from anorexia nervosa. Again, however, there is no evidence of benefits from excess consumption of calcium by people who do not already have an impaired calcium status.

One of the most persistent beliefs about food among athletes is that milk should be avoided because of a condition called **"cotton mouth,"** a sensation of dryness in the mouth that can be distracting to an athlete. Apparently, however, there is no relationship between milk consumption and the development of a dry mouth. Some athletes also report an unpleasant accumulation of oral mucus after drinking milk. This effect also remains unconfirmed.

PRECOMPETITION MEALS

Many experts believe that the type of food athletes eat before competition influences their performance. There is no "magic" precompetition meal, but there are some generally agreed upon recommendations. A precompetition meal should be taken 1 to 4 hours before competing; it should provide between 300 and 1000 kcals; and it should be relatively low in fat and high in complex carbohydrates such as bread, cereal, and vegetables. The recommended timing allows for the complete digestion of the food and absorption of its nutrients before competition. This ensures that when competition begins, blood is not being diverted to the gastrointestinal tract but is fully available to carry oxygen and nutrients to the muscles.

Liquid meals may offer advantages to athletes who have trouble digesting regular meals. They are quickly digested, leave little residue, provide substantial amounts of energy, and can be taken within an hour of competition.

Caffeine and Athletic Performance

Coffee or other caffeine-containing foods increase the release of fatty acids into the blood and thereby increase the utilization of fat as an energy source. Research investigating the potential of this action of caffeine as an aid to athletic performance has produced equivocal results.[5] Although caffeine may enhance performance and endurance, it can also cause anxiety, fluid loss, and increased heart rate, which might counteract any benefits. The International Olympic Committee does not approve the use of caffeine to aid athletic performance.

SPECIAL ERGOGENIC FOODS

Over the years certain foods and nutrients have developed reputations as **ergogenic** (energy-producing) foods that can enhance athletic performance. Purported ergogenic foods and nutrients include the following:

- Wheat germ
- Wheat germ oil
- Paprika
- Honey
- Bee pollen
- Sunflower seeds
- Kelp
- Vitamins C, D, and E
- Brewer's yeast
- Fructose
- Lecithin

Investigations of these foods and nutrients have revealed no evidence that they offer special benefits to adequately nourished athletes or other people. Some of these foods and nutrients are specially packaged and promoted for use by athletes and sold at exorbitant prices. All of the evidence suggests that buying such special preparations is at best a waste of money.

The list of specific foods, nutrients, and other substances that are promoted as having special benefits for athletes is likely to vary over the years, with new "miracle" products emerging as rapidly as the older supposed miracles fall into disuse often to appear again years later. Readers are cautioned to regard all products promoted in this way with considerable skepticism. They should be wary of both the testimony of successful athletes and of "scientific" claims that have never been published in reputable scientific journals. Many athletes who use these products genuinely believe that they have significant benefits, but the benefits may well be psychological rather than physiological. To date, no special physiological benefits of products marketed in this way have been documented.

Benefits of Moderate Exercise and Possible Adverse Consequences of Excessive Exercise Throughout the Life Cycle

BENEFITS OF MODERATE EXERCISE DURING THE LIFE CYCLE

Childhood
- Establish lifelong exercise and health habits

Adolescence
- Prevent and treat obesity and eating disorders
- Establish lifelong exercise and health habits

Adulthood
- Weight control
- Prevent and treat many diseases
- Promote mental health and feelings of well-being

Pregnancy
- Control of excessive weight gain
- More favorable nutrient profile as a result of an increased energy intake
- Possibly less constipation and varicose veins

Lactation
- Promote return to prepregnancy weight
- Possibly improve postpartum mental status

Elderly
- Favorable effects on age-related physiological changes
- Prevent and treat osteoporosis
- Socialization

POSSIBLE ADVERSE CONSEQUENCES OF STRENUOUS EXERCISE DURING THE LIFE CYCLE

Childhood
- Inability to meet energy needs and compromised growth and development

Adolescence
- Inadequate energy intake
- Oxidation of dietary protein for energy
- Oligomenorrhea or amenorrhea
- Negative calcium balance and reduced bone mass
- Sports anemia
- Anorexia athletica

Adulthood
- Possible increased need for riboflavin and vitamin B_6

Pregnancy
- Low weight gain
- Low-birth-weight infant

Lactation
- Excessive rate of weight loss, which compromises milk production and infant growth

Elderly
- Exercise-related injuries leading to disability and other complications

Modified from Kris-Etherton PM: *Nutr Today* 21:6, 1986.

CONSEQUENCES OF EXCESSIVE PHYSICAL EXERCISE

The people most commonly affected by excessive physical exercise are young women who combine excessive exercise with restricted food intake to maintain a low body weight. These women can suffer from the cessation of menstruation (amenorrhea), infrequent or scanty menstrual periods (oligomenorrhea), delayed onset of menstruation, and decreased bone mass. The long-term consequences of these effects of excessive exercise and dietary restriction are unknown but in all probability are significant.

Among athletes, excessive exercise is most common among gymnasts, ballet dancers, divers, and cyclists. Many affected athletes suffer from reduced hormone levels and increased losses of bone minerals.

Another cause for concern is the tendency of athletes who exercise excessively to suffer a variety of "overuse injuries." These are forms of damage caused by performing the same movement many times a day, day after day. Common examples are shoulder injuries among baseball pitchers and swimmers and knee injuries among runners.

The overall message about exercise for the general public not involved in competitive sports is that it is beneficial *in moderation,* but it should not be indulged in to excess. Competitive athletes must obviously train intensively to have any hope of succeeding in their sport, but they too must beware of the dangers of excessive exercise.

ISSUES AND OPINIONS

Steroid Substitutes: The New Drug Scourge of Athletics

The types of drugs most widely associated with drug abuse in athletics are the **anabolic steroids.** The use of anabolic steroids is banned by national and international athletics authorities, and in 1990 it also became a federal crime to possess them. The threat of up to 5 years of imprisonment if caught in possession of anabolic steroids has led many athletes to turn to a variety of **steroid substitutes** instead. Because these drugs are banned by athletic authorities, athletes who use them are risking their career in athletics, but they are not risking criminal charges.

Some top-ranking athletes, including a U.S. hammer thrower, a U.S. shot putter, and a German sprinter, have already been caught and punished for using nonsteroid drugs that can enhance athletic performance. The two were sent home early from the 1992 Olympics after testing positive for the drug clenbuterol, and one was not allowed to attend the Olympics after testing positive for the same drug. The key properties of clenbuterol and the other main nonsteroid drugs being misused by athletes are summarized in the following paragraphs.

Clenbuterol is a veterinary drug used in Europe to build up muscle mass and strength in livestock before exhibition. It is not approved in the United States, even for use on animals, but some athletes use it in an attempt to build up their own muscle mass and strength. Clenbuterol can cause serious short-term side effects in humans, including headache, dizziness, nausea, rapid heart rate, muscle tremors, fevers, and chills. The long-term effects of clenbuterol use are unknown but are likely to be significant.

Gamma hydroxybutyric acid, or GHB, is a new drug being illegally marketed as a steroid substitute. It is claimed to stimulate the production of human growth hormone, which in turn promotes the development of muscles. It is also promoted as a "street drug" and as an aid to sleep. GHB is now being used by many athletes and teenagers, but it is an extremely dangerous compound. Large numbers of people have been hospitalized from its use, suffering from a range of side effects including drowsiness, dizziness, vomiting, tremors, seizures, low heartbeat, low blood pressure, and severe difficulties with breathing.

Human growth hormone is being used directly as a steroid substitute in the hope that it promotes the growth of muscle tissue. It is a natural hormone required to promote normal growth, but it is approved as a drug only for the treatment of dwarfism. It has not been proved that human growth hormone can actually increase muscle mass when used by normal adolescents and adults. Because the use of human growth hormone is currently undetectable, it has reportedly become the most commonly abused drug in modern athletics. The risks of using this drug include abnormal growth and possibly cancer. The former Los Angeles Raiders football player Lyle Alzado died in 1992 of a rare form of brain cancer, which he believed was caused by his use of human growth hormone and steroids.

Erythropoietin is another natural human hormone. It increases the number of circulating red blood cells and thereby increases the delivery of oxygen to the muscles of athletes using it. Its use appears to be associated with an increased risk of blood clots, which can cause heart attacks or stroke. The thickening of the blood induced by erythropoietin can be made worse by the loss of fluid experienced by endurance athletes such as marathon runners.

The increasing abuse of steroid substitutes in athletics is of great concern to both the athletics community and the medical profession. Everyone involved with athletics, apart from the drug abusers, wants to see fair competition between athletes who are not assisted by banned drugs. Of much greater concern, however, are the considerable health risks of drug abuse, especially to youngsters whose healthy interest in athletics may lead them into situations in which they feel pressure to experiment with drugs. One particular concern about the new steroid substitutes is that little is known about their effects on humans. The dangers of anabolic steroids are well known, and all anabolic steroids have been approved for use in humans to treat certain medical conditions. By taking steroid substitutes that are not approved for human use or are only approved for specific problems in humans, many athletes are taking a risky leap into the unknown.

From Napier K: *Nutritional supplements for athletes? calories, not capsules, enhance performance*, New York, 1993, American Council on Science and Health.

BY NOW YOU SHOULD KNOW

- Water probably has a greater effect on athletic performance than any other nutrient.
- Guidelines for the good nutrition of athletes are essentially the same as those for good nutrition in general: consume a mixed diet with the appropriate proportion of carbohydrate, fat, and protein and that supplies sufficient energy to maintain a healthy weight.
- Athletes should drink fluids containing carbohydrate and sometimes sodium before, during, and after competition.
- Athletes have an increased need for energy to meet the energy cost of their activities. Their need for many other nutrients, particularly those involved in energy metabolism, increases in proportion to their increased need for energy.
- Athletes may have a greater need for protein than nonathletes, but their needs are easily met by the typical North American diet. There are no advantages to consuming more than the recommended amount of protein.
- Many products marketed as dietary aids for athletes cannot deliver the enhanced performance the advertising suggests.
- Thirst is not an adequate gauge of water needs for athletes. An athlete should consume sufficient water to compensate for water loss. Water should be consumed (on its own or within appropriate beverages) before, during, and after exercise.
- Vitamin and mineral supplements do not supply energy for, or significantly enhance the performance of, an already well-nourished athlete. Iron supplements are only beneficial to athletes who are already anemic.
- A precompetition meal should be taken 1 to 4 hours before an event. The composition of the meal should be chosen to allow the food to leave the stomach before the start of the event.
- Amenorrhea and bone loss can occur in female athletes who exercise strenuously and restrict their dietary intake.
- Exercise should be performed in moderation, just as food should be consumed in moderation.

~ STUDY QUESTIONS ~

1. At the beginning of the event, a marathon runner weighed 135 pounds. At the end of the event he weighed 129 pounds. How many cups of fluid would the runner need to consume to make up for the weight loss?
2. Explain why water is an essential nutrient and why it is especially significant to athletes.
3. What is the difference between the aerobic metabolism of glucose and the anaerobic metabolism of glucose? Why are these two forms of glucose metabolism of relevance to sprinters?
4. Summarize the arguments against the use of amino acid or protein supplements by athletes.
5. What are the primary fuels for muscle during exercise?

~ CRITICAL ANALYSIS ~

1. The nutrient needs of athletes differ from those of non athletes mainly in the amounts of carbohydrate, protein, and water needed to support the increased level of activity. Using your body weight, you can calculate the needs of an athlete based on the recommendations in this chapter.

   The recommendation for carbohydrate intake is normally expressed as 50% to 60% of total caloric intake. For the non athlete, this translates to 3 to 4 g of carbohydrate per kilogram of body weight. The recommendation for the athlete is 8 g/kg of body weight because of the enhanced energy requirement (this must be adjusted downward for sports and training that entail short bursts of anaerobic activity). Calculate the carbohydrate needs of an athlete using your body weight.

______ ÷ 2.2 = ______
(Body weight in lbs) (Body weight in kg)

______ × 8 g carbohydrate per kilogram body weight = ______
(Body weight in kg) (Daily need for carbohydrate in grams)

2. Now calculate the needs of this athlete for protein. In this chapter it was stated that strength athletes needed approximately 0.9 g of protein per kilogram of body weight, whereas endurance athletes need 1.2 to 1.6 g/kg of body weight. Try it both ways.

______ × 0.9 and 1.6 g of protein per kilogram body weight = ______
(Body weight in kg) (Daily need for protein in grams)

3. What is the need for fat? (No, it is not "none.") Although more careful calculations may be necessary for athletes in endurance training and events, one reasonable way to calculate the need for fat is as follows:
   a. Convert the daily needs for carbohydrate and protein in grams to calories (that is, multiply the grams of protein and carbohydrate each by 4 kcal/g).
   b. Calculate the estimated daily energy needs of the athlete.

c. Subtract the calories of carbohydrate and protein needed from the estimated daily energy needs.

The remainder is the daily calories that can be supplied by fat. Calculation of estimated daily energy needs is shown in Chapter 6. Remember to choose an appropriate activity factor. Also, remember that all such calculations yield estimates of energy expenditure and nutrition needs. Once these estimates have been implemented, they may need to be adjusted. For example, if the athlete follows your recommendations and is unintentionally losing or gaining weight, your recommendations for energy and nutrients may need to be revised upward or downward.

REFERENCES

1. Gisolfi CV, Duchman SM: Guidelines for optimal replacement beverages for different athletic events, *Med Sci Sports Exerc* 24:79, 1992.
2. Maughan R: Fluid balance and exercise, *Int J Sports Med* 13:S132, 1991.
3. Nielsen BG and others: Fluid balance in exercise dehydration and rehydration with different glucose-electrolyte drinks, *Eur J Appl Physiol* 55:318, 1986.
4. Lemon PWR, Proctor DN: Protein intake and athletic performance, *Sports Med* 12:313, 1991.
5. Costell DL, Hargreaves M: Carbohydrate nutrition and fatigue, *Sports Med* 13:86, 1992.
6. Eichner TR: Sports anemia, iron supplements and blood doping, *Med Sci Sports Exerc* 24:S315, 1992.
7. Corley G, Demarest-Litchford M, Bazarre TL: Nutrition knowledge and dietary practices of college coaches, *J Am Diet Assoc* 90(3):705, 1990.
8. Holt WS Jr: Nutrition and athletes, *Am Fam Physician* 47(8):1757, 1993.

ADDITIONAL READINGS

Berning J, Steen S, editors: *Sports nutrition for the 90's: the health professional's handbook,* Gaithersburg, Md, 1991, Aspen.

Coleman E: *Eating for endurance,* Palo Alto, Calif, 1992, Bell.

Coleman E: *Diet, exercise, and fitness: continuing education course,* San Marcos, Calif, 1993, Nutrition Dimensions.

Helm K, Berning J, Steen S: *Sports nutrition for the 90's: continuing education course,* Gaithersburg, Md, 1993, Aspen.

Probart CK, Bird PJ, Parker KA: Diet and athletic performance, *Clin Nutr* 77(4):757, 1993.

Wolinsky I, Hickson JF Jr, editors: *Nutrition in exercise and sport,* ed 2, Boca Raton, 1994, CRC Press.

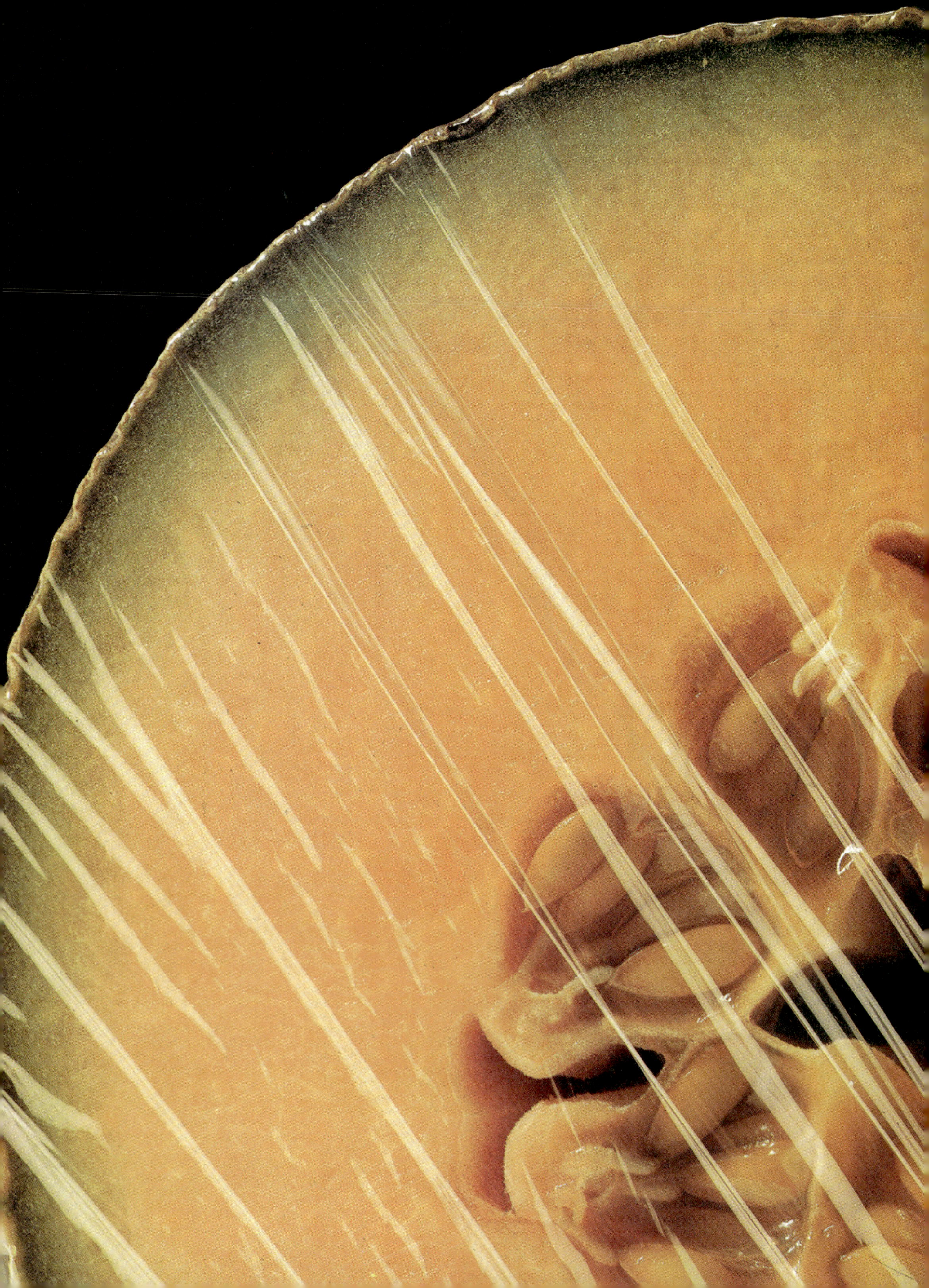

C H A P T E R 1 9

F O O D S A F E T Y

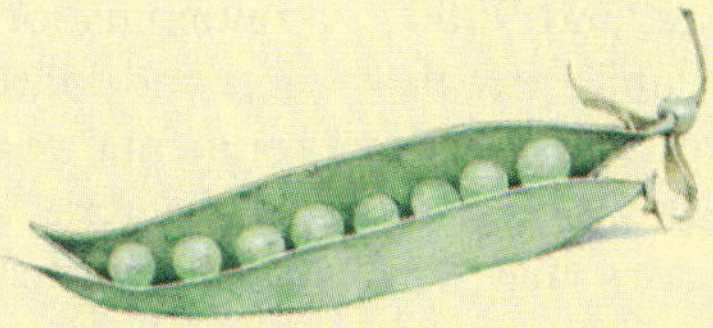

The earlier chapters of this book focused on the nutrients required to promote good health throughout life; the sources of those nutrients; the consequences of failure to consume adequate amounts of nutrients; and the effect of food processing, storage, and preparation on the stability of the nutrients. Of equal, or in some respects greater and more immediate, public concern is the question of the safety of the food supply. The Centers for Disease Control (CDC) estimates that from 1 in 10 to 1 in 30 persons each year suffer from some degree of diarrhea or more severe gastrointestinal distress attributable to contaminants in our food supply. This occurs in spite of significant advances in our knowledge of the cause and control of food-borne diseases. Food safety can be compromised at almost any point throughout the whole food delivery system from production to consumption.

This chapter provides a brief overview of the ways in which food can become a source of illness. It also considers the precautions that can be taken to minimize the possibility of becoming infected and the steps that regulatory agencies, particularly the Food and Drug Administration (FDA), take to ensure the safety of our food supply. In addition to the FDA, the Environmental Protection Agency (EPA), the U.S. Department of Agriculture (USDA), and the U.S. Public Health Service Department of Health and Human Services (DHHS) also have responsibility for the safety of some aspects of our food supply.

The basis for concern about food-borne diseases is evident from estimates that they cause between 24 and 81 million illnesses, 6 million acute illnesses, and 9000 deaths in the United States each year. Public health officials note that because only one in every 10 to 25 cases is severe enough to warrant medical attention and is thus reported, the actual number of cases may be much higher.[1] Almost half of all food-borne illnesses are attributed to meat and poultry products. The economic cost of food-borne illness has been estimated at $5 billion to $17 billion per year in the United States and $1.3 billion in Canada in medical care and lost productivity. These illnesses tend to hit hardest those individuals with immature or weakened defense mechanisms such as young infants, the ill, the elderly, alcoholics, and victims of AIDS or other conditions in which the immune system is compromised.[1]

> Food-borne diseases cause more than 6 million acute illnesses and 9000 deaths in the United States each year.

Food hazards worldwide are ranked by the FDA in the following order of importance:

- Microbiological pathogens
- Nutritional imbalance
- Environmental contaminants
- Natural toxicants
- Pesticide residues
- Food additives

The size of the problem associated with each category of hazard is far greater in developing than in industrialized countries, but the order of ranking seems to be universal. In contrast to this view of scientists, consumers rank food safety risks in the following way:

- Pesticide residues
- Hormone residues
- Chemical residues
- Food additives
- Irradiated foods
- Microbiological organisms

FOOD PATHOGENS

The majority of food pathogens are microorganisms that enter the food system somewhere between the farm and the human stomach. Problems of microbial contamination are associated primarily with raw products and ingredients, improper food handling, or environmental contamination.

Bacteria account for over 90% of food-borne illnesses. Bacteria that cause food-borne illnesses can be divided into two categories: those that cause food-borne *infections* (60%) and those that cause food-borne *intoxications* (40%). Within the first category the presence of bacterial growth in the food is itself the cause of illness. Within the second category, the presence of toxins produced by bacteria is the cause of illness. Table 19-1 shows some of the most significant types of bacteria in each category. The majority of food-borne diseases are caused by the first category of bacteria, which causes illness simply by infecting food rather than developing toxins in it.

Many hundreds of microorganisms are found in food, but only about a dozen are capable of causing food-borne infections. Many of the others, such as those used to produce fermented foods, are not only harmless but actually perform useful functions. Food-borne infections result when harmful microorganisms, such as *Salmonella typhimurium,* multiply to such an extent that significant numbers survive passage through the stomach and enter the intestine. The presence of the microorganisms in the intestine either irritates the intestinal mucosa or causes the production of an **enterotoxin** (a toxin produced in the intestine). Because cooking food kills most of these microorganisms, food should be safe after being heated to at least 155° F (68° C), unless it is recontaminated. Such recontamination can occur when cooked meat comes into contact with the juice of raw

> Of food-borne diseases reported to the Centers for Disease Control over a 5-year period, 75% were attributed to food service establishments, 20% to homes, and fewer than 0.05% to food processing plants. The most common symptom is diarrhea.

TABLE 19-1

Most common pathogens causing food-borne illness

	CAUSE	SYMPTOMS	STATISTICS	NOTORIOUS CASES	HOW TO AVOID
FOOD-BORNE INFECTIONS					
Salmonella typhimurium	Improperly cooked or thawed meats, poultry, eggs; unpasteurized cheese and milk; chocolate made from contaminated cocoa beans	Abdominal cramps, diarrhea, nausea, vomiting, fever	CDC estimates 800,000 to 4 million cases annually; only 1% to 5% are reported	1985, Illinois: more than 200,000 cases from milk contaminations after pasteurization; deaths unknown	Thaw food properly; cook food thoroughly, avoid unpasteurized dairy products and foods containing raw eggs
Listeria monocytogenes	Undercooked meat and poultry; soft cheese, paté, unpasteurized milk	Fever, headache, stiff neck, miscarriage	1990: 1850 cases, 425 deaths	1985, California: 142 cases, 48 deaths from Mexican-style soft cheese	Cook food thoroughly, avoid soft cheeses during pregnancy
Campylobacter jejuni	Undercooked poultry; unpasteurized milk	Abdominal pain, nausea, low-grade fever, headache, muscle pain	1989: 7970 cases, no deaths	1981, Arizona: 190 cases from unpasteurized milk	Cook food thoroughly, avoid unpasteurized dairy products
Escherichia coli	Improperly handled, undercooked beef, especially ground beef; unpasteurized milk	Abdominal cramps, diarrhea	1993: 500 cases, 4 deaths	1993, Northwestern United States: at least 500 cases and 4 deaths from tainted, undercooked hamburgers	Cook food thoroughly, avoid unpasteurized milk
FOOD-BORNE INTOXICANTS					
Clostridium botulinum	Improper home canning. Insufficient heat for processing. Honey fed to infants	Abdominal pain, weakness, headache, double vision, other neurological symptoms	1991: 121 cases, 4 deaths	1985, Vancouver: 37 cases, no deaths, from rehydrated garlic served by a restaurant	Process foods at high temperatures, use proper canning methods
Staphylococcus aureus	Contamination by food preparer from infected wounds or coughing and sneezing	Nausea, vomiting, diarrhea	No good estimates, rarely fatal	No significant outbreaks	Wash hands before handling food, refrigerate food promptly

Modified from Food Safety Bugaboo: *Eating well,* Charlotte, Vt, 1993, Camden House Publishing.

meat, for example. Symptoms of abdominal pain, diarrhea, gastroenteritis, vomiting, or fever usually occur 12 to 18 hours after consuming infected food and last from 1 to 7 days. Spore-forming bacteria, such as *Clostridium botulinum,* may withstand higher cooking temperatures.

Food intoxication results from ingesting food containing preformed toxins. These food-borne toxins, such as those produced by *Staphylococcus aureus* and *Clostridium botulinum,* can cause severe nausea and vomiting 2 to 4 hours or less after the affected food is consumed. With the exception of the heat-labile toxin produced by *Clostridium botulinum,* the toxins are not degraded by heat; therefore cooking food that is affected by other toxins does not prevent illness. Symptoms, including vomiting, abdominal cramps, sweating, chills, and weak pulse and respiration, occur in 30 minutes to 4 hours and last up to 2 days. Whether an illness is caused by food-borne infection or food-borne toxins, sufficient quantities of food containing the microorganisms or toxin must be eaten to overcome the **resistance threshold** of the individual.[3]

Many of the organisms responsible for food-borne illnesses grow in the intestinal tracts of animals as well as humans. Thus livestock are capable of contaminating both the meat that their bodies produce and any meat from uncontaminated animals that comes in contact with their intestinal contents during the butchering process. Similarly, shellfish harvested from off-shore waters that are subject to human and animal pollutants concentrate the microorganisms from the environment and can become a potent source of infective microorganisms. Vegetables produced in the ground close to areas where runoff water may carry microorganisms from animal feces are another common source of pathogens that cause human illness.

Animal foods sold by retail outlets often have a high incidence of contamination with *Salmonella* and *Campylobacter organisms,* and *Listeria monocytogenes.* Fortunately these microorganisms are killed by thorough cooking.

CONTAMINATION

In general, cross-contamination occurs either through the fecal-oral route or the raw to processed route. This may involve food handlers who do not wash their hands properly, fecal contamination from gut contents during processing, or the transfer of organisms on cutting boards or utensils from raw to cooked foods.

CONTAMINATION DURING PROCESSING

In food processing plants microorganisms can enter food by contact with water, air, workers, and equipment. Procedures should be in place to protect against this hazard, but these procedures are sometimes ineffective because of mishap or mistakes. Once a microorganism comes in contact with food, it grows only if there is sufficient water and nutrients available for it and if the temperature, pH level, and other environmental factors are suitable. The pathogen also multiplies sufficiently to cause disease only if given sufficient time to do so. The best protection against microbial contamination of food is to keep the microbes out of the food in the first place. If microbes are introduced, however, it is critical to destroy them by the processing methods as quickly and as completely as possible. Major methods used include heat treatment such as pasteurization and canning, dehydration, freezing, refrigeration, specialized packaging, and approved antimicrobial preservatives.

Steps necessary to prevent or control microbial growth during food processing are set out in ***Good Manufacturing Practices (GMP),*** a set of guidelines for the food industry. These guidelines set out standards for the design and construction of food processing plants and equipment to ensure that they are easy to clean and sanitize. They also set standards for employee hygiene, the treatment of water, cleaning and sanitizing procedures for plants and equipment, management of unavoidable pests, and many other aspects of food processing.

The **Hazard Analysis and Critical Control Points (HACCP) System** that was originally designed by the National Aeronautical Space Administration (NASA) is used by the food industry to prevent problems with the growth of botulism-causing organisms. It is based on the premise that if one begins with good-quality food ingredients, monitors each processing step, identifies critical control points where hazards may occur, and keeps these critical points under control, the finished product should be safe and of high quality. Food processing plants are also monitored visually, biologically, and chemically to identify the sites in plants where contamination is most likely to occur. In addition to the steps taken by food processors themselves through GMP and HACCP to control microbial contamination, local, state, national, and international government regulatory agencies are also involved in inspecting food processing plants (Table 19-2).

Microorganisms can be controlled by drying to remove water needed for growth, freezing, or refrigerating to temperatures too low for growth; by fermenting to produce acids, alcohol, or gases that interfere with metabolism; or by using chemical preservatives, heat, or irradiation. If a food containing harmful microorganisms is discovered at the point of sale, it is recalled and extensive efforts are made to notify the consumer of the brand, package size, production code date, and type of hazard involved.

Microorganisms can be controlled by
- Drying
- Freezing or refrigerating
- Fermenting
- Use of alcohols or gases to inhibit growth
- Chemical preservatives
- Heat
- Irradiation

CONTAMINATION AT RETAIL OUTLETS

Foods classified as **shelf stable** have been processed by sterilization to destroy all preexisting microorganisms. They can be stored at room temperature and should contain no microbial infections unless the packaging has been damaged. Consumers should always ensure that the packaging of such foods is undamaged before they buy them. **Perishable** foods, on the other hand, are susceptible to the introduction and growth of pathogens. Again, consumers should only buy perishable

TABLE 19-2

Government agencies with responsibilities for inspecting food processing plants

AGENCY	RESPONSIBILITY
United States Department of Agriculture (USDA)	Responsible for inspecting plants that process red meat, poultry, and eggs. These processing facilities are under continuous inspection when these products are being processed. The live animal through the finished product is inspected to ensure safety of the final foods.
Food and Drug Administration (FDA)	Responsible for inspecting all other foods sold in interstate commerce. The FDA usually tries to inspect each food processing plant once or twice a year. It inspects plants that have problems more often. Generally, 90% to 95% of the processing plants comply with the Federal Food, Drug and Cosmetic Act plus the Good Manufacturing Practices.
National Marine Fisheries Service (NMFS)	Has a voluntary inspection program for fish and seafood. The FDA works closely with NMFS and has the final enforcement authority for these foods.
Environmental Protection Agency (EPA)	Responsible for water safety, waste treatment, and pest management involved with food processing plants.
State, local, and international agencies	The FDA, USDA, NMFS, EPA and local and state health and agricultural departments help ensure that food processing plants manufacture safe foods. Governments of many other nations have memoranda of understanding with our regulatory agencies to ensure the safety of foods imported from those countries. International cooperation is becoming more common as the world takes on a global interdependent nature.

From Burgess WD, editor: *Producer through consumer: partners to a safe food supply,* West Lafayette, Ind, 1993, Purdue University, Cooperative Extension Service.

products in undamaged packaging, but they must also check the "sell by" date, which should appear on the packaging.

CONTAMINATION IN THE HOME

The greatest risk of contamination with pathogens occurs in the home. Food hygiene at home is not subject to any governmental regulations or regular inspections and can often be far from satisfactory. Because many pathogenic microorganisms do not change the taste, smell, or appearance of food in which they are growing until they have reached large numbers, it is important to keep them out of the food and to keep food in conditions of temperature (Figure 19-1), acidity, and water activity that do not favor microbial growth. Basic common-sense techniques to achieve good food hygiene practices at home are summarized in Table 19-3.

COMMON PATHOGENS

SALMONELLA

"Salmonellae," a generic name for about 2000 related bacteria, are responsible for over one third of food-borne outbreaks. Beef, turkey, and homemade ice cream are the most frequently reported carriers. The *Salmonella typhimurium* strain was involved in the largest outbreak in U.S. history, and *Salmonella enteritidis* outbreaks from contaminated shell eggs, especially those eaten raw or partially cooked, are increasing rapidly. Salmonellae are destroyed by ordinary heating and pasteurization procedures.

STAPHYLOCOCUS AUREUS

Staphylococcus aureus, found in or on the nose, throat, hair, or skin of 50% of healthy people, accounts for almost one fourth of food-borne illness outbreaks. Cooked protein foods such as meat, fish, and poultry; dairy products; salads; and custards support the growth of staphylococci. *S. aureus* causes illness within 2 to 6 hours after infection. Keeping foods below 40° F (4° C) or above 140° F (60° C) limits growth sufficiently to prevent food poisoning problems.

Trichinosis caused by *Trichinella spiralis,* a worm that infects pork, was once a major health problem but is now rare (less than 100 cases per year).

FIGURE 19-1

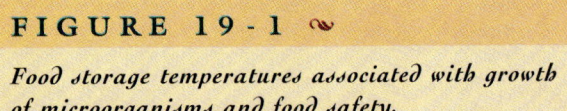

Food storage temperatures associated with growth of microorganisms and food safety.

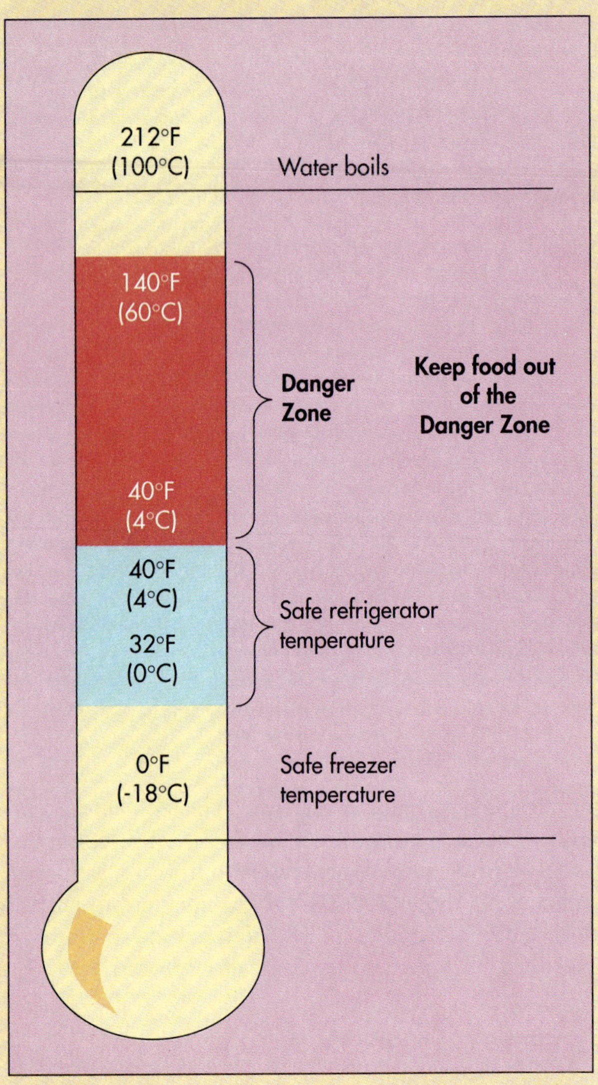

EMERGING FOOD-BORNE PATHOGENS

Many of the pathogens causing food-borne illnesses have been known for some time, but some have been recognized only recently and new pathogens continue to be discovered. That mysteries remain in this field is emphasized by the fact that between 1973 and 1987 the agents responsible for food-borne illness were identified in only 62% of reported cases. This section reviews some of the more recently discovered emerging food-borne pathogens.

Listeria monocytogenes is a deadly food-borne pathogen that for a long time was considered harmless. It is now known to be responsible for 1850 cases of listeriosis and 425 deaths per year in the United States alone. It has the unusual ability to grow at temperatures as low as 40° F (4° C) and thrives at normal refrigeration temperatures. It also survives freezing temperatures and grows at a wide range of pH values—from 4.4 to 9.8. It is also very heat resistant, with a temperature of at least 160° F (70° C) for 2 minutes required to significantly reduce its numbers. It is especially virulent in pregnant women and their fetuses, the elderly, and immunosuppressed persons. The foods most likely to be contaminated with *L. monocytogenes* are those that are kept at lower-than-normal refrigeration temperatures, have an extended shelf-life, and do not require further heating. These include cooked and pressed meats, prepared salads, cooked prepared meals, cooked seafood and seafood products, unpasteurized milk and milk products, and soft cheeses. Listeriosis is common in the third trimester of pregnancy when it often leads to premature delivery or stillbirth. In late-onset listeriosis the most common complication is meningitis in the young infant at several weeks of age.[4]

Escherichia coli 0157:H7 was first identified in 1982 and since then has been associated with at least 16 major outbreaks of infection from this organism and 22 deaths. The CDC estimates that there are at least 20,000 cases of E. coli infection a year. The organism grows in the intestinal tract of both mammals and humans. It can be carried from animal to animal, from animal to human, from animal to human within food, and from person to person through close contact or via food. It can survive refrigeration and freezer storage, multiply slowly at 44° F (6° C), and be destroyed by cooking at 160° F (70° C). It causes excessively bloody diarrhea, acute renal failure, and even stroke. The incubation period is 4 to 9 days, and the disease normally lasts 4 to 10 days. This bacterium is found in up to 4% of retail raw meat and poultry samples, in undercooked hamburgers, in unpasteurized milk, and in apple cider. A 1993 outbreak caused four deaths among people who ate inadequately cooked hamburger in a U.S. restaurant, which led to the formation of toxins in the body. This outbreak prompted a concerted effort to develop a vaccine that protects cows from infection with *E. coli* 0157:H7, to conduct studies to determine what makes dairy cows so susceptible to the infection, and to develop a more rapid test for identifying the problem.[5] In the meantime, restaurants have been urged to adopt cooking procedures that destroy the organism.

Salmonella enteritidis has been associated with the consumption of raw or partially cooked eggs or egg-containing foods, most of which have been stored at room temperature, and raw or undercooked chicken. The rate of infections from this organism has been increasing steadily since the mid-1980s possibly because of the importation of infected birds.[6,7]

Campylobacter jejuni is becoming known as the leading cause of bacterial gastroenteritis, affecting 2.8

TABLE 19-3

Techniques to reduce pathogen contamination of food in the home

OBJECTIVE	TECHNIQUE
To keep pathogens out of your food	Always wash your hands before preparing or serving foods. Wear gloves or avoid handling food if you have any cuts or abrasions on your hand. Avoid breathing, coughing, or sneezing on food, especially if you have a cold. Keep your kitchen and food preparation equipment clean. Keep raw and cooked foods separate—use separate cutting boards. Never place cooked food on a plate that held the raw food, unless it is thoroughly washed first. Wash fruits and vegetables carefully.
To keep pathogens from growing	Cook meats thoroughly to kill microbial contaminants. Thaw frozen foods in the refrigerator or the microwave. Use or cook at once. Foods thawed on the counter present a food safety risk because the outside of the food thaws faster than the inside and may reach a temperature sufficient to support microbial growth. Never leave perishable foods at room temperature for more than 2 hours. Food pathogens grow rapidly at temperatures between 40° F and 140° F (4° C). Keep hot food hot (at least 165° F [72° C]). and cold foods cold (at least 40° F [4° C]).
To avoid pathogens in food	Do not use canned goods that are swollen, dented, or otherwise damaged. Check expiration date on foods—do not use out-of-date food. Do not consume raw eggs or fish. Do not eat moldy or spoiled foods.

million people a year. It causes symptoms similar to those caused by other enteric pathogens: diarrhea, abdominal pain, fever, and bloody stools. Although it occurs as a result of contamination of both beef and poultry during evisceration, it is much more likely to thrive in poultry (50% to 80% of which are contaminated).

***Yersinia enterocolitica** 0:3* is the cause of **yersinosis,** which has symptoms similar to those of appendicitis. It is found only in pork, where it is concentrated in lymphoid tissue such as tonsils and in pig feces. It can grow at temperatures as low as 32° F (0° C).

Clostridium perfringens is generally found in meat and poultry. It causes abdominal pain and diarrhea 8 to 24 hours after consumption of an infected meal.

Clostridium botulinum produces a deadly neurotoxin in a low-acid, oxygen-free (anaerobic) environment such as that found in canned vegetables with a low acid content. It is also present in some honeys. There is a 10% death rate among afflicted people, and symptoms occur 1 to 2 days after consuming the contaminated food. The neurotoxin is heat labile and is destroyed by heating at temperatures above 176° F (80° C) for 10 minutes.

Vibrio vulnificus is a member of the genus known for cholera and gastroenteritis outbreaks caused by seafood. It is attracted to the chitin in the outer shell of lobster, crab, and shrimp. It causes septicemia, which results in death in 2 days in over 50% of those affected. Oysters taken from the Gulf of Mexico from March to October contain naturally occurring *V. vulnificus,* which is particularly harmful to alcoholics and those with liver disease, weakened immune systems, and disorders of iron metabolism.

FUNGI

The most common fungi in the food supply are the **molds** found almost everywhere in nature. Most fungi are harmless and some are even beneficial, but a few harmful types are a threat to the safety of food. Under certain environmental conditions some molds produce poisonous substances called **mycotoxins.** Some mycotoxins are known carcinogens, and others have been implicated in birth defects.

Aflatoxins are the most lethal naturally occurring mycotoxins and are not destroyed by cooking or processing. They can impair the immune system and cause cancer. They are produced by the mold *Aspergillus flavus,* which grows on peanuts, corn, and cottonseed, especially when these have been damaged during harvest and are stored under warm, humid conditions. Aflatoxins can also appear in the milk of cattle that have been fed moldy grain. Other dangerous mycotoxins include **ergot,** produced by a fungus that grows on rye and other grains; **patulin,** a potential carcinogen produced

TABLE 19-4

Proper treatment of food once mold growth appears

FOOD ITEM	TREATMENT
Bread	Most store-bought breads and baked goods have a preservative to prevent mold growth for several days. Throw away if molded.
Apples	Trim away all signs of rot.
Jellies, jams, syrups	Lift out carefully, then use another clean spoon to remove and discard a larger portion from the surrounding area. If the mold is extensive, throw the food away.
Hard cheeses	Studies show that aflatoxin does not develop on hard cheeses under refrigeration. If they have been properly refrigerated, trim off the mold if it is not too extensive. For a margin of safety, trim off ½ inch extra cheese around and underneath the affected area. Keep the knife out of the mold itself. Rewrap in fresh packaging.
Soft and semisoft cheeses and other dairy products	Throw away soft cheeses such as cream cheese or Brie. Yogurt and sour cream should also be discarded.
Peanuts and other nuts	Throw away; do not eat moldy nuts.
Meats	Throw away visibly molded foods such as hot dogs, lunch meats, and cooked chicken. You can safely remove mold from old-fashioned dry, salt-cured hams and bacon if followed by a thorough washing.
Fruits and vegetables	Trim mold from firm vegetables and fruits. Cut an extra ½ inch from around and beneath the area of mold. Throw away molded small fruits, soft fruits, berries, and soft vegetables. If you use dry corn to make cornmeal or for animal feed, check carefully and do not use if it is moldy.

From Patrick R: *Beware the fungus among us,* Baton Rouge, La, 1993, Pennington Biomedical Research Center.

by molds found in rotten apples; and **fumonisin B-1,** produced by a mold that grows on corn. Once mold starts to grow, it does so quickly in the presence of air. Table 19-4 provides guidelines on the use of foods once mold growth has appeared.

IRRADIATION

Since the irradiation of food was proposed as a way to inactivate organisms responsible for food spoilage or food-borne illness, controversy has continued about the safety of the technique.

During the irradiation process the food is passed through a chamber in which it is bombarded with gamma rays. The gamma rays are released from rods of radioactive cobalt-60 or cesium-137 embedded in the chamber wall. Because these rays can kill most bacteria, insects, and molds normally responsible for many food-borne diseases, irradiation can make foods safe for an extended time. The technique does not make the food radioactive and does not form any harmful compounds in the food.

The level of exposure of the food to radiation is measured in rads (radiant absorbed dose), with a *gray* being the term used to designate 1000 rads and a kilogray being 1,000,000 rads. One kilogray considerably limits the viability of many organisms, and 4.75 to 8.0 kilograys kills *Salmonella* organisms, but larger doses of radiation are required to kill fungi and viruses.

Food irradiation is generally considered an effective, safe, and economical way of preserving food. It has received the endorsement of scientists and approval of government regulatory agencies. Because of the public's long-standing fear of anything associated with radioactivity, however, food retailers have had difficulty promoting the sale of irradiated food products. All individual foods that have been treated by gamma irradiation must carry the universal green "radura" symbol shown in Figure 19-2, although processed foods containing irradiated products need not carry this symbol. Other commercial deterrents to the use of irradiation are the high cost of the irradiation facilities and the detailed precautions required to prevent any risk of leaks or sabotage. Because these deterrents mean that only a small number of irradiation plants are likely to be constructed, they lead to the additional drawback of high transport costs in taking food to and from the plants. Currently, there is only one food irradiation facility in the United States.[18] To be a feasible means of controlling *Salmonella* and *Campylobacter* organisms in poultry (which accounted for 4 million cases of illness in 1992), a great many irradiation plants must be constructed throughout the country.

By 1994 the FDA had approved the use of irradiation in the treatment of spices (which often arrive contaminated with insects and bacteria); fresh pork (in

FIGURE 19-2

The "radura" symbol must be carried by all foods treated with gamma radiation, although it need not be carried by processed foods, which include irradiated ingredients.

which the control of *Trichinella spiralis* is essential); fresh produce such as potatoes, onions, tomatoes, mushrooms, and strawberries; and uncooked packaged poultry (40% of which is now contaminated with *Salmonella* organisms). Several states such as Maine, New Jersey, and New York, which have not yet been convinced of the safety and feasibility of food irradiation, have banned the sale of any irradiated food products other than spices. Some food processors and retailers have announced that they will not use any irradiated ingredients in their products. On the other hand, food irradiation has been approved in 37 countries for more than 40 products. Belgium, Holland, and France make most use of irradiation, using it on up to 10,000 tons of food each year.

Many factors contribute to concern about the advisability of approving the use of irradiated food products. For example, it is impossible to monitor the level of irradiation to which a food has been subjected. In addition, there are concerns about the possible formation of compounds of unknown toxicity as a result of the irradiation process. There is only minimal concern about possible effects of irradiation on the nutritive value of foods because any nutritive losses are similar to those caused by cooking or freezing. Food scientists maintain that irradiated food products are safe, even though the process causes the formation of "radiolytic" products that do not occur naturally in food. They believe that the radiolytic products are identical to those produced during cooking or other heat treatment of food.

PESTICIDES

The control of pests in agriculture production is essential to produce the quantities of high-quality and relatively low-cost food that we desire and have become accustomed to. The pests that must be controlled include animals such as insects and rodents; plant weeds; and microbial pathogens such as viruses, bacteria, and fungi, which adversely affect the quality of food products. The major method of controlling these organisms is the use of pesticides (pest killers), which can be chemical or biologic, natural, or synthetic. The most commonly used pesticides are the weed control agents known as herbicides (plant killers), followed by fungicides (fungus killers) and insecticides (insect killers). Rodentocides (rodent killers) and nematicides (worm killers) are used less frequently. Although the use of pesticides is usually attributed to agricultural practices, over half of all pesticide use is by hospitals, restaurants, termite control companies, and other nonagricultural users.

Although sulfur was used earlier than 1000 BC as an insecticide, the widespread use of insecticides began only in the late 1950s with the discovery and use of dichlorodiphenyltrichloroethane (DDT) and the development of aerial spraying and commercial sprayers. It was soon recognized that the protection of animals and humans required a system of integrated pest management (IPM), which considered the effects of a pesticide on the entire ecological system in which pests lived. The options available to control pests in an IPM program include the following:

- Physical methods such as temperature, light, and sound
- Cultural methods such as modified planting and harvesting times or modified tillage procedures
- Genetic methods to breed pest-resistant plants and animals or predators able to destroy specific pests
- Careful management of water and fertilizer use
- Biological control methods that rely on predators, parasites, and pathogens to control or destroy pests
- The use of chemical pesticides to control, reduce, or destroy pests
- Various preventive methods to prevent pests from becoming established in the environment

Because all pesticides are designed to destroy some organism, none is completely safe and without risk. The decision to use a pesticide should follow careful consideration of the risks and benefits. Such risk and benefit analyses are not easy to perform, particularly when vocal individuals who oppose pesticide use may think that their views are not adequately represented. The popular press, with the help of politicians and advocacy groups, has done much to "fan the fires" of anxiety among the public about the dangers of pesticides in the environment. The most widely publicized recent "exposés" have been the daminozide (ALAR) scare and the cranberry scare in which apples and cranberries were removed from sale for a short time because of concern about excessive chemical residues. Both of these scares raised considerable public anxiety about the possible carcinogenic properties of pesticides and chemicals used in fruit production. In contrast to the public's view of pesticides as the number one food safety issue, however, the scientific community generally views the risks from pesticide use as minimal.

> *In contrast to the public's view of pesticides as the number one food safety issue, the scientific community generally views the risks from pesticide use as minimal.*

The Environmental Protection Agency (EPA) has the final control over what level of exposure (usually referred to as the **tolerance level**) is safe, without health risk, and appropriate in both the short and long term. In arriving at a decision the EPA considers the **no observable effect level (NOEL)**, which is the highest dose at which no adverse effect is seen in animals, and the **acceptable daily intake (ADI),** which is 1% of the NOEL and is regarded as the maximal daily exposure that results in no appreciable risk to humans. The EPA bases its final judgment on what the available scientific information indicates about the benefits relative to the risks of using the chemical. It establishes criteria for how each pesticide can be used, on what crops it can be used, and in what amounts, in addition to who can apply it (usually certified and licensed applicators) and at what time in the growing season it can be applied. As a result of these regulatory controls, only small quantities of pesticide appear in our food supply.[8,9]

Until recently, regulatory agencies based their recommendations on acceptable levels of pesticides on information derived from studies of adults, which were extrapolated to the whole population. A National Academy of Sciences report in 1993 recommended that the federal government change some of its policies to provide greater protection to infants and children.[10] It pointed out that the current system does not take into account differences in pesticide exposure between adults and children. Nor does it consider that infants and children have growth rates and diets different from those of adults.

A "safe" level of intake of a pesticide is usually set at 1⁄100 or 1⁄1000 of the level at which the risk is estimated to be "negligible" compared with the benefits. In spite of attempts to document the levels considered acceptable or nonacceptable, there is considerable public debate about the rationale used, particularly in relation to the possible carcinogenic effects of several pesticides and other chemicals in the environment. The EPA has established **permissible tolerance levels** for the total residue of over 300 pesticides in food or feed in the United States. Monitoring of the food supply by the FDA (including both domestically produced and imported foods) has shown that the residues exceed these levels in less than 1% of the samples tested. In more than two thirds of samples no pesticides were detectable. Foods found to contain more than the permissible tolerance level of a pesticide are removed from the food supply until the shipper or producer provides evidence that the food meets acceptable standards.

The use of pesticides on a large number of food products including apples, grapes, tomatoes, citrus fruits, and pineapple is threatened by a 1992 court ruling that the EPA's efforts to set these negligible risk tolerance levels were in violation of the **Delaney clause.** This clause was part of a 1958 amendment to the Food, Drug and Cosmetic Act of 1938, the basic statute that governs food regulation in the United States. The Delaney clause states that "no food or color additive may be deemed safe that has been found to cause cancer when ingested by man or animals." This forced EPA to revert to a **zero tolerance** standard for pesticide residues in food unless the Food, Drug and Cosmetic Act is amended or administrative changes are pursued by EPA.[9, 11]

ANTIBIOTICS

Antibiotics are chemicals synthesized by certain microorganisms that inhibit the growth of other microorganisms. They were originally used in medicine to control bacterial and fungal diseases in humans. Adding antibiotics to animal feed at levels below that used for medicinal purposes has a growth-promoting or growth-enhancing effect on the animals. The mechanism of this effect is unknown, although several theories have been proposed. The currently favored theory is that antibiotics reduce the number of nutrient-requiring microorganisms living in the animals' gastrointestinal tracts, thus releasing additional nutrients to promote the growth of the animals. More than 100 antibiotics have been approved for use in animal feed in the United States, including penicillins, sulfonamides, and tetracyclines. This use of antibiotics accounts for almost half of the antibiotics used. It is estimated that two thirds to three fourths of all domestic animals raised for food in the United States have been treated with antibiotics at some time.

The widespread addition of antibiotics to animal feed has provoked concern about the safety of the practice and possible effects of antibiotic residues within food. One of the major concerns is the possibility that certain pathogenic microorganisms may develop a resistance to certain widely used antibiotics and thus be difficult to control in humans. There is also concern about possible allergic reactions to antibiotic residues in food, which may vary in severity from rashes to potentially fatal **anaphylactic shock.**

To minimize the risk of undesirable effects from the use of antibiotics in animal feed, the FDA regulates the allowable dose in animal feed, the time for which the antibiotic must be withdrawn from feed before slaughter, and the tolerance levels for antibiotics in animal products. The USDA Food Safety and Inspection Service is responsible for analyzing samples of meat and poultry to ensure that they comply with FDA standards.

HORMONES

Hormones are increasingly used in animal husbandry to modify animal metabolism, giving rise to considerable public concern and controversy. Implants of steroid hormones are used to produce larger and leaner animals. The protein hormone **bovine Somatotropin (bST),** or bovine growth hormone **(bGH),** was approved in 1993 for administration to dairy cattle, increasing their milk production efficiency by as much as 20%. The use of a growth hormone, pST, to produce leaner pork products is under consideration.

FDA regulations require that the amount of any hormone administered to an animal must not exceed 1% of the amount normally produced by the animal. Because only a fraction of any orally administered hormone is absorbed by the animal, the possibility that people eating the eventual products will ingest significantly increased amounts is negligible. Because the hormones used may be produced by genetic engineering, however, some consumers are more concerned about the added hormone than about its naturally produced counterpart.

Because bST is a protein, almost 90% of it is destroyed by denaturation resulting from the heat used in pasteurization of milk. Naturally occurring bST has been studied for over 60 years, and bST produced by genetic engineering has been available since 1980. Scientists agree that administering extra bST to dairy cows does not alter the taste, composition, safety, or nutritional quality of the milk produced. They also find that the level of bST in milk is the same in milk produced by supplemented and unsupplemented cows. bST, whether supplemental or naturally present, increases the production of another protein hormone called insulin-like growth factor (IGF-1). This bovine hormone is digested when consumed, however, and there is no evidence to suggest that it is biologically active in humans.[12] The safety of the use of bST has been confirmed by a wide range of government and professional organizations. Because there are no identifiable differences in milk produced from bST-supplemented and unsupplemented cows, the FDA has ruled that it is unnecessary to label milk produced by supplemented cows.

Scientists agree that administering extra bST to dairy cows does not alter the taste, composition, safety, or nutritional quality of the milk produced. They also find that the level of bST in milk is the same in milk produced by supplemented or unsupplemented cows.

NATURAL TOXICANTS

The Food, Drug and Cosmetic Act states that a food is *adulterated* if it contains any poisonous or deleterious substance that may render it injurious to health.[11] If, however, the substance is present in the food naturally or is technologically unavoidable, rather than having been added, the food is not considered adulterated if the amount of the substance present does not ordinarily render it injurious to health.

Contrary to popular opinion, many foods that have traditionally been considered free from any harmful components contain small amounts of naturally occurring chemicals that have toxic properties when consumed in large amounts. Few of these traditional foods are consumed in sufficient quantities to be cause for any concern. Other less traditional foods such as herbal teas, particularly those made from comfrey, sassafras, and chamomile, contain toxicants at levels that are cause for concern. In particular, they have been associated with problems such as anaphylactic shock, cancer, and cardiac arrhythmias.

Natural toxicants not considered a threat to health in the amounts consumed in most Western diets include the following:

- **Glucosinolates** are found primarily in foods of the cruciferous family (cabbage, brussels sprouts, cauliflower, and turnips). At high concentrations (seldom found in modern varieties of vegetables) these can be digested to chemicals that promote goiter. At lower concentrations, however, they may protect against certain cancers, especially of the colon and rectum.

Adulterated Food Characteristics

- Contains poisonous or deleterious substances, filth, or decomposed or diseased material
- Has had material substance subtracted or omitted
- Has had inferiority concealed
- Has been handled so that it contains adulterants

- **Oxalates** are found in rhubarb, tea, cocoa, and spinach. They are metabolic precursors of kidney stones and interfere with the absorption of calcium when taken in high amounts.
- **Cyanogenic glycosides** are found in several hundred plants, including lima beans, cassava, apple seeds, apricot kernels, and several grains. They break down during digestion to yield hydrogen cyanide. Hydrogen cyanide is a highly toxic chemical capable of causing neurological damage. Its presence is usually not a threat because cultures that consume large amounts of foods that can produce it have found ways to prepare the foods that prevent hydrogen cyanide formation or have bred new, safe varieties of plants such as lima beans.
- **Solanine** is a compound, chemically classified as **glycoalkaloid,** found near the green skin of some potatoes (where they have been exposed to the light) and in potato sprouts. It is a toxic compound that interferes with the nervous system. Potatoes containing over 20 mg of solanine cannot be used commercially. If the green parts of potatoes are removed, however, the remaining unaffected parts are safe to eat.
- **Biologically active amines** such as tyramine are found in some foods, notably aged cheeses, red wine, chicken, liver, and pickled herring. These amines are normally metabolized by pathways beginning with the action of the enzyme **monoamine oxidase.**[12] Drugs that inhibit the activity of monoamine oxidase are prescribed for the treatment of depression and other psychiatric disorders. People taking these monoamine oxidase inhibitors are at risk of high blood pressure, headaches, and intracerebral hemorrhage if they eat foods containing large amounts of biologically active amines. **Heterocyclic amines** are produced when some foods are cooked, especially if exposed to flames. **Nitrosamines** are formed from nitrates and nitrites in foods, either during drying and cooking or when the food is in the gastrointestinal tract. These heterocyclic amines and nitrosamines are known carcinogens that may be responsible for some cancers of the esophagus and stomach. Vegetables are the main source of dietary nitrates and nitrites, but nitrites are also used as food additives to preserve the color of meats, inhibit oxidation, and prevent toxicity resulting from *Clostridium botulinum.*

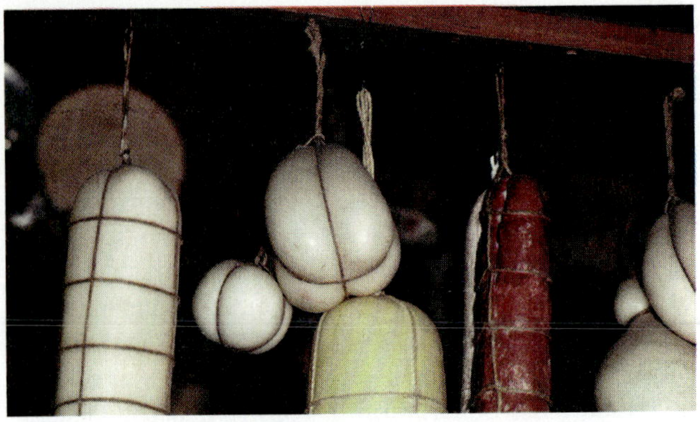

Cured meats rely on nitrites to preserve their color. The National Cancer Institute advises moderation because these foods pose some cancer risk.

Even though they are not considered to pose any threat to health, many of these natural toxicants are present in food in considerably greater amounts than are pesticide residues.

ENVIRONMENTAL CONTAMINANTS

Environmental contaminants can enter the food supply from exposure of the food to air, water or soil that has been contaminated by industrial wastes, and other environmental pollutants. Many of the chemicals concerned, such as mercury, DDT, and lead, are not degraded by plant or animal metabolism. Once they enter the food chain, they tend to accumulate in specific parts of the body such as the liver, brain, or storage lipids. The most common environmental contaminants are the "heavy" metals (so called because of their high atomic weight), particularly mercury, lead, and cadmium.

The highest concentrations of mercury are found in tuna and swordfish, although fruit, meats, and dairy products also contain detectable amounts. Lead enters the food chain primarily through water that becomes contaminated by lead pipes and solder. The amount of lead in the environment has been greatly reduced by measures such as the shift from leaded to unleaded gas, the banning of lead-based house paints, and control of the disposal of batteries containing lead. Nevertheless, detectable levels of lead are still found in many foods. Cadmium is a highly toxic mineral that enters the food supply via the soil. Its most obvious effect is kidney dysfunction. Fruits and vegetables grown on soils that have been heavily fertilized with superphosphate fertilizers have higher cadmium levels than those grown on soil with less exposure to these fertilizers.[14]

FOOD ADDITIVES

The use of additives in food is governed by the Food, Drug and Cosmetic Act. This act was first passed as the Pure Food and Drug Act in 1906, when it focused on the manufacture and sale of adulterated and misbranded foods. A 1938 amendment to the act was designed to protect the health of the public while at the same time improving the food supply through the use of beneficial additives. It required any company wishing to use an additive to provide proof of its safety, and it permitted the addition to food of substances that are safe at the levels required for their intended use. The amended act defined a food as *illegal* or *adulterated* if it bears or contains a poisonous or deleterious substance that may render it injurious to health, whether that substance is added or is naturally occurring. A 1960 amendment to the act addressed the risk-benefit balance of the use of substances that add color to food, drugs, or cosmetics. This amendment permits companies to apply for "tolerances" for the use of any color that is scientifically considered safe under normal conditions of use.

Food additives are all substances added (intentionally or unintentionally) to basic food products. They include anything added during the production, processing, treatment, packaging, transport, and storage of a food. In general, food additives are used to decrease the risk of contamination by certain microbes, maintain or improve nutritional quality, enhance appearance, increase shelf life, reduce waste, or contribute to convenience.

All food additives present in food sold to the public must now be approved for safety by the FDA or, in the case of meat and poultry, the USDA. Before an additive is approved it must be demonstrated that it does the following:

- Serves a useful purpose
- Does not disguise faulty processing, conceal damage or spoilage, or in any way deceive the consumer
- Does not decrease the nutritional value of the product
- Could not be replaced by good manufacturing practices

The FDA also evaluates the minimal amounts of additives required to fulfill their intended purpose. The main classes of food additives and their functions are shown in Table 19-5. For regulatory purposes the FDA categorizes food additives into the following six groups[14]:

- Those described as **generally recognized as safe (GRAS),** meaning that they have been used for many years without any known adverse effects (for example, salt, sugar, and vinegar).
- **Regulated food additives** that have been found to be safe on the basis of rigorous screening by the FDA. This group includes additives used to improve or enhance the color of food and nitrates used in curing ham, bacon, and corned beef to inhibit the formation of the botulism toxin.
- **Prior sanction additives,** that is, those approved by the FDA before the implementation of the Delaney clause, which required that no additive known to be carcinogenic at any level in any animal may be approved. If the safety of such additives is questioned, they must be subjected to further review.
- **Indirect food additives** added unintentionally during processing.
- **Radiation-induced additives,** which are chemical compounds formed in food as the result of radiation.
- **Feed additives,** which are chemicals present in food because they have been added to the rations of animals used for human food.

FOOD PACKAGING

Food packaging is designed to protect food against chemical, physical, or biological damage during storage, transportation, and retailing. It protects against the entrance and loss of moisture, oxygen, or other gases; against physical damage resulting from light, dirt, dust, and mechanical stresses; and against contamination by microorganisms and insects. Packaging material must be strong enough to prevent damage and contamination; must not convey odors, flavors, or toxic chemicals to the food; and must be resistant to any heating, freezing, and refrigeration during processing and storage. Recently, emphasis has also been placed on the ability of packaging to prevent tampering with the food and on the biodegradable qualities of the materials used in packaging.

The major packaging materials include glass, paper, metal, and plastics, each of which has its own merits and limitations. Plastics often best meet consumers' desires for convenience, adaptability, and long shelf life without the use of additives. However, they may be opposed on environmental grounds and also raise concerns about the migration of chemicals from the packaging material to the food, which might affect the safety, flavor, or odor of the food.[15] The FDA is responsible for regulating the safety of packaging materials.

TABLE 19-5

Additive classes and functions

ADDITIVE CLASS	FUNCTION
Anticaking/free-flowing agents	Prevent lumping and caking by absorbing moisture
Antimicrobial agents	Prevent the growth of bacteria, molds, fungi, and yeast
Antioxidants	Prevent flavor and color changes and retard rancidity and deterioration from exposure to oxygen
Colors and adjuncts	Provide, preserve, or enhance the color of a food
Curing and pickling agents	Impart a unique flavor or color to a food; often increase shelf life and stability
Dough conditioners	Modify starch and gluten to improve baking quality of yeast-leavened dough
Drying agents	Absorb moisture
Emulsifiers	Prevent the separation of oil and water in food
Enzymes	Improve food processing and the quality of finished foods
Firming agents	Maintain the shape or crispness in fruits and vegetables
Flavor enhancers	Supplement, enhance, or modify the original flavor or aroma of a food without contributing flavors of their own
Flavoring agents and adjuvants	Impart or help impart a taste or an aroma in food
Flour treating agents	Improve the color or baking qualities of flour
Formulation aids	Promote or produce a desired physical state or texture
Fumigants	Control insects or pests
Humectants	Promote retention of moisture
Leavening agents	Produce or stimulate CO_2 production in baked goods
Lubricants and release agents	Prevent sticking of food to contact surfaces
Nonnutritive sweeteners	Provide less than 2% of the caloric value of sucrose per equivalent unit of sweetening capacity when used to sweeten foods
Nutritive sweeteners	Provide greater than 2% of the caloric value of sucrose per equivalent unit of sweetening capacity when used to sweeten foods
Oxidizing and reducing agents	Produce a more stable product
pH control agents	Change or maintain active acidity or alkalinity
Processing aids	Enhance the appeal or utility of a food or food component
Propellants, aerating agents, and gases	Supply force to expel a product
Sequestrants	Increase product quality and stability by combining with metal ions to form a soluble metal complex
Solvents and vehicles	Extract or dissolve another substance
Stabilizers and thickeners	Produce viscous solutions or dispersions to impart body, improve consistency, or stabilize emulsions
Surface active agents	Modify surface properties of liquid food components
Surface-finishing agents	Increase palatability, preserve gloss, and inhibit discoloration
Synergists	Produce a total effect different from or greater than the sum of the effects produced by the individual food ingredients
Texturizers	Affect the feel or appearance of the food

From Burgess WD, editor: *Producer through consumer: Partner to a safe food supply,* West Lafayette, Ind, 1993, Purdue University, Cooperative Extension Service.

IMPORTED FOODS

Government agencies must ensure that imported foods meet domestic standards of wholesomeness and safety. They must also ensure that imported foods are not adulterated or misbranded at their point of entry into the United States. Imported food is considered *adulterated* if it is filthy, putrid, decomposed, or spoiled; contains harmful microorganisms; or contains any other harmful substances such as pesticides, residues, heavy metals, or industrial chemicals. It is considered *misbranded* if it does not comply with relevant standards of identity, contains substances not listed on the label, or does not contain some of the substances listed on the label.

The 1993 accord reached among 103 nations to revise the 1947 General Agreement on Tariffs and Trade (GATT) includes provisions that will strengthen food safety standards worldwide. It is possible, however, that this accord will lead to a weakening of the current stringent requirements within the United States and Canada. The food safety standards of different countries are being steadily harmonized on the basis of internationally accepted scientific principles. It is proposed to base this harmonization on the food safety standards set by the **Codex Alimentarius,** a United Nations organization founded in 1982 and funded by the World Health Organization and the Food and Agricultural Organization.

Common Errors in Interpreting Scientific Reports

SCIENTIFIC TERMS	LAY INTERPRETATION
Contributes to	Causes
Suggests	Means
Indicates	Proves
Is associated with	Causes
Some scientists believe	All scientists agree
At least in some people	Probably in all people
Animal studies show	Human studies indicate
High intakes increase X	Low intakes decrease X
Reduced or low	Eliminated or none
Increased or high	As much as possible

RISK ASSESSMENT

Risk assessment in food safety issues is a major concern of the USDA and the FDA, the agencies primarily responsible for the safety of the food supply.[17] Risk assessment is essentially the process of estimating the probability that an adverse event will occur. When information on the direct risks to humans is available, as in the case of reportable food-borne illnesses, risk assessment can be fairly precise. However, when human data are unavailable, as in the case of pesticide residues, potential health risks can be estimated only by extrapolating from high-dose animal experiments to humans. The results of such indirect risk assessments are much less reliable than those based on human data. Scientists use many conservative assumptions and "worse-case" estimates to ensure that a risk is not underestimated. Although scientists are now debating how to improve risk assessment, most agree that a more pressing problem is how the estimates of risk are communicated to the public. If they report that a food additive, for example, carries a lifetime one-in-a-million risk of causing cancer, they are concerned that this is interpreted literally to mean that out of 250 million Americans, 250 develop cancer from the specific risk concerned. In reality, because any officially determined risk is based on various worst-case assumptions, the actual risk is much lower and may even be zero. Common errors on the part of the public or the media in the interpretation of scientific reports are indicated in the box above.

BIOTECHNOLOGY IN FOOD PRODUCTION

The widespread use of biotechnology to transfer desirable characteristics between different species of plants and animals has given rise to public anxiety about the safety of both the procedures and the bioengineered products that result. Biotechnology is defined in the broadest sense as the production of any article of commerce by biological processes other than traditional agriculture or those that occur without human intervention. Cross-breeding of both animals and plants and the preservation of food through fermentation by microbiological enzymes are long-standing and widely accepted examples of biotechnology. The more recent introduction of genetic engineering (also known as *gene cloning* and *recombinant DNA technology*) to improve both animal and plant species has met with considerable resistance and caution. In general, genetic engineering involves transferring genes among organisms, allowing selected organisms to be "programmed" to make proteins they normally do not produce. The proteins encoded by the transferred genes can be the desired product itself, or they can change the engineered organism's characteristics in a more subtle way by increasing its yield and resistance to pests.

The benefits of biotechnology to agriculture include increased crop and livestock survival, enhanced nutritional quality of foods, increased industrial productivity, and reduced need for pesticides and herbicides. Examples of the application of biotechnology in the food supply include the development of a tomato that ripens more slowly, giving it a longer shelf life while retaining the characteristic fresh tomato flavor, and the production of pork from hogs injected with porcine somatotropin (pST), which has a lower fat and high lean content and is produced with 15% to 35% greater efficiency in the use of feed. Similarly, the FDA-approved chymotrypsin, usually known as *rennin* (used in making cheese), can be produced in large quantities by bacteria without the impurities associated with the chymotrypsin extracted from the stomach of veal calves.[19,21]

The greatest concerns about the use of biotechnology in food production are focused on the following possibilities:

- It may give rise to new food allergens by changing the chemical characteristics of foods.
- It may make the food more susceptible to microbial contamination or a better substrate for the production of toxins.
- It may reduce the nutritional value of the food.
- It may lead to the formation of substances in the food whose toxic properties have not been characterized.

It is proposed that foods that represent any safety or health risk or have undergone a significant change in composition should carry a label indicating that the food has been produced using genetic engineering. The FDA does not routinely conduct premarket reviews of all new plant varieties because of the limited nature of most modifications, but it does conduct a review whenever the

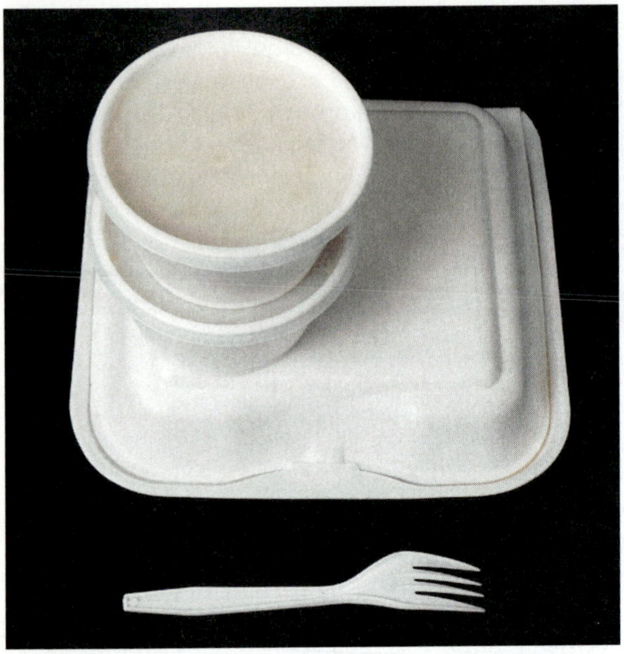

Packaging is evaluated on its ability to protect food and more recently on its environmental impact.

nature of the change raises a safety question that the FDA must resolve to protect public health. The FDA has a comprehensive protocol for the safety assessment of new varieties.[22]

There is general agreement that biotechnology has much to offer in the worldwide battle against hunger and disease. It is important, however, to avoid both the overeager introduction of the new methods and, at the other extreme, inappropriate caution simply because the methods are new.[20]

FUTURE CONCERNS REGARDING FOOD SAFETY

Both the food industry and the FDA have tried to identify food safety issues they believe will attract the attention of the scientific community in the next decade. The FDA, aware of its responsibility to ensure the safety of the U. S. food supply, is trying to identify sensitive techniques to provide reasonable certainty that foods cause no harm. It is also concerned about issues raised by the proliferation of new packaging materials and techniques; the increased use of macronutrient substitutes in low-calorie and reduced-calorie foods; and the imminent increase in the so-called designer or novel foods. The opportunities for growth of microbial organisms in the controlled-atmosphere and low-oxygen packaging being developed present a regulatory challenge. Similarly, the internationalization of the food industry will require sophisticated sampling and surveillance of imported packaged foods.[23] The food industry has identified microbiological food safety, pesticide residue controls, risk assessment, and the federal government's role in food safety as the issues of greatest concern.

ISSUES AND OPINIONS

Designing Foods by Using Biotechnology

by Terry D. Etherton
Professor, The Pennsylvania State University

The last 15 years have seen some of the most remarkable biological science discoveries in the history of humankind. These scientific advances have been used widely to develop novel biotechnologies that will markedly affect food production. Numerous benefits will be realized by integrating these emerging biotechnologies into agriculture; they will increase productivity, enhance productive efficiency (unit of food produced per unit of resource input), alter food composition, and result in foods that are more nutritious and of higher quality. Based on current projections, many of these technologies will be integrated into food production and food processing systems between now and the end of the decade.*

The development and use of these novel technologies for food production and processing have many important implications for the consumer. In addition, it is important that technological innovation continues in agricultural research to enable food production to keep pace with the expanding world population. To illustrate this point, it has been estimated that the amount of food needed over the next 40 years to feed the growing population is equal to the amount previously produced in the history of humankind.† Some of the biotechnologies under development and the benefits they will provide to the consumer are discussed in detail in a recent publication from the U.S. Congress, Office of Technology Assessment.*

WHAT IS BIOTECHNOLOGY?

Although biotechnology has been touted as a recent development, it has been used for thousands of years to produce foods such as bread, fermented foods, and beverages. Biotechnology, broadly defined, involves the use of any living organisms or processes to make or modify products, to improve plants or animals, or to develop microorganisms for specific uses.* The modern era of biotechnology began in 1973 when scientists cut a gene (a small piece of DNA) out of a cell from *Xenopus* and "spliced" it into a tiny bacterial chromosome (plasmid). The ability to specifically cut and recombine genes led to the development of what is now known as *recombinant DNA technology.* Although the terms *biotechnology* and *genetic engineering* are frequently used interchangeably, biotechnology is more than simply splicing genes. It is a vast array of techniques and processes that includes recombinant DNA technology, molecular biology, protein purification and sequencing, protein engineering, animal and plant cell culture, root culture, monoclonal antibody technology, and cell fusion techniques. Biotechnology has been applied not only to food production and processing, but also to the development of human and veterinary diagnostic and health care products and novel approaches for degrading toxic and solid waste materials, to an increase in mineral and oil recovery, and the production of fuels that will be alternatives to petroleum-derived fuels.

EMERGING PLANT BIOTECHNOLOGIES

The application of biotechnology to crop agriculture has resulted in a rapid increase in the number of genetically modified crops. The ability to genetically modify crops has resulted in varieties that are more resistant to specific herbicides, which allows the application of more effective, environmentally acceptable, and cost-

* U.S. Congress, Office of Technology Assessment: *A new technological era for American agriculture,* OTA-F474, Washington, DC, 1992, U.S. Government Printing Office.
† Bauman DE: *J Dairy Sci* 75:3432, 1992.

effective chemicals to control weeds. In addition, a number of transgenic plants have been developed that contain genes to control insects and diseases in ways that may obviate or reduce the need for chemical control. Genetically engineered crops have been developed in which oil content is increased or certain fatty acids in the seed oil have been eliminated. The technology is at hand to reduce processing costs of certain plant products by eliminating allergenic or off-flavor components. Research is ongoing to develop plants to produce industrial feedstocks and even human pharmaceutical products.

EMERGING ANIMAL BIOTECHNOLOGIES

A number of biotechnologies are being developed that will have a marked impact on animal agriculture. With respect to food production, these biotechnologies have been developed to improve efficiency of animal production and reduce carcass fat.[‡] The need to alter carcass composition (increase muscle and decrease fat) is important for two reasons: (1) as animals grow, the proportion of fat in body weight gain increases, which adversely affects both growth rate and feed efficiency (resulting in a negative economic impact), and (2) dietary, total, and saturated fats play a large role in the risk of chronic disease. Because the risk of chronic disease increases as total fat and saturated fat intake increases, it is imperative to develop and implement new strategies to reduce carcass fat that are more cost-effective and efficient than the current practice of trimming excess carcass fat.

The two animal biotechnologies that are projected to be among the first commercially used in the United States are bovine somatotropin (bST) and porcine somatotropin (pST). In November 1993 the Food and Drug Administration (FDA) approved the commercial use of bST for dairy farmers. When administered to dairy cows, bST increases milk production 15% and enhances productive efficiency (about a 10% increase in milk and feed).[†] When pST is administered to growing pigs, growth rate increases by 10% to 20% and carcass fat content can be reduced by as much as 70%. This change in growth rate is accompanied by a marked increase in muscle growth (maximal increase, 50%) and productive efficiency (body weight gain and feed efficiency are increased by 15% to 35%). Despite stories that have appeared in the popular press, the scientific evidence overwhelmingly shows that these biotechnologies are safe for the consumer and target animals.[‡]

SUMMARY

As the world population continues to expand, advances in technology that increase productivity and efficiency of food production will be imperative to keep pace with the increasing population. Many new and beneficial biotechnologies will be approved for use in the United States in this decade. These biotechnologies are safe and efficacious and thus will benefit society.

† Bauman DE: *J Dairy Sci* 75:3432, 1992.

‡ Etherton TD, Kris-Etherton PM, Mills EW: *J Am Diet Assoc* 93:177, 1993.

BY NOW YOU SHOULD KNOW

- Foods contain a variety of chemicals and nutrients. The chemicals may occur naturally or be added intentionally or unintentionally during processing and preparation.
- Food pathogens are the most common causes of food-borne illnesses.
- Food can become contaminated with pathogens during storage and preparation in the home.
- Various governmental agencies are responsible for regulating the production and marketing of food to ensure the safety of the food supply.
- Scientific experts consider pesticide residues, environmental contaminants, and food additives to present minimal risks to consumers but consider that the activities of food pathogens present great risks to consumers.
- New technologies, such as food irradiation and biotechnology, offer tremendous opportunities to ensure the safety of the food supply and maximize the quality of the food supply.
- Consumers consider pesticide residues to be their most important food safety concern, whereas food scientists rank food-borne pathogens the greatest threat to health.

STUDY QUESTIONS

1. Identify the major agents responsible for causing food-borne illnesses.
2. Distinguish between food-borne bacterial infection and intoxication.
3. What governmental agencies have responsibility for monitoring the safety of our food supply?
4. Identify the following terms: *acceptable dietary intake, no observable effect level, radura symbol, natural toxicants, food irradiation, Delaney clause,* and *Good Manufacturing Practices.*
5. What are the major categories of pesticides used in agriculture?
6. What are the purpose and the basis of concern about the use of antibiotics and hormones in feeding animals used for food? Are they warranted?

~ CRITICAL ANALYSIS ~

1. Many restaurants offer salad bars that are in fact much more than salad bars. The variety of foods offered allows for some interesting strategies for assuring food safety and sanitation. However, the informed and alert diner also should be a major line of defense against food-borne illness. Consider the following foods and their conditions on a food bar. In the space next to each of the foods, write whether you would consider that food safe to eat. If the food is unsafe, state why.

FOOD	SAFE/UNSAFE (IF UNSAFE, WHY)
1. Potato salad in a bowl surrounded by water from melted ice	____________
2. Well-done meat balls kept in a steam table tray with a cover	____________
3. Cream of vegetable soup that is lukewarm upon tasting it	____________
4. Ranch salad dressing in a tall container; the container is in a bed of ice but the ice surrounds only the very bottom portion of the container	____________
5. Shredded carrots in a container surrounded by ice	____________
6. Raw fish wrapped in seaweed	____________
7. Pizza bread topped with cheese that does not feel hot	____________
8. Soft-serve ice cream or yogurt that melts (i.e., does not hold its shape) as it is dispensed from the machine	____________

~ REFERENCES ~

1. Lechowich RV: Current concerns in food safety. In Finley JW, Robinson SF, Armstrong DJ, editors: *Food safety assessment,* American Chemical Society Symposium Series No 484, Washington DC, 1992, American Chemical Society.
2. Foster EM: Is there a food safety crisis? *Food Technol* 37:(8):82, 1982.
3. Burgess WD, editor: *Producer through consumer: partners to a safe food supply,* West Lafayette, Ind, 1993, Purdue University Cooperative Extension Service.
4. Rigby D: Food-borne listeriosis—a review, *J N Z Diet Assoc* 47(1):24, 1993.
5. Doyle MP: *Escherichia coli* O157:H7 and its significance in foods, *Int J Food Microbiol* 12:289, 1991.
6. Watier L, Richardson S, Herbert B: *Salmonella einteritidis infection in France and the United States:* characterization by a deterministic model, *Am J Public Health* 83(12):1694, 1993.
7. St. Louis ME and others: The emergence of grade A eggs as a major source of *Salmonella enteritidis* infections: new implications for the control of salmonellosis, *JAMA* 14:2103, 1988.
8. National Research Council: *Regulating pesticides in food: the Delaney paradox,* Washington DC, 1987, National Academy Press.
9. Institute of Food Technologists: The risk/benefit concept as applied to food, *Food Technol* 42(3):119, 1988.
10. Board of Environmental Studies and Toxicology: *Pesticides in the diets of infants and children,* Washington, DC, 1993, National Academy of Sciences.
11. Winter CK: Pesticide residues and the Delaney clause, *Food Technol* 47(7):81, 1993.
12. Daughaday WH, Barbano DM: Bovine somatotropin supplementation in dairy cows, *JAMA* 264:1003, 1990.
13. Ames BN, Magaw R, Gold LS: Ranking possible carcinogenic hazards, *Science* 236:271, 1987.
14. Hatchcock IN, Rader J: Food additives, contaminants and natural toxins. In Shils ME, Olson JA, Shike M, editors: *Modern nutrition in health and disease,* ed 8, Philadelphia, 1994, Lea & Febiger.
15. Middlekauff RD: Regulating the safety of food, *Food Technol* 43(9):296, 1989.

16. Fox RA: Plastic packaging—the consumer preference of tomorrow, *Food Technol* 43(12):84, 1989.

17. Expert Panel on Food Safety and Nutrition, Institute of Food Technology: Government regulation of food safety: interaction of scientific and societal forces, *Food Technol* 46(1):73, 1992.

18. Pazczola D: Irradiated poultry makes U.S. debut in Midwest and Florida markets, *Food Technol* 47(11):89, 1993.

19. Council on Scientific Affairs: American Medical Association, Biotechnology and the American agricultural industry, *JAMA* 265:1429, 1991.

20. Hall RL: Food safety and biotechnology, *Nutr Today* 26(3):15, 1991.

21. Etherton TD: The efficacy and safety of growth hormone for animal agriculture, *J Clin Endocrinol Metabol* 72:957A, 1991.

22. Kessler DA and others: The safety of foods developed by biotechnology, *Science* 256:1747, 1992.

23. Life Sciences Research Office: *Emerging issues in food safety and quality for the next decade* Bethesda, Md, 1991, Federation of American Societies for Experimental Biology.

ADDITIONAL READINGS

Expert Panel on Food Safety and Nutrition, Institute of Food Technologists: Bacteria associated with food-borne diseases, *Food Technol* 42(4):1, 1988.

Finley JW, Robinson SF, Armstrong DJ, editors: *Food safety assessment,* Washington DC, 1992, American Chemical Society.

Food and Drug Administration: Backgrounder statement: biotechnology of food, *Nutr Today* 29:28, 1994.

Food and Drug Administration: Genetically engineered foods: fears and facts, *FDA Consumer* 27:10, 1993.

Giese J: Antimicrobials: assuring food safety, *Food Technol* 48(6):102, 1994.

Hatchcock JN: Nutritional toxicology: basic principles and actual problems, *Food Addit Contam* 7:512, 1990.

National Research Council: Toxicants occurring naturally in foods, Washington DC, 1973, National Academy Press.

Trebole E: *Food safety, additives, and contaminants,* San Marcos, Calif, 1991, Nutrition Dimension.

World Health Organization, Consultation on Food Irradiation: *Safety and nutritional adequacy of irradiated food,* Geneva, Switzerland, 1994, World Health Organization.

Appendixes

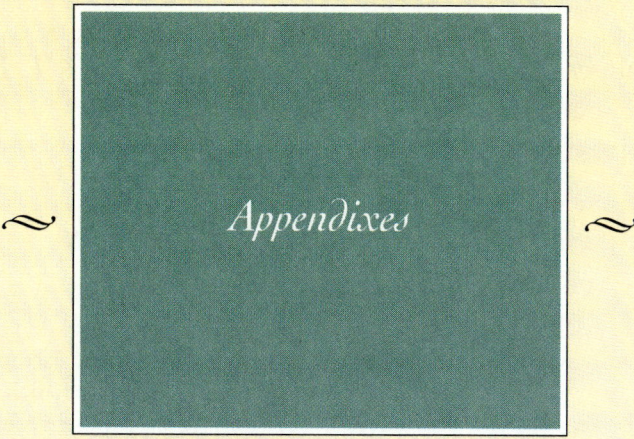

APPENDIX A

CHEMISTRY AND LIFE

If we examine the human body to find out what it is made of and how it works, we soon discover distinct parts that play specific roles in keeping the body alive and working properly. The most obvious parts of the body are its **organs,** such as the brain, heart, lungs, and stomach. An organ is defined as a distinct part of the body that performs some specific function. Several different organs often work together within a **system,** such as the digestive system or the circulatory system. On closer look with the aid of microscopes, it can be found that every organ is composed of living **cells,** each one a tiny self-contained unit of life. Cells differ in size, shape, and in the chemical processes that occur within them. A collection of cells of the same type is known as a *tissue,* and most organs contain several different kinds of tissue. When cells are examined in detail with electron microscopes and by chemical analysis, we find that they are intricate chemical machines. Cells are made entirely of chemicals, and everything they do is sustained by a network of interconnected chemical reactions, known collectively as the **metabolism** of the cell. All chemicals are derived from **atoms,** and all atoms are composed of **subatomic particles** known as **protons, neutrons** and **electrons** (Figure A-1).

PRINCIPLES OF CHEMISTRY

ATOMS, MOLECULES, AND IONS

The fundamental particles of chemistry are the 92 different types of atoms that occur naturally. Any substance composed of only one type of atom is called an **element,** and the names of the different elements and therefore of the different kinds of atoms are listed in the Periodic Table (Figure 1-1). Atoms themselves are composed of the three kinds of subatomic particles known as **protons, neutrons,** and **electrons.** The protons and neutrons are clustered together in the central **nucleus** of an atom, and the electrons move around within regions of space known as orbitals, which surround the nucleus. The protons carry a positive electric charge of +1 and the electrons carry a negative electric charge of –1. Because all atoms have equal numbers of protons and electrons, all atoms are electrically neutral overall, meaning that their positive and negative charges cancel out each other. An atom of any element is identified by the number of protons it contains, (known as the element's **atomic number**). For example, hydrogen has an atomic number of 1 (all hydrogen atoms contain one proton), whereas carbon has an atomic number of 6 (all carbon atoms contain six protons).

Two other kinds of particles derived from atoms are found in chemicals, including foods. **Molecules** are particles that contain two or more atoms chemically bonded together. **Ions** are particles that, unlike atoms, have an overall electric charge because of an imbalance in the number of protons and electrons they contain. Ions can be derived from either atoms or molecules when the atoms or molecules either lose electrons (to become positively charged ions) or gain electrons (to become negatively charged ions). All of the foods we consume and all of the chemicals the body makes from these foods are composed of a mixture of atoms, molecules, and ions. In nutrition and other biological sciences, the term *molecules* is often loosely used to refer to particles that may be true molecules, individual atoms, or ions. This less rigorous usage prevents the awkwardness of constantly distinguishing among atoms, molecules, and ions.

ENERGY

In addition to containing protons, neutrons, and electrons, atoms (and therefore molecules and ions) contain the more subtle property known as **energy.** Energy is formally defined as "the ability to do work." Physicists say work is done when a **force** is applied through some distance. This means that the energy of a system is a property of the system that is able to "make changes

FIGURE A-1

Deconstruction of the body into systems, organs, tissues, cells, chemicals, atoms, protons, neutrons, and electrons.

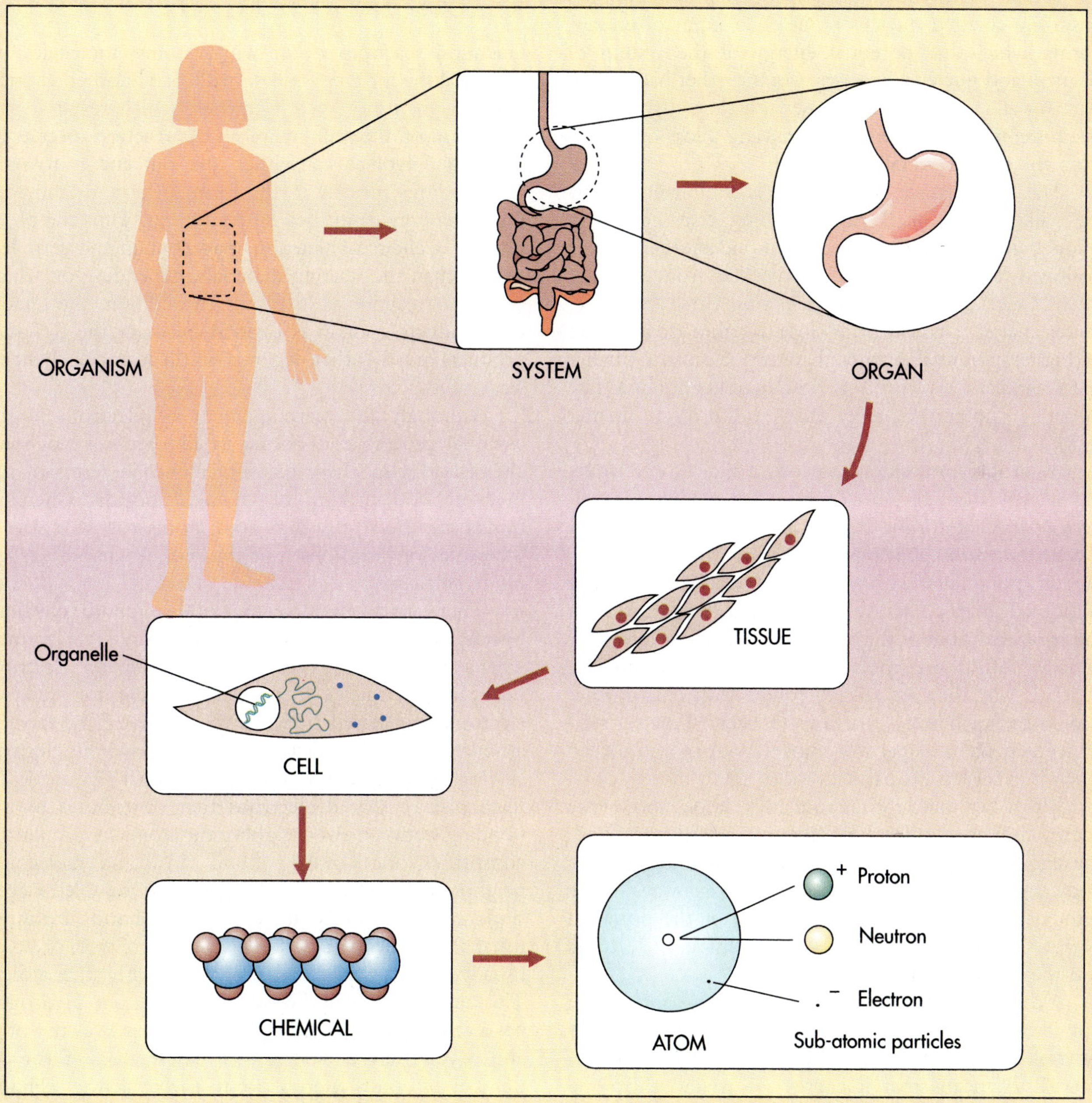

happen" through the application of forces. The energy released from our food is able to make our muscles move, for example, or keep us warm by making the chemical particles within us move about more quickly.

The concept of energy is perhaps best understood by comparing systems that contain a lot of energy with those that contain less. First, we must appreciate that there are two basic forms of energy: **kinetic energy** and **potential energy.** Kinetic energy is simply the energy things possess because they are moving. So anything that is moving, such as an electron moving within an atom or a ball rolling along the ground, contains kinetic energy. Potential energy is the energy systems contain because of the *positions* of their parts. In chemistry, potential energy is always associated with the arrangements of protons and electrons. Electrons, being negatively charged, are attracted toward protons, which are positively charged. This is the well-known "like attracts unlike" (or attraction of opposites) rule concerning electric charges. Movement *against* this force of attraction requires an input of energy, which increases the potential energy of the system. Thus moving an electron away from the positively charged nucleus requires an input of energy, during which the potential energy of the system of electron and nucleus increases. On the other hand, if an electron and nucleus move closer together, their collective potential energy decreases, causing a loss of energy from the system overall.

The "like attracts unlike" rule is complemented by the "like repels like" rule, meaning that negatively charged electrons are repelled from one another, just as positively charged protons are repelled from one another. Once again, movement *against* these forces requires energy. Two electrons close together are in a state of higher potential energy than two electrons further apart. Similarly, two protons close together are in a state of higher potential energy than two protons further apart.

All atoms, molecules, and ions contain some **internal energy** from the movement of their electrons (kinetic energy) and from the way in which their negatively charged electrons and positively charged nuclei are arranged (potential energy). Chemicals also contain some additional kinetic energy, known as **heat energy,** from the *overall* motion of the atoms, molecules, or ions they contain. All atoms, molecules, and ions are moving, which is why they are able to collide with one another and so cause chemical reactions to occur. When a substance is heated, its particles move about more quickly; when it is cooled, its particles move about more slowly.

When we talk throughout this book about the energy contained in food, the energy released from food, the energy required to make certain chemicals of the body, and so on, the energy concerned is always in the form of the kinetic energy of motion or the potential energy stored within the relative positioning of electrons and the atomic nuclei they surround.

Although energy is a rather abstract concept, in one way it behaves very ordinarily: it cannot be created or destroyed. This is known as the **law of conservation of energy.** It means that if energy is given out by one system, such as a collection of chemicals, it must be transferred to another system. Energy never appears from nowhere and never disappears into nothing.

Energy is commonly measured in either **calories** or **kilocalories** (kcal), with 1 kcal equal to 1000 calories. The kilocalorie, however, is also referred to as the **Calorie** (with a capital C). Thus a meal supplying 600 Calories, for example, supplies 600,000 calories, or 600 kcal. One other unit for measuring energy is the *joule.* 1 calorie = 4.18 joules; 1 kcal = 4.18 kilojoules (kJ); 1 Calorie = 4.18 kJ. Although the joule is being used increasingly in Europe and Canada, the United States has not adopted it as the unit of measurement of energy and continues to use calories, kilocalories, and Calories instead.

REACTIONS AND BONDS

Chemical reactions occur when atoms, molecules, or ions of different types collide with one another, causing rearrangements of their electrons, which result in the formation of different chemicals. As reactions occur, the chemicals involved can either give out energy to their surroundings, usually in the form of heat, or they can take in energy from their surroundings. Thus the products of a chemical reaction may contain more or less energy than the starting materials, depending on which particular reaction is involved. In addition, the energy the products contain is divided between the different products in a way that depends on their precise chemical structures.

Although the rearrangement of electrons is the essential process that occurs in all chemical reactions, chemists discuss these rearrangements in terms of the breaking and making of chemical **bonds.** Chemical bonds are the forces that hold atoms together within molecules or hold ions together within what are called *ionic compounds.*

There are two fundamental kinds of bonds: **covalent bonds** and **ionic bonds.** Covalent bonds are formed when atoms are held together by *sharing* electrons between their nuclei. In a water molecule, for example, electrons are shared between the nuclei of the oxygen atom and the two hydrogen atoms present; this electron sharing holds the entire molecule together (Figure A-2). Each pair of shared electrons that contributes to the bonding between two neighboring atoms in a molecule constitutes one covalent bond. In some molecules, neighboring atoms are held together by double or even triple covalent bonds, although single bonds are more usual. Each element and therefore each type of atom usually forms a fixed number of bonds with other atoms. This number is called the **valency** of an atom. Hydrogen has a valency of 1, for example; carbon has a valency of 4; and oxygen has a valency of 2. These atoms form the number of bonds appropriate to their valencies (Figure A-2).

The second basic type of bonding is ionic bonding (Figure A-3). An ionic bond is the force of attraction between oppositely charged ions. These ions are formed when one or more electrons are *transferred* from one atom (or group of atoms) onto some other atom (or group of atoms). This process of electron transfer creates positively charged ions that are derived from the particles that have lost electrons and negatively charged ions that are derived from the particles that have gained electrons. These oppositely charged ions are then held together tightly within the solid structure of an ionic compound. When ionic compounds dissolve in water, however, their

FIGURE A-2

Covalent bonds are formed when electrons are shared among different atoms.

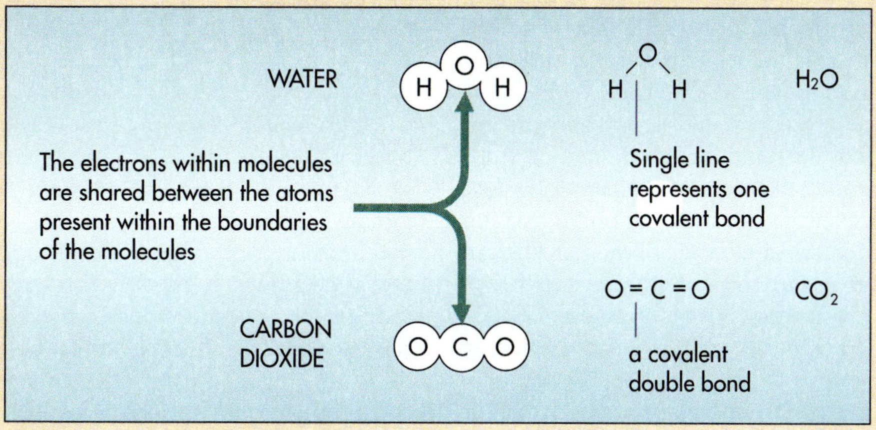
WATER
H O H
H O H
H₂O
The electrons within molecules are shared between the atoms present within the boundaries of the molecules
Single line represents one covalent bond
O = C = O
CO₂
CARBON DIOXIDE
O C O
a covalent double bond

FIGURE A-3

Ionic bonds are the strong forces of attraction between oppositely charged ions.

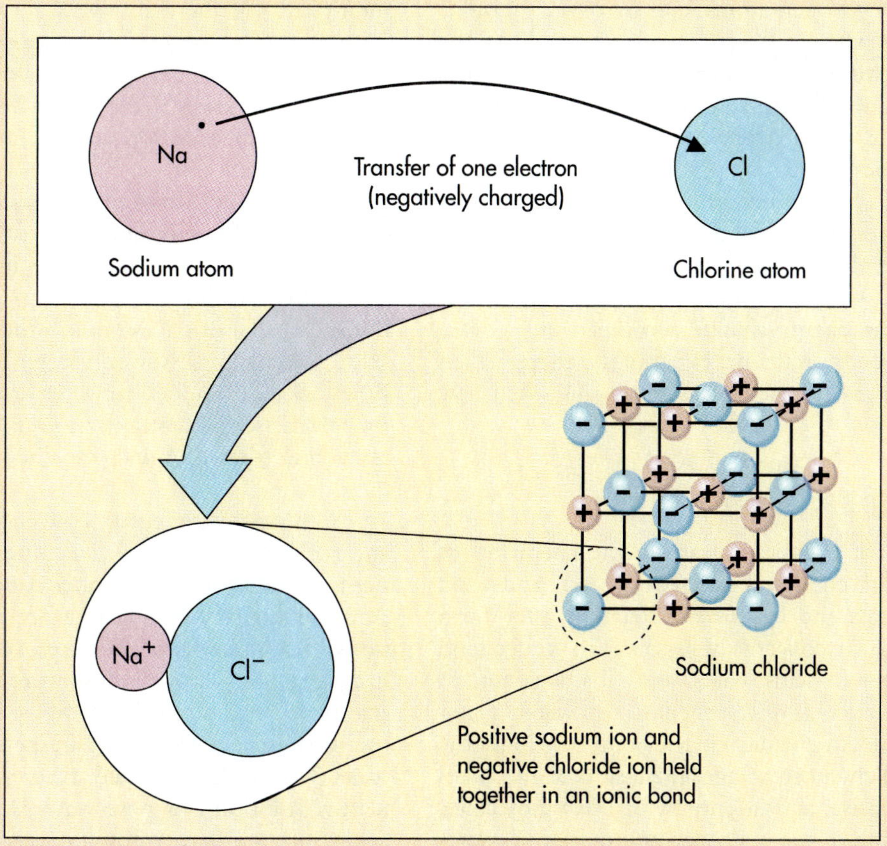
Na
Transfer of one electron (negatively charged)
Cl
Sodium atom
Chlorine atom
Na+
Cl−
Sodium chloride
Positive sodium ion and negative chloride ion held together in an ionic bond

individual ions separate and move about freely within the solution.

Many of the chemicals within food exist in the form of ions, particularly many of the essential minerals. Ions can have a single, double, or triple positive or negative charge, depending on the type of ion. The size of charge on an ion is equal to its valency, and many elements can participate in both covalent and ionic bonding, depending on the circumstances. Oxygen, for example, whose valency is 2, can participate in covalent bonding within many molecules (such as water), but oxygen atoms can also gain two electrons to form doubly charged O^{2-} ions. A further complication is that ions can contain many atoms that are themselves bonded together by covalent bonds. Phosphate ions (PO_4^{3-}, for example) contain a phosphorus atom covalently bonded to four oxygen atoms, whereas the whole cluster of atoms carries a triple negative charge overall.

The simplest way to represent atoms, molecules, or ions is to use their chemical **formulas.** A chemical formula simply lists the symbols for the atoms or ions present in any substance, accompanied by subscript numbers indicating the proportions in which the atoms or ions are present. Thus water molecules (formula H_2O) contain two hydrogen atoms bonded to an oxygen atom; sodium chloride (NaCl), which is an ionic compound, contains one sodium ion for each chloride ion; and glucose molecules, $C_6H_{12}O_6$, contain six carbon atoms, 12 hydrogen atoms, and six oxygen atoms.

During any chemical reaction, some or all of the existing bonds within the **reactants** (the chemicals that react together) may be broken, allowing new bonds to form and create the products of a reaction. Thus all reactions can be viewed simply as rearrangements of chemical bonds, which are in turn always caused by rearrangements of the electrons involved in the bonds. It is a general rule that breaking bonds always requires an input of energy, whereas forming bonds always gives out energy. Thus the energy change accompanying a reaction overall depends on the net effect of the energy taken in to break bonds and the energy given out when new bonds form.

ACIDS, BASES, AND SALTS

Two key types of chemicals, both in the chemistry of nutrition and in chemistry in general, are acids and bases. When acids and bases react together, they form compounds known collectively as salts. To understand the main features of acids, bases, and salts, it is best to begin with some details of the chemistry of water. Water is the most abundant chemical in the body, providing the medium in which most of the chemistry of life takes place. Water consists almost entirely of H_2O molecules, but a tiny portion of the hydrogen and oxygen in water occurs in the form of hydrogen ions (H^+) and hydroxide ions (OH^-). These ions are formed by the reversible splitting of water molecules as summarized by the following equation:

$$H_2O \rightleftharpoons H^+ + OH^-$$

This *equilibrium* process lies heavily in favor of water molecules, with the concentrations of the H^+ and OH^- ions in pure water being a tiny 0.0000001 moles/L (that is, 1×10^{-7} mol/L). Notice that this is the concentration of *both* the H^+ and the OH^- ions; so the concentrations of the ions are exactly equal. Although the concentrations of these ions are small, they can have a great influence on many chemical processes in the body, including the rates of key reactions and the three-dimensional structures of key molecules such as proteins. Acids and bases can alter the concentrations of hydrogen and hydroxide ions in water-based (**aqueous**) solutions in opposite ways.

Acids can be defined in various ways, but the most useful definition for the chemistry of nutrition is that acids are substances that release hydrogen ions. This means that acids that dissolve in water upset the balance of hydrogen and hydroxide ions, increasing the concentration of H^+ ions while at the same time decreasing the concentration of OH^- ions. There is an interesting relationship between the concentrations of these two ions in aqueous solutions: when the concentrations are multiplied together, the result always equals 1×10^{-14}. Thus if the hydrogen ion concentration rises, the hydroxide ion concentration *must* also fall by an appropriate amount. However, if the hydrogen ion concentration falls, the hydroxide ion concentration *must* rise by an appropriate amount.

For the purposes of the chemistry of nutrition, **bases** can be defined as substances that either release hydroxide ions or react with hydrogen ions in a way that increases the hydroxide ion concentration within aqueous solutions. Thus bases are essentially the chemical *opposites* of acids. Bases that dissolve in water are known as **alkalis.** When alkalis are added to water or to aqueous solutions, they decrease the concentration of hydrogen ions at the same time that they increase the concentration of hydroxide ions.

Solutions with equal concentrations of hydrogen and hydroxide ions, as well as pure water, are said to be **neutral.** Solutions with higher concentrations of hydrogen ions than hydroxide ions are **acidic**, whereas solutions with higher concentrations of hydroxide ions than hydrogen ions are **alkaline** (or **basic**). The level of acidity or alkalinity of aqueous solutions, including all the solutions in the body, is measured using the **pH** scale. To use the pH scale, three facts must be known: neutral solutions, or pure water, have a pH value of 7, acidic solutions have pH values less than 7 (the lower the value the more acidic the solution is), and alkaline

FIGURE A-4

The main organic functional groups relevant to the chemistry of nutrition.

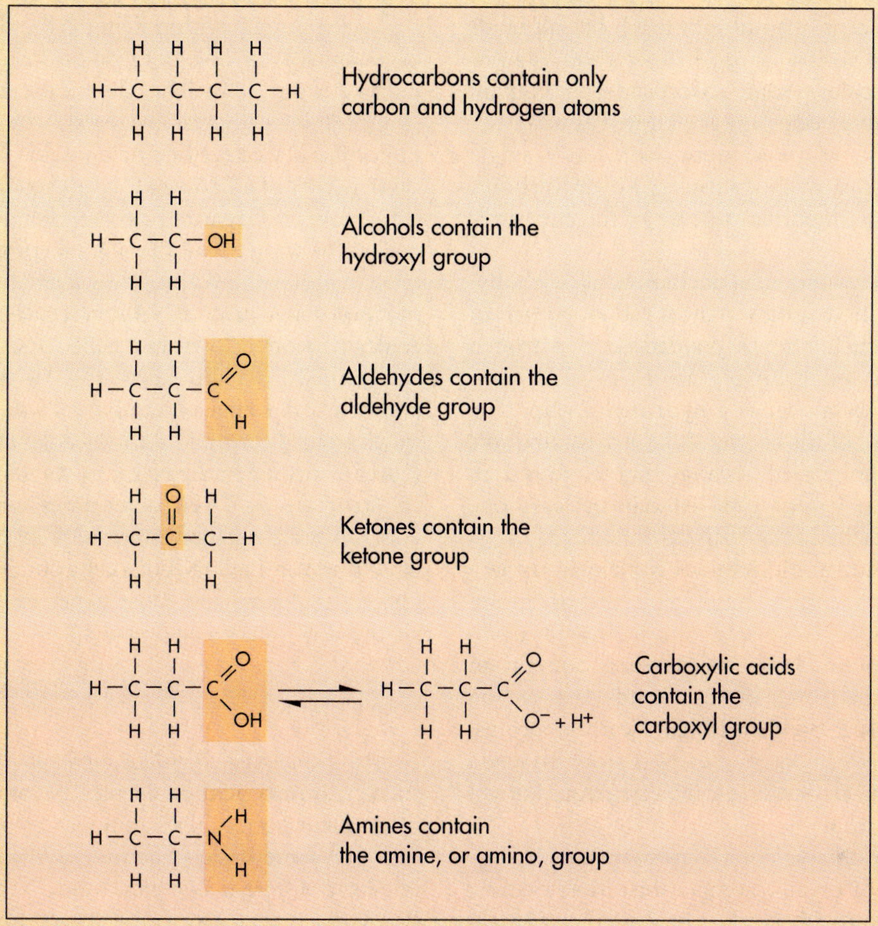
Hydrocarbons contain only carbon and hydrogen atoms
Alcohols contain the hydroxyl group
Aldehydes contain the aldehyde group
Ketones contain the ketone group
Carboxylic acids contain the carboxyl group
Amines contain the amine, or amino, group

solutions have pH values greater than 7 (the higher the value the more alkaline the solution is).

Technically, the pH level of a solution is defined as "the negative logarithm, to the base 10, of the hydrogen ion concentration." This means that when the hydrogen ion concentration is written in "standard form" such as 1×10^{-7} mol/L, the pH value has the same magnitude but opposite sign to the final subscript (pH = +7 in this case). It is not necessary to remember this definition, however, to make use of the pH scale.

Most of the chemistry of the body occurs at pH values close to neutrality, or in other words close to pH 7. One major exception is the chemistry that occurs within the stomach because the stomach contents are acidic, with a pH value of about 1 or 2.

When acids and bases (including alkalis) react together, they **neutralize** each other and form compounds known as **salts.** Common **table salt,** the salt sodium chloride (Figure A-3), is formed when hydrochloric acid is neutralized by reaction with the alkali sodium hydroxide. Although commonly referred to simply as "salt," sodium chloride is in fact just one member of an enormous range of compounds that are all known as salts.

ORGANIC CHEMICALS

The chemicals that form most of the structure of living things are known as **organic compounds,** which, in its broadest chemical sense, means compounds containing the elements carbon (although carbon dioxide is not usually considered an organic compound). In biology, the term *organic* is often used more generally to refer to anything derived from living things. Chains and rings of bonded carbon atoms form the basic structural "skeletons" of carbohydrates, proteins, lipids, and vitamins—four of the six classes of nutrients. The only nutrients that are not organic compounds are water and the various minerals. The student of nutrition spends a lot of time considering the properties of organic compounds and needs to be familiar with the main types of organic compounds and the main chemical groups they contain (Figure A-4).

The simplest organic compounds are the **hydrocarbons,** which consist of chains or rings of carbon atoms with hydrogen atoms attached. Pure hydrocarbons are not found in significant quantities in food, but all lipids and some vitamins contain large hydrocarbon regions within their molecules. Some hydrocarbons contain carbon-carbon double bonds and are known as **unsaturated** hydrocarbons, whereas those with only single carbon-carbon bonds are called **saturated** hydrocarbons. This distinction is an important feature of the chemistry of fats and oils.

Many organic compounds, including all carbohydrates, contain carbon atoms that are bonded to an oxygen atom, which in turn is bonded to a hydrogen atom. The oxygen and hydrogen atoms in such compounds form what is known as a **hydroxyl** group. The characteristic feature of the chemicals known as **alcohols** (such as the alcohol called *ethanol* that is found in alcoholic beverages) is that they contain at least one hydroxyl group attached to a hydrocarbon chain.

Compounds known as **aldehydes** contain an oxygen atom attached by a double bond to a carbon atom, which is itself bonded to at least one hydrogen atom. The related compounds known as **ketones** contain an oxygen atom attached by a double bond to a carbon atom, which is itself bonded to two carbon atoms. Aldehydes and ketones contain a carbon atom attached by a double bond to an oxygen atom, a structure known as the **carbonyl group.**

Acids can be inorganic compounds (such as hydrochloric acid, HCl) or organic compounds. Most organic acids are **carboxylic acids,** so called because they contain a **carboxyl group,** which consists of a carbon atom bonded to a hydroxyl group, and they are joined by a double bond to an oxygen atom. This chemical group is acidic because a hydrogen ion is readily detached from it (Figure A-4).

Proteins are made by the bonding together of smaller molecules called *amino acids,* and all amino acids contain a carboxyl group, but they also contain an **amino** group. The amino, or **amine,** group consists of a nitrogen atom bonded to two hydrogen atoms. It is a basic (or alkaline) group because it can combine with hydrogen ions (forming an NH_3^+ group), thus removing them from solution. Thus amino acids contain both an acidic carboxyl group and a basic amino group.

These various chemical groups are examples of what are called the **functional groups** of organic chemistry, chemical groups that can be attached to the "carbon skeletons" of organic compounds in many different ways and combinations to form an enormous range of different organic compounds. All of the functional groups have not been discussed, but the key ones involved in the chemistry of nutrition have been dealt with. We can now turn our attention from the basic principles of chemistry to the specific chemical processes involved in life, which must be sustained by the nutrients in food.

THE CHEMISTRY OF LIFE

The chemistry of life, known as **biochemistry,** occurs largely within living cells, although parts of it occur outside of cells because of the action of chemicals released from cells. The chemical centerpiece of every living cell is its **genetic material,** which consists of giant molecules of **deoxyribonucleic acid** (**DNA**). The chemical structure of DNA stores a cell's **genetic information,** which can be regarded as the chemical "instructions" needed to bring about the manufacture of a specific set of protein molecules within the cell and in a smaller number of **ribonucleic acid** (**RNA**) molecules. The protein molecules "encoded" within a cell's DNA are the chemicals that actually facilitate all of the chemical reactions that allow the cell to live and grow, *including* all the reactions involved in allowing DNA molecules to specify what proteins are formed in the cell. The ways in which the chemical structure of DNA determines what proteins a cell contains are described more fully in Chapter 5. In general, however, the DNA of a cell contains distinct portions known as **genes,** and most genes are able to direct the synthesis of one specific protein.

PROTEINS

Proteins are long chainlike molecules made when many smaller **amino acid** molecules become linked together by covalent bonds. The amino acids found in proteins all have the same basic structure, as shown in Figure A-5, but have different chemical "side" chains (indicated as R_1, R_2, etc.) attached to the central carbon atom. Figure A-5 also illustrates the way in which these amino acids can join up to form a protein chain. Twenty different amino acids are used in protein synthesis, and a protein can contain up to several hundred amino acid molecules joined in a specific sequence to form the protein chain. Once a protein chain has been formed, it automatically folds into a specific three-dimensional structure in a way that is determined by the amino acid sequence of the newly formed protein.

After folding, a protein may be immediately ready to perform its specific task in the life of the cell. Many proteins, however, must be further modified before they become functional. The modifications include the addition of sugar groups to form **glycoproteins,** the addition of phosphate groups to form **phosphoproteins,** the combination with metal ions to form **metalloproteins,** the addition of lipids to form **lipoproteins,** and the aggregation of two or more protein chains (identical or different) to form **multisubunit proteins.** This list is not comprehensive, but it includes the main kinds of modifications that proteins undergo.

Once formed, folded, and chemically modified if appropriate, proteins perform a wide variety of roles within cells, but most of that variety is encompassed within nine main categories of activity:

FIGURE A-5

The general structure of amino acids, the formation of a protein chain, and the folding of the original chain into a specific three-dimensional structure.

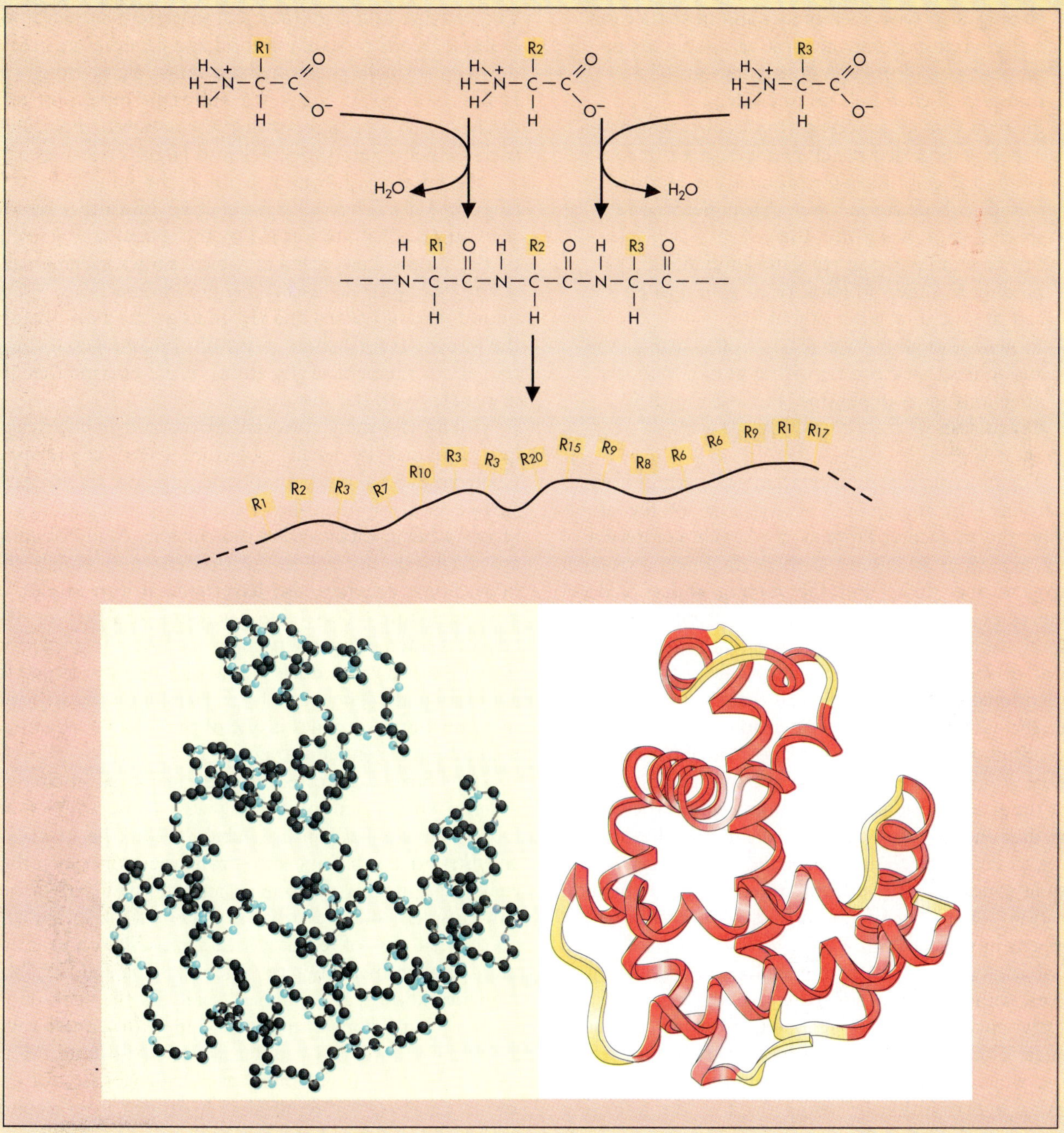

- Proteins can act as enzymes, the molecules that control the chemistry of the cell by catalyzing (greatly speeding up) the reactions needed within cells.
- Proteins can perform structural roles, forming much of the physical framework of living things.
- Proteins can form contractile structures, which can undergo cycles of contraction and relaxation to allow cells and organisms to change shape and move.
- Proteins can act as carrier molecules, binding to specific other chemicals and transporting them around the body.
- Proteins can act as messenger molecules, such as hormones, being made in some cells of the body and released to travel to other cells, bind

to them, and bring about some appropriate response.

- Proteins can act as "gates" and "pumps" embedded in cell membranes, permitting specific chemicals to cross membranes and in some cases actively transporting chemicals across the membranes to build up high concentrations of the transported chemicals on one side.
- Proteins can act as receptor molecules, which may be embedded in cell membranes or free within the cell. Receptor proteins can bind to specific substances in a way that initiates some specific responses within the cell.
- Proteins can perform regulatory functions, binding to other proteins, or to genes, to either activate them or inhibit them.
- Proteins can perform defensive roles, such as the antibodies that circulate within blood, bind to infectious microorganisms, and assist in their destruction.

The function that a protein molecule can perform is determined by the *spatial arrangement* of the atoms within the molecule. Proteins are largely composed of only five types of atoms: carbon, hydrogen, oxygen, nitrogen, and sulfur; but the varying amino acid sequences of proteins allow them to fold into an almost infinite variety of structures, each with these various types of atoms arranged in a specific way in three-dimensional space. The chemicals that the proteins must interact with also have specific spatial arrangements of the atoms they contain. It is the match between the spatial arrangement of atoms at the surface of a protein and the spatial arrangement of atoms within the chemicals they interact with that actually allows the interactions to take place. This basic principle is crucial to the way in which enzymes are able to catalyze the chemical reactions of life, a process central to everything that happens in the cell.

Each enzyme can bind selectively to certain molecules, known as the **substrates** of the enzyme, and greatly encourage some reaction involving the substrates. This reaction converts the substrates into **products,** which are then released from the enzyme. This process is conventionally summarized by the following general equation:

$$E + S \longrightarrow ES \longrightarrow E + P$$

where E represents the enzyme, S the substrates, ES the **enzyme-substrate complex** formed when the substrates bind to the enzyme, and P the products. Enzymes are **catalysts** in that they encourage specific chemical reactions while remaining unchanged themselves. Because an enzyme is left unchanged by its act of catalysis, one enzyme molecule can go through many cycles of substrate binding, reaction catalysis, and product release. In this way, a small number of enzyme molecules can quickly bring about major chemical changes.

Many enzymes bind to only one substrate molecule. The enzyme called *amylase* that is present in saliva, for example, binds to starch in food and catalyzes its breakdown into smaller carbohydrate units. Many other enzymes bind to at least two substrate molecules and catalyze some reaction between the substrate molecules, such as their joining together into larger molecules.

All enzymes, however, work in the same basic way (Figure A-6). They all have specific **binding sites** on their surface that are formed by the spatial arrangement of the atoms they contain, which allows specific substrates to bind via weak chemical interactions. Once bound, the substrates quickly undergo reaction because the process of reaction is greatly encouraged by the spatial arrangement of the atoms of the enzyme that are in contact with the substrate.

Many enzymes, however, are assisted in their catalytic activities by small molecules called **coenzymes.** Coenzymes also bind to specific sites on the enzyme surface in a way that allows them to participate in the reaction being catalyzed by the enzyme. Many vitamins are chemicals needed to form coenzymes within the body. Some enzymes also have mineral ions as part of their structure. These ions become attached to the enzymes after the protein chain has been formed, and their presence is essential for the enzymes concerned to work properly. The need for certain minerals to form fully functional enzymes is one of the reasons why these minerals are essential nutrients.

It is often easy to tell from the name of an enzyme exactly what reaction it catalyzes. The name of an enzyme always ends in *ase* (which allows the names of enzymes to be distinguished from the names of other chemicals, such as substrates), and the first part of the name usually indicates what substrates the enzyme acts on or what type of reaction it catalyzes. Thus a protease is an enzyme that binds to other proteins and catalyzes their breakdown. A deaminase catalyzes the removal of amino groups from a substrate. A dehydrogenase catalyzes the removal of hydrogen from its substrate. More specifically, the enzyme alcohol dehydrogenase, for example, catalyzes the removal of hydrogen from alcohol molecules.

Sometimes the name of an enzyme also indicates where in the body it acts. A gastric protease, for example, is an enzyme in the stomach that breaks down protein molecules during digestion. Hepatic lysine deaminase is an enzyme in the liver that catalyzes the deamination of the amino acid lysine. Thus the names of enzymes can be revealing. In some cases, however, the origins of enzyme names are rooted in historical or technical terms that may not be commonly used in everyday language. In the two preceding examples, it is necessary to know that

FIGURE A-6

The general principles of enzyme- substrate interaction and enzyme catalysis.

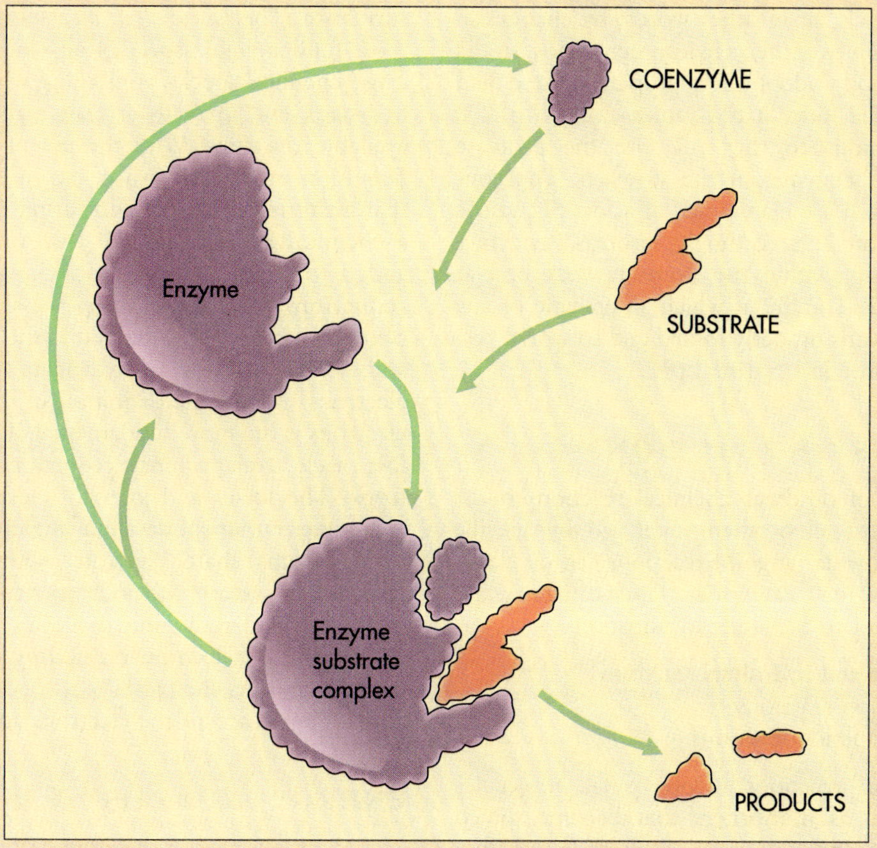

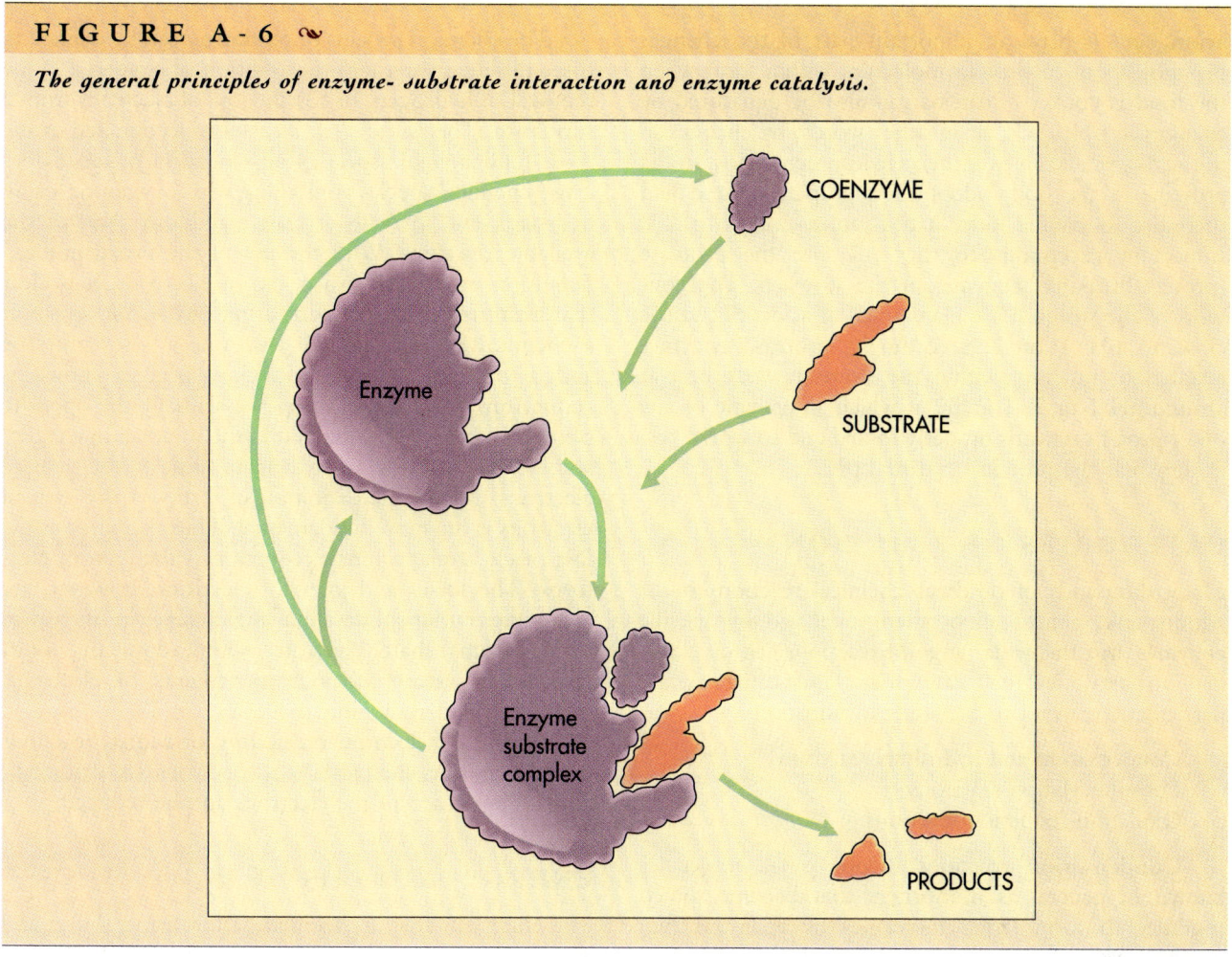

gastric refers to the stomach and *hepatic* refers to the liver. The origins of the names of some other enzymes are much more obscure.

Enzymes are crucial to almost every aspect of the chemistry of life because they catalyze all of the chemical reactions involved, but the vital importance of enzymes should not cause us to forget the many other things that proteins do, summarized in the preceding list. Many of these other functions of proteins are relevant to nutrition. For example, some proteins in cell membranes allow specific nutrients to cross the membranes or may actively transport specific nutrients across the membranes. Receptor proteins, especially ones embedded in cell membranes, are involved in generating the sensation of taste and in allowing hormones to control the rate of metabolism, in addition to many other important roles.

Hormones are of great importance to many aspects of nutrition, and many hormones are proteins. In general, a hormone is a substance produced in what is called an **endocrine gland,** such as the pituitary or thyroid gland. After being released from the endocrine gland, hormone molecules travel in the blood, bind to specific receptors on certain cells, elicit some specific response. The hormone **insulin,** for example, is a protein produced by specific cells of the pancreas. It is released into the blood and is carried to almost every cell in the body. It binds to protein receptors specific for insulin in the cell membranes and assists in the uptake of the nutrient glucose into the cells from the blood. Similarly, **thyroxin,** a hormone produced in the thyroid gland, is carried to other cells of the body where it helps regulate the rate at which the cells generate and use their supplies of energy.

Although enzymes and other proteins can last a relatively long time in the body (one enzyme molecule catalyzing its reaction many thousands of times, for example), existing proteins are continually being broken down and replaced. Proteins are also sensitive to changes in temperature and pH levels. The proteins of the human body work best at temperatures close to the normal body temperature of about 98.6° F (37° C). At temperatures above 104° F (40° C), proteins begin to undergo damaging changes as a result of a process called **denaturation.** During denaturation the crucial folded structure of a protein becomes disrupted, causing the protein chain to partially or fully unravel, which prevents the protein from performing its normal role. When caused by high temperatures, this is called **heat denatur-**

ation, and it plays an important part in the changes brought about in protein molecules within food when the food is cooked. Proteins can also be denatured by changes in pH levels, or in other words, by changes in the acidity or alkalinity of their environment. Most of the proteins in the body adopt their properly folded and therefore functional form at pH values close to pH 7. Important exceptions to that rule are the protease (protein-breaking) enzymes in the stomach. The contents of the stomach are maintained at acidic pH values close to pH 1 or 2; accordingly, protease enzymes adapted to function within the stomach work best at around pH 1 or 2. The pH at which an enzyme or any other protein remains properly folded and so works best is known as the protein's **optimal pH.**

CATEGORIES OF REACTIONS

Many thousands of different chemical reactions occur within cells, almost all of them catalyzed by specific enzymes, but this wide range of reactions can be classified into only a few main categories. Three categories are particularly relevant to the study of nutrition:

- Condensation and hydrolysis reactions
- Phosphorylation reactions
- Oxidation-reduction reactions

Condensation reactions involve small molecules known in general as **monomers** that become joined together to form larger molecules by reactions that involve the formation of water (hence the term *condensation*). The joining together of amino acids to form a protein chain is a key example of a condensation reaction (Figure A-5). Simple sugars can also join together in condensation reactions to form large chainlike carbohydrates such as starch and cellulose, as is considered in Chapter 3. When condensation reactions join a great many monomers into large molecules or **macromolecules,** the monomers have joined to form **polymers.** Condensation polymerization (the formation of polymers by condensation reactions) is the way in which all of the large macromolecules of the cell are formed. The reverse process, in which water molecules combine with a polymer during its breakdown into smaller parts and ultimately into individual monomers, is called **hydrolysis.** Hydrolysis reactions catalyzed by digestive enzymes play a major role in converting the molecules in food into smaller molecules that can be absorbed into the body.

Phosphorylation reactions involve the transfer of a phosphate group (PO_4^{3-}) from one chemical to another. Phosphorylation reactions are important in the trapping and use of energy by cells. They are also involved in processes that regulate proteins, activating (switching on) or inhibiting (switching off) the proteins' activities as appropriate.

The chemical process of **oxidation** can be defined in three different ways: (1) the addition of oxygen, (2) the removal of hydrogen, or (3) the loss of electrons from a substance. The *loss of electrons* is now recognized as the most fundamental aspect of all oxidation processes because chemical species combining with oxygen or losing hydrogen end up with at least a reduced *share* of the available electrons. With the use of the broad modern definition of oxidation as a loss of electrons, it is clear that *oxidation can occur without the presence of oxygen.* If a chemical is oxidized, the electrons it loses must be added to some other chemical in a process known as **reduction.** Because reduction is essentially the opposite of oxidation, it can be defined as the removal of oxygen, and/or the addition of hydrogen, and/or the gain of electrons. Again, the definition in terms of the gain of electrons is the more fundamental. Thus oxidation is the loss of electrons, whereas reduction is the gain of electrons. The losses and gains of electrons, however, are sometimes rather subtle, involving changes in the way in which atoms share electrons within covalent bonds rather than clearly obvious movements of electrons. Oxidation and reduction processes are always coupled together into **oxidation-reduction,** or **redox,** reactions because as one chemical loses electrons (is oxidized), another must accept the electrons and be reduced.

ENERGY AND LIFE

The chemicals that are formed within living things and are required to sustain living things are in a higher energy state than the simple raw materials from which they are formed. Figure 1-3 summarizes this fundamental fact. It shows that the input of energy from the sun is needed to convert carbon dioxide (CO_2), water (H_2O), and a wide variety of minerals into the many different chemicals within plants. This energy-trapping process within plants is called **photosynthesis.** Animals get supplies of high-energy raw materials either by eating plants directly or by eating other animals that are themselves ultimately sustained by plant food. The high-energy chemicals within food, however, cannot be directly converted into the high-energy chemicals of the body. Instead, they must be broken down into simpler starting materials and then *rebuilt* into the chemicals of the body. During this breaking-down process the energy trapped within food would be lost as heat if cells did not possess some mechanism for trapping and storing it until required. Cells are in fact equipped with a range of complicated chemical mechanisms for the trapping and storage of the energy released from food. The most important high-energy storage compound is called **adenosine triphosphate (ATP).**

ATP is formed when adenosine diphosphate (ADP) and phosphate ions (P_i) combine in a condensation reaction. Its formation requires an input of energy

FIGURE A-7

How the energy released by the respiration of food is trapped within ATP and can later be used to power the manufacture of the high-energy chemicals of the body.

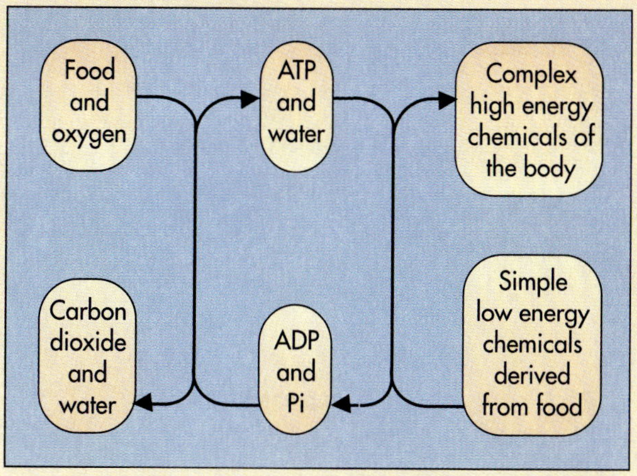

because ATP and water (the products of the formation reaction) are in a higher energy state than ADP and P_i (the starting materials). Thus ATP can be made only if its formation is chemically *coupled* to a reaction that gives out enough energy to power the formation of ATP. This coupling happens during the process known as **respiration,** when cells oxidize food molecules to generate carbon dioxide and water. In essence, this process reverses the energy-trapping process of photosynthesis within plants and thus releases energy, much of which can be captured within ATP (Figure A-7). Notice that the formation of ATP is an example of a phosphorylation reaction, one of the crucial categories of reaction types identified earlier.

The formation and use of ATP are two of the chemical centerpieces of the study of nutrition. Much of the food we eat is oxidized to release energy that is then trapped within the chemical structure of ATP. The ATP energy stores are used to drive forward all of the energy-requiring processes within the body, such as the synthesis of new proteins, new carbohydrates, and new lipids. Because we also need energy to allow us to move, the chemical changes in our muscles that make them move are also major consumers of the ATP supplies generated by the respiration of food.

METABOLISM

The sum of the chemical processes within a cell, or a multicellular organism such as a human, is known as its **metabolism.** The overall effect of human metabolism is to use the raw materials available in food to build and maintain the chemicals of our bodies and provide us with the energy we need. Metabolism is divided into two main categories of process: **catabolism** and **anabolism.** Catabolism is the *breaking down* of food molecules by reactions that release energy, which can be trapped and stored within ATP. Anabolism is the *building up,* or synthesis, of the molecules of the body by reactions that require the energy stored within ATP to be used to make them happen. Thus catabolic reactions give out energy, some of which is trapped within ATP, whereas anabolic reactions take in energy, which is largely provided by the hydrolysis of ATP.

THE BIOLOGY OF THE CELL

All organisms are made up of cells. Complex multicellular organisms such as humans contain many billions of individual cells, whereas the simplest organisms are free-living single cells. Cells are membrane-bound entities, separated from one another and from the environment by their thin lipid-based membranes. Although there are many different types of cells, each with its own specialized structures and activities, all cells share certain basic features (Figure A-8).

The **cell membrane** serves much the same function for the cell as the lining of the intestinal tract does for the body. It controls the entry of nutrients and other substances into the cell. It is composed of a double layer of lipid molecules joined back to back, with various protein molecules embedded within this **lipid bilayer.** The cell membrane is a selective and semipermeable barrier between the cell **cytoplasm** inside and the extracellular environment outside. It allows certain substances to pass through it freely and other substances to pass through only when appropriate, and it presents an impenetrable barrier to many other substances.

Within the cell are certain specialized structures called **organelles,** each one able to perform some specific function in the life of the cell. The **mitochondrion** is a membrane-bound organelle in which most of the ATP supplies of a cell are formed during catabolism; hence it is colloquially known as the "powerhouse" of the cell. Each cell contains many mitochondria; the amount depends on how much energy must flow through a cell. Muscle cells, for example, which must generate large quantities of ATP to power muscular contraction, contain large numbers of mitochondria.

Lysosomes are small membrane-bound organelles responsible for breaking down complex molecules taken in from the environment into simpler molecules capable of being used by the cell. Lysosomes perform an analogous function to digestion in humans and contain specialized enzymes to catalyze the reactions involved. They can also break down and destroy invading microorganisms and can even destroy the cell itself once it has

FIGURE A-8

The basic features of cell structure.

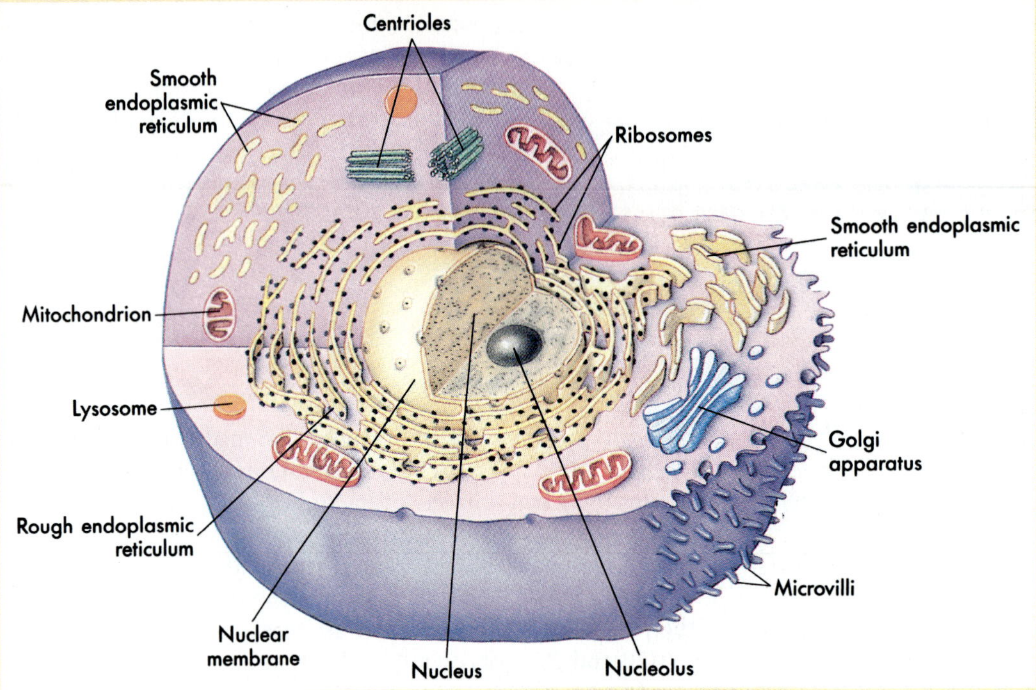

outlived its usefulness or pathologically, during certain diseases.

The genetic material (DNA) of the cell is found within a large membrane-bound organelle known as the cell **nucleus.** The all-important genes embodied in the DNA never leave the nucleus (apart from when the nucleus itself breaks down during cell division), but they are constantly used to direct the manufacture of the proteins a cell needs, as described in Chapter 5. The role of most of the genes is to direct the synthesis of specific proteins, but the process of protein synthesis itself occurs in the cytoplasm on small granules of protein and RNA known as **ribosomes.** It is here that amino acids within the cell are linked into new protein chains, whose amino acid sequences are determined by the chemical structure of the genes within the nucleus. Many of the ribosomes are found attached to an extensive network of membranes within the cell (and which is also attached to the nuclear membrane) known as the **endoplasmic reticulum** (**ER**). All of the membranes within the cell, such as those of the ER, nucleus, mitochondria, and lysosomes, have the same basic lipid bilayer structure, containing embedded proteins, as the outer cell membrane itself. What distinguishes these various membranes from one another and gives them different properties is the particular types of lipids they contain and the particular types of proteins that are embedded within them.

APPENDIX B

DAILY VALUES ESTABLISHED BY THE FOOD AND DRUG ADMINISTRATION AS STANDARDS FOR NUTRIENT LABELING PURPOSES

DAILY VALUES ESTABLISHED BY THE FOOD AND DRUG ADMINISTRATION AS STANDARDS FOR NUTRIENT LABELING PURPOSES

REFERENCE DAILY INTAKES (RDIs)*†§

NUTRIENT	REFERENCE AMOUNT
Vitamin A‖	5000 International Units (IU)
Vitamin C‖	60 mg
Thiamin	1.5 mg
Riboflavin	1.7 mg
Niacin	20 mg
Calcium‖	1 g
Iron‖	18 mg
Vitamin D	400 IU
Vitamin E	30 IU
Vitamin B_6	2 mg
Folic acid	0.4 mg
Vitamin B_{12}	6 μg
Phosphorus	1 g
Iodine	150 μg
Magnesium	400 mg
Zinc	15 mg
Copper	2 mg
Biotin	0.3 mg
Pantothenic acid	10 mg

DAILY REFERENCE VALUES (DRVs)†§

NUTRIENT	BASIS FOR CALCULATING DAILY REFERENCE VALUE
Total fat	30% of calories
Saturated fat	10% of calories
Carbohydrate	60% of calories
Dietary fiber	11.5 g of fiber per each 1000 calories
Protein	10% of calories for adults and children over 4 years

NUTRIENT	2000 CALORIES	2500 CALORIES
Total fat‖	65 g	80 g
Saturated fat‖	20 g	25 g
Cholesterol‖	300 mg	300 mg
Sodium‖	2.4 mg	2.4 mg
Total carbohydrate‖	300 g	375 g
Dietary fiber‖	25 g	30 g
Protein‖	50 g	65 g
Potassium	3.5 mg	3.5 mg

* Based on the National Academy of Sciences' 1968 Recommended Dietary Allowances (same as USRDA used until 1994). Values are highest RDAs except for pregnancy and lactation.

† The DRV for protein does not apply to certain populations. An RDI for protein has been established for these groups: infants under 1 yr, 14 g; children 1-4 yr, 16 g; pregnant women, 50 g; and nursing mothers, 66 g.

‡ Daily Value (DV) as used on label includes both RDIs for vitamins and minerals and DRVs for macronutrients and electrolytes.

§ Some DVs have been rounded to make label reading easier for consumers.

‖ Percentages of DVs must be declared on label. Percentages of DV for other nutrients may be provided voluntarily.

APPENDIX C

RECOMMENDED NUTRIENT INTAKES FOR CANADIANS

SUMMARY EXAMPLES OF RECOMMENDED NUTRIENT INTAKES FOR CANADIANS

				FAT-SOLUBLE VITAMINS		
AGE	SEX	WEIGHT (kg)	PROTEIN (g/day)[a]	VITAMIN A (RE/day)[b]	VITAMIN D (μg/day)[c]	VITAMIN E (mg/day)[d]
MONTHS						
0-4	Both	6	12[f]	400	10	3
5-12	Both	9	12	400	10	3
YEARS						
1	Both	11	13	400	10	3
2-3	Both	14	16	400	5	4
4-6	Both	18	19	500	5	5
7-9	M	25	26	700	2.5	7
	F	25	26	700	2.5	6
10-12	M	34	34	800	2.5	8
	F	36	36	800	5	7
13-15	M	50	49	900	5	9
	F	48	46	800	5	7
16-18	M	62	58	1000	5	10
	F	53	47	800	2.5	7
19-24	M	71	61	1000	2.5	10
	F	58	50	800	2.5	7
25-49	M	74	64	1000	2.5	9
	F	59	51	800	2.5	6
50-74	M	73	63	1000	5	7
	F	63	54	800	5	6
75+	M	69	59	1000	5	6
	F	64	55	800	5	5
PREGNANT (ADDITIONAL)						
First trimester			5	0	2.5	2
Second trimester			20	0	2.5	2
Third trimester			24	0	2.5	2
LACTATING (ADDITIONAL)			20	400	2.5	3

NOTE: Recommended intakes of energy and of certain nutrients are not listed in this table because of the nature of the variables upon which they are based. The figures for energy are estimates of average requirements for expected patterns of activity. For nutrients not shown, the following amounts are recommended based on at least 2000 kcal/day and body weights as given: thiamin, 0.4 mg/1000 kcal (0.48 mg/5000 kJ); riboflavin, 0.5 mg/1000 kcal (0.6 mg/5000 kJ); niacin, 7.2 niacin equivalents (NE)/1000 kcal (8.6 NE/5000 kJ); vitamin B_6, 15 μg, as pyridoxine per gram of protein. Recommended intakes during periods of growth are taken as appropriate for individuals representative of the midpoint in each age group. All recommended intakes are designed to cover individual variations in essentially all of a healthy population subsisting on a variety of common foods available in Canada.

From Health and Welfare Canada: *Nutrition recommendations: the report of the Scientific Review Committee*, Ottawa, 1990, Canadian Government Publishing Centre.

SUMMARY EXAMPLES OF RECOMMENDED NUTRIENT INTAKES FOR CANADIANS *(continued)*

WATER-SOLUBLE VITAMINS			MINERALS					
VITAMIN C (mg/day)[e]	FOLATE (μg/day)	VITAMIN B_{12} (μg/day)	CALCIUM (mg/day)	PHOSPHORUS (mg/day)	MAGNESIUM (mg/day)	IRON (mg/day)	IODINE (μg/day)	ZINC (mg/day)
20	25	0.3	250	150	20	0.3[g]	30	2[h]
20	40	0.4	400	200	32	7	40	3
20	40	0.5	500	300	40	6	55	4
20	50	0.6	550	350	50	6	65	4
25	70	0.8	600	400	65	8	85	5
25	90	1.0	700	500	100	8	110	7
25	90	1.0	700	500	100	8	95	7
25	120	1.0	900	700	130	8	125	9
25	130	1.0	1100	800	135	8	110	9
30	175	1.0	1100	900	185	10	160	12
30	170	1.0	1000	850	180	13	160	9
40	220	1.0	900	1000	230	10	160	12
30	190	1.0	700	850	200	12	160	9
40	220	1.0	800	1000	240	9	160	12
30	180	1.0	700	850	200	13	160	9
40	230	1.0	800	1000	250	9	160	12
30	185	1.0	700	850	200	13[i]	160	9
40	230	1.0	800	1000	250	9	160	12
30	195	1.0	800	850	210	8	160	9
40	215	1.0	800	1000	230	9	160	12
30	200	1.0	800	850	210	8	160	9
0	200	0.2	500	200	15	0	25	6
10	200	0.2	500	200	45	5	25	6
10	200	0.2	500	200	45	10	25	6
25	100	0.2	500	200	65	0	50	6

[a]The primary units are grams per kilogram of body weight. The figures shown here are examples.

[b]One retinol equivalent (RE) corresponds to the biological activity of 1 μg of retinol, 6 μg of beta-carotene, or 12 μg of other carotenes.

[c]Expressed as cholecalciferol or ergocalciferol.

[d]Expressed as δ-α-tocopherol equivalents, relative to which β- and γ-tocopherol and α-tocotrienol have activities of 0.5, 0.1, and 0.3, respectively.

[e]Cigarette smokers should increase intake by 50%.

[f]Based on the assumption that the protein is from breast milk or is of the same biological value as that of breast milk, and that between 3 and 9 months of age, adjustment for the quality of the protein is made.

[g]Based on the assumption that breast milk is the source of iron.

[h]Based on the assumption that breast milk is the source of zinc.

[i]After menopause, the recommended intake is 8 mg/day.

AVERAGE ENERGY REQUIREMENTS FOR CANADIANS

AGE	SEX	AVERAGE HEIGHT (cm)	AVERAGE WEIGHT (kg)	REQUIREMENTS[a] (kcal/kg)[b]	(MJ/kg)[b]	(kcal/day)	(MJ/day)	(kcal/cm)	(MV/cm)
MONTHS									
0-2	Both	55	4.5	120-100	0.50-0.42	500	2.0	9	0.04
3-5	Both	63	7.0	100-95	0.42-0.40	700	2.8	11	0.05
6-8	Both	69	8.5	95-97	0.40-0.41	800	3.4	11.5	0.05
9-11	Both	73	9.5	97-99	0.41	950	3.8	12.5	0.05
YEARS									
1	Both	82	11	101	0.42	1100	4.8	13.5	0.06
2-3	Both	95	14	94	0.39	1300	5.6	13.5	0.06
4-6	Both	107	18	100	0.42	1800	7.6	17	0.07
7-9	M	126	25	88	0.37	2200	9.2	17.5	0.07
	F	125	25	76	0.32	1900	8.0	15	0.06
10-12	M	141	34	73	0.30	2500	10.4	17.5	0.07
	F	143	36	61	0.25	2200	9.2	15.5	0.06
13-15	M	159	50	57	0.24	2800	12.0	17.5	0.07
	F	157	48	46	0.19	2200	9.2	14	0.06
16-18	M	172	62	51	0.21	3200	13.2	18.5	0.08
	F	160	53	40	0.17	2100	8.8	13	0.05
19-24	M	175	71	42	0.18	3000	12.6		
	F	160	58	36	0.15	2100	8.8		
25-49	M	172	74	36	0.15	2700	11.3		
	F	160	59	32	0.13	1900	8.0		
50-74	M	170	73	31	0.13	2300	9.7		
	F	158	63	29	0.12	1800	7.6		
75+	M	168	69	29	0. 12	2000	8.4		
	F	155	64	23	0.10	1500	6.3		

[a]Requirements can be expected to vary within a range of ±30%.

[b]First and last figures are averages at the beginning and at the end of the 3-month period.

From Health and Welfare Canada: *Nutrition recommendations: the report of the Scientific Review Committee,* Ottawa, 1990, Canadian Government Publishing Centre.

APPENDIX D

NUTRIENT ANALYSIS: INSTRUCTIONS FOR KEEPING FOOD RECORDS

To assess the nutritive adequacy of your diet, it is necessary to have a complete record of all food and beverages consumed during at least a 3-day period. To do this:

RECORD DIETARY INTAKE

Select three 24-hour periods that you think are representative of your normal dietary intake and activity. Most students include two weekdays and one weekend day to represent an average week's dietary intake and activity. Record everything you consume each 24-hour period starting at midnight.

Before you begin recording, look over the food composition tables in Appendix E. Become aware of the detail necessary to accurately identify a food item (for example, method of cooking and units of measurement).

List all foods and beverages consumed at and between meals for the 3 days. Record everything you put into your mouth and swallow (including vitamin and mineral supplements). Do not forget such items as gravy, jams, jellies, sauces, salad dressing, nuts, candy, margarine, butter, sugar, milk on cereal or fruit, and social beverages. Record foods immediately after eating. Do not rely on your memory. List separately the different foods that compose one dietary item. For example, for a ham sandwich, list bun, ham, butter, mustard, and lettuce. Record time of day the food was eaten—this helps you remember all foods. Describe the food in as complete detail as possible, for example, include the following:

Methods of preparation	Raw, broiled, fried, baked
Form of food	Canned, frozen
	Buttered toast
	Whole milk
	Yogurt with fruit
	Meat trimmed of fat
	Cake with frosting

Some dishes may have foods prepared differently. For example, a vegetable salad may be composed of raw spinach, cooked beans, and raw onions; potatoes may be french-fried, baked, or creamed.

Estimate the serving size.

By volume	Cups, tablespoons
By weight	Ounces, pounds
By unit	1 biscuit
	1 frankfurter
	1 medium apple

Express amounts of foods as specifically and accurately as possible. Indicate serving sizes of meats as ounces or measure the dimensions (for example, hamburger, 3 oz, or beef, one piece, 2″ × 3″ × 1/2″ thick). Express fruits, vegetables, and fats in terms of standard measuring cups or measuring spoons (for example, cole slaw, 1/2 cup; margarine, 1 teaspoon). Some items may be expressed as pieces or slices. Drinks should be recorded in fluid ounces or measuring cups.

Usual serving sizes are

Cereal	1 oz (dry weight)
Meat	3 oz
Fruit juice	6 oz
Vegetables	4 oz

CALCULATE DIETARY SCORE

Evaluate your food intake for each day recorded by calculating a dietary score. Categorize the food you ate according to one of the four food groups listed. All foods do not fall into these food groups. Group others as "miscellaneous." Each time you eat *one serving* of a food, write the specific food under the food group that includes the specific food. Do not list more than two servings for dairy or meat or more than four servings for fruits and vegetables or breads and cereals. Thus intake that exceeds the maximal intake is not counted. You may list combination dishes in different food groups, for example: pizza—cheese = milk and milk group, tomato sauce = fruits and vegetable group, and

FORM D-1

Example of food record.

MEAL	TIME	FOOD	DESCRIPTION	AMOUNT	SCORE
Breakfast	6:30 AM	Branflakes	With raisins	3/4 Cup	
		Sugar	Brown	1 T	
		Milk	2% fat	3/4 Cup	
		Coffee	Black	1 Cup	
Snack	10:00 AM	Orange	Frozen,	6 oz	
		juice	reconstituted		
		Crackers	Graham	2	
Lunch	2:15 PM	Vegetable	Instant	1 Cup	
		soup			
		Tomato	Raw & sliced	1/2 Medium	
		Bread	Whole-wheat	1 Thin slice	
		Milk	Chocolate	1/2 Pint	
Snack	3:30 PM	Coke	Diet/	8 oz	
			decaffeinated		
		Corn Chips	1 Bag	1 oz	
Dinner	6:15 PM				

crust = bread and cereal group. See Canada's Food Guide (Figure 2-5) for examples of food categories and serving sizes.

EVALUATE NUTRIENT INTAKE

Record the foods and amounts for each of the 3 days, and look up the quantity of each nutrient in each food. Combine identical foods eaten on all 3 days (for example, if you have 1½ cups of whole milk for breakfast, 2 cups for lunch, and 3 cups for dinner, total the amount and record the category as "whole milk, 6½ cups"). This saves space and calculations. Do this only when foods are identical. This helps you recognize the major contributions of each food group.

Information on labels may also be used to supplement food composition data. Remember that labels list the daily values in each serving of only some nutrients.

Example

If label says one serving has 10% U.S. RDA for iron, you find that the U.S. RDA for iron is 18 mg. Thus $0.10 \times 18 = 1.8$ mg of iron per serving.

COMPARE AVERAGE NUTRIENT CONSUMPTION TO THE RDAs

Total the 3-day intake for each nutrient, and then calculate the 3-day average. Compare the RDAs appropriate for your age and sex (see inside front and back cover of the text) with your 3-day averages (without supplements) for nutrient intake. Calculate the percent RDA for each nutrient.

Example

If your average vitamin A intake was 6000 IU and the RDA is 5000 IU, then the percent RDA for vitamin A is:

$$\frac{\text{Your intake}}{\text{RDA}} = \frac{6000}{5000} \times 100 = 120\% \text{ RDA}$$

If the percent RDA was less than 77 (without vitamin or mineral supplements), select at least two foods that would significantly improve your intake with a single serving of the food. Also choose foods you are likely to eat. If the percent RDA was more than 77 (without vitamin or mineral supplements), list the foods that were the major contributors of that nutrient in *your* diet.

APPENDIX E

FOOD COMPOSITION TABLES

WT, weight; **KCAL**, kcalories; **PROT**, protein; **CARB**, carbohydrate; **FIBR**, fiber; **FAT**, fat; **SATF**, saturated fat;

MONO, monsaturated fat; **POLY**, polyunsaturated fat; **CHOL**, cholesterol; **SOD**, sodium; **POT**, potassium;

FOOD NAME	PORTION	WT (g)	KCAL	PROT (g)	CARB (g)	FIBR (g)	FAT (g)	SATF (g)	MONO (g)	POLY (g)
BABY FOODS										
BABY FOOD-CEREAL-OATMEAL-MILK	OUNCE	28.4	33	1	4	0.7	1	0.4	0.8	0.9
BABY FOOD-CEREAL-RICE-MILK	OUNCE	28.4	33	1	5	0.3	1	t	t	t
BABY FOOD-DESSERT-BANANAS & TAPIOCA	OUNCE	28.4	16	t	4	0.7	0	0	0	0
BABY FOOD-DESSERT-CUSTARD CHOCOLATE-USDA	OUNCE	28.4	24	1	5	0.1	1	0.3	0.2	t
BABY FOOD-DESSERT-CUSTARD-VANILLA	OUNCE	28.4	24	t	5	0.1	1	0.3	0.2	t
BABY FOOD-DESSERT-MANGO/TAPIOCA	OUNCE	28.4	23	t	6	0	t	0	0	0
BABY FOOD-DESSERT-ORANGE PUDDING	OUNCE	28.4	23	t	5	0.1	t	0.2	0.1	t
BABY FOOD-DESSERT-PAPAYA/APPLE/TAPIOCA	OUNCE	28.4	20	t	5	0.1	0	0	0	0
BABY FOOD-DESSERT-PLUMS & TAPIOCA	OUNCE	28.4	20	0	6	0.3	0	0	0	0
BABY FOOD-DESSERT-PRUNES & TAPIOCA	OUNCE	28.4	20	t	5	0.7	0	0	0	0
BABY FOOD-EGG YOLKS	SERVING	28.4	58	3	t	0	5	1.5	1.8	0.5
BABY FOOD-FRUIT JUICE-APPLE	FL OZ	31	14	0	4	0.3	0	0	0	0
BABY FOOD-FRUIT JUICE-APPLE BLUEBERRY	OUNCE	28.4	17	t	5	0.1	t	0	0	0
BABY FOOD-FRUIT JUICE-APPLE PEACH-USDA	FL OZ	31	13	0	3	0.3	0	0	0	0
BABY FOOD-FRUIT JUICE-APPLE PRUNE-USDA	FL OZ	31	23	t	6	0.5	0	0	0	0
BABY FOOD-FRUIT JUICE-MIXED FRUIT-USDA	FL OZ	31	14	0	4	0.3	0	0	0	0
BABY FOOD-FRUIT JUICE-ORANGE	FL OZ	31	14	t	3	0.3	t	0	0	0
BABY FOOD-FRUIT-APPLESAUCE	OUNCE	28.4	12	t	3	0.7	0	0	0	0
BABY FOOD-FRUIT-PEACHES	OUNCE	28.4	20	t	5	0.7	0	0	0	0
BABY FOOD-FRUIT-PEARS	OUNCE	28.4	12	t	3	0.3	0	0	0	0
BABY FOOD-FRUIT-PEARS & PINEAPPLE	OUNCE	28.4	12	t	3	0.3	0	0	0	0
BABY FOOD-MEAT-BEEF	OUNCE	28.4	30	4	0	0	2	0.7	0.6	0.1
BABY FOOD-MEAT-BEEF & EGG NOODLES-STR	OUNCE	28.4	15	1	2	0.1	1	0.2	0.2	t
BABY FOOD-MEAT-BEEF STEW	OUNCE	28.4	14	1	2	0.3	t	0.2	0.1	t
BABY FOOD-MEAT-CHICKEN STEW-STR	OUNCE	28.4	22	2	2	0.2	1	0.3	0.5	0.2
BABY FOOD-MEAT-LAMB	OUNCE	28.4	29	4	0	0	1	0.7	0.5	0.1
BABY FOOD-MEAT-LIVER	OUNCE	28.4	29	4	t	0	1	0.4	0.2	t
BABY FOOD-MEAT-PORK	OUNCE	28.4	35	4	0	0	2	0.7	1	0.2
BABY FOOD-MEAT-VEAL	OUNCE	28.4	29	4	0	0	1	0.7	0.6	0.1
BABY FOOD-VEGETABLES-BEANS-GREEN	OUNCE	28.4	7	t	2	0.4	0	0	0	0
BABY FOOD-VEGETABLES-BEANS-GREEN/BU-STR	OUNCE	28.4	9	t	2	0.7	t	t	0	t
BABY FOOD-VEGETABLES-CARROTS-STR-USDA	OUNCE	28.4	8	t	2	0.7	0	0	0	0
BABY FOOD-VEGETABLES-GARDEN	OUNCE	28.4	11	1	2	0.7	t	0	0	0
BABY FOOD-VEGETABLES-PEAS	OUNCE	28.4	11	1	2	0.7	t	0	0	0
BABY FOOD-VEGETABLES-SQUASH	OUNCE	28.4	7	t	2	0.7	t	0	0	0
BABY FOOD-VEGETABLES-SWEET POTATOES	OUNCE	28.4	16	t	4	0.7	0	0	0	0
BEVERAGES										
ALE-MILD-AMERICAN	CUP	230	98	1	8	0	0	0	0	0
BEER-BUDWEISER	FL OZ	30	13	t	1	0.2	0	0	0	0
BEER-LIGHT	FL OZ	29.5	8	t	t	0	0	0	0	0
BEER-MICHELOB	FL OZ	30	13	t	1	0.1	0	0	0	0
BEER-NATURAL LIGHT	FL OZ	30	8	t	1	0	0	0	0	0
BEER-REGULAR	FL OZ	29.7	12	t	1	0.1	0	0	0	0
BRANDY-CALIFORNIA	ITEM	30	73	*	*	0	0	0	0	0
BRANDY-COGNAC-PONY	ITEM	30	73	0	0	0	0	0	0	0
CARNATION INSTANT BREAKFAST-CHOCOLATE	ITEM	36	130	7	23	*	1	*	*	*
CARNATION INSTANT BREAKFAST-EGGNOG	ITEM	34	130	7	23	*	0	0	0	0
CARNATION INSTANT BREAKFAST-VANILLA	ITEM	35	130	7	24	*	0	0	0	0
CHAMPAGNE-DOMESTIC-GLASSFUL	ITEM	120	84	t	3	0	0	0	0	0
CHOCOLATE BEVERAGE POWDER-DRY MILK ADDED	OUNCE	28.4	100	5	20	0.5	1	0.5	0.3	0
CHOCOLATE BEVERAGE POWDER-NO DRY MILK	OUNCE	28.4	99	1	26	12	1	0.5	0.3	t
CIDER-FERMENTED	FL OZ	30	12	t	t	0	0	0	0	0

t= Trace of nutrient present **= Not available*

MAG, magnesium; **IRON,** iron; **ZINC,** zinc; **VITA,** vitamin A; **VITC,** vitamin C; **THIA,** thiamin; **RIBO,** riboflavin; **NIAC,** niacin; **VB6,** vitamin B-6; **FOL,** folate; **VB12,** vitamin B-12; **CALC,** calcium; **PHOS,** phosphorus; **SEL,** selenium; **VE-a,** alpha tocopherol equivalents.

CHOL (mg)	SOD (mg)	POT (mg)	MAG (mg)	IRON (mg)	ZINC (mg)	VITA (RE)	VITC (mg)	THIA (mg)	RIBO (mg)	NIAC (mg)	VB6 (mg)	FOL (µg)	VB12 (µg)	CALC (mg)	PHOS (mg)	SEL (µg)	VE-a (mg)
0	13	58	10	3.4	0.3	6	t	0.14	0.16	1.7	0.02	3	0.09	62	45	1	0.2
0	13	54	13	3.5	0.2	6	t	0.13	0.14	1.5	0.03	2	0.09	68	50	1	0.2
0	3	25	3	0.1	t	1	5	t	0.01	0.1	0.03	2	0	1	2	0	0.2
0	7	24	3	0.1	0.1	1	t	t	0.03	t	t	1	t	17	14	0	0.1
0	8	19	2	0.1	0.1	2	t	t	0.02	t	0.01	2	t	16	13	0	0.1
0	1	17	1	t	t	19	35	0.01	0.01	0.1	0.03	1	0	1	2	0	0.2
0	6	24	2	t	t	3	3	0.01	0.02	t	0.01	2	0	9	8	0	0.1
0	1	22	1	0.1	t	2	32	t	0.01	t	0.01	1	0	2	2	0	0.2
0	2	24	1	0.1	t	3	t	t	0.01	0.1	0.01	t	0	2	2	0	0.2
0	1	50	3	0.1	t	13	t	0.01	0.02	0.1	0.02	t	0	4	4	0	0.2
223	11	22	2	0.8	0.5	107	t	0.02	0.08	t	0.05	26	0.44	22	81	5	0.5
0	1	28	1	0.2	t	1	18	t	0.01	t	0.01	0	0	1	2	0	0.2
0	0	20	1	0.1	t	1	8	0.01	0.01	t	0.01	1	0	1	2	0	0.2
0	t	30	1	0.2	t	2	18	t	t	0.1	0.01	t	0	1	1	0	0.2
0	2	46	2	0.3	t	1	21	t	t	0.1	0.01	0	0	3	5	0	0.2
0	1	31	2	0.1	t	1	20	0.01	t	t	0.01	2	0	2	2	0	0.2
0	0	57	3	0.1	t	2	19	0.01	0.01	0.1	0.02	8	0	4	3	0	0.2
0	1	20	1	0.1	t	0	11	t	0.01	t	0.01	1	0	1	2	0	0.2
0	2	46	2	0.1	t	5	9	t	0.01	0.2	t	1	0	2	3	0	0.2
0	1	37	2	0.1	t	1	7	t	0.01	0.1	t	1	0	2	3	0	0.2
0	1	33	2	0.1	t	1	8	0.01	0.01	0.1	0.01	1	0	3	2	0	0.2
4	23	62	5	0.4	0.7	16	1	t	0.04	0.8	0.04	2	0.4	2	24	3	0.1
2	8	13	2	0.1	0.1	31	t	0.01	0.01	0.2	0.01	1	0.03	3	8	3	0.1
4	98	40	3	0.2	0.2	95	1	t	0.02	0.4	0.02	2	0.15	3	12	3	0.1
8	114	26	3	0.2	0.1	50	1	0.01	0.02	0.3	0.01	t	0.04	10	14	3	0.1
0	18	58	4	0.4	0.8	7	t	0.01	0.06	0.8	0.04	1	0.62	2	27	4	0.1
52	21	64	4	1.5	0.8	3247	6	0.01	0.51	2.4	0.1	96	0.61	1	58	7	0.1
14	12	63	3	0.3	0.6	3	1	0.04	0.06	0.6	0.06	1	0.28	1	27	4	0.1
11	18	61	4	0.4	0.6	4	1	0.01	0.05	1	0.04	2	0.37	2	28	3	0.1
0	1	45	7	0.2	0.1	13	2	0.01	0.02	0.1	0.01	10	0	11	6	0	0.2
0	1	45	7	0.4	0.1	13	2	0.01	0.03	0.1	0.01	8	0	18	6	170	0.2
0	11	56	3	0.1	t	325	2	0.01	0.01	0.1	0.02	4	0	6	6	0	0.2
0	10	48	6	0.2	0.1	172	2	0.02	0.02	0.2	0.03	11	0	8	8	0	0.2
0	1	32	4	0.3	0.1	16	2	0.02	0.02	0.3	0.02	7	0	6	12	0	0.2
0	1	51	3	0.1	t	57	2	t	0.02	0.1	0.02	4	0	7	4	0	0.2
0	6	75	4	0.1	0.1	183	3	0.01	0.01	0.1	0.03	3	0	4	7	0	0.2
0	16	*	*	0.2	*	0	0	0	0.07	0.5	*	*	*	30	41	1	*
0	2	7	2	t	0	0	0	t	0.01	0.1	0.02	2	0.01	1	4	0	0
0	1	5	1	t	t	0	0	t	0.01	0.1	0.01	1	t	1	4	0	0
0	2	7	2	t	0	0	0	t	0.01	0.1	0.02	2	0.01	1	4	0	0
0	2	5	1	t	t	0	0	t	0.01	0.1	0.01	1	0	1	4	0	0
0	1	7	2	t	t	0	0	t	0.01	0.1	0.02	2	0.01	1	4	*	0
0	*	*	*	*	*	*	*	*	*	*	*	*	*	*	*	*	*
0	t	1	0	t	t	0	0	t	t	t	0	0	0	0	1	*	0
*	136	422	80	4.5	3	525	27	0.3	0.07	5	0.4	0	0.6	100	150	*	5
0	196	266	80	4.5	3	525	27	0.3	0.07	5	0.4	0	0.6	100	150	*	5
0	145	382	80	4.5	3	525	27	0.3	0.07	5	0.4	0	0.6	100	150	*	5
0	*	*	*	*	*	*	*	*	*	*	*	*	*	*	*	*	*
2	147	227	23	0.5	0.3	3	1	0.04	0.21	0.2	t	12	0.68	167	155	*	0.1
0	60	168	28	0.9	0.4	1	t	0.01	0.04	0.1	t	2	0	11	36	*	0.1
0	0	36	1	0.1	t	0	t	0.01	0.01	t	0.01	t	0	2	2	*	t

WT, weight; **KCAL**, kcalories; **PROT**, protein; **CARB**, carbohydrate; **FIBR**, fiber; **FAT**, fat; **SATF**, saturated fat;

MONO, monsaturated fat; **POLY**, polyunsaturated fat; **CHOL**, cholesterol; **SOD**, sodium; **POT**, potassium;

FOOD NAME	PORTION	WT (g)	KCAL	PROT (g)	CARB (g)	FIBR (g)	FAT (g)	SATF (g)	MONO (g)	POLY (g)
COCKTAIL-DAIQUIRI	ITEM	100	186	t	7	0	t	t	t	t
COCKTAIL-EGGNOG	ITEM	123	335	4	18	0	16	1.8	1.3	0.3
COCKTAIL-GIN RICKEY	ITEM	120	150	0	1	0	0	0	0	0
COCKTAIL-HIGHBALL	FL OZ	29	26	0	0	0	0	0	0	0
COCKTAIL-MANHATTAN	FL OZ	28.5	64	t	1	0	0	0	0	0
COCKTAIL-MARTINI	FL OZ	28.2	63	0	t	0	0	0	0	0
COCKTAIL-MINT JULEP	ITEM	300	212	0	3	0	0	0	0	0
COCKTAIL-OLD FASHIONED	ITEM	100	180	0	4	0	0	0	0	0
COCKTAIL-PINA COLADA-HOME RECIPE	FL OZ	31.4	58	t	9	0.1	1	0.3	0.1	0.1
COCKTAIL-PLANTERS PUNCH	ITEM	100	175	t	8	0	0	0	0	0
COCKTAIL-RUM SOUR	ITEM	100	165	0	0	0	0	0	0	0
COCKTAIL-TOM COLLINS	FL OZ	29.6	16	0	t	0	0	0	0	0
COFFEE SUBSTITUTE-PREPARED	FL OZ	30.3	2	t	t	0	0	0	0	0
COFFEE-BREWED	FL OZ	29.6	1	t	t	0	0	t	0	t
COFFEE-INSTANT-PREPARED	CUP	239	5	t	1	0	0	t	0	t
CORDIALS/LIQUEUR-54 PROOF	FL OZ	34	97	t	12	0	0	0	0	0
FRUIT PUNCH DRINK-CANNED	FL OZ	31	15	0	4	0	0	t	t	t
FRUIT PUNCH-POWDERED-PREPARED WITH WATER	CUP	262	97	0	25	*	t	t	t	t
GATORADE-THIRST QUENCHING DRINK	FL OZ	30.1	8	0	2	0	0	0	0	0
HOT COCOA-PREPARED WITH MILK-HOME RECIPE	CUP	250	218	9	26	3	9	5.6	2.7	0.3
LIQUEURS-ANISETTE	ITEM	20	74	0	7	0	0	0	0	0
LIQUEURS-APRICOT BRANDY	ITEM	20	64	t	6	0	0	0	0	0
LIQUEURS-BENEDICTINE	ITEM	20	69	*	7	0	0	0	0	0
LIQUEURS-CREME DE MENTHE	FL OZ	33.6	125	0	14	0	t	t	t	0.1
LIQUEURS-CURACAO	ITEM	20	54	*	6	0	0	0	0	0
OVALTINE-CHOCOLATE FLAVOR-PREPARED/MILK	CUP	265	227	10	29	0.2	9	5.5	2.6	0.4
OVALTINE-MALT FLAVOR-PREPARED WITH MILK	CUP	265	228	10	29	0.1	8	5.4	2.5	0.4
POSTUM-INSTANT GRAIN BEVERAGE-DRY MIX	OUNCE	28.4	103	2	24	0	t	0	0	0
SANKA-DECAFFEINATED COFFEE-PREPARED	FL OZ	29.8	t	0	t	0	0	0	0	0
SODA-CLUB-CARBONATED	FL OZ	29.6	0	0	0	0	0	0	0	0
SODA-COLA TYPE-CARBONATED	FL OZ	30.8	13	0	3	0	0	t	0	0
SODA-CREAM FLAVORED-CARBONATED	FL OZ	30.9	16	0	4	0	0	0	0	0
SODA-DIET COLA-NUTRASWEET-CARBONATED	FL OZ	29.6	t	t	t	0	0	0	0	0
SODA-DR. PEPPER TYPE COLA-CARBONATED	FL OZ	30.8	13	0	3	0	t	t	0	0
SODA-GINGER ALE-CARBONATED	FL OZ	30.5	10	0	3	0	0	0	0	0
SODA-GRAPE-CARBONATED	FL OZ	31	13	0	3	0	0	0	0	0
SODA-ROOT BEER-CARBONATED	FL OZ	30.8	13	0	3	0	0	0	0	0
SODA-TAB-LOW CALORIE COLA-CARBONATED	CUP	236	0	0	0	0	0	0	0	0
SODA-TONIC WATER/QUININE-CARBONATED	FL OZ	30.5	10	0	3	0	0	0	0	0
TANG-INSTANT BREAKFAST DRINK-ORANGE-DRY	OUNCE	28.4	104	0	26	*	0	0	0	0
TEA-BREWED	FL OZ	29.6	t	0	t	0	0	t	0	t
TEA-HERBAL-BREWED	FL OZ	29.6	t	0	t	0	0	t	0	t
TEA-INSTANT-PREPARED-SWEETENED	CUP	259	88	t	22	0	0	t	t	t
TEA-INSTANT-PREPARED-UNSWEETENED	CUP	237	2	0	t	0	0	0	0	0
WATER-MINERAL-PERRIER	CUP	237	0	0	0	0	0	0	0	0
WATER-MUNICIPAL TAP	CUP	237	0	0	0	0	0	0	0	0
WHISKEY/GIN/RUM/VODKA-100 PROOF	FL OZ	27.8	82	0	0	0	0	0	0	0
WHISKEY/GIN/RUM/VODKA-80 PROOF	FL OZ	27.8	64	0	0	0	0	0	0	0
WHISKEY/GIN/RUM/VODKA-86 PROOF	FL OZ	27.8	70	0	t	0	0	0	0	0
WHISKEY/GIN/RUM/VODKA-90 PROOF	FL OZ	27.7	73	0	0	0	0	0	0	0
WHISKEY/GIN/RUM/VODKA-94 PROOF	FL OZ	27.8	77	0	0	0	0	0	0	0
WINE COOLER-WHITE WINE AND 7UP	SERVING	102	55	t	6	0	0	0	0	0
WINE-CALIFORNIA/RED-GLASSFUL	ITEM	102	85	t	3	0	0	0	0	0
WINE-DESSERT	FL OZ	30	46	t	4	0	0	0	0	0
WINE-MADEIRA-GLASSFUL	ITEM	100	105	t	1	0	0	0	0	0
WINE-MUSCATEL/PORT-GLASSFUL	ITEM	100	158	t	14	0	0	0	0	0
WINE-RED-TABLE	FL OZ	29.5	21	t	1	0	0	0	0	0
WINE-ROSE-TABLE	FL OZ	29.5	21	t	t	0	0	0	0	0
WINE-SAUTERNE-GLASSFUL	ITEM	100	84	t	4	0	0	0	0	0
WINE-SHERRY-DRY-GLASSFUL	ITEM	60	84	t	5	0	0	0	0	0
WINE-VERMOUTH-DRY-GLASSFUL	ITEM	100	105	0	1	0	0	0	0	0
WINE-VERMOUTH-SWEET-GLASSFUL	ITEM	100	167	0	12	0	0	0	0	0
WINE-WHITE-TABLE	FL OZ	29.5	20	t	t	0	0	0	0	0

t = Trace of nutrient present ** = Not available*

MAG, magnesium; **IRON,** iron; **ZINC,** zinc; **VITA,** vitamin A; **VITC,** vitamin C; **THIA,** thiamin; **RIBO,** riboflavin; **NIAC,** niacin; **VB6,** vitamin B-6; **FOL,** folate; **VB12,** vitamin B-12; **CALC,** calcium; **PHOS,** phosphorus; **SEL,** selenium; **VE-a,** alpha tocopherol equivalents.

CHOL (mg)	SOD (mg)	POT (mg)	MAG (mg)	IRON (mg)	ZINC (mg)	VITA (RE)	VITC (mg)	THIA (mg)	RIBO (mg)	NIAC (mg)	VB6 (mg)	FOL (µg)	VB12 (µg)	CALC (mg)	PHOS (mg)	SEL (µg)	VE-a (mg)
0	5	21	2	0.2	0.1	1	2	0.01	t	t	0.01	2	0	3	6	*	t
94	75	178	16	0.7	0.6	25	0	0.04	0.11	0	0.07	15	0.57	44	74	*	0.2
0	19	12	1	0	0.1	t	4	0.01	0	0	t	1	0	2	1	*	t
0	4	1	t	t	t	0	0	t	0	t	0	0	0	1	1	*	*
0	1	7	1	t	t	0	0	t	t	t	0	t	0	1	2	*	0
0	1	5	1	t	t	0	0	0	t	t	t	t	0	1	1	*	0
0	0	6	t	0.1	0.1	0	0	0.02	0.01	t	t	0	0	t	10	*	0
0	1	2	0	t	t	0	0	0.01	t	t	t	0	0	0	4	*	0
0	2	22	3	0.1	t	t	1	0.01	t	t	0.01	3	0	3	2	*	t
0	*	*	*	0.1	*	0	8	0.1	0	0	*	*	*	4	3	*	*
0	1	2	0	t	t	0	0	0.01	t	t	t	0	0	0	4	*	0
0	5	2	t	t	t	0	1	t	0	t	t	t	0	1	t	*	t
0	1	7	1	t	t	0	0	t	0	0.1	t	t	0	1	2	*	0
0	1	16	1	t	t	0	0	0	0	0.1	0	t	0	1	t	0	0
0	7	86	10	0.1	0.1	0	0	0	t	0.7	0	0	0	7	7	0	0
0	1	1	0	t	t	0	0	t	t	t	0	0	0	0	0	*	0
0	7	8	1	0.1	t	1	9	0.01	0.01	t	0	t	0	2	t	0	0
0	37	3	3	0.1	0.1	t	31	0	0.01	t	0	t	0	42	52	*	*
0	12	3	t	t	t	0	0	t	0	0	0	0	0	0	3	*	0
33	123	480	56	0.8	1.2	96	2	0.1	0.44	0.4	0.11	12	0.87	298	270	*	0.3
0	*	*	*	*	*	*	*	*	*	*	*	*	*	*	*	*	*
0	2	11	1	t	t	t	3	0.01	t	t	t	1	0	1	1	*	t
0	*	*	*	*	*	*	*	*	*	*	*	*	*	*	*	*	*
0	2	0	0	t	t	0	0	0	0	t	0	0	0	0	0	*	*
0	*	*	*	*	*	*	*	*	*	*	*	*	*	*	*	*	*
34	228	600	52	4.8	1.1	700	29	0.63	0.97	12.7	0.77	29	0.87	392	302	*	0.4
37	201	576	47	4.5	1.1	770	30	0.67	1.16	11.9	0.75	29	0.87	371	308	*	0.3
0	28	896	*	1.9	*	0	0	0.17	0.08	6.8	*	*	*	77	189	*	*
0	0	10	1	t	t	0	0	0	0	t	0	0	0	1	1	*	0
0	6	0	0	t	t	0	0	0	0	0	0	0	0	1	0	*	0
0	1	t	t	t	t	0	0	0	0	0	0	0	0	1	4	*	0
0	4	t	t	t	t	0	0	0	0	0	0	0	0	2	0	*	0
0	2	0	t	t	t	0	0	t	0.01	0	0	0	0	1	3	*	*
0	3	t	0	t	t	0	0	0	0	0	0	0	0	1	3	*	0
0	2	t	t	0.1	t	0	0	0	0	0	0	0	0	1	0	*	0
0	5	t	t	t	t	0	0	0	0	0	0	0	0	1	0	*	0
0	4	t	t	t	t	0	0	0	0	0	0	0	0	2	0	*	0
0	30	*	*	*	*	*	*	*	*	*	*	*	*	*	30	*	*
0	1	0	0	t	t	0	0	0	0	0	0	0	0	t	0	*	0
0	13	81	*	t	*	535	107	0	0	0	*	*	*	71	76	*	*
0	1	11	1	t	t	0	0	0	t	0	0	2	0	0	t	0	*
0	t	3	t	t	t	0	0	t	t	0	0	t	0	1	0	*	0
0	8	49	5	0.1	0.1	0	0	0	0.05	0.1	0.01	10	0	5	3	0	0
0	7	47	5	t	0.1	0	0	0	0.01	0.1	0.01	1	0	5	2	0	0
0	3	0	1	0	0	0	0	0	0	0	0	0	0	32	0	*	0
0	7	1	2	t	0.1	0	0	0	0	0	0	0	0	5	0	*	0
0	0	0	0	t	t	0	0	t	t	t	0	0	0	0	1	*	0
0	0	1	0	t	t	0	0	t	0	0	0	0	0	0	1	0	0
0	t	1	0	t	t	0	0	t	0	t	0	0	0	0	1	0	0
0	1	0	0	0	0	0	0	0	0	0	0	0	0	0	0	0	0
0	0	0	0	t	t	0	0	t	t	t	0	0	0	0	1	*	0
0	7	41	5	0.2	0.1	t	2	t	t	t	0.01	t	0	6	7	*	t
0	10	116	11	1	0.1	0	0	0.01	0.03	0.1	0.04	1	0.01	8	13	*	0
0	3	28	3	0.1	t	0	0	0.01	0.01	0.1	0	t	0	2	3	*	0
0	5	92	9	0.2	0.1	0	0	0.02	0.02	0.2	0	t	0	8	9	*	0
0	4	75	4	1.6	0.1	0	0	0.01	0.01	0.2	0.05	2	0	8	9	*	0
0	19	41	4	0.1	t	0	0	t	0.01	t	0.01	1	0	2	4	*	0
0	1	29	3	0.1	t	0	0	t	0.01	t	0.01	t	t	2	4	*	0
0	2	89	10	0.4	0.1	0	0	t	0.02	0.1	0.02	1	0.01	8	14	*	0
0	2	45	6	0.2	t	0	0	0.01	0.01	0.1	0.01	1	0.01	5	8	3	0
0	4	75	10	0.4	0.1	0	0	0.01	0.01	0.2	0.02	1	0.01	8	14	5	0
0	9	92	9	0.2	0.1	0	0	0.02	0.02	0.2	0	t	0	8	9	*	0
0	1	24	3	0.1	t	0	0	t	t	t	t	t	0	3	4	*	0

WT, weight; **KCAL,** kcalories; **PROT,** protein; **CARB,** carbohydrate; **FIBR,** fiber; **FAT,** fat; **SATF,** saturated fat;

MONO, monsaturated fat; **POLY,** polyunsaturated fat; **CHOL,** cholesterol; **SOD,** sodium; **POT,** potassium;

FOOD NAME	PORTION	WT (g)	KCAL	PROT (g)	CARB (g)	FIBR (g)	FAT (g)	SATF (g)	MONO (g)	POLY (g)
BREADS										
BAGEL-EGG-3 INCH DIAMETER	ITEM	55	163	6	31	1.2	1	*	*	*
BAGEL-WATER-3 INCH DIAMETER	ITEM	55	163	6	31	1.2	1	0.2	0.4	0.6
BISCUITS-BAKING POWDER-FROM HOME RECIPE	ITEM	28.4	105	2	13	0.4	5	1.2	2	1.2
BISCUITS-BAKING POWDER-PREPARED FROM MIX	ITEM	28.4	104	2	13	0.5	5	3.3	1.3	0.2
BREAD STICKS-VIENNA TYPE	ITEM	35	106	3	20	1	1	*	*	*
BREAD-CRACKED WHEAT-ENRICHED	SLICE	25	66	2	13	1.3	1	0.1	0.2	0.2
BREAD-FRENCH-ENRICHED	SLICE	35	98	3	18	0.8	1	0.2	0.4	0.4
BREAD-ITALIAN-ENRICHED	SLICE	30	85	3	17	0.8	0	0	0	0
BREAD-MELBA TOAST-PLAIN	SLICE	4.67	16	1	3	0.3	0	0	0	0
BREAD-MELBA TOAST-WHEAT	SLICE	4.67	16	1	3	0.3	0	0	0	0
BREAD-MIXED GRAIN-UNTOASTED	SLICE	25	64	2	12	1.6	1	*	*	*
BREAD-PITA	ITEM	38	105	4	21	0.6	1	0.1	t	0.1
BREAD-PUMPERNICKEL	SLICE	32	82	3	15	1.9	1	*	*	*
BREAD-RAISIN-ENRICHED	SLICE	25	70	2	13	0.6	1	0.2	0.3	0.2
BREAD-RYE-AMERICAN-LIGHT	SLICE	25	66	2	12	1.6	1	*	*	*
BREAD-VIENNA-ENRICHED	SLICE	25	70	2	13	0.8	1	0.2	0.3	0.3
BREAD-WHEAT-FIRM	SLICE	21	59	2	11	2.4	1	0.1	0.2	0.3
BREAD-WHEAT-TOASTED	SLICE	22	68	2	12	2.5	2	0.2	0.3	0.8
BREAD-WHITE-FIRM	SLICE	23	61	2	11	0.4	1	0.2	0.3	0.3
BREAD-WHITE-FIRM-ENRICHED-TOASTED	SLICE	20	65	2	12	0.5	1	0.2	0.3	0.3
BREAD-WHITE-SOFT-ENRICHED-CRUMBS	CUP	45	120	4	22	1.2	2	0.3	0.5	0.5
BREAD-WHOLE WHEAT-FIRM	SLICE	25	61	2	11	2.8	1	0.1	0.2	0.3
BREAD-WHOLE WHEAT	SLICE	25	67	2	12	2.8	2	0.2	0.3	0.8
BREADCRUMBS-DRY-GRATED-ENRICHED	CUP	100	390	13	73	3.7	5	1	1.6	1.4
CORNBREAD-HOME RECIPE	SLICE	45	108	2	16	1.2	4	1.5	1.9	1.1
CRACKERS-ANIMAL	ITEM	1.9	9	t	1	t	t	0.1	0.1	t
CRACKERS-CHEDDAR SNACKS	ITEM	1.6	7	t	1	0.1	t	*	*	*
CRACKERS-CHEESE	ITEM	1	5	t	1	t	t	0.1	0.1	t
CRACKERS-CHEESE SNACKS	ITEM	1.13	6	t	1	t	t	0.1	0.1	t
CRACKERS-GRAHAM-PLAIN	ITEM	7	28	1	5	0.2	1	0.1	0.3	0.2
CRACKERS-GRAHAM-SUGAR-HONEY	ITEM	7	30	1	5	0.1	1	0.1	0.4	0.1
CRACKERS-OYSTER	ITEM	0.45	2	t	t	t	t	0	0	0
CRACKERS-RITZ	ITEM	3.33	18	t	2	0.1	1	*	*	*
CRACKERS-RY KRISP-NATURAL	ITEM	2.1	8	t	2	0.3	t	0	0	0
CRACKERS-RYE WAFERS	ITEM	6.5	23	1	5	1.1	0	0	0	0
CRACKERS-SALTINES	ITEM	2.75	13	t	2	0.1	t	0.1	0.1	0.1
CRACKERS-SESAME AND WHEAT-RALSTON	ITEM	1.9	9	t	1	0.2	t	*	*	*
CRACKERS-SNACKERS-RALSTON	ITEM	3.5	18	t	2	0.1	1	*	*	*
CRACKERS-TRISCUITS	ITEM	4.5	21	t	3	0.2	1	0.2	0.2	0.2
CRACKERS-WHEAT THINS	ITEM	1.8	9	t	1	0.1	t	*	*	*
FRENCH TOAST-FROM HOME RECIPE	SLICE	65	153	6	17	2	7	0.5	0.9	0.5
MUFFIN-BLUEBERRY-FROM HOME RECIPE	ITEM	40	110	3	17	0.9	4	1.1	1.4	0.7
MUFFIN-BRAN-FROM HOME RECIPE	ITEM	40	112	3	17	2.5	5	1.2	1.4	0.8
MUFFIN-CORN-FROM HOME RECIPE	ITEM	40	125	3	19	1	4	1.2	1.6	0.9
MUFFIN-ENGLISH-PLAIN-TOASTED	ITEM	53	154	5	30	1.5	1	0.3	0.4	0.4
MUFFIN-ENGLISH-PLAIN	ITEM	56	133	4	26	1.3	1	1.9	2.6	1.5
MUFFIN-PLAIN-FROM HOME RECIPE	ITEM	40	120	3	17	0.9	4	1	1.7	1
MUFFIN-SOY	ITEM	40	119	4	17	0.8	4	*	*	*
PANCAKES-BUCKWHEAT-FROM MIX	ITEM	27	55	2	6	0.6	2	0.8	0.9	0.4
PANCAKES-PLAIN-FROM HOME RECIPE	ITEM	27	60	2	9	0.5	2	0.5	0.8	0.5
PANCAKES-PLAIN-FROM MIX	ITEM	27	59	2	8	0.4	2	0.7	0.7	0.3
ROLL-BROWN & SERVE-ENRICHED	ITEM	26	85	2	14	1	2	0.4	0.7	0.5
ROLL-CINNAMON	ITEM	26	100	2	14	0.7	4	0.6	1.2	0.5
ROLL-CROISSANT-SARA LEE	ITEM	26	109	2	11	0.6	6	3.3	1.6	0.3
ROLL-HAMBURGER/HOTDOG-COMMERCIAL	ITEM	40	114	3	20	1	2	0.5	0.8	0.6
ROLL-HARD-COMMERCIAL-ENRICHED	ITEM	50	155	5	30	1.5	2	0.4	0.6	0.5
ROLL-SUBMARINE/HOAGIE-ENRICHED	ITEM	135	390	12	75	3.8	4	0.9	1.4	1.4
ROLL-WHOLE WHEAT-HOMEMADE	ITEM	35	90	4	18	1.8	1	0.4	0.6	1.4
WAFFLES-ENRICHED-FROM HOME RECIPE	ITEM	75	245	7	26	1.1	13	2.3	2.8	1.4
WAFFLES-FROZEN	ITEM	37	103	2	16	0.9	4	*	*	*
WAFFLES-OAT BRAN-NO CHOLESTEROL-EGGO	ITEM	39	110	3	16	2	4	0.7	1.1	2.1

t = Trace of nutrient present   ** = Not available*

MAG, magnesium; **IRON,** iron; **ZINC,** zinc; **VITA,** vitamin A; **VITC,** vitamin C; **THIA,** thiamin; **RIBO,** riboflavin; **NIAC,** niacin; **VB6,** vitamin B-6; **FOL,** folate; **VB12,** vitamin B-12; **CALC,** calcium; **PHOS,** phosphorus; **SEL,** selenium; **VE-a,** alpha tocopherol equivalents.

CHOL (mg)	SOD (mg)	POT (mg)	MAG (mg)	IRON (mg)	ZINC (mg)	VITA (RE)	VITC (mg)	THIA (mg)	RIBO (mg)	NIAC (mg)	VB6 (mg)	FOL (μg)	VB12 (μg)	CALC (mg)	PHOS (mg)	SEL (μg)	VE-a (mg)
8	198	41	11	1.5	0.3	24	0	0.21	0.16	1.9	0.02	13	0.05	23	37	*	*
0	198	41	11	1.5	0.3	0	0	0.21	0.16	1.9	0.02	13	0	23	37	18	*
0	175	33	6	0.4	*	0	0	0.08	0.08	0.7	*	*	*	34	49	5	1
1	221	33	3	0.6	0.1	37	0	0.1	0.07	1.8	0.01	2	0.04	34	99	5	1
0	548	33	*	0.3	*	0	0	0.02	0.03	0.3	*	*	*	16	31	*	*
0	108	33	9	0.7	*	0	0	0.1	0.1	0.8	0.02	*	0	16	32	11	t
0	193	30	7	1.1	0.2	0	0	0.16	0.12	1.4	0.02	13	0	39	28	10	t
0	152	22	*	0.7	*	0	0	0.12	0.07	1	0.02	11	0	5	23	8	t
0	30	11	2	0.1	0.1	0	0	0.01	0.01	0.1	t	1	0	5	10	*	t
0	30	11	3	0.1	0.1	0	0	0.01	0.01	0.1	0.01	1	0	5	10	*	t
0	103	55	12	0.8	0.3	0	0	0.1	0.1	1	0.03	16	0	26	53	11	t
0	215	45	8	0.9	0.3	0	0	0.17	0.08	1.4	0.04	22	0	31	38	*	t
0	173	139	22	0.9	0.4	0	0	0.11	0.17	1.1	0.05	*	0	23	70	14	0
0	94	60	6	0.8	0.2	0	0	0.08	0.16	1	0.01	9	0	26	23	*	*
0	174	51	6	0.7	0.3	0	0	0.1	0.08	0.8	0.02	10	0	20	36	9	*
0	138	22	5	0.8	0.2	0	0	0.12	0.09	1	0.01	9	0	28	20	7	t
0	153	42	23	0.8	0.4	0	0	0.07	0.05	0.9	0.05	13	0	17	63	11	t
0	91	87	24	0.7	0.6	t	0	0.06	0.04	0.8	0.05	13	0.03	20	64	11	t
0	118	26	5	0.7	0.1	0	0	0.11	0.07	0.9	0.01	8	0	29	25	6	t
0	117	28	5	0.6	0.1	0	0	0.07	0.06	0.8	0.01	8	0	22	23	6	t
0	231	50	9	1.3	0.3	0	0	0.21	0.14	1.7	0.02	16	0	57	49	13	0.1
0	159	44	23	0.9	0.4	0	0	0.09	0.05	1	0.05	14	0	18	65	11	t
0	89	85	23	0.7	0.6	11	0	0.07	0.04	0.8	0.05	12	0.03	20	63	11	t
0	736	152	32	3.6	*	0	0	0.35	0.35	4.8	*	*	*	122	141	20	*
0	126	42	8	0.7	0.2	7	0	0.08	0.08	0.7	0.03	5	0.08	49	44	5	0.6
0	8	2	t	0.1	t	0	0	0.01	0.01	0.1	0	t	t	t	1	0	t
*	14	2	t	0.1	t	t	0	0.01	0.01	0.1	t	t	0.01	1	2	1	t
t	12	2	t	t	t	t	0	t	t	0.1	t	t	0.01	1	2	0	t
t	10	2	t	0.1	t	t	0	0.01	0.01	t	t	t	0.04	1	1	1	t
0	33	28	4	0.3	0.1	0	0	0.01	0.04	0.3	0.01	1	0	3	11	1	t
0	33	12	2	0.2	0.1	0	0	0.02	0.02	0.2	0.01	1	0	3	8	1	t
0	5	1	t	t	t	0	0	t	t	t	0	t	0	t	t	0	t
0	32	3	*	0.1	*	*	*	0.01	0.01	0.1	*	*	*	5	8	*	t
0	19	10	3	0.1	0.1	*	*	0.01	0.01	t	0.01	1	*	1	7	1	t
0	57	39	*	0.3	*	0	0	0.02	0.02	0.1	*	*	*	4	25	1	t
1	37	3	1	0.1	t	0	0	0.13	0.01	0.1	t	t	0	1	3	4	t
0	17	4	1	0.1	t	0	0	0.01	0.01	0.1	t	t	0.01	1	3	1	t
0	24	4	t	0.1	t	t	0	0.01	0.02	0.2	t	t	t	1	3	1	t
0	24	6	3	0.2	0.1	0	0	0.02	0.01	0.2	0.01	1	0.04	1	9	1	t
0	*	*	*	*	*	*	*	*	*	*	*	*	*	*	*	0	t
t	257	86	12	1.3	0.6	22	0	0.12	0.16	1	0.04	18	0.29	72	85	*	0.4
21	252	46	10	0.6	*	18	0	0.09	0.1	0.7	*	*	*	34	53	*	*
21	168	99	35	1.3	1.1	40	2	0.1	0.11	1.3	0.11	17	0.09	54	111	*	*
21	192	54	18	0.7	*	25	0	0.1	0.1	0.7	*	*	*	42	68	*	*
0	414	364	12	1.8	0.5	0	0	0.24	0.21	2.4	0.03	21	0	105	73	15	0.1
0	358	314	11	1.6	0.4	0	0	0.26	0.18	2.1	0.02	18	0	91	63	15	0.9
21	176	50	11	0.6	*	8	0	0.09	0.12	0.9	*	*	*	42	60	*	*
0	*	*	52	0.9	*	40	0	0.08	0.1	0.5	*	*	*	35	56	*	*
20	160	66	5	0.4	0.2	12	0	0.04	0.05	0.2	0.06	3	0.36	59	91	2	*
20	160	33	5	0.4	0.2	6	0	0.06	0.07	0.5	0.06	3	0.36	27	38	2	*
20	160	43	5	0.3	0.2	8	0	0.04	0.06	0.3	0.06	3	0.36	36	71	3	*
0	144	25	5	0.8	0.2	0	0	0.1	0.06	0.9	0.02	10	*	20	23	8	0.2
0	96	36	5	0.5	0.1	4	t	0.07	0.07	0.4	0.02	6	t	8	22	5	0.3
29	140	40	7	1	0.2	8	0	0.28	0.1	1.2	0.02	9	0.05	12	32	*	0.1
0	241	37	8	1.2	0.2	0	0	0.2	0.13	1.6	0.01	15	*	54	33	12	t
0	312	49	12	1.2	0.3	0	0	0.2	0.12	1.7	0.02	30	0	24	46	15	t
0	761	122	*	3	*	0	0	0.54	0.32	4.5	0.05	*	*	58	115	41	0.1
0	197	102	40	0.8	0.6	0	0	0.12	0.05	1.1	0.08	16	0.05	34	98	16	t
45	445	129	17	1.5	0.7	28	0	0.18	0.24	1.5	0.05	14	0.37	154	135	11	*
0	256	78	8	1.8	0.3	95	0	0.17	0.2	1.9	0.1	1	*	30	141	*	*
0	220	194	39	1.8	0.7	100	0	0.15	0.17	0.8	0.2	16	0.6	20	135	*	0.6

WT, weight; **KCAL**, kcalories; **PROT**, protein; **CARB**, carbohydrate; **FIBR**, fiber; **FAT**, fat; **SATF**, saturated fat;

MONO, monsaturated fat; **POLY**, polyunsaturated fat; **CHOL**, cholesterol; **SOD**, sodium; **POT**, potassium;

FOOD NAME	PORTION	WT (g)	KCAL	PROT (g)	CARB (g)	FIBR (g)	FAT (g)	SATF (g)	MONO (g)	POLY (g)
BREAKFAST CEREALS										
CEREAL-100% BRAN	CUP	66	178	8	48	19.5	3	0.6	0.6	1.9
CEREAL-100% NATURAL-PLAIN	CUP	104	489	12	65	3.8	22	15.1	4.3	2
CEREAL-40% BRAN FLAKES-KELLOGGS	CUP	39	127	5	31	5.5	1	0	0	0
CEREAL-40% BRAN FLAKES-POST	CUP	47	152	5	37	6.5	1	0	0	0
CEREAL-ALL BRAN	CUP	85.2	212	12	63	25.5	2	0.2	0.2	0.8
CEREAL-ALPHA BITS	CUP	28.4	111	2	25	0.3	1	0.1	0.2	0.3
CEREAL-APPLE JACKS	CUP	28.4	110	2	26	0.2	t	0	0	0
CEREAL-BRAN BUDS	CUP	85.2	220	12	65	23.6	2	0.3	0.3	1.1
CEREAL-BRAN CHEX	CUP	49	156	5	39	7.9	1	0.2	0.2	0.7
CEREAL-BRAN FLAKES-RALSTON	CUP	49	159	6	39	6	1	0	0	0
CEREAL-C.W. POST-PLAIN	CUP	97	432	9	69	2.2	15	11.3	1.7	1.4
CEREAL-C.W. POST-WITH RAISINS	CUP	103	446	9	74	2	15	11	1.7	1.4
CEREAL-CAP'N CRUNCH	CUP	37	156	2	30	0.4	3	2.2	0.4	0.5
CEREAL-CAP'N CRUNCH-CRUNCHBERRIES	CUP	35	146	2	29	0.4	3	1.9	0.4	0.5
CEREAL-CHEERIOS	CUP	22.7	89	3	16	0.9	1	0.3	0.5	0.6
CEREAL-COCOA KRISPIES	CUP	36	139	2	32	0.2	1	0	0	0
CEREAL-COCOA PEBBLES	CUP	32.5	133	2	28	0.2	2	1	0.6	0.1
CEREAL-CORN BRAN	CUP	36	125	2	30	6.8	1	*	*	*
CEREAL-CORN CHEX	CUP	28.4	111	2	25	0.5	t	0	0	0
CEREAL-CORN FLAKES-KELLOGGS	CUP	22.7	88	2	20	0.5	t	0	0	0
CEREAL-CORN FLAKES-LOW SODIUM	CUP	25	100	2	22	0.3	t	0	0	0
CEREAL-CORN FLAKES-RALSTON	CUP	25	98	2	22	0.5	t	0	0	0
CEREAL-CORN GRITS-REGULAR-ENRICHED-HOT	CUP	242	145	3	32	0.6	t	0.1	0.1	0.2
CEREAL-CORN GRITS-REGULAR-UNENRICHED-HOT	CUP	242	145	3	32	0.6	t	0.1	0.1	0.2
CEREAL-CORN-SHREDDED-ADDED SUGAR	CUP	25	95	2	22	1.5	0	0	0	0
CEREAL-CRACKLIN BRAN	CUP	60	229	6	41	9.1	9	5.6	0.8	1.5
CEREAL-CRACKLIN OAT BRAN-KELLOGGS	SERVING	28.4	110	3	20	2	4	1	3	0
CEREAL-CREAM OF RICE-COOKED	CUP	244	127	2	28	0.4	t	0	0	0
CEREAL-CREAM OF WHEAT-INSTANT	CUP	241	153	4	32	2.2	1	0	0	0
CEREAL-CREAM OF WHEAT-PACKET SIZE	ITEM	150	132	3	29	2	t	0	0	0
CEREAL-CREAM OF WHEAT-REGULAR-HOT	CUP	251	133	4	28	1.9	1	0	0	0
CEREAL-CRISP RICE-LOW SODIUM	CUP	26	105	1	24	0.4	t	0	0	0
CEREAL-CRISPY RICE	CUP	28.4	112	2	25	1	t	0	0	0
CEREAL-CRISPY WHEATS AND RAISINS	CUP	43	150	3	35	2	1	0	0	0
CEREAL-FARINA-COOKED-ENRICHED-HOT	CUP	233	117	3	25	3.3	t	t	t	0.1
CEREAL-FORTIFIED OAT FLAKES	CUP	48	177	9	35	1.2	1	0	0	0
CEREAL-FROOT LOOPS-GENERAL MILLS	CUP	28.4	111	2	25	0.3	1	0	0	0
CEREAL-FROSTED FLAKES-KELLOGGS	CUP	35	133	2	32	0.8	t	0	0	0
CEREAL-FROSTED FLAKES-RALSTON	CUP	38	149	2	34	0.8	1	0	0	0
CEREAL-FROSTED MINI WHEATS-KELLOGGS	ITEM	7.1	26	1	6	0.5	t	0	0	0
CEREAL-FROSTED RICE KRISPIES-KELLOGGS	CUP	28.4	109	1	26	0.1	t	0	0	0
CEREAL-GRANOLA-HOMEMADE	CUP	122	594	15	67	12.8	33	5.8	9.4	17.2
CEREAL-GRANOLA-NATURE VALLEY	CUP	113	503	12	76	4.2	20	13	2.9	2.8
CEREAL-GRAPE NUTS FLAKES-POST	CUP	32.5	116	3	27	2.1	t	0	0	0
CEREAL-GRAPE NUTS-POST	CUP	114	407	13	94	5.5	t	0	0	0
CEREAL-HEARTLAND NATURAL-PLAIN	CUP	115	499	12	79	5.4	18	9.5	3.5	3.7
CEREAL-HONEY BRAN	CUP	35	119	3	29	3.9	1	0	0	0
CEREAL-HONEY NUT CHEERIOS-GENERAL MILLS	CUP	33	125	4	27	1.3	1	0.1	0.3	0.3
CEREAL-HONEYCOMB-POST	CUP	22	86	1	20	0.3	t	t	0.1	0.2
CEREAL-KING VITAMAN	CUP	21	85	1	18	0.3	1	0.7	0.2	0.2
CEREAL-KIX	CUP	18.9	74	2	16	0.3	t	0.1	0.1	0.2
CEREAL-LIFE-PLAIN/CINNAMON	CUP	44	162	8	32	1.4	1	0	0	0
CEREAL-LUCKY CHARMS	CUP	32	125	3	26	0.6	1	0.2	0.4	0.5
CEREAL-MALT O MEAL-COOKED	CUP	240	122	4	26	0.6	t	0	0	0
CEREAL-MAYPO-COOKED-HOT	CUP	240	170	6	32	1.2	2	*	*	*
CEREAL-NUTRI GRAIN-BARLEY	CUP	41	153	5	34	2.4	t	0	0	0
CEREAL-NUTRI GRAIN-CORN	CUP	42	160	3	36	2.6	1	0.1	0.2	0.5
CEREAL-NUTRI GRAIN-RYE	CUP	40	144	4	34	2.6	t	0	0	0
CEREAL-NUTRI GRAIN-WHEAT	CUP	44	158	4	37	2.8	1	0	0	0
CEREAL-OAT BRAN-COOKED	CUP	219	88	7	25	1.8	2	0.4	0.6	0.7
CEREAL-OAT BRAN-KELLOGGS	SERVING	28.4	100	4	22	1.5	1	*	*	*
CEREAL-OAT BRAN-QUAKER	CUP	85	270	18	51	12.3	6	0.8	1.7	2.1

t = Trace of nutrient present ** = Not available*

MAG, magnesium; **IRON,** iron; **ZINC,** zinc; **VITA,** vitamin A; **VITC,** vitamin C; **THIA,** thiamin; **RIBO,** riboflavin; **NIAC,** niacin; **VB6,** vitamin B-6; **FOL,** folate; **VB12,** vitamin B-12; **CALC,** calcium; **PHOS,** phosphorus; **SEL,** selenium; **VE-a,** alpha tocopherol equivalents.

CHOL (mg)	SOD (mg)	POT (mg)	MAG (mg)	IRON (mg)	ZINC (mg)	VITA (RE)	VITC (mg)	THIA (mg)	RIBO (mg)	NIAC (mg)	VB6 (mg)	FOL (µg)	VB12 (µg)	CALC (mg)	PHOS (mg)	SEL (µg)	VE-a (mg)
0	457	824	312	8.1	5.7	0	63	1.6	1.8	20.9	2.1	47	6.3	46	801	20	1.5
0	45	514	125	3.1	2.4	6	0	0.31	0.56	2.4	0.19	31	0.13	181	383	*	0.7
0	363	248	71	11.2	5.1	516	0	0.5	0.6	6.9	0.7	138	2.1	19	192	4	0.2
0	431	251	102	7.5	2.5	622	0	0.6	0.7	8.3	0.8	166	2.5	21	296	5	0.2
0	961	1051	318	13.5	11.2	1125	45	1.11	1.28	15	1.53	301	0	69	794	25	1.3
0	219	110	17	1.8	1.5	375	0	0.4	0.4	5	0.5	100	1.5	8	51	10	t
0	125	23	6	4.5	3.7	375	15	0.4	0.4	5	0.5	100	0	3	30	18	0.1
0	523	1425	271	13.5	11.2	1125	45	1.11	1.28	15	1.53	301	0	57	740	25	0.9
0	455	394	126	7.8	2.1	11	26	0.6	0.26	8.6	0.9	173	2.6	29	327	10	0.6
0	456	191	118	7.8	2	649	26	0.6	0.7	8.6	0.9	173	2.6	27	273	*	1
0	167	198	67	15.4	1.6	1284	0	1.3	1.5	17.1	1.7	342	5.1	47	224	*	0.7
0	160	260	74	16.4	1.6	1364	0	1.3	1.5	18.1	1.9	364	5.5	51	232	*	0.7
0	278	48	15	9.8	4	5	0	0.66	0.71	8.6	1	238	2.34	6	47	*	0.2
0	243	49	14	9	3.6	5	0	0.59	0.67	8.1	0.93	128	2.51	11	47	*	0.2
0	246	81	31	3.6	0.6	300	12	0.3	0.34	4	0.41	5	1.2	39	107	10	0.2
0	275	53	12	2.3	1.9	477	19	0.5	0.5	6.3	0.6	127	0.02	6	47	*	t
0	155	54	13	2.1	1.7	430	0	0.42	0.49	5.7	0.59	115	1.72	6	25	*	t
0	310	70	18	12.2	4	8	0	0.37	0.7	10.9	0.86	232	1.39	41	52	2	*
0	271	23	4	1.8	0.1	14	15	0.4	0.07	5	0.5	100	1.5	3	11	2	0.1
0	281	21	3	1.4	0.1	300	12	0.3	0.34	4	0.41	80	0	1	14	1	t
0	3	18	3	0.6	0.1	10	0	t	0.05	0.1	0.02	2	0	11	12	1	t
0	239	22	3	0.6	0.1	10	13	0.1	0	1.1	0.02	2	0	2	10	1	0.1
0	0	53	10	1.6	0.2	*	*	0.24	0.15	2	0.06	2	0	0	29	24	t
0	0	53	10	1.6	0.2	*	*	0.24	0.15	2	0.06	2	0	0	29	24	t
0	247	*	4	0.6	0.1	0	13	0.33	0.05	4.4	0.45	88	1.33	1	10	2	0.1
0	487	355	116	3.8	3.2	794	32	0.8	0.9	10.6	1.1	212	0	40	241	10	0.7
0	140	160	60	1.8	1.5	180	15	0.38	0.43	5	0.5	100	1.5	20	150	*	1.2
0	2	49	7	0.5	0.4	0	0	0	0	1	0.07	7	0	7	42	*	*
0	6	48	14	12	0.4	0	0	0.2	0.1	1.8	0.03	11	0	59	43	*	t
0	241	55	9	8.1	0.2	1250	0	0.4	0.2	5	0.5	100	0	40	20	*	0.7
0	2	43	10	10.3	0.3	0	0	0.25	0	1.5	0.04	10	0	50	42	*	t
0	3	20	10	0.8	0.4	0	0	0	0.05	0.4	0.04	3	0	17	27	4	t
0	208	27	12	0.7	0.5	0	1	0.11	0.03	2	0.04	3	0.08	5	31	4	t
0	204	174	35	6.8	0.5	569	0	0.6	0.6	7.6	0.8	15	2.3	71	117	6	11.4
0	0	30	5	1.2	0.2	*	*	0.19	0.12	1.3	0.02	5	0	5	28	*	2
0	429	343	58	13.7	1.5	636	0	0.6	0.7	8.4	0.9	169	2.5	68	176	10	0.3
0	145	26	7	4.5	3.7	375	15	0.4	0.4	5	0.5	100	0	3	24	18	0.1
0	284	22	3	2.2	0.1	463	19	0.5	0.5	6.2	0.6	124	0	1	26	*	*
0	247	24	3	1	0.8	503	20	0.5	0.6	6.7	0.7	3	2	4	9	*	*
0	2	24	56	0.4	0.4	94	4	0.09	0.11	1.3	0.13	25	0	2	19	*	t
0	240	21	5	1.8	0.3	375	15	0.4	0.4	5	0.5	100	0	1	27	4	t
0	12	612	141	4.8	4.5	10	1	0.73	0.31	2.1	0.43	99	0	76	494	3	5.7
0	232	389	116	3.8	2.2	8	0	0.39	0.19	0.8	0.09	85	0	71	354	37	3.4
0	250	113	36	5.2	0.7	430	0	0.42	0.49	5.7	0.59	115	1.72	13	97	10	0.1
0	792	381	76	5	2.5	1500	0	1.48	1.71	20.1	2.05	402	6.04	43	286	34	0.3
0	294	385	147		3	7	1	0.36	0.16	1.6	0.19	64	0	75	416	*	0.8
0	202	151	46	5.6	0.9	463	19	0.5	0.5	6.2	0.6	23	1.9	16	132	*	0.8
0	299	115	39	5.2	0.9	437	17	0.4	0.5	5.8	0.6	22	1.7	23	122	*	0.2
0	166	70	8	1.4	1.2	291	0	0.3	0.3	3.9	0.4	78	1.2	4	22	*	0.1
0	161	26	7	12.7	0.2	717	33	0.92	1.06	12.9	1.18	286	4.13	2	27	*	6.7
0	226	30	8	5.4	0.2	250	10	0.25	0.28	3.3	0.34	67	1	24	26	*	t
0	229	197	14	11.6	1.5	3	1	0.95	1	11.6	0.08	37	0	154	238	*	0.3
0	227	66	27	5.1	0.6	424	17	0.4	0.5	5.6	0.6	6	1.7	36	88	*	0.2
0	2	31	5	9.5	0.2	0	0	0.4	0.3	5.9	0.02	6	0	5	23	*	0.3
0	9	211	51	8.4	1.5	702	28	0.7	0.8	9.4	0.9	9	2.8	125	248	*	*
0	277	108	32	1.5	5.4	543	22	0.5	0.6	7.2	0.7	145	2.2	11	126	27	10.8
0	276	98	27	0.9	5.5	556	22	0.5	0.6	7.4	0.8	148	2.2	1	120	3	t
0	272	72	31	1.1	5.3	530	21	0.5	0.6	7	0.7	141	2.1	8	104	*	t
0	299	120	34	1.2	5.8	583	23	0.6	0.7	7.7	0.8	155	2.3	12	164	7	t
0	2	201	88	1.9	1.2	0	0	0.35	0.07	0.3	0.06	13	0	22	261	*	0.4
0	270	115	40	4.5	3.8	180	*	0.38	0.43	5	0.5	*	1.5	*	150	*	*
0	15	540	180	5.4	3.6	1028	0	0.9	0.31	15	1.49	48	5.18	60	600	*	2

WT, weight; **KCAL**, kcalories; **PROT**, protein; **CARB**, carbohydrate; **FIBR**, fiber; **FAT**, fat; **SATF**, saturated fat;

MONO, monsaturated fat; **POLY**, polyunsaturated fat; **CHOL**, cholesterol; **SOD**, sodium; **POT**, potassium;

FOOD NAME	PORTION	WT (g)	KCAL	PROT (g)	CARB (g)	FIBR (g)	FAT (g)	SATF (g)	MONO (g)	POLY (g)
CEREAL-OAT BRAN-RAISIN/SPICE-HOT	OUNCE	28.4	100	3	19	3.8	1	*	*	*
CEREAL-OATMEAL-COOKED	CUP	234	145	6	25	2.1	2	0.4	0.8	0.9
CEREAL-OATMEAL-RAW	CUP	81	311	13	54	4.6	5	0.9	1.8	2.1
CEREAL-OATS-APPLE/CINNAMON-QUAKER-PACKET	ITEM	149	135	4	26	1.4	2	0.3	0.6	0.7
CEREAL-OATS-BRAN/RAISIN-QUAKER-PACKET	ITEM	195	158	5	30	1.8	2	0.3	0.7	0.8
CEREAL-OATS-CINNAMON/SPICE-QUAKER-PACKET	ITEM	161	177	5	35	1.5	2	0.3	0.7	0.8
CEREAL-OATS-MAPLE/SUGAR-QUAKER-PACKET	ITEM	155	163	5	32	1.4	2	0.3	0.7	0.8
CEREAL-OATS-PLAIN-QUAKER-INSTANT-PACKET	ITEM	177	104	4	18	1.6	2	0.3	0.6	0.7
CEREAL-OATS-PUFFED-ADDED SUGAR	CUP	25	100	3	19	2.7	1	0.2	0.1	0.5
CEREAL-PRODUCT 19-KELLOGGS	CUP	33	126	3	27	0.4	t	0	0	0
CEREAL-RAISIN BRAN-KELLOGGS	CUP	49.2	154	5	37	5.3	1	0.1	0.1	0.5
CEREAL-RAISIN BRAN-POST	CUP	56.8	174	5	43	6	1	0.2	0.2	0.5
CEREAL-RAISIN BRAN-RALSTON	CUP	56	178	4	47	7.1	t	0	0	0
CEREAL-RALSTON-COOKED-HOT	CUP	253	134	6	28	4.2	1	0	0	0
CEREAL-RICE CHEX	CUP	25.2	100	1	23	0.2	t	0	0	0
CEREAL-RICE KRISPIES-KELLOGGS	CUP	28.4	112	2	25	0.1	t	0	0	0
CEREAL-RICE-PUFFED-ADDED SUGAR	CUP	28.4	115	1	26	0.2	0	0	0	0
CEREAL-RICE-PUFFED-PLAIN	CUP	14	56	1	13	0.1	t	0	0	0
CEREAL-ROMAN MEAL-COOKED	CUP	241	147	7	33	2.3	1	*	*	*
CEREAL-SPECIAL K-KELLOGGS	CUP	21.3	83	4	16	0.2	t	0	0	0
CEREAL-SUGAR CORN POPS-KELLOGGS	CUP	28.4	108	1	26	0.2	t	0	0	0
CEREAL-SUGAR SMACKS-KELLOGGS	CUP	37.9	141	3	33	0.5	1	0	0	0
CEREAL-SUPER SUGAR CRISP-POST	CUP	33	123	2	30	0.5	t	0	0	0
CEREAL-TASTEEOS	CUP	24	94	3	19	0.8	1	0	0	0
CEREAL-TEAM	CUP	42	164	3	36	0.4	1	0	0	0
CEREAL-TOASTIES-POST	CUP	22.7	88	2	20	0.4	t	0	0	0
CEREAL-TOTAL-GENERAL MILLS	CUP	33	116	3	26	2.4	1	0.1	0.1	0.3
CEREAL-TRIX-GENERAL MILLS	CUP	28.4	109	2	25	0.3	t	0	0	0
CEREAL-WHEAT CHEX	CUP	46	169	5	38	3.4	1	0.5	0.1	0.3
CEREAL-WHEAT FLAKES-ADDED SUGAR	CUP	30	105	3	24	2.7	0	0	0	0
CEREAL-WHEAT GERM-BROWN SUGAR AND HONEY	CUP	113	426	25	69	5.7	9	1.6	1.3	5.5
CEREAL-WHEAT GERM-TOASTED	CUP	113	432	33	56	14.6	12	2.1	1.7	7.5
CEREAL-WHEAT-PUFFED-ADDED SUGAR	SERVING	38	138	6	30	2.1	t	*	0.1	0.1
CEREAL-WHEAT-PUFFED-PLAIN	CUP	12	44	2	10	0.4	t	0	0	0
CEREAL-WHEAT-ROLLED-COOKED-HOT	CUP	240	180	5	41	2.9	1	0.2	0.1	0.5
CEREAL-WHEAT-SHREDDED-BISCUIT	ITEM	23.6	83	3	19	2.2	t	0	0	0
CEREAL-WHEAT-WHOLE MEAL-COOKED-HOT	CUP	245	110	4	23	1.6	1	0.2	0.1	0.5
CEREAL-WHEATENA-COOKED	CUP	243	136	5	29	2.6	1	*	*	*
CEREAL-WHEATIES	CUP	29	101	3	23	2	1	0.1	0.1	0.2
CEREAL-WHOLE WHEAT NATURAL	CUP	242	150	5	33	2.7	1	0.2	0.2	0.4
OATS-ROLLED OR OATMEAL-DRY	CUP	81	311	13	54	3.8	5	0.9	1.6	1.9
COMBINATION FOODS										
BEEF POTPIE-HOME RECIPE-1/3 OF 9" PIE	SLICE	210	515	21	39	3.9	30	7.9	12.9	7.4
BEEF STEW-WITH VEGETABLES	CUP	245	220	16	15	3.2	11	4.9	4.5	0.5
BEEF-RAVIOLIOS-CANNED WITH MEAT SAUCE	OUNCE	28.4	28	1	4	0.2	1	0.1	0.2	0.3
BURRITO-BEANS AND CHEESE	ITEM	93	189	8	28	8.3	6	3.4	1.2	0.9
CHEESE SOUFFLE-HOME RECIPE	CUP	95	207	9	6	0.1	16	6.6	5.8	2.5
CHICKEN A LA KING-COOKED-HOME RECIPE	CUP	245	470	27	12	1.2	34	12.9	13.4	6.2
CHICKEN AND NOODLES-COOKED-HOME RECIPE	CUP	240	365	22	26	1.3	18	5.9	7.1	3.5
CHICKEN CHOW MEIN-CANNED	CUP	250	95	7	18	0.9	0	0	0	0
CHICKEN CHOW MEIN-HOME RECIPE	CUP	250	255	31	10	0.5	10	2.4	3.4	3.1
CHICKEN POTPIE-BAKED-HOME RECIPE	SLICE	232	545	23	42	4.2	31	11	13.5	5.5
CHILI CON CARNE-WITH BEANS-CANNED	CUP	255	340	19	31	5	16	7.5	7.2	1
CHILI WITH BEANS-CANNED	CUP	255	286	15	30	6.9	14	6	6	0.9
CHIMICHANGA-BEEF	ITEM	174	425	20	43	4.3	20	8.5	8.1	1.1
CHOP SUEY-WITH BEEF AND PORK-HOME RECIPE	CUP	250	300	26	13	*	17	8.5	6.2	0.7
CORN DOG-PLAIN	ITEM	175	460	17	56	2.8	19	5.2	9.1	3.5
ENCHILADA-CHEESE	ITEM	163	320	10	29	3.2	19	10.6	6.3	0.8
ENCHIRITO-CHEESE/BEEF/BEAN	ITEM	193	344	18	34	3.4	16	8	6.5	0.3
HAMBURGER-BACON AND CHEESE-GENERIC	ITEM	150	464	25	29	1.8	27	*	*	*
HOT DOG-PLAIN WITH BUN-GENERIC	ITEM	98	242	10	18	0.9	15	5.1	6.9	1.7
MACARONI & CHEESE-BAKED-HOME RECIPE	CUP	200	430	17	40	*	22	11.9	7.3	1

t = Trace of nutrient present ** = Not available*

MAG, magnesium; **IRON,** iron; **ZINC,** zinc; **VITA,** vitamin A; **VITC,** vitamin C; **THIA,** thiamin; **RIBO,** riboflavin; **NIAC,** niacin; **VB6,** vitamin B-6; **FOL,** folate; **VB12,** vitamin B-12; **CALC,** calcium; **PHOS,** phosphorus; **SEL,** selenium; **VE-a,** alpha tocopherol equivalents.

CHOL (mg)	SOD (mg)	POT (mg)	MAG (mg)	IRON (mg)	ZINC (mg)	VITA (RE)	VITC (mg)	THIA (mg)	RIBO (mg)	NIAC (mg)	VB6 (mg)	FOL (μg)	VB12 (μg)	CALC (mg)	PHOS (mg)	SEL (μg)	VE-a (mg)
0	10	100	43	0.7	0.8	0	t	0.06	0.05	1.2	0.08	24	0	16	148	*	0
0	1	132	56	1.6	1.2	7	*	0.26	0.05	0.3	0.05	9	0	20	178	20	3.5
0	3	284	120	3.4	2.5	10	0	0.59	0.11	0.6	0.1	26	0	42	384	22	0.2
0	222	107	34	6.1	0.7	435	0	0.48	0.28	5.1	0.7	137	0	158	117	13	0.9
0	247	236	57	7.6	1.4	479	0	0.56	0.63	8.1	0.76	155	0	173	206	17	1.2
0	280	104	51	6.7	1	475	0	0.56	0.34	5.7	0.77	153	0	172	146	14	1
0	280	102	42	6.4	0.9	451	0	0.53	0.32	5.4	0.74	145	0	162	143	13	0.9
0	286	100	43	6.3	0.9	455	0	0.53	0.29	5.5	0.74	150	0	163	133	15	1.1
0	294	*	28	4	0.7	275	13	0.33	0.38	4.4	0.45	6	1.33	44	102	6	0.2
0	378	51	12	21	0.5	1748	70	1.7	2	23.3	2.3	466	7	4	47	*	34.9
0	359	256	64	6	5	500	0	0.49	0.59	6.7	0.69	133	2.02	17	183	5	1.1
0	370	350	97	9	3	750	0	0.74	0.85	10	1.02	201	3.01	27	238	6	1.3
0	486	287	84	6.7	1.7	556	2	0.6	0.6	7.4	0.7	148	2.2	27	247	6	*
0	4	153	59	1.6	1.4	0	0	0.2	0.18	2.1	0.11	18	0.11	14	148	*	2
0	211	29	6	1.6	0.3	2	13	0.33	0.01	4.4	0.45	89	1.34	4	25	4	t
0	340	30	10	1.8	0.5	375	15	0.4	0.4	5	0.5	100	0	4	34	4	t
0	21	43	8	0	1.5	300	15	0	0	0	0.5	99	1.48	3	14	2	0.2
0	t	16	4	0.1	0.1	0	0	0.02	0.01	0.4	0.01	3	0	1	14	1	0.1
0	3	302	109	2.1	1.8	0	0	0.24	0.12	3.1	0.11	24	0	30	215	*	*
0	199	37	12	3.4	2.8	280	11	0.28	0.32	3.8	0.38	75	0.01	6	41	13	0.1
0	103	17	2	1.8	1.5	375	15	0.4	0.4	5	0.5	100	0	1	28	*	t
0	100	56	18	2.4	0.4	500	20	0.49	0.57	6.7	0.68	134	0	4	41	*	*
0	29	123	20	2.1	1.7	437	0	0.4	0.5	5.8	0.6	116	1.7	7	60	26	0.1
0	183	71	26	3.8	0.7	318	13	0.31	0.36	4.2	0.43	9	1.27	11	96	10	0.2
0	259	71	19	2.6	0.6	556	22	0.5	0.6	7.4	0.8	7	2.2	6	65	7	0.1
0	238	26	3	0.6	0.1	300	0	0.3	0.34	4	0.41	80	1.2	1	10	*	0.1
0	409	123	37	21	0.8	1748	70	1.7	2	23.3	2.3	466	7	56	137	*	34.9
0	181	27	6	4.5	0.1	371	15	0.37	0.43	5	0.51	3	1.51	6	19	*	0.1
0	308	174	58	7.3	1.2	0	24	0.6	0.17	8.1	0.8	162	2.4	18	182	*	0.2
0	368	81	33	4.8	0.7	330	16	0.4	0.45	5.3	0.54	9	1.59	12	83	3	0.1
0	3	803	272	7.7	14.1	0	0	1.41	0.7	4.7	0.83	298	0	38	971	*	20.5
0	5	1070	362	10.3	18.8	50	7	1.89	0.93	6.3	1.11	398	0	51	1295	*	15.9
0	2	132	55	1.8	0.9	0	0	0.08	0.09	4.1	0.07	12	0	11	135	*	*
0	t	42	17	0.6	0.3	0	0	0.02	0.03	1.3	0.02	4	0	3	43	*	0.1
0	535	202	53	1.7	1.2	0	0	0.17	0.07	2.2	*	26	*	19	182	*	2.5
0	t	77	40	0.7	0.6	0	0	0.07	0.06	1.1	0.06	12	0	10	86	*	0.1
0	535	118	54	1.2	1.2	0	0	0.15	0.05	1.5	*	27	*	17	127	*	2.6
0	5	187	49	1.4	1.7	0	0	0.02	0.05	1.3	0.05	17	0	10	146	58	*
0	363	108	32	4.6	0.7	384	15	0.4	0.4	5.1	0.5	9	1.5	44	100	3	0.1
0	1	171	54	1.5	1.2	0	0	0.17	0.12	2.2	0.18	27	0	17	167	58	2.6
0	3	284	120	3.4	2.5	20	0	0.59	0.11	0.6	0.1	26	0	42	384	43	1.2
44	596	334	*	3.8	*	344	6	0.3	0.3	5.5	*	*	*	29	149	*	1.2
72	1006	613	*	2.9	*	480	17	0.15	0.17	4.7	*	*	t	29	184	*	0.5
*	131	46	*	0.3	*	50	t	0.03	0.02	0.4	*	*	*	5	*	*	t
14	583	248	40	1.1	0.8	118	1	0.11	0.36	1.8	0.13	41	0.45	107	90	*	0.9
137	346	115	14	1	1	152	0	0.05	0.23	0.2	0.06	14	0.35	191	185	*	1.4
186	759	404	*	2.5	*	226	12	0.1	0.42	5.4	*	*	*	127	358	*	0.9
96	600	149	*	2.2	*	80	0	0.05	0.17	4.3	*	*	*	26	247	*	0.2
98	722	418	*	1.3	*	30	13	0.05	0.1	1	*	*	*	45	85	*	0
98	717	473	*	2.5	*	56	10	0.08	0.23	4.3	*	*	*	58	293	*	0
72	593	343	*	3	*	618	5	0.34	0.31	5.5	*	*	*	70	232	32	0.9
38	1354	594	*	4.3	*	30	*	0.08	0.18	3.3	0.26	*	*	82	321	*	*
43	1330	932	115	8.8	5.1	86	4	0.12	0.27	0.9	0.34	58	0.03	119	393	*	1.4
9	910	587	62	4.6	5	15	5	0.48	0.64	5.8	0.27	31	1.52	63	123	*	4.5
64	1052	425	*	4.8	*	120	33	0.28	0.38	5	*	*	*	60	248	*	0
79	972	262	17	6.2	1.3	36	0	0.29	0.71	4.2	0.1	60	0.44	101	166	*	1.3
44	784	240	50	1.3	2.5	186	1	0.09	0.42	1.9	0.39	34	0.74	324	133	*	1.7
49	1251	560	71	2.4	2.8	134	5	0.18	0.69	3	0.21	254	1.63	217	224	*	*
68	660	339	35	3.7	5.3	75	2	0.15	0.27	4.9	0.24	26	1.8	116	302	23	0.1
44	671	143	13	2.3	2	0	t	0.24	0.27	3.7	0.05	30	0.51	24	97	*	*
68	1086	240	36	1.6	1.8	258	1	0.15	0.31	1.5	0.15	17	0.46	362	322	*	1

WT, weight; **KCAL,** kcalories; **PROT,** protein; **CARB,** carbohydrate; **FIBR,** fiber; **FAT,** fat; **SATF,** saturated fat;

MONO, monsaturated fat; **POLY,** polyunsaturated fat; **CHOL,** cholesterol; **SOD,** sodium; **POT,** potassium;

FOOD NAME	PORTION	WT (g)	KCAL	PROT (g)	CARB (g)	FIBR (g)	FAT (g)	SATF (g)	MONO (g)	POLY (g)
MACARONI & CHEESE-ENRICHED-CANNED	CUP	240	230	9	26	1.4	10	4.2	3.1	1.4
MACARONI & CHEESE-ENRICHED-HOME RECIPE	CUP	200	430	17	40	1.2	22	8.9	8.8	2.9
MEAT LOAF-WITH CELERY AND ONIONS	SERVING	87.6	213	16	5	0.1	14	5.3	5.9	0.6
MIXED FRUIT-CANNED-HEAVY SYRUP PACK	CUP	255	184	1	48	2.9	t	t	t	0.1
MIXED FRUIT-FROZEN-SWEETENED	CUP	250	245	4	61	3	t	0.1	0.1	0.2
NACHOS-CHEESE	SERVING	113	345	9	36	2.2	19	7.8	8	2.2
PEAS & CARROTS-CANNED-DIETARY-LOW SODIUM	CUP	255	96	6	22	7.1	1	0.1	0.1	0.3
PEAS AND CARROTS-CANNED	CUP	255	97	6	22	8.6	1	0.1	0.1	0.3
PEAS AND CARROTS-FROZEN-BOILED	CUP	160	77	5	16	7.1	1	0.1	0.1	0.3
PEAS AND ONIONS-CANNED	CUP	120	61	4	10	4.3	t	0.1	t	0.2
PEAS AND ONIONS-FROZEN-BOILED	CUP	180	81	5	16	4.7	t	0.1	t	0.2
PIZZA-CHEESE-BAKED	SLICE	63	140	8	21	1.6	3	1.5	1	0.5
PIZZA-CHEESE/MEAT/VEGETABLE	SLICE	79	184	13	21	1.8	5	1.5	2.5	0.9
PIZZA-PEPPERONI-BAKED	SLICE	71	181	10	20	1.5	7	2.2	3.1	1.2
PORK AND BEANS WITH FRANKFURTERS-CANNED	CUP	257	365	17	40	12.8	17	6.1	7.3	2.2
PORK AND BEANS WITH SWEET SAUCE-CANNED	CUP	253	281	13	53	14	4	1.4	1.6	0.5
PORK AND BEANS WITH TOMATO SAUCE-CANNED	CUP	253	248	13	49	13.8	3	1	1.1	0.3
RICE-FRIED (NASI GORENG)	OUNCE	28.3	55	1	7	t	2	0.3	0.5	1.1
SALAD-CARROT RAISIN-HOME RECIPE	CUP	268	306	4	56	16.7	12	6.8	12.8	23.4
SALAD-CHEF-WITH HAM AND CHEESE	SERVING	200	196	13	7	2.4	13	7	4.1	0.7
SALAD-CHICKEN	CUP	205	502	26	17	2.2	36	4.3	7.2	10.1
SALAD-COLESLAW	TBSP	8	6	t	1	0.3	t	t	0.1	0.1
SALAD-CRAB	SERVING	100	145	12	5	0.3	9	1	1.7	3.5
SALAD-FRUIT-CANNED-JUICE PACK	CUP	249	125	1	33	1.6	t	t	t	t
SALAD-FRUIT-CANNED-WATER PACK	CUP	245	74	1	19	4.5	t	t	t	0.1
SALAD-GREEN SALAD-TOSSED	SERVING	207	32	3	7	2.1	t	t	t	0.1
SALAD-MACARONI	SERVING	28.4	51	1	5	0.3	3	0.2	0.4	0.7
SALAD-MANDARIN ORANGE GELATIN	SERVING	28.4	23	t	6	0.6	0	0	0	0
SALAD-POTATO	CUP	250	358	7	28	5.3	21	3.6	6.2	9.3
SALAD-TACO	SERVING	198	279	13	24	2.8	15	6.8	5.2	1.8
SALAD-THREE BEAN-ALEX	SERVING	28.4	33	1	7	2.1	t	*	*	*
SALAD-THREE BEAN-CANNED-DEL MONTE	OUNCE	28.4	22	1	5	1.5	t	0	0	0
SALAD-WALDORF GELATIN	SERVING	28.4	27	2	5	0.3	t	0	0	0
SANDWICH-BLT-WITH MAYONNAISE	ITEM	148	282	7	29	2.9	16	6.8	5.5	4.9
SANDWICH-CHICKEN/SALAD/MAYONNAISE	OUNCE	28.3	81	6	3	0.4	5	0.6	1	1.4
SANDWICH-CLUB	ITEM	315	590	36	42	4.2	21	14.5	11.6	10.5
SANDWICH-HAM AND CHEESE	ITEM	146	353	21	33	3.3	16	6.4	6.7	1.4
SANDWICH-ROAST BEEF-PLAIN	ITEM	139	346	22	34	3.4	14	3.6	6.8	1.7
SANDWICH-ROAST BEEF-WITH CHEESE	ITEM	176	402	32	27	2.7	18	9	3.7	3.5
SANDWICH-STEAK	ITEM	204	459	30	52	5.2	14	3.8	5.4	3.4
SANDWICH-SUBMARINE-ROAST BEEF	ITEM	216	411	29	44	4.4	13	7.1	1.8	2.6
SANDWICH-SUBMARINE-WITH COLDCUTS	ITEM	228	456	22	51	5.1	19	6.8	8.2	2.3
SANDWICH-TUNA/SALAD/MAYONNAISE	OUNCE	28.3	64	5	5	0.3	3	0.4	0.7	1.1
SPAGHETTI IN SAUCE/CHEESE-FRANCO	OUNCE	28.4	11	1	5	*	t	*	*	*
SPAGHETTI/TOMATO/CHEESE-CANNED	CUP	250	190	6	39	2.5	2	0.5	0.3	0.4
SPAGHETTI/TOMATO/CHEESE-FROM HOME RECIPE	CUP	250	260	9	37	2.5	9	2	5.4	0.7
SPAGHETTI/TOMATO/MEAT-CANNED	CUP	250	260	12	29	2.8	10	2.2	3.3	3.9
SPAGHETTI/TOMATO/MEAT-FROM HOME RECIPE	CUP	248	330	19	39	2.7	12	3.3	6.3	0.9
SPINACH SOUFFLE	CUP	136	219	11	3	0.8	18	7.2	6.8	3.1
TACO	ITEM	171	370	21	27	2.7	21	11.4	6.6	1
TUNA-SALAD-CELERY/MAYONNAISE/PICKLE/EGG	CUP	205	350	30	7	1	22	4.3	6.3	6.7
VEGETABLES-MIXED-CANNED-DRAINED	CUP	163	77	4	15	8.1	t	0.1	t	0.2
VEGETABLES-MIXED-FROZEN-BOILED	CUP	182	107	5	24	6.9	t	0.1	t	0.1
DAIRY PRODUCTS										
CHEESE FOOD-AMERICAN-PASTEURIZED PROCESS	OUNCE	28.4	93	6	2	0	7	4.4	2	0.2
CHEESE SPREAD-AMERICAN-PROCESSED	OUNCE	28.4	82	5	2	0	6	3.8	1.8	0.2
CHEESE-AMERICAN-PASTEURIZED PROCESS	OUNCE	28.4	106	6	t	0	9	5.6	2.5	0.3
CHEESE-BLUE	OUNCE	28.4	100	6	1	0	8	5.3	2.2	0.2
CHEESE-BLUE-CRUMBLED-UNPACKED	CUP	135	477	29	3	0	39	25.2	10.5	1.1
CHEESE-BRICK	OUNCE	28.4	105	7	1	0	8	5.3	2.4	0.2
CHEESE-BRIE	OUNCE	28.4	95	6	t	0	8	4.9	2.3	0.2
CHEESE-CAMEMBERT-WEDGE	ITEM	38	114	8	t	0	9	5.8	2.7	0.3
CHEESE-CARAWAY	OUNCE	28.4	107	7	1	0	8	5.3	2.4	0.2

t = Trace of nutrient present   * *= Not available*

MAG, magnesium; **IRON**, iron; **ZINC**, zinc; **VITA**, vitamin A; **VITC**, vitamin C; **THIA**, thiamin; **RIBO**, riboflavin; **NIAC**, niacin; **VB6**, vitamin B-6; **FOL**, folate; **VB12**, vitamin B-12; **CALC**, calcium; **PHOS**, phosphorus; **SEL**, selenium; **VE-a**, alpha tocopherol equivalents.

CHOL (mg)	SOD (mg)	POT (mg)	MAG (mg)	IRON (mg)	ZINC (mg)	VITA (RE)	VITC (mg)	THIA (mg)	RIBO (mg)	NIAC (mg)	VB6 (mg)	FOL (µg)	VB12 (µg)	CALC (mg)	PHOS (mg)	SEL (µg)	VE-a (mg)
42	729	139	*	1	*	52	0	0.12	0.24	1	*	*	*	199	182	*	0.4
42	1086	240	52	1.8	*	172	0	0.2	0.4	1.8	*	*	*	362	322	28	0.3
107	103	182	14	1.9	3.1	12	1	0.05	0.15	3.2	0.16	11	1.52	23	112	1	0.1
0	10	214	13	0.9	0.2	49	176	0.04	0.1	1.5	0.09	8	0	3	26	1	0.7
0	8	327	14	0.7	0.1	81	188	0.04	0.09	1	0.06	19	0	18	30	1	*
18	816	172	55	1.3	1.8	92	1	0.19	0.37	1.5	0.2	10	0.82	272	276	*	3
0	10	256	37	1.9	1.5	1471	17	0.19	0.14	1.5	0.22	47	0	58	116	3	0.1
0	663	255	36	1.9	1.5	1471	17	0.19	0.14	1.5	0.22	47	0	59	117	*	0.1
0	109	253	26	1.5	0.7	1242	13	0.36	0.1	1.9	0.14	42	0	37	78	*	0.2
0	530	115	19	1	0.7	19	4	0.12	0.08	1.5	0.23	32	0	20	61	*	t
0	67	211	23	1.6	0.5	63	12	0.27	0.12	1.9	0.16	36	0	25	61	*	0.2
9	336	110	16	0.6	0.8	74	1	0.18	0.16	2.5	0.04	59	0.33	116	113	*	*
21	382	178	18	1.5	1.1	101	2	0.21	0.17	2	0.09	27	0.36	101	131	*	0.8
14	267	153	8	0.9	0.5	54	2	0.14	0.23	3.1	0.05	53	0.19	65	75	*	*
15	1105	604	72	4.5	4.8	39	6	0.15	0.14	2.3	0.12	77	0	123	267	*	0.6
18	850	673	86	4.2	3.8	28	8	0.12	0.15	0.9	0.22	95	0	154	266	*	0.6
17	1113	759	88	8.3	14.8	62	8	0.13	0.12	1.3	0.18	57	0	141	297	*	0.6
7	126	41	4	2.2	0.1	70	0	0.01	0.01	0.5	0.02	3	0.02	6	15	*	0.4
33	377	928	42	3	0.5	1100	12	0.16	0.16	1	0.68	28	0.14	96	130	*	16
46	567	415	28	1.2	1.7	740	24	0.34	0.24	2.2	0.21	46	0.47	227	251	19	0.7
67	1395	521	40	3.7	2	30	2	0.47	0.42	7.7	0.34	39	0.2	128	207	*	5.6
1	2	15	1	t	t	7	3	0.01	0.01	t	0.01	2	0	4	3	*	0.4
69	487	260	26	0.6	2.8	9	2	0.06	0.06	1.3	0.12	35	4.74	38	129	*	1.4
0	13	288	21	0.6	0.4	149	8	0.03	0.04	0.9	0.07	6	0	28	36	1	*
0	7	191	12	0.7	0.2	108	5	0.04	0.05	0.9	0.08	6	0	17	22	1	*
0	53	356	22	1.3	0.4	235	48	0.06	0.1	1.2	0.16	77	0	26	80	1	0.5
1	148	21	3	0.3	0.1	4	1	0.03	0.02	0.2	0.02	2	0.01	5	12	*	0.2
0	14	9	*	*	*	*	*	*	*	*	*	*	*	*	*	*	*
171	1323	635	39	1.6	0.8	82	25	0.19	0.15	2.2	0.35	17	0.39	48	130	*	5.9
44	763	416	52	2.3	2.7	78	4	0.1	0.35	2.5	0.21	40	0.64	192	143	*	2.3
*	107	63	*	*	*	*	*	*	*	*	*	*	*	*	*	*	*
0	101	38	6	0.3	0.1	8	1	0.01	0.01	0.1	0.01	10	0.01	10	16	*	0.3
0	16	14	5	0.1	0.1	5	1	0.01	0.01	t	0.02	2	0.01	5	10	*	0.3
44	1222	274	27	1.5	1.8	174	13	0.16	0.14	1.6	0.23	26	0.55	53	89	*	1.9
9	75	27	6	0.3	0.3	11	t	0.02	0.04	0.8	0.05	5	0.03	7	26	*	0.8
93	2601	583	58	4.3	3.9	350	27	0.38	0.41	10.2	0.5	55	1.17	103	394	*	4.1
58	772	290	16	3.3	1.4	77	3	0.31	0.49	2.7	0.2	71	0.54	130	152	*	1.1
52	792	316	31	4.2	3.4	21	2	0.38	0.31	5.9	0.27	40	1.22	54	239	*	0.2
77	1634	345	40	5.1	5.4	46	0	0.38	0.46	5.9	0.34	41	2.05	183	401	*	0.4
73	798	525	49	5.2	4.5	44	6	0.4	0.37	7.3	0.37	89	1.57	91	297	*	0.4
73	845	330	67	2.8	4.4	50	6	0.42	0.42	6	0.32	45	1.82	41	193	*	5.2
35	1650	394	68	2.5	2.6	79	12	1	0.8	5.5	0.13	54	1.09	189	287	*	5.4
3	93	31	5	1.4	0.1	11	t	0.02	0.04	0.9	0.03	6	0.21	10	34	*	0.7
*	114	*	*	0.2	*	11	0	0.03	0.02	0.3	*	*	*	3	*	*	*
4	955	303	28	2.8	*	186	10	0.35	0.28	4.5	*	*	*	40	88	25	*
4	955	408	*	2.3	*	216	13	0.25	0.18	2.3	*	*	*	80	135	*	*
39	1220	245	28	3.3	*	200	5	0.15	0.18	2.3	*	*	*	53	113	*	*
75	1009	665	*	3.7	*	1590	22	0.25	0.3	4	*	*	*	124	236	22	*
184	763	201	38	1.3	1.3	675	3	0.09	0.31	0.5	0.12	62	1.36	230	231	*	1.8
57	802	473	71	2.4	3.9	147	2	0.15	0.45	3.2	0.24	23	1.04	221	203	*	1.7
68	434	*	*	2.7	*	118	2	0.08	0.23	10.3	*	*	*	41	291	*	0
0	243	474	26	1.7	0.7	1899	8	0.08	0.08	0.9	0.13	39	0	44	69	1	1
0	64	308	40	1.5	0.9	778	6	0.13	0.22	1.6	0.14	35	0	46	93	1	*
18	337	79	9	0.2	0.9	78	0	0.01	0.13	t	0.04	2	0.32	163	130	6	0.2
16	381	69	8	0.1	0.7	67	0	0.01	0.12	t	0.03	2	0.11	159	202	6	0.2
27	406	46	6	0.1	0.9	103	0	0.01	0.1	t	0.02	2	0.2	174	211	3	0.2
21	396	73	7	0.1	0.8	61	0	0.01	0.11	0.3	0.05	10	0.35	150	110	6	0.2
102	1884	346	31	0.4	3.6	292	0	0.04	0.52	1.4	0.22	49	1.64	712	523	27	0.9
27	159	38	7	0.1	0.7	92	0	t	0.1	t	0.02	6	0.36	191	128	3	0.2
28	178	43	6	0.1	0.7	57	0	0.02	0.15	0.1	0.07	18	0.47	52	53	*	0.2
27	320	71	8	0.1	0.9	105	0	0.01	0.19	0.2	0.09	24	0.49	147	132	8	0.2
26	196	26	6	0.2	0.8	90	0	0.01	0.13	0.1	0.02	5	0.08	191	139	*	0.2

WT, weight; **KCAL**, kcalories; **PROT**, protein; **CARB**, carbohydrate; **FIBR**, fiber; **FAT**, fat; **SATF**, saturated fat;

MONO, monsaturated fat; **POLY**, polyunsaturated fat; **CHOL**, cholesterol; **SOD**, sodium; **POT**, potassium;

FOOD NAME	PORTION	WT (g)	KCAL	PROT (g)	CARB (g)	FIBR (g)	FAT (g)	SATF (g)	MONO (g)	POLY (g)
CHEESE-CHEDDAR-CUT PIECES	OUNCE	28.4	114	7	t	0	9	6	2.7	0.3
CHEESE-CHEDDAR-INCH CUBES	ITEM	17.2	69	5	t	0	6	3.6	1.6	0.2
CHEESE-CHEDDAR-LOWFAT-LOW SODIUM-PAULY	OUNCE	28.4	83	9	1	0	5	1.3	0.6	0.1
CHEESE-CHEDDAR-SHREDDED	CUP	113	455	28	1	0	38	23.8	10.6	1.1
CHEESE-CHESHIRE	OUNCE	28.4	110	7	1	0	9	5.5	2.5	0.2
CHEESE-COLBY	OUNCE	28.4	112	7	1	0	9	5.7	2.6	0.3
CHEESE-COTTAGE-1% LOWFAT-UNPACKED	CUP	226	164	28	6	0	2	1.5	0.7	0.1
CHEESE-COTTAGE-2% LOWFAT-UNPACKED	CUP	226	203	31	8	0	4	2.8	1.2	0.1
CHEESE-COTTAGE-4% FAT-LARGE CURD-UNPACK	CUP	225	232	28	6	0	10	6.4	2.9	0.3
CHEESE-COTTAGE-4% FAT-SMALL CURD-UNPACK	CUP	210	217	26	6	0	9	6	2.7	0.3
CHEESE-COTTAGE-DRY CURD-UNCREAMED	CUP	145	123	25	3	0	1	0.4	0.2	t
CHEESE-COTTAGE-WITH FRUIT-UNPACKED	CUP	226	279	22	30	0	8	4.9	2.2	0.2
CHEESE-CREAM	OUNCE	28.4	100	2	1	0	10	6.3	2.8	0.4
CHEESE-EDAM	OUNCE	28.4	101	7	t	0	8	5	2.3	0.2
CHEESE-FETA	OUNCE	28.4	75	4	1	0	6	4.2	1.3	0.2
CHEESE-FONTINA	OUNCE	28.4	110	7	t	0	9	5.4	2.5	0.5
CHEESE-GARLIC-LOWFAT-LOW SODIUM-PAULY	OUNCE	28.4	80	8	0	0	6	3	*	2.5
CHEESE-GJETOST	OUNCE	28.4	132	3	12	0	8	5.4	2.2	0.3
CHEESE-GOUDA	OUNCE	28.4	101	7	1	0	8	5	2.2	0.2
CHEESE-GRUYERE	OUNCE	28.4	117	8	t	0	9	5.4	2.9	0.5
CHEESE-LIMBURGER	OUNCE	28.4	93	6	t	0	8	4.8	2.4	0.1
CHEESE-MONTEREY JACK	OUNCE	28.4	106	7	t	0	9	5.4	2.5	0.3
CHEESE-MONTEREY JACK-LOWFAT-LOW SODIUM	OUNCE	28.4	80	8	0	0	6	3	*	2.5
CHEESE-MOZZARELLA-MADE FROM SKIM MILK	OUNCE	28.4	72	7	1	0	5	2.9	1.3	0.1
CHEESE-MOZZARELLA-MADE FROM WHOLE MILK	OUNCE	28.4	80	6	1	0	6	3.7	1.9	0.2
CHEESE-MUENSTER	OUNCE	28.4	104	7	t	0	9	5.4	2.5	0.2
CHEESE-NEUFCHATEL	OUNCE	28.4	74	3	1	0	7	4.2	1.9	0.2
CHEESE-PARMESAN-GRATED	CUP	100	456	42	4	0	30	19.1	8.7	0.7
CHEESE-PIMENTO-PROCESSED	OUNCE	28.4	106	6	t	0	9	5.6	2.5	0.3
CHEESE-PORT DU SALUT	OUNCE	28.4	100	7	t	0	8	4.7	2.7	0.2
CHEESE-PROVOLONE	OUNCE	28.4	100	7	1	0	8	4.8	2.1	0.2
CHEESE-RICOTTA-MADE WITH PART SKIM MILK	CUP	246	340	28	13	0	20	12.1	5.7	0.6
CHEESE-RICOTTA-MADE WITH WHOLE MILK	CUP	246	428	28	7	0	32	20.4	8.9	1
CHEESE-ROMANO	OUNCE	28.4	110	9	1	0	8	4.9	2.2	0.2
CHEESE-ROQUEFORT	OUNCE	28.4	105	6	1	0	9	5.5	2.4	0.4
CHEESE-SWISS	OUNCE	28.4	107	8	1	0	8	5	2.1	0.3
CHEESE-SWISS-LOWFAT-LOW SODIUM-PAULY	OUNCE	28.4	97	9	1	0	7	5.1	2.1	0.3
CHEESE-SWISS-PASTEURIZED PROCESS	OUNCE	28.4	95	7	1	0	7	4.6	2	0.2
CHEESE-TILSIT	OUNCE	28.4	96	7	1	0	7	4.8	2	0.2
CREAM-COFFEE-TABLE-LIGHT-FLUID	CUP	240	469	6	9	0	46	28.9	13.4	1.7
CREAM-HALF & HALF-MILK AND CREAM-FLUID	CUP	242	315	7	10	0	28	17.3	8	1
CREAM-IMITATION-LIQUID-NON DAIRY-FROZEN	CUP	245	333	2	28	0	24	4.8	18.5	0.1
CREAM-IMITATION-NON DAIRY-POWDERED	CUP	94	514	5	52	0	33	30.6	0.9	t
CREAM-MOCHA MIX-NON DAIRY	TBSP	15	20	1	1	t	2	0.8	0.8	0.8
CREAM-SOUR-CULTURED	CUP	230	493	7	10	0	48	30	13.9	1.8
CREAM-SOUR-HALF & HALF	TBSP	15	20	t	1	0	2	1.1	0.5	0.1
CREAM-SOUR-IMITATION	OUNCE	28.4	59	1	2	0	6	5	0.2	t
CREAM-SOUR-IMITATION-NONFAT DRY MILK	CUP	235	415	8	11	0	39	31.2	5	1.2
CREAM-WHIPPED-IMITATION-NON DAIRY-FROZEN	CUP	75	239	1	17	0	19	16.3	1.2	0.4
CREAM-WHIPPED-IMITATION-NON DAIRY-POWDER	CUP	80	151	3	13	0	10	8.6	0.7	0.2
CREAM-WHIPPED-IMITATION-PRESSURIZED	CUP	60	154	2	7	0	13	8.3	3.9	0.5
CREAM-WHIPPED-IMITATION-PRESSURIZED	CUP	70	184	1	11	0	16	13.2	1.4	0.2
CREAM-WHIPPING-HEAVY-UNWHIPPED-FLUID	CUP	238	821	5	7	0	88	54.8	25.4	3.3
CREAM-WHIPPING-LIGHT-UNWHIPPED-FLUID	CUP	239	699	5	7	0	74	46.2	21.7	2.1
MILK-1% FAT-LOWFAT-FLUID	CUP	244	102	8	12	0	3	1.6	0.8	0.1
MILK-1% FAT-NONFAT MILK SOLIDS ADDED	CUP	245	104	9	12	0	2	1.5	0.7	0.1
MILK-1% FAT-PROTEIN FORTIFIED	CUP	246	119	10	14	0	3	1.8	0.8	0.1
MILK-2% FAT-FLUID-PROTEIN FORTIFIED	CUP	246	137	10	14	0	5	3	1.4	0.2
MILK-2% FAT-LOWFAT-FLUID	CUP	244	121	8	12	0	5	2.9	1.4	0.2
MILK-2% FAT-NONFAT MILK SOLIDS ADDED	CUP	245	125	9	12	0	5	2.9	1.4	0.2
MILK-BUTTERMILK-CULTURED-FLUID	CUP	245	99	8	12	0	2	1.3	0.6	0.1
MILK-BUTTERMILK-DRIED-SWEET CREAM	CUP	120	464	41	59	0	7	4.3	2	0.3
MILK-CHOCOLATE-1% FAT-FLUID	CUP	250	158	8	26	0.2	3	1.5	0.8	0.1
MILK-CHOCOLATE-2% FAT-FLUID	CUP	250	179	8	26	0.2	5	3.1	1.5	0.2

t = Trace of nutrient present ** = Not available*

MAG, magnesium; **IRON**, iron; **ZINC**, zinc; **VITA**, vitamin A; **VITC**, vitamin C; **THIA**, thiamin; **RIBO**, riboflavin; **NIAC**, niacin; **VB6**, vitamin B-6; **FOL**, folate; **VB12**, vitamin B-12; **CALC**, calcium; **PHOS**, phosphorus; **SEL**, selenium; **VE-a**, alpha tocopherol equivalents.

CHOL (mg)	SOD (mg)	POT (mg)	MAG (mg)	IRON (mg)	ZINC (mg)	VITA (RE)	VITC (mg)	THIA (mg)	RIBO (mg)	NIAC (mg)	VB6 (mg)	FOL (µg)	VB12 (µg)	CALC (mg)	PHOS (mg)	SEL (µg)	VE-a (mg)
30	176	28	8	0.2	0.9	90	0	0.01	0.11	t	0.02	5	0.23	204	145	5	0.2
18	107	17	5	0.1	0.5	55	0	0.01	0.07	t	0.01	3	0.14	124	88	3	0.1
14	68	32	8	0.2	0.9	18	0	0.01	0.01	t	0.02	5	0.24	200	137	*	0.1
119	701	111	31	0.8	3.5	359	0	0.03	0.42	0.1	0.08	21	0.94	815	579	18	0.7
29	198	27	6	0.1	0.8	84	0	0.01	0.08	t	0.02	5	0.23	182	131	*	0.2
27	171	36	7	0.2	0.9	88	0	t	0.11	t	0.02	5	0.23	194	129	16	0.2
10	918	193	12	0.3	0.9	25	0	0.05	0.37	0.3	0.15	28	1.43	138	302	52	1.5
19	918	217	14	0.4	1	47	0	0.05	0.42	0.3	0.17	30	1.61	155	340	52	1.5
34	911	189	11	0.3	0.8	110	0	0.05	0.37	0.3	0.15	27	1.4	135	297	52	1.4
31	850	177	11	0.3	0.8	103	0	0.04	0.34	0.3	0.14	26	1.31	126	277	48	1.3
10	19	47	6	0.3	0.7	13	0	0.04	0.21	0.2	0.12	21	1.2	46	151	34	0.9
25	915	151	9	0.3	0.7	84	0	0.04	0.29	0.2	0.12	22	1.12	108	236	4	*
31	85	34	2	0.3	0.2	122	0	0.01	0.06	t	0.01	4	0.12	23	30	1	0.2
25	274	53	8	0.1	1.1	78	0	0.01	0.11	t	0.02	5	0.44	207	152	1	0.2
25	316	18	5	0.2	0.8	36	0	0.04	0.24	0.3	0.12	9	0.48	140	96	*	0.2
33	227	18	4	0.1	1	100	0	0.01	0.06	t	0.02	2	0.48	156	98	*	0.2
20	95	*	*	*	*	*	*	*	*	*	*	*	*	*	*	*	*
27	170	399	20	0.1	0.3	78	0	0.09	0.39	0.2	0.08	1	0.69	113	126	*	0.2
32	232	34	8	0.1	1.1	55	0	0.01	0.1	t	0.02	6	0.44	198	155	0	0.2
31	95	23	10	t	1.1	104	0	0.02	0.08	t	0.02	3	0.45	287	172	1	0.2
26	227	36	6	t	0.6	109	0	0.02	0.14	t	0.02	16	0.3	141	111	*	0.2
25	152	23	8	0.2	0.9	81	0	t	0.11	t	0.02	5	0.23	212	126	13	0.2
20	95	*	*	*	*	*	*	*	*	*	*	*	*	*	*	*	*
16	132	24	7	0.1	0.8	50	0	0.01	0.09	t	0.02	2	0.23	183	131	3	0.2
22	106	19	5	0.1	0.6	68	0	t	0.07	t	0.02	2	0.19	147	105	3	0.2
27	178	38	8	0.1	0.8	96	0	t	0.09	t	0.02	3	0.42	203	133	*	0.2
22	113	32	2	0.1	0.2	96	0	t	0.06	t	0.01	3	0.08	21	39	*	0.2
79	1862	107	51	1	3.2	211	0	0.05	0.39	0.3	0.11	8	1.4	1376	807	24	0.6
27	405	46	6	0.1	0.8	108	1	0.01	0.1	t	0.02	2	0.2	174	211	6	0.2
35	151	39	7	0.1	0.7	114	0	t	0.07	t	0.02	5	0.43	184	102	*	0.2
20	248	39	8	0.2	0.9	69	0	0.01	0.09	t	0.02	3	0.42	214	141	*	0.2
76	307	308	36	1.1	3.3	319	0	0.05	0.46	0.2	0.05	32	0.72	669	449	*	1.6
124	207	257	28	0.9	2.9	362	0	0.03	0.48	0.3	0.11	30	0.83	509	389	*	1.6
29	340	25	12	0.2	0.7	49	0	0.01	0.11	t	0.02	2	0.32	302	215	*	0.2
26	513	26	8	0.2	0.6	89	0	0.01	0.17	0.2	0.04	14	0.18	188	111	*	0.2
26	74	31	10	0.1	1.1	72	0	0.01	0.1	t	0.02	2	0.48	272	171	2	0.2
19	32	32	10	t	1.1	72	0	0.01	0.11	t	0.02	2	0.48	273	172	*	0.2
24	388	61	8	0.2	1	69	0	t	0.08	t	0.01	2	0.35	219	216	2	0.2
29	213	18	4	0.1	1	89	0	0.02	0.1	0.1	0.02	6	0.6	198	142	*	0.2
159	95	292	21	0.1	0.7	519	2	0.08	0.36	0.1	0.08	6	0.53	231	192	1	2
89	98	314	25	0.2	1.2	315	2	0.09	0.36	0.2	0.09	6	0.8	254	230	1	2
0	194	466	0	0.1	t	66	0	0	0	0	0	0	0	22	157	*	*
0	170	763	4	1.1	0.5	57	0	0	0.16	0	0	0	0	21	397	*	*
0	5	20	*	*	*	*	*	*	*	*	*	*	*	*	*	*	*
102	123	331	26	0.1	0.6	546	2	0.08	0.34	0.2	0.04	25	0.69	268	195	*	*
6	6	19	2	t	0.1	20	t	0.01	0.02	t	t	2	0.05	16	14	*	t
0	29	46	2	0.1	0.3	0	0	0	0	0	0	0	0	1	13	*	0
0	240	380	*	0.1	*	6	2	0.09	0.38	0.2	*	*	*	266	205	*	*
0	19	14	1	0.1	t	194	0	0	0	0	0	0	0	5	6	*	*
8	53	121	8	t	0.2	87	1	0.02	0.09	t	0.02	3	0.21	72	69	*	*
46	78	88	6	t	0.2	165	0	0.02	0.04	t	0.03	2	0.18	61	54	*	*
0	43	13	1	t	t	99	0	0	0	0	0	0	0	4	13	*	*
326	89	179	17	0.1	0.6	1051	1	0.05	0.26	0.1	0.06	9	0.43	154	149	*	2
265	82	231	17	0.1	0.6	809	1	0.06	0.3	0.1	0.07	9	0.47	166	146	*	2
10	123	381	34	0.1	1	150	2	0.1	0.41	0.2	0.11	12	0.9	300	235	3	0.1
10	128	397	35	0.1	1	150	2	0.1	0.42	0.2	0.11	13	0.94	313	245	3	0.1
10	143	444	39	0.2	1.1	150	3	0.11	0.47	0.2	0.12	15	1.05	349	273	3	0.1
19	145	447	40	0.2	1.1	150	3	0.11	0.48	0.2	0.13	15	1.05	352	276	6	0.1
18	122	377	33	0.1	1	150	2	0.1	0.4	0.2	0.11	12	0.89	297	232	7	0.1
18	128	397	35	0.1	1	150	2	0.1	0.42	0.2	0.11	13	0.94	313	245	7	0.1
9	257	371	27	0.1	1	24	2	0.08	0.38	0.1	0.08	12	0.54	285	219	3	1
83	621	1910	131	0.4	4.8	79	7	0.47	1.9	1.1	0.41	57	4.59	1421	1119	*	0
7	152	426	33	0.6	1	150	2	0.1	0.42	0.3	0.1	12	0.86	287	256	3	0.2
17	150	422	33	0.6	1	150	2	0.09	0.41	0.3	0.1	12	0.85	284	254	3	0.2

WT, weight; **KCAL**, kcalories; **PROT**, protein; **CARB**, carbohydrate; **FIBR**, fiber; **FAT**, fat; **SATF**, saturated fat;

MONO, monsaturated fat; **POLY**, polyunsaturated fat; **CHOL**, cholesterol; **SOD**, sodium; **POT**, potassium;

FOOD NAME	PORTION	WT (g)	KCAL	PROT (g)	CARB (g)	FIBR (g)	FAT (g)	SATF (g)	MONO (g)	POLY (g)
MILK-CHOCOLATE-WHOLE-FLUID	CUP	250	208	8	26	0.2	8	5.3	2.5	0.3
MILK-CONDENSED-SWEETENED-CANNED	CUP	306	982	24	166	0	27	16.8	7.4	1
MILK-EGGNOG-COMMERCIAL	CUP	254	342	10	34	0	19	11.3	5.7	0.9
MILK-EVAPORATED-SKIM-CANNED	CUP	255	199	19	29	0	1	0.3	0.2	t
MILK-EVAPORATED-WHOLE-CANNED	CUP	252	338	17	25	0	19	11.6	5.9	0.6
MILK-GOAT-WHOLE-FLUID	CUP	244	168	9	11	0	10	6.5	2.7	0.4
MILK-HUMAN-WHOLE-MATURE	CUP	246	171	3	17	0	11	4.9	4.1	1.2
MILK-IMITATION	CUP	244	150	4	15	0	8	1.9	4.9	1.2
MILK-INDIAN BUFFALO-WHOLE	CUP	244	236	9	13	0	17	11.2	4.4	0.4
MILK-MALTED-CHOCOLATE FLAVOR-PREPARED	CUP	265	229	9	30	0.1	9	5.5	2.6	0.4
MILK-MALTED-NATURAL FLAVOR-PREPARED	CUP	265	237	10	27	0.2	10	6	2.8	0.6
MILK-NONFAT/SKIM-FLUID	CUP	245	86	8	12	0	t	0.3	0.1	t
MILK-NONFAT/SKIM-INSTANTIZED-DRIED	CUP	68	244	24	36	0	t	0.3	0.1	t
MILK-NONFAT/SKIM-INSTANTIZED-ENVELOPE	ITEM	91	326	32	48	0	1	0.4	0.2	t
MILK-NONFAT/SKIM-MILK SOLIDS ADDED	CUP	245	90	9	12	0	1	0.4	0.2	t
MILK-NONFAT/SKIM-PROTEIN FORTIFIED	CUP	246	100	10	14	0	1	0.4	0.2	t
MILK-SHEEP-WHOLE-FLUID	CUP	245	264	15	13	0	17	11.3	4.2	0.8
MILK-SOY-FLUID	CUP	240	79	7	4	3.1	5	0.5	0.8	2
MILK-WHOLE-DRY	CUP	128	635	34	49	0	34	21.4	10.1	0.9
MILK-WHOLE-LOW SODIUM	CUP	244	149	8	11	0	8	5.3	2.4	0.3
MILK-WHOLE-REGULAR-3.3% FAT-FLUID	CUP	244	150	8	11	0	8	5.1	2.4	0.3
MILKSHAKE-CHOCOLATE-THICK	ITEM	300	356	9	64	0.8	8	5	2.3	0.3
MILKSHAKE-VANILLA-THICK	ITEM	313	350	12	56	0.2	9	5.9	2.7	0.4
WHEY-ACID-DRY	TBSP	2.9	10	t	2	0	t	t	t	t
WHEY-ACID-FLUID	CUP	246	59	2	13	0	t	0.1	0.1	t
WHEY-SWEET-DRY	TBSP	7.5	26	1	6	0	t	0.1	t	t
WHEY-SWEET-FLUID	CUP	246	66	2	13	0	1	0.6	0.2	t
YOGURT-FRUIT FLAVORS-LOWFAT-ADDED SOLIDS	CUP	227	231	10	43	0.8	2	1.6	0.7	0.1
YOGURT-ORIGINAL COFFEE-LOWFAT-DANNON	SERVING	227	200	10	34	0	3	1.8	0.8	0.1
YOGURT-PLAIN-LOWFAT-MILK SOLIDS ADDED	CUP	227	144	12	16	0	4	2.3	1	0.1
YOGURT-PLAIN-NONFAT-MILK SOLIDS ADDED	CUP	227	127	13	17	0	t	0.3	0.1	t
YOGURT-PLAIN-WHOLE MILK-NO SOLIDS	CUP	227	139	8	11	0	7	4.8	2	0.2
DESSERTS										
BROWNIES WITH NUTS-HOME RECIPE	ITEM	20	95	1	10	0.5	6	1.5	3	1.2
BROWNIES-COMMERCIALLY PREPARED	ITEM	60	243	3	39	1.3	10	3.1	3.8	2.6
CAKE-ANGEL FOOD-PREPARED FROM MIX	SLICE	53	142	4	32	t	t	*	*	*
CAKE-CHEESECAKE-COMMERCIAL	SLICE	85	257	5	24	1.8	16	6.7	6	2.9
CAKE-COFFEE-PREPARED FROM MIX	SLICE	72	230	5	38	2.4	7	2	2.7	1.5
CAKE-DEVILS FOOD WITH ICING-FROM MIX	SLICE	69	235	3	40	1.5	8	3.1	2.8	1.1
CAKE-GINGERBREAD-PREPARED FROM MIX	SLICE	63	175	2	32	1.8	4	1.1	1.8	1.1
CAKE-PINEAPPLE UPSIDE DOWN-HOME RECIPE	SLICE	70	221	2	35	1.2	9	1.9	3.9	2.1
CAKE-POUND-HOME RECIPE	SLICE	33	160	2	16	0.1	10	5.9	3	0.6
CAKE-SHEET-NO ICING-HOME RECIPE	SLICE	86	315	4	48	1	12	3.3	4.9	2.6
CAKE-SPONGE-HOME RECIPE	SLICE	66	188	5	36	0	3	1.1	1.3	0.5
CAKE-STRAWBERRY SHORTCAKE	SERVING	175	344	5	61	2.1	9	*	*	*
CAKE-STREUSEL TYPE-WITH ICING-FROM MIX	SLICE	50	172	2	25	0.9	8	*	*	*
CAKE-WHITE/CHOCOLATE ICING-HOME RECIPE	SLICE	71	271	3	42	0.8	11	3	2.9	1.3
CAKE-YELLOW/CHOCOLATE ICING-HOME RECIPE	SLICE	69	268	3	40	0.6	11	3	3	1.4
COOKIE-CHOCOLATE CHIP-BAKED FROM MIX	ITEM	10.5	50	1	7	0.3	2	0.7	0.9	0.6
COOKIE-CHOCOLATE CHIP-FROM HOME RECIPE	ITEM	10	46	1	6	0.3	3	0.6	1.2	0.8
COOKIE-FIG BAR-COMMERCIAL	ITEM	14	53	1	11	0.6	1	0.2	0.3	0.2
COOKIE-GINGERSNAP-FROM HOME RECIPE	ITEM	7	34	t	5	0.3	2	*	*	*
COOKIE-MACAROON	ITEM	19	90	1	13	0.4	5	*	*	*
COOKIE-OATMEAL/RAISIN-PREPARED FROM MIX	ITEM	13	62	1	9	0.4	3	0.5	0.8	0.5
COOKIE-PEANUT BUTTER-FROM MIX	ITEM	10	50	1	6	0.2	3	0.6	1.2	0.7
COOKIE-SANDWICH-CHOCOLATE/VANILLA	ITEM	10	50	1	7	0.2	2	0.6	1	0.6
COOKIE-SUGAR-FROM MIX	ITEM	20	99	1	13	0.3	5	*	*	*
COOKIE-VANILLA WAFER	ITEM	4	19	t	3	t	1	0.1	0.2	0.1
CUPCAKE WITH CHOCOLATE ICING	ITEM	36	130	2	21	0.4	5	2	1.7	0.7
CUPCAKE-NO ICING	ITEM	25	90	1	14	0.3	3	0.8	1.2	0.7
CUSTARD-BAKED	CUP	265	305	14	29	1	15	6.8	5.4	0.7
DANISH PASTRY-CHEESE	ITEM	91	353	6	29	0.6	25	5.1	15.6	2.4
DANISH PASTRY-FRUIT	ITEM	94	335	5	45	1.8	16	3.3	10.1	1.6

t = Trace of nutrient present ** = Not available*

MAG, magnesium; **IRON**, iron; **ZINC**, zinc; **VITA**, vitamin A; **VITC**, vitamin C; **THIA**, thiamin; **RIBO**, riboflavin; **NIAC**, niacin; **VB6**, vitamin B-6; **FOL**, folate; **VB12**, vitamin B-12; **CALC**, calcium; **PHOS**, phosphorus; **SEL**, selenium; **VE-a**, alpha tocopherol equivalents.

CHOL (mg)	SOD (mg)	POT (mg)	MAG (mg)	IRON (mg)	ZINC (mg)	VITA (RE)	VITC (mg)	THIA (mg)	RIBO (mg)	NIAC (mg)	VB6 (mg)	FOL (μg)	VB12 (μg)	CALC (mg)	PHOS (mg)	SEL (μg)	VE-a (mg)
30	149	417	33	0.6	1	91	2	0.09	0.41	0.3	0.1	12	0.84	280	251	3	0.2
104	389	1136	78	0.6	2.9	302	8	0.28	1.27	0.6	0.16	34	1.36	868	775	3	0
149	138	420	47	0.5	1.2	268	4	0.09	0.48	0.3	0.13	2	1.14	330	278	3	*
10	293	847	69	0.7	2.3	300	3	0.12	0.79	0.4	0.14	23	0.61	740	497	3	0
73	267	764	61	0.5	1.9	184	5	0.12	0.8	0.5	0.13	20	0.41	658	509	3	0
28	122	499	34	0.1	0.7	135	3	0.12	0.34	0.7	0.11	1	0.16	326	270	*	0
34	42	126	8	0.1	0.4	178	12	0.03	0.09	0.4	0.03	13	0.11	79	34	4	2.2
0	191	279	16	1	2.9	0	0	0.03	0.22	0	0	0	0	79	181	*	2.6
46	127	434	76	0.3	0.5	130	5	0.13	0.33	0.2	0.06	14	0.89	412	286	*	*
34	172	499	47	0.5	1.1	80	3	0.13	0.44	0.6	0.14	16	0.91	304	265	3	0.2
37	223	529	52	0.3	1.1	94	3	0.2	0.59	1.3	0.19	22	1.03	354	303	3	*
4	126	406	28	0.1	1	150	2	0.09	0.34	0.2	0.1	13	0.93	302	247	7	0.1
12	373	1160	80	0.2	3	484	4	0.28	1.19	0.6	0.24	34	2.72	837	670	*	*
17	499	1552	107	0.3	4	648	5	0.38	1.59	0.8	0.31	45	3.63	1120	896	22	*
5	130	418	36	0.1	1	150	2	0.1	0.43	0.2	0.11	13	0.95	316	255	3	0.1
5	144	446	40	0.2	1.1	150	3	0.11	0.48	0.2	0.12	15	1.05	352	275	3	0.1
66	108	334	45	0.2	1.3	108	10	0.16	0.87	1	0.15	17	1.74	474	387	*	0
0	29	338	46	1.4	0.6	7	0	0.39	0.17	0.4	0.1	4	0	10	118	*	t
124	475	1702	108	0.6	4.3	354	11	0.36	1.54	0.8	0.39	47	4.16	1168	993	*	0.2
33	6	617	12	0.1	0.9	95	2	0.05	0.26	0.1	0.08	12	0.88	246	209	3	0.1
33	120	370	33	0.1	0.9	92	2	0.09	0.4	0.2	0.1	12	0.87	291	228	3	0.1
32	333	672	48	0.9	1.4	78	0	0.14	0.67	0.4	0.08	15	0.95	396	378	5	*
37	299	572	37	0.3	1.2	107	0	0.09	0.61	0.5	0.13	21	1.63	457	361	5	*
t	28	66	6	t	0.2	1	t	0.02	0.06	t	0.02	1	0.07	59	39	*	t
1	118	352	24	0.2	1.1	5	t	0.1	0.34	0.2	0.1	5	0.44	253	191	*	*
t	80	155	13	0.1	0.2	1	t	0.04	0.17	0.1	0.04	1	0.18	59	70	*	t
5	132	396	20	0.2	0.3	12	t	0.09	0.39	0.2	0.08	2	0.68	115	112	*	*
10	133	442	33	0.2	1.7	31	2	0.08	0.4	0.2	0.09	21	1.06	345	271	11	*
11	140	498	37	0.2	1.9	30	2	0.1	0.46	0.2	0.1	24	1.2	389	306	*	0.1
14	159	531	40	0.2	2	45	2	0.1	0.49	0.3	0.11	25	1.28	415	326	11	*
4	174	579	43	0.2	2.2	5	2	0.11	0.53	0.3	0.12	28	1.39	452	355	11	*
29	105	351	26	0.1	1.3	84	1	0.07	0.32	0.2	0.07	17	0.84	274	215	11	*
0	50	38	3	0.4	*	7	0	0.04	0.03	0.2	*	*	*	8	30	1	0.5
9	153	83	16	1.3	0.6	3	3	0.07	0.13	0.6	0.03	4	0.15	25	87	3	*
0	142	52	6	0.5	0.1	0	0	0.06	0.12	0.6	0.01	5	0.02	50	63	3	1.4
57	189	83	9	0.4	0.4	43	4	0.03	0.11	0.4	0.05	15	0.42	48	75	*	1.5
*	310	78	*	1.2	*	24	0	0.14	0.15	1.3	*	*	*	44	125	5	1.9
33	180	90	*	1	*	20	0	0.07	0.1	0.6	*	4	*	41	72	4	1.9
1	90	173	14	0.9	0.3	0	0	0.09	0.11	0.8	0.05	5	0.07	57	63	4	*
20	167	119	12	1.1	0.4	54	4	0.11	0.08	0.7	0.04	8	0.06	50	44	*	0.6
68	58	20	*	0.5	*	16	0	0.05	0.06	0.4	*	2	*	6	24	2	0.9
1	382	68	12	0.9	0.3	30	0	0.13	0.15	1.1	0.02	6	0.09	55	88	6	2.3
162	164	59	7	1.1	0.8	25	0	0.09	0.13	0.7	0.04	15	0.33	25	65	4	1.8
*	*	*	*	2	*	86	89	0.17	0.21	1.3	*	*	*	73	84	*	*
*	214	55	7	0.7	0.2	6	0	0.06	0.06	0.5	0.02	5	0.1	27	99	*	0.4
3	200	77	14	0.7	0.3	4	0	0.07	0.11	0.7	0.02	4	0.06	70	127	5	1.9
36	191	73	13	0.8	0.3	10	0	0.08	0.1	0.7	0.02	6	0.12	57	61	4	1.9
6	38	14	3	0.2	0.1	6	0	0.01	0.02	0.2	t	1	*	3	7	1	0.3
5	21	21	4	0.2	t	1	0	0.02	0.02	0.1	t	1	0.01	3	8	1	0.3
0	45	41	4	0.3	0.1	3	0	0.02	0.02	0.2	0.02	1	0	10	8	1	0.4
0	20	14	1	0.2	t	1	0	0.01	0.01	0.1	t	1	0.01	3	4	1	0.2
0	6	88	*	0.2	*	0	0	0.01	0.03	0.1	*	*	*	5	16	1	0.5
0	37	23	4	0.3	0.1	2	0	0.02	0.02	0.2	0.01	2	*	4	14	1	0.3
3	57	19	4	0.2	0.8	3	0	0.02	0.02	0.4	0.01	2	0.01	12	24	*	0.3
0	63	4	5	0.2	0.1	0	0	0.02	0.03	0.2	t	t	0	3	24	1	0.3
*	109	14	2	0.4	0.1	3	0	0.04	0.02	0.5	0.01	2	*	21	38	1	0.5
3	10	3	1	0.1	*	1	0	0.01	0.01	0.1	*	*	*	2	3	0	0.1
15	120	42	*	0.4	*	12	0	0.05	0.06	0.4	*	*	*	47	71	3	0.1
0	113	21	*	0.3	*	8	0	0.05	0.05	0.4	*	*	*	40	59	2	0.7
278	209	387	*	1.1	*	87	1	0.11	0.5	0.3	*	*	*	297	310	3	*
20	320	116	16	1.9	0.6	43	3	0.27	0.21	2.6	0.06	15	0.23	70	80	*	3.2
19	333	110	14	1.4	0.5	24	2	0.29	0.21	1.8	0.06	15	0.23	22	69	*	2.3

WT, weight; **KCAL,** kcalories; **PROT,** protein; **CARB,** carbohydrate; **FIBR,** fiber; **FAT,** fat; **SATF,** saturated fat;

MONO, monsaturated fat; **POLY,** polyunsaturated fat; **CHOL,** cholesterol; **SOD,** sodium; **POT,** potassium;

FOOD NAME	PORTION	WT (g)	KCAL	PROT (g)	CARB (g)	FIBR (g)	FAT (g)	SATF (g)	MONO (g)	POLY (g)
DANISH PASTRY-PLAIN	ITEM	65	250	4	29	0.6	14	4.7	6.1	3.2
DOUGHNUTS-CAKE-PLAIN	ITEM	25	104	1	12	0.3	6	1.2	1.2	2
DOUGHNUTS-YEAST-GLAZED	ITEM	50	205	3	22	1.1	11	3	5.8	3.3
ECLAIR-CUSTARD WITH CHOCOLATE ICING	ITEM	100	239	6	23	0.5	14	*	*	*
FROZEN YOGURT-FRUIT VARIETIES	CUP	226	216	7	42	*	2	*	*	*
FRUIT BAR-OAT BRAN-NUTS-HEALTH VALLEY	ITEM	43	150	4	28	2.9	4	*	*	*
GRANOLA BAR	ITEM	24	109	2	16	1	4	*	*	*
ICE CREAM SUNDAE-CARAMEL	ITEM	165	323	8	53	*	10	4.8	3.2	1.1
ICE CREAM SUNDAE-HOT FUDGE	ITEM	165	297	6	50	1.2	9	5.3	2.4	0.8
ICE CREAM SUNDAE-STRAWBERRY	ITEM	165	289	7	48	0.7	8	4	2.9	1.1
ICE CREAM-FRENCH VANILLA-SOFT SERVE	CUP	173	377	7	38	0	23	13.5	5.9	0.7
ICE CREAM-VANILLA-HARDENED-10% FAT	CUP	133	269	5	32	0	14	8.9	3.6	0.3
ICE CREAM-VANILLA-RICH-HARDENED-16% FAT	CUP	148	349	4	32	0	24	14.7	6.8	0.9
ICE MILK-VANILLA-HARDENED-4.3% FAT	CUP	131	184	5	29	0	6	3.5	1.4	0.1
ICE MILK-VANILLA-SOFT SERVE-2.6% FAT	CUP	175	223	8	38	0	5	2.9	1.2	0.1
PIE-APPLE-FROM HOME RECIPE	SLICE	135	323	3	49	2.2	14	3.9	6.4	3.6
PIE-BANANA CREAM-FROM HOME RECIPE	SLICE	130	285	6	40	1.4	12	3.8	4.7	2.3
PIE-BLUEBERRY-FROM HOME RECIPE	SLICE	135	325	3	47	1.7	15	3.5	6.2	3.6
PIE-BOSTON CREAM-HOME RECIPE	SLICE	69	210	3	34	1	6	1.9	2.5	1.3
PIE-CHERRY-FROM HOME RECIPE	SLICE	135	350	4	52	1.1	15	4	6.4	3.6
PIE-CUSTARD-FROM HOME RECIPE	SLICE	130	285	8	30	2.1	14	4.8	5.5	2.5
PIE-LEMON MERINGUE-FROM HOME RECIPE	SLICE	120	300	4	47	1.4	11	3.7	4.8	2.3
PIE-MINCE-FROM HOME RECIPE	SLICE	135	365	3	56	2	16	4	6.6	3.6
PIE-PEACH-FROM HOME RECIPE	SLICE	135	345	3	52	1.8	14	3.5	6.2	3.6
PIE-PECAN-FROM HOME RECIPE	SLICE	118	495	6	61	4.1	27	4	14.4	6.3
PIE-PUMPKIN-FROM HOME RECIPE	SLICE	130	275	5	32	3.5	15	5.4	5.4	2.4
PUDDING-BANANA CREAM-INSTANT MIX-JELLO	OUNCE	28.4	106	0	27	0	0	0	0	0
PUDDING-BUTTERSCOTCH-INSTANT MIX-JELLO	OUNCE	28.4	105	0	27	0	0	0	0	0
PUDDING-CHOCOLATE-COOKED-FROM MIX & MILK	CUP	260	320	9	59	0	8	4.3	2.6	2
PUDDING-CHOCOLATE-INSTANT-FROM MIX	CUP	260	325	8	63	0	7	3.6	2.2	0.3
PUDDING-CHOCOLATE-SUGAR FREE-2% MILK	SERVING	133	100	5	14	0.3	3	*	*	*
PUDDING-LEMON-INSTANT MIX-JELLO	OUNCE	28.4	105	t	27	0.3	t	0	0	0
PUDDING-RICE WITH RAISINS	CUP	265	387	10	71	1.4	8	*	*	*
PUDDING-TAPIOCA CREAM-HOME RECIPE-STARCH	CUP	165	220	8	28	0.6	8	4.1	2.5	0.5
PUDDING-VANILLA (BLANCMANGE)-HOME RECIPE	CUP	255	285	9	41	0	10	6.2	2.5	0.2
PUDDING-VANILLA-SUGAR FREE-WITH 2% MILK	SERVING	133	90	4	12	0.2	2	*	*	*
SHERBET-ORANGE-2% FAT	CUP	193	270	2	59	0	4	2.4	1	0.1
TURNOVER-APPLE	OUNCE	28.4	85	1	11	0.2	5	1.3	2.3	1.4
TURNOVER-CHERRY	OUNCE	28.4	84	1	11	0.2	5	1.1	1.9	1.1
TWINKIE-HOSTESS	ITEM	42	143	1	26	*	4	*	*	*
EGGS										
EGG SUBSTITUTE-FROZEN	CUP	240	384	27	8	0	27	4.6	5.8	15
EGG SUBSTITUTE-LIQUID	CUP	251	211	30	2	0	8	1.7	2.3	4
EGG SUBSTITUTE-POWDER	SERVING	28.4	126	16	6	0	4	1.1	1.5	0.5
EGG-DUCK-WHOLE-FRESH-RAW	ITEM	70	130	9	1	0	10	2.6	4.6	0.9
EGG-FRIED IN BUTTER-WHOLE-LARGE-CHICKEN	ITEM	46	92	6	1	0	7	1.9	2.8	1.3
EGG-HARD COOKED-NO SHELL-LARGE-CHICKEN	ITEM	50	77	6	1	0	5	1.6	2	0.7
EGG-POACHED-WHOLE-LARGE-CHICKEN	ITEM	50	74	6	1	0	5	1.5	1.9	0.7
EGG-RAW-WHITE-LARGE-CHICKEN	ITEM	33.4	17	4	t	0	0	0	0	0
EGG-RAW-WHOLE-LARGE-CHICKEN	ITEM	50	75	6	1	0	5	1.6	1.9	0.7
EGG-RAW-YOLK-LARGE-CHICKEN	ITEM	16.6	59	3	t	0	5	1.6	2	0.7
EGG-SCRAMBLED-WITH MILK & BUTTER-CHICKEN	ITEM	61	101	7	1	0	7	2.2	2.9	1.3
OMELET-TWO EGG-HAM AND CHEESE	ITEM	120	266	19	2	0	20	7.3	7.5	2.9
FAST FOODS										
ARBY'S-BEEF AND CHEESE SANDWCH	ITEM	176	402	32	27	1.1	18	9	3.7	3.5
ARBY'S-CHICKEN BREAST SANDWICH	ITEM	184	493	23	48	1.6	25	5.1	9.6	10.3
ARBY'S-CLUB SANDWICH	ITEM	252	560	30	43	2.3	30	11.6	9.3	8.4
ARBY'S-HAM AND CHEESE SANDWICH	ITEM	146	353	21	33	1	16	6.4	6.7	1.4
ARBY'S-ROAST BEEF SANDWICH	ITEM	139	346	22	34	1	14	3.6	6.8	1.7
ARBY'S-SUPER ROAST BEEF SANDWICH	ITEM	234	501	25	50	1.6	22	8.5	8.2	5.4
ARBY'S-TURKEY DELUXE	ITEM	236	510	28	46	*	24	*	*	*

t = Trace of nutrient present   ** = Not available*

MAG, magnesium; **IRON,** iron; **ZINC,** zinc; **VITA,** vitamin A; **VITC,** vitamin C; **THIA,** thiamin; **RIBO,** riboflavin; **NIAC,** niacin; **VB6,** vitamin B-6; **FOL,** folate; **VB12,** vitamin B-12; **CALC,** calcium; **PHOS,** phosphorus; **SEL,** selenium; **VE-a,** alpha tocopherol equivalents.

CHOL (mg)	SOD (mg)	POT (mg)	MAG (mg)	IRON (mg)	ZINC (mg)	VITA (RE)	VITC (mg)	THIA (mg)	RIBO (mg)	NIAC (mg)	VB6 (mg)	FOL (µg)	VB12 (µg)	CALC (mg)	PHOS (mg)	SEL (µg)	VE-a (mg)
0	249	61	10	1.2	0.5	11	0	0.16	0.15	1.5	*	*	*	69	66	*	*
10	139	27	6	0.4	0.1	2	0	0.06	0.05	0.4	0.01	2	*	11	55	2	0.2
13	117	34	10	0.6	*	5	0	0.1	0.1	0.8	*	11	*	16	33	4	0.4
*	82	122	*	0.7	*	68	0	0.04	0.16	0.1	*	*	*	80	112	*	*
*	*	*	24	0	*	0	0	0.01	0.26	0	*	*	*	200	200	*	*
0	5	230	40	1.4	0.8	0	10	0.19	0.06	0.7	0.06	19	0	25	134	*	3
*	67	78	*	0.8	*	*	*	0.07	0.03	*	*	*	0	14	67	*	*
26	208	338	30	0.2	0.9	56	4	0.07	0.31	1	0.05	13	0.64	201	231	*	1
22	190	413	35	0.6	1	46	2	0.07	0.31	1.1	0.13	10	0.68	216	238	*	0.7
23	99	292	26	0.3	0.7	48	2	0.07	0.3	1	0.08	20	0.69	173	167	*	0.8
153	153	338	25	0.4	2	199	1	0.08	0.45	0.2	0.1	9	1	236	199	2	0.1
59	116	257	18	0.1	1.4	133	1	0.05	0.33	0.1	0.06	3	0.63	176	134	2	0.1
88	108	221	16	0.1	1.2	207	1	0.04	0.28	0.1	0.05	2	0.54	151	115	3	0.1
18	105	265	19	0.2	0.6	52	1	0.08	0.35	0.1	0.09	3	0.88	176	129	2	0.1
13	163	412	29	0.3	0.9	44	1	0.12	0.54	0.2	0.13	5	1.37	274	202	3	1
0	207	115	11	1.2	0.2	5	2	0.15	0.11	1.2	0.04	7	0	12	31	15	2.2
40	252	264	*	1	*	66	1	0.11	0.22	1	*	*	*	86	107	15	*
0	361	88	9	1.4	*	8	4	0.15	0.11	1.4	*	*	0	15	31	15	2.2
0	128	61	*	0.7	*	28	0	0.09	0.11	0.8	*	*	*	46	70	5	*
0	410	142	9	0.9	*	118	0	0.16	0.12	1.4	*	*	0	19	34	15	2.2
*	373	178	*	1.2	*	60	0	0.11	0.27	0.8	*	*	*	125	147	15	2.1
0	223	53	7	0.9	0.3	33	4	0.1	0.12	0.7	0.03	11	0.19	16	48	13	1.9
0	604	240	24	1.9	*	0	1	0.14	0.12	1.4	*	*	*	38	51	15	2.2
0	361	21	9	1.2	*	198	4	0.15	0.14	2	*	*	0	14	39	15	2.2
0	260	145	*	3.7	*	40	0	0.26	0.14	1	*	*	*	55	122	12	*
0	278	208	17	1	*	320	0	0.11	0.18	1	*	*	*	66	90	15	2.1
0	190	1	*	t	*	0	0	0	0	0	*	*	*	1	111	*	*
0	244	1	*	t	*	0	0	0	0	0	*	*	*	1	102	*	*
32	335	354	*	0.8	*	68	2	0.05	0.39	0.3	*	*	*	265	247	*	*
28	322	335	*	1.3	*	68	2	0.08	0.39	0.3	*	*	*	374	237	*	*
*	310	*	*	0.7	*	40	*	0.06	0.26	*	*	*	*	150	300	*	*
0	190	1	*	t	*	0	0	0	0	0	*	*	*	1	111	*	*
*	188	469	*	1.1	*	35	0	0.08	0.37	0.5	*	*	*	260	249	*	*
80	257	223	*	0.7	*	60	2	0.07	0.3	0.2	*	*	*	173	180	*	*
36	165	352	*	0	*	82	2	0.08	0.41	0.3	*	*	*	298	232	*	*
*	380	*	*	*	*	40	*	0.03	0.17	*	*	*	*	150	200	*	*
14	88	198	15	0.3	1.3	39	4	0.03	0.09	0.1	0.03	14	0.16	103	74	*	*
1	109	14	3	0.3	0.1	2	t	0.03	0.02	0.3	0.01	1	0.03	4	11	*	0.5
4	124	20	3	0.2	0.1	12	t	0.02	0.02	0.2	0.01	1	0	4	14	*	0.5
21	189	*	*	0.5	*	8	0	0.06	0.06	0.5	*	*	*	19	*	*	*
5	479	512	36	4.8	2.4	324	1	0.29	0.93	0.3	0.32	39	0.81	175	172	*	1.3
3	444	828	22	5.3	3.3	542	0	0.28	0.75	0.3	0.01	37	0.75	133	304	*	1.4
162	227	211	18	0.9	0.5	105	t	0.06	0.5	0.2	0.04	35	1	92	136	*	0.2
619	102	156	12	2.7	1	279	0	0.11	0.28	0.1	0.18	56	3.78	45	154	*	0.6
211	162	61	5	0.7	0.5	114	0	0.03	0.24	t	0.07	18	0.42	25	89	12	*
213	62	63	5	0.6	0.5	84	0	0.03	0.26	t	0.06	22	0.56	25	86	12	0.4
212	140	60	5	0.7	0.6	95	0	0.03	0.22	t	0.06	18	0.4	25	89	12	0.4
0	55	48	4	t	0	0	0	t	0.15	t	t	1	0.07	2	4	5	0
213	63	60	5	0.7	0.6	95	0	0.03	0.25	t	0.07	23	0.5	25	89	22	0.4
213	7	16	1	0.6	0.5	323	0	0.03	0.11	t	0.07	24	0.52	23	81	7	0.3
215	171	84	7	0.7	0.6	119	t	0.03	0.27	t	0.07	18	0.47	44	104	*	1.3
445	598	182	17	1.7	1.8	273	4	0.18	0.57	0.8	0.19	38	1.08	153	286	33	0.1
77	1634	345	40	5.1	5.4	58	0	0.38	0.46	5.9	0.34	41	2.05	183	401	*	0.4
91	1019	330	46	3.5	1.7	15	0	0.45	0.39	14.8	0.65	32	0.34	111	290	*	2.6
100	1610	466	46	3.6	3.1	127	28	0.68	0.43	7	0.4	44	0.94	200	433	*	3.3
58	772	290	16	3.3	1.4	96	3	0.31	0.49	2.7	0.2	71	0.54	130	152	*	1.1
52	792	316	31	4.2	3.4	63	2	0.38	0.31	5.9	0.27	40	1.22	54	239	*	0.2
40	798	503	58	6.4	10.7	0	0	0.53	0.6	9.4	0.48	41	4.29	115	402	*	0.4
70	1220	*	*	2.7	*	*	*	0.45	0.34	8	*	*	*	80	*	*	*

WT, weight; **KCAL,** kcalories; **PROT,** protein; **CARB,** carbohydrate; **FIBR,** fiber; **FAT,** fat; **SATF,** saturated fat;

MONO, monsaturated fat; **POLY,** polyunsaturated fat; **CHOL,** cholesterol; **SOD,** sodium; **POT,** potassium;

FOOD NAME	PORTION	WT (g)	KCAL	PROT (g)	CARB (g)	FIBR (g)	FAT (g)	SATF (g)	MONO (g)	POLY (g)
ARBYS-SOUP-BOSTON CLAM CHOWDER	SERVING	227	207	10	18	1.4	11	4	5	2
ARBYS-SOUP-CREAM OF BROCCOLI	SERVING	227	180	9	19	1.8	8	5	2	1
ARBYS-SOUP-FRENCH ONION	SERVING	227	67	2	7	0.9	3	1	2	1
ARBYS-SOUP-LUMBERJACK MIXED VEGETABLE	SERVING	227	89	2	13	1.3	4	2	1	1
ARBYS-SOUP-OLD FASHIONED CHICKEN NOODLE	SERVING	227	99	6	15	0.7	2	1	1	1
ARBYS-SOUP-PILGRIM CLAM CHOWDER	SERVING	227	193	10	18	1.9	11	4	5	2
ARBYS-SOUP-ROAST BEEF AND VEGETABLE	SERVING	227	96	5	14	0.5	3	1	1	1
ARBYS-SOUP-SPLIT PEA AND HAM	SERVING	227	200	8	21	3.9	10	5	1	1
ARBYS-SOUP-TOMATO FLORENTINE	SERVING	227	84	3	15	0.5	2	1	1	1
ARBYS-SOUP-WISCONSIN CHEESE	SERVING	227	287	9	19	1.8	19	8	8	3
ARTHUR TREACHER-CHICKEN SANDWICH	ITEM	156	413	16	44	*	19	*	*	6.7
BEEF BURGER-FAST FOOD	OUNCE	28.3	72	5	7	t	3	*	*	*
BUN-HAMBURGER/HOTDOG-FAST FOOD	OUNCE	28.3	98	3	16	0	2	*	*	*
BURGER KING-BACON DOUBLE CHEESE-DELUXE	SERVING	195	592	33	28	1.1	39	16	14	6
BURGER KING-BARBECUE BACON DOUBLE CHEESE	ITEM	174	536	32	31	0.8	31	14	13	2
BURGER KING-BK BROILER	ITEM	168	379	24	31	1.8	18	3	8	3.8
BURGER KING-BK BROILER SAUCE	SERVING	14	90	0	0	0	10	1	2	5
BURGER KING-CHICKEN TENDERS	PIECE	90	39	3	2	0.3	2	0.5	0.8	0.5
BURGER KING-CROISSANT-EGG AND CHEESE	ITEM	127	369	13	24	2.1	25	14.1	7.5	1.4
BURGER KING-CROISSANT-EGG/CHEESE/HAM	ITEM	152	475	19	24	*	34	17.5	11.4	2.4
BURGER KING-DOUBLE CHEESEBURGER	ITEM	172	483	30	29	1.4	27	13	11	2
BURGER KING-FISH TENDERS	SERVING	99	267	12	18	1.1	16	3	7	4
BURGER KING-MUSHROOM SWISS DOUBLE CHEESE	ITEM	176	473	31	27	*	27	12	11	2
BURGER KING-RANCH DIP SAUCE	SERVING	28	171	0	2	*	18	3	4	10
BURGER KING-SWEET & SOUR SAUCE	SERVING	28	45	0	11	t	0	0	0	0
BURGER KING-TARTAR DIP SAUCE	SERVING	28	174	0	3	t	18	3	4	11
BURGER KING-TATER TENDERS	SERVING	71	213	2	25	*	12	3	6	3
BURGER KING-WHOPPER HAMBURGER	ITEM	261	630	26	50	2.5	36	16.5	13.8	2.2
CHEESE BURGER-FAST FOOD	OUNCE	28.3	78	6	7	0.1	3	1.7	1.7	0.2
CHICKEN-BREAST AND WING-BREADED-FRIED	SERVING	163	494	36	20	0.3	30	7.8	12.2	6.8
CHICKEN-BREAST-FAST FOOD	OUNCE	28.3	73	8	3	0	4	0.6	0.9	0.5
CHICKEN-DRUMSTICK & THIGH-BREADED-FRIED	SERVING	148	430	30	16	0.2	27	7.1	10.9	6.3
CHICKEN-DRUMSTICK-FAST FOOD	OUNCE	28.3	59	7	4	0	2	0.9	1.2	0.7
CHICKEN-FRIED-FAST FOOD-VARIOUS PORTIONS	OUNCE	28.3	82	5	6	0	5	1.1	1.7	1
CHICKEN-MEAT-SHAPED-FRIED-FAST FOOD	OUNCE	28.3	82	5	5	0	5	*	*	*
CHICKEN-SHOULDER-FAST FOOD	OUNCE	28.3	92	5	3	0	6	*	*	*
CHICKEN-THIGH-FAST FOOD	OUNCE	28.3	104	7	3	0	7	1.2	1.7	1
CHICKEN-WING-FAST FOOD	OUNCE	28.3	92	8	3	0	5	*	*	*
CHURCHS CHICKEN-WHITE MEAT	ITEM	100	327	21	10	*	23	*	*	*
COLESLAW-FAST FOOD	OUNCE	28.3	24	1	3	0	1	0.2	0.4	0.8
DAIRY QUEEN-BANANA SPLIT	ITEM	383	540	10	91	*	15	*	*	*
DAIRY QUEEN-DIP ICE CREAM CONE-REGULAR	ITEM	156	300	7	40	*	13	*	*	*
DAIRY QUEEN-FLOAT	ITEM	397	330	6	59	*	8	*	*	*
DAIRY QUEEN-ICE CREAM CONE-REGULAR	ITEM	142	226	5	33	*	8	4.9	2.5	0.5
DAIRY QUEEN-ICE CREAM SUNDAE-REGULAR	ITEM	177	319	6	53	2.2	10	5.6	2.6	0.9
DAIRY QUEEN-MALT-REGULAR	ITEM	418	600	15	89	*	20	*	*	*
DOUBLE CHEESE BURGER-FAST FOOD	OUNCE	28.3	66	4	7	0.1	3	2.2	1.9	0.2
FAST FOOD-PIZZA WITH CHEESE	OUNCE	28.4	63	3	9	0.6	1	0.7	0.4	0.2
FAST FOOD-PIZZA WITH PEPPERONI	OUNCE	28.4	72	4	8	0.6	3	0.9	1.3	0.5
FISH CAKE-FRIED-WITH BUN-FAST FOOD	OUNCE	28.3	85	3	8	0	5	0.4	0.8	0.5
FRANKFURTER-CONEY DOG-FAST FOOD	OUNCE	28.3	69	3	7	0	3	3.1	4	0.8
FRANKFURTER-HOT DOG-FAST FOOD	OUNCE	28.3	78	3	7	0	4	3.1	4	0.8
HAMBURGER-DOUBLE PATTY-EVERYTHING ON IT	OUNCE	28.4	68	4	5	0.3	3	1.3	1.3	0.4
HARDEE-BACON AND EGG BISCUIT	SERVING	124	410	15	35	0.6	24	5	14	5
HARDEE-BACON EGG AND CHEESE BISCUIT	SERVING	137	460	17	35	0.7	28	8	15	5
HARDEE-BIG COUNTRY BREAKFAST-COUNTRY HAM	SERVING	254	670	29	52	*	38	9	21	8
HARDEE-BIG COUNTRY BREAKFAST-SAUSAGE	SERVING	274	850	33	51	*	57	16	31	11
HARDEE-BIG COUNTRY BREAKFAST-WITH BACON	SERVING	217	660	24	51	0	40	10	22	8
HARDEE-BIG COUNTRY BREAKFAST-WITH HAM	SERVING	251	620	28	51	*	33	7	19	8
HARDEE-BIG ROAST BEEF SANDWICH	SERVING	134	300	18	32	0.9	11	5	5	2
HARDEE-BIG TWIN HAMBURGER	SERVING	173	450	23	34	1.7	25	11	9	5
HARDEE-BISCUIT N GRAVY	SERVING	221	440	9	45	*	24	6	14	5
HARDEE-CHICKEN N PASTA SALAD	SERVING	414	230	27	23	*	3	1	1	1

t= Trace of nutrient present **= Not available*

MAG, magnesium; **IRON**, iron; **ZINC**, zinc; **VITA**, vitamin A; **VITC**, vitamin C; **THIA**, thiamin; **RIBO**, riboflavin; **NIAC**, niacin; **VB6**, vitamin B-6; **FOL**, folate; **VB12**, vitamin B-12; **CALC**, calcium; **PHOS**, phosphorus; **SEL**, selenium; **VE-a**, alpha tocopherol equivalents.

CHOL (mg)	SOD (mg)	POT (mg)	MAG (mg)	IRON (mg)	ZINC (mg)	VITA (RE)	VITC (mg)	THIA (mg)	RIBO (mg)	NIAC (mg)	VB6 (mg)	FOL (µg)	VB12 (µg)	CALC (mg)	PHOS (mg)	SEL (µg)	VE-a (mg)
28	1157	319	20	1.4	0.7	100	4	0.06	0.22	0.9	0.12	9	9.38	170	143	*	0.1
3	1113	455	55	0.8	0.7	50	9	0.11	0.42	0.8	0.18	46	0.59	237	193	*	1.4
0	1248	106	2	0.6	0.6	10	2	0.03	0.02	0.6	0.05	14	0	25	11	*	0.3
4	1075	268	6	1.9	2.7	250	9	0.06	0.1	1.9	0.15	14	0.3	41	91	*	0.4
25	929	78	5	0.7	0.4	200	1	0.05	0.06	1.3	0.03	2	0.14	16	34	*	0.1
28	1157	379	19	2	1.1	350	4	0.06	0.16	1.3	0.15	9	9.67	134	126	*	0.2
10	996	211	5	1	1.4	300	5	0.03	0.05	1	0.07	10	0.3	16	39	*	0.3
30	1029	272	36	2	3	300	1	0.11	0.09	2.4	0.2	4	0.23	32	168	*	0.1
2	910	221	10	1.6	0.2	100	12	0.09	0.09	1.3	0.12	15	0.1	45	58	*	2.3
31	1129	441	7	1.3	1.1	90	2	0.03	0.24	0.7	0.05	7	0	252	241	*	0.4
*	708	279	27	1.7	*	37	19	0.17	0.24	8.1	*	*	*	59	147	*	*
*	55	46	*	0.3	*	8	t	0.02	0.04	0.8	*	*	*	3	25	*	*
*	22	31	*	0.2	*	0	t	0.07	0.02	0.4	*	*	*	9	13	*	*
111	804	463	38	4	6.4	71	8	0.3	0.39	8.1	0.37	31	3.24	156	373	*	1.5
105	795	429	36	4	6.5	49	4	0.29	0.39	8.3	0.35	27	3.34	158	379	*	0.6
53	764	324	29	3.2	3.2	44	6	0.27	0.26	5.2	0.24	38	1.52	74	153	*	2.6
7	95	*	*	*	*	*	*	*	*	*	*	*	*	*	*	*	*
8	90	249	22	1	0.7	25	0	0.14	0.12	6.2	0.32	9	0.3	9	234	*	0.3
216	551	174	22	2.2	1.8	300	t	0.19	0.38	1.5	0.1	36	0.78	244	349	*	0.7
213	1080	272	26	2.1	2.2	135	11	0.52	0.3	3.2	0.23	36	1.01	144	336	*	*
100	851	344	31	3	4	100	6	0.22	0.31	4.9	0.24	31	1.81	189	305	*	1.8
28	870	176	33	1.7	0.6	20	t	0.23	0.17	2.3	0.06	23	1.05	60	191	*	1.3
95	746	*	*	4.1	*	*	*	*	*	*	*	*	*	*	*	*	*
0	208	*	*	*	*	*	*	*	*	*	*	*	*	*	*	*	*
0	52	9	2	0.1	t	0	0	t	t	0.1	t	t	0	1	3	*	0
16	302	14	1	0.3	0.1	26	t	t	0.01	t	0.08	2	0.06	7	8	*	3.9
3	318	*	*	*	*	*	*	*	*	*	*	*	*	*	*	*	*
104	990	520	50	6	5.3	192	13	0.02	0.03	5.2	0.31	31	2.81	104	312	*	3.9
12	198	68	6	0.6	0.7	9	t	0.02	0.05	0.6	0.04	7	0.31	25	33	*	0.1
149	975	566	38	1.5	1.6	58	0	0.14	0.3	12	0.57	9	0.67	60	307	*	1
24	142	85	8	0.2	0.3	9	1	0.02	0.05	2	0.16	1	0.09	4	52	*	0.1
165	756	446	37	1.6	3.2	67	0	0.14	0.43	7.2	0.33	10	0.83	36	240	*	1.3
26	133	74	6	0.3	0.8	7	t	0.02	0.06	1.4	0.1	2	0.09	4	41	*	0.1
25	153	71	7	0.3	0.6	7	t	0.02	0.05	1.6	0.12	2	0.09	4	39	*	0.2
*	141	40	*	0.3	*	6	t	0.01	0.01	0.8	*	*	*	4	34	*	*
*	150	74	*	0.1	*	4	t	0.02	0.04	1.9	*	*	*	4	32	*	*
26	139	68	6	0.1	0.7	6	t	0.02	0.07	1.4	0.09	2	0.08	4	37	*	0.1
*	198	54	*	0.2	*	7	1	0.02	0.04	1.5	*	*	*	5	31	*	*
*	498	186	*	1	*	48	1	0.1	0.18	7.2	*	*	*	94	*	*	*
1	77	45	4	0.5	t	8	t	0.01	t	t	0.02	9	0.01	10	9	*	0.4
30	*	*	*	1.8	*	225	18	0.6	0.6	0.8	*	*	0.9	350	250	*	*
20	*	*	*	0.4	*	90	0	0.09	0.34	0	*	*	0.6	200	150	*	*
20	*	*	*	0	*	30	0	0.12	0.17	0	*	*	0.6	200	200	*	*
38	126	233	21	0.2	0.8	87	2	0.07	0.36	0.4	0.09	7	0.28	212	192	*	*
23	204	443	37	0.7	1.1	75	3	0.07	0.34	1.2	0.14	11	0.73	232	255	*	1.6
50	*	*	*	3.6	*	225	4	0.12	0.6	0.8	*	*	1.8	500	400	*	*
17	50	85	6	0.6	0.9	8	t	0.02	0.04	0.8	0.05	5	0.42	3	31	*	0.1
4	151	49	7	0.3	0.4	33	1	0.08	0.07	1.1	0.02	26	0.15	52	51	*	0.3
6	107	61	3	0.4	0.2	22	1	0.05	0.09	1.2	0.02	21	0.07	26	30	*	*
20	167	52	8	0.5	0.7	6	t	0.02	0.04	1.4	0.03	12	0.85	14	34	*	0.3
15	242	49	3	1	0.6	7	1	0.07	0.07	1.1	0.03	1	0.33	12	30	*	0.1
15	219	48	3	0.6	0.6	5	t	0.01	0.01	0.6	0.03	1	0.33	6	33	*	0.1
15	99	71	6	0.7	0.7	1	t	0.05	0.05	1	0.07	6	0.51	13	39	*	0.1
155	990	180	25	2.2	1.4	116	3	0.33	0.45	3	0.14	14	0.47	253	358	*	1.2
165	1220	200	27	2.4	1.5	129	3	0.37	0.49	3.3	0.15	15	0.52	279	396	*	1.3
345	2870	710	*	*	*	*	*	*	*	*	*	*	*	*	*	*	*
340	1980	670	*	*	*	*	*	*	*	*	*	*	*	*	*	*	*
305	1540	530	23	2.5	2.5	333	0	0.31	0.8	1.8	0.34	53	1.5	78	347	*	4.7
325	1780	620	*	*	*	*	*	*	*	*	*	*	*	*	*	*	*
45	880	320	33	3.7	6.1	0	0	0.3	0.34	5.4	0.28	24	2.45	66	230	*	0.2
55	580	280	35	4	4.6	17	3	0.28	0.31	6.7	0.27	34	2.27	80	197	*	0.9
15	1250	210	*	*	*	*	*	*	*	*	*	*	*	*	*	*	*
55	380	620	*	9	*	*	*	*	*	*	*	*	*	*	*	*	*

WT, weight; **KCAL**, kcalories; **PROT**, protein; **CARB**, carbohydrate; **FIBR**, fiber; **FAT**, fat; **SATF**, saturated fat;

MONO, monsaturated fat; **POLY**, polyunsaturated fat; **CHOL**, cholesterol; **SOD**, sodium; **POT**, potassium;

FOOD NAME	PORTION	WT (g)	KCAL	PROT (g)	CARB (g)	FIBR (g)	FAT (g)	SATF (g)	MONO (g)	POLY (g)
HARDEE-CRISPY CURLS	SERVING	85	300	4	36	*	16	3	8	5
HARDEE-GRILLED CHICKEN SANDWICH	SERVING	192	310	24	34	2.2	9	1	3	5
HARDEE-HAM & EGG BISCUIT	SERVING	138	370	15	35	1.1	19	4	12	4
HARDEE-HAM EGG & CHEESE BISCUIT	SERVING	151	420	18	35	0.8	23	6	13	4
HARDEE-MUSHROOM N SWISS HAMBURGER	SERVING	186	490	30	33	*	27	13	12	2
HARDEE-REGULAR ROAST BEEF SANDWICH	SERVING	114	260	15	31	0.8	9	4	4	2
HARDEE-THE LEAN ONE SANDWICH	ITEM	220	420	27	37	*	18	8	8	2
HARDEE-THREE PANCAKES	SERVING	137	280	8	56	1.4	2	1	1	1
JACK IN THE BOX-BREAKFAST JACK SANDWICH	ITEM	121	301	18	28	*	13	*	*	*
JACK IN THE BOX-JUMBO JACK CHEESEBURGER	ITEM	272	628	32	45	*	35	15	12.6	2
JACK IN THE BOX-JUMBO JACK HAMBURGER	ITEM	246	551	28	45	*	29	11.4	12.6	2.4
JACK IN THE BOX-MOBY JACK SANDWICH	ITEM	141	455	17	38	*	26	*	*	*
JACK IN THE BOX-ONION RINGS-BAG	ITEM	83	275	4	31	1.3	16	7	6.7	0.7
KFC-CHICKEN HOT WINGS	PIECE	119	63	4	3	0.1	4	0.8	10.3	0.7
KFC-CHICKEN SANDWICH	SERVING	166	482	21	39	1.4	27	6	3.9	9
KFC-CRISPY CHICKEN-BREAST	PIECE	135	342	33	12	0.1	20	5	4.7	2
KFC-CRISPY CHICKEN-DRUMSTICK	PIECE	69	204	14	6	t	14	3	3.7	2
KFC-CRISPY CHICKEN-THIGH	PIECE	119	406	20	14	0.1	30	8	7	4
KFC-CRISPY CHICKEN-WING	PIECE	65	254	12	9	0.1	19	4	5.7	3
LONG JOHN SILVER-BATTERED SHRIMP-9 PIECE	PIECE	357	95	3	10	1.8	5	1.1	3.2	0.6
LONG JOHN SILVER-BREADED SHRIMP	PIECE	420	51	1	6	2.1	2	0.5	1.6	0.3
LONG JOHN SILVER-CATFISH FILLET	SERVING	373	860	28	90	0.1	42	10	26	6
LONG JOHN SILVER-CHICKEN PLANK-4 PIECE	SERVING	415	940	39	94	*	44	10	29	5
LONG JOHN SILVER-CHICKEN-LIGHT HERB	SERVING	498	630	35	85	0	17	3	5	7
LONG JOHN SILVER-CLAM CHOWDER WITH COD	SERVING	198	140	11	10	1.7	6	2	3	2
LONG JOHN SILVER-CLAM DINNER	SERVING	363	980	21	122	0	45	10	30	6
LONG JOHN SILVER-COLE SLAW	SERVING	98	140	1	20	2.3	6	1	2	4
LONG JOHN SILVER-FISH & CHICKEN ENTREE	SERVING	398	870	35	91	*	40	9	26	5
LONG JOHN SILVER-FISH & MORE ENTREE	SERVING	381	800	31	88	1.7	37	8	23	5
LONG JOHN SILVER-FISH AND FRYES-3 PIECE	SERVING	358	810	42	77	*	38	9	27	2
LONG JOHN SILVER-FISH SANDWICH PLATTER	SERVING	379	870	26	108	4.1	38	8	22	7
LONG JOHN SILVER-FRIES	SERVING	85	220	3	30	2.9	10	3	7	1
LONG JOHN SILVER-GARDEN SALAD	SERVING	246	170	9	13	2.1	9	0.8	1	0.8
LONG JOHN SILVER-GUMBO-COD & SHRIMP BOBS	SERVING	198	120	9	4	3	8	2	3	3
LONG JOHN SILVER-HOMESTYLE FISH SANDWICH	SERVING	196	510	22	58	2.1	22	5	13	3
LONG JOHN SILVER-HOMESTYLE FISH-3 PIECE	SERVING	456	960	43	97	2	44	10	29	5
LONG JOHN SILVER-HOMESTYLE FISH-6 PIECE	SERVING	513	1260	49	124	2.3	64	14	43	6
LONG JOHN SILVER-HUSHPUPPIES	PIECE	24	70	2	10	*	2	1	1	1
LONG JOHN SILVER-LIGHT FISH-LEMON	SERVING	291	320	24	49	2.4	4	1	1	1
LONG JOHN SILVER-LIGHT FISH-PAPRIKA	SERVING	284	300	24	45	1.3	2	1	1	1
LONG JOHN SILVER-MIXED VEGETABLES	SERVING	113	60	2	9	5.9	2	1	1	1
LONG JOHN SILVER-OCEAN CHEF SALAD	SERVING	321	250	24	19	*	9	2	2	2
LONG JOHN SILVER-RICE PILAF	SERVING	142	210	5	43	0.8	2	1	1	1
LONG JOHN SILVER-SEAFOOD PLATTER	SERVING	400	970	30	109	5.3	46	10	30	6
LONG JOHN SILVER-SEAFOOD SALAD	SERVING	337	270	16	36	1.3	7	1	2	3
LONG JOHN SILVER-SEAFOOD SALAD-SCOOP	SERVING	142	210	14	26	0.6	5	1	2	3
LONG JOHN SILVER-SHRIMP & FISH DINNER	SERVING	348	770	25	85	7.3	37	8	23	5
LONG JOHN SILVER-SHRIMP FISH & CHICKEN	SERVING	380	840	31	89	*	40	9	26	5
LONG JOHN SILVER-SHRIMP SCAMPI	SERVING	529	610	25	87	0	18	3	6	7
MCDONALDS-APPLE BRAN MUFFIN	SERVING	85	190	5	46	4.5	0	0	0	0
MCDONALDS-APPLE DANISH	SLICE	115	390	6	51	1.6	18	3.5	10.8	2
MCDONALDS-APPLE PIE	SERVING	83	260	2	30	1.1	15	4.8	9.1	0.9
MCDONALDS-BACON AND EGG BISCUIT	SERVING	156	440	18	33	0.8	26	8.2	16.1	2
MCDONALDS-BACON BITS	SERVING	3	16	1	t	0	1	0	1.2	0
MCDONALDS-BARBEQUE (BARBECUE) SAUCE	SERVING	32	50	t	12	1.9	1	0.1	0.2	0.2
MCDONALDS-BIG MAC HAMBURGER	ITEM	215	560	25	43	*	32	10.1	20.1	1.5
MCDONALDS-BISCUIT WITH SPREAD	SERVING	75	260	5	32	1	13	3.4	8.6	0.6
MCDONALDS-CHEESEBURGER	ITEM	116	310	15	31	*	14	5.2	7.7	0.9
MCDONALDS-CHEF SALAD	SERVING	283	230	21	8	*	13	5.9	6.5	0.9
MCDONALDS-CHICKEN MCNUGGETS-6 PIECE	SERVING	113	290	19	17	*	16	4.1	10.4	1.8
MCDONALDS-CHOCOLATE MILKSHAKE-LOWFAT	SERVING	293	320	12	66	*	2	0.8	0.9	0.1
MCDONALDS-CHUNKY CHICKEN SALAD	SERVING	250	140	23	5	1	3	0.9	2	0.5
MCDONALDS-CINNAMON AND RAISIN DANISH	ITEM	110	440	6	58	*	21	4.2	13	1.6
MCDONALDS-COOKIE-CHOCOLATY	SERVING	56	330	4	42	1.1	16	5	10.2	0.4

t = Trace of nutrient present ** = Not available*

MAG, magnesium; **IRON**, iron; **ZINC**, zinc; **VITA**, vitamin A; **VITC**, vitamin C; **THIA**, thiamin; **RIBO**, riboflavin; **NIAC**, niacin; **VB6**, vitamin B-6; **FOL**, folate; **VB12**, vitamin B-12; **CALC**, calcium; **PHOS**, phosphorus; **SEL**, selenium; **VE-a**, alpha tocopherol equivalents.

CHOL (mg)	SOD (mg)	POT (mg)	MAG (mg)	IRON (mg)	ZINC (mg)	VITA (RE)	VITC (mg)	THIA (mg)	RIBO (mg)	NIAC (mg)	VB6 (mg)	FOL (µg)	VB12 (µg)	CALC (mg)	PHOS (mg)	SEL (µg)	VE-a (mg)
0	840	370	*	*	*	*	*	*	*	*	*	*	*	*	*	*	*
60	890	410	44	3	2.7	413	t	0.43	0.59	4.2	0.1	31	0.47	542	611	*	3.4
160	1050	210	26	2.8	1.6	127	9	0.56	0.54	3.9	0.21	39	0.73	95	234	*	1.9
170	1270	230	30	2.7	1.7	142	4	0.4	0.54	3.7	0.17	17	0.57	308	436	*	1.5
70	940	370	*	*	*	*	*	*	*	*	*	*	*	*	*	*	*
35	730	260	28	3.1	5.2	0	0	0.26	0.29	4.6	0.24	20	2.09	56	196	*	0.2
85	760	510	*	*	*	*	*	*	*	*	*	*	*	*	*	*	*
15	890	240	25	1.9	0.9	63	1	0.22	0.39	1.4	0.1	14	0.42	341	411	*	1.6
182	1037	190	24	2.5	1.8	133	3	0.41	0.47	5.1	0.14	*	1.1	177	310	*	*
110	1666	499	49	4.6	4.8	220	5	0.52	0.38	11.3	0.31	*	3.05	273	411	*	*
80	1134	492	44	4.5	4.2	74	4	0.47	0.34	11.6	0.3	*	2.68	134	261	*	*
56	837	246	30	1.7	1.1	72	1	0.3	0.21	4.5	0.12	*	1.1	167	263	*	*
14	430	129	15	0.9	0.4	2	1	0.09	0.1	0.9	0.06	11	0.12	73	86	*	0.6
25	113	218	22	1.5	2.1	63	t	0.05	0.15	7.7	0.49	4	0.33	18	175	*	0.9
47	1060	297	41	3.1	1.5	14	0	0.4	0.35	13.4	0.59	29	0.31	100	261	*	2.3
114	790	347	40	1.6	1.5	20	0	0.11	0.17	18.4	0.77	5	0.46	21	312	*	0.6
71	324	157	16	0.9	2	17	0	0.06	0.16	4.1	0.24	6	0.22	8	120	*	0.5
129	688	280	29	1.8	3	35	0	0.11	0.29	8.2	0.4	10	0.36	16	221	*	0.6
67	422	115	12	0.8	1.1	25	0	0.04	0.09	4.3	0.27	2	0.18	10	97	*	0.6
14	163	94	132	10.3	4.2	242	5	0.3	0.5	9.9	0.36	34	3.4	214	764	*	14.1
6	85	41	156	12.1	5	285	6	0.35	0.58	11.6	0.43	39	3.99	252	899	*	16.6
65	990	1180	121	4.6	3.4	317	11	0.2	0.49	9.7	0.87	67	9.41	200	1017	*	5.7
70	1660	1320	*	*	*	*	*	*	*	*	*	*	*	*	*	*	*
85	2170	790	95	4.8	3.6	120	0	0.32	0.65	26.3	1.05	10	0.75	214	782	*	1.3
20	590	380	17	1.7	0.9	74	4	0.05	0.14	1.2	0.13	8	8.44	117	110	*	0.2
15	1200	870	41	56.7	6.2	365	47	0.34	0.91	7.2	0.26	54	201	209	572	*	4.5
15	260	190	13	0.5	0.1	225	30	0.04	0.03	0.3	0.13	37	0.03	36	23	*	4.4
70	1520	1290	*	*	*	*	*	*	*	*	*	*	*	*	*	*	*
70	1390	1260	131	3.3	2.1	71	5	0.39	0.5	12.3	0.72	46	5.17	133	769	*	7.7
85	1630	1340	*	*	*	*	*	*	*	*	*	*	*	*	*	*	*
55	1110	1050	94	6.4	2.3	65	2	0.87	0.65	11.1	0.42	89	2.29	238	488	*	5.7
5	60	390	29	0.6	0.3	0	9	0.15	0.02	2.8	0.2	25	0	16	79	*	0.2
5	380	20	40	1.7	1.1	239	26	0.14	0.15	11.4	0.56	66	0.27	42	217	*	0.9
25	740	310	41	2.3	0.8	300	21	0.12	0.08	2	0.17	47	0.24	100	105	*	1.7
45	780	470	48	18	1.2	33	1	0.45	0.34	5.7	0.22	46	1.19	123	252	*	2.9
100	1890	1540	157	3.9	2.6	85	6	0.47	0.59	14.7	0.87	56	6.19	159	920	*	9.3
130	1590	1660	177	4.4	2.9	96	7	0.53	0.67	16.6	0.98	62	6.97	179	1035	*	10.4
5	25	65	*	*	*	*	*	*	*	*	*	*	*	*	*	*	*
75	900	470	56	2.3	1.4	80	10	0.29	0.15	3.4	0.34	46	0.58	40	238	*	3.1
70	650	460	98	2.4	1.6	53	4	0.29	0.37	9.2	0.54	35	3.86	99	573	*	5.8
0	330	120	24	0.9	0.5	75	4	0.08	0.13	0.9	0.08	21	t	29	56	*	0.8
80	1340	160	*	*	*	*	*	*	*	*	*	*	*	*	*	*	*
0	570	140	17	1.8	0.6	60	1	0.15	0.02	1.5	0.08	5	0.01	17	45	*	0.8
70	1540	1100	114	4.1	2.2	59	13	0.42	0.37	8.2	0.88	37	1.68	109	484	*	4.3
90	670	100	86	3.2	5.2	129	20	0.13	0.16	3.7	0.27	47	2.89	148	444	*	7.4
90	570	100	36	1.4	2.2	250	8	0.05	0.07	1.6	0.11	20	1.22	63	187	*	3.1
80	1250	1030	82	3.5	1.6	28	17	0.37	0.21	6.6	0.64	35	1.06	54	422	*	4.4
80	1450	1170	*	*	*	*	*	*	*	*	*	*	*	*	*	*	*
220	2120	560	203	13.6	6.2	364	11	0.13	0.2	13.6	0.55	10	5.57	299	1156	*	12.9
0	230	202	55	0.6	1.2	1	1	0.02	0.08	0.4	0.37	77	0.78	31	178	*	0.4
26	370	69	8	1.4	0.2	35	16	0.28	0.2	2.2	0.03	3	0	14	31	*	3.8
0	240	50	6	0.7	0.2	0	11	0.06	0.02	0.3	0.02	2	0	11	22	*	2.7
253	1230	237	31	2.6	1.7	160	0	0.36	0.33	2.5	0.17	18	0.59	185	451	*	1.5
0	95	4	3	0	0.1	0	0	0	0	0	t	4	0.04	0	7	*	0.2
0	340	56	6	0.3	0.1	30	2	0.01	0.01	0.2	0.02	1	0	13	6	*	1.8
103	950	237	38	4	4.7	106	2	0.48	0.41	6.8	0.27	21	1.8	256	314	*	*
1	730	100	14	1.3	0.7	0	0	0.23	0.11	1.7	0.03	6	0.1	75	168	*	1.8
53	750	223	21	2.3	2.1	118	2	0.29	0.21	3.9	0.12	18	0.94	199	177	*	0.5
128	490	*	*	1.5	*	411	14	0.31	0.29	3.6	*	*	*	256	*	*	*
65	520	*	*	1	*	0	0	0.11	0.12	9	*	*	*	13	*	*	*
10	240	*	*	0.8	*	92	0	0.13	0.5	0.4	*	*	*	332	*	*	*
78	230	436	37	1	2.9	366	20	0.22	0.17	8.5	0.6	27	0.63	34	257	*	10.8
35	430	*	*	1.8	*	33	3	0.32	0.24	2.8	*	*	*	35	*	*	*
4	280	72	20	2.2	0.5	0	0	0.18	0.21	2.5	0.03	5	0.07	24	71	*	1.4

WT, weight; **KCAL**, kcalories; **PROT**, protein; **CARB**, carbohydrate; **FIBR**, fiber; **FAT**, fat; **SATF**, saturated fat;

MONO, monsaturated fat; **POLY**, polyunsaturated fat; **CHOL**, cholesterol; **SOD**, sodium; **POT**, potassium;

FOOD NAME	PORTION	WT (g)	KCAL	PROT (g)	CARB (g)	FIBR (g)	FAT (g)	SATF (g)	MONO (g)	POLY (g)
MCDONALDS-COOKIE-MCDONALDLAND	SERVING	56	290	4	47	0.6	9	1.9	6.8	0.5
MCDONALDS-CROUTONS	SERVING	11	50	1	7	0.5	2	0.5	1.3	0.1
MCDONALDS-EGG MCMUFFIN	ITEM	138	290	18	28	1.4	11	3.8	6.1	1.3
MCDONALDS-ENGLISH MUFFIN	SERVING	59	170	5	27	1.6	5	2.4	1.7	0.5
MCDONALDS-FILET O FISH	ITEM	142	440	14	38	1.1	26	5.2	10.2	10.8
MCDONALDS-FRENCH FRIES-LARGE	SERVING	122	400	6	46	4.2	22	9.1	11.6	0.9
MCDONALDS-FRENCH FRIES-MEDIUM	SERVING	97	320	4	36	3.4	17	7.2	9.2	0.7
MCDONALDS-FRENCH FRIES-REGULAR ORDER	SERVING	68	220	3	26	*	12	5.1	6.5	0.5
MCDONALDS-GARDEN SALAD	SERVING	213	110	7	6	1.8	7	2.9	3.2	0.5
MCDONALDS-HAMBURGER	ITEM	102	260	12	31	*	10	3.6	5.1	0.8
MCDONALDS-HASHBROWN POTATO	SERVING	55	130	1	15	1.1	7	3.2	3.7	0.4
MCDONALDS-HONEY SAUCE	SERVING	14	45	0	12	*	0	0	0	0
MCDONALDS-HOT CAKES WITH SYRUP	SERVING	176	410	8	74	*	9	3.7	3.1	2.5
MCDONALDS-HOT CARAMEL SUNDAE	SERVING	174	270	7	59	1	3	1.5	1.2	0.1
MCDONALDS-HOT FUDGE SUNDAE	SERVING	169	240	7	51	1.3	3	2.4	0.8	0.1
MCDONALDS-HOT MUSTARD SAUCE	SERVING	30	70	1	8	0.3	4	0.5	1.2	1.9
MCDONALDS-ICED CHEESE DANISH	SERVING	110	390	7	42	*	22	6	12.1	1.8
MCDONALDS-McCHICKEN SANDWICH	SERVING	190	490	19	40	1.6	29	5.4	11.5	11.6
MCDONALDS-McDLT HAMBURGER	ITEM	234	580	26	36	*	37	11.5	16.7	8.5
MCDONALDS-MCLEAN DELUXE HAMBURGER	SERVING	206	320	22	35	2.4	10	4	5	1
MCDONALDS-MILKSHAKE-CHOCOLATE-LOWFAT	SERVING	293	320	12	66	*	2	1	1	0
MCDONALDS-MILKSHAKE-STRAWBERRY-LOWFAT	SERVING	293	320	11	67	*	1	1	1	0
MCDONALDS-MILKSHAKE-VANILLA-LOWFAT	SERVING	293	290	11	60	0	1	1	1	0
MCDONALDS-PORK SAUSAGE	SERVING	48	180	8	0	0	16	5.9	8.5	1.9
MCDONALDS-QUARTER POUND CHEESEBURGER	ITEM	194	520	29	35	*	29	11.2	16.5	1.5
MCDONALDS-QUARTER POUNDER HAMBURGER	ITEM	166	410	23	34	*	21	8.1	11.4	1.2
MCDONALDS-RASPBERRY DANISH	ITEM	117	410	6	62	*	16	3.1	10.2	1.1
MCDONALDS-SALAD DRESSING-PEPPERCORN	OUNCE	28.4	160	0	2	0	18	2	4	10
MCDONALDS-SALAD DRESSING-RED FRENCH	OUNCE	28.4	80	0	10	0	4	0	2	2
MCDONALDS-SAUSAGE AND EGG BISCUIT	ITEM	180	520	20	33	*	35	11.2	20	2.5
MCDONALDS-SAUSAGE BISCUIT	ITEM	123	440	13	32	1.4	29	9.3	17.2	2.5
MCDONALDS-SAUSAGE MCMUFFIN	ITEM	117	370	17	27	1.1	22	7.8	11.7	2.4
MCDONALDS-SAUSAGE MCMUFFIN WITH EGG	ITEM	167	440	23	28	1.6	27	9.5	14.2	3.2
MCDONALDS-SCRAMBLED EGGS	SERVING	98	140	12	1	0	10	3.3	5	1.4
MCDONALDS-SIDE SALAD	SERVING	115	60	4	3	1.2	3	1.5	1.6	0.3
MCDONALDS-STRAWBERRY MILKSHAKE-LOWFAT	SERVING	293	320	11	67	*	1	0.6	0.6	0.1
MCDONALDS-STRAWBERRY SUNDAE	SERVING	171	210	6	49	0.7	1	0.6	0.4	t
MCDONALDS-SWEET AND SOUR SAUCE	SERVING	32	60	t	14	t	t	t	0.1	0.1
MCDONALDS-VANILLA MILKSHAKE-LOWFAT	SERVING	293	290	11	60	*	1	0.6	0.7	0.1
MCDONALDS-VANILLA-FROZEN YOGURT	SERVING	80	100	4	22	*	1	0.4	0.3	0.1
PIZZA-BEEF/CHICKEN/ONION	OUNCE	28.3	73	6	7	t	2	*	*	*
PIZZA-BEEF/ONION	OUNCE	28.3	73	4	8	0.1	3	*	*	*
PIZZA-CHICKEN CURRY/PEAS	OUNCE	28.3	82	4	9	0.2	3	*	*	*
PIZZA-CHICKEN/MUSHROOM/TOMATO	OUNCE	28.3	61	5	7	0.1	1	*	*	*
PIZZA-CHICKEN/PINEAPPLE	OUNCE	28.3	81	4	6	0.1	4	*	*	*
PIZZA-COMBINATION SUPREME	OUNCE	28.3	51	4	7	0.2	1	1.3	1.5	0.4
PIZZA-CURRY BEEF/PEAS	OUNCE	28.3	71	5	7	0.2	3	0.9	1.6	1
PIZZA-ONION/TOMATO/GREEN PEPPER/MUSHROOM	OUNCE	28.3	45	3	7	0.2	1	*	*	*
PIZZA-PEPPERONI/BEEF/SALAMI/MUSHROOM/ETC	OUNCE	28.3	83	5	5	0.1	5	*	*	*
PIZZA-SHRIMP/CUCUMBER	OUNCE	28.3	69	4	7	0.1	3	*	*	*
PIZZA-SHRIMP/SQUID/MUSHROOM	OUNCE	28.3	70	5	7	0.1	2	*	*	*
POTATOES-FRENCH FRIED-FAST FOOD	OUNCE	28.3	91	1	10	0	5	1.8	1.9	0.8
POTATOES-MASHED-FAST FOOD	OUNCE	28.3	26	1	5	0	t	0.3	0.5	0.3
RAX-GRILLED CHICKEN SANDWICH	ITEM	190	440	24	36	1.6	19	2.9	4.5	5.4
SALAD-FAST FOOD	OUNCE	28.3	34	t	3	0	2	*	*	*
SPAGHETTI-VEGETABLES/SAUCE/CHEESE	OUNCE	28.3	28	4	3	0.3	t	*	*	*
SUBWAY SANDWICH-HAM AND CHEESE-ON WHEAT	ITEM	194	673	39	86	6	22	7	8	4
SUBWAY-BMT SANDWICH-ON HONEY WHEAT ROLL	ITEM	220	1011	45	88	6	57	20	25	7
SUBWAY-BMT SANDWICH-ON ITALIAN ROLL	ITEM	213	982	44	83	5	55	20	24	7
SUBWAY-CLUB SANDWICH-ON HONEY WHEAT	ITEM	220	722	47	89	6	23	7	9	4
SUBWAY-CLUB SANDWICH-ON ITALIAN ROLL	ITEM	213	693	46	83	5	22	7	8	4
SUBWAY-COLD CUT COMBO SANDWICH-ITALIAN	ITEM	184	853	46	83	5	40	12	15	10
SUBWAY-COLD CUT COMBO SANDWICH-ON WHEAT	ITEM	191	883	48	88	6	41	12	15	10

t = Trace of nutrient present ** = Not available*

MAG, magnesium; **IRON**, iron; **ZINC**, zinc; **VITA**, vitamin A; **VITC**, vitamin C; **THIA**, thiamin; **RIBO**, riboflavin; **NIAC**, niacin; **VB6**, vitamin B-6; **FOL**, folate; **VB12**, vitamin B-12; **CALC**, calcium; **PHOS**, phosphorus; **SEL**, selenium; **VE-a**, alpha tocopherol equivalents.

CHOL (mg)	SOD (mg)	POT (mg)	MAG (mg)	IRON (mg)	ZINC (mg)	VITA (RE)	VITC (mg)	THIA (mg)	RIBO (mg)	NIAC (mg)	VB6 (mg)	FOL (µg)	VB12 (µg)	CALC (mg)	PHOS (mg)	SEL (µg)	VE-a (mg)
0	300	38	13	2.1	0.3	0	0	0.25	0.18	2.5	0.03	4	0.07	9	91	*	1.4
0	140	20	5	0.4	0.1	0	t	0.05	0.03	0.4	0.01	3	0	6	15	*	0.1
226	740	213	33	2.8	1.8	150	1	0.47	0.33	3.7	0.16	44	0.8	256	319	*	1.8
9	270	74	12	1.6	0.4	37	0	0.33	0.14	2.5	0.1	51	t	151	60	*	0.1
50	1030	150	27	1.8	0.9	44	t	0.3	0.15	2.7	0.1	20	0.82	165	229	*	*
16	200	866	40	0.9	0.6	0	15	0.24	0	3.3	0.32	40	0.15	18	162	*	0.3
12	150	692	32	0.7	0.5	0	12	0.19	0	2.6	0.25	32	0.12	14	129	*	0.2
9	110	484	22	0.5	0.4	0	8	0.14	0	1.8	0.18	22	0.08	10	90	*	*
83	160	450	35	1.3	1	391	14	0.1	0.16	0.6	0.49	57	0.23	149	188	*	0.8
37	500	215	23	2.3	2.1	46	2	0.28	0.16	3.8	0.12	17	0.84	122	110	*	0.4
9	330	238	9	0.3	0.2	0	2	0.06	0.02	0.9	0.07	4	0	6	39	*	0.1
0	0	*	*	0.1	*	0	t	0	0.01	t	*	*	*	*	*	*	*
21	640	187	25	2.1	0.6	52	5	0.32	0.33	2.8	0.12	9	0.19	114	501	*	*
13	180	414	51	0.1	1.1	87	0	0.08	0.35	0.3	0.38	19	0.66	222	198	*	1.2
6	170	274	32	0.5	1.3	64	0	0.08	0.35	0.3	0.07	7	0.6	235	178	*	1.1
5	250	26	5	0.2	0.1	2	t	0.01	0.01	0.2	0.01	1	0	15	7	*	1.2
47	420	*	*	1.4	*	38	1	0.29	0.23	2.1	*	*	*	33	*	*	*
43	780	340	47	2.6	1.7	31	2	0.96	0.21	8.9	0.67	33	0.35	143	299	*	2.7
109	990	*	*	3.9	*	226	7	0.39	0.36	6.9	*	*	*	225	*	*	*
60	670	290	35	3.8	3.2	67	10	0.35	0.31	5.8	0.26	48	1.48	93	170	*	2.7
10	240	*	*	*	*	*	*	*	*	*	*	*	*	332	*	*	*
10	170	*	*	*	*	*	*	*	*	*	*	*	*	327	*	*	*
10	170	643	48	0.2	2.4	38	2	0.12	0.59	0.3	0.13	31	1.54	327	394	*	0.1
48	350	*	*	0.7	*	0	0	0.27	0.1	2.3	*	*	*	8	*	*	*
118	1150	341	41	3.7	5.7	211	3	0.37	0.39	6.7	0.23	23	2.15	295	382	*	*
86	660	322	37	3.7	5.1	67	3	0.36	0.29	6.7	0.27	23	1.88	142	249	*	*
26	310	*	*	1.5	*	35	3	0.33	0.21	2.1	*	*	*	14	*	*	*
14	170	22	0	0.1	t	6	0	t	0.01	t	t	1	0.04	3	4	*	2.4
0	220	22	0	0.1	t	6	0	t	0.01	t	t	1	0.04	3	4	*	2.4
275	1250	319	25	3.2	2.2	88	t	0.53	0.35	4	0.2	40	1.37	116	490	*	*
49	1080	196	20	2	1.5	0	0	0.49	0.21	4	0.11	9	0.5	83	443	*	3.1
64	830	179	20	2.3	1.7	72	1	0.6	0.29	4.8	0.13	48	0.5	235	273	*	1.6
263	980	255	29	3.3	2.4	150	0	0.64	0.42	4.8	0.19	68	0.72	263	390	*	2.3
399	290	102	10	2.1	1.1	156	1	0.07	0.26	0.1	0.08	27	1.68	57	136	*	2.9
41	85	219	12	0.7	0.3	217	7	0.05	0.08	0.3	0.06	40	0	76	26	*	0.4
10	170	*	*	0.1	*	92	0	0.13	0.48	0.3	*	*	*	327	*	*	*
5	95	263	19	0.2	1.2	64	1	0.07	0.29	0.3	0.07	9	0.54	190	127	*	0.6
0	190	10	2	0.2	t	65	1	0	0.01	0.1	t	t	0	11	3	*	0
10	170	*	*	0.1	*	92	0	0.13	0.48	0.3	*	*	*	327	*	*	*
3	80	*	*	0.2	*	38	0	0.04	0.18	0.4	*	*	*	112	*	*	*
*	267	49	*	0.7	*	23	1	0.03	0.02	1.3	*	*	*	73	53	*	*
*	132	50	*	0.2	*	23	t	0.01	0.02	0.9	*	*	*	21	36	*	*
*	146	45	*	0.2	*	30	t	0.02	0.03	1.7	*	*	*	19	37	*	*
*	167	44	*	0.2	*	23	t	0.01	0.01	0.8	*	*	*	24	37	*	*
*	267	37	*	0.4	*	25	1	0.03	0.03	2.1	*	*	*	86	114	*	*
6	165	45	6	0.2	0.3	10	1	0.02	0.02	1.8	0.04	7	0.08	27	39	*	0.3
8	130	47	7	0.2	0.7	29	1	0.02	0.02	3.6	0.06	2	0.37	24	38	*	0.7
*	136	43	*	0.2	*	9	t	0.01	0.02	1.6	*	*	*	25	33	*	*
*	367	61	*	0.2	*	22	t	0.02	t	3.1	*	*	*	76	59	*	*
*	143	46	*	0.2	*	12	t	0.01	0.01	2.3	*	*	*	25	48	*	*
*	160	33	*	0.2	*	13	t	0.01	0.01	0.9	*	*	*	22	38	*	*
3	17	130	10	0.6	0.1	6	t	0.02	0.01	0.4	0.07	8	0	2	20	*	0.1
1	82	48	5	0.8	0.1	15	t	0.02	0.01	0.2	0.06	2	0.02	3	14	*	0.2
88	1050	340	47	3.6	1.7	16	0	0.46	0.4	15.3	0.67	33	0.35	114	299	*	2.7
*	128	40	*	0.7	*	4	1	0.02	0.01	t	*	*	*	5	14	*	*
*	84	52	*	0.3	*	4	t	0.01	0.01	0.2	*	*	*	4	10	*	*
73	2508	918	*	*	*	*	*	*	*	*	*	*	*	*	*	*	*
133	3199	1002	*	*	*	*	*	*	*	*	*	*	*	*	*	*	*
133	3139	917	66	4.3	6.1	67	5	0.27	0.34	5.1	0.48	63	2.33	64	308	*	5.1
84	2777	1055	40	3.2	1.4	83	15	0.49	0.35	9.3	0.46	43	0.44	96	247	*	4.2
84	2717	971	66	3.1	2.5	74	20	0.48	0.33	12.5	0.58	47	0.95	58	384	*	1.3
166	2218	876	28	2.9	2.7	87	17	0.36	0.33	3.8	0.2	39	1.23	227	315	*	0.9
166	2278	1010	29	3	2.8	90	18	0.37	0.35	3.9	0.21	41	1.28	235	327	*	0.9

WT, weight; **KCAL**, kcalories; **PROT**, protein; **CARB**, carbohydrate; **FIBR**, fiber; **FAT**, fat; **SATF**, saturated fat;

MONO, monsaturated fat; **POLY**, polyunsaturated fat; **CHOL**, cholesterol; **SOD**, sodium; **POT**, potassium;

FOOD NAME	PORTION	WT (g)	KCAL	PROT (g)	CARB (g)	FIBR (g)	FAT (g)	SATF (g)	MONO (g)	POLY (g)
SUBWAY-HAM & CHEESE SANDWICH-ON ITALIAN	ITEM	184	643	38	81	5	18	7	8	4
SUBWAY-MEATBALL SANDWICH-ON ITALIAN ROLL	ITEM	215	918	42	96	3	44	17	17	4
SUBWAY-MEATBALL-ON HONEY WHEAT ROLL	ITEM	224	947	44	101	*	45	17	18	4
SUBWAY-ROAST BEEF SANDWICH-ITALIAN ROLL	ITEM	184	689	42	84	5	23	8	9	4
SUBWAY-ROAST BEEF SANDWICH-ON WHEAT ROLL	ITEM	189	717	41	89	6	24	8	9	4
SUBWAY-SALAD DRESSING-BUTTERMILK RANCH	SERVING	56.7	348	1	2	0	37	5	7	24
SUBWAY-SALAD DRESSING-LITE ITALIAN	SERVING	56.7	23	1	4	0	1	4	6.4	15.9
SUBWAY-SEAFOOD/CRAB SANDWICH-ON ITALIAN	ITEM	210	986	29	94	*	57	11	15	28
SUBWAY-SEAFOOD/CRAB SANDWICH-ON WHEAT	ITEM	219	1015	31	100	2.5	58	11	16	28
SUBWAY-SPICY ITALIAN SANDWICH-ON ITALIAN	ITEM	213	1043	42	83	5	63	23	28	7
SUBWAY-STEAK & CHEESE SANDWICH-ITALIAN	ITEM	213	765	43	83	6	32	12	12	4
SUBWAY-TURKEY BREAST SANDWICH-WHEAT ROLL	ITEM	192	674	42	88	7	20	6	7	7
TACO BELL-BEAN BURRITO	ITEM	168	332	17	43	6.4	12	5.6	4.2	0.6
TACO BELL-BEEF BURRITO	ITEM	110	262	13	29	1.3	10	5.2	3.7	0.4
TACO BELL-BEEFY TOSTADA	ITEM	225	334	16	30	5.2	17	11.5	3.5	0.5
TACO BELL-BURRITO SUPREME	ITEM	225	457	21	43	5	22	7.7	7.4	1.7
TACO BELL-DOUBLE BEEF BURRITO SUPREME	ITEM	255	457	24	42	5.7	22	10.1	15.4	2.1
TACO BELL-ENCHIRITO	ITEM	213	382	20	31	*	20	9.3	*	1.5
TACO BELL-MEXICAN PIZZA	SERVING	223	575	21	40	5.8	37	11.4	8.2	9.7
TACO BELL-NACHOS	SERVING	106	346	7	38	1.4	19	5.7	10	1.6
TACO BELL-NACHOS BELLGRANDE	SERVING	287	649	22	61	*	35	12.3	*	2.6
TACO BELL-PINTOS & CHEESE	SERVING	128	190	9	19	4.9	9	3.6	4.9	0.8
TACO BELL-SOFT TACO	ITEM	92.1	228	12	18	2.6	12	5.4	3.7	1.2
TACO BELL-TACO BELLGRANDE	ITEM	163	355	18	18	4.5	23	10.9	6.6	1.3
TACO BELL-TACO LIGHT	ITEM	170	410	19	18	*	29	11.6	*	5.4
TACO BELL-TACO SALAD WITH SALSA/NO SHELL	SERVING	530	520	31	30	7	31	14.4	19.2	1.7
TACO BELL-TACO SALAD WITH SALSA/SHELL	SERVING	595	941	36	63	7.9	61	18.7	21.6	12.1
TACO BELL-TACO SALAD-NO SALSA-NO SHELL	SERVING	530	502	30	26	7	31	14.4	19.2	1.7
TACO BELL-TACO-REGULAR	ITEM	171	370	21	27	1.2	21	11.4	6.6	1
TACO BELL-TOSTADA-REGULAR	ITEM	144	223	10	27	4	10	5.4	3.1	0.7
WENDYS-BACON AND CHEESE POTATO	SERVING	347	450	15	57	9.9	18	37.1	38.2	14.1
WENDYS-BIG CLASSIC-QUARTER POUND BURGER	SERVING	277	570	27	46	2.3	33	15.9	14.8	4.3
WENDYS-BROCCOLI AND CHEESE POTATO	SERVING	377	400	9	59	*	16	*	*	*
WENDYS-CHEESE POTATO	SERVING	348	470	13	57	3.6	21	12.1	9.3	4
WENDYS-CHEESE SAUCE	SERVING	56	40	1	5	0.2	2	1.9	1.1	0.3
WENDYS-CHEESE TORTELLINI/SPAGHETTI SAUCE	SERVING	112	120	4	24	1	1	2.8	2.2	0.9
WENDYS-CHICKEN CLUB SANDWICH	SERVING	231	500	30	42	2.3	24	5.5	8.5	8
WENDYS-CHICKEN SALAD	SERVING	56	120	7	4	0.2	8	3	2.8	3
WENDYS-CHILI	SERVING	255	220	21	23	6	7	3	5.7	1.1
WENDYS-DOUBLE HAMBURGER	ITEM	226	540	34	40	2.3	27	10.5	10.3	2.8
WENDYS-FRENCH FRIES-REGULAR SIZE	SERVING	134	440	5	53	4.6	23	8.5	9.1	3.6
WENDYS-KIDS MEAL HAMBURGER	SERVING	104	260	14	30	1.3	9	3.5	4.8	0.8
WENDYS-REFRIED BEANS	SERVING	56	70	4	10	3	3	1	2.2	1
WENDYS-SEAFOOD SALAD	SERVING	56	110	4	7	0.2	7	1	4.5	4
WENDYS-SINGLE CHEESEBURGER/EVERYTHING	SERVING	252	490	29	35	2.7	27	10.8	11.2	4.6
WENDYS-SINGLE HAMBURGER	ITEM	218	511	26	40	2.8	27	10.4	11.4	2.2
WENDYS-SINGLE HAMBURGER/EVERYTHING	SERVING	234	420	25	35	2.7	21	6.7	9.4	4.4
WENDYS-SPANISH RICE	SERVING	56	70	2	13	0.7	1	0.1	0.3	1
WENDYS-TACO SALAD WITH TACO CHIPS	SERVING	791	660	40	46	10.5	37	28.8	28.7	15.4
WENDYS-TRIPLE HAMBURGER	ITEM	259	693	50	29	*	42	15.9	18.2	2.7
WENDYS-TUNA SALAD	SERVING	56	100	8	4	0.3	6	1	0.8	3
FATS & OILS										
BUTTER-REGULAR-PAT	ITEM	5	36	t	t	0	4	2.5	1.2	0.2
BUTTER-REGULAR-STICK	ITEM	113	813	1	t	0	92	57.3	26.6	3.4
BUTTER-REGULAR-TABLESPOON	TBSP	14	100	t	t	0	11	7.1	3.3	0.4
BUTTER-UNSALTED-PAT	ITEM	5	36	t	t	0.1	4	2.5	1.2	0.2
FAT-ANIMAL-CHICKEN-FOR COOKING	TBSP	12.8	115	0	0	0	13	3.8	5.7	2.7
FAT-ANIMAL-LARD (PORK)	CUP	205	1849	0	0	0	205	80.4	92.5	23
MARGARINE-DIET/LOW CALORIE-MAZOLA	TBSP	14	50	0	0	0	6	1	2.1	2.6
MARGARINE-IMITATION-40% FAT	TSP	4.8	17	0	0	0	2	0.4	0.8	0.7
MARGARINE-IMITATION-SPREAD-60% FAT	TSP	4.8	26	0	0	0	3	0.6	1.5	0.7
MARGARINE-NO STICK-SPRAY-MAZOLA	SERVING	0.72	6	0	0	0	1	0.1	0.2	0.4

t = Trace of nutrient present ** = Not available*

MAG, magnesium; **IRON,** iron; **ZINC,** zinc; **VITA,** vitamin A; **VITC,** vitamin C; **THIA,** thiamin; **RIBO,** riboflavin; **NIAC,** niacin; **VB6,** vitamin B-6; **FOL,** folate; **VB12,** vitamin B-12; **CALC,** calcium; **PHOS,** phosphorus; **SEL,** selenium; **VE-a,** alpha tocopherol equivalents.

CHOL (mg)	SOD (mg)	POT (mg)	MAG (mg)	IRON (mg)	ZINC (mg)	VITA (RE)	VITC (mg)	THIA (mg)	RIBO (mg)	NIAC (mg)	VB6 (mg)	FOL (μg)	VB12 (μg)	CALC (mg)	PHOS (mg)	SEL (μg)	VE-a (mg)
73	1710	834	50	2.2	2.8	174	17	0.53	0.39	3.6	0.34	45	0.76	304	527	*	3.8
88	2022	1210	47	5	6.2	72	19	0.33	0.39	9.4	0.4	35	3.21	78	263	*	1
88	2082	1498	*	*	*	*	*	*	*	*	*	*	*	*	*	*	*
83	2288	910	57	3.7	5.3	58	5	0.23	0.29	4.4	0.42	54	2.01	55	266	*	4.4
75	2348	994	59	3.8	5.4	59	5	0.24	0.3	4.5	0.43	56	2.07	56	273	*	4.5
6	492	17	1	0.1	0.1	48	0	0.01	0.01	t	0.01	4	0.12	8	15	*	2.3
0	952	13	t	0.1	0.1	14	0	0.01	0.01	t	0.01	3	0.09	6	3	*	4.9
56	2027	641	62	4.4	5.3	107	5	0.51	0.38	7	0.26	91	6.54	230	336	*	2.5
56	1967	557	*	*	*	*	*	*	*	*	*	*	*	*	*	*	*
137	2282	880	*	*	*	*	*	*	*	*	*	*	*	*	*	*	*
82	1556	909	43	4.2	6.8	119	6	0.33	0.46	5.1	0.38	36	2.54	231	456	*	0.8
67	2520	605	*	*	*	*	*	*	*	*	*	*	*	*	*	*	*
79	1030	405	t	3.8	3	240	3	0.28	0.6	3.9	0.21	73	1	144	143	*	1.9
33	746	370	41	3.1	2.4	42	1	0.12	0.46	3.2	0.16	20	0.99	42	88	*	0.9
75	870	490	68	2.5	3.2	383	4	0.09	0.5	2.9	0.26	t	1.13	190	173	*	2
126	367	350	52	3.8	5.9	216	8	0.45	0.92	6.2	0.27	43	1.53	146	245	*	2.1
57	1053	431	87	4	5.9	286	9	0.43	2.19	3.7	0.35	132	2.18	145	548	*	2.3
54	1243	*	*	2.8	*	290	28	0.26	0.42	2.3	*	*	*	269	*	*	*
52	1031	408	63	3.7	2.3	295	31	0.32	0.33	3	0.27	113	0.2	257	360	*	2.5
9	399	159	43	0.9	2.6	169	2	0.01	0.16	0.7	0.12	16	0.62	191	439	*	2.8
36	997	674	*	3.5	*	341	58	0.1	0.34	2.2	*	*	*	297	*	*	*
16	642	399	50	1.4	1.1	132	51	0.05	0.15	0.4	0.19	98	0.08	156	175	*	1.4
32	516	178	31	2.3	1.4	64	1	0.39	0.22	2.7	0.16	40	0.31	116	132	*	0.9
56	472	334	54	1.9	2.4	254	5	0.11	0.29	2	0.28	71	0.55	182	234	*	1.6
56	594	316	*	2.4	*	199	5	0.2	0.33	2.5	*	*	*	155	*	*	*
80	1431	1151	111	5.1	9.1	908	76	0.26	0.64	3.2	0.78	99	4.29	367	567	*	6
80	1662	1212	125	7.1	10.3	888	77	0.51	0.75	4.8	0.88	111	4.82	398	637	*	6.8
80	1056	988	111	4.5	9.1	572	74	0.25	0.5	3.2	0.78	99	4.29	331	567	*	6
57	802	473	71	2.4	3.9	257	2	0.15	0.45	3.2	0.24	23	1.04	221	203	*	0.8
30	543	403	59	1.9	1.9	187	1	0.1	0.33	1.3	0.17	75	0.68	211	116	*	1.4
10	1125	1580	167	15.3	7	266	77	1.04	0.81	14.5	1.94	75	2.26	713	1015	*	4.9
85	1075	590	49	4.8	6.4	162	9	0.35	0.5	8	0.38	51	2.92	304	491	*	2.9
0	470	1555	*	*	*	*	*	*	*	*	*	*	*	*	*	*	*
0	580	1435	72	2.3	2.4	288	34	0.22	0.43	3.5	0.57	31	0.3	417	398	*	2.3
0	300	70	10	0.1	0.2	24	t	0.03	0.11	0.1	0.03	3	0.22	114	88	*	0.1
5	280	110	14	1.3	0.6	110	4	0.12	0.18	1.2	0.09	12	0.17	75	92	*	0.9
75	950	515	42	14.4	1.5	87	16	0.51	0.37	16	0.48	45	0.46	101	259	*	4.4
0	215	60	8	0.5	0.7	22	1	0.02	0.08	1.8	0.13	6	0.14	13	58	*	2.4
45	750	495	53	6.3	4.1	146	19	0.16	0.26	4.8	0.23	41	1.46	55	228	*	1.8
122	791	569	49	6	5.7	31	1	0.36	0.39	7.6	0.54	27	4.07	102	314	*	1.1
25	265	855	46	1	0.5	0	14	0.24	0.04	4.4	0.32	39	0	26	125	*	0.3
35	545	205	22	2.5	2.2	7	1	0.23	0.2	3.8	0.14	25	1	63	110	*	0.5
0	215	210	25	1.2	0.5	0	2	0.08	0.04	0.2	0.09	71	0	25	72	*	0.5
0	455	40	14	0.5	0.9	21	3	0.02	0.03	0.6	0.05	8	0.48	25	74	*	1.2
90	1155	495	44	4.3	4.3	136	11	0.4	0.42	6.5	0.3	55	1.8	234	348	*	3.2
86	825	479	43	4.9	4.9	93	3	0.42	0.38	7.3	0.33	36	2.38	96	233	*	1.1
70	865	495	40	4.3	3.7	76	11	0.4	0.35	6.6	0.29	54	1.68	105	193	*	3
0	440	130	9	0.7	0.2	24	9	0.05	0.02	0.6	0.06	4	0	15	17	*	0.3
35	1110	1330	166	9.2	13.6	1478	67	0.4	0.93	15.2	1.16	147	6.41	532	847	*	9
142	713	785	55	8.3	10.8	47	1	0.31	0.56	11	0.62	31	4.92	65	393	*	*
0	290	90	10	0.6	0.2	15	1	0.02	0.04	3.8	0.05	4	0.68	9	62	*	0.5
11	41	1	t	t	t	8	0	0	t	t	0	t	0.01	1	1	0	0.1
248	937	29	2	0.2	0.1	855	0	0.01	0.04	t	t	3	0.14	27	26	3	1.8
31	116	4	t	t	t	105	0	t	0.01	t	0	t	0.02	3	3	0	0.2
11	1	1	t	t	t	38	0	0	t	t	0	t	0.01	1	1	*	0.1
11	0	0	0	0	0	0	0	0	0	0	0	0	0	0	0	*	2.7
195	t	t	t	0	0.2	0	0	0	0	0	0	0	0	t	0	86	2.5
0	130	1	t	0	t	130	0	0	0	0	0	0	0	0	t	0	0.1
0	46	1	t	0	0	48	t	0	t	t	0	t	t	1	1	*	0.4
0	48	1	t	0	0	48	t	0	t	t	0	t	t	1	1	*	0.4
0	0	*	*	0	*	0	0	0	0	0	*	*	*	0	0	*	*

WT, weight; **KCAL,** kcalories; **PROT,** protein; **CARB,** carbohydrate; **FIBR,** fiber; **FAT,** fat; **SATF,** saturated fat;

MONO, monsaturated fat; **POLY,** polyunsaturated fat; **CHOL,** cholesterol; **SOD,** sodium; **POT,** potassium;

FOOD NAME	PORTION	WT (g)	KCAL	PROT (g)	CARB (g)	FIBR (g)	FAT (g)	SATF (g)	MONO (g)	POLY (g)
MARGARINE-REGULAR-HARD-UNSALTED	TSP	4.7	34	0	0	0	4	0.7	1.7	1.2
MARGARINE-REGULAR-SOFT-UNSALTED	TSP	4.7	34	0	0	0	4	0.6	1.8	1.2
MARGARINE-SOYBEAN-SOFT-TUB-UNSALTED	TSP	4.7	34	0	0	0	4	0.6	1.7	1.3
MARGARINE-WHIPPED	TBSP	9	70	0	0	0	8	1.4	2.5	3.1
MAYONNAISE-IMITATION-MILK CREAM	TBSP	15	15	t	2	0	1	0.4	0.3	0.1
MAYONNAISE-LIGHT-LOW CALORIE-KRAFT	TBSP	14	40	0	1	0	4	0.5	0.6	1.4
MAYONNAISE-SOYBEAN-COMMERCIAL	TBSP	14	99	t	t	0	11	1.6	3.1	5.7
OIL-VEGETABLE-CORN	CUP	218	1927	0	0	0	218	27.7	52.7	128
OIL-VEGETABLE-OLIVE	CUP	216	1909	0	0	0	216	30.7	159	18.2
OIL-VEGETABLE-PEANUT	CUP	216	1909	0	0	0	216	36.4	99.9	69.2
OIL-VEGETABLE-SAFFLOWER	CUP	218	1927	0	0	0	218	20.5	26.3	162
OIL-VEGETABLE-SESAME	TBSP	13.6	120	0	0	0	14	1.9	5.4	5.7
OIL-VEGETABLE-SOYBEAN	CUP	218	1927	0	0	0	218	31.8	93.8	82
SALAD DRESSING-BLUE CHEESE	TBSP	15.3	77	1	1	0.1	8	1.5	1.9	4.3
SALAD DRESSING-BLUE CHEESE-LOW CALORIE	TBSP	16	10	0	1	0	1	0.5	0.3	0
SALAD DRESSING-CAESAR	TBSP	15	70	0	1	t	7	*	*	*
SALAD DRESSING-FRENCH	TBSP	15.6	67	t	3	0.1	6	1.5	1.2	3.4
SALAD DRESSING-FRENCH-LOW CALORIE	TBSP	16.3	22	0	4	0.1	1	0.1	0.2	0.5
SALAD DRESSING-ITALIAN	TBSP	14.7	69	0	2	0.1	7	1	1.7	4.1
SALAD DRESSING-ITALIAN-LOW CALORIE	TBSP	15	16	0	1	0.1	2	0.2	0.3	0.9
SALAD DRESSING-MAYONNAISE TYPE	TBSP	14.7	57	0	4	0	5	0.7	1.3	2.6
SALAD DRESSING-MAYONNAISE-LOW CALORIE	TBSP	16	20	0	2	0	2	0.4	0.4	1
SALAD DRESSING-MIRACLE WHIP LIGHT	TBSP	14	45	0	2	0	4	*	*	*
SALAD DRESSING-OIL/VINEGAR-HOME RECIPE	TBSP	15.6	70	0	t	0	8	1.4	2.3	3.8
SALAD DRESSING-RANCH STYLE	TBSP	15	54	t	1	0	6	0.7	1.4	2.7
SALAD DRESSING-RUSSIAN	TBSP	15.3	76	t	2	0	8	1.1	1.8	4.5
SALAD DRESSING-RUSSIAN-LOW CALORIE	TBSP	16.3	23	t	5	0.2	1	0.1	0.2	0.4
SALAD DRESSING-THOUSAND ISLAND	TBSP	15.6	59	0	2	0.6	6	0.9	1.3	3.1
SALAD DRESSING-THOUSAND-LOW CALORIE	TBSP	15.3	24	t	3	0.3	2	0.2	0.4	1
SANDWICH SPREAD-COMMERCIAL	TBSP	15.3	60	t	3	t	5	0.8	1.1	3.1
SHORTENING-VEGETABLE-SOYBEAN/COTTONSEED	CUP	205	1812	0	0	0	205	51.2	89	52.2
VEGETABLE SPRAY-PAM-BUTTER FLAVORED	SERVING	0.9	7	0	0	0	1	0.1	0.2	0.5
VEGETABLE SPRAY-PAM-UNFLAVORED	SERVING	0.9	7	0	0	0	1	0.1	0.2	0.5
FISH										
FISH STICKS-BREADED-FROZEN-COOKED	OUNCE	28.4	77	4	7	0.7	3	0.9	1.4	0.9
FISH-ANCHOVY-FILLET-CANNED	ITEM	4	8	1	0	0	t	0.1	0.2	0.1
FISH-BLUEFISH-BAKED WITH BUTTER	ITEM	155	246	41	0	0	8	1.8	1.8	3.9
FISH-CARP-COOKED-DRY HEAT	SERVING	85	138	19	0	0	6	1.2	2.5	1.6
FISH-CATFISH-BREADED-FRIED	SERVING	85	195	15	7	0.8	11	2.8	4.8	2.8
FISH-CLAMS-BREADED-FRIED	SERVING	85	172	12	9	0.3	9	2.3	3.9	2.4
FISH-CLAMS-CANNED-SOLIDS AND LIQUIDS	OUNCE	28.4	13	2	1	0	t	0.1	0	0
FISH-CLAMS-COOKED-MOIST HEAT	SERVING	85	126	22	4	0	2	0.2	0.1	0.5
FISH-CLAMS-RAW-MEAT ONLY	SERVING	85	63	11	2	0	1	0.1	0.1	0.2
FISH-COD-ATLANTIC-COOKED-DRY HEAT	PIECE	180	189	41	0	0	2	0.3	0.2	0.5
FISH-CRAB CAKE	ITEM	60	93	12	t	t	5	0.9	1.7	1.4
FISH-CRAB MEAT-KING-CANNED-UNPACKED	CUP	135	135	24	1	0	3	0.6	0.6	2
FISH-CRAB-ALASKA KING-RAW	SERVING	85	71	16	0	0	1	0.1	0.1	0.1
FISH-CRAB-BLUE-CANNED	CUP	135	134	28	0	0	2	0.3	0.3	0.6
FISH-CRAB-BLUE-COOKED-MOIST HEAT	CUP	135	138	27	0	0	2	0.3	0.4	0.9
FISH-CRAB-DEVILED	CUP	240	451	27	32	2.3	23	4.8	9.6	7.1
FISH-CRAB-IMITATION-SURIMI	SERVING	85	87	10	9	0	1	0.2	0.2	0.6
FISH-CRAB-IMPERIAL	CUP	220	323	32	9	0	17	4.2	6.7	4.8
FISH-CRAB-STEAMED-PIECES	CUP	155	150	30	0	0	2	0.2	0.3	0.8
FISH-CRAYFISH-COOKED-MOIST HEAT	SERVING	85	97	20	0	0	1	0.2	0.3	0.3
FISH-CROAKER-BREADED-FRIED	SERVING	85	188	16	6	0.3	11	3	4.5	2.5
FISH-EEL-COOKED-DRY HEAT	SERVING	85	201	20	0	0	13	2.6	7.8	1
FISH-FLATFISH-COOKED-DRY HEAT	SERVING	85	100	21	0	0	1	0.3	0.3	0.4
FISH-GEFILTEFISH-COMMERCIAL-WITH BROTH	PIECE	42	35	4	3	t	1	0.2	0.3	0.1
FISH-GROUPER-COOKED-DRY HEAT	SERVING	85	100	21	0	0	1	0.3	0.2	0.3
FISH-HADDOCK-BREADED-FRIED	PIECE	85	140	17	5	0.3	5	1.4	2.2	1.2
FISH-HADDOCK-BROILED	SERVING	85	95	21	0	0	1	0.1	0.1	0.3
FISH-HALIBUT-ALL TYPES-BROILED IN BUTTER	PIECE	125	214	32	0	0	9	*	*	*
FISH-HALIBUT-COOKED-BROILED	SERVING	85	119	23	0	0	2	0.4	0.8	0.8

t = Trace of nutrient present ** = Not available*

MAG, magnesium; **IRON,** iron; **ZINC,** zinc; **VITA,** vitamin A; **VITC,** vitamin C; **THIA,** thiamin; **RIBO,** riboflavin; **NIAC,** niacin; **VB6,** vitamin B-6; **FOL,** folate; **VB12,** vitamin B-12; **CALC,** calcium; **PHOS,** phosphorus; **SEL,** selenium; **VE-a,** alpha tocopherol equivalents.

CHOL (mg)	SOD (mg)	POT (mg)	MAG (mg)	IRON (mg)	ZINC (mg)	VITA (RE)	VITC (mg)	THIA (mg)	RIBO (mg)	NIAC (mg)	VB6 (mg)	FOL (µg)	VB12 (µg)	CALC (mg)	PHOS (mg)	SEL (µg)	VE-a (mg)
0	t	1	t	0	0	47	t	0	t	t	0	t	t	1	1	0	0.6
0	1	2	t	0	0	47	t	0	t	t	0	t	t	1	1	0	0.5
0	1	2	t	0	0	47	t	0	t	t	0	t	t	1	1	0	0.1
0	97	2	t	0	0	310	0	0	0	0	t	t	0.01	2	2	0	1.1
6	76	15	1	0.1	t	t	t	t	0.02	t	t	t	0.04	11	9	*	0.1
5	15	1	0	0	t	1	0	0	t	0	0	t	0.01	0	0	*	2.9
8	78	5	t	0.1	t	12	0	0	0	0	0.08	1	0.04	2	4	*	2.9
0	0	0	0	0	0	0	0	0	0	0	0	0	0	0	0	*	31.1
0	t	0	t	0.8	0.1	0	0	0	0	0	0	0	0	t	3	*	25.7
0	t	t	t	0.1	t	0	0	0	0	0	0	0	0	t	0	*	25.1
0	0	0	0	0	0	0	0	0	0	0	0	0	0	0	0	*	74.2
0	0	0	0	0	0	0	0	0	0	0	0	0	0	0	0	*	0.2
0	0	0	0	0	0	0	0	0	0	0	0	0	0	0	0	*	17.7
9	167	6	0	0	0	10	t	0	0.02	0	0.01	1	0.04	12	11	*	0.9
4	177	5	*	0	*	9	0	0	0.01	0	*	*	*	10	8	*	8
*	*	*	*	*	*	*	*	*	*	*	*	*	*	*	*	*	7
2	214	12	0	0.1	t	3	0	t	t	0	t	1	0.02	2	2	*	0.8
1	128	13	0	0.1	t	0	0	0	0	0	0	0	0	2	2	*	0.2
0	116	2	t	0	t	4	0	0	0	0	t	1	0.02	1	1	*	0.7
1	118	2	0	0	t	0	0	0	0	0	0	0	0	0	1	*	0
4	104	1	t	0	t	10	0	0	0	0	t	1	0.03	2	4	*	0.6
2	44	1	*	0	*	12	*	0	0	0	*	*	*	3	4	*	5
5	95	*	*	*	*	*	*	*	*	*	*	*	*	*	*	*	4
0	t	1	0	0	0	0	0	0	0	0	0	0	0	2	1	*	0.6
4	97	1	t	t	t	13	0	t	t	t	t	1	0.03	2	4	*	0.6
0	133	24	t	0.1	0.1	32	1	0.01	0.01	0.1	0.01	2	0.05	3	6	*	0.9
1	141	26	t	0.1	t	3	1	t	t	0	t	1	0.02	3	6	*	0.1
5	109	18	t	0.1	t	15	0	0	0	0	t	1	0.03	2	3	*	0.6
2	153	17	t	0.1	t	15	0	0	0	0	t	1	0.03	2	3	*	0.2
12	153	5	0	0	0	0	0	0	0	0	0	0	0	0	0	*	0.6
0	0	0	0	0	0	0	0	0	0	0	0	0	0	0	0	*	27.9
0	0	0	*	0	*	0	0	*	*	*	*	*	*	0	0	*	*
0	0	0	*	0	*	0	0	*	*	*	*	*	*	0	0	*	*
32	165	74	7	0.2	0.2	9	0	0.04	0.05	0.6	0.02	5	0.51	6	51	3	*
3	147	22	3	0.2	0.1	1	0	t	0.02	0.8	0.01	1	0.04	9	10	2	t
108	161	*	43	1.1	*	24	*	0.17	0.16	2.9	*	*	1.64	45	445	47	*
72	54	363	32	1.4	1.6	8	1	0.12	0.06	1.8	0.19	15	1.25	44	451	26	1.8
69	238	289	23	1.2	0.7	7	0	0.06	0.11	1.9	0.16	14	1.62	37	184	*	1.8
52	309	277	12	11.8	1.2	77	9	0.09	0.21	1.8	0.05	16	34.2	54	160	*	1.7
18	15	40	*	1.2	0.3	*	*	t	0.03	0.3	*	*	5.4	16	39	46	0.6
57	95	534	16	23.8	2.3	145	19	0.13	0.36	2.9	0.09	16	84.1	78	287	*	1.7
29	48	267	8	11.9	1.2	77	11	0.07	0.18	1.5	0.05	14	42	39	144	16	0.2
99	141	440	76	0.9	1	25	2	0.16	0.14	4.5	0.51	15	1.89	25	248	81	0.1
90	198	195	20	0.7	2.5	49	2	0.05	0.05	1.7	0.1	25	3.56	63	128	13	1.2
135	675	149	29	1.1	5.8	*	*	0.11	0.11	2.6	*	*	13.5	61	246	30	1.7
36	711	173	42	0.5	5.1	6	6	0.04	0.04	0.9	0.13	37	7.65	39	186	19	*
120	450	505	53	1.1	5.4	3	4	0.11	0.11	1.9	0.2	57	0.62	136	351	30	1.4
135	376	437	45	1.2	5.7	3	4	0.14	0.07	4.5	0.24	69	9.86	140	278	30	1.4
223	2081	398	64	2.9	5.5	330	14	0.19	0.26	3.6	0.31	88	8.69	113	329	53	5.3
17	715	77	37	0.3	0.3	17	0	0.03	0.02	0.2	0.03	1	1.36	11	240	19	0.1
275	1602	288	57	2	6.4	211	11	0.13	0.26	2.4	0.31	83	10.6	132	365	48	3.5
82	1662	406	53	1.2	11.8	14	12	0.08	0.09	2.1	0.28	79	17.8	92	434	34	1.5
151	58	298	26	2.7	1.4	19	3	0.15	0.07	2.5	0.15	3	2.94	26	281	*	1.3
71	296	289	35	0.7	0.4	19	0	0.08	0.11	3.7	0.22	15	1.79	27	184	*	2.3
137	55	297	22	0.5	1.8	966	2	0.16	0.04	3.8	0.07	15	2.45	22	235	43	4.5
58	89	292	49	0.3	0.5	9	0	0.07	0.1	1.9	0.2	8	2.13	15	246	*	*
13	220	38	4	1	0.3	11	t	0.03	0.03	0.4	0.03	1	0.35	10	31	*	0
40	45	403	32	1	0.4	43	0	0.07	0.01	0.3	0.3	9	0.59	18	121	*	*
42	150	296	*	1	*	*	2	0.03	0.06	2.7	*	*	1.1	34	210	41	0.5
63	74	339	43	1.2	0.4	16	0	0.03	0.04	3.9	0.29	11	1.18	36	205	25	0.5
75	168	656	*	1	*	255	*	0.06	0.09	10.4	*	*	*	20	310	41	0.5
35	59	490	91	0.9	0.5	46	0	0.06	0.08	6.1	0.34	12	1.16	51	242	51	*

WT, weight; **KCAL,** kcalories; **PROT,** protein; **CARB,** carbohydrate; **FIBR,** fiber; **FAT,** fat; **SATF,** saturated fat;

MONO, monsaturated fat; **POLY,** polyunsaturated fat; **CHOL,** cholesterol; **SOD,** sodium; **POT,** potassium;

FOOD NAME	PORTION	WT (g)	KCAL	PROT (g)	CARB (g)	FIBR (g)	FAT (g)	SATF (g)	MONO (g)	POLY (g)
FISH-HERRING-ATLANTIC-BROILED	SERVING	85	173	20	0	0	10	2.2	4.1	2.3
FISH-HERRING-ATLANTIC-RAW	SERVING	85	134	15	0	0	8	1.7	3.2	1.8
FISH-HERRING-CANNED-SOLIDS AND LIQUIDS	SERVING	100	208	20	0	0	14	*	*	2
FISH-HERRING-PICKLED-BISMARCK TYPE	ITEM	50	131	7	5	0	9	1.2	6	0.8
FISH-LOBSTER NEWBURG	CUP	250	485	46	13	0	27	30.1	14.9	2.3
FISH-LOBSTER THERMIDOR	SERVING	157	405	29	15	0	27	18.9	9.4	1.5
FISH-LOBSTER-COOKED-MOIST HEAT	OUNCE	28.4	28	6	t	0	t	t	t	t
FISH-LOBSTER-NORTHERN-RAW	OUNCE	28.4	26	5	t	0	t	0.1	0.1	t
FISH-MACKEREL-ATLANTIC-CANNED	CUP	190	296	44	0	0	12	3.4	5.2	0.2
FISH-MACKEREL-ATLANTIC-RAW	OUNCE	28.4	58	5	0	0	4	0.9	1.2	1.4
FISH-MACKEREL-COOKED-DRY HEAT	SERVING	85	223	20	0	0	15	3.6	6	3.7
FISH-MULLET-COOKED-DRY HEAT	SERVING	85	128	21	0	0	4	1.2	1.2	0.8
FISH-MUSSELS-BLUE-RAW	CUP	150	129	18	6	0	3	0.6	0.8	0.9
FISH-OCEAN PERCH-BREADED-FRIED	PIECE	85	195	16	6	0.1	11	2.7	4.4	2.3
FISH-OCEAN PERCH-COOKED-DRY HEAT	SERVING	85	103	20	0	0	2	0.3	0.7	0.5
FISH-OYSTER-EASTERN-CANNED	CUP	248	171	18	10	0	6	1.6	0.6	1.8
FISH-OYSTER-EASTERN-COOKED-MOIST HEAT	SERVING	85	117	12	7	0	4	1.1	0.4	1.3
FISH-OYSTERS-BREADED-FRIED	SERVING	85	167	7	10	0.1	11	2.7	4	2.8
FISH-OYSTERS-EASTERN-RAW-MEAT ONLY	CUP	248	171	18	10	0	6	1.6	0.6	1.8
FISH-OYSTERS-PACIFIC-RAW	SERVING	85	69	8	4	0	2	0.4	0.3	0.8
FISH-PERCH-COOKED-DRY HEAT	SERVING	85	100	21	0	0	1	0.2	0.2	0.4
FISH-PIKE-COOKED-DRY HEAT	SERVING	85	96	21	0	0	1	0.1	0.2	0.2
FISH-POLLOCK-ATLANTIC-RAW	SERVING	85	78	17	0	0	1	0.1	0.1	0.4
FISH-POLLOCK-COOKED-DRY HEAT	SERVING	85	96	20	0	0	1	0.2	0.1	0.4
FISH-POMPANO-COOKED-DRY HEAT	SERVING	85	179	20	0	0	10	3.8	2.8	1.2
FISH-RED SNAPPER-COOKED-DRY HEAT	SERVING	85	109	22	0	0	1	0.3	0.3	0.5
FISH-RED SNAPPER-RAW	SERVING	85	85	17	0	0	1	0.2	0.2	0.4
FISH-ROCKFISH-COOKED-DRY HEAT	SERVING	100	121	24	0	0	2	0.5	0.4	0.6
FISH-SALMON PATTY	SERVING	100	239	16	16	1	12	3.5	5.3	3.6
FISH-SALMON-BROILED OR BAKED-WITH BUTTER	SERVING	100	182	27	0	0	7	1.4	2.7	2.7
FISH-SALMON-COOKED-MOIST HEAT	SERVING	85	157	23	0	0	6	1.2	2.2	1.9
FISH-SALMON-PINK-CANNED-SOLIDS & LIQUIDS	SERVING	85	118	17	0	0	5	1.3	1.5	1.7
FISH-SALMON-SMOKED	SERVING	100	117	18	0	0	4	0.9	2	1
FISH-SARDINES-ATLANTIC-CANNED IN OIL	ITEM	12	25	3	0	0	1	0.2	0.5	0.6
FISH-SARDINES-CANNED IN TOMATO SAUCE	ITEM	38	68	6	0	0.1	5	1.2	1.4	1.6
FISH-SCALLOPS-BAY AND SEA-STEAMED	OUNCE	28.4	32	7	1	0	t	*	*	*
FISH-SCALLOPS-FROZEN-BREADED-FRIED	ITEM	15	32	3	2	0.1	2	0.4	0.7	0.4
FISH-SCALLOPS-RAW	SERVING	85	75	14	2	0	1	0.1	t	0.2
FISH-SEA BASS-COOKED-DRY HEAT	SERVING	85	105	20	0	0	2	0.6	0.5	0.8
FISH-SHAD-BAKED-BUTTER/MARGARINE & BACON	SERVING	100	201	23	0	0	11	2.5	2.2	5.9
FISH-SHRIMP-CANNED MEAT	CUP	128	154	30	1	0	3	0.5	0.4	1
FISH-SHRIMP-COOKED-MOIST HEAT	SERVING	85	84	18	0	0	1	0.2	0.2	0.4
FISH-SHRIMP-FRENCH FRIED	SERVING	85	206	18	10	0.5	10	1.8	3.2	3.8
FISH-SMELT-ATLANTIC-CANNED	ITEM	20	40	4	0	0	3	*	*	*
FISH-SMELT-COOKED-DRY HEAT	SERVING	85	105	19	0	0	3	0.5	0.7	1
FISH-SOLE/FLOUNDER-BAKED	SERVING	127	148	31	0	0	2	0.5	0.4	0.5
FISH-SQUID-COOKED-FRIED	SERVING	85	149	15	7	0.3	6	1.6	2.3	1.8
FISH-SQUID-RAW	SERVING	85	78	13	3	0	1	0.3	0.1	0.4
FISH-STURGEON-STEAMED	SERVING	100	135	21	0	0	5	1.2	2.5	0.9
FISH-SURIMI	SERVING	85	84	13	6	0	1	0.2	0.1	0.4
FISH-SWORDFISH-BROILED-BUTTER/MARGARINE	SERVING	100	174	28	0	0	6	2	3.4	2.2
FISH-SWORDFISH-COOKED-DRY HEAT	SERVING	85	132	22	0	0	4	1.2	1.7	1
FISH-TILEFISH-COOKED-DRY HEAT	SERVING	85	125	21	0	0	4	0.7	1.1	1.1
FISH-TROUT-BROOK-COOKED	SERVING	100	196	24	t	0	11	1.5	2.8	2.6
FISH-TROUT-RAINBOW-COOKED-DRY HEAT	SERVING	85	128	22	0	0	4	0.7	1.1	1.3
FISH-TUNA-BLUEFIN-COOKED-DRY HEAT	SERVING	85	156	25	0	0	5	1.4	1.8	1.6
FISH-TUNA-CANNED IN OIL-DRAINED SOLIDS	SERVING	85	168	25	0	0	7	1.3	2.5	2.5
FISH-TUNA-DIETETIC-LOW SODIUM-DRAINED	OUNCE	28.4	36	8	t	0	1	0.1	0.2	0.2
FISH-TUNA-LIGHT-CANNED IN WATER-DRAINED	SERVING	85	111	25	0	0	t	0.1	0.1	0.1
FISH-TUNA-WHITE-ALBACORE-CANNED IN WATER	SERVING	85	116	23	0	0	2	0.6	0.6	0.8
FISH-TUNA-YELLOWFIN-RAW	SERVING	85	92	20	0	0	1	0.2	0.1	0.2
FISH-WHITE PERCH-FRIED FILET	ITEM	65	108	13	0	0	5	*	*	*
FISH-WHITEFISH-LAKE-BAKED-STUFFED	SERVING	100	215	15	6	0.6	14	*	*	*
FISH-WHITING-COOKED-DRY HEAT	SERVING	85	98	20	0	0	1	0.3	0.3	0.5

t = Trace of nutrient present   ** = Not available*

MAG, magnesium; **IRON,** iron; **ZINC,** zinc; **VITA,** vitamin A; **VITC,** vitamin C; **THIA,** thiamin; **RIBO,** riboflavin; **NIAC,** niacin; **VB6,** vitamin B-6; **FOL,** folate; **VB12,** vitamin B-12; **CALC,** calcium; **PHOS,** phosphorus; **SEL,** selenium; **VE-a,** alpha tocopherol equivalents.

CHOL (mg)	SOD (mg)	POT (mg)	MAG (mg)	IRON (mg)	ZINC (mg)	VITA (RE)	VITC (mg)	THIA (mg)	RIBO (mg)	NIAC (mg)	VB6 (mg)	FOL (μg)	VB12 (μg)	CALC (mg)	PHOS (mg)	SEL (μg)	VE-a (mg)
66	98	356	35	1.2	1.1	26	1	0.1	0.25	3.5	0.3	10	11.2	63	258	52	0.9
51	76	278	27	0.9	0.8	24	1	0.08	0.2	2.7	0.26	9	11.6	49	201	85	0.9
98	*	*	*	1.8	*	*	*	0.18	*	*	*	*	*	147	297	58	*
7	435	35	4	0.6	0.3	129	0	0.02	0.07	1.7	0.09	1	2.14	39	45	50	0.5
376	573	428	56	2.3	4.2	530	1	0.18	0.28	1.6	0.17	32	4.11	218	480	188	2.6
236	360	388	35	1.9	2.6	295	0	0.15	0.51	4.8	0.11	20	2.58	290	451	118	1.7
20	108	100	10	0.1	0.8	7	0	t	0.02	0.3	0.02	3	0.88	17	53	23	0.3
27	84	78	8	0.1	0.9	6	0	t	0.01	0.4	0.02	3	0.26	14	41	21	*
150	720	369	70	3.9	1.9	248	2	0.08	0.4	11.7	0.4	10	13.2	458	572	89	3.2
20	26	89	22	0.5	0.2	14	t	0.05	0.09	2.6	0.11	t	2.47	3	62	*	0.4
64	71	341	83	1.3	0.8	46	t	0.14	0.35	5.8	0.39	1	16.2	13	236	30	1.9
54	60	389	28	1.2	0.7	36	1	0.09	0.09	5.4	0.42	8	0.21	26	207	*	2.1
42	429	479	51	5.9	2.4	72	12	0.24	0.32	2.4	0.08	63	18	39	296	84	1.1
32	128	242	*	1.1	*	*	*	0.1	0.1	1.6	*	*	0.85	28	192	20	1.1
46	82	298	33	1	0.5	12	1	0.11	0.11	2.1	0.23	9	0.98	117	235	30	1.6
136	278	568	134	16.6	226	223	12	0.37	0.41	3.1	0.24	22	47.5	112	344	149	2.6
93	190	389	93	11.4	155	145	7	0.25	0.28	2.1	0.08	15	32.5	76	236	51	*
69	355	208	49	5.9	74.1	77	3	0.13	0.17	1.4	0.05	12	13.3	53	135	*	1.9
136	277	568	135	16.6	226	222	12	0.34	0.41	3.3	0.12	25	47.5	111	344	141	2
43	90	143	19	4.3	14.1	69	7	0.06	0.2	1.7	0.04	9	13.6	7	138	56	0.7
98	67	292	32	1	1.2	9	1	0.07	0.1	1.6	0.12	5	1.87	87	218	30	1.6
43	42	281	34	0.6	0.7	20	3	0.06	0.07	2.4	0.12	15	1.96	62	239	32	1.4
60	73	303	57	0.4	0.4	9	0	0.04	0.16	2.8	0.24	3	2.71	51	188	*	*
82	99	329	62	0.2	0.5	20	0	0.06	0.07	1.4	0.06	3	3.57	5	410	*	*
54	65	541	27	0.6	0.6	31	0	0.58	0.13	3.2	0.2	15	1.02	36	290	*	0.9
40	48	444	31	0.2	0.4	30	1	0.05	t	0.3	0.39	5	2.98	34	171	*	*
31	54	355	27	0.2	0.3	26	1	0.04	t	0.2	0.34	4	2.55	27	169	*	*
44	77	520	34	0.5	0.5	66	1	0.04	0.08	3.9	0.27	10	1.2	12	228	39	*
64	96	89	34	1.2	0.8	20	4	0.12	0.22	4	0.07	13	3	78	104	*	2.1
47	116	443	32	1.2	0.7	48	2	0.16	0.06	9.8	0.22	5	2.71	18	418	48	1.4
42	50	454	32	0.8	0.4	15	1	0.16	0.17	7.1	0.39	4	3.06	39	248	26	1.2
47	471	277	29	0.7	0.8	14	0	0.02	0.16	5.6	0.26	13	5.85	181	279	45	1.2
23	784	175	18	0.9	0.3	26	0	0.02	0.1	4.7	0.28	2	3.26	11	164	61	1.4
17	61	48	5	0.4	0.2	8	0	0.01	0.03	0.6	0.02	1	1.07	46	59	6	*
23	157	130	13	0.9	0.5	27	t	0.02	0.09	1.6	0.05	9	3.42	91	139	*	0.2
15	75	135	*	0.9	*	*	*	*	*	*	*	*	*	33	96	15	*
9	70	50	9	0.1	0.2	3	t	0.01	0.02	0.2	0.02	3	0.2	6	35	12	0.1
28	137	274	48	0.2	0.8	13	3	0.01	0.06	1	0.13	14	1.3	20	186	65	*
45	74	279	45	0.3	0.4	54	0	0.11	0.13	1.6	0.39	5	0.26	11	211	*	1
69	79	377	*	0.6	*	9	*	0.13	0.26	8.6	*	*	*	24	313	*	2
222	216	269	53	3.5	1.6	23	3	0.04	0.05	3.5	0.14	2	1.44	75	299	41	3.6
166	190	155	29	2.6	1.3	56	2	0.03	0.03	2.2	0.11	3	1.26	33	116	54	3.2
150	292	191	34	1.1	1.2	48	1	0.11	0.12	2.6	0.08	7	1.59	57	185	27	0.8
*	*	*	*	0.3	*	*	*	*	*	*	*	*	*	72	74	10	0.1
77	66	316	32	1	1.8	15	0	0.63	0.12	1.5	0.15	4	3.37	66	251	105	1.7
86	133	436	74	0.4	0.8	14	4	0.1	0.15	2.8	0.31	11	3.19	23	368	160	1.5
221	260	237	33	0.9	1.5	9	4	0.05	0.39	2.2	0.05	5	1.04	33	213	*	1.9
198	37	209	28	0.6	1.3	9	4	0.02	0.35	1.9	0.05	4	1.1	27	188	*	1
75	108	364	35	2	0.5	243	0	0.08	0.09	9.8	0.22	17	2.6	40	263	49	0.6
26	122	95	37	0.2	0.3	17	0	0.02	0.02	0.2	0.03	1	1.36	8	240	*	*
4	478	354	33	1.3	1.4	616	3	0.04	0.05	10.9	0.36	3	1.9	7	275	47	1.2
43	98	314	29	0.9	1.3	35	1	0.04	0.1	10	0.32	2	1.72	5	287	*	1
54	50	435	28	0.3	0.5	18	0	0.12	0.16	3	0.26	15	2.13	22	201	*	*
69	79	302	35	1.1	1.3	96	1	0.12	0.06	2.5	0.44	17	3.25	218	272	*	0.8
62	29	539	33	2.1	1.2	19	3	0.07	0.19	5.9	0.39	15	2.98	73	273	*	0.7
42	43	275	54	1.1	0.7	643	0	0.24	0.26	9	0.45	2	9.25	9	277	85	0.9
15	301	176	26	1.2	0.8	20	0	0.03	0.1	10.5	0.09	5	1.87	11	264	61	1.4
10	11	74	9	0.3	0.1	7	*	0.01	0.01	3.5	0.11	0	0.4	1	63	33	1
15	303	267	25	2.7	0.4	20	0	0.03	0.1	10.5	0.32	4	1.87	10	158	61	*
35	333	241	29	0.5	0.4	20	0	t	0.04	4.9	0.37	4	1.87	3	227	61	*
38	32	377	43	0.6	0.4	15	1	0.37	0.04	8.3	0.77	2	0.44	14	162	85	0.4
*	*	*	*	0.7	*	0	0	0.04	0.05	2.7	*	*	*	9	113	16	0.8
*	195	291	*	0.5	*	601	0	0.11	0.11	2.3	*	*	*	*	246	*	*
71	113	369	23	0.4	0.5	29	0	0.06	0.05	1.4	0.15	13	2.21	53	242	*	*

WT, weight; **KCAL**, kcalories; **PROT**, protein; **CARB**, carbohydrate; **FIBR**, fiber; **FAT**, fat; **SATF**, saturated fat;

MONO, monsaturated fat; **POLY**, polyunsaturated fat; **CHOL**, cholesterol; **SOD**, sodium; **POT**, potassium;

FOOD NAME	PORTION	WT (g)	KCAL	PROT (g)	CARB (g)	FIBR (g)	FAT (g)	SATF (g)	MONO (g)	POLY (g)
FROZEN DINNERS										
BEEF AND GREEN PEPPERS-STOUFFER DINNER	ITEM	220	225	10	18	*	11	*	*	*
BEEF AND SPINACH PASTA SHELLS-STOUFFER	ITEM	255	290	19	28	*	11	*	*	*
BEEF BURGUNDY-FROZEN DINNER-EFFICIENC	ITEM	142	144	17	6	*	5	*	*	*
BEEF CUBES IN WINE SAUCE-HORMEL ENTREE	OUNCE	28.4	52	4	1	*	4	1.9	1.6	0.1
BEEF DINNER-SWANSON FROZEN DINNER	ITEM	326	320	25	34	3.3	9	9.6	12.7	4.1
BEEF SHORT RIBS IN BARBECUE SAUCE-HORMEL	OUNCE	28.4	54	5	1	0.8	3	1.7	1.4	0.2
BEEF SIRLOIN TIPS-LE MENU FROZEN DINNER	ITEM	326	400	29	27	*	19	*	*	*
BEEF STEW-HORMEL ENTREE	OUNCE	28.4	29	2	2	*	1	0.5	0.5	t
BEEF STROGANOFF-FROZEN DINNER-EFFICIENC	ITEM	170	192	20	8	*	8	*	*	*
BEEF TERIYAKI-LIGHT AND ELEGANT	ITEM	227	240	18	37	*	3	*	*	*
CHICKEN AND BROCCOLI-LIGHT AND ELEGANT	ITEM	270	290	19	30	*	11	*	*	*
CHICKEN AND DUMPLINGS WITH GRAVY-HORMEL	OUNCE	28.4	31	3	2	0.3	1	0.4	0.6	0.2
CHICKEN BURGUNDY-CLASSIC LITE DINNER	ITEM	319	240	23	24	*	5	*	*	*
CHICKEN CACCIATORE-STOUFFER DINNER	ITEM	319	310	25	29	2.9	11	8.4	12.2	9.7
CHICKEN CHOW MEIN-LEAN CUISINE DINNER	ITEM	319	250	14	36	*	5	*	*	*
CHICKEN CREPES/MUSHROOM SAUCE-STOUFFER	ITEM	234	390	30	19	2.3	22	7.3	3.8	0.9
CHICKEN DINNER-SWANSON FROZEN DINNER	ITEM	326	660	26	64	6.2	33	7.4	10.5	6.9
CHICKEN DIVAN-STOUFFER FROZEN DINNER	ITEM	241	335	21	14	1	22	9.2	8.2	3.3
CHICKEN FLORENTINE-LE MENU FROZEN DINNER	ITEM	354	510	28	35	6.7	28	8	11.4	7.5
CHICKEN KIEV-LE MENU FROZEN DINNER	ITEM	234	500	21	35	4.4	30	5.3	7.6	5
CHICKEN PARMIGIANA-LE MENU FROZEN DINNER	ITEM	333	390	26	28	*	19	*	*	*
CHICKEN PASTA SHELLS-STOUFFER DINNER	ITEM	255	400	26	24	3	22	2.5	3.2	2
CHICKEN-GLAZED-WITH RICE-LEAN CUISINE	ITEM	241	270	26	23	*	8	*	*	*
CHICKEN-SWEET AND SOUR-BUDGET GOURMET	SERVING	284	350	18	53	1.7	7	1.3	1.7	3.3
CORN SOUFFLE-STOUFFER FROZEN SIDE DISH	ITEM	113	155	4	19	*	7	*	*	*
EGG ROLL-BEEF AND SHRIMP-FROZEN-LA CHOY	ITEM	12	27	1	4	0.1	1	0.1	0.2	0.1
FETTUCINI ALFREDO-STOUFFER FROZEN DINNER	ITEM	142	270	8	19	*	18	*	*	*
FETTUCINI-CHICKEN-BUDGET GOURMET	SERVING	284	400	23	29	*	21	*	*	*
FILET OF FISH DIVAN-LEAN CUISINE DINNER	ITEM	351	270	31	16	*	10	*	*	*
FILET OF FISH FLORENTINE-LEAN CUISINE	ITEM	255	240	26	13	*	9	*	*	*
FISH AND CHIPS-VAN DE KAMPS DINNER	ITEM	224	500	16	45	4.7	30	6.2	7	6.9
FLOUNDER FILET-LE MENU FROZEN DINNER	ITEM	298	350	22	27	*	17	*	*	*
GLAZED CHICKEN-LIGHT AND ELEGANT	ITEM	227	230	24	25	*	4	*	*	*
HAM-BANQUET FROZEN DINNER	ITEM	284	369	17	48	2.6	12	2	3.4	3.1
LASAGNA-SAUSAGE-BUDGET GOURMET	SERVING	284	284	20	38	3.8	20	9	5.8	0.9
LINGUINI WITH CLAM SAUCE-STOUFFER DINNER	ITEM	298	285	17	36	*	8	*	*	*
MACARONI AND CHEESE-LIGHT AND ELEGANT	ITEM	255	300	15	37	*	9	*	*	*
MANICOTTI-CHEESE/MEAT-BUDGET GOURMET	SERVING	284	450	20	33	2.4	26	11.1	6	1.3
MEATBALLS AND NOODLES-STOUFFER DINNER	ITEM	312	475	25	33	*	27	*	*	*
MEATLOAF-BANQUET FROZEN DINNER	ITEM	312	412	21	29	5.4	24	7.5	9.1	2.9
MEXICAN DINNER-SWANSON FROZEN DINNER	ITEM	454	590	20	64	6.7	29	9.5	13	8.5
NOODLES ROMANOFF-STOUFFER FROZEN DINNER	ITEM	113	170	6	16	*	9	*	*	*
OCEAN FISH WITH LEMON SAUCE-EFFICIENC	SERVING	113	262	14	3	0.9	21	1.6	0.9	1.5
ORIENTAL BEEF-LEAN CUISINE FROZEN DINNER	ITEM	245	250	18	28	*	7	*	*	*
PEPPER STEAK WITH RICE-BUDGET GOURMET	SERVING	284	300	15	39	1.4	9	5.8	8.2	11.8
PORK LOIN AND GRAVY-HORMEL ENTREE	OUNCE	28.4	40	5	1	*	2	0.9	0.7	0.3
QUICHE LORRAINE-FROZEN DINNER-MRS SMITHS	ITEM	269	720	34	54	0.8	41	*	*	*
SALISBURY STEAK-LEAN CUISINE	ITEM	269	280	25	11	*	15	*	*	*
SCALLOPED POTATOES AND HAM-HORMEL ENTREE	OUNCE	28.4	28	2	3	0.6	1	0.6	0.4	0.1
SCALLOPS/VEGETABLES/RICE-LEAN CUISINE	ITEM	312	220	17	32	*	3	*	*	*
SEAFOOD GUMBO-HORMEL ENTREE	OUNCE	28.4	10	1	1	*	t	t	t	t
SHRIMP CREOLE-LIGHT AND ELEGANT	ITEM	283	200	11	31	2.2	2	2.9	5.6	5.1
SIRLOIN TIP/VEGETABLES-BUDGET GOURMET	SERVING	284	310	16	21	2.6	18	1.9	2	0.4
SOLE-LIGHT-VAN DE KAMP'S FROZEN DINNER	ITEM	142	293	16	17	1.9	18	0.4	0.3	0.5
SPAGHETTI-BEEF AND MUSHROOM-LEAN CUISINE	ITEM	326	280	15	38	*	7	*	*	*
SPAGHETTI-LIGHT AND ELEGANT	ITEM	290	290	16	40	*	8	*	*	*
SWEDISH MEATBALLS IN SAUCE-HORMEL ENTREE	SERVING	28.4	44	3	2	0.1	3	1.7	1.1	0.2
SWISS STEAK IN GRAVY-HORMEL ENTREE	OUNCE	28.4	34	4	1	0.4	2	0.7	1	0.2
TUNA NOODLE CASSEROLE-STOUFFER DINNER	ITEM	163	200	10	18	0.5	9	*	*	*
TURKEY & GRAVY-FROZEN	CUP	240	160	14	11	2.7	6	2	2.3	1.1
TURKEY BREAST-LE MENU FROZEN DINNER	ITEM	319	470	27	36	*	24	*	*	*
TURKEY PIE-STOUFFER FROZEN DINNER	ITEM	284	460	20	35	*	26	*	*	*

t = Trace of nutrient present ** = Not available*

MAG, magnesium; **IRON**, iron; **ZINC**, zinc; **VITA**, vitamin A; **VITC**, vitamin C; **THIA**, thiamin; **RIBO**, riboflavin; **NIAC**, niacin; **VB6**, vitamin B-6; **FOL**, folate; **VB12**, vitamin B-12; **CALC**, calcium; **PHOS**, phosphorus; **SEL**, selenium; **VE-a**, alpha tocopherol equivalents.

CHOL (mg)	SOD (mg)	POT (mg)	MAG (mg)	IRON (mg)	ZINC (mg)	VITA (RE)	VITC (mg)	THIA (mg)	RIBO (mg)	NIAC (mg)	VB6 (mg)	FOL (μg)	VB12 (μg)	CALC (mg)	PHOS (mg)	SEL (μg)	VE-a (mg)
*	960	420	*	2.3	*	136	0	0.08	0.16	3.9	*	*	*	0	*	*	*
*	1315	485	*	*	*	*	*	*	*	*	*	*	*	*	*	*	*
411	147	*	0.6	*	449	0	0.04	0.24	4.1	*	*	*	5	*	*	*	*
15	106	71	4	0.5	1.3	*	t	0.77	0.05	0.5	0.02	4	0.41	3	23	*	*
84	1085	616	42	4	4.7	1140	6	0.14	0.27	4.9	0.52	24	2.1	36	283	*	2
15	176	92	5	0.7	1.7	11	t	0.01	0.07	0.7	0.03	11	0.52	3	28	*	0.8
*	1100	*	*	*	*	*	*	*	*	*	*	*	*	*	*	*	*
7	106	51	3	0.2	0.5	*	t	0.01	0.02	0.3	0.01	6	0.15	4	15	*	t
*	785	316	*	2.9	*	68	2	0.05	0.32	2.9	*	*	*	23	*	*	*
*	625	215	*	5.6	*	24	2	0.4	0.1	2.5	*	*	*	30	152	*	*
*	805	180	*	1.6	*	75	1	0.11	0.21	1.8	*	*	*	204	240	*	*
9	116	45	3	0.2	0.2	65	t	0.01	0.03	0.6	0.04	11	0.06	5	29	*	0
*	*	*	*	*	*	*	*	*	*	*	*	*	*	*	*	*	*
166	1135	300	73	3.9	4.1	176	33	0.24	0.42	18.2	0.95	22	0.57	75	398	*	2.9
25	1030	270	*	*	*	*	*	*	*	*	*	*	*	*	*	*	*
76	1040	420	50	2.6	1.1	910	33	0.15	0.19	8	0.46	28	0.19	54	192	*	0.9
111	1610	602	60	2.7	2.6	323	12	0.33	0.39	10.3	0.45	30	0.36	112	295	*	2.8
86	830	415	52	1.7	2	221	20	0.13	0.44	4.6	0.29	41	0.74	269	295	*	0.9
121	985	653	66	2.9	2.9	351	13	0.36	0.42	11.2	0.49	33	0.39	122	320	*	3.1
80	745	432	43	1.9	1.9	232	9	0.24	0.28	7.4	0.33	22	0.26	80	212	*	2
*	900	*	*	*	*	*	*	*	*	*	*	*	*	*	*	*	*
165	1060	350	47	3.7	2.2	177	28	0.3	0.43	7.5	0.35	28	0.39	59	226	*	1.3
55	810	380	*	*	*	*	*	*	*	*	*	*	*	*	*	*	*
40	640	429	45	0.7	1.4	80	2	0.12	0.34	3	0.38	13	0.17	60	163	*	1.3
*	510	190	*	0.4	*	94	0	0.08	0.16	0.8	*	34	*	48	*	*	*
2	81	15	1	0.1	0.1	12	2	0.01	0.01	0.1	0.01	1	0.02	2	5	*	0.1
*	1195	240	*	*	*	*	*	*	*	*	*	*	*	*	*	*	*
100	740	*	*	1.8	*	350	2	0.15	0.43	6	*	*	*	200	*	*	*
85	780	850	*	*	*	*	*	*	*	*	*	*	*	*	*	*	*
100	700	540	*	*	*	*	*	*	*	*	*	*	*	*	*	*	*
33	551	785	53	2.2	1	18	11	0.24	0.14	4.3	0.41	23	0.68	35	271	*	2.8
*	1125	*	*	*	*	*	*	*	*	*	*	*	*	*	*	*	*
*	655	300	*	4.8	*	31	*	0.21	0.07	7.7	*	*	*	18	348	*	*
36	1590	125	38	2.5	2.5	1311	57	0.57	0.23	3.4	0.48	21	0.45	151	278	*	4.4
80	950	591	54	2.7	3.7	183	18	0.45	0.43	4	0.28	23	0.91	400	348	*	1.1
*	1010	115	*	*	*	*	*	*	*	*	*	*	*	*	*	*	*
*	1015	210	*	2	*	60	t	0.34	0.43	1.5	*	*	*	238	334	*	*
50	920	484	45	2.7	2.3	280	10	0.45	0.51	4	0.23	31	0.72	450	376	*	2
*	1620	395	*	*	*	*	*	*	*	*	*	*	*	*	*	*	*
79	1991	468	64	4.3	3.4	427	8	0.16	0.22	4.2	0.36	48	1.21	84	243	*	1.7
44	1865	603	75	5.1	3.6	93	7	0.35	0.3	3.8	0.3	135	0.83	198	340	*	4
*	675	95	*	0.8	*	61	*	0.08	0.16	0.8	*	*	*	88	*	*	*
16	370	224	22	0.7	0.5	0	0	0.17	0.18	2.8	0.13	18	0.22	15	93	*	1.2
35	1150	270	*	*	*	*	*	*	*	*	*	*	*	*	*	*	*
25	800	729	49	0.7	6	60	2	0.15	0.17	3	0.59	22	3.9	40	350	*	4
9	133	82	5	0.2	0.4	*	t	2.61	0.04	0.9	0.06	10	0.07	2	32	*	*
95	1965	610	*	2.7	*	67	0	0.33	1.01	6	*	*	*	97	*	*	*
95	800	650	*	*	*	*	*	*	*	*	*	*	*	*	*	*	*
4	146	68	4	0.1	0.2	8	1	0.05	0.03	0.4	0.02	6	0.06	8	23	*	0.4
20	1200	360	*	*	*	*	*	*	*	*	*	*	*	*	*	*	*
6	146	82	5	0.2	0.1	*	t	0.01	0.02	0.2	0.03	6	0.09z	8	16	*	*
293	1045	200	88	2.5	2.4	889	1	0.22	0.03	3.3	0.32	14	1.91Z	54	225	*	6.5
40	570	504	35	0.4	4.4	150	2	0.15	0.17	4	0.44	16	1.87	60	195	*	0.4
45	412	453	39	0.9	0.6	10	21	0.13	0.13	3.3	0.25	36	1.35	39	200	*	0.7
20	1450	580	*	*	*	*	*	*	*	*	*	*	*	*	*	*	*
*	700	273	*	6	*	157	10	0.25	0.15	3.4	*	*	*	100	252	*	*
8	165	87	6	0.5	0.4	11	t	1.07	0.06	0.5	0.03	9	0.18	15	39	*	0.1
8	110	86	5	0.5	0.6	76	t	0.02	0.05	0.9	0.04	27	0.32	5	15	*	0.1
*	670	210	*	1.2	*	54	*	0.17	0.23	3.5	*	*	*	98	*	*	*
43	1328	146	20	2.2	1.7	20	0	0.06	0.31	4.3	0.23	10	0.58	33	194	*	2
*	1165	*	*	*	*	*	*	*	*	*	*	*	*	*	*	*	*
*	1735	270	*	*	*	*	*	*	*	*	*	*	*	*	*	*	*

WT, weight; **KCAL,** kcalories; **PROT,** protein; **CARB,** carbohydrate; **FIBR,** fiber; **FAT,** fat; **SATF,** saturated fat;

MONO, monsaturated fat; **POLY,** polyunsaturated fat; **CHOL,** cholesterol; **SOD,** sodium; **POT,** potassium;

FOOD NAME	PORTION	WT (g)	KCAL	PROT (g)	CARB (g)	FIBR (g)	FAT (g)	SATF (g)	MONO (g)	POLY (g)
TURKEY TETRAZZINI-STOUFFER FROZEN DINNER	ITEM	170	240	12	17	*	14	*	*	*
TURKEY-SLICED-LIGHT AND ELEGANT	ITEM	227	230	20	25	*	5	*	*	*
VEAL PARMIGIANA-EFFICIENC ENTREE	ITEM	213	296	24	17	1.6	14	9	7.6	4.8
VEAL STEAK-CLASSIC LITE FROZEN DINNER	ITEM	312	280	25	27	5.8	8	5.9	6.9	3.6
VEGETABLE LASAGNA-LE MENU FROZEN DINNER	ITEM	312	400	15	30	5.1	24	9.4	6.7	4.2
FRUITS										
APPLES-RAW-PEELED	ITEM	128	73	t	19	2.4	t	0.1	t	0.1
APPLES-RAW-PEELED-BOILED	CUP	171	91	t	23	4.1	1	0.1	t	0.2
APPLES-RAW-SLICED-WITH SKIN	CUP	110	65	t	17	2.4	t	0.1	t	0.1
APPLESAUCE-CANNED-SWEETENED	CUP	255	194	t	51	3.1	t	0.1	t	0.1
APPLESAUCE-CANNED-UNSWEETENED	CUP	244	105	t	28	3.7	t	t	t	t
APRICOT-RAW-WITHOUT PIT	ITEM	35.3	17	t	4	0.7	t	t	0.1	t
APRICOTS-CANNED-JUICE PACK	CUP	248	119	2	31	2.8	t	t	t	t
APRICOTS-DRIED-SULFURED-COOKED-NO SUGAR	CUP	250	213	3	55	19.5	t	t	0.2	0.1
APRICOTS-DRIED-SULFURED-UNCOOKED	CUP	130	309	5	80	10.1	1	t	0.3	0.1
AVOCADO-RAW-CALIFORNIA	ITEM	173	306	4	12	6.1	30	4.5	19.4	3.5
BANANAS-RAW-PEELED	ITEM	114	105	1	27	1.8	1	0.2	t	0.1
BLACKBERRIES-FROZEN-UNSWEETENED	CUP	151	97	2	24	7.6	1	t	0.1	0.4
BLACKBERRIES-RAW	CUP	144	75	1	18	8.9	1	0.1	0.2	0.3
BLUEBERRIES-CANNED-HEAVY SYRUP PACK	CUP	256	225	2	57	2.8	1	0.1	0.1	0.3
BLUEBERRIES-FROZEN-UNSWEETENED	CUP	155	79	1	19	4.9	1	t	0.1	0.6
BLUEBERRIES-RAW	CUP	145	81	1	21	3.3	1	0.1	0.2	0.3
BOYSENBERRIES-FROZEN-UNSWEETENED	CUP	132	66	1	16	5.2	t	t	t	0.2
CHERRIES-SWEET-RAW	ITEM	6.8	5	t	1	0.1	t	t	t	t
CRANAPPLE JUICE-CANNED	CUP	253	170	t	43	0	0	0	0	0
CRANBERRY JUICE COCKTAIL-BOTTLED	CUP	253	144	0	36	0	t	0	0	0
CRANBERRY SAUCE-CANNED-SWEETENED	CUP	277	418	1	108	3.2	t	0.1	0.1	0.2
DATES-DOMESTIC-NATURAL AND DRY-WHOLE	ITEM	8.3	23	t	6	0.7	t	0	0	0
FIGS-DRIED-UNCOOKED	CUP	199	507	6	130	18.5	2	0.5	0.5	1.1
FRUIT COCKTAIL-CANNED-JUICE PACK	CUP	248	114	1	29	1.5	t	t	t	t
FRUIT ROLL UP-CHERRY	ITEM	14.4	50	0	12	*	1	*	*	*
GRAPE DRINK-CANNED	CUP	253	154	1	38	0	t	0.1	t	0.1
GRAPEFRUIT-CANNED-JUICE PACK	CUP	249	92	2	23	1.6	t	t	t	0.1
GRAPEFRUIT-PINK & RED-RAW	ITEM	246	74	1	19	3.2	t	t	t	0.1
GRAPEFRUIT-WHITE-RAW	ITEM	236	78	2	20	2.5	t	t	t	0.1
GRAPES-RAW-SLIP SKIN (AMERICAN) TYPE	CUP	92	58	1	16	1.5	t	0.1	t	0.1
JUICE APPLE-CANNED OR BOTTLED	CUP	248	116	t	29	0.5	t	t	t	0.1
JUICE-APPLE-FROZEN-DILUTED	CUP	239	112	t	28	0.6	t	t	t	0.1
JUICE-GRAPE-CANNED & BOTTLED	CUP	253	154	1	38	0	t	0.1	t	0.1
JUICE-GRAPE-FROZEN CONCENTRATE	ITEM	216	387	1	96	0.6	1	0.2	t	0.2
JUICE-GRAPEFRUIT-CANNED-SWEETENED	CUP	250	115	1	28	0	t	t	t	0.1
JUICE-GRAPEFRUIT-CANNED-UNSWEETENED	CUP	247	94	1	22	0.4	t	t	t	0.1
JUICE-GRAPEFRUIT-FROZEN CONCENTRATE	ITEM	207	302	4	72	0	1	0.1	0.1	0.2
JUICE-LEMON-CANNED & BOTTLED	CUP	244	51	1	16	0.7	1	0.1	t	0.2
JUICE-LEMON-FROZEN-SINGLE STRENGTH	CUP	244	54	1	16	0.7	1	0.1	t	0.2
JUICE-LEMON-RAW	CUP	244	61	1	21	0.7	0	0	0	0
JUICE-ORANGE GRAPEFRUIT-CANNED	CUP	247	106	1	25	0.5	t	t	t	t
JUICE-ORANGE GRAPEFRUIT-FROZEN-DILUTED	CUP	248	110	1	26	0	0	0	0	0
JUICE-ORANGE-CANNED	CUP	249	104	1	25	0.3	t	t	0.1	0.1
JUICE-ORANGE-CANNED-FROZEN CONCENTRATE	ITEM	213	339	5	81	1.7	t	0.1	0.1	0.1
JUICE-PINEAPPLE-CANNED	CUP	250	140	1	35	0.3	t	t	t	0.1
JUICE-PINEAPPLE-FROZEN-DILUTED	CUP	250	130	1	32	0.3	t	t	t	t
JUICE-PRUNE-CANNED & BOTTLED	CUP	256	182	2	45	2.6	t	t	0.1	t
LEMONADE-CANNED-FROZEN CONCENTRATE	ITEM	219	425	0	112	5.6	0	0	0	0
LEMONADE-FROZEN CONCENTRATE-DILUTED	CUP	248	105	0	28	0.6	0	0	0	0
LEMONS-RAW-UNPEELED	ITEM	108	22	1	12	1	t	t	t	0.1
MELONS-CANTALOUPE-RAW-CUBED PIECES	CUP	160	56	1	13	1.3	t	0	0	0
MELONS-CASABA-RAW	CUP	170	44	2	11	2	t	0	0	0
MELONS-HONEYDEW-RAW-CUBED PIECES	CUP	170	60	1	16	1.5	t	0	0	0
NECTARINES-RAW	ITEM	136	67	1	16	2.2	1	0.1	0.2	0.3
ORANGES-RAW-ALL COMMON VARIETIES-WHOLE	ITEM	131	62	1	15	3.1	t	t	t	t
PAPAYA NECTAR-CANNED	CUP	250	143	t	36	1.2	t	0.1	0.1	0.1
PAPAYAS-RAW	CUP	140	55	1	14	1.3	t	0.1	0.1	t

t = Trace of nutrient present ** = Not available*

MAG, magnesium; **IRON,** iron; **ZINC,** zinc; **VITA,** vitamin A; **VITC,** vitamin C; **THIA,** thiamin; **RIBO,** riboflavin; **NIAC,** niacin; **VB6,** vitamin B-6; **FOL,** folate; **VB12,** vitamin B-12; **CALC,** calcium; **PHOS,** phosphorus; **SEL,** selenium; **VE-a,** alpha tocopherol equivalents.

CHOL (mg)	SOD (mg)	POT (mg)	MAG (mg)	IRON (mg)	ZINC (mg)	VITA (RE)	VITC (mg)	THIA (mg)	RIBO (mg)	NIAC (mg)	VB6 (mg)	FOL (μg)	VB12 (μg)	CALC (mg)	PHOS (mg)	SEL (μg)	VE-a (mg)
*	620	200	*	0.6	*	41	*	0.12	0.24	2.4	*	*	*	72	*	*	*
*	1020	280	*	1	*	171	1	0.12	0.14	4.6	*	*	*	18	121	*	*
162	973	466	49	2.3	3.6	123	6	0.3	0.38	6.8	0.43	25	1.21	97	401	*	2.6
60	1738	932	81	3.6	4.2	241	33	0.36	0.43	6.5	0.53	62	0.85	171	299	*	2.7
39	1135	519	82	3.2	1.5	723	62	0.23	0.47	3.3	0.34	78	0.2	296	274	*	2.5

CHOL (mg)	SOD (mg)	POT (mg)	MAG (mg)	IRON (mg)	ZINC (mg)	VITA (RE)	VITC (mg)	THIA (mg)	RIBO (mg)	NIAC (mg)	VB6 (mg)	FOL (μg)	VB12 (μg)	CALC (mg)	PHOS (mg)	SEL (μg)	VE-a (mg)
0	0	144	4	0.1	0.1	6	5	0.02	0.01	0.1	0.06	1	0	5	9	1	0.3
0	2	150	5	0.3	0.1	8	t	0.03	0.02	0.2	0.08	1	0	9	13	1	0.1
0	0	126	5	0.2	t	6	6	0.02	0.02	0.1	0.05	3	0	8	8	1	0.6
0	8	156	7	0.9	0.1	3	4	0.03	0.07	0.5	0.07	2	0	9	17	1	0.2
0	5	183	7	0.3	0.1	7	3	0.03	0.06	0.5	0.06	1	0	7	17	1	0.2
0	t	104	3	0.2	0.1	92	4	0.01	0.01	0.2	0.02	3	0	5	7	0	0.3
0	9	409	24	0.7	0.3	420	12	0.05	0.05	0.9	0.13	4	0	30	50	1	2.2
0	9	1222	42	4.2	0.7	591	4	0.02	0.08	2.4	0.29	0	0	40	104	*	*
0	13	1791	61	6.1	1	941	3	0.01	0.2	3.9	0.2	13	0	59	152	*	*
0	21	1097	70	2	0.7	106	14	0.19	0.21	3.3	0.48	113	0	19	73	*	3.7
0	1	451	33	0.4	0.2	9	10	0.05	0.11	0.6	0.66	22	0	7	22	1	0.3
0	2	211	33	1.2	0.4	17	5	0.04	0.07	1.8	0.09	51	0	44	45	1	1.1
0	0	282	29	0.8	0.4	24	30	0.04	0.06	0.6	0.08	49	0	46	30	1	0.9
0	9	102	9	0.8	0.2	16	3	0.09	0.14	0.3	0.09	4	0	14	26	2	1.7
0	2	84	8	0.3	0.1	13	4	0.05	0.06	0.8	0.09	10	0	12	17	1	1.6
0	9	129	7	0.2	0.2	15	19	0.07	0.07	0.5	0.05	9	0	9	15	1	*
0	2	183	21	1.1	0.3	9	4	0.07	0.05	1	0.07	84	0	36	36	1	0.6
0	0	15	1	t	t	1	t	t	t	t	t	t	0	1	1	0	t
0	5	68	5	0.2	0.1	0	81	0.01	0.05	0.2	0.05	1	0	18	8	1	*
0	10	46	5	0.4	0.2	0	90	0.02	0.02	0.1	0.05	1	0	8	5	1	*
0	80	72	8	0.6	0.1	6	11	0.04	0.06	0.3	0.04	*	0	11	17	1	*
0	t	54	3	0.1	t	t	0	0.01	0.01	0.2	0.02	1	0	3	3	*	*
0	22	1417	117	4.4	1	26	2	0.14	0.18	1.4	0.45	15	0	287	135	*	0
0	10	236	17	0.5	0.2	76	7	0.03	0.04	1	0.13	6	0	20	35	1	0.5
0	5	45	*	*	*	*	*	*	*	*	*	*	0	*	*	*	*
0	8	334	25	0.6	0.1	2	t	0.07	0.09	0.7	0.16	7	0	23	28	*	*
0	19	420	26	0.5	0.2	0	84	0.07	0.05	0.6	0.05	22	0	37	30	1	0.6
0	0	312	20	0.3	0.2	64	91	0.1	0.05	0.5	0.1	23	0	36	22	1	0.6
0	0	350	21	0.1	0.2	2	79	0.09	0.05	0.6	0.1	24	0	28	18	1	0.6
0	2	176	5	0.3	t	9	4	0.09	0.05	0.3	0.1	4	0	13	9	1	0.6
0	7	296	8	0.9	0.1	t	2	0.05	0.04	0.2	0.07	t	0	16	18	2	t
0	17	301	12	0.6	0.1	*	1	0.01	0.04	0.1	0.08	1	0	14	17	2	t
0	8	334	25	0.6	0.1	2	t	0.07	0.09	0.7	0.16	7	0	23	28	1	*
0	15	160	32	0.8	0.3	6	179	0.11	0.2	0.9	0.32	10	0	28	32	2	*
0	5	405	25	0.9	0.2	0	67	0.1	0.06	0.8	0.05	26	0	20	28	1	0.1
0	2	378	25	0.5	0.2	2	72	0.1	0.05	0.6	0.05	26	0	17	27	1	0.1
0	6	1002	78	1	0.4	7	248	0.3	0.16	1.6	0.32	26	0	56	101	1	0.1
0	51	249	20	0.3	0.1	4	61	0.1	0.02	0.5	0.11	25	0	27	22	1	*
0	2	217	20	0.3	0.1	3	77	0.14	0.03	0.3	0.15	23	0	20	20	1	*
0	2	303	15	0.1	0.1	5	112	0.07	0.02	0.2	0.12	32	0	17	15	1	*
0	7	390	25	1.1	0.2	29	72	0.14	0.07	0.8	0.06	35	0	20	35	1	0.1
0	2	439	24	0.2	0.2	27	102	0.15	0.02	0.7	0.06	*	0	20	32	1	0.1
0	6	436	27	1.1	0.2	44	86	0.15	0.07	0.8	0.22	136	0	21	36	1	0.1
0	7	1435	73	0.7	0.4	59	294	0.6	0.14	1.5	0.33	331	0	67	122	1	*
0	3	335	33	0.7	0.3	1	27	0.14	0.06	0.6	0.24	58	0	43	20	2	*
0	3	340	23	0.8	0.3	3	30	0.18	0.05	0.5	0.19	27	0	28	20	2	0.1
0	10	707	36	3	0.5	1	11	0.04	0.18	2	0.56	1	0	31	64	1	*
0	4	153	*	0.4	*	4	66	0.05	0.06	0.7	*	*	0	9	13	1	*
0	0	40	*	0.1	*	1	17	0.01	0.02	0.2	*	12	0	2	3	1	*
0	3	157	13	0.8	0.1	3	83	0.05	0.04	0.2	0.12	11	0	66	16	1	0.3
0	14	494	18	0.3	0.3	516	68	0.06	0.03	0.9	0.18	27	0	18	27	1	0.2
0	20	357	14	0.7	0.3	5	27	0.1	0.03	0.7	0.2	29	0	9	12	1	0.2
0	17	461	12	0.1	*	7	42	0.13	0.03	1	0.1	*	0	10	17	1	0.2
0	0	288	11	0.2	0.1	100	7	0.02	0.06	1.4	0.03	5	0	7	22	1	1.2
0	0	237	13	0.1	0.1	27	70	0.11	0.05	0.4	0.08	40	0	52	18	2	0.3
0	13	78	8	0.9	0.4	28	8	0.02	0.01	0.4	0.02	5	0	25	0	1	1.9
0	4	359	14	0.1	0.1	282	87	0.04	0.05	0.5	0.03	53	0	34	7	1	*

WT, weight; **KCAL**, kcalories; **PROT**, protein; **CARB**, carbohydrate; **FIBR**, fiber; **FAT**, fat; **SATF**, saturated fat;

MONO, monsaturated fat; **POLY**, polyunsaturated fat; **CHOL**, cholesterol; **SOD**, sodium; **POT**, potassium;

FOOD NAME	PORTION	WT (g)	KCAL	PROT (g)	CARB (g)	FIBR (g)	FAT (g)	SATF (g)	MONO (g)	POLY (g)
PEACHES-CANNED-HEAVY SYRUP PACK	CUP	256	189	1	51	1.1	t	t	0.1	0.1
PEACHES-RAW-SLICED	CUP	170	73	1	19	2.7	t	t	0.1	0.1
PEACHES-RAW-WHOLE	ITEM	87	37	1	10	1.4	t	t	t	t
PEAR NECTAR-CANNED	CUP	250	150	t	39	1.6	t	t	t	t
PEARS-CANNED-HEAVY SYRUP PACK	CUP	255	189	1	49	2.4	t	t	0.1	0.1
PEARS-RAW-BARTLETT WITH SKIN	ITEM	166	98	1	25	4.3	1	t	0.1	0.2
PINEAPPLE GRAPEFRUIT DRINK	CUP	253	129	1	32	0	t	t	t	0.1
PINEAPPLE ORANGE DRINK	CUP	253	134	1	32	0	0	0	0	0
PINEAPPLE-BITS-CANNED IN SYRUP	CUP	252	131	1	34	1.9	t	t	t	0.1
PINEAPPLE-FROZEN-SWEETENED	CUP	245	208	1	54	5.4	t	t	t	0.1
PINEAPPLE-RAW-DICED	CUP	155	76	1	19	1.9	1	0.1	0.1	0.2
PLUMS-PURPLE-CANNED-HEAVY SYRUP PACK	CUP	258	230	1	60	1.1	t	t	0.2	0.1
PLUMS-RAW-JAPANESE & HYBRID	ITEM	66	36	1	9	1.4	t	t	0.3	0.1
PLUMS-RAW-PRUNE TYPE	ITEM	28.4	20	0	6	0.6	0	0	0	0
POMEGRANATES-RAW	ITEM	154	105	1	26	1.1	t	0.1	t	0.1
PRUNES-CANNED-HEAVY SYRUP PACK	CUP	234	246	2	65	8.6	t	t	0.3	0.1
PRUNES-DRIED-COOKED-WITH SUGAR	CUP	238	295	3	78	7.6	1	t	0.3	0.1
PRUNES-DRIED-COOKED-WITHOUT SUGAR	CUP	212	227	2	60	7.5	t	t	0.3	0.1
PRUNES-DRIED-UNCOOKED	CUP	161	385	4	101	11	1	0.1	0.5	0.2
RAISINS-SEEDLESS	CUP	145	435	5	115	7.7	1	0.2	t	0.2
RAISINS-SEEDLESS-PACKET	ITEM	14	42	t	11	0.7	t	t	t	t
RASPBERRIES-CANNED-HEAVY SYRUP PACK	CUP	256	234	2	60	6.5	t	t	t	0.2
RASPBERRIES-FROZEN-SWEETENED	CUP	250	258	2	65	11	t	t	t	0.2
RASPBERRIES-RAW	CUP	123	60	1	14	5.5	1	t	0.1	0.4
RHUBARB-COOKED FROM RAW-ADDED SUGAR	CUP	270	380	1	97	5.4	0	0	0	0
STRAWBERRIES-CANNED-HEAVY SYRUP PACK	CUP	254	234	1	60	3.1	1	t	0.1	0.3
STRAWBERRIES-FROZEN-SWEETENED-SLICED	CUP	255	245	1	66	19.8	t	t	t	0.2
STRAWBERRIES-FROZEN-SWEETENED-WHOLE	CUP	255	199	1	54	5.6	t	t	t	0.2
STRAWBERRIES-FROZEN-UNSWEETENED	CUP	149	52	1	14	3.9	t	t	t	0.1
STRAWBERRIES-RAW-WHOLE	CUP	149	45	1	11	3.9	1	t	0.1	0.3
TANGERINES-CANNED-LIGHT SYRUP PACK	CUP	252	154	1	41	1.4	t	t	t	0.1
TANGERINES-RAW-PEELED	ITEM	84	37	1	9	1.7	t	t	t	t
WATERMELON-RAW	CUP	160	51	1	12	0.6	1	*	*	*
GRAINS										
BISQUICK MIX-DRY	CUP	112	480	8	76	3	16	*	*	*
CORN CHIPS	OUNCE	28.4	155	2	17	1.7	9	1.5	3.4	4.3
CORN GRITS-DRY	CUP	156	579	14	124	18.6	2	0.3	0.5	0.8
CORNMEAL-DEGERMED-ENRICHED-COOKED	CUP	240	878	20	186	1.9	4	0.5	1	1.7
CROUTONS-HERB SEASONED	CUP	30	100	4	20	1.4	0	0	0	0
FLOUR-WHEAT-ENRICHED-SIFTED	CUP	115	419	12	88	3.1	1	0.2	0.1	0.5
FLOUR-WHEAT-WHITE-FOR BREAD	CUP	137	495	16	99	4.5	2	0.3	0.2	1
MACARONI-COOKED-FIRM STAGE-HOT	CUP	130	183	6	37	2.1	1	0.1	0.1	0.4
NOODLES-EGG-COOKED	CUP	160	213	8	40	3	2	0.5	0.7	0.7
NOODLES-EGG-SPINACH-COOKED	CUP	160	211	8	39	0.4	3	0.6	0.8	0.6
NOODLES-RAMEN-ORIENTAL	CUP	227	207	6	31	2	9	0.4	0.4	0.4
OAT BRAN-RAW	CUP	94	231	16	62	12.5	7	1.3	2.2	2.6
OATS-WHOLE GRAIN-UNCOOKED	CUP	156	607	26	104	20.8	11	1.9	3.4	4
PASTA-FRESH-PLAIN-COOKED	OUNCE	28.4	38	1	7	0.3	t	t	t	0.1
POPCORN-POPPED-OIL & SALT	CUP	9	40	1	5	0.4	2	1.5	0.2	0.2
POPCORN-POPPED-PLAIN	CUP	6	25	1	5	0.4	0	0	0	0
POPCORN-POPPED-SUGAR COATED	CUP	35	135	2	30	1.4	1	0.5	0.2	0.4
PRETZEL-DUTCH-TWISTED	ITEM	16	60	2	12	*	1	*	*	*
PRETZEL-THIN-STICK	ITEM	0.3	1	t	t	*	t	0	0	0
PRETZEL-THIN-TWISTED	ITEM	6	24	1	5	*	t	*	*	*
RICE CAKE-LOW SODIUM	ITEM	9.31	35	1	8	0.2	t	1.2	0.1	t
RICE CAKE-REGULAR	ITEM	9.31	35	1	8	0.2	t	1.2	0.1	t
RICE-BROWN-LONG GRAIN-COOKED	CUP	195	216	5	45	3.3	2	0.4	0.6	0.6
RICE-BROWN-LONG GRAIN-RAW	CUP	185	685	15	143	10.7	5	1.1	2	1.9
RICE-WHITE-INSTANT-HOT	CUP	165	162	3	35	1.3	t	0.1	0.1	0.1
RICE-WHITE-LONG GRAIN-COOKED	CUP	205	264	6	57	2.1	1	0.2	0.2	0.2
RICE-WHITE-LONG GRAIN-RAW	CUP	185	675	13	148	1.9	1	0.3	0.4	0.3
RICE-WILD-COOKED	CUP	164	166	7	35	2.6	1	0.1	0.1	0.4
RYE-WHOLE-DRY	CUP	169	566	25	118	8.9	4	0.5	0.5	0.9

t = Trace of nutrient present   ** = Not available*

MAG, magnesium; **IRON,** iron; **ZINC,** zinc; **VITA,** vitamin A; **VITC,** vitamin C; **THIA,** thiamin; **RIBO,** riboflavin; **NIAC,** niacin; **VB6,** vitamin B-6; **FOL,** folate; **VB12,** vitamin B-12; **CALC,** calcium; **PHOS,** phosphorus; **SEL,** selenium; **VE-a,** alpha tocopherol equivalents.

CHOL (mg)	SOD (mg)	POT (mg)	MAG (mg)	IRON (mg)	ZINC (mg)	VITA (RE)	VITC (mg)	THIA (mg)	RIBO (mg)	NIAC (mg)	VB6 (mg)	FOL (µg)	VB12 (µg)	CALC (mg)	PHOS (mg)	SEL (µg)	VE-a (mg)
0	15	235	13	0.7	0.1	85	7	0.03	0.06	1.6	0.05	8	0	8	28	1	*
0	0	335	12	0.2	0.2	91	11	0.03	0.07	1.7	0.03	6	0	9	20	1	0.2
0	0	171	6	0.1	0.1	47	6	0.02	0.04	0.9	0.02	3	0	4	10	1	0.1
0	10	33	8	0.7	0.2	t	3	0.01	0.03	0.3	0.04	3	0	13	8	1	t
0	13	166	10	0.6	0.2	0	3	0.03	0.06	0.6	0.04	3	0	13	18	1	0.3
0	0	208	10	0.4	0.2	3	7	0.03	0.07	0.2	0.03	12	0	18	18	1	0.8
0	56	139	15	0.8	0.1	0	68	0.05	0.05	0.6	2.02	25	0	15	10	2	0.2
0	8	121	15	0.7	0.2	134	63	0.08	0.05	0.5	0.12	28	0	13	10	2	0
0	3	266	40	1	0.3	4	19	0.23	0.06	0.7	0.19	12	0	36	17	3	0.3
0	5	245	25	1	0.3	7	20	0.25	0.07	0.7	0.18	26	0	22	10	2	0.2
0	2	175	22	0.6	0.1	4	24	0.14	0.06	0.7	0.14	16	0	11	11	1	0.2
0	50	234	13	2.2	0.2	67	1	0.04	0.1	0.8	0.07	7	0	24	33	1	*
0	0	114	5	0.1	0.1	21	6	0.03	0.06	0.3	0.05	1	0	3	7	0	0.5
0	0	48	2	0.1	t	8	1	0.01	0.01	0.1	0.02	1	0	3	5	0	0.2
0	5	399	5	0.5	0.2	0	9	0.05	0.05	0.5	0.16	9	0	5	12	1	0.8
0	7	529	35	1	0.4	187	7	0.08	0.29	2	0.48	t	0	40	61	1	*
0	4	741	45	2.5	0.5	68	6	0.05	0.22	1.6	0.48	t	0	51	78	1	*
0	4	708	43	2.4	0.5	65	6	0.05	0.21	1.5	0.46	t	0	48	75	1	*
0	6	1200	73	4	0.9	320	5	0.13	0.26	3.2	0.43	6	0	82	127	1	*
0	17	1089	48	3	0.4	1	5	0.23	0.13	1.2	0.36	5	0	71	141	1	1
0	2	105	5	0.3	t	t	t	0.02	0.01	0.1	0.04	t	0	7	14	0	0.1
0	9	241	31	1.1	0.4	9	22	0.05	0.08	1.1	0.11	27	0	27	23	1	1.2
0	3	285	33	1.6	0.5	15	41	0.05	0.11	0.6	0.09	65	0	38	43	1	0.8
0	0	187	22	0.7	0.6	16	31	0.04	0.11	1.1	0.07	32	0	27	15	1	0.4
0	5	548	32	1.6	0.2	22	16	0.05	0.14	0.8	0.05	14	0	211	41	1	0.5
0	9	218	22	1.2	0.2	7	80	0.05	0.09	0.1	0.12	01	0	33	29	1	0.4
0	8	249	18	1.5	0.1	6	106	0.04	0.13	1	0.08	38	0	28	32	1	0.5
0	3	250	15	1.2	0.1	7	101	0.04	0.2	0.7	0.07	10	0	28	31	1	0.5
0	3	221	16	1.1	0.2	7	61	0.03	0.06	0.7	0.04	25	0	24	19	1	0.3
0	1	247	15	0.6	0.2	4	85	0.03	0.1	0.3	0.09	26	0	21	28	1	0.2
0	15	197	20	0.9	0.6	212	50	0.13	0.11	1.1	0.11	12	0	18	25	1	*
0	1	132	10	0.1	0.2	77	26	0.09	0.02	0.1	0.06	17	0	12	8	1	*
0	3	186	18	0.3	0.1	59	15	0.13	0.03	0.3	0.23	4	0	13	14	1	*
*	1400	*	*	*	*	*	*	*	*	*	*	*	*	*	*	*	0.3
0	164	43	22	0.4	0.4	11	1	0.05	0.03	0.6	0.05	2	0	37	55	2	1.9
0	1	213	42	6.1	0.6	0	0	1	0.59	7.7	0.23	7	0	3	114	*	0.2
0	7	389	96	9.9	1.7	98	0	1.72	0.98	12.1	0.62	115	0	12	202	6	0.4
0	372	39	11	1.5	0.3	0	0	0.13	0.2	1.7	0	0	0	29	42	*	0.3
0	2	123	25	5.3	0.8	0	0	0.9	0.57	6.8	0.05	30	0	17	124	5	t
0	2	136	34	6	1.2	0	0	1.11	0.7	10.4	0.05	40	0	21	133	*	*
0	1	41	23	1.8	0.7	0	0	0.27	0.13	2.2	0.05	1	0	1	71	32	t
53	11	45	30	2.5	1	10	0	0.3	0.13	2.4	0.06	11	0.14	19	110	*	*
52	20	59	38	1.7	1	17	0	0.39	0.2	2.4	0.18	34	0.22	30	91	*	12.7
36	829	69	17	1.8	0.6	221	t	0.16	0.1	1.4	0.07	8	0.01	18	70	*	0.2
0	4	532	221	5.1	2.9	0	0	1.1	0.21	0.9	0.16	49	0	55	690	*	1.6
0	3	669	276	7.4	6.2	0	0	1.19	0.22	1.5	0.19	87	0	84	816	*	1.7
10	2	7	5	0.3	0.2	2	0	0.06	0.04	0.3	0.01	2	0.04	2	18	*	0.1
0	174	*	16	0.2	0.4	*	0	*	0.01	0.2	*	*	*	1	19	2	*
0	0	*	*	0.2	0.5	*	0	*	0.01	0.1	0.01	*	0	1	17	1	*
0	0	*	*	0.5	*	*	0	*	0.02	0.4	*	*	*	2	47	7	*
0	258	21	4	0.2	0.2	0	0	0.05	0.04	0.7	t	3	0	4	21	*	t
0	5	t	t	t	t	0	0	t	t	t	0	t	0	t	t	*	0
0	97	6	1	0.1	0.1	0	0	0.02	0.02	0.3	t	1	0	2	5	*	t
0	t	26	3	0.2	0.1	0	t	t	t	0.1	0.01	1	0	7	10	*	t
0	11	27	3	0.2	0.1	0	t	t	t	0.1	0.01	1	0	7	10	*	t
0	9	83	83	0.8	1.2	0	0	0.19	0.05	3	0.28	8	0	20	161	76	1.3
0	13	413	265	2.7	3.7	0	0	0.74	0.17	9.4	0.94	36	0	43	616	*	1.3
0	5	7	8	1	0.4	0	0	0.12	0.08	1.5	0.02	6	0	13	23	33	0.2
0	4	80	26	2.3	0.9	0	0	0.33	0.03	3	0.19	7	0	23	95	41	0.2
0	9	213	46	8	2	0	0	1.07	0.09	7.8	0.3	16	0	52	213	37	0.2
0	6	166	53	1	2.2	0	0	0.09	0.14	2.1	0.22	43	0	5	134	*	0.3
0	10	4462	204	4.5	6.3	0	0	0.53	0.42	7.2	0.5	101	0	56	632	*	2.2

WT, weight; **KCAL**, kcalories; **PROT**, protein; **CARB**, carbohydrate; **FIBR**, fiber; **FAT**, fat; **SATF**, saturated fat;

MONO, monsaturated fat; **POLY**, polyunsaturated fat; **CHOL**, cholesterol; **SOD**, sodium; **POT**, potassium;

FOOD NAME	PORTION	WT (g)	KCAL	PROT (g)	CARB (g)	FIBR (g)	FAT (g)	SATF (g)	MONO (g)	POLY (g)
SHAKE 'N BAKE-PACKAGE-GENERAL FOODS	OUNCE	28.4	116	2	18	*	4	*	*	*
SORGHUM-WHOLE-DRY	CUP	192	651	22	143	28.6	6	0.9	1.9	2.6
SPAGHETTI-COOKED-TENDER STAGE-HOT	CUP	140	155	5	32	2.2	1	*	*	*
STUFFING MIX-DRY FORM	CUP	30	111	4	22	*	1	*	*	*
STUFFING MIX-PREPARED	CUP	140	501	9	50	*	31	*	*	*
TACO SHELLS	ITEM	11	50	1	7	0.9	2	0.3	1.2	0.5
TORTILLA CHIPS-DORITOS	OUNCE	28.4	139	2	19	1.9	7	1.4	3.2	1.8
MEATS										
BACON BITS	TBSP	6	27	2	2	0.6	2	0.2	0.4	0.8
BACON-PORK-BROILED/PAN-FRIED/ROASTED	SLICE	6.3	36	2	t	0	3	1.1	1.5	0.4
BARBECUE LOAF-PORK AND BEEF	SLICE	23	40	4	1	*	2	0.7	1	0.2
BEEF CUTS-LEAN AND FAT-SIMMERED/ROASTED	SLICE	85	297	21	0	0	23	9.5	10.2	0.9
BEEF CUTS-LEAN ONLY-SIMMERED/ROASTED	SLICE	85	347	19	0	0	30	12.3	13.7	1
BEEF-DRIED-CURED-CHIPPED	SERVING	71	117	21	1	0	3	1.1	1.1	0.1
BEEF-HEART-COOKED-SIMMERED	SLICE	85	149	25	t	0	5	1.4	1.1	1
BEEF-LIVER-FRIED IN MARGARINE	SLICE	85	184	23	7	0	7	2.4	1.5	1.5
BEEF-POT ROAST-CHUCK-ARM CUT-COOKED	SLICE	100	231	33	0	0	10	3.8	4.4	0.4
BEEF-POT ROAST-CHUCK-BLADE CUT-COOKED	SLICE	100	270	31	0	0	15	6.2	6.8	0.5
BEEF-RIB STEAK-COOKED	ITEM	100	221	28	0	0	11	4.8	4.9	0.3
BEEF-STEAK-CHICKEN FRIED	ITEM	100	389	18	12	0	30	6.6	7.4	1.1
BEEF-TENDERLOIN STEAK-BROILED	ITEM	100	204	28	0	0	9	3.6	3.6	0.4
BEERWURST-BEER SALAMI-BEEF	SLICE	6	20	1	t	0	2	0.8	0.8	0.1
BEERWURST-BEER SALAMI-PORK	SLICE	6	14	1	t	0	1	0.4	0.5	0.1
BOCKWURST-RAW-PORK-LINK	ITEM	65	200	9	t	0	18	6.6	8.5	1.9
BOLOGNA-CURED PORK-4 BY 1/8 INCH SLICE	SLICE	23	57	4	t	0	5	1.6	2.3	0.5
BRATWURST-PORK-COOKED-LINK	ITEM	85	256	12	2	0	22	7.9	10.4	2.3
BRAUNSCHWEIGER-LIVER SAUSAGE-CURED PORK	SLICE	18	65	2	1	0	6	2	2.7	0.7
BRISKET-LEAN-COOKED	SLICE	100	241	29	0	0	13	4.6	5.8	0.4
CANADIAN BACON-PORK-GRILLED	SLICE	23.3	43	6	t	0	2	0.7	0.9	0.2
CHEESEFURTER-PORK AND BEEF	ITEM	43	141	6	1	0	13	4.5	5.9	1.3
CHITTERLINGS-PORK-SIMMERED	OUNCE	28.4	86	3	0	0	8	2.9	2.8	2.1
CHORIZO-PORK AND BEEF-LINK	ITEM	60	273	15	1	0	23	8.6	11	2.1
CORNED BEEF HASH-CANNED	CUP	220	400	19	24	*	25	11.9	10.9	0.5
CORNED BEEF LOAF-JELLIED	SLICE	28.4	44	7	0	0	2	0.7	0.8	0.1
CORNED BEEF-CANNED	SERVING	85	213	23	1	0	13	5.3	5.1	0.5
FRANKFURTER (HOT DOG)-NO BUN-BEEF & PORK	ITEM	57	183	6	1	0	17	6.1	7.8	1.6
FROG LEGS-FRIED-FLOUR COATED	ITEM	24	70	4	2	0.2	5	0.7	1.2	0.7
HAM AND CHEESE LOAF/ROLL	SLICE	28.4	74	5	t	0.5	6	2.1	2.6	0.6
HAM AND CHEESE SPREAD	TBSP	15	37	2	t	*	3	1.3	1.1	0.2
HAM SALAD SPREAD	TBSP	15	32	1	2	0	2	0.8	1.1	0.4
HAM-BOILED-REGULAR-11% FAT-LUNCHEON MEAT	SLICE	28.4	52	5	1	0	3	1	1.4	0.3
HAM-CANNED-CHOPPED-LUNCHEON MEAT	SLICE	21	50	3	t	0	4	1.3	1.9	0.4
HAM-CANNED-EXTRA LEAN-4% FAT	CUP	140	190	30	1	0	7	2.2	3.5	0.6
HAM-CANNED-PORK-ROASTED-13% FAT	CUP	140	316	29	1	0	21	7.1	9.9	2.5
HAM-DEVILED-CANNED-LUNCHEON MEAT	TBSP	13	45	2	0	0	4	1.5	1.8	0.4
HAM-EXTRA LEAN-5% FAT-ROASTED	CUP	140	203	29	2	0	8	2.5	3.7	0.8
HAM-LEAN ONLY-ROASTED	CUP	140	220	35	0	0	8	2.6	3.5	0.9
HAM-MINCED-PORK	SLICE	21	55	3	t	0	4	1.5	2	0.5
HAM-ROASTED-REGULAR-11% FAT-BONELESS	CUP	140	249	32	0	0	13	4.4	6.2	2
HAMBURGER PATTY-BROILED-EXTRA LEAN BEEF	ITEM	85	218	22	0	0	14	5.5	6.1	0.5
HAMBURGER PATTY-BROILED-MEDIUM-LEAN BEEF	ITEM	85	231	21	0	0	16	6.2	6.9	0.6
HAMBURGER-GROUND-REGULAR-BAKED	SERVING	85	244	20	0	0	18	7	7.8	0.7
HAMBURGER-GROUND-REGULAR-FRIED	SERVING	85	260	20	0	0	19	7.5	8.4	0.7
HEADCHEESE-PORK	SLICE	28.4	60	5	t	0	4	1.4	2.3	0.5
ITALIAN SAUSAGE-PORK-LINK	ITEM	67	216	13	1	0	17	6.1	8	2.2
KIELBASA-PORK AND BEEF	SLICE	26	81	3	1	0	7	2.6	3.4	0.8
KNOCKWURST-PORK AND BEEF-LINK	ITEM	68	209	8	1	0	19	6.9	8.7	2
LAMB CHOP-RIB-BROILED-LEAN AND FAT	SERVING	85	307	19	0	0	25	10.8	10.3	2
LAMB CHOP-RIB-BROILED-LEAN ONLY	SERVING	57	134	16	0	0	7	2.7	3	0.7
LAMB-LEG-ROASTED-LEAN AND FAT	SLICE	85	219	22	0	0	14	5.9	5.9	1
LAMB-LEG-ROASTED-LEAN ONLY	SLICE	71	136	20	0	0	6	2	2.4	0.4
LAMB-SHOULDER-ROASTED-LEAN AND FAT	SLICE	85	235	19	0	0	17	7.2	6.9	1.4
LAMB-SHOULDER-ROASTED-LEAN ONLY	SLICE	64	131	16	0	0	7	2.6	2.8	0.6

t = Trace of nutrient present ** = Not available*

MAG, magnesium; **IRON,** iron; **ZINC,** zinc; **VITA,** vitamin A; **VITC,** vitamin C; **THIA,** thiamin; **RIBO,** riboflavin; **NIAC,** niacin; **VB6,** vitamin B-6; **FOL,** folate; **VB12,** vitamin B-12; **CALC,** calcium; **PHOS,** phosphorus; **SEL,** selenium; **VE-a,** alpha tocopherol equivalents.

CHOL (mg)	SOD (mg)	POT (mg)	MAG (mg)	IRON (mg)	ZINC (mg)	VITA (RE)	VITC (mg)	THIA (mg)	RIBO (mg)	NIAC (mg)	VB6 (mg)	FOL (µg)	VB12 (µg)	CALC (mg)	PHOS (mg)	SEL (µg)	VE-a (mg)
*	984	57	*	0.7	*	62	t	0.16	0.18	2.2	*	*	*	14	44	*	*
0	12	672	*	8.5	*	0	0	0.46	0.27	5.6	*	*	0	54	551	*	*
0	1	85	24	1.3	0.7	0	0	0.2	0.11	1.5	0.09	17	0	11	70	85	0.1
*	399	52	*	1	*	0	0	0.07	0.08	1	*	*	*	37	57	*	*
*	1254	126	*	2.2	*	91	0	0.13	0.17	2.1	*	*	*	92	136	*	*
0	20	27	11	0.3	0.1	5	0	0.03	0.02	0.2	0.04	3	0	16	25	*	0.5
0	180	51	21	0.5	0.2	5	0	0.03	0.03	t	0.1	4	0	30	59	*	1.2
0	165	9	6	0.3	0.1	0	t	0.03	0.02	0.1	0.01	8	0.07	8	18	*	0.4
5	101	31	2	0.1	0.2	0	2	0.04	0.02	0.5	0.02	t	0.11	1	21	1	t
9	307	76	4	0.3	0.6	2	4	0.08	0.06	0.5	0.06	2	0.39	13	30	3	*
78	50	244	18	2.2	4.7	0	0	0.07	0.18	2.9	0.26	6	2.03	8	164	25	0.1
78	55	186	14	1.9	4.5	0	0	0.05	0.15	2.4	0.2	5	1.91	8	147	25	0.1
65	2464	315	23	3.2	3.7	*	0	0.05	0.23	2.7	*	*	1.31	4	124	38	*
164	54	198	21	6.4	2.7	0	1	0.12	1.31	3.5	0.18	2	12.2	5	213	48	0.5
410	90	309	20	5.3	4.6	9216	19	0.18	3.52	12.3	1.22	187	95	9	392	48	0.5
101	66	289	24	3.8	8.7	0	0	0.08	0.29	3.7	0.33	11	3.4	9	268	6	0.1
106	71	263	23	3.7	10.3	0	0	0.08	0.28	2.7	0.29	6	2.47	13	235	6	0.1
80	69	394	27	2.6	7	0	0	0.11	0.22	4.8	0.4	8	3.32	13	208	6	0.1
97	815	126	30	2.3	4.9	8	0	0.11	0.14	2.7	0.5	11	3.27	11	110	*	0.1
84	63	419	30	3.6	5.6	0	0	0.13	0.3	3.9	0.38	8	0.44	7	238	*	0.2
4	62	10	1	0.1	0.1	0	1	t	0.01	0.2	0.01	t	0.12	1	6	2	t
4	74	15	1	t	0.1	0	2	0.03	0.01	0.2	0.02	t	0.05	t	6	2	t
38	718	176	12	0.4	1	4	0	0.27	0.11	2.7	0.15	4	0.53	10	95	10	*
14	272	65	3	0.2	0.5	0	8	0.12	0.04	0.9	0.06	1	0.21	3	32	4	t
51	473	180	12	1.1	2	0	1	0.43	0.16	2.7	0.18	2	0.81	38	126	25	*
28	206	36	2	1.7	0.5	759	2	0.05	0.28	1.5	0.06	8	3.62	2	30	2	0.1
93	72	287	23	2.8	6.9	0	0	0.07	0.22	3.8	0.3	8	2.55	6	239	5	0.1
14	360	91	5	0.2	0.4	0	5	0.19	0.05	1.6	0.11	1	0.18	3	69	3	0.1
29	465	89	5	0.5	1	16	8	0.11	0.07	1.3	0.05	1	0.74	25	76	10	0.1
41	11	2	3	1.1	1.4	0	0	0	0.02	t	t	1	0.29	8	13	*	0.1
53	741	239	11	1	2.1	0	0	0.38	0.18	3.1	0.32	1	1.2	5	90	10	0.1
50	1188	440	*	4.4	*	*	*	0.02	0.2	4.6	*	*	*	29	147	*	0.1
13	270	29	3	0.6	1.2	0	2	0	0.03	0.5	0.03	2	0.36	3	21	7	0.1
73	855	116	12	1.8	3	0	t	0.02	0.2	2.9	0.11	3	1.38	17	94	21	0.1
29	639	95	6	0.7	1.1	0	15	0.11	0.07	1.5	0.08	2	0.74	6	49	5	0.1
32	119	65	6	0.3	0.3	0	1	0.03	0.06	0.3	0.03	6	0.11	5	39	*	0.5
16	381	84	5	0.3	0.6	7	7	0.17	0.05	1	0.07	1	0.23	17	72	*	t
9	179	24	3	0.1	0.3	14	1	0.05	0.03	0.3	0.02	t	0.11	33	74	*	0
6	137	23	2	0.1	0.2	0	1	0.07	0.02	0.3	0.02	t	0.11	1	18	*	0
16	373	94	5	0.3	0.6	0	8	0.24	0.07	1.5	0.1	1	0.24	2	70	13	0
10	287	60	3	0.2	0.4	0	0	0.11	0.04	0.7	0.07	1	0.15	1	29	10	0
42	1589	487	29	1.3	3.1	0	39	1.45	0.35	6.9	0.63	7	0.99	8	293	66	0.4
87	1317	500	24	1.9	3.5	0	20	1.15	0.36	7.4	0.42	7	1.48	11	340	66	0.4
10	160	*	2	0.3	0.2	0	*	0.02	0.01	0.2	0.04	*	0.09	1	12	2	0
74	1684	402	20	2.1	4	0	29	1.06	0.28	5.6	0.56	5	0.91	11	275	66	0.4
77	1858	442	31	1.3	3.6	0	t	0.95	0.36	7	0.66	6	0.98	10	318	66	0.4
15	261	65	3	0.2	0.4	0	6	0.15	0.04	0.9	0.06	t	0.2	2	33	10	*
83	2100	573	30	1.9	3.5	0	32	1.02	0.46	8.6	0.43	4	0.98	12	393	66	0.4
71	60	266	18	2	4.6	6	0	0.05	0.23	4.2	0.23	8	1.84	6	137	20	0.3
74	65	256	18	1.8	4.6	9	0	0.04	0.18	4.4	0.22	8	2	9	134	20	0.3
74	51	188	13	2.1	4.2	0	0	0.03	0.14	4	0.2	7	1.99	8	117	*	0.3
75	71	255	17	2.1	4.3	0	0	0.03	0.17	5	0.2	8	2.3	10	145	*	0.3
23	357	9	3	0.3	0.4	*	6	0.01	0.05	0.3	0.05	1	0.3	5	17	5	*
52	618	204	12	1	1.6	0	1	0.42	0.16	2.8	0.22	3	0.87	16	114	22	0.1
17	280	71	4	0.4	0.5	0	5	0.06	0.06	0.7	0.05	1	0.42	11	39	4	t
39	687	136	8	0.6	1.1	0	18	0.23	0.1	1.9	0.11	1	0.8	7	67	10	0
84	64	230	20	1.6	3.4	0	0	0.08	0.19	6	0.09	12	2.16	16	151	14	0.1
52	49	178	17	1.3	3	0	0	0.06	0.14	3.7	0.09	12	1.5	9	121	10	0.1
79	56	266	20	1.7	3.7	*	*	0.09	0.23	5.6	0.13	17	2.2	9	162	14	t
63	48	240	19	1.5	3.5	*	*	0.08	0.21	4.5	0.12	16	1.87	6	146	12	t
78	56	214	19	1.7	4.4	*	*	0.08	0.2	5.2	0.11	18	2.24	17	156	14	0.1
56	44	170	16	1.4	3.9	*	*	0.06	0.17	3.7	0.1	16	1.73	12	128	11	0.1

WT, weight; **KCAL,** kcalories; **PROT,** protein; **CARB,** carbohydrate; **FIBR,** fiber; **FAT,** fat; **SATF,** saturated fat;

MONO, monsaturated fat; **POLY,** polyunsaturated fat; **CHOL,** cholesterol; **SOD,** sodium; **POT,** potassium;

FOOD NAME	PORTION	WT (g)	KCAL	PROT (g)	CARB (g)	FIBR (g)	FAT (g)	SATF (g)	MONO (g)	POLY (g)
LIVER CHEESE-PORK	SLICE	38	116	6	1	0	10	3.4	4.7	1.3
LIVERWURST-LIVER SAUSAGE-PORK	SLICE	18	59	3	t	0	5	1.9	2.4	0.5
MORTADELLA-PORK AND BEEF	SLICE	15	47	2	t	0	4	1.4	1.7	0.5
OLIVE LOAF-PORK	SLICE	28.4	67	3	3	0	5	1.7	2.2	0.6
PEPPERONI-PORK AND BEEF	SLICE	5.5	27	1	t	0	2	0.9	1.2	0.2
PIMENTO/PICKLE LOAF-PORK	SLICE	28.4	74	3	2	*	6	2.2	2.7	0.7
POLISH SAUSAGE-PORK	ITEM	227	740	32	4	0	65	23.4	30.6	7
PORK CHOP-LOIN-BROILED-LEAN AND FAT	ITEM	82	284	19	0	0	22	8.1	10.2	2.5
PORK CHOP-LOIN-BROILED-LEAN ONLY	ITEM	66	169	18	0	0	10	3.5	4.5	1.2
PORK-CENTER LOIN-ROASTED-LEAN AND FAT	ITEM	88	268	22	0	0	19	6.9	8.8	2.2
PORK-CENTER LOIN-ROASTED-LEAN ONLY	SLICE	72	173	21	0	0	9	3.3	4.2	1.1
PORK-FEET-PICKLED	OUNCE	28.4	58	4	t	0	5	1.6	2.2	0.5
PORK-FEET-SIMMERED	OUNCE	28.4	55	5	0	0	4	1.2	1.7	0.4
PORK-KIDNEYS-BRAISED	CUP	140	211	36	0	0	7	2.1	2.2	0.5
PORK-LIVER-BRAISED	OUNCE	28.4	47	7	1	0	1	0.4	0.2	0.3
PORK-SHOULDER-ROASTED-LEAN ONLY	CUP	140	342	36	0	0	21	7.2	9.4	2.6
PORK-SPARERIBS-BRAISED	OUNCE	28.4	113	8	0	0	9	3.3	4	1
PORK-TENDERLOIN-ROASTED-LEAN ONLY	OUNCE	28.4	47	8	0	0	1	0.5	0.6	0.2
PORK-TONGUE-BRAISED	SERVING	85	230	21	0	0	16	5.5	7.5	1.6
POTTED MEAT-CANNED-BEEF/CHICKEN/TURKEY	TBSP	13	30	2	0	0	2	0.8	0.9	0.1
RABBIT-STEWED-BONELESS-SKINLESS	SERVING	85	175	26	0	0	7	2.1	1.9	1.4
ROAST BEEF-BOTTOM ROUND-COOKED-LEAN ONLY	SLICE	78	173	25	0	0	8	2.7	3.4	0.3
ROAST BEEF-BOTTOM ROUND-LEAN AND FAT	SLICE	85	222	25	0	0	13	4.8	5.7	0.5
ROAST BEEF-RIB-BROILED-LEAN AND FAT	SLICE	85	308	18	0	0	26	10.8	11.4	0.9
ROAST BEEF-RIB-BROILED-LEAN ONLY	SLICE	51	122	14	0	0	7	3	3.1	0.2
SALAMI-COOKED-BEEF-4 BY 1/8 INCH SLICE	SLICE	23	60	3	1	0	5	2.1	2.2	0.2
SALAMI-DRY OR HARD-PORK-SLICE	SLICE	10	41	2	t	0	3	1.2	1.6	0.4
SAUSAGE-LINK-COOKED-PORK	ITEM	13	48	3	t	0	4	1.4	1.8	0.5
SAUSAGE-PATTY-COOKED-FRESH PORK	ITEM	27	100	5	t	0	8	2.9	3.8	1
SAUSAGE-VIENNA-CANNED-BEEF AND PORK	ITEM	16	45	2	t	0	4	1.5	2	0.3
STEAK-SIRLOIN-BROILED-LEAN AND FAT	ITEM	85	238	23	0	0	15	6.4	6.9	0.6
STEAK-SIRLOIN-BROILED-LEAN ONLY	ITEM	56	116	17	0	0	5	2	2.2	0.2
STEAK-TOP ROUND-BROILED-LEAN AND FAT	SLICE	85	179	26	0	0	7	2.8	3.1	0.3
STEAK-TOP ROUND-BROILED-LEAN ONLY	SLICE	68	130	22	0	0	4	1.5	1.7	0.2
SWEETBREADS-CALF-BRAISED	SERVING	85	143	28	0	0	3	*	*	*
THURINGER/CERVELAT-PORK	SLICE	23	77	4	t	0	7	2.8	3	0.3
VEAL-LEG-TOP ROUND-PAN FRIED	SERVING	85	179	27	0	0	7	2.7	2.8	0.5
VEAL-RIB-SEPARABLE LEAN ONLY-BRAISED	SERVING	85	185	29	0	0	7	2.2	2.2	0.6
VEAL-SHOULDER-ARM-LEAN ONLY-ROASTED	SERVING	85	139	22	0	0	5	2	1.8	0.4
VENISON-DRIED-SALTED	SERVING	100	142	31	0	0	1	*	*	0.1
VENISON-ROASTED	SLICE	100	146	30	0	0	2	2.1	1.1	1.9
MISCELLANEOUS										
BAKING POWDER-LOW SODIUM	TSP	4.3	7	t	2	*	0	0	0	0
BAKING POWDER-NO CALCIUM SULFATE	TSP	3	4	t	1	*	0	0	0	0
BAKING POWDER-STRAIGHT PHOSPHATE	TSP	3.8	5	t	1	*	0	0	0	0
BAKING POWDER-WITH CALCIUM SULFATE	TSP	2.9	3	t	1	*	0	0	0	0
BAKING SODA	TSP	3	0	0	0	0	0	0	0	0
CHEWING GUM-CANDY COATED	ITEM	1.7	5	0	2	0	t	0	0	0
CHEWING GUM-WRIGLEYS	ITEM	3	10	0	2	0	0	0	0	0
GELATIN DESSERT-PREPARED	CUP	240	140	4	34	0	0	0	0	0
GELATIN-D ZERTA-LOW CALORIE-PREPARED	CUP	240	16	4	0	0	0	0	0	0
GELATIN-DRY-ENVELOPE	ITEM	7	25	6	0	0	0	0	0	0
GELATIN-JELLO-SUGAR FREE-PREPARED	CUP	240	16	2	0	0	0	0	0	0
OLIVES-GREEN-PICKLED-CANNED	ITEM	4	4	t	t	0.1	1	0.1	0.4	t
OLIVES-MISSION-RIPE-CANNED	ITEM	3	5	t	t	0.1	1	0.1	0.4	t
PICKLE RELISH-HAMBURGER-HEINZ	OUNCE	28.4	30	0	7	*	0	0	0	0
PICKLE RELISH-HOT DOG-HEINZ	OUNCE	28.4	35	0	8	*	0	0	0	0
PICKLE RELISH-SWEET-CHOPPED	TBSP	15	20	0	5	0.3	0	0	0	0
PICKLE-DILL-CUCUMBER-MEDIUM SIZED	ITEM	65	5	0	1	0.8	0	0	0	0
PICKLE-FRESH PACK-CUCUMBER-SLICED	ITEM	7.5	5	0	2	0.1	0	0	0	0
PICKLE-SWEET/GHERKIN-SMALL-WHOLE	ITEM	15	20	0	5	0.2	0	0	0	0
POPSICLE	ITEM	95	70	0	18	0	0	0	0	0

t = Trace of nutrient present ** = Not available*

MAG, magnesium; **IRON,** iron; **ZINC,** zinc; **VITA,** vitamin A; **VITC,** vitamin C; **THIA,** thiamin; **RIBO,** riboflavin; **NIAC,** niacin; **VB6,** vitamin B-6; **FOL,** folate; **VB12,** vitamin B-12; **CALC,** calcium; **PHOS,** phosphorus; **SEL,** selenium; **VE-a,** alpha tocopherol equivalents.

CHOL (mg)	SOD (mg)	POT (mg)	MAG (mg)	IRON (mg)	ZINC (mg)	VITA (RE)	VITC (mg)	THIA (mg)	RIBO (mg)	NIAC (mg)	VB6 (mg)	FOL (µg)	VB12 (µg)	CALC (mg)	PHOS (mg)	SEL (µg)	VE-a (mg)
66	466	86	5	4.1	1.4	1996	1	0.08	0.85	4.5	0.18	40	9.33	3	79	6	0.1
28	215	36	2	1.2	0.5	760	2	0.05	0.19	1.5	0.03	5	2.42	5	41	3	0.1
8	187	25	2	0.2	0.3	0	4	0.02	0.02	0.4	0.02	t	0.22	3	15	2	t
11	421	84	5	0.2	0.4	6	3	0.08	0.07	0.5	0.07	1	0.36	31	36	4	0.1
4	112	19	1	0.1	0.1	0	0	0.02	0.01	0.3	0.01	t	0.14	1	7	1	t
11	394	97	5	0.3	0.4	2	4	0.08	0.07	0.6	0.05	1	0.34	27	40	4	*
159	1989	538	32	3.3	4.4	0	2	1.14	0.34	7.8	0.43	5	2.22	27	309	66	0.4
77	54	287	20	0.7	2	2	t	0.69	0.29	4.3	0.31	4	0.81	5	193	14	0.1
63	49	276	19	0.6	1.9	2	t	0.64	0.28	3.9	0.3	4	0.71	5	184	11	0.1
80	56	284	17	0.9	1.8	2	t	0.73	0.21	4.4	0.35	1	0.53	5	173	28	0.1
66	50	261	15	0.8	1.6	2	t	0.65	0.19	3.9	0.32	1	0.43	4	158	23	0.1
26	262	67	1	0.2	0.4	0	0	t	0.01	0.1	0.11	1	0.18	9	10	*	0.1
28	9	42	1	0.1	0.3	0	0	t	0.02	0.1	0.03	t	0.05	13	14	*	0.1
673	111	200	25	7.4	5.8	109	15	0.55	2.22	8.1	0.65	57	10.9	18	337	294	0.6
101	14	43	4	5.1	1.9	1531	7	0.07	0.62	2.4	0.16	46	5.3	3	68	20	0.1
136	106	493	28	2.1	5.9	3	t	0.82	0.51	6	0.56	7	1.23	11	323	43	0.2
34	26	91	7	0.5	1.3	1	0	0.12	0.11	1.6	0.1	1	0.31	13	74	5	t
26	19	153	7	0.4	0.9	1	t	0.27	0.11	1.3	0.12	2	0.16	3	82	9	0.1
124	93	201	17	4.2	3.9	0	1	0.27	0.43	4.5	0.2	3	2.03	16	148	*	0.3
15	156	*	*	*	*	*	*	0	0.03	0.2	*	*	*	*	*	2	0
73	32	255	17	2	2	0	0	0.05	0.15	6.1	0.29	8	5.53	17	192	*	1.6
75	40	240	20	2.7	4.3	0	0	0.06	0.2	3.2	0.28	9	1.93	4	212	19	0.1
81	43	248	20	2.8	4.4	0	0	0.06	0.21	3.3	0.29	9	2.04	5	217	20	0.1
73	52	257	17	1.8	4.3	0	0	0.07	0.15	2.7	0.25	5	2.37	10	140	20	0.1
41	38	192	13	1.3	3.5	0	0	0.04	0.11	2.1	0.15	4	1.49	5	109	12	0.1
15	270	52	3	0.5	0.5	0	4	0.02	0.04	0.7	0.05	t	1.11	2	26	4	t
8	226	38	2	0.1	0.4	0	0	0.09	0.03	0.6	0.06	t	0.28	1	23	2	t
11	168	47	2	0.2	0.3	0	0	0.1	0.03	0.6	0.04	t	0.22	4	24	4	t
22	349	97	5	0.3	0.7	0	0	0.2	0.07	1.2	0.09	1	0.47	9	50	3	t
8	152	16	1	0.1	0.3	0	0	0.01	0.02	0.3	0.02	1	0.16	2	8	8	0
77	54	306	24	2.6	4.9	15	0	0.1	0.22	3.3	0.34	8	2.26	9	185	29	0.1
50	37	226	18	1.9	3.7	3	0	0.07	0.17	2.4	0.25	6	1.6	6	137	19	0.1
72	51	365	26	2.4	4.6	0	0	0.1	0.22	5	0.46	10	2.08	5	203	29	0.1
57	42	301	21	2	3.8	0	0	0.08	0.18	4.1	0.38	8	1.69	4	167	23	0.1
*	*	*	*	*	*	*	*	0.05	0.14	2.5	*	*	*	*	*	*	*
17	286	62	3	0.6	0.6	0	5	0.04	0.08	1	0.06	t	1.27	3	26	3	t
89	64	362	26	0.8	2.8	0	t	0.06	0.3	1	0.41	13	1.23	5	237	10	t
123	84	270	22	1.2	5.1	0	0	0.05	0.26	6.7	0.29	14	1.3	20	186	10	t
93	77	302	23	1	3.7	0	0	0.06	0.28	7	0.25	15	1.33	23	192	*	0.3
*	*	*	*	1.9	*	*	*	0.09	0.34	10	*	*	*	60	298	*	*
82	70	336	29	3.5	4.5	0	0	0.37	0.28	7.4	0.26	7	6.22	20	264	*	t
0	t	471	*	0	*	0	0	0	0	0	*	*	*	207	314	*	*
0	329	5	*	0	*	0	0	0	0	0	*	*	*	58	87	*	*
0	312	6	*	0	*	0	0	0	0	0	*	*	*	239	359	*	*
0	290	4	*	0	*	0	0	0	0	0	*	*	*	183	45	*	*
0	821	*	*	*	*	0	0	0	0	0	0	0	0	*	*	*	0
0	t	0	0	0	0	0	0	0	0	0	0	0	0	t	0	*	0
0	0	0	0	0	0	0	0	0	0	0	0	0	0	3	0	*	0
0	0	0	0	0	0	0	0	0	0	0	0	0	0	5	46	16	0
0	20	3	2	t	0.1	0	0	0	0	0	t	0	0	6	0	*	0
0	8	180	0	0.4	0	0	4	0	0	0	0	0	0	0	0	2	0
0	120	*	*	*	*	*	*	*	*	*	*	*	*	*	*	*	*
0	81	2	1	0.1	t	1	0	0	0	t	0	t	0	2	1	0	0.1
0	19	1	1	t	t	1	0	0	0	t	0	t	0	3	t	0	0.1
0	325	*	*	0.2	*	*	*	*	*	*	*	*	*	6	4	0	*
0	200	*	*	0.2	*	*	*	*	*	*	*	*	*	6	4	0	*
0	124	30	1	0.1	t	2	1	0	t	0	t	1	0	3	2	0	t
0	928	130	8	0.7	0.2	7	4	0	0.01	0	0.01	1	0	17	14	0	0.1
0	50	15	t	0.2	t	1	1	0	0	0	t	t	0	3	2	0	t
0	128	30	t	0.2	t	1	1	0	0	0	t	t	0	2	2	0	t
0	0	4	0	0	0	0	0	0	0	0	0	0	0	0	0	*	0

WT, weight; **KCAL**, kcalories; **PROT**, protein; **CARB**, carbohydrate; **FIBR**, fiber; **FAT**, fat; **SATF**, saturated fat;

MONO, monsaturated fat; **POLY**, polyunsaturated fat; **CHOL**, cholesterol; **SOD**, sodium; **POT**, potassium;

FOOD NAME	PORTION	WT (g)	KCAL	PROT (g)	CARB (g)	FIBR (g)	FAT (g)	SATF (g)	MONO (g)	POLY (g)
VANILLA-PURE	TSP	4.7	14	0	1	0	0	0	0	0
VINEGAR-CIDER	TBSP	15	0	0	1	0	0	0	0	0
VINEGAR-DISTILLED	CUP	240	29	0	12	0	0	0	0	0
YEAST-BAKER'S-DRY-ACTIVE-PACKAGE	SERVING	7	20	3	3	2.2	0	0	0	0
YEAST-BREWER'S-DRY	TBSP	8	25	3	3	2.5	0	0	0	0
NUTS & SEEDS										
ALMOND BUTTER-PLAIN	TBSP	16	101	2	3	1.8	9	0.9	6.1	2
NUT-FILBERT/HAZEL-DRIED-CHOPPED	CUP	115	727	15	18	9.8	72	5.3	56.5	6.9
NUT-WALNUT-PERSIAN/ENGLISH	CUP	120	770	17	22	5.8	74	6.7	17	47
NUTS-ALMONDS-UNBLANCHED-SHELLED-CHOPPED	CUP	130	766	26	27	12.1	68	6.4	44.1	14.2
NUTS-ALMONDS-UNBLANCHED-SHELLED-SLIVERED	CUP	115	677	23	24	10.7	60	5.7	39	12.6
NUTS-BEECHNUTS-DRIED	OUNCE	28.4	164	2	10	2.6	14	1.6	6.2	5.7
NUTS-BRAZIL-DRIED-SHELLED	CUP	140	918	20	18	10.8	93	22.6	32.2	33.8
NUTS-BUTTERNUTS-DRIED	OUNCE	28.4	174	7	3	2.4	16	0.4	3	12.1
NUTS-CASHEWS-DRY ROASTED	CUP	137	786	21	45	10	64	12.5	37.4	10.7
NUTS-CASHEWS-OIL ROASTED	CUP	130	749	21	37	7.8	63	12.4	36.9	10.6
NUTS-HICKORY-DRIED	OUNCE	28.4	187	4	5	2.4	18	2	9.3	6.2
NUTS-MACADAMIA-DRIED	CUP	134	941	11	18	12.4	99	14.8	77.9	1.7
NUTS-MACADAMIA-OIL ROASTED	CUP	134	962	10	17	9.3	103	15.4	80.9	1.8
NUTS-MIXED-DRY ROASTED	CUP	137	814	24	35	11.6	71	9.5	43	14.8
NUTS-MIXED-OIL ROASTED	CUP	142	876	24	30	12.8	80	12.4	45	18.9
NUTS-PEANUTS-OIL ROASTED	CUP	144	837	38	27	12.8	71	9.9	35.2	22.4
NUTS-PEANUTS-OIL ROASTED-SALTED	CUP	144	837	38	27	12.8	71	9.9	35.2	22.4
NUTS-PEANUTS-SPANISH-DRIED	CUP	146	828	38	24	11.7	72	10	35.7	22.7
NUTS-PECANS-DRIED-HALVES	CUP	108	720	8	20	7	73	5.9	45.5	18.1
NUTS-PECANS-OIL ROASTED	CUP	110	754	8	18	8.5	78	6.3	48.8	19.4
NUTS-PISTACHIO-DRIED	CUP	128	739	26	32	13.8	62	7.8	41.8	9.4
NUTS-PISTACHIO-DRY ROASTED	CUP	128	776	19	35	13.8	68	8.6	45.6	10.2
NUTS-SOYBEAN KERNELS-ROASTED	CUP	108	489	40	33	9.2	26	3.4	6	13.8
NUTS-WALNUT-BLACK-DRIED-CHOPPED	CUP	125	759	30	15	8.1	71	4.5	15.9	46.9
NUTS-WALNUTS-FINELY GROUND	CUP	80	486	20	10	5.2	45	2.9	10.2	29.9
PEANUT BUTTER-CHUNK STYLE	TBSP	16.1	95	4	3	1.1	8	1.5	3.8	2.3
PEANUT BUTTER-LOW SODIUM-PETER PAN	TBSP	16	95	5	3	1.7	9	1.4	4	2.5
PEANUT BUTTER-OLD FASHIONED	TBSP	16	95	4	3	1.1	8	1.5	3.8	2.7
PEANUT BUTTER-SMOOTH TYPE	TBSP	16	94	4	3	1	8	1.5	3.8	2.3
SEEDS-BREADFRUIT-ROASTED	OUNCE	28.4	59	2	11	8	1	0.2	0.1	0.4
SEEDS-PUMPKIN/SQUASH-DRIED	CUP	138	747	34	25	14.8	63	12	19.7	28.8
SEEDS-PUMPKIN/SQUASH-ROASTED	CUP	64	285	12	34	29.4	12	2.4	3.9	5.7
SEEDS-SESAME-DRIED-WHOLE	CUP	144	825	26	34	21.6	72	10	27	31.4
SEEDS-SESAME-ROASTED-WHOLE	OUNCE	28.4	161	5	7	5.3	14	1.9	5.2	6
SEEDS-SUNFLOWER-DRIED	CUP	144	821	33	27	9.8	71	7.5	13.6	47.1
SEEDS-SUNFLOWER-OIL ROASTED	CUP	135	830	29	20	9.2	78	8.1	14.8	51.2
POULTRY										
CHICK-BREAST-NO SKIN-ROASTED	ITEM	172	284	53	0	0	6	1.7	2.1	1.3
CHICK-THIGH-NO SKIN-ROASTED	ITEM	52	109	14	0	0	6	1.6	2.2	1.3
CHICKEN FRANKFURTER	ITEM	45	116	6	3	0	9	2.5	3.8	1.8
CHICKEN ROLL-LIGHT	SLICE	28.4	45	6	1	0	2	0.6	0.8	0.5
CHICKEN SPREAD-CANNED	TBSP	13	25	2	1	0	2	1.7	0.8	0.1
CHICKEN-BACK-FRIED-FLOUR COATED	ITEM	144	477	40	9	0.2	30	8.1	11.8	6.9
CHICKEN-BACK-STEWED	ITEM	122	316	27	0	0	22	6.1	8.7	4.9
CHICKEN-BREAST-NO SKIN-FRIED	ITEM	172	322	58	1	0	8	2.2	3	1.8
CHICKEN-BREAST-ROASTED	ITEM	196	386	58	0	0	15	4.3	5.9	3.3
CHICKEN-BREAST-STEWED	ITEM	220	404	60	0	0	16	4.6	6.4	3.5
CHICKEN-BREAST-WITH SKIN-FRIED IN BATTER	ITEM	280	728	70	25	*	37	9.9	15.3	8.6
CHICKEN-BREAST-WITH SKIN-FRIED IN FLOUR	ITEM	196	436	62	3	0.1	17	4.8	6.9	3.8
CHICKEN-CANNED-BONELESS-WITH BROTH	ITEM	142	234	31	0	0	11	3.1	4.5	2.5
CHICKEN-CAPON-ROASTED	ITEM	1274	2914	369	0	0	148	41.6	60.5	32.1
CHICKEN-DRUMSTICK-WITH SKIN-FRIED/FLOUR	ITEM	49	120	13	1	0	7	1.8	2.7	1.6
CHICKEN-GIBLETS-FRIED-FLOUR COATED	CUP	145	402	47	6	*	20	5.5	6.4	4.9
CHICKEN-GIBLETS-SIMMERED	CUP	145	228	38	1	0	7	2.2	1.7	1.6
CHICKEN-GIZZARD-SIMMERED	CUP	145	222	39	2	0	5	1.5	1.4	1.5

t = Trace of nutrient present ** = Not available*

MAG, magnesium; **IRON,** iron; **ZINC,** zinc; **VITA,** vitamin A; **VITC,** vitamin C; **THIA,** thiamin; **RIBO,** riboflavin; **NIAC,** niacin; **VB6,** vitamin B-6; **FOL,** folate; **VB12,** vitamin B-12; **CALC,** calcium; **PHOS,** phosphorus; **SEL,** selenium; **VE-a,** alpha tocopherol equivalents.

CHOL (mg)	SOD (mg)	POT (mg)	MAG (mg)	IRON (mg)	ZINC (mg)	VITA (RE)	VITC (mg)	THIA (mg)	RIBO (mg)	NIAC (mg)	VB6 (mg)	FOL (µg)	VB12 (µg)	CALC (mg)	PHOS (mg)	SEL (µg)	VE-a (mg)
0	0	0	*	0	*	0	0	0	0	0	*	*	0	0	*	*	*
0	t	15	3	0.1	t	0	0	0	0	0	0	0	0	1	1	13	0
0	2	36	0	1.4	0	0	0	0	0	0	0	0	0	14	22	74	0
0	1	140	4	1.1	*	0	0	0.16	0.38	2.6	0.14	286	0	3	90	0	t
0	9	152	18	1.4	0.6	0	0	1.25	0.34	3	0.2	313	0	17	140	0	t
0	2	121	48	0.6	0.5	0	t	0.02	0.1	0.5	0.01	10	0	43	84	*	1.5
0	3	512	328	3.8	2.8	8	1	0.58	0.13	1.3	0.7	83	0	216	359	2	27.3
0	12	602	203	2.9	3.3	15	4	0.46	0.18	1.3	0.67	79	0	113	380	23	3.1
0	14	952	385	4.8	3.8	0	1	0.27	1.01	4.4	0.15	76	0	346	676	5	31.1
0	13	842	340	4.2	3.4	0	1	0.24	0.9	3.9	0.13	68	0	306	598	5	27.6
0	11	289	0	0.7	0.1	0	4	0.09	0.11	0.2	0.19	32	0	t	0	2	*
0	3	840	315	4.8	6.4	0	1	1.4	0.17	2.3	0.35	6	0	246	840	2260	9
0	0	119	67	1.1	0.9	3	1	0.11	0.04	0.3	0.16	19	0	15	127	2	*
0	22	774	356	8.2	7.7	0	0	0.27	0.27	1.9	0.35	95	0	62	671	7	0.8
0	22	689	332	5.3	6.2	0	0	0.55	0.23	2.3	0.33	88	0	53	554	88	0.2
0	t	124	49	0.6	1.2	4	1	0.25	0.04	0.3	0.06	11	0	17	95	2	1.5
0	7	493	155	3.2	2.3	0	0	0.47	0.15	2.9	0.26	21	0	94	182	7	4.7
0	9	441	157	2.4	1.5	1	0	0.29	0.15	2.7	0.27	21	0	60	268	7	4.7
0	16	817	308	5.1	5.2	2	1	0.27	0.27	6.4	0.41	69	0	96	596	7	8.2
0	16	825	333	4.6	7.2	3	1	0.71	0.32	7.2	0.34	118	0	153	659	7	8.5
0	8	982	266	2.6	9.6	0	0	0.36	0.16	20.6	0.37	181	0	127	744	55	10
0	624	982	266	2.6	9.6	0	0	0.36	0.16	20.6	0.37	181	0	127	744	55	10
0	26	1029	245	6.7	4.8	0	0	0.93	0.2	17.6	0.51	350	0	134	549	7	12.2
0	1	423	138	2.3	5.9	14	2	0.92	0.14	1	0.2	42	0	39	314	3	3.4
0	1	395	142	2.3	6.1	*	2	0.34	0.11	1	0.21	43	0	37	324	6	1.4
0	7	1399	203	8.7	1.7	30	9	1.05	0.22	1.4	0.32	74	0	173	644	7	6.7
0	8	1242	166	4.1	1.7	31	9	0.54	0.32	1.8	0.33	76	0	90	609	7	6.7
0	4	1588	187	4.8	3.9	22	2	0.11	0.16	1.9	0.32	244	0	149	392	*	*
0	2	655	252	3.8	4.3	37	4	0.27	0.14	0.9	0.69	82	0	72	580	24	1.1
0	1	419	161	2.5	2.7	24	3	0.18	0.09	0.6	0.44	52	0	46	371	15	0.7
0	78	121	26	0.3	0.4	0	0	0.02	0.02	2.2	0.07	15	0	7	51	1	1
0	5	110	28	0.3	0.5	0	0	0.02	0.02	2.2	0.06	13	0	5	60	2	1.1
0	75	110	30	0.3	0.5	0	0	0.01	0.01	2.3	0.06	13	0	5	60	2	1
0	77	115	25	0.3	0.4	*	0	0.02	0.02	2.1	0.06	13	0	5	52	2	1.1
0	8	307	18	0.3	0.3	8	2	0.12	0.07	2.1	0.12	17	0	24	50	4	*
0	24	1114	738	20.7	10.3	53	3	0.29	0.44	2.4	0.12	79	0	59	1620	*	1.4
0	12	588	168	2.1	6.6	4	t	0.02	0.03	0.2	0.02	6	0	35	59	*	0.6
0	16	674	505	21	11.2	1	0	1.14	0.36	6.5	1.14	139	0	1404	906	*	3.3
0	3	135	101	4.2	2	t	0	0.23	0.07	1.3	0.23	28	0	281	181	*	0.6
0	4	992	509	9.8	7.3	7	2	3.29	0.36	6.5	1.81	327	0	168	1015	111	71.7
0	4	652	171	9.1	7	7	2	0.43	0.38	5.6	1.07	316	0	76	1538	104	66.8
146	126	440	50	1.8	1.7	11	0	0.12	0.2	23.6	1.02	6	0.58	26	392	46	0.6
49	46	124	12	0.7	1.3	10	0	0.04	0.12	3.4	0.18	4	0.16	6	95	21	0.2
45	617	38	5	0.9	0.5	17	0	0.03	0.05	1.4	0.14	2	0.11	43	48	10	0.1
14	166	65	5	0.3	0.2	7	0	0.02	0.04	1.5	0.06	1	0.04	12	45	*	0.1
7	50	14	2	0.3	0.2	3	0	t	0.02	0.4	0.02	t	0.02	16	12	*	t
128	130	325	33	2.3	3.6	53	0	0.15	0.34	10.5	0.44	12	0.4	35	239	25	0.5
96	78	178	20	1.5	2.4	113	0	0.05	0.18	5.3	0.18	6	0.22	22	146	25	0.4
156	136	474	54	2	1.9	12	0	0.14	0.22	25.4	1.1	8	0.62	28	424	31	0.6
166	138	480	54	2.1	2	55	0	0.13	0.23	24.9	1.08	6	0.64	28	420	53	0.7
166	136	390	48	2	2.1	54	0	0.09	0.25	17.2	0.64	6	0.46	28	344	53	0.8
238	770	564	68	3.5	2.7	57	0	0.32	0.41	29.5	1.2	16	0.82	56	516	30	1
176	150	506	58	2.3	2.1	29	0	0.16	0.26	26.9	1.14	8	0.68	32	456	21	0.7
78	714	196	17	2.3	2	100	3	0.02	0.18	9	0.5	6	0.42	20	350	20	0.4
1098	626	3252	308	18.9	22.1	260	0	0.89	2.17	114	5.5	70	4.14	182	3140	227	4.5
44	44	112	11	0.7	1.4	12	0	0.04	0.11	3	0.17	4	0.16	6	86	5	0.2
647	164	478	37	15	9.1	5195	13	0.14	2.21	15.9	0.88	550	19.3	26	414	25	2
570	85	229	30	9.3	6.6	3234	12	0.13	1.38	6	0.49	545	14.7	18	331	25	2
281	97	259	29	6	6.4	82	2	0.04	0.35	5.8	0.17	77	2.81	14	225	25	*

WT, weight; **KCAL**, kcalories; **PROT**, protein; **CARB**, carbohydrate; **FIBR**, fiber; **FAT**, fat; **SATF**, saturated fat;

MONO, monsaturated fat; **POLY**, polyunsaturated fat; **CHOL**, cholesterol; **SOD**, sodium; **POT**, potassium;

FOOD NAME	PORTION	WT (g)	KCAL	PROT (g)	CARB (g)	FIBR (g)	FAT (g)	SATF (g)	MONO (g)	POLY (g)
CHICKEN-HEART-SIMMERED	CUP	145	268	38	t	0	12	3.3	2.9	3.3
CHICKEN-LEG-NO SKIN-ROASTED	ITEM	95	182	26	0	0	8	2.2	2.9	1.9
CHICKEN-LEG-NO SKIN-STEWED	ITEM	101	187	27	0	0	8	2.2	3	1.9
CHICKEN-LEG-ROASTED	ITEM	114	265	30	0	0	15	4.2	6	3.4
CHICKEN-LIVER PATE-CANNED	TBSP	13	26	2	1	0	2	0.5	0.7	0.3
CHICKEN-LIVER-SIMMERED	CUP	140	219	34	1	0	8	2.6	1.9	1.3
CHICKEN-THIGH-FRIED-FLOUR COATED	ITEM	62	162	17	2	t	9	2.5	3.6	2.1
CHICKEN-THIN SLICED-SMOKED-LAND O FROST	SERVING	28.4	60	5	1	0	4	1	1.4	0.8
CHICKEN-WING-FRIED-FLOUR COATED	ITEM	32	103	8	1	0	7	1.9	2.8	1.6
CHICKEN-WING-ROASTED	ITEM	34	99	9	0	0	7	1.9	2.6	1.4
CHICKEN-WING-STEWED	ITEM	40	100	9	0	0	7	1.9	2.6	1.4
DUCK-FLESH & SKIN-ROASTED	ITEM	764	2574	145	0	0	217	73.9	98.6	27.9
DUCK-NO SKIN-ROASTED	ITEM	442	890	104	0	0	50	18.4	16.4	6.3
GOOSE-FLESH & SKIN-ROASTED	ITEM	1548	4721	389	0	0	339	106	159	39
GOOSE-LIVER PATE-SMOKED-CANNED	TBSP	13	60	1	1	0	6	*	*	*
GOOSE-NO SKIN-ROASTED	ITEM	1182	2813	342	0	0	150	53.9	51.3	18.3
TURKEY HAM-CURED THIGH MEAT	SLICE	28.4	37	5	t	0	1	0.5	0.3	0.4
TURKEY LOAF-BREAST	SERVING	28.4	31	6	0	0	t	0.1	0.1	0.1
TURKEY PASTRAMI	SLICE	28.4	40	5	t	0	2	1	0.6	0.5
TURKEY ROLL-LIGHT	OUNCE	28.4	42	5	t	0	2	0.6	0.7	0.5
TURKEY ROLL-LIGHT AND DARK	OUNCE	28.4	42	5	1	0	2	0.6	0.7	0.5
TURKEY-BREAST-NO SKIN-ROASTED	ITEM	612	826	184	0	0	5	1.4	0.8	1.2
TURKEY-DARK MEAT-NO SKIN-ROASTED	CUP	140	262	40	0	0	10	3.4	2.3	3
TURKEY-GIBLETS-SIMMERED	CUP	145	242	39	3	0	7	2.2	1.7	1.7
TURKEY-GIZZARD-SIMMERED	CUP	145	236	43	1	0	6	1.6	1.1	1.6
TURKEY-LIGHT MEAT-NO SKIN-ROASTED	CUP	140	219	42	0	0	5	1.4	0.8	1.2
TURKEY-LIGHT/DARK MEAT-NO SKIN-ROASTED	CUP	140	238	41	0	0	7	2.3	1.5	2
TURKEY-LIVER-SIMMERED	CUP	140	237	34	5	0	8	2.6	2.1	1.5
TURKEY-THIN SLICED-SMOKED-LAND O FROST	SERVING	28.4	50	5	1	0	3	0.8	0.9	0.7
SAUCES & DIPS										
CATSUP-TOMATO-HEINZ LITE	TBSP	15	8	t	2	*	0	0	0	0
CATSUP-TOMATO-LOW SODIUM-HEINZ	TBSP	15	8	t	2	*	0	0	0	0
DIP-BACON AND HORSERADISH-KRAFT	TBSP	15	30	1	2	*	3	*	*	*
DIP-BUTTERMILK-KRAFT	TBSP	15	40	1	1	*	4	*	*	*
DIP-CLAM-KRAFT	TBSP	15	30	1	2	*	2	*	*	*
DIP-FRENCH ONION-KRAFT	TBSP	15	30	1	2	*	2	*	*	*
DIP-GARLIC-KRAFT	TBSP	15	30	1	2	*	2	*	*	*
DIP-GREEN ONION-KRAFT	TBSP	15	25	1	2	*	2	*	*	*
DIP-GUACAMOLE-KRAFT	TBSP	15	25	1	2	*	2	*	*	*
DIP-JALAPENO BEAN-FRITOS	OUNCE	28.4	33	2	3	1.9	1	0.2	0.4	0.9
DIP-JALAPENO PEPPER-KRAFT	TBSP	15	25	1	2	*	2	*	*	*
GRAVY-BEEF-CANNED	CUP	233	123	9	11	0.1	5	2.7	2.2	0.2
GRAVY-BROWN-FROM DRY-PREPARED WITH WATER	CUP	258	75	2	13	t	2	0.8	0.7	0.1
GRAVY-CHICKEN-CANNED	CUP	238	188	5	13	2.1	14	3.4	6.1	3.4
GRAVY-MUSHROOM-CANNED	CUP	238	119	3	13	1	6	1	2.8	2.4
GRAVY-PORK-FROM DRY-PREPARED WITH WATER	CUP	258	77	2	13	*	2	0.7	0.9	0.2
GRAVY-TURKEY-CANNED	CUP	238	121	6	12	*	5	1.5	2.1	1.2
HORSERADISH-PREPARED	TBSP	15	6	t	1	0.3	0	0	0	0
MUSTARD-BROWN-PREPARED	CUP	250	228	15	13	2.1	16	7.7	14	30.8
MUSTARD-LOW SODIUM-FEATHERWEIGHT	TSP	5	4	t	t	*	t	*	*	*
MUSTARD-YELLOW-PREPARED	TSP	5	5	t	t	0.1	t	0	0	0
SAUCE-BARBECUE-READY TO SERVE	CUP	250	188	5	32	2.3	5	0.7	1.9	1.7
SAUCE-BEARNAISE-FROM DRY MIX-MILK/BUTTER	CUP	255	701	8	18	0.1	68	41.8	19.9	3
SAUCE-CHEESE-FROM DRY MIX-MILK/BUTTER	CUP	279	307	16	23	0.1	17	9.3	5.3	1.6
SAUCE-CHILI-BOTTLED	TBSP	15	16	t	4	*	0	0	0	0
SAUCE-CHILI-LOW SODIUM	TBSP	14.2	8	0	2	*	0	0	0	0
SAUCE-CURRY-FROM DRY MIX-MADE WITH MILK	CUP	272	269	11	26	0.9	15	6	5.1	2.8
SAUCE-HOLLANDAISE-DRY MIX-MADE WITH MILK	CUP	255	703	8	18	0.1	68	41.9	20	2.9
SAUCE-MARINARA-CANNED	CUP	250	170	4	26	*	8	1.2	4.3	2.3
SAUCE-MUSHROOM-DRY MIX-MADE WITH MILK	CUP	267	227	11	24	0.5	10	5.4	3.3	1.1
SAUCE-PICANTE-CANNED	FL OZ	16	9	t	2	*	1	0	0	0
SAUCE-SALSA WITH GREEN CHILIES-CANNED	FL OZ	16	10	t	2	*	1	0	0	0
SAUCE-SOUR CREAM-FROM MIX-WITH MILK	CUP	314	509	19	45	*	30	16.1	9.9	2.8

t = Trace of nutrient present ** = Not available*

MAG, magnesium; **IRON**, iron; **ZINC**, zinc; **VITA**, vitamin A; **VITC**, vitamin C; **THIA**, thiamin; **RIBO**, riboflavin; **NIAC**, niacin; **VB6**, vitamin B-6; **FOL**, folate; **VB12**, vitamin B-12; **CALC**, calcium; **PHOS**, phosphorus; **SEL**, selenium; **VE-a**, alpha tocopherol equivalents.

CHOL (mg)	SOD (mg)	POT (mg)	MAG (mg)	IRON (mg)	ZINC (mg)	VITA (RE)	VITC (mg)	THIA (mg)	RIBO (mg)	NIAC (mg)	VB6 (mg)	FOL (µg)	VB12 (µg)	CALC (mg)	PHOS (mg)	SEL (µg)	VE-a (mg)
350	70	192	29	13.1	10.6	12	3	0.1	1.07	4.1	0.47	116	10.6	27	289	71	1.7
89	87	230	23	1.2	2.7	18	0	0.07	0.22	6	0.35	8	0.31	12	174	13	0.3
90	78	192	21	1.4	2.8	18	0	0.06	0.22	4.9	0.22	8	0.23	11	151	13	0.4
105	99	256	26	1.5	3	46	0	0.08	0.24	7.1	0.37	8	0.35	14	199	16	0.4
51	50	12	2	1.2	0.3	28	1	0.01	0.18	1	0.03	42	1.05	1	23	*	t
883	71	196	29	11.9	6.1	6886	22	0.21	2.45	6.2	0.82	1077	27.1	20	437	99	3.4
60	55	147	15	0.9	1.6	18	0	0.06	0.15	4.3	0.21	5	0.19	8	116	11	0.2
21	182	49	5	0.4	0.5	0	0	0	0.03	1.6	0.07	2	0.06	0	39	*	0.1
26	25	57	6	0.4	0.6	12	0	0.02	0.04	2.1	0.13	1	0.09	5	48	6	0.1
29	28	62	7	0.4	0.6	16	0	0.01	0.04	2.3	0.14	1	0.1	5	51	6	0.1
28	27	56	6	0.5	0.7	16	0	0.02	0.04	1.9	0.09	1	0.07	5	48	6	0.1
640	454	1560	124	20.6	14.2	483	0	1.33	2.06	36.9	1.4	50	2.26	86	1190	*	5.3
396	286	1114	88	11.9	11.5	103	0	1.15	2.08	22.5	1.1	44	1.76	52	898	*	3.1
1416	1084	5092	341	43.8	40.6	325	0	1.19	5	64.5	5.73	31	6.35	201	4180	*	26.8
20	91	18	2	0.7	0.1	130	t	0.01	0.04	0.3	0.01	8	1.22	9	26	*	0
1138	898	4586	296	33.9	499	142	0	1.09	4.61	48.2	5.5	142	5.56	165	3652	*	21
16	283	92	5	0.8	0.8	0	0	0.02	0.07	1	0.07	2	0.07	3	54	*	0.2
12	406	79	6	0.1	0.3	0	0	0.01	0.03	2.4	0.1	1	0.57	2	65	*	0.1
15	297	74	4	0.5	0.6	0	0	0.02	0.07	1	0.08	1	0.07	3	57	*	0.1
12	139	71	5	0.4	0.4	0	0	0.03	0.06	2	0.09	1	0.07	11	52	*	0.1
16	166	77	5	0.4	0.6	0	0	0.03	0.08	1.4	0.08	1	0.07	9	48	*	0.1
510	318	1784	178	9.4	10.6	0	0	0.26	0.8	45.9	3.42	38	2.36	76	1370	49	0.6
119	110	406	34	3.3	6.3	0	0	0.09	0.35	5.1	0.5	13	0.52	45	286	35	0.9
606	86	290	25	9.7	5.3	2629	3	0.07	1.31	6.5	0.47	501	34.8	19	296	*	0.2
336	79	306	27	7.9	6	81	2	0.05	0.47	4.5	0.17	75	2.76	22	186	*	3.4
97	89	426	39	1.9	2.9	0	0	0.09	0.18	9.6	0.75	8	0.52	27	307	*	0.1
107	99	418	37	2.5	4.3	0	0	0.09	0.26	7.6	0.64	10	0.52	35	298	35	0.9
876	89	272	21	10.9	4.3	5288	3	0.07	1.99	8.3	0.73	932	66.5	15	381	*	4
23	283	80	7	0.4	0.8	0	0	0	0.03	1.2	0.12	2	0.1	40	58	*	0.1
0	110	54	*	0.1	*	21	2	0.01	0.01	0.2	*	*	*	7	8	0	*
0	90	54	*	0.1	*	21	2	0.01	0.01	0.2	*	*	*	7	8	0	*
0	100	*	*	*	*	*	*	*	*	*	*	*	*	*	*	*	*
3	135	*	*	*	*	*	*	*	*	*	*	*	*	*	*	*	*
5	115	*	*	*	*	*	*	*	*	*	*	*	*	*	*	*	*
0	120	*	*	*	*	*	*	*	*	*	*	*	*	*	*	*	*
0	80	*	*	*	*	*	*	*	*	*	*	*	*	*	*	*	*
0	85	*	*	*	*	*	*	*	*	*	*	*	*	*	*	*	*
0	108	*	*	*	*	*	*	*	*	*	*	*	*	*	*	*	*
1	163	77	9	0.4	0.1	4	0	0.02	0.03	1.1	0.03	20	0	7	23	6	0.3
0	80	*	*	*	*	*	*	*	*	*	*	*	*	*	*	*	*
7	1305	189	5	1.6	2.3	0	0	0.08	0.08	1.5	0.02	5	0.23	14	70	*	*
3	1076	57	10	0.2	0.3	0	0	0.04	0.09	0.8	0	0	0	66	44	*	*
5	1373	260	5	1.1	1.9	264	0	0.04	0.1	1.1	0.02	5	0.24	48	69	*	1.7
0	1357	252	5	1.6	1.7	0	0	0.08	0.15	1.6	0.05	29	0	17	36	*	t
3	1235	57	10	0.3	0.3	0	2	0.05	0.06	0.8	0.03	3	0.16	31	44	*	*
5	1373	259	5	1.7	1.9	0	0	0.05	0.19	3.1	0.02	5	0	10	69	*	*
0	165	44	3	0.1	0.1	0	3	t	t	t	0.01	t	0	9	5	*	t
0	3268	325	46	4.5	0.8	0	2	0.07	0.02	0.4	0.09	11	0	310	335	*	4.4
0	1	7	*	0.1	*	*	*	*	*	*	*	*	*	4	4	3	0.1
0	65	7	2	0.1	*	*	*	*	*	*	*	*	*	4	4	0	0.1
0	2032	435	45	2.3	0.5	218	18	0.08	0.05	2.3	0.19	10	0	48	50	*	3.3
189	1265	298	26	0.3	0.8	757	2	0.08	0.26	0.3	0.08	10	0.51	230	186	*	*
53	1566	554	47	0.3	1	117	2	0.15	0.56	0.3	0.14	13	1.12	570	437	*	*
0	201	56	*	0.1	*	21	2	0.01	0.01	0.2	*	*	*	3	8	0	*
0	10	*	*	*	*	*	*	*	*	*	*	*	*	*	*	*	*
35	1276	495	46	1.1	1.1	41	3	0.11	0.54	0.5	0.11	16	1.09	484	280	*	*
189	1134	309	26	0.2	0.8	696	2	0.08	0.33	0.2	0.08	10	0.51	240	194	*	*
0	1573	1060	60	2	0.7	240	32	0.11	0.15	4	0.62	34	0	45	88	*	*
34	1535	494	37	0.5	1.3	94	2	0.19	0.8	4.8	0.19	40	0.8	302	166	*	0.7
0	218	77	*	0.3	*	23	9	0.02	0.01	0.2	*	*	*	4	8	*	*
0	111	87	*	0.3	*	39	9	0.02	0.01	0.3	*	*	*	4	9	*	*
91	1007	733	44	0.6	1.4	144	3	0.13	0.7	0.6	0.13	16	0.94	546	*	*	*

WT, weight; **KCAL**, kcalories; **PROT**, protein; **CARB**, carbohydrate; **FIBR**, fiber; **FAT**, fat; **SATF**, saturated fat;

MONO, monsaturated fat; **POLY**, polyunsaturated fat; **CHOL**, cholesterol; **SOD**, sodium; **POT**, potassium;

FOOD NAME	PORTION	WT (g)	KCAL	PROT (g)	CARB (g)	FIBR (g)	FAT (g)	SATF (g)	MONO (g)	POLY (g)
SAUCE-SOY	TBSP	18	10	1	2	0	t	t	t	t
SAUCE-SOY-TAMARI	TBSP	18	11	2	1	0	t	t	t	t
SAUCE-SPAGHETTI-TOMATO BASED-CANNED	CUP	249	271	5	40	*	12	1.7	6.1	3.3
SAUCE-STEAK-HEINZ 57	TBSP	15	15	t	3	*	t	0	0	0
SAUCE-STROGANOFF-FROM MIX-PREPARED	CUP	296	272	12	34	1.2	11	6.8	3	0.4
SAUCE-SWEET/SOUR-FROM MIX-PREPARED	CUP	313	294	1	73	1.9	t	t	t	t
SAUCE-TABASCO	TSP	5	0	t	t	0	0	0	0	0
SAUCE-TACO-CANNED	FL OZ	16	11	t	2	*	1	*	*	*
SAUCE-TARTAR-REGULAR	TBSP	14	75	0	1	*	8	1.5	1.8	4.1
SAUCE-TERIYAKI-BOTTLED-READY TO SERVE	TBSP	18	15	1	3	t	0	0	0	0
SAUCE-TERIYAKI-FROM MIX-PREPARED-WATER	CUP	283	130	4	28	0.1	1	0.1	0.2	0.5
SAUCE-TOMATO-CANNED-LOW SODIUM-S&W	CUP	226	90	4	18	3.4	0	0	0	0
SAUCE-TOMATO-CANNED-SALT ADDED	CUP	245	74	3	18	3.7	t	0.1	0.1	0.2
SAUCE-TOMATO-SPANISH-CANNED	CUP	244	81	4	18	3.7	1	0.1	0.1	0.3
SAUCE-TOMATO-WITH HERBS/CHEESE-CANNED	CUP	244	144	5	25	3.7	5	1.5	0.9	2
SAUCE-TOMATO-WITH MUSHROOMS-CANNED	CUP	245	86	4	21	3.7	t	t	t	0.1
SAUCE-TOMATO-WITH ONIONS-CANNED	CUP	245	103	4	24	3.7	t	0.1	0.1	0.2
SAUCE-WHITE-DEHYDRATED-PREPARED-MILK	CUP	264	240	10	21	0.1	14	6.4	4.7	1.7
SAUCE-WHITE-MEDIUM-WITH ENRICHED FLOUR	CUP	250	405	10	22	0.4	31	19.3	7.8	0.8
SAUCE-WORCESTERSHIRE	TBSP	15	12	t	3	0	0	0	0	0
TOMATO CATSUP	TBSP	15	15	0	4	0.2	0	0	0	0
SOUPS										
SOUP-BEAN WITH BACON-CANNED-WITH WATER	CUP	253	173	8	23	3.2	6	1.5	2.2	1.8
SOUP-BEEF BROTH-CANNED-READY TO EAT	CUP	240	17	3	t	0	1	0.3	0.2	t
SOUP-BEEF BROTH-DEHYDRATED-CUBED	ITEM	3.6	6	1	1	0	t	0.1	0.1	t
SOUP-BEEF NOODLE-CANNED-PREPARED-WATER	CUP	244	84	5	9	1.5	3	1.2	1.2	0.5
SOUP-BEEF-CHUNKY-CANNED-READY TO SERVE	CUP	240	170	12	20	*	5	2.6	2.1	0.2
SOUP-BLACK BEAN-CANNED-PREPARED-WATER	CUP	247	116	6	20	*	2	0.4	0.5	0.5
SOUP-CHEESE-CANNED-PREPARED WITH MILK	CUP	251	230	9	16	2	15	9.1	4.1	0.4
SOUP-CHICKEN AND DUMPLINGS-CANNED-MILK	CUP	241	96	6	6	0.7	6	1.3	2.5	1.3
SOUP-CHICKEN BROTH-CANNED-PREPARED-WATER	CUP	244	39	5	1	0	1	0.4	0.6	0.3
SOUP-CHICKEN NOODLE-CANNED-WITH WATER	CUP	241	75	4	9	1.5	2	0.7	1.1	0.6
SOUP-CHICKEN NOODLE-LOW SODIUM	CUP	240	91	5	10	1.4	2	0.7	1.1	0.6
SOUP-CHICKEN NOODLE-PREPARED FROM DRY	CUP	252	53	3	7	0.2	1	0.3	0.5	0.4
SOUP-CHICKEN-CHUNKY-CANNED-READY TO EAT	CUP	251	178	13	17	0.8	7	2	3	1.4
SOUP-CHICKEN-CHUNKY-LOW SODIUM	CUP	251	173	13	15	*	5	*	*	*
SOUP-CHICKEN/RICE-CANNED-READY TO SERVE	CUP	240	127	12	13	1.4	3	1	1.4	0.7
SOUP-CHILI-BEEF-CANNED-PREPARED-WATER	CUP	250	170	7	22	*	7	3.4	2.8	0.3
SOUP-CLAM CHOWDER-MANHATTAN STYLE-WATER	CUP	244	78	2	12	2.1	2	0.4	0.4	1.3
SOUP-CLAM CHOWDER-NEW ENGLAND-WITH MILK	CUP	248	163	9	17	1.5	7	3	2.3	1.1
SOUP-CLAM CHOWDER-NEW ENGLAND-WITH WATER	CUP	244	95	5	12	1.5	3	0.4	1.2	1.1
SOUP-CONSOMME-CANNED-PREPARED WITH WATER	CUP	241	29	5	2	*	0	0	0	*
SOUP-CORN-CANNED-LOW SODIUM-CAMPBELLS	SERVING	305	191	3	31	*	5	*	*	*
SOUP-CRAB-CANNED-READY TO SERVE	CUP	244	76	5	10	*	2	0.4	0.7	0.4
SOUP-CREAM OF ASPARAGUS-CANNED-WITH MILK	CUP	248	161	6	16	0.8	8	3.3	2.1	2.2
SOUP-CREAM OF CELERY-CANNED-WITH MILK	CUP	248	164	6	15	0.8	10	3.9	2.5	2.7
SOUP-CREAM OF CHICKEN-CANNED-WITH MILK	CUP	248	191	7	15	0.5	12	4.6	4.5	1.6
SOUP-CREAM OF CHICKEN-CANNED-WITH WATER	CUP	244	117	3	9	0.5	7	2.1	3.3	1.5
SOUP-CREAM OF MUSHROOM-CANNED-WITH MILK	CUP	248	203	6	15	0.5	14	5.1	3	4.6
SOUP-CREAM OF MUSHROOM-CANNED-WITH WATER	CUP	244	129	2	9	0.9	9	2.4	1.7	4.2
SOUP-CREAM OF POTATO-CANNED-WITH MILK	CUP	248	148	6	17	0.5	6	3.8	1.7	0.6
SOUP-CREAM OF SHRIMP-CANNED-WITH MILK	CUP	248	164	7	14	0.2	9	5.8	2.7	0.3
SOUP-ESCAROLE-CANNED-READY TO SERVE	CUP	248	27	2	2	*	2	0.5	0.8	0.4
SOUP-GAZPACHO-CANNED-READY TO SERVE	CUP	244	57	9	1	*	2	0.3	0.5	1.3
SOUP-LENTIL WITH HAM-CANNED-READY TO EAT	CUP	248	139	9	20	*	3	1.1	1.3	0.3
SOUP-MINESTRONE-CANNED-PREPARED-WATER	CUP	241	82	4	11	1.9	3	0.6	0.7	1.1
SOUP-ONION-CANNED-PREPARED WITH WATER	CUP	241	58	4	8	*	2	0.3	0.7	0.7
SOUP-ONION-DEHYDRATED-PACKET	SERVING	39	115	5	21	2.2	2	0.5	1.4	0.3
SOUP-ONION-DEHYDRATED-PREPARED-WATER	CUP	246	27	1	5	0.4	1	0.1	0.3	0.1
SOUP-OYSTER STEW-CANNED-PREPARED-MILK	CUP	245	134	6	10	*	8	5.1	2.1	0.3
SOUP-OYSTER STEW-CANNED-PREPARED-WATER	CUP	241	58	2	4	*	4	2.5	0.9	0.2
SOUP-PEA GREEN-CANNED-PREPARED WITH MILK	CUP	254	239	13	32	2.8	7	4	2.2	0.5

t = Trace of nutrient present   ** = Not available*

MAG, magnesium; **IRON,** iron; **ZINC,** zinc; **VITA,** vitamin A; **VITC,** vitamin C; **THIA,** thiamin; **RIBO,** riboflavin; **NIAC,** niacin; **VB6,** vitamin B-6; **FOL,** folate; **VB12,** vitamin B-12; **CALC,** calcium; **PHOS,** phosphorus; **SEL,** selenium; **VE-a,** alpha tocopherol equivalents.

CHOL (mg)	SOD (mg)	POT (mg)	MAG (mg)	IRON (mg)	ZINC (mg)	VITA (RE)	VITC (mg)	THIA (mg)	RIBO (mg)	NIAC (mg)	VB6 (mg)	FOL (µg)	VB12 (µg)	CALC (mg)	PHOS (mg)	SEL (µg)	VE-a (mg)
0	1029	32	6	0.4	0.1	0	0	0.01	0.02	0.6	0.03	3	0	3	20	*	0
0	1005	38	7	0.4	0.1	0	0	0.01	0.03	0.7	0.04	3	0	4	23	*	0
0	1235	956	60	1.6	0.5	306	28	0.14	0.15	3.8	0.88	54	0	70	90	*	*
0	265	*	*	*	*	*	*	*	*	*	*	*	*	*	*	0	*
39	1829	672	39	1.3	1.1	127	1	0.86	0.77	0.8	0.12	9	0.59	521	302	*	*
0	779	66	9	1.6	0.1	0	0	0.01	0.1	0.9	0.31	2	0	41	188	*	1.4
0	22	3	1	t	t	3	3	0	0.01	0	0.01	1	0	t	1	*	t
0	128	88	*	0.3	*	4	6	0.02	0.01	0.3	*	*	*	6	10	*	*
9	98	11	*	0.1	*	3	0	0	0	0	*	*	*	3	4	*	7
0	690	41	11	0.3	t	0	0	0.01	0.01	0.2	0.02	4	0	5	28	*	0.1
0	4791	216	85	2.8	0.1	0	0	0.03	0.09	1.3	0.14	28	0	113	215	*	1.2
0	65	838	43	1.7	0.6	221	30	0.16	0.14	2.6	0.36	20	0	32	72	2	2.9
0	1482	908	47	1.9	0.6	240	32	0.16	0.14	2.8	0.38	23	0	34	78	*	*
0	1152	900	46	8.5	0.8	242	21	0.18	0.15	3.2	0.43	33	0	42	117	*	*
*	1325	869	46	2.1	0.9	240	25	0.19	0.3	3	0.05	20	0	90	132	*	*
0	1107	931	47	2.2	0.5	233	30	0.18	0.27	3.1	0.33	23	0	32	78	*	*
0	1350	1012	47	2.3	0.6	208	31	0.18	0.33	3	0.65	55	0	42	96	*	*
34	797	443	264	0.3	0.5	92	3	0.08	0.45	0.5	0.07	16	1.06	425	256	*	3.9
33	796	348	38	0.5	0.5	115	2	0.12	0.43	0.7	0.06	12	0.7	288	233	*	3.7
0	147	120	2	0.9	t	5	27	0	0.03	0	0	0	0	15	9	*	0
0	156	54	4	0.1	t	21	2	0.01	0.01	0.2	0.02	1	0	3	8	0	0.3
3	952	403	44	2.1	1	89	2	0.09	0.03	0.6	0.04	32	0.05	81	132	8	*
0	782	130	5	0.4	0	0	0	0.01	0.05	1.9	0.02	5	0.17	14	31	8	*
t	864	15	2	0.1	t	1	0	0.01	0.01	0.1	0.01	1	0.04	2	8	0	t
5	952	99	6	1.1	1.5	63	t	0.07	0.06	1.1	0.04	4	0.2	15	46	8	0.8
14	866	336	5	2.3	2.6	261	7	0.06	0.15	2.7	0.13	13	0.61	31	120	8	*
0	1198	273	42	2.2	1.4	49	1	0.08	0.05	0.5	0.09	25	0.02	45	107	8	*
48	1020	340	20	0.8	0.7	147	1	0.06	0.33	0.5	0.08	10	0.44	288	250	8	0.4
34	860	116	5	0.6	0.4	52	0	0.02	0.07	1.8	0.04	2	0.16	15	60	8	0
1	776	210	2	0.5	0.2	0	0	0.01	0.07	3.4	0.02	5	0.24	9	73	8	*
7	1106	55	5	0.8	0.4	72	t	0.05	0.06	1.4	0.03	2	0.15	17	36	8	0.1
7	36	106	5	1.2	0.4	109	t	0.17	0.14	2.6	0.03	2	0.14	17	36	8	0.1
3	1283	30	8	0.5	0.2	6	t	0.07	0.06	0.9	0.01	2	0	33	33	8	*
30	887	176	8	1.7	1	130	1	0.09	0.17	4.4	0.05	5	0.25	24	113	8	0.1
*	78	264	*	1.8	*	94	2	0.13	0.25	4.8	*	*	*	28	*	8	*
12	888	108	10	1.9	1	586	4	0.02	0.1	4.1	0.05	4	0.31	35	72	8	0.1
13	1035	525	30	2.1	1.4	151	4	0.06	0.08	1.1	0.16	18	0.32	43	148	8	*
2	578	188	12	1.6	1	96	4	0.03	0.04	0.8	0.1	10	4.05	27	42	8	0.2
22	992	300	23	1.5	0.8	40	4	0.07	0.24	1	0.13	10	10.3	187	157	8	0.1
5	915	146	7	1.5	0.8	1	2	0.02	0.04	1	0.08	4	8	44	54	8	0.1
0	636	154	0	0.5	0.4	0	1	0.02	0.03	0.7	0.02	3	0	10	31	8	*
*	33	164	*	0.8	*	93	6	0.1	0.15	1.9	*	*	*	28	*	8	*
10	1234	326	88	1.2	1.5	50	0	0.2	0.07	1.3	0.12	15	0.2	66	88	8	*
22	1041	359	20	0.9	0.9	83	4	0.1	0.28	0.9	0.06	30	0.5	175	153	8	0.8
32	1009	310	22	0.7	0.2	68	1	0.07	0.25	0.4	0.06	9	0.5	186	151	8	1
27	1046	273	18	0.7	0.7	94	1	0.07	0.26	0.9	0.07	8	0.55	180	152	8	0.2
10	986	88	2	0.6	0.6	56	t	0.03	0.06	0.8	0.02	2	0.1	34	37	8	0.2
20	1076	270	20	0.6	0.6	38	2	0.08	0.28	0.9	0.06	10	0.5	178	156	8	1.3
2	1031	101	5	0.5	0.6	0	1	0.05	0.09	0.7	0.02	5	0.05	46	50	*	1.2
22	1060	323	17	0.5	0.7	67	1	0.08	0.24	0.6	0.09	9	0.5	166	160	8	0.1
35	1036	248	22	0.6	0.8	54	1	0.06	0.23	0.5	0.45	10	1.04	164	337	8	3.3
2	3864	265	5	0.7	2.2	217	4	0.07	0.05	2.3	0.22	35	0.5	32	79	8	*
0	1183	224	7	1	0.2	20	3	0.05	0.02	0.9	0.15	10	0	24	37	8	*
7	1319	357	22	2.7	0.7	36	4	0.17	0.11	1.4	0.22	50	0.3	42	184	8	*
2	911	313	7	0.9	0.7	234	1	0.05	0.04	0.9	0.1	16	0	34	55	8	*
0	1053	68	2	0.7	0.6	0	1	0.03	0.02	0.6	0.05	15	0	27	12	8	*
2	3493	260	25	0.6	0.2	1	1	0.11	0.24	2	0.04	6	0	55	126	0	t
0	849	64	5	0.1	0.1	0	t	0.03	0.06	0.5	0	1	0	12	30	*	*
32	1040	235	21	1	10.3	45	4	0.07	0.23	0.3	0.06	10	2.63	167	162	8	*
15	981	48	5	1	10.3	7	3	0.02	0.04	0.2	0.01	2	2.19	22	48	8	*
18	1048	377	55	2	1.8	58	3	0.16	0.27	1.3	0.1	8	0.44	173	238	8	0.2

WT, weight; **KCAL**, kcalories; **PROT**, protein; **CARB**, carbohydrate; **FIBR**, fiber; **FAT**, fat; **SATF**, saturated fat;

MONO, monsaturated fat; **POLY**, polyunsaturated fat; **CHOL**, cholesterol; **SOD**, sodium; **POT**, potassium;

FOOD NAME	PORTION	WT (g)	KCAL	PROT (g)	CARB (g)	FIBR (g)	FAT (g)	SATF (g)	MONO (g)	POLY (g)
SOUP-PEA GREEN-CANNED-PREPARED/WATER	CUP	250	165	9	27	2.8	3	1.4	1	0.4
SOUP-PEA GREEN-LOW SODIUM-CANNED-WATER	CUP	250	165	9	27	0.8	3	1.4	1	0.4
SOUP-PEA-SPLIT-CANNED-PREPARED-WATER	CUP	253	189	10	28	2.8	4	1.8	1.8	0.6
SOUP-PEPPERPOT-CANNED-PREPARED/WATER	CUP	241	103	6	9	*	5	2.1	2	0.4
SOUP-TOMATO BEEF & NOODLE-CANNED/WATER	CUP	244	139	4	21	1.5	4	1.6	1.7	0.7
SOUP-TOMATO BISQUE-CANNED-PREPARED/MILK	CUP	251	198	6	29	*	7	3.1	1.9	1.2
SOUP-TOMATO BISQUE-LOW SODIUM-WITH WATER	CUP	247	123	2	24	*	3	0.5	0.7	1.1
SOUP-TOMATO RICE-CANNED-PREPARED/WATER	CUP	247	119	2	22	1.7	3	0.5	0.6	1.4
SOUP-TOMATO VEGETABLE-PREPARED FROM DRY	CUP	253	56	2	10	1.1	1	0.4	0.3	0.1
SOUP-TOMATO-CANNED-PREPARED WITH MILK	CUP	248	161	6	22	0.8	6	2.9	1.6	1.1
SOUP-TOMATO-CANNED-PREPARED WITH WATER	CUP	244	85	2	17	0.9	2	0.4	0.4	1
SOUP-TURKEY NOODLE-CANNED-PREPARED/WATER	CUP	244	68	4	9	0.7	2	0.6	0.8	0.5
SOUP-TURKEY NOODLE-LOW SODIUM-WITH WATER	CUP	244	68	4	9	*	2	0.6	0.8	0.5
SOUP-TURKEY VEGETABLE-CANNED-WATER	CUP	241	72	3	9	1	3	0.9	1.3	0.7
SOUP-TURKEY-CHUNKY-CANNED-READY TO SERVE	CUP	236	135	10	14	2.5	4	1.2	1.8	1.1
SOUP-VEGETABLE BEEF-CANNED-LOW SODIUM	SERVING	305	165	12	18	1.2	4	1.1	1	0.1
SOUP-VEGETABLE BEEF-CANNED-WITH WATER	CUP	245	78	6	10	1	2	0.9	0.8	0.1
SOUP-VEGETABLE-CANNED-LOW SODIUM	CUP	240	98	2	14	3.1	0	0	0	0
SOUP-VEGETARIAN-CANNED-PREPARED-WATER	CUP	241	72	2	12	1.2	2	0.3	0.8	0.7
SOUP-VICHYSSOISE-CANNED-PREPARED/MILK	CUP	248	148	6	17	*	6	3.8	1.7	0.6
SUGARS & SWEETS										
APPLE BUTTER	TBSP	20	37	t	9	0.2	t	t	t	t
CANDY-ALMOND JOY	OUNCE	28.4	151	2	19	0.3	8	1.7	2.5	1.7
CANDY-BIT O HONEY	OUNCE	28.4	121	1	21	*	4	1.7	1.6	0.2
CANDY-CARAMELS-PLAIN/CHOCOLATE	OUNCE	28.4	115	1	22	0.8	3	1.6	1.1	0.1
CANDY-CHOCOLATE COATED PEANUTS	OUNCE	28.4	160	5	11	*	12	4	4.7	2.1
CANDY-CHOCOLATE-SEMISWEET	CUP	170	860	7	97	8.8	61	36.2	19.8	1.7
CANDY-FONDANT-UNCOATED	OUNCE	28.4	105	0	25	0	1	0.1	0.3	0.1
CANDY-FUDGE-CHOCOLATE-PLAIN	OUNCE	28.4	115	1	21	0.4	3	1.3	1.4	0.6
CANDY-GUM DROPS	OUNCE	28.4	100	0	25	0	0	0	0	0
CANDY-HARD	OUNCE	28.4	110	0	28	0	0	0	0	0
CANDY-JELLY BEANS	ITEM	2.8	7	0	3	0	0	0	0	0
CANDY-KIT KAT BAR	ITEM	43	210	3	25	0.6	11	5.6	3.8	0.4
CANDY-LIFE SAVERS	ITEM	2	8	0	2	0	t	0	0	0
CANDY-LOLLIPOP	ITEM	28.4	108	0	28	0	0	0	0	0
CANDY-M & M-PLAIN-PACKAGE	ITEM	45	220	3	31	*	10	*	*	*
CANDY-MILK CHOCOLATE BAR-NO SUGAR	ITEM	10.1	60	1	5	*	4	*	*	*
CANDY-MILK CHOCOLATE WITH ALMONDS	OUNCE	28.4	151	3	15	1.3	10	4.1	3.9	1.4
CANDY-MILK CHOCOLATE WITH PEANUTS	OUNCE	28.4	154	4	13	*	11	5.2	5	1.8
CANDY-MILK CHOCOLATE-PLAIN	OUNCE	28.4	145	2	16	*	9	5.5	3	0.3
CANDY-MILKY WAY BAR	ITEM	60	260	3	43	0.1	9	5.1	3.6	0.3
CANDY-PEANUT BRITTLE	OUNCE	28.4	123	2	20	0.5	4	1.9	1.8	0.6
CANDY-PEANUT BUTTER CUP	PIECE	17	92	2	9	0.8	5	2.8	1.8	0.8
CANDY-SNICKERS BAR	ITEM	57	270	6	33	1.4	13	4.7	5	2
CHOCOLATE-BITTER-FOR BAKING	OUNCE	28.4	145	3	8	4.3	15	8.9	4.9	0.4
COCONUT CREAM-RAW	CUP	240	792	9	16	1.6	83	73.8	3.5	0.9
COCONUT MILK-RAW	CUP	240	552	6	13	1.1	57	50.7	2.4	0.6
HONEY-STRAINED/EXTRACTED	TBSP	21	65	0	17	0.1	0	0	0	0
ICING-CAKE-CHOCOLATE-PREPARED FROM MIX	CUP	275	1035	9	185	*	38	23.4	11.7	1
ICING-CAKE-FUDGE-PREPARED FROM MIX/WATER	CUP	245	830	7	183	*	16	5.1	6.7	3.1
ICING-CAKE-WHITE-BOILED	CUP	94	295	1	75	0	0	0	0	0
ICING-CAKE-WHITE-UNCOOKED	CUP	319	1200	2	260	0	21	12.7	5.1	0.5
ICING-CAKE-WHITE/COCONUT-BOILED	CUP	166	605	3	124	*	13	11	0.9	0
JAM/PRESERVES-STRAWBERRY-LOW CALORIE	TSP	6	8	0	2	0.1	0	0	0	0
JAMS/PRESERVES-REGULAR	TBSP	20	55	0	14	0.2	0	0	0	0
JAMS/PRESERVES-REGULAR-PACKET SIZE	ITEM	14	40	0	10	0.1	0	0	0	0
JELLIES-REGULAR	TBSP	18	50	0	13	0	0	0	0	0
JELLIES-REGULAR-PACKET SIZE	ITEM	14	40	0	10	0	0	0	0	0
MARSHMALLOWS	OUNCE	28.4	90	1	23	0	0	0	0	0
MOLASSES-CANE-BLACKSTRAP	TBSP	20	45	0	11	0	0	0	0	0
MOLASSES-CANE-LIGHT	TBSP	20	50	0	13	0	0	0	0	0
NUTS-COCONUT-DRIED-FLAKED-CANNED	CUP	77	341	3	32	4.4	24	21.6	1	0.3

t = Trace of nutrient present ** = Not available*

MAG, magnesium; **IRON**, iron; **ZINC**, zinc; **VITA**, vitamin A; **VITC**, vitamin C; **THIA**, thiamin; **RIBO**, riboflavin; **NIAC**, niacin; **VB6**, vitamin B-6; **FOL**, folate; **VB12**, vitamin B-12; **CALC**, calcium; **PHOS**, phosphorus; **SEL**, selenium; **VE-a**, alpha tocopherol equivalents.

CHOL (mg)	SOD (mg)	POT (mg)	MAG (mg)	IRON (mg)	ZINC (mg)	VITA (RE)	VITC (mg)	THIA (mg)	RIBO (mg)	NIAC (mg)	VB6 (mg)	FOL (µg)	VB12 (µg)	CALC (mg)	PHOS (mg)	SEL (µg)	VE-a (mg)
0	988	190	39	2	1.7	20	2	0.11	0.07	1.2	0.05	2	0	28	124	8	0.1
0	33	190	39	2	1.7	20	2	0.11	0.07	1.2	0.05	2	0	28	124	8	0.1
8	1008	399	48	2.3	1.3	44	1	0.15	0.08	1.5	0.07	3	0	22	213	8	0.1
10	970	152	5	0.9	1.2	87	1	0.05	0.05	1.2	0.06	10	0.17	23	42	8	*
5	917	221	8	1.1	0.8	53	0	0.08	0.09	1.9	0.09	7	0.19	17	56	8	0.8
22	1108	604	25	0.9	0.6	110	7	0.11	0.27	1.3	0.14	21	0.44	186	174	8	*
4	30	417	9	0.8	0.6	72	6	0.07	0.07	1.2	0.09	15	0	40	60	8	*
2	815	330	5	0.8	0.5	76	15	0.06	0.05	1.1	0.08	14	0	22	33	8	0.8
0	1146	103	20	0.6	0.2	20	6	0.06	0.05	0.8	0.05	10	0	8	29	*	t
17	932	449	22	1.8	0.3	108	68	0.13	0.25	1.5	0.16	21	0.44	159	149	8	*
0	871	263	8	1.8	0.2	69	66	0.09	0.05	1.4	0.11	15	0	12	34	8	2.5
5	815	75	5	0.9	0.6	29	t	0.07	0.06	1.4	0.04	2	0.15	12	48	8	*
5	42	75	5	0.9	0.6	29	t	0.07	0.06	1.4	0.04	2	0.15	12	48	8	*
2	905	175	4	0.8	0.6	244	0	0.03	0.04	1	0.05	5	0.17	17	40	8	0.2
9	923	361	24	1.9	2.1	716	6	0.04	0.11	3.6	0.31	11	2.12	50	104	8	*
6	57	455	8	1.4	1.9	553	11	0.24	0.33	4.2	0.1	13	0.39	49	50	8	5007
5	960	174	5	1.1	1.6	189	2	0.04	0.05	1	0.08	11	0.31	17	42	8	0.3
0	38	185	7	1	0.5	371	3	0.05	0.05	1.2	0.06	11	0	19	35	8	0.5
0	823	209	7	1.1	0.5	300	1	0.05	0.05	0.9	0.06	11	0	21	35	8	0.3
22	1060	323	17	0.5	0.7	67	1	0.08	0.24	0.6	0.09	9	0.5	166	160	8	*
0	0	50	2	0.1	t	0	t	t	t	t	0.01	t	0	3	4	*	t
1	22	114	13	0.3	0.4	3	t	0.02	0.1	0.2	0.02	4	0.18	60	68	1	0.3
*	*	*	*	0.3	*	*	*	0	0.13	1.4	*	*	*	13	*	1	t
0	74	54	1	0.4	0.2	0	0	0.01	0.05	0.1	0.01	2	0.04	42	35	1	t
0	16	143	*	0.4	*	0	0	0.1	0.05	2.1	*	*	*	33	84	1	0.2
0	3	553	192	4.4	2.6	9	0	0.02	0.14	0.9	0.07	5	0	51	255	6	1.2
0	60	1	t	0.3	0	0	0	0	0	0	0	0	0	4	2	1	0
0	54	42	13	0.3	0.1	0	0	0.01	0.03	0.1	0.01	1	0.06	22	24	1	0.2
0	10	1	t	0.1	t	0	0	0	0	0	0	0	0	2	0	1	t
0	9	1	*	0.5	*	0	0	0	0	0	*	*	*	6	2	1	t
0	t	0	*	t	*	0	0	0	*	*	*	*	*	t	t	0	*
3	38	129	19	0.6	0.4	9	0	0.03	0.11	0.1	0.02	3	0.07	65	78	2	0.3
0	1	0	*	t	*	0	0	0	0	0	*	*	*	t	t	0	*
0	*	*	*	0	*	0	0	0	0	0	*	*	*	0	0	1	*
*	*	*	*	*	*	*	*	*	*	*	*	*	*	*	*	2	0.5
*	10	*	*	*	*	*	*	*	*	*	*	*	*	*	*	1	*
5	23	125	27	0.5	0.4	21	0	0.02	0.12	0.2	0.01	4	0.15	65	77	1	0.3
*	19	138	*	0.4	*	15	0	0.07	0.07	1.4	*	*	*	49	83	1	0.3
0	28	109	16	0.3	*	24	0	0.02	0.1	0.1	*	2	*	65	65	1	0.2
4	114	157	20	0.4	0.4	4	t	0.02	0.14	0.3	0.02	4	0.22	79	79	2	0.7
0	9	43	11	0.6	0.3	2	0	0.02	0.01	1.3	0.02	14	0	11	35	1	0.5
3	55	68	15	0.2	0.2	1	0	0.05	0.03	0.8	0.03	17	0.04	15	41	1	0.2
9	145	189	37	0.5	0.6	3	0	0.03	0.1	1.7	0.06	29	0.17	66	102	2	0.6
0	1	235	82	1.9	0.3	6	0	0.01	0.07	0.4	0.01	3	0	22	109	*	0.3
0	10	781	41	5.5	2.3	0	7	0.07	0	2.1	0.07	34	0	26	293	*	1.8
0	37	630	89	3.9	1.6	0	7	0.06	0	1.8	0.08	39	0	39	240	*	1.8
0	1	11	1	0.1	t	0	0	0	0.01	0.1	t	0	0	1	1	1	0
0	882	536	*	3.3	*	174	1	0.06	0.28	0.6	*	*	*	165	305	3	*
0	568	238	*	2.7	*	0	0	0.05	0.2	0.7	*	*	*	96	218	3	*
0	134	17	*	0	*	0	0	0	0.03	0	*	*	*	2	2	1	*
0	156	57	*	0	*	258	0	0	0.06	0	*	*	*	48	38	3	*
0	195	277	*	0.8	*	0	0	0.02	0.07	0.3	*	*	*	10	50	2	*
0	6	5	t	t	t	t	1	t	t	t	t	1	0	1	t	0	t
0	2	18	1	0.2	t	0	0	0	0.01	0	t	2	0	4	2	0	t
0	1	12	1	0.1	t	0	0	0	0	0	t	1	0	3	1	0	t
0	3	14	1	0.3	t	0	1	0	0.01	0	t	t	0	4	1	0	t
0	2	11	1	0.2	t	0	1	0	0	0	t	t	0	3	1	0	t
0	11	2	1	0.5	t	0	0	0	0	0	0	0	0	5	2	0	0
0	18	585	9	3.2	0.1	0	0	0.02	0.04	0.4	0.04	0	0	137	17	13	0.1
0	3	183	9	0.9	0.1	0	0	0.01	0.01	0	0.04	0	0	33	9	13	0.1
0	15	249	38	1.4	1.2	0	0	0.02	0.02	0.2	0.18	5	0	11	79	*	0.5

WT, weight; **KCAL**, kcalories; **PROT**, protein; **CARB**, carbohydrate; **FIBR**, fiber; **FAT**, fat; **SATF**, saturated fat;

MONO, monsaturated fat; **POLY**, polyunsaturated fat; **CHOL**, cholesterol; **SOD**, sodium; **POT**, potassium;

FOOD NAME	PORTION	WT (g)	KCAL	PROT (g)	CARB (g)	FIBR (g)	FAT (g)	SATF (g)	MONO (g)	POLY (g)
NUTS-COCONUT-DRIED-SHREDDED	CUP	93	466	3	44	3.9	33	29.3	1.4	0.4
NUTS-COCONUT-RAW-SHREDDED	CUP	80	283	3	12	7.2	27	23.8	1.1	0.3
SORGHUM	TBSP	21	55	0	14	0	0	0	0	0
SUGAR-BROWN-PRESSED DOWN	CUP	220	820	0	212	0	0	0	0	0
SUGAR-EQUAL-PACKET SIZE	ITEM	1	4	0	1	0	0	0	0	0
SUGAR-SWEET & LOW-PACKET SIZE	ITEM	1	4	0	1	0	0	0	0	0
SUGAR-WHITE-GRANULATED	TBSP	12	45	0	12	0	0	0	0	0
SUGAR-WHITE-POWDERED-SIFTED	CUP	100	385	0	100	0	0	0	0	0
SYRUP-CHOCOLATE FLAVORED-FUDGE-THICK	FL OZ	38	125	2	20	*	5	3.1	1.6	0.1
SYRUP-CHOCOLATE FLAVORED-THIN	FL OZ	38	83	1	22	0.1	t	0.2	0.1	t
SYRUP-CORN-TABLE BLENDS-LIGHT AND DARK	TBSP	21	60	0	15	0	0	0	0	0
SYRUP-PANCAKE-KARO	TBSP	20.5	60	0	15	0	0	0	0	0
SYRUP-PANCAKE-LIGHT-AUNT JEMIMA	FL OZ	39	60	0	15	0	0	0	0	0
VEGETABLES										
ALFALFA SEEDS-SPROUTED-RAW	CUP	33	10	1	1	0.7	t	t	t	0.1
AMARANTH-BOILED-DRAINED	CUP	132	28	3	5	12.5	t	0.1	0.1	0.1
AMARANTH-RAW	CUP	28	7	1	1	2.7	t	t	t	t
ARTICHOKES-BOILED-DRAINED	ITEM	120	60	4	13	4	t	t	t	0.1
ASPARAGUS-CANNED-DIETARY PACK-LOW SODIUM	CUP	244	34	4	5	3.9	t	0.1	t	0.2
ASPARAGUS-CANNED-SPEARS-DRAINED SOLIDS	CUP	242	46	5	6	3.5	2	0.4	0.1	0.7
ASPARAGUS-FROZEN-BOILED-DRAINED-SPEARS	CUP	180	50	5	9	2.2	1	0.2	t	0.3
ASPARAGUS-FROZEN-BOILED-DRAINED-TIPS	CUP	180	50	5	9	2.2	1	0.2	t	0.3
ASPARAGUS-RAW-BOILED-DRAINED-SPEARS	CUP	180	45	5	8	2.2	1	0.1	t	0.2
ASPARAGUS-RAW-BOILED-DRAINED-TIPS	CUP	180	45	5	8	2.2	1	0.1	t	0.2
BALSAM PEAR-LEAFY TIPS-BOILED-DRAINED	CUP	58	20	2	4	1.2	t	t	t	t
BALSAM PEAR-PODS-BOILED-DRAINED	CUP	124	24	1	5	2.5	t	t	t	t
BAMBOO SHOOTS-BOILED-DRAINED	CUP	120	14	2	2	2.2	t	0.1	t	0.1
BAMBOO SHOOTS-CANNED-DRAINED	CUP	131	25	2	4	3.4	1	0.1	t	0.2
BAMBOO SHOOTS-RAW	CUP	151	41	4	8	3.9	t	0.1	t	0.2
BEANS-ADZUKI-BOILED	CUP	230	294	17	57	14.3	t	0.1	7.2	2.1
BEANS-ADZUKI-CANNED-SWEETENED	CUP	296	702	11	163	13.7	t	0	0	0
BEANS-BAKED BEANS-CANNED	CUP	254	236	12	52	19.6	1	0.3	0.1	0.5
BEANS-BAKED BEANS-HOME RECIPE	CUP	253	382	14	54	19.5	13	4.9	5.4	1.9
BEANS-BLACK-COOKED-BOILED	CUP	172	227	15	41	7.2	1	0.2	0.1	0.4
BEANS-FRENCH-COOKED-BOILED	CUP	177	228	13	43	14.9	1	0.1	0.1	0.8
BEANS-GARBANZO-CANNED-RECONSTITUTED	SERVING	28.4	28	1	5	1.4	1	0.1	0.2	0.3
BEANS-GARBANZO-DRY-RAW	CUP	200	720	41	122	*	10	*	*	*
BEANS-GREAT NORTHERN-DRY-COOKED-DRAINED	CUP	180	210	14	38	9.7	1	4.4	5.5	1.7
BEANS-GREEN-CANNED-DIETARY-LOW SODIUM	CUP	136	26	2	6	1.8	t	t	t	0.1
BEANS-GREEN-FROZEN-BOILED-FRENCH STYLE	CUP	135	35	2	8	2.2	t	t	t	0.1
BEANS-KIDNEY-CANNED-DIETARY-LOW SODIUM	CUP	255	230	15	42	12.5	1	0	0	0
BEANS-LIMA-BABY-FROZEN-BOILED-DRAINED	CUP	180	189	12	35	13	1	0.1	t	0.3
BEANS-LIMA-CANNED-DIETARY-LOW SODIUM	CUP	248	186	11	34	10.4	1	0.2	t	0.4
BEANS-LIMA-CANNED-SOLIDS & LIQUIDS	CUP	248	186	11	34	10.4	1	0.2	t	0.4
BEANS-LIMA-FROZEN-BOILED-DRAINED	CUP	170	170	10	32	8.3	1	0.1	t	0.3
BEANS-LIMA-RAW-BOILED-DRAINED	CUP	170	209	12	40	12.2	1	0.1	t	0.3
BEANS-MUNG-SPROUTED-BOILED	CUP	125	26	3	5	2.7	t	t	t	t
BEANS-MUNG-SPROUTED-RAW	CUP	104	31	3	6	1.6	t	t	t	0.1
BEANS-NAVY PEA-DRY-COOKED-DRAINED	CUP	190	225	15	40	9.3	1	0.2	0.1	0.3
BEANS-NAVY-SPROUTED-BOILED	OUNCE	28.4	22	2	4	1.4	t	t	t	0.1
BEANS-PINTO-FROZEN-BOILED	OUNCE	28.4	46	3	9	1.4	t	t	t	0.1
BEANS-RED KIDNEY-CANNED-SOLIDS & LIQUIDS	CUP	255	230	15	42	12.5	1	1.2	3.5	3.1
BEANS-REFRIED	CUP	253	271	16	47	11.6	3	1	1.2	0.3
BEANS-REFRIED-CANNED-SAUSAGE-OLD EL PASO	CUP	200	388	14	26	6	26	6.9	7.9	2.3
BEANS-SHELLIE-CANNED	CUP	245	74	4	15	12	t	0.1	t	0.3
BEANS-SMALL WHITE-BOILED	CUP	179	254	16	46	7.9	1	0.3	0.1	0.5
BEANS-SNAP-GREEN-CANNED-DRAINED-CUTS	CUP	135	27	2	6	1.8	t	t	t	0.1
BEANS-SNAP-GREEN-DIETETIC-LOW SODIUM	OUNCE	28.4	4	t	1	0.4	t	0	0	0
BEANS-SNAP-GREEN-FROZEN-BOILED-CUTS	CUP	135	35	2	8	2.2	t	t	t	0.1
BEANS-SNAP-GREEN-RAW-BOILED	CUP	125	44	2	10	2.3	t	0.1	t	0.2
BEANS-SNAP-YELLOW/WAX-CANNED	CUP	136	27	2	6	1.8	t	t	t	0.1
BEANS-SNAP-YELLOW/WAX-FROZEN-BOILED	CUP	135	35	2	8	2.2	t	t	t	0.1

t = Trace of nutrient present ** = Not available*

MAG, magnesium; **IRON,** iron; **ZINC,** zinc; **VITA,** vitamin A; **VITC,** vitamin C; **THIA,** thiamin; **RIBO,** riboflavin; **NIAC,** niacin; **VB6,** vitamin B-6; **FOL,** folate; **VB12,** vitamin B-12; **CALC,** calcium; **PHOS,** phosphorus; **SEL,** selenium; **VE-a,** alpha tocopherol equivalents.

CHOL (mg)	SOD (mg)	POT (mg)	MAG (mg)	IRON (mg)	ZINC (mg)	VITA (RE)	VITC (mg)	THIA (mg)	RIBO (mg)	NIAC (mg)	VB6 (mg)	FOL (µg)	VB12 (µg)	CALC (mg)	PHOS (mg)	SEL (µg)	VE-a (mg)
0	244	313	47	1.8	1.7	0	1	0.03	0.02	0.4	0.25	8	0	14	99	16	0.7
0	16	285	26	1.9	0.9	0	3	0.05	0.02	0.4	0.04	21	0	12	90	11	0.6
0	2	37	t	2.6	t	0	0	0.03	0.02	0	0	0	0	35	5	26	0.1
0	66	757	44	7.5	0.6	0	0	0.02	0.07	0.4	0.09	0	0	187	42	3	0
0	0	0	0	0	0	0	0	0	0	0	0	0	0	0	0	0	0
0	4	3	0	0	0	0	0	0	0	0	0	0	0	0	0	0	0
0	t	0	0	0	t	0	0	0	0	0	0	0	0	0	0	0	0
0	1	3	0	0.1	0	0	0	0	0	0	0	0	0	0	0	1	0
0	27	107	*	0.5	0.3	18	0	0.02	0.08	0.2	*	*	*	48	60	*	*
0	20	106	21	0.6	0.3	0	0	0.01	0.03	0.2	t	2	0	6	35	*	t
0	15	1	t	0.8	t	0	0	0	0	0	0	0	0	9	3	3	0
0	35	1	t	0.8	t	0	0	0	0	0	0	0	0	9	3	0	0
0	18	7	1	0.1	t	0	0	t	0.01	0	0	0	0	1	4	0	0
0	2	26	9	0.3	0.3	5	3	0.03	0.04	0.2	0.01	12	0	11	23	*	t
0	28	846	73	3	1.2	366	54	0.03	0.18	0.7	0.23	75	0	276	95	*	11.2
0	5	171	15	0.7	0.3	82	12	0.01	0.04	0.2	0.05	24	0	60	14	*	2.4
0	114	425	72	1.6	0.6	22	12	0.08	0.08	1.2	0.13	61	0	54	103	*	0.2
0	849	373	22	1.4	1.2	115	40	0.13	0.22	2.1	0.24	208	0	34	93	3	0.9
0	944	416	24	4.4	1	128	45	0.15	0.24	2.3	0.27	231	0	39	104	9	0.9
0	7	392	23	1.2	1	147	44	0.12	0.19	1.9	0.04	242	0	41	99	7	2.5
0	7	392	23	1.2	1	148	44	0.12	0.19	1.9	0.04	242	0	41	99	7	2.5
0	7	558	34	1.2	0.9	149	49	0.18	0.22	1.9	0.25	177	0	43	110	7	3.6
0	7	558	34	1.2	0.9	149	49	0.18	0.22	1.9	0.25	177	0	43	110	7	3.6
0	8	349	55	0.6	0.2	100	32	0.09	0.16	0.6	0.44	51	0	24	45	*	0.3
0	7	396	20	0.5	1	14	41	0.06	0.07	0.3	0.05	63	0	11	45	*	0.6
0	5	640	4	0.3	0.6	0	0	0.02	0.06	0.4	0.12	3	0	14	24	*	1.2
0	9	105	5	0.4	0.9	1	1	0.03	0.03	0.2	0.18	4	0	11	33	*	1.3
0	6	805	5	0.8	1.7	3	6	0.23	0.11	0.9	0.36	11	0	20	89	*	1.6
0	18	1224	120	4.6	4.1	1	0	0.27	0.15	1.7	0.22	279	0	63	385	*	0.5
0	646	353	91	3.3	4.6	3	0	0.3	0.17	1.9	0.25	316	0	66	220	*	1.9
0	1008	752	81	0.7	3.6	43	8	0.39	0.15	1.1	0.34	61	0	127	264	*	*
13	1068	907	110	5	1.8	t	3	0.34	0.12	1	0.23	122	0.03	155	275	*	0.5
0	1	611	121	3.6	1.9	1	0	0.42	0.1	0.9	0.12	256	0	47	241	*	*
0	11	655	99	1.9	1.1	1	2	0.23	0.11	1	0.19	132	0	111	181	*	*
0	113	55	9	0.7	0.3	1	1	t	0.01	0.1	*	*	0	11	30	*	1
0	52	1594	*	13.8	*	10	*	0.62	0.3	4	*	*	0	300	662	4	6
0	12	749	86	4.9	1.8	0	0	0.25	0.13	1.3	1.01	63	0	90	266	23	0.4
0	3	148	18	1.2	0.4	*	6	0.02	0.08	0.3	*	43	0	32	26	1	t
0	18	151	28	1.1	0.8	72	11	0.07	0.1	0.6	0.08	11	0	61	32	1	0.2
0	10	673	10	4.6	1.9	1	8	0.13	0.1	1.5	1.12	36	0	74	278	5	0
0	52	740	101	3.5	1	31	10	0.13	0.1	1.4	0.21	28	0	50	202	1	0
0	10	668	84	3.9	1.6	43	22	0.07	0.11	1.3	0.15	40	0	70	176	3	1.6
0	618	668	84	3.9	1.6	43	22	0.07	0.11	1.3	0.15	40	0	70	176	4	0.7
0	90	694	58	2.3	0.7	32	22	0.12	0.1	1.8	0.21	111	0	38	153	1	0
0	29	969	126	4.2	1.3	63	17	0.24	0.16	1.8	0.33	45	0	54	221	9	0
0	13	126	18	0.8	0.6	1	14	0.06	0.13	1	0.07	37	0	15	35	*	t
0	6	155	22	0.9	0.4	2	14	0.09	0.13	0.8	0.09	63	0	14	56	*	t
0	13	790	97	5.1	1.8	0	0	0.27	0.13	1.3	1.06	67	0	95	281	21	0.6
0	4	90	32	0.6	0.3	t	5	0.11	0.07	0.4	0.06	30	0	5	29	4	0.1
0	24	183	15	0.8	0.2	0	t	0.08	0.03	0.2	0.06	10	0	15	28	*	t
0	833	673	10	4.6	1.9	1	8	0.13	0.1	1.5	1.12	36	0	74	278	9	0
0	1073	994	99	4.5	3.5	0	15	0.12	0.14	1.2	0.25	211	0	116	213	*	2.1
16	624	600	88	4.2	1.8	0	6	0.29	0.14	0.6	0.31	254	0	88	258	*	1.7
0	818	267	37	2.4	0.7	56	8	0.08	0.13	0.5	0.12	44	0	71	74	*	*
0	4	828	122	5.1	2	0	0	0.42	0.11	0.5	0.23	245	0	131	302	*	0.3
0	339	147	18	1.2	0.4	47	7	0.02	0.08	0.3	0.05	43	0	35	34	1	t
0	t	24	3	0.2	0.1	10	1	0.01	0.01	0.1	*	*	0	7	6	0	t
0	18	151	28	1.1	0.8	72	11	0.07	0.1	0.6	0.08	11	0	61	32	1	0.2
0	4	374	31	1.6	0.5	84	12	0.09	0.12	0.8	0.07	42	0	58	49	1	t
0	341	148	18	1.2	0.4	48	7	0.02	0.08	0.3	0.05	43	0	35	26	1	0.4
0	18	151	28	1.1	0.8	72	11	0.07	0.1	0.6	0.08	11	0	61	32	1	0.2

WT, weight; **KCAL**, kcalories; **PROT**, protein; **CARB**, carbohydrate; **FIBR**, fiber; **FAT**, fat; **SATF**, saturated fat;

MONO, monsaturated fat; **POLY**, polyunsaturated fat; **CHOL**, cholesterol; **SOD**, sodium; **POT**, potassium;

FOOD NAME	PORTION	WT (g)	KCAL	PROT (g)	CARB (g)	FIBR (g)	FAT (g)	SATF (g)	MONO (g)	POLY (g)
BEANS-SNAP-YELLOW/WAX-RAW-BOILED	CUP	125	44	2	10	2.3	t	0.1	t	0.2
BEET GREENS-BOILED-DRAINED	CUP	145	39	4	8	4.4	t	t	0.1	0.1
BEETS-CANNED-DIETARY PACK-LOW SODIUM	CUP	246	71	2	17	2.7	t	t	t	0.1
BEETS-SLICED-BOILED-DRAINED	CUP	170	53	2	11	3.4	t	t	t	t
BEETS-SLICED-CANNED-DRAINED	CUP	170	53	2	12	2.9	t	t	t	0.1
BEETS-WHOLE-BOILED-DRAINED	ITEM	50	16	1	3	1.1	t	t	t	t
BEETS-WHOLE-CANNED	CUP	246	71	2	17	2.7	t	t	t	0.1
BROCCOLI-FROZEN-BOILED-DRAINED	CUP	185	52	6	10	7.3	t	t	t	0.1
BROCCOLI-RAW	CUP	88	25	3	5	2.5	t	t	t	0.1
BROCCOLI-RAW-BOILED-DRAINED	CUP	155	43	5	8	4	1	0.1	t	0.3
BRUSSELS SPROUTS-FROZEN-BOILED	CUP	155	65	6	13	4.5	1	0.1	t	0.3
BRUSSELS SPROUTS-RAW-BOILED	CUP	156	61	4	14	6.7	1	0.2	0.1	0.4
BURDOCK ROOT-BOILED-DRAINED	ITEM	166	146	3	35	*	t	*	*	*
CABBAGE-CELERY-RAW	CUP	76	12	1	2	0.8	t	t	t	0.1
CABBAGE-COMMON-BOILED-DRAINED	CUP	145	31	1	7	4	t	t	t	0.2
CABBAGE-COMMON-RAW-SHREDDED	CUP	90	22	1	5	1.8	t	t	t	0.1
CABBAGE-COMMON-RAW-SLICED	CUP	70	17	1	4	1.5	t	t	t	0.1
CABBAGE-RED-RAW-SHREDDED	CUP	70	19	1	4	1.4	t	t	t	0.1
CABBAGE-SAVOY-RAW-SHREDDED	CUP	70	19	1	4	1.5	t	t	t	t
CABBAGE-WHITE MUSTARD-BOILED	CUP	170	20	3	3	2.7	t	t	t	0.1
CABBAGE-WHITE MUSTARD-RAW	CUP	70	9	1	2	0.7	t	t	t	0.1
CARROT JUICE-CANNED	CUP	246	98	2	23	5.9	t	0.1	t	0.2
CARROT-RAW-SCRAPED-SHREDDED	CUP	110	47	1	11	3.5	t	t	t	0.1
CARROT-RAW-SCRAPED-WHOLE	ITEM	72	31	1	7	2.3	t	t	t	0.1
CARROTS-BOILED-DRAINED-SLICED	CUP	156	70	2	16	5.8	t	0.1	t	0.1
CARROTS-CANNED-DIETARY PACK-LOW SODIUM	CUP	246	57	2	12	2.7	t	0.1	t	0.2
CARROTS-CANNED-SLICED-DRAINED	CUP	146	34	1	8	2.2	t	0.1	t	0.1
CARROTS-FROZEN-BOILED-DRAINED	CUP	146	53	2	12	5.4	t	t	t	0.1
CAULIFLOWER-FROZEN-BOILED	CUP	180	34	3	7	3.2	t	0.1	t	0.2
CAULIFLOWER-RAW-BOILED-DRAINED	CUP	124	30	2	6	2.7	t	t	t	0.1
CAULIFLOWER-RAW-CHOPPED	CUP	100	24	2	5	2.4	t	0	0	0
CELERY-PASCAL-RAW-DICED	CUP	120	19	1	4	1.9	t	t	t	0.1
CELERY-PASCAL-RAW-STALK	ITEM	40	6	t	1	0.6	t	t	t	t
CHARD-SWISS-BOILED-DRAINED	CUP	175	35	3	7	3.7	t	t	0	0.1
CHARD-SWISS-RAW	CUP	36	7	1	1	0.6	t	0	0	0
CHICORY GREENS-RAW-CHOPPED	CUP	180	41	3	8	4.3	1	0.1	t	0.2
CHICORY ROOTS-RAW	ITEM	60	44	1	11	1.4	t	t	t	0.1
CHIVES-FREEZE DRIED	TBSP	0.2	1	t	t	t	t	t	t	t
CHIVES-RAW-CHOPPED	TBSP	3	1	t	t	0.1	t	t	t	t
COLLARDS-FROZEN-BOILED-DRAINED	CUP	170	61	5	12	5.2	1	*	*	*
COLLARDS-RAW-BOILED-DRAINED	CUP	128	35	2	8	2.1	t	t	t	0.1
CORN FRITTER	ITEM	35	132	3	14	0.6	8	2	3.2	1.9
CORN-CREAMED-CANNED-DIETARY-LOW SODIUM	CUP	256	184	4	46	3.1	1	0.2	0.3	0.5
CORN-EAR-FROZEN-BOILED-DRAINED	ITEM	126	117	4	28	2.7	1	0.1	0.3	0.4
CORN-FROZEN-BOILED-DRAINED-KERNELS	CUP	165	134	5	34	3.5	t	t	t	0.1
CORN-KERNELS FROM ONE EAR-BOILED-DRAINED	ITEM	77	83	3	19	2.9	1	0.2	0.3	0.5
CORN-SWEET-CANNED-DRAINED	CUP	165	134	4	31	2.3	2	0.3	0.5	0.8
CORN-SWEET-CANNED-LOW SODIUM	CUP	256	156	5	38	2.1	1	0.2	0.3	0.5
CORN-SWEET-CANNED-VACUUM PACKED	CUP	210	166	5	41	9.5	1	0.2	0.3	0.5
CORN-SWEET-CREAM STYLE-CANNED	CUP	256	184	4	46	3.1	1	0.2	0.3	0.5
CORN-WITH RED AND GREEN PEPPERS-CANNED	CUP	227	170	5	41	5.1	1	0.2	0.4	0.6
CRESS-GARDEN-RAW	CUP	50	16	1	3	0.6	t	t	0.1	0.1
CUCUMBER-RAW-SLICED	CUP	104	14	1	3	1	t	t	t	0.1
CUCUMBER-RAW-WHOLE	ITEM	301	39	2	9	3	t	0.1	t	0.2
DANDELION GREENS-BOILED	CUP	105	35	2	7	4.1	1	0.1	t	0.4
EGGPLANT-BOILED-DRAINED	CUP	96	27	1	6	2.7	t	t	t	0.1
ENDIVE-RAW-CHOPPED	CUP	50	9	1	2	1.2	t	t	t	t
FRIJOLES-BEANS WITH CHEESE	CUP	167	226	11	29	*	8	4.1	2.6	0.7
GARLIC-RAW-CLOVE	ITEM	3	4	t	1	0.1	t	t	0	t
GINGER ROOT-RAW-SLICED	CUP	96	66	2	15	0.7	1	0.2	0.1	0.1
GOURD-WHITE FLOWERED-BOILED	CUP	146	22	1	5	1.6	t	t	t	t
HUMMUS	CUP	246	421	12	50	0	21	3.1	8.8	7.8
JERUSALEM ARTICHOKES-RAW	CUP	150	114	3	26	2	t	0	t	t

t = Trace of nutrient present   ** = Not available*

MAG, magnesium; **IRON,** iron; **ZINC,** zinc; **VITA,** vitamin A; **VITC,** vitamin C; **THIA,** thiamin; **RIBO,** riboflavin; **NIAC,** niacin; **VB6,** vitamin B-6; **FOL,** folate; **VB12,** vitamin B-12; **CALC,** calcium; **PHOS,** phosphorus; **SEL,** selenium; **VE-a,** alpha tocopherol equivalents.

CHOL (mg)	SOD (mg)	POT (mg)	MAG (mg)	IRON (mg)	ZINC (mg)	VITA (RE)	VITC (mg)	THIA (mg)	RIBO (mg)	NIAC (mg)	VB6 (mg)	FOL (µg)	VB12 (µg)	CALC (mg)	PHOS (mg)	SEL (µg)	VE-a (mg)
0	4	374	31	1.6	0.5	84	12	0.09	0.12	0.8	0.07	42	0	58	48	1	0.4
0	349	1318	99	2.8	0.7	740	36	0.17	0.42	0.7	0.19	21	0	165	60	*	2.2
0	113	349	39	1.7	0.6	2	10	0.03	0.09	0.4	0.14	71	0	34	39	3	0.1
0	83	530	63	1.1	0.4	2	9	0.05	0.02	0.5	0.05	90	0	19	53	1	0.1
0	466	252	29	3.1	0.4	2	7	0.02	0.07	0.3	0.1	51	0	26	29	1	0.1
0	25	156	19	0.3	0.1	1	3	0.02	0.01	0.1	0.02	27	0	6	12	1	t
0	647	349	39	1.7	0.6	2	10	0.03	0.09	0.4	0.14	71	0	34	39	1	0.1
0	44	333	37	1.1	0.6	350	74	0.1	0.15	0.8	0.24	104	0	94	102	3	0.9
0	24	286	22	0.8	0.4	136	82	0.06	0.11	0.6	0.14	63	0	42	58	1	0.4
0	40	453	37	1.3	0.6	215	116	0.09	0.18	0.9	0.22	78	0	71	92	3	0.7
0	36	504	37	1.2	0.6	92	71	0.16	0.18	0.8	0.45	157	0	37	84	1	1.3
0	33	495	31	1.9	0.5	112	97	0.17	0.12	0.9	0.28	94	0	56	87	1	1.3
0	7	597	65	1.3	0.6	0	4	0.07	0.1	0.5	0.46	32	0	82	154	*	*
0	7	181	10	0.2	0.2	91	21	0.03	0.04	0.3	0.18	60	0	59	22	2	0.1
0	28	297	22	0.6	0.2	13	35	0.08	0.08	0.3	0.09	29	0	48	36	3	2.4
0	16	221	14	0.5	0.2	11	43	0.05	0.03	0.3	0.09	51	0	42	21	2	1.5
0	13	172	11	0.4	0.1	9	33	0.04	0.02	0.2	0.07	40	0	33	16	2	1.2
0	8	144	11	0.3	0.1	3	40	0.04	0.02	0.2	0.15	15	0	36	29	2	0.1
0	20	161	20	0.3	0.2	70	22	0.05	0.02	0.2	0.13	56	0	25	29	2	0.1
0	58	631	19	1.8	0.3	437	44	0.05	0.11	0.7	0.28	69	0	158	49	4	1.2
0	46	176	13	0.6	0.1	210	32	0.03	0.05	0.4	0.14	46	0	74	26	2	0.1
0	71	718	34	1.1	0.4	6335	21	0.23	0.14	1	0.53	9	0	59	103	*	t
0	39	355	17	0.6	0.2	3094	10	0.11	0.06	1	0.16	15	0	30	48	2	0.5
0	25	233	11	0.4	0.1	2025	7	0.07	0.04	0.7	0.11	10	0	19	32	2	0.3
0	103	354	20	1	0.5	3830	4	0.05	0.09	0.8	0.38	22	0	48	47	2	0.7
0	96	426	22	1.5	0.7	3239	7	0.05	0.07	1	0.28	20	0	62	49	3	1
0	352	261	12	0.9	0.4	2010	4	0.03	0.04	0.8	0.16	13	0	37	35	2	0.6
0	86	231	15	0.7	0.4	2584	4	0.04	0.05	0.6	0.19	16	0	41	38	3	0.6
0	32	250	16	0.7	0.2	4	56	0.07	0.1	0.6	0.16	74	0	31	43	1	0.1
0	8	400	14	0.5	0.3	2	69	0.08	0.06	0.7	0.25	63	0	34	44	1	t
0	15	355	14	0.6	0.2	2	72	0.08	0.06	0.6	0.23	66	0	29	46	1	t
0	104	344	13	0.5	0.2	16	8	0.06	0.05	0.4	0.1	34	0	48	30	0	0.4
0	35	115	4	0.2	0.1	5	3	0.02	0.02	0.1	0.04	11	0	16	10	0	0.1
0	313	961	150	4	0.6	549	32	0.06	0.15	0.6	0.15	15	0	102	58	70	2.6
0	64	198	31	0.8	0.1	113	6	0.01	0.03	0.1	0.03	3	0	21	12	*	0.5
0	81	756	54	1.6	0.8	720	43	0.11	0.18	0.9	0.19	197	0	180	85	*	*
0	30	174	13	0.5	0.2	1	3	0.02	0.02	0.2	0.15	14	0	25	37	*	0.6
0	t	6	1	t	t	14	1	t	t	t	t	t	0	2	1	*	129
0	t	8	2	t	t	19	2	t	0.01	t	0.01	t	0	2	2	*	t
0	85	427	51	1.9	0.5	1017	45	0.08	0.2	1.1	0.19	129	0	357	46	1	*
0	21	168	9	0.2	0.1	349	16	0.03	0.07	0.4	0.07	8	0	29	10	1	2.9
25	167	47	8	0.6	0.2	14	1	0.06	0.07	0.6	0.02	11	0.06	22	54	*	1.1
0	8	343	44	1	1.4	26	12	0.06	0.14	2.5	0.16	115	0	8	131	1	0.1
0	5	316	37	0.8	0.8	27	6	0.22	0.09	1.9	0.28	38	0	4	95	1	0.1
0	8	228	30	0.5	0.6	41	4	0.11	0.12	2.1	0.16	33	0	4	78	1	0.1
0	13	192	25	0.5	0.4	17	5	0.17	0.06	1.2	0.05	36	0	2	79	1	0.1
0	533	322	33	1.4	0.6	26	14	0.05	0.13	2	0.08	80	0	8	107	1	0.1
0	8	392	41	0.9	0.9	31	17	0.07	0.16	2.4	0.1	98	0	10	131	1	0.1
0	572	390	48	0.9	1	51	17	0.09	0.15	2.5	0.12	104	0	10	134	1	0.1
0	730	343	44	1	1.4	26	12	0.06	0.14	2.5	0.16	115	0	8	131	1	0.1
0	788	347	57	1.8	0.8	52	20	0.05	0.18	2.2	0.22	77	0	11	141	1	0.1
0	8	304	19	0.7	0.1	465	35	0.04	0.13	0.5	0.12	40	0	40	38	*	0.4
0	2	155	11	0.3	0.2	5	5	0.03	0.02	0.3	0.05	15	0	15	18	1	0.2
0	6	448	33	0.8	0.7	15	14	0.09	0.06	0.9	0.16	42	0	42	51	1	0.5
0	46	244	25	1.9	0.3	1229	19	0.14	0.18	0.5	0.17	13	0	147	44	1	2.6
0	3	238	13	0.3	0.1	6	1	0.07	0.02	0.6	0.08	14	0	6	21	*	t
0	11	157	8	0.4	0.4	103	3	0.04	0.04	0.2	0.01	71	0	26	14	*	0.5
36	882	605	85	2.2	1.7	46	2	0.14	0.33	1.5	0.19	111	0.68	188	175	*	*
0	1	12	1	0.1	t	0	1	0.01	t	t	0.04	t	0	5	5	0	0
0	13	398	41	0.5	0.3	0	5	0.02	0.03	0.7	0.15	11	0	17	26	*	0.7
0	3	248	16	0.4	1	0	12	0.04	0.03	0.6	0.06	6	0	35	19	*	*
0	600	428	71	3.9	2.7	5	19	0.23	0.13	1	0.98	146	0	123	275	*	0
0	6	644	26	5.1	0.2	3	6	0.3	0.09	2	0.12	20	0	21	117	*	0.3

WT, weight; **KCAL**, kcalories; **PROT**, protein; **CARB**, carbohydrate; **FIBR**, fiber; **FAT**, fat; **SATF**, saturated fat;

MONO, monsaturated fat; **POLY**, polyunsaturated fat; **CHOL**, cholesterol; **SOD**, sodium; **POT**, potassium;

FOOD NAME	PORTION	WT (g)	KCAL	PROT (g)	CARB (g)	FIBR (g)	FAT (g)	SATF (g)	MONO (g)	POLY (g)
KALE-FROZEN-BOILED-DRAINED	CUP	130	39	4	7	3.8	1	0.1	t	0.3
KALE-RAW-BOILED-DRAINED	CUP	130	42	2	7	4.3	1	0.1	t	0.3
KOHLRABI-BOILED-DRAINED	CUP	165	48	3	11	3.3	t	t	t	0.1
KOHLRABI-RAW	CUP	140	38	2	9	2.5	t	t	t	0.1
LEEKS-BOILED-DRAINED	ITEM	124	38	1	9	4	t	t	t	0.1
LEEKS-RAW	ITEM	124	76	2	18	2.5	t	0.1	t	0.2
LENTILS-SPROUTED-RAW	CUP	77	82	7	17	6.2	t	t	0.1	0.2
LENTILS-WHOLE-COOKED	CUP	198	231	18	40	9.8	1	0.1	0.1	0.3
LETTUCE-BUTTERHEAD-HEAD	ITEM	163	21	2	4	1.6	t	t	t	0.2
LETTUCE-BUTTERHEAD-LEAVES	SLICE	15	2	t	t	0.2	t	t	t	t
LETTUCE-ICEBERG-RAW-CHOPPED	CUP	55	7	1	1	0.6	t	t	t	0.1
LETTUCE-ICEBERG-RAW-HEAD	ITEM	539	70	5	11	5.4	1	0.1	t	0.5
LETTUCE-ICEBERG-RAW-LEAVES	PIECE	20	3	t	t	0.2	t	t	t	t
LETTUCE-LOOSELEAF-RAW	CUP	55	10	1	2	0.8	t	t	t	0.1
LETTUCE-ROMAINE-RAW-SHREDDED	CUP	56	9	1	1	1	t	t	t	0.1
LOTUS ROOT-BOILED-DRAINED	OUNCE	28.4	19	t	5	0.9	t	t	t	t
LOTUS ROOT-RAW	ITEM	115	64	3	20	3.5	t	t	t	t
MISO-FERMENTED SOYBEANS	CUP	275	567	33	77	9.9	17	2.4	3.7	9.4
MUSHROOMS-BOILED-DRAINED	ITEM	12	3	t	1	0.3	t	t	t	t
MUSHROOMS-CANNED-DRAINED	ITEM	12	3	t	1	0.2	t	t	t	t
MUSHROOMS-RAW-CHOPPED	CUP	70	18	1	3	0.9	t	t	t	0.1
MUSTARD GREENS-BOILED-DRAINED	CUP	140	21	3	3	2.7	t	t	0.2	0.1
NATTO-FERMENTED SOYBEANS	CUP	280	468	47	32	9.7	21	4.5	6.8	17.4
NUTS-CHESTNUTS-CHINESE-DRIED	OUNCE	28.4	103	2	23	2.2	1	0.1	0.3	0.1
NUTS-CHESTNUTS-CHINESE-RAW	OUNCE	28.4	64	1	14	2.2	t	t	0.2	0.1
NUTS-CHESTNUTS-ROASTED	OUNCE	28.4	68	1	15	2.2	t	0.1	0.2	0.1
OKRA-RAW-BOILED-DRAINED	CUP	160	51	3	12	2	t	0.1	t	0.1
ONION RINGS-FROZEN-PREPARED-HEATED	ITEM	10	41	1	4	0.4	3	0.9	1.1	0.5
ONIONS-MATURE-BOILED-DRAINED	CUP	210	92	3	21	1.7	t	0.1	0.1	0.2
ONIONS-MATURE-RAW-CHOPPED	CUP	160	61	2	14	2.6	t	t	t	0.1
ONIONS-YOUNG GREEN	ITEM	5	1	t	t	0.1	t	t	0	0
PARSLEY-RAW-CHOPPED	TBSP	4	1	t	t	0.2	t	t	t	t
PARSNIPS-SLICED-BOILED-DRAINED	CUP	156	126	2	31	7.6	t	0.1	0.2	0.1
PEAS-BLACKEYE/COWPEAS-BOILED-DRAINED	CUP	165	179	13	30	15.8	1	0.3	0.1	0.4
PEAS-BLACKEYE/COWPEAS-FROZEN-BOILED	CUP	170	224	14	40	9.8	1	0.3	0.1	0.5
PEAS-BLACKEYE/COWPEAS-RAW-BOILED	CUP	165	160	5	34	11	1	0.2	0.1	0.3
PEAS-EDIBLE PODDED-RAW	CUP	145	61	4	11	3.8	t	0.1	t	0.1
PEAS-GREEN-CANNED-DIETARY-LOW SODIUM	CUP	170	117	8	21	5.8	1	0.1	0.1	0.3
PEAS-GREEN-CANNED-DRAINED	CUP	170	117	8	21	5.8	1	0.1	0.1	0.3
PEAS-GREEN-FROZEN-BOILED-DRAINED	CUP	160	125	8	23	6.1	t	0.1	t	0.2
PEAS-SPLIT-DRY-COOKED	CUP	200	230	16	42	10.5	1	0.1	0.2	0.3
PEAS-SWEET-CANNED IN WATER-DIETETIC	OUNCE	28.4	12	1	2	0.6	t	0	0	0
PEPPERS-HOT CHILI-CANNED	CUP	136	34	1	8	2.1	t	t	t	0.1
PEPPERS-HOT CHILI-RAW	CUP	150	60	3	14	3.6	t	t	t	0.2
PEPPERS-HOT-RED-DRIED	TSP	2	5	0	1	0.7	0	0	0	0
PEPPERS-JALAPENO-CANNED-CHOPPED	CUP	136	33	1	1	2	1	0.1	t	0.4
PEPPERS-SWEET-BOILED-DRAINED	ITEM	73	20	1	5	0.7	t	t	t	0.1
PEPPERS-SWEET-RAW	ITEM	74	20	1	5	1.2	t	t	t	0.1
PIMIENTOS-4 OUNCE CAN OR JAR	ITEM	113	31	1	7	2.6	1	0.1	t	0.4
POI-TARO ROOT PRODUCT	CUP	240	269	1	65	4.8	t	0.1	t	0.1
POTATO CHIPS-SALT ADDED	ITEM	2	11	t	1	t	1	0.2	0.1	0.4
POTATO PANCAKES-HOME RECIPE	ITEM	76	495	5	26	1.4	13	3.4	5.4	2.5
POTATO PUFFS-FROZEN-HEATED	ITEM	7	16	t	2	0.2	1	0.4	0.3	0.1
POTATO SKIN-BAKED	ITEM	58	115	2	27	3	t	t	t	t
POTATO-AU GRATIN-HOME RECIPE	CUP	245	323	12	28	4.4	19	11.6	5.3	0.7
POTATO-AU GRATIN-PREPARED FROM MIX	OUNCE	28.4	26	1	4	0.5	1	0.7	0.3	t
POTATO-BAKED-FLESH & SKIN-WHOLE	ITEM	202	220	5	51	4.9	t	0.1	t	0.1
POTATO-BAKED-PEELED AFTER BAKING	ITEM	156	145	3	34	3.7	t	t	t	0.1
POTATO-BOILED-PEELED AFTER BOILING	ITEM	136	118	3	27	2	t	t	t	0.1
POTATO-BOILED-PEELED BEFORE BOILING	ITEM	135	116	2	27	1.5	t	t	t	0.1
POTATO-CANNED-DRAINED	ITEM	35	21	t	5	0.9	t	t	t	t
POTATO-FRENCH FRIED-PREPARED FROM FROZEN	ITEM	5	11	t	2	0.2	t	0.2	0.2	t
POTATO-FRENCH FRIED-PREPARED FROM RAW	ITEM	5	14	t	2	0.2	1	0.2	0.2	t
POTATO-HASH BROWN-PREPARED FROM RAW	CUP	156	239	4	12	3.1	22	8.5	9.7	2.5

t = Trace of nutrient present ** = Not available*

MAG, magnesium; **IRON,** iron; **ZINC,** zinc; **VITA,** vitamin A; **VITC,** vitamin C; **THIA,** thiamin; **RIBO,** riboflavin; **NIAC,** niacin; **VB6,** vitamin B-6; **FOL,** folate; **VB12,** vitamin B-12; **CALC,** calcium; **PHOS,** phosphorus; **SEL,** selenium; **VE-a,** alpha tocopherol equivalents.

CHOL (mg)	SOD (mg)	POT (mg)	MAG (mg)	IRON (mg)	ZINC (mg)	VITA (RE)	VITC (mg)	THIA (mg)	RIBO (mg)	NIAC (mg)	VB6 (mg)	FOL (µg)	VB12 (µg)	CALC (mg)	PHOS (mg)	SEL (µg)	VE-a (mg)
0	20	417	23	1.2	0.2	826	33	0.06	0.15	0.9	0.11	19	0	179	36	1	10.4
0	30	296	23	1.2	0.3	962	53	0.07	0.09	0.7	0.18	17	0	94	36	1	10.4
0	35	561	31	0.7	0.5	7	89	0.07	0.03	0.6	0.25	20	0	41	74	*	2.7
0	28	490	27	0.6	t	6	87	0.07	0.03	0.6	0.21	23	0	34	64	1	t
0	12	108	17	1.4	0.1	6	5	0.03	0.03	0.2	0.14	30	0	37	21	0	1.1
0	25	223	35	2.6	0.1	12	15	0.07	0.04	0.5	0.29	80	0	73	43	0	1.1
0	8	248	29	2.5	1.2	4	13	0.18	0.1	0.9	0.15	77	0	19	133	8	1
0	4	731	71	6.6	2.5	2	3	0.34	0.15	2.1	0.35	358	0	37	356	20	0.2
0	8	419	21	0.5	0.3	158	13	0.1	0.1	0.5	0.08	119	0	52	38	2	0.9
0	1	39	2	t	t	15	1	0.01	0.01	t	0.01	11	0	5	3	0	0.1
0	5	87	5	0.3	0.1	18	2	0.03	0.02	0.1	0.02	31	0	11	11	0	0.2
0	49	852	49	2.7	1.2	178	21	0.25	0.16	1	0.22	302	0	102	108	5	2.3
0	2	32	2	0.1	t	7	1	0.01	0.01	t	0.01	11	0	4	4	0	0.1
0	5	145	6	0.8	0.2	105	10	0.03	0.04	0.2	0.03	27	0	37	14	0	0.2
0	4	162	3	0.6	0.1	146	13	0.06	0.06	0.3	0.03	76	0	20	25	0	0.2
0	13	103	6	0.3	0.1	0	8	0.04	t	0.1	0.06	2	0	7	22	*	t
0	46	639	27	1.3	0.4	0	51	0.18	0.25	0.5	0.21	15	0	52	115	*	t
0	10030	451	116	7.5	9.1	25	0	0.27	0.69	2.4	0.59	91	0	182	421	*	*
0	t	43	1	0.2	0.1	0	t	0.01	0.04	0.5	0.01	2	0	1	10	1	t
0	51	16	2	0.1	0.1	0	0	0.01	t	0.2	0.01	1	0	1	8	5	t
0	3	259	7	0.9	0.5	0	2	0.07	0.31	2.9	0.07	15	0	4	73	9	0.1
0	22	283	21	1	0.2	424	35	0.06	0.09	0.6	0	103	0	103	58	1	2.8
0	20	697	322	10.4	8.5	0	0	0.07	0.5	1.1	0.36	22	0	103	182	*	t
0	2	206	39	0.7	0.4	9	17	0.07	0.08	0.4	0.19	31	0	8	44	2	0.1
0	1	127	24	0.4	0.2	6	10	0.05	0.05	0.2	0.12	19	0	5	27	2	0.1
0	1	135	26	0.4	0.3	t	11	0.04	0.03	0.4	0.12	21	0	5	29	2	0.1
0	8	515	91	0.7	0.9	92	26	0.21	0.09	1.4	0.3	73	0	101	90	1	1.1
0	38	13	2	0.2	t	2	t	0.03	0.01	0.4	0.01	1	0	3	8	*	0.1
0	6	349	23	0.5	0.4	0	11	0.09	0.05	0.3	0.27	32	0	46	74	7	0.3
0	5	251	16	0.4	0.3	0	10	0.07	0.03	0.2	0.19	30	0	32	53	3	0.5
0	t	13	1	0.1	t	25	2	t	0.01	t	t	1	0	3	2	0	t
0	2	21	2	0.2	t	21	4	t	t	0.1	t	7	0	5	2	0	0.1
0	16	574	46	0.9	0.4	0	20	0.13	0.08	1.1	0.15	91	0	58	108	1	1.6
0	7	693	83	2.4	1.3	105	3	0.11	0.18	1.8	0.08	173	0	46	197	0	0.2
0	9	638	85	3.6	2.4	13	5	0.44	0.11	1.2	0.16	240	0	40	208	*	0.2
0	7	690	86	1.9	1.7	130	4	0.17	0.24	2.3	0.11	210	0	211	84	*	0.2
0	6	290	35	3	0.4	20	87	0.22	0.12	0.9	0.23	61	0	62	77	1	0.2
0	3	294	29	1.6	1.2	131	16	0.21	0.13	1.2	0.11	75	0	34	114	2	t
0	372	294	29	1.6	1.2	131	16	0.21	0.13	1.2	0.11	75	0	34	114	1	t
0	139	269	46	2.5	1.5	107	16	0.45	0.16	2.4	0.18	94	0	38	144	1	0.2
0	8	592	72	3.4	2.1	8	1	0.3	0.18	1.8	0.1	129	0	22	178	3	0.2
0	1	27	5	0.6	0.2	16	3	0.02	0.02	0.2	*	*	0	6	17	0	1
0	1595	254	19	0.7	0.2	83	92	0.03	0.07	1.1	0.21	14	0	10	24	*	0.9
0	10	510	38	1.8	0.5	116	364	0.14	0.14	1.4	0.42	35	0	26	68	*	1
0	20	20	3	0.3	0.1	130	0	0	0.02	0.2	t	t	0	5	4	0	t
0	1990	185	16	3.8	0.3	231	18	0.04	0.07	0.7	0.28	18	0	35	23	0	0.9
0	1	121	7	0.3	0.1	43	54	0.04	0.02	0.3	0.17	11	0	7	13	0	0.5
0	1	131	7	0.3	0.1	47	66	0.05	0.02	0.4	0.18	16	0	7	14	0	0.5
0	35	311	6	1.7	0.2	260	107	0.02	0.07	0.5	0.19	14	0	8	19	*	1
0	28	439	58	2.1	0.5	5	10	0.31	0.1	2.6	0.66	51	0	37	94	*	0.5
0	9	26	1	t	t	0	1	t	0	0.1	0.01	1	0	1	3	0	0.1
93	388	538	24	1.2	0.7	9	t	0.1	0.1	1.6	0.29	22	0.22	21	78	*	1.1
0	52	27	1	0.1	t	t	t	0.01	0.01	0.2	0.02	1	0	2	3	*	0.3
0	12	332	25	4.1	0.3	0	8	0.07	0.06	1.8	0.36	13	0	20	59	*	t
56	1061	970	49	1.6	1.7	93	24	0.16	0.28	2.4	0.43	20	0.49	292	277	*	1.6
*	125	62	4	0.1	0.1	9	1	0.01	0.02	0.3	0.01	2	0	24	27	*	*
0	16	844	55	2.8	0.7	*	26	0.22	0.07	3.3	0.7	22	0	20	115	1	0.1
0	8	610	39	0.6	0.5	0	20	0.16	0.03	2.2	0.47	14	0	8	78	1	t
0	5	515	30	0.4	0.4	0	18	0.14	0.03	2	0.41	14	0	7	60	1	t
0	7	443	26	0.4	0.4	0	10	0.13	0.03	1.8	0.36	12	0	10	54	1	t
0	91	80	5	0.4	0.1	0	2	0.02	0.01	0.3	0.07	2	0	2	10	1	0.1
0	2	23	1	0.1	t	0	1	0.01	t	0.1	0.01	1	0	t	4	0	t
0	11	43	2	0.1	t	0	1	0.01	t	0.2	0.01	1	0	1	6	0	t
0	37	501	31	1.3	0.5	0	9	0.12	0.03	3.1	0.43	12	0	13	66	*	0.3

WT, weight; **KCAL**, kcalories; **PROT**, protein; **CARB**, carbohydrate; **FIBR**, fiber; **FAT**, fat; **SATF**, saturated fat;

MONO, monsaturated fat; **POLY**, polyunsaturated fat; **CHOL**, cholesterol; **SOD**, sodium; **POT**, potassium;

FOOD NAME	PORTION	WT (g)	KCAL	PROT (g)	CARB (g)	FIBR (g)	FAT (g)	SATF (g)	MONO (g)	POLY (g)
POTATO-HASH BROWN-PREPARED FROM FROZEN	CUP	156	340	5	44	1.5	18	7	8	2.1
POTATO-HUSH PUPPIES	SERVING	78	256	5	35	1.9	12	2.7	7.8	0.4
POTATO-MASHED-FROM DEHYDRATED-WITH MILK	CUP	210	166	4	28	1.2	5	1.4	1.4	1.3
POTATO-MASHED-FROM RAW-WITH MILK	CUP	210	162	4	37	1.2	1	0.7	0.3	0.1
POTATO-MASHED-HOME RECIPE-MILK/BUTTER	CUP	210	223	4	35	3.2	9	2.2	3.7	2.5
POTATO-O'BRIEN-HOME RECIPE	CUP	194	157	5	30	*	2	1.6	0.7	0.1
POTATO-SCALLOPED-HOME RECIPE	CUP	245	211	7	26	4.4	9	5.5	2.6	0.4
POTATO-SCALLOPED-PREPARED FROM MIX	OUNCE	28.4	26	1	4	0.5	1	0.7	0.3	0.1
PUMPKIN PIE MIX-CANNED	CUP	270	281	3	71	*	t	0.2	t	t
PUMPKIN-BOILED-DRAINED-MASHED	CUP	245	49	2	12	6.7	t	0.1	t	t
PUMPKIN-CANNED	CUP	245	83	3	20	5	1	0.4	0.1	t
PUMPKIN-RAW-CUBED	CUP	116	30	1	8	2	t	0.1	t	t
RADISH-DAIKON-SLICED-BOILED-DRAINED	CUP	147	25	1	5	2.9	t	0.1	0.1	0.2
RADISHES-RAW	ITEM	4.5	1	t	t	0.1	t	t	t	t
RUTABAGAS-BOILED-DRAINED	CUP	170	58	2	13	2.5	t	t	t	0.1
SAUERKRAUT-CANNED	CUP	236	45	2	10	6.1	t	0.1	t	0.1
SEAWEED-AGAR-DRIED	SERVING	28.4	87	2	23	0.9	t	t	t	t
SEAWEED-IRISHMOSS-RAW	OUNCE	28.4	14	t	3	1	t	t	t	t
SEAWEED-KELP (KOMBU)-RAW	OUNCE	28.4	12	t	3	1.2	t	0.1	t	t
SEAWEED-LAVER (NORI)-RAW	OUNCE	28.4	10	2	1	1	t	t	t	t
SEAWEED-SPIRULINA-DRIED	OUNCE	28.4	82	16	7	1.4	2	0.8	0.2	0.6
SEAWEED-WAKAME-RAW	OUNCE	28.4	13	1	3	1.2	t	t	t	0.1
SHALLOTS-FREEZE DRIED	TBSP	0.9	3	t	1	0.1	t	t	t	t
SHALLOTS-RAW	TBSP	10	7	t	2	*	t	t	t	t
SOYBEANS-DRY-COOKED	CUP	180	234	20	19	*	10	*	*	*
SOYBEANS-GREEN-BOILED-DRAINED	CUP	180	254	22	20	*	12	1.3	1.3	6.4
SOYBEANS-SPROUTED-STEAMED	CUP	94	76	8	6	1	4	0.5	0.5	2.3
SPINACH-CANNED-DIETARY PACK-LOW SODIUM	CUP	234	45	5	7	5.1	1	0.1	t	0.4
SPINACH-CANNED-DRAINED	CUP	214	50	6	7	6.8	1	0.2	t	0.4
SPINACH-CANNED-SOLIDS AND LIQUIDS	CUP	234	45	5	7	5.1	1	0.1	t	0.4
SPINACH-FROZEN-BOILED-CHOPPED	CUP	205	57	6	11	4.5	t	0.1	t	0.2
SPINACH-LEAF-FROZEN-BOILED-DRAINED	CUP	190	53	6	10	4	t	0.1	t	0.2
SPINACH-RAW-BOILED-DRAINED	CUP	180	41	5	7	4	t	0.1	t	0.2
SPINACH-RAW-CHOPPED	CUP	56	12	2	2	1.5	t	t	t	0.1
SQUASH-ACORN-BAKED	CUP	205	115	2	30	4.3	t	0.1	t	0.1
SQUASH-BUTTERNUT-BAKED	CUP	205	82	2	22	3.5	t	t	t	0.1
SQUASH-HUBBARD-BOILED-MASHED	CUP	236	71	3	15	4.2	1	0.2	0.1	0.4
SQUASH-SUMMER-BOILED-SLICED	CUP	180	36	2	8	2.5	1	0.1	t	0.2
SQUASH-WINTER-BAKE-MASHED	CUP	205	80	2	18	5.7	1	0.3	0.1	0.5
SQUASH-ZUCCHINI-FROZ-BOILED	CUP	223	38	3	8	3.2	t	0.1	t	0.1
SQUASH-ZUCCHINI-ITALIA-CANNED	CUP	227	66	2	16	7	t	0.1	t	0.1
SQUASH-ZUCCHINI-RAW-BOILED	CUP	180	29	1	7	2.3	t	t	t	t
SQUASH-ZUCCHINI-RAW-SLICED	CUP	130	18	2	4	2	t	t	t	0.1
SUCCOTASH-BOILED-DRAINED	CUP	192	221	10	47	14	2	0.3	0.3	0.7
SWEET POTATO-BAKED-PEELED	ITEM	114	117	2	28	3.4	t	t	t	0.1
SWEET POTATO-BOILED-MASHED	CUP	328	344	5	80	9.8	1	0.2	t	0.4
SWEET POTATO-CANDIED	PIECE	105	144	1	29	1.1	3	1.4	0.7	0.2
SWEET POTATO-CANNED-MASHED	CUP	255	258	5	59	4.6	1	0.1	t	0.2
SWEET POTATO-CANNED-VACUUM PACK	CUP	200	182	3	42	4.8	t	0.1	t	0.2
TARO ROOT-COOKED-SLICED	CUP	132	187	1	46	6	t	t	t	0.1
TARO ROOT-RAW-SLICED	CUP	104	111	2	28	*	t	t	t	0.1
TEMPEH-SOYBEAN PRODUCT	CUP	166	330	32	28	*	13	1.8	2.8	7.2
TOFU-FRIED	PIECE	13	35	2	1	0.2	3	0.4	0.6	1.5
TOFU-OKARA	CUP	122	94	4	15	5	2	0.2	0.4	0.9
TOFU-RAW-FIRM	CUP	252	365	40	11	3	22	3.2	4.9	12.4
TOFU-SOYBEAN CURD	PIECE	120	86	9	3	1.4	5	2.6	4.4	4.8
TOMATO JUICE-CANNED	CUP	244	42	2	10	2.9	t	t	t	0.1
TOMATO JUICE-LOW SODIUM	CUP	244	42	2	10	2.8	t	t	t	0.1
TOMATO PASTE-CANNED-LOW SODIUM	CUP	262	220	10	49	11.3	2	0.3	0.4	0.9
TOMATO PASTE-CANNED-SALT ADDED	CUP	262	220	10	49	11.3	2	0.3	0.4	0.9
TOMATO POWDER	OUNCE	28.4	86	4	21	0.7	t	t	t	0.1
TOMATO PUREE-CANNED-LOW SODIUM	CUP	250	103	4	25	5.8	t	t	t	0.1
TOMATO PUREE-CANNED-SALT ADDED	CUP	250	103	4	25	5.8	t	t	t	0.1

t = Trace of nutrient present ** = Not available*

MAG, magnesium; **IRON**, iron; **ZINC**, zinc; **VITA**, vitamin A; **VITC**, vitamin C; **THIA**, thiamin; **RIBO**, riboflavin; **NIAC**, niacin; **VB6**, vitamin B-6; **FOL**, folate; **VB12**, vitamin B-12; **CALC**, calcium; **PHOS**, phosphorus; **SEL**, selenium; **VE-a**, alpha tocopherol equivalents.

CHOL (mg)	SOD (mg)	POT (mg)	MAG (mg)	IRON (mg)	ZINC (mg)	VITA (RE)	VITC (mg)	THIA (mg)	RIBO (mg)	NIAC (mg)	VB6 (mg)	FOL (µg)	VB12 (µg)	CALC (mg)	PHOS (mg)	SEL (µg)	VE-a (mg)
0	54	680	26	2.3	0.5	0	10	0.17	0.03	3.8	0.2	39	0	24	112	1	0.3
135	965	188	16	1.4	0.4	9	0	0	0.02	2	0.1	21	0.18	69	190	*	1.8
4	491	704	34	1.3	0.5	19	6	0.06	0.11	1.7	0.42	15	0	65	92	1	0.1
4	636	628	39	0.6	0.6	4	14	0.19	0.08	2.4	0.49	17	0.11	55	100	1	0.1
4	620	607	38	0.5	0.6	42	13	0.18	0.08	2.3	0.47	17	0	55	97	1	0.1
7	421	516	35	0.9	0.6	93	32	0.15	0.11	2	0.41	16	0.16	70	97	*	*
29	821	926	47	1.4	1	47	26	0.17	0.23	2.6	0.44	21	0	140	154	*	1.1
*	97	58	4	0.1	0.1	6	1	0.01	0.02	0.3	0.01	t	0	10	16	*	*
0	562	373	43	2.9	0.7	2241	9	0.04	0.32	1	0.43	95	0	100	122	*	*
0	3	564	22	1.4	0.6	265	12	0.08	0.19	1	0.11	21	0	37	74	*	2.5
0	12	505	56	3.4	0.4	5404	10	0.06	0.13	0.9	0.14	30	0	64	86	*	2.5
0	1	1	14	0.9	0.4	186	10	0.06	0.13	0.7	0.06	16	0	24	51	1	1.2
0	19	419	13	0.2	0.2	0	22	0	0.03	0.2	0.06	26	0	25	35	1	0.7
0	1	10	t	t	t	t	1	0	t	t	t	1	0	1	1	0	0
0	31	488	36	0.8	0.5	0	37	0.12	0.06	1.1	0.15	26	0	71	83	*	0.3
0	1560	401	31	3.5	0.4	5	35	0.05	0.05	0.3	0.31	56	0	71	47	24	3.9
0	29	320	219	6.1	1.7	0	0	t	0.06	0.1	0.09	165	0	178	15	2	1.6
0	19	18	41	2.5	0.6	3	3	t	0.13	0.2	0.02	52	0	20	45	*	0.3
0	66	25	34	0.8	0.3	3	1	0.01	0.04	0.1	t	51	0	48	12	2	0.2
0	14	101	1	0.5	0.3	148	11	0.03	0.13	0.4	0.05	42	0	20	17	1	0.3
0	298	387	55	8.1	0.6	16	3	0.68	1.04	3.6	0.1	27	0	34	34	2	1
0	248	14	30	0.6	0.1	10	1	0.02	0.07	0.5	t	56	0	43	23	1	0.3
0	1	15	1	0.1	t	51	t	t	t	t	0.02	1	0	2	3	*	*
0	1	33	2	0.1	t	125	1	0.01	t	t	0.04	3	0	4	6	*	t
0	4	972	*	4.9	*	5	0	0.38	0.16	1.1	*	*	0	131	322	*	*
0	25	970	108	4.5	1.6	29	31	0.47	0.28	2.3	0.11	201	0	261	284	90	0
0	9	334	56	1.2	1	1	8	0.19	0.05	1	0.1	75	0	56	127	47	t
0	746	538	131	3.7	1	1505	32	0.04	0.25	0.6	0.19	136	0	194	75	3	t
0	57	740	162	4.9	1	1878	31	0.03	0.3	0.8	0.21	209	0	271	94	2	t
0	746	538	131	3.7	1	1505	32	0.04	0.25	0.6	0.19	136	0	194	75	3	t
0	176	611	141	3.1	1.4	1596	25	0.12	0.34	0.9	0.3	220	0	299	98	2	3.9
0	164	566	131	2.9	1.3	1479	23	0.11	0.32	0.8	0.28	204	0	277	91	2	3.6
0	126	839	157	6.4	1.4	1474	18	0.17	0.43	0.9	0.44	262	0	245	101	2	3.4
0	44	312	44	1.5	0.3	376	16	0.04	0.11	0.4	0.11	108	0	55	27	1	1
0	9	896	87	1.9	0.4	88	22	0.34	0.03	1.8	0.4	38	0	90	93	2	0.2
0	8	582	60	1.2	0.3	1435	31	0.15	0.04	2	0.25	39	0	84	55	2	0.2
0	12	505	32	0.7	0.2	946	15	0.1	0.07	0.8	0.24	23	0	24	33	2	0.3
0	2	346	44	0.6	0.7	52	10	0.08	0.07	0.9	0.12	36	0	48	69	6	0.2
0	2	896	16	0.7	0.5	730	20	0.17	0.05	1.4	0.15	57	0	29	41	6	0.2
0	4	433	29	1.1	0.4	96	8	0.09	0.09	0.9	0.1	17	0	38	56	7	0.3
0	850	622	31	1.5	0.6	123	5	0.1	0.09	1.2	0.35	69	0	39	66	*	0.3
0	5	455	40	0.6	0.3	43	8	0.07	0.07	0.8	0.14	30	0	23	72	6	0.2
0	4	322	29	0.5	0.3	44	12	0.09	0.04	0.5	0.12	29	0	20	42	4	0.2
0	33	787	102	2.9	1.2	56	16	0.32	0.18	2.6	0.22	63	0	33	225	*	0.7
0	11	397	23	0.5	0.3	2487	28	0.08	0.15	0.7	0.28	26	0	32	63	1	5.2
0	42	602	32	1.8	0.9	5594	56	0.17	0.46	2.1	0.8	36	0	70	88	2	15
0	73	198	12	1.2	0.2	440	7	0.02	0.04	0.4	0.04	12	0.03	27	27	1	4.6
0	191	536	61	3.4	0.5	3857	13	0.07	0.23	2.4	0.17	27	0	76	133	2	1.1
0	106	624	44	1.8	0.4	1596	53	0.07	0.11	1.5	0.38	33	0	44	98	2	0.9
0	20	638	40	1	0.4	0	7	0.14	0.04	0.7	0.44	25	0	24	100	*	3.3
0	11	615	34	0.6	0.2	0	5	0.1	0.03	0.6	0.29	23	0	45	87	*	*
0	10	609	116	3.8	3	114	0	0.22	0.18	7.7	0.5	86	1.66	154	342	*	*
0	2	19	8	0.6	0.3	0	0	0.02	0.01	t	0.01	3	0	48	37	0	t
0	11	259	32	1.6	0.7	0	0	0.02	0.02	0.1	0.14	32	0	98	73	*	*
0	35	597	237	26.4	4	43	1	0.4	0.26	1	0.23	74	0	517	479	5	*
0	8	50	115	2.3	1	0	0	0.07	0.04	0.1	0.06	21	0.05	154	151	2	1.1
0	881	537	27	1.4	0.3	137	45	0.11	0.08	1.6	0.27	49	0	22	46	1	0.5
0	24	537	27	1.4	0.3	137	45	0.11	0.08	1.6	0.27	49	0	22	46	1	0.5
0	172	2442	134	7.8	2.1	647	111	0.41	0.5	8.4	1	59	0	92	207	3	*
0	2070	2442	134	7.8	2.1	647	111	0.41	0.5	8.4	1	59	0	92	207	3	4.4
0	38	547	51	1.3	0.5	490	33	0.26	0.22	2.6	0.13	34	0	47	84	*	0.2
0	50	1050	60	2.3	0.6	340	88	0.18	0.14	4.3	0.38	28	0	38	100	3	0.6
0	998	1050	60	2.3	0.6	340	88	0.18	0.14	4.3	0.38	28	0	38	100	3	0.6

WT, weight; **KCAL**, kcalories; **PROT**, protein; **CARB**, carbohydrate; **FIBR**, fiber; **FAT**, fat; **SATF**, saturated fat;

MONO, monsaturated fat; **POLY**, polyunsaturated fat; **CHOL**, cholesterol; **SOD**, sodium; **POT**, potassium;

FOOD NAME	PORTION	WT (g)	KCAL	PROT (g)	CARB (g)	FIBR (g)	FAT (g)	SATF (g)	MONO (g)	POLY (g)
TOMATO-CANNED-DIETARY PACK-LOW SODIUM	CUP	240	48	2	10	1.7	1	0.1	0.1	0.2
TOMATO-COOKED-STEWED-HOME RECIPE	CUP	101	80	2	13	1	3	0.5	1.1	0.9
TOMATO-RED-CANNED-STEWED	CUP	255	66	2	17	2	t	0.1	0.1	0.1
TOMATO-RED-CANNED-WHOLE	CUP	240	48	2	10	1.9	1	0.1	0.1	0.2
TOMATO-RED-CANNED-WITH GREEN CHILIES	CUP	241	36	2	9	0.9	t	t	t	0.1
TOMATO-RED-RAW-BOILED	CUP	240	65	3	14	2.1	1	0.1	0.2	0.4
TOMATO-RED-RIPE-RAW	ITEM	123	26	1	6	1.6	t	0.1	0.1	0.2
TOMATOES-GREEN-RAW	ITEM	123	30	1	6	0.6	t	t	t	0.1
TURNIP GREENS-FROZEN-BOILED	CUP	164	49	5	8	5.1	1	0.2	t	0.3
TURNIP GREENS-RAW-BOILED	CUP	144	29	2	6	4.5	t	0.1	t	0.1
TURNIPS-BOILED-DRAINED-DICED	CUP	156	28	1	8	3.1	t	t	t	0.1
VEGETABLE JUICE-CANNED	CUP	242	46	2	11	2.7	t	t	t	0.1
VEGETABLE JUICE-SNAP E TOM-TOMATO	CUP	243	46	2	9	1.9	0	0	0	0
VEGETABLE JUICE-V8 COCKTAIL-LOW SODIUM	CUP	243	51	0	10	2.7	0	0	0	0
VEGETABLE JUICE-V8-REGULAR	CUP	243	49	0	10	2.4	0	0	0	0
WATERCHESTNUTS-CHINESE-CANNED	CUP	140	70	1	17	*	t	t	t	t
WATERCHESTNUTS-CHINESE-RAW	CUP	124	131	2	30	*	t	t	t	t
WATERCRESS-RAW	CUP	34	4	1	t	0.4	t	t	t	t
YAM-MOUNTAIN-HAWAII-STEAMED	CUP	145	119	3	29	5.6	t	t	t	0.1
YAMS-BOILED OR BAKED-DRAINED	CUP	136	158	2	38	3.3	t	t	t	0.1

t = Trace of nutrient present ** = Not available*

MAG, magnesium; **IRON**, iron; **ZINC**, zinc; **VITA**, vitamin A; **VITC**, vitamin C; **THIA**, thiamin; **RIBO**, riboflavin; **NIAC**, niacin; **VB6**, vitamin B-6; **FOL**, folate; **VB12**, vitamin B-12; **CALC**, calcium; **PHOS**, phosphorus; **SEL**, selenium; **VE-a**, alpha tocopherol equivalents.

CHOL (mg)	SOD (mg)	POT (mg)	MAG (mg)	IRON (mg)	ZINC (mg)	VITA (RE)	VITC (mg)	THIA (mg)	RIBO (mg)	NIAC (mg)	VB6 (mg)	FOL (μg)	VB12 (μg)	CALC (mg)	PHOS (mg)	SEL (μg)	VE-a (mg)
0	31	530	29	1.5	0.4	144	36	0.11	0.07	1.8	0.22	19	0	62	46	2	0.5
0	460	249	15	1.1	0.2	68	18	0.11	0.08	1.1	0.09	11	0	26	38	1	0.3
0	648	609	31	1.9	0.4	140	34	0.12	0.09	1.8	0.04	14	0	84	51	2	0.6
0	391	530	29	1.5	0.4	144	36	0.11	0.07	1.8	0.22	19	0	62	46	2	0.5
0	966	258	27	0.6	0.3	94	15	0.08	0.05	1.5	0.25	22	0	48	34	2	0.5
0	26	670	34	1.3	0.3	178	55	0.17	0.14	1.8	0.23	31	0	14	74	1	0.8
0	11	273	14	0.6	0.1	76	24	0.07	0.06	0.8	0.1	19	0	6	30	1	0.4
0	16	251	12	0.6	0.1	79	29	0.07	0.05	0.6	0.1	11	0	16	34	*	0.5
0	25	367	43	3.2	0.7	1309	36	0.09	0.12	0.8	0.11	65	0	249	56	1	3.7
0	42	292	32	1.2	0.2	792	40	0.07	0.1	0.6	0.26	171	0	197	42	1	3.3
0	78	211	13	0.3	0.3	0	18	0.04	0.04	0.5	0.11	14	0	34	30	1	t
0	883	467	27	1	0.5	283	67	0.1	0.07	1.8	0.34	51	0	27	41	1	0.8
0	1298	688	27	1.9	0.5	103	10	0.1	0.07	2.4	0.34	51	0	37	41	*	0.5
0	58	571	*	1.5	*	437	53	0.05	0.07	1.9	*	*	0	39	*	1	*
0	819	513	27	1.5	0.5	342	49	0.05	0.05	1.7	0.34	51	0	29	41	1	0.8
0	12	164	6	1.2	0.5	1	2	0.02	0.03	0.5	0.22	8	0	6	28	*	*
0	17	724	27	0.1	0.6	0	5	0.17	0.25	1.2	0.41	20	0	14	78	*	*
0	14	112	8	0.1	t	160	15	0.03	0.04	0.1	0.04	3	0	40	20	*	0.3
0	18	717	15	0.6	0.5	0	0	0.13	0.02	0.2	0.3	18	0	11	57	1	6.6
0	11	911	25	0.7	0.3	0	17	0.13	0.04	0.8	0.31	22	0	19	66	1	6.2

APPENDIX F

FOOD COMPOSITION TABLES FOR CANADIANS*

	PORTION	WT (g)	KCAL	PROT (g)	CARB (g)	FAT (g)	CHOL (mg)	SATF (g)	MONO (g)
DAIRY PRODUCTS									
Cottage cheese, dry curd, 0.4% butterfat	250 ml	153	129	26	3	tr†	10	tr	tr
Processed food		45	149	9	4	11	29	7	
Cheddar, cold pack									
Coffee whitener	15 ml	15	20	tr	2	1	0	tr	
Skim milk	250 ml	259	90	9	13	tr	5	tr	
Evaporated milk 2% butterfat, undiluted	250 ml	268	246	20	30	5	21	3	
MEAT									
Creton	15 ml	13	59	2	tr	5	11	2	
Wieners, beef, and pork	1	37	95	5	3	7	37	2	
Beaver, roasted		90	223	26	0	12	90	5	
VEGETABLES									
Asparagus, boiled, drained	4 spears	60	15	2	3	tr	0	tr	
Brussels sprouts	250 ml	165	64	4	14	tr	0	tr	
Applehead	250 ml	93	19	2	3	tr	0	tr	
Greens, frozen, cooked									
Parsnips, boiled, drained	250 ml	165	134	2	32	tr	0	tr	
Turnips, boiled, drained, mashed	250 ml	243	44	2	12	tr	0	tr	
GRAIN PRODUCTS									
Bread, white	1 slice	28	76	2	14	tr	tr	tr	
Calcium carbonate added to flour									
Bran flakes	200 ml	40	139	4	30	tr	0	tr	
Corn flakes	200 ml	19	70	1	16	tr	0	tr	
Rice, white, short-grained, cooked	250 ml	73	202	4	45	tr	0	tr	
Wheat flour	250 ml	133	484	14	101	1	0	tr	
Macaroni, enriched, cooked	250 ml	148	164	5	34	1	0	tr	
Egg noodles, enriched, cooked	250 ml	70	211	7	39	2	0	tr	
Red River cereal, cooked	125 ml	125	82	3	16	tr	0	tr	
Oats, puffed (Cheerios)	250 ml	24	92	3	17	2	tr	0	
FRUIT									
Apple juice	250 ml	262	123	tr	31	tr	0	tr	
Canned or bottled									
Vitamin C added									
Grapes, Canadian type (slip skin)	10	24	15	tr	4	tr	0	tr	

From Health and Welfare Canada: *Nutrient value of some common foods,* Ottawa, Canada KIA 059, revised 1988, reprinted 1993; Canadian Government Publishing Center.

* Ninety percent of the data on 3211 foods in the Canadian Nutrient File (CNF) has been derived from USDA Handbook Nos 8-1 through 8-14. Foods shown in this appendix are representative of foods for which some nutrient values differ from USDA values. These include (1) foods typically Canadian, (2) cereal products subject to Canada's mandatory enrichment standards, and (3) enriched fruit juices.

† *tr,* Trace.

POLY (g)	SOD (mg)	POT (mg)	IRON (mg)	VITA (RE)	VITC (mg)	THIA (mg)	RIBO (mg)	NIAC (mg)	CALC (mg)	FIBR (g)
tr	20	50	0.4	12	0	0.04	0.22	5.1	49	
tr	435	163	0.4	91	0	0.01	0.2	2.2	224	
tr	12	29	tr		0	0	tr	1		
tr	133	429	0.1	153	3	0.09	0.36	2.3	320	
tr	296	851	0.6	210	44	0.12	0.84	5.1	738	
tr	37	25	0.3	tr		0.05	0.02	0.8	2	
1	507	31		14		0.02	0.04	1.8	35	
2	37	331	1.4	0		0.07	0.34	15	19	
tr	2	186	0.4	50	16	0.06	0.07	0.9	41	0.9
tr	35	523	2	119	102	0.18	0.13	1.8	59	5
tr	2	206	0.8	7	tr	tr	tr		5	0.3
tr	17	606	1	0	21	0.14	0.08	1.6	61	5.8
tr	92	262	0.4	0		0.06	0.04	0.8	41	3
tr	142	29	0.7	0	0	0.08	0.05	1.2	46	0.4
tr	291	175	5.3	4	0	0.8	0.04	2.7	1	3.9
tr	185	21	2.5	0	0	0.38	tr	1.2	tr	tr
tr	692	52	0.4	0	0	0.04	0.02	1.4	19	0.6
tr	125	0	5.2			0.63	0.4	8.4	21	3.9
tr	1	90	2.2	0	0	0.21	0.38	2.6	12	1.2
tr	3	74	2.5	35	0	0.24	0.43	3.3	17	—
tr	7	0	0.4	1	0	0.04	tr	1.1	13	2.4
tr	214	86	3.2	0	0	0.02	0.02	1.9	28	0.8
tr	8	312	1	0	87	0.06	0.05	0.3	18	
tr	tr	46	tr	2	tr	0.02	0.01	tr	3	0.3

A P P E N D I X G

FOOD SOURCES OF NUTRIENTS IN RELATION TO THE DAILY VALUES

FOOD SOURCES OF NUTRIENTS IN RELATION TO DAILY VALUES (DVs)

NUTRIENT	SOURCES* EXCELLENT (75% DV)	SIGNIFICANT (50% DV)	GOOD (25% DV)	FAIR (10% DV)
Vitamin A	Cantaloupe Carrots Liver Sweet potatoes Spinach Turnip greens		Apricots	Broccoli Brussels sprouts Green peas Pumpkin Milk
Vitamin C	Cauliflower (raw) Brussels sprouts (raw) Oranges Spinach (raw) Strawberries	Asparagus Broccoli Carrots Cantaloupe Red cabbage Tangerines	Cabbage Cooked spinach Grapefruit Tomato	Apples Blueberries Green peas Peaches Radishes Sauerkraut
Vitamin B_6	Super fortified cereals		Beef liver Chicken breast Garbanzo beans Soybeans	Alfalfa sprouts Avocado Bananas Beef Potatoes Spinach Tomato sauce Tuna
Folate	Liver Sugar-fortified cereals		Asparagus Cooked lentils Navy beans	Artichokes Avocado Broccoli Brussels sprouts Cauliflower Green peas Okra Orange juice Spinach
Vitamin B_{12}	Beef liver Clams Lamb Salmon		Veal Swordfish	Eggs Cottage cheese Scallops

* Because they are frequently consumed, some foods that are fair or good sources of a particular nutrient may actually make greater contributions to the overall dietary intake of a nutrient than those that qualify as significant or excellent sources.

FOOD SOURCES OF NUTRIENTS IN RELATION TO DAILY VALUES (DVs) *(continued)*

NUTRIENT	SOURCES* EXCELLENT (75% DV)	SIGNIFICANT (50% DV)	GOOD (25% DV)	FAIR (10% DV)
Calcium			Buttermilk Milk Sardines Swiss cheese Yogurt	Beet greens Broccoli Canned salmon Processed cheese Spinach Tofu
Magnesium			Canned salmon Lima beans Spinach	Broccoli Ice cream Lettuce Milk Peanut butter Tomato Whole wheat bread
Iron	Pork liver		Beef liver Oysters Raisin Bran (enriched) Soybeans	Bagel Chick peas Kidney beans Noodles Potatoes Rice Spinach Tuna Turkey
Zinc		Calf liver Oysters	Beef Beef or pork liver Veal	Chicken Pork

APPENDIX H

EXCHANGE SYSTEM LISTS

MILK EXCHANGE LIST

SKIM MILK (12 g carbohydrate, 8 g protein, 0 g fat, 90 kcal)

1 MILK EXCHANGE	
1 cup	Skim or nonfat milk (½% and 1%)
⅓ cup	Powdered (nonfat dry, before adding liquid)
½ cup	Canned, evaporated skim milk
1 cup	Buttermilk made from skim milk
1 cup	Yogurt made from skim milk (plain, unflavored)

LOW-FAT MILK (12 g carbohydrate, 8 g protein, 5 g fat, 120 kcal)

1 MILK EXCHANGE, 1 FAT EXCHANGE	
1 cup	2% fat-fortified milk
1 cup	Plain nonfat yogurt

WHOLE MILK (12 g carbohydrate, 8 g protein, 8 g fat, 150 kcal)

1 MILK EXCHANGE, 2 FAT EXCHANGES	
1 cup	Whole milk
½ cup	Buttermilk made from whole milk
1 cup	Custard-style yogurt made from whole milk (plain, unflavored)

VEGETABLE EXCHANGE LIST

(5 g carbohydrate, 2 g protein, 0 fat, 25 kcal)

1 EXCHANGE IS
½ CUP OF COOKED VEGETABLES OR VEGETABLE JUICE;
1 CUP OF RAW VEGETABLES

Artichoke (medium)
Beans (green, wax)
Beets
Broccoli
Brussels sprouts
Cabbage
Carrots
Cauliflower
Celery
Eggplant
Green pepper
Greens
Onions
Pea pods
Rhubarb
Sauerkraut
Squash, summer
String beans (green, yellow)
Tomatoes
Tomato juice
Turnips
Vegetable juice

FRUIT EXCHANGE LIST

(15 g carbohydrate, 0 g protein, 0 g fat, 60 kcal)

1 FRUIT EXCHANGE

1	Apple (2″ diameter)
4 rings	Dried apple
½ cup	Apple juice
½ cup	Applesauce (unsweetened)
7 halves	Apricots, fresh
½ cup	Apricots, canned
4 medium	Apricots, dried
½	Banana, 9″ long
¾ cup	Blackberries
¾ cup	Blueberries
1 cup	Raspberries
1¼ cup	Strawberries
⅓ melon	Cantaloupe (5″ diameter)
12 large	Cherries (large, raw)
½ cup	Cherries, canned
½ cup	Cider
⅓ cup	Cranberry juice
2½ medium	Dates
2	Figs, fresh (2″ diameter)
1½	Figs, dried
½	Grapefruit
½ cup	Grapefruit juice
14	Grapes
⅓ cup	Grape juice
⅛	Honeydew melon (7″ diameter)
1	Kiwi (large)
¾ cup	Mandarin oranges
½ small	Mango
1 small	Nectarine (1½″ diameter)
1 small	Orange (2½″ diameter)
½ cup	Orange juice
1 medium or ¾ cup	Peach, fresh (2¾″ diameter)
½ cup or 2 halves	Peach, canned
1 small or ½ large	Pear, fresh
½ cup or 2 halves	Pear, canned
¾ cup	Pineapple, raw
⅓ cup	Pineapple, canned
½ cup	Pineapple juice
1 medium	Plums (2″)
3	Prunes, dried
⅓ cup	Prune juice
2 T	Raisins
1 medium	Tangerine (2½″ diameter)
1¼ cups	Watermelon (cubes)

STARCH/BREAD EXCHANGE LIST

(15 g carbohydrate, 3 g protein, 0 g fat, 80 kcal)

1 STARCH/BREAD EXCHANGE

BREAD	
1 slice	White (including French and Italian)
1 slice	Whole wheat
1 slice	Rye or pumpernickel
1 slice	Raisin (untoasted)
2 (⅔ oz)	Bread sticks (crisp, 4″ long, ½″ wide)
½ (1 oz)	Bagel, small
½	English muffin
1	Plain roll
½ (1 oz)	Frankfurter roll
½ (1 oz)	Hamburger bun
3 T	Dried bread crumbs
1	Tortilla (6″)
½	Pita (6″ diameter)
CEREAL/GRAINS/PASTA	
½ cup	Bran flakes
¾ cup	Other ready-to-eat unsweetened cereal
1½ cup	Puffed cereal (unfrosted)
½ cup	Cereal (cooked)
⅓ cup	Rice or barley (cooked)
3 T	Grapenuts
½ cup	Shredded wheat
3 T	Wheat germ
½ cup	Pasta (cooked spaghetti, noodles, macaroni)
2½ cups	Cornmeal (dry)
2½ T	Flour (dry)
CRACKERS/SNACKS	
3	Graham (2½″ square)
¾ oz	Matzoh (4″ × 6″)
24	Oyster
4	Rye crisp (2″ × 3½″)
6	Saltines
8	Animal
5 slices	Melba toast
3 cups	Popcorn
¾ oz	Pretzels
DRIED BEANS/PEAS/LENTILS	
⅓ cup	Dried beans, such as kidney, white, split, blackeye (cooked)
⅓ cup	Lentils (cooked)
STARCHY VEGETABLES	
½ cup	Corn
1 cup	Corn on the cob (6″ long)
½ cup	Lima beans
½ cup	Peas, green
1 small	Potato, white (3 oz baked)
½ cup	Potato, mashed
¾ cup	Winter squash, acorn, or butternut
⅓ cup	Yam or sweet potato

STARCH GROUP (WITH FAT)

1 STARCH/BREAD EXCHANGE 1 FAT EXCHANGE

1	Biscuit (2½″ across)
½ cup	Chow mein noodles
1 (2 oz)	Cornbread (2″ cube)
6	Cracker, round butter type
10 (1½ oz)	French fries (2″ to 3½″ long)
1	Muffin, plain, small
2	Pancake (4″ across)
¼ cup	Stuffing, bread (prepared)
2	Taco shell (6″ across)
1	Waffle (4½″ sq)
4-6 (1 oz)	Whole wheat crackers (Triscuits)

MEAT EXCHANGE LIST

(15 g carbohydrate, 3 g protein, 0 fat, 80 kcal)
LEAN (0 g carbohydrate, 7 g protein, 3 g fat, 55 kcal)

1 MEAT EXCHANGE

Beef	1 oz	Baby beef (lean, chipped beef, chuck, flank steak, tenderloin, plate ribs, round [bottom, top]), all cuts rump, spare ribs, tripe
Pork	1 oz	Leg (whole rump, center shank), ham (center slices). USDA good or choice grades such as round, sirloin, flank, and tenderloin
Veal	1 oz	Leg, loin, rib, shank, shoulder, chops, roasts, all cuts except cutlets (ground or cubed)
Poultry	1 oz	Chicken, turkey, cornish hen
Fish	2 oz	Fresh or frozen, any type canned salmon, tuna, mackerel, crab, lobster
	1 oz	Clams, oysters, scallops, shrimp
	3 oz	Sardines, drained
Cheeses	1 oz	Cottage, farmer's cheese or pot cheese (low-fat)
	2 T	Grated Parmesan
Dried beans and peas	½ cup	Cooked

MEDIUM FAT (0 g carbohydrate, 7 g protein, 5 g fat, 75 kcal)

1 MEAT EXCHANGE 1 FAT EXCHANGE

Beef	1 oz	All ground beef, roast (rib, chuck, rump), steak (cubed, porterhouse, T-bone), meat loaf
Lamb	1 oz	Leg, rib, sirloin, loin (roast and chops), shank, shoulder
Pork	1 oz	Loin (all cuts tenderloin), chops, roast, Boston butt, cutlets
Poultry	1 oz	Capon, duck (domestic), goose, ground turkey
Veal	1 oz	Cutlets
Organ meats	1 oz	All types
Cheeses	¼ cup	Cottage (creamed), mozzarella (made with skim milk), ricotta, farmer's, neufchatel
	3 tbsp	Parmesan
	1	Egg

HIGH FAT (0 g carbohydrate, 7 g protein, 8 g fat, 100 kcal)

1 MEAT EXCHANGE, 1½ FAT EXCHANGE

Beef	1 oz	Brisket, corned beef, ground beef (commercial), chuck (ground commercial), roasts (rib), steaks (club and rib). Most USDA prime cuts of beef
Lamb	1 oz	Patties (ground lamb)
Pork	1 oz	Spare ribs, loin (back ribs), pork (ground), country-style ham, deviled ham, pork sausage
Cheeses	1 oz	All regular cheeses (American, blue, brick, camembert, cheddar, gouda, limburger, muenster, swiss, monterey), all processed cheeses
Cold cuts	1 oz	Bologna, salami, pimento loaf
Frankfurter	1 oz	(Turkey, chicken)
Peanut butter	1 oz	
Sausage	1 oz	(Polish, Italian)

FAT EXCHANGE LIST

(0 g carbohydrate, 0 g protein, 5 g fat, 45 kcal)

1 FAT EXCHANGE

1/8 medium	Avocado
1 strip	Bacon, crisp
1 tsp	Butter, margarine
2 T	Cream, light
2 T	Cream, sour
1 T	Cream, heavy
1 T	Cream, cottage
DRESSING	
1 T	Oil varieties
2 tsp	Mayonnaise type
1 T	Reduced calorie (mayonnaise type)
1 T	Gravy, meat
OLIVES	
10 small or 5 large	
NUTS	
6	Almonds, whole, dry-roasted
2 large	Pecans, whole
20 small or 10 large	Peanuts, Spanish, whole
10	Peanuts, Virginia, whole
2 whole	Walnuts
1 T	Cashews, dry roasted
1 T	Seeds (pine, sunflower)
2 tsp	Pumpkin seeds
1 T	Other
OIL	
1 tsp	Corn, cottonseed, safflower, soy, sunflower, olive, peanut

FREE FOODS

A free food is any food or drink that contains less than 20 kcal/serving. You can eat as much as you want of those items that have no serving size specified. You may eat two or three servings per day of those items that have a specific serving size. Be sure to spread them out through the day.

DRINKS
Bouillon or broth without fat
Bouillon, low-sodium
Carbonated drinks, sugar-free
Carbonated water
Club soda
Cocoa powder, unsweetened (1 T)
Coffee/tea
Drink mixes, sugar-free
Tonic water, sugar-free

NONSTICK PAN SPRAY

FRUIT
Cranberries, unsweetened (1/2 cup)
Rhubarb,
unsweetened (1/2 cup)

VEGETABLES
(raw, 1 cup)
Cabbage
Celery
Chinese cabbage
Cucumber
Green onion
Hot peppers
Mushrooms (fresh)
Radishes
Zucchini

SALAD GREENS
Endive
Escarole
Lettuce
Romaine
Spinach

SWEET SUBSTITUTES
Candy, hard, sugar-free
Gelatin, sugar-free
Gum, sugar-free
Jam/jelly, sugar-free (2 tsp)
Pancake syrup, sugar-free (1-2 T)
Sugar substitutes
(saccharin, aspartame)
Whipped topping (2 T)

CONDIMENTS
Catsup (1 T)
Horseradish
Mustard
Pickles, dill, unsweetened
Salad dressing, low-calorie (2 T)
Taco sauce (3 T)
Vinegar

SEASONINGS
Basil (fresh)
Celery seeds
Cinnamon
Chili powder
Chives
Curry
Dill
Flavoring extracts
(e.g., vanilla, almond, walnut, peppermint, butter, lemon)
Garlic
Garlic powder
Herbs
Hot pepper sauce
Lemon
Lemon juice
Lemon pepper
Lime
Lime juice
Mint
Onion powder
Oregano
Paprika
Pepper
Pimento
Soy sauce
Soy sauce, low-sodium (lite)
Spices
Wine, used in cooking (1/4 cup)
Worcestershire sauce

APPENDIX I

STANDARDS FOR TRICEPS SKINFOLD MEASUREMENTS

Triceps skinfold in millimeters for persons 6 months to 19 years of age—number examined, mean, standard deviation, and selected percentiles by sex and age: United States, 1976-1980

Sex and age	Number of examined persons	Mean	Standard deviation	Percentile								
				5TH	10TH	15TH	25TH	50TH	75TH	85TH	90TH	95TH
MALE												
6-11 months	179	10.4	3.1	6.5	7.0	7.0	8.0	10.0	12.0	14.0	15.0	16.0
1 year	370	10.4	2.7	6.5	7.0	7.5	8.5	10.0	12.0	13.0	14.0	15.5
2 years	375	10.2	2.9	6.0	7.0	7.0	8.0	10.0	12.0	13.0	14.5	15.0
3 years	418	10.0	2.6	6.5	7.0	7.5	8.0	9.5	11.5	12.5	13.0	15.0
4 years	404	9.6	3.0	6.0	6.5	7.0	7.5	9.0	11.0	12.0	13.0	15.0
5 years	397	8.9	2.9	5.5	6.0	6.5	7.0	8.0	10.5	11.5	12.5	14.5
6 years	133	9.3	4.4	5.0	5.5	6.0	6.5	8.0	10.5	12.0	13.0	17.5
7 years	148	9.2	4.0	5.0	5.5	6.0	6.5	8.5	11.0	12.0	15.0	17.5
8 years	147	10.5	4.9	5.5	6.0	6.0	7.0	9.0	12.0	16.5	17.0	22.0
9 years	145	10.6	5.7	5.0	5.0	6.0	7.0	9.0	12.5	16.0	19.0	23.0
10 years	157	12.6	6.6	5.0	6.0	6.5	7.5	11.0	16.5	20.0	22.0	26.0
11 years	155	13.3	7.7	4.5	5.5	6.0	7.5	10.5	17.0	22.0	25.0	30.0
12 years	145	12.4	6.4	5.0	6.0	6.0	8.0	11.0	15.0	18.0	21.5	26.5
13 years	173	11.2	7.0	5.0	5.5	6.0	7.0	9.0	12.5	16.5	20.5	22.5
14 years	186	10.4	5.8	4.0	5.0	5.5	6.0	9.0	13.0	15.0	17.0	23.0
15 years	184	10.1	7.2	5.0	5.0	6.0	6.0	7.5	11.0	14.5	18.0	22.0
16 years	178	10.9	6.6	4.5	5.0	5.5	6.5	8.0	13.0	18.5	20.5	25.5
17 years	173	8.5	4.6	4.0	4.5	5.0	5.5	7.0	10.5	12.5	15.0	18.0
18 years	164	11.1	6.6	4.0	5.0	5.0	6.0	9.5	14.5	17.5	19.0	22.5
19 years	148	10.9	6.1	5.0	5.5	6.0	6.5	9.0	13.0	16.0	18.5	23.0
FEMALE												
6-11 months	177	9.9	2.6	6.5	7.0	7.0	8.0	10.0	11.5	12.5	13.0	14.5
1 year	336	10.6	3.3	6.0	7.0	7.5	8.0	10.5	12.0	13.5	15.0	16.5
2 years	336	10.6	3.0	6.0	7.0	7.5	8.0	10.5	12.5	13.5	15.0	16.0
3 years	366	10.3	2.9	6.0	7.0	7.0	8.0	10.0	12.0	12.5	13.5	16.5
4 years	396	10.4	3.1	6.0	6.5	7.5	8.0	10.0	12.0	13.0	14.0	15.5
5 years	364	10.6	3.2	6.0	7.0	7.5	8.5	10.5	12.5	14.0	14.5	16.0
6 years	135	11.0	3.9	6.0	7.0	7.5	8.0	10.0	12.0	14.5	16.0	18.5
7 years	157	11.5	4.5	6.0	7.0	7.5	9.0	10.5	13.0	15.0	18.0	20.0
8 years	123	11.9	5.2	6.0	6.5	7.0	8.5	11.0	14.0	16.0	18.0	21.0
9 years	149	14.3	6.5	7.0	7.5	8.5	10.0	13.0	16.0	20.0	23.0	27.0
10 years	136	14.5	5.9	7.0	8.0	8.0	10.0	13.5	18.0	21.0	22.5	24.5
11 years	140	15.7	6.9	8.0	8.5	9.0	11.0	14.0	19.5	21.5	23.0	29.5
12 years	147	15.1	6.0	7.5	8.0	9.0	11.5	13.5	18.5	21.5	23.0	27.0
13 years	162	15.9	7.9	6.0	7.5	9.0	10.5	15.0	19.0	22.0	25.0	30.0
14 years	178	17.6	7.5	8.0	10.0	10.5	12.0	17.0	21.5	25.0	29.5	32.0
15 years	145	17.1	7.1	8.5	9.5	10.0	11.5	16.5	20.5	24.5	26.0	32.1
16 years	170	19.5	7.2	11.0	11.5	12.0	14.0	18.0	23.0	27.0	30.5	33.1
17 years	134	19.8	7.8	9.5	11.0	11.5	14.0	20.0	24.5	26.5	28.5	34.5
18 years	170	19.9	7.6	11.0	12.0	12.5	14.0	18.0	23.5	27.0	32.5	35.0
19 years	158	20.4	7.6	10.5	11.5	13.0	15.0	19.0	25.0	28.0	30.0	33.5

From National Center for Health Statistics: *Anthropometric Reference Data and Prevalence of Overweight, United States, 1976-1980,* Vital and Health Statistics Series 11, No 238, Washington, DC, 1987, U.S. Department of Health and Human Services.

Triceps skinfold in millimeters for males 18 to 74 years of age—number examined, mean, standard deviation, and selected percentiles by race and age: United States, 1976-1980

Race and age	Number of examined persons	Mean	Standard deviation	Percentile								
				5TH	10TH	15TH	25TH	50TH	75TH	85TH	90TH	95TH
ALL RACES*												
18-74 years	5916	12.9	6.7	5.0	6.0	6.5	8.0	12.0	16.0	19.5	22.0	25.5
18-24 years	988	11.6	6.5	4.5	5.0	6.0	6.5	10.0	15.0	17.5	20.0	24.5
25-34 years	1067	12.9	7.0	4.5	5.5	6.5	7.5	11.5	16.5	20.0	23.0	26.0
35-44 years	745	13.8	7.1	5.0	6.0	7.0	9.0	12.5	17.0	20.0	23.0	27.0
45-54 years	690	13.5	6.7	5.5	6.5	7.0	9.0	12.0	16.5	20.0	22.0	25.5
55-64 years	1227	13.2	6.3	5.0	6.0	7.5	9.0	12.0	16.0	19.5	21.5	25.5
65-74 years	1199	12.7	6.1	5.0	6.0	7.0	8.0	11.5	16.0	18.5	21.0	25.0
WHITE												
18-74 years	5148	13.0	6.6	5.0	6.0	7.0	8.0	12.0	16.0	19.5	22.0	25.5
18-24 years	846	11.9	6.5	4.5	5.0	6.0	7.0	10.0	15.0	18.0	20.0	25.0
25-34 years	901	13.1	6.9	5.0	6.0	7.0	8.0	12.0	16.5	20.0	22.5	26.0
35-44 years	653	13.9	7.0	5.5	6.5	7.0	9.0	12.5	17.0	21.0	23.0	27.0
45-54 years	617	13.4	6.5	5.5	6.5	7.5	9.0	12.0	16.5	20.0	21.0	25.0
55-64 years	1086	13.1	5.9	5.5	6.5	7.5	9.0	12.0	16.0	19.0	21.0	24.5
65-74 years	1045	12.9	6.0	5.0	6.5	7.0	8.0	12.0	16.0	19.0	21.0	25.0
BLACK												
18-74 years	649	12.1	7.8	4.0	4.5	5.0	6.5	10.0	16.0	19.0	23.0	27.0
18-24 years	121	9.7	6.4	4.0	4.0	4.5	5.0	7.5	13.0	15.0	18.5	21.5
25-34 years	139	11.5	7.5	3.5	4.0	5.0	6.0	10.0	15.5	19.0	23.0	24.5
35-44 years	70	13.0	8.1	*	5.0	6.5	9.0	11.0	16.0	18.5	20.0	*
45-54 years	62	15.0	8.7	*	5.5	6.0	9.0	13.0	18.0	25.5	27.5	*
55-64 years	129	12.9	7.8	3.5	4.5	5.5	7.0	10.5	17.5	22.0	25.0	29.0
65-74 years	128	11.6	6.7	4.0	4.5	5.5	7.0	10.0	14.5	16.0	19.5	27.5

* Includes all other races not shown as separate categories.

Triceps skinfold in millimeters for females 18 to 74 years of age—number examined, mean, standard deviation, and selected percentiles by race and age: United States, 1976-1980

Race and age	Number of examined persons	Mean	Standard deviation	Percentile								
				5TH	10TH	15TH	25TH	50TH	75TH	85TH	90TH	95TH
ALL RACES*												
18-74 years	6588	24.9	9.8	11.0	13.0	15.0	17.5	24.0	31.0	35.1	38.0	43.0
18-24 years	1066	20.7	8.6	10.0	11.5	12.5	15.0	19.0	25.0	29.5	32.0	37.0
25-34 years	1170	23.6	9.9	10.0	13.0	14.0	16.5	22.0	29.0	33.5	36.6	43.5
35-44 years	844	26.3	9.8	12.0	14.5	16.5	19.5	25.0	32.6	37.0	40.5	44.5
45-54 years	763	27.5	9.7	12.5	15.0	17.0	20.5	27.0	34.0	38.0	40.5	45.0
55-64 years	1329	27.2	9.5	12.0	15.0	17.5	21.0	26.5	33.0	37.0	40.0	43.6
65-74 years	1416	25.7	9.0	12.0	14.5	16.5	19.0	25.0	31.0	35.0	37.6	42.0
WHITE												
18-74 years	5,686	24.7	9.5	11.5	13.5	15.0	17.5	23.5	30.5	35.0	37.5	42.5
18-24 years	892	20.8	8.5	10.5	11.5	13.0	15.0	19.0	25.0	29.0	32.0	37.1
25-34 years	1000	23.3	9.4	10.5	13.0	14.0	16.5	22.0	28.5	33.0	36.0	42.1
35-44 years	726	26.1	9.6	12.0	14.5	16.0	19.0	24.5	32.0	36.5	40.0	44.0
45-54 years	647	27.2	9.4	13.0	15.0	16.5	20.5	27.0	33.0	37.0	40.0	43.1
55-64 years	1176	27.0	9.4	12.5	15.0	17.5	21.0	26.0	32.6	36.5	39.1	43.1
65-74 years	1245	25.5	8.8	12.0	14.5	16.5	19.0	25.0	30.5	34.0	37.0	41.1
BLACK												
18-74 years	782	26.6	11.6	10.0	12.0	14.0	17.5	25.5	35.0	39.0	42.5	48.0
18-24 years	147	20.6	8.8	8.0	10.0	11.0	14.0	19.0	27.0	31.0	35.0	37.0
25-34 years	145	25.5	12.2	8.0	11.0	13.0	16.0	24.0	32.0	37.0	47.0	49.5
35-44 years	103	28.7	11.4	9.0	14.0	15.5	20.5	29.5	36.6	40.5	45.0	48.0
45-54 years	100	31.6	11.8	10.5	16.0	20.0	23.5	31.5	40.0	43.5	48.5	53.1
55-64 years	135	29.5	10.8	12.0	14.0	18.0	22.0	28.5	38.5	42.0	43.0	46.0
65-74 years	152	29.0	10.5	11.5	14.5	17.0	21.5	29.0	37.0	38.6	44.0	47.5

* Includes all other races not shown as separate categories.

APPENDIX J

SELECTED SOURCES OF RELIABLE NUTRITION INFORMATION

AGENCIES

AMERICAN COUNCIL ON SCIENCE AND HEALTH
1995 Broadway, 16th Floor
New York, NY 10023-5860
212-362-7044

AMERICAN DENTAL ASSOCIATION
211 E. Chicago Avenue
Chicago, IL 60611-2678
312-440-2500

AMERICAN DIABETES ASSOCIATION
1660 Duke Street
Alexandria, VA 22314
212-947-9707

AMERICAN DIETETIC ASSOCIATION
Publications Department
216 W. Jackson Boulevard
Chicago, IL 60606-6995
312-899-0400
800-366-1655 (Hotline)

AMERICAN HEART ASSOCIATION
Box BHG, National Center
7320 Greenville Avenue
Dallas, TX 75231
800-527-6941

AMERICAN ASSOCIATION OF FAMILY AND CONSUMER SCIENCES
Division of Public Affairs
1555 King Street
Alexandria, VA 22314
703-706-4600

AMERICAN INSTITUTE OF NUTRITION
9650 Rockville Pike
Bethesda, MD 20814-3998
301-530-7050

AMERICAN NATIONAL RED CROSS
Food and Nutrition Consultant
National Headquarters
431 18th Street, NW
Washington, DC 20006
202-737-8300

AMERICAN PUBLIC HEALTH ASSOCIATION
1015 15th Street, NW
Washington, DC 20005
202-467-5000

AMERICAN SCHOOL FOOD SERVICE
1600 Duke Street, 7th Floor
Alexandria, VA 22314
303-200-8484

CANADIAN DIETETIC ASSOCIATION
480 University Avenue, Suite 601
Toronto, Ontario M5G 1U2
Canada
416-596-0857

FOOD AND AGRICULTURAL ORGANIZATION
United Nations International Publishers (UNIPUB)
345 Park Avenue South
New York, NY 10016
212-686-4707
or
Liason Office for North America
1001 22nd Street, NW
Washington, D.C. 20437

FOOD AND DRUG ADMINISTRATION (FDA)
Parklane Building
5600 Fishers Lane
Rockville, MD 20852
301-443-3170

FOOD AND NUTRITION INFORMATION CENTER (FNIC)
National Agricultural Library
Room 304
10301 Baltimore Boulevard
Beltsville, MD 20705
301-344-3719

U.S. DEPARTMENT OF AGRICULTURE AGRICULTURAL RESEARCH SERVICE
Survey Systems/Food Consumption Laboratory
301-436-8457
Product Quality and Development Institute
Family Economics Research/Nutrition Education
301-436-5090
6505 Bellcrest Road
Federal Center Building
Hyattsville, MD 20782

INSTITUTE OF FOOD TECHNOLOGISTS
221 N. Lasalle Street, Suite 300
Chicago, IL 60601
312-782-8424

INTERNATIONAL LIFE SCIENCES INSTITUTE (ILSI)
1126 16th Street, Suite 111
Washington, DC 20036
202-659-0074

NATIONAL DAIRY COUNCIL
O'Hare International Center
10255 West Higgins Road, Suite 900
Rosemond, IL 60018
312-696-1020

NATIONAL FOUNDATION—MARCH OF DIMES
1275 Mamaroneck Avenue
White Plains, NY 10605
914-428-7100

NATIONAL LIVESTOCK AND MEAT BOARD
444 N. Michigan Avenue
Chicago, IL 60611
312-467-5520

PENN STATE NUTRITION CENTER
417 E. Calder Way
Pennsylvania State University
University Park, PA 16801-5663
814-865-6323

SOCIETY FOR NUTRITION EDUCATION
2001 Killebrew Drive, Ste 340
Minneapolis, MN 55425-1882
415-444-7133

SUPERINTENDENT OF DOCUMENTS
U.S. GOVERNMENT PRINTING OFFICE
Washington, DC 20402
202-783-3238

U.S. DEPARTMENT OF AGRICULTURE (USDA)
COOPERATIVE EXTENSION SERVICE
Home Economics
14th Street, SW and Independence Avenue
Washington, DC 20250
202-720-2791

AGENCIES *(continued)*

USDA OFFICE OF COMMUNICATION
Washington, DC 20250

NATIONAL SCHOOL LUNCH PROGRAM AND SCHOOL BREAKFAST PROGRAM
The Policy & Program Development Branch
Child Nutrition Division
Food and Nutrition Service USDA
3101 Park Center Drive
Alexandria, VA 22302
703-305-2620

WORLD HEALTH ORGANIZATION
Regional Office
525 23rd Street, NW
Washington, DC 20037
518-436-9686

PERIODIC NUTRITION UPDATES

ACHS News and Views
American Council on Science and Health
1995 Broadway, 16th Floor
New York, NY 10023-5860
6 issues/yr

Dairy Council Digests
National Dairy Council
O'Hare International Center
10255 W. Higgins Road, Suite 900
Rosemond, IL 60018

Dietetic Currents
Ross Laboratories
625 Cleveland Avenue
Columbus, OH 43216

Food and Nutrition News
National Livestock and Meat Board
444 N. Michigan Avenue
Chicago, IL 60611

Journal of the American Dietetic Association
Publications Department
216 W. Jackson Boulevard
Chicago, IL 60606-6995
12 issues/yr

Nutrition Action
Center for Science in the Public Interest (CSPI)
1875 Connecticut Ave., NW, Suite 300
Washington, DC 20009
10 issues/yr

Nutrition Forum
P.O. Box 747924
Regal Park, NY 11374
12 issues/yr

Nutrition and the M.D.
Raven Press
1185 Avenue of the Americans
New York, NY 10036
12 issues/yr

Nutrition Research Newsletter
P.O. Box 700
Palisades, NY 10964
12 issues/yr

Nutrition Reviews
International Life Sciences Institute (ILSI)
Springer Verlag, NY
175 Fifth Avenue
New York, NY 10010
12 issues/yr

Nutrition Today
Williams & Wilkins
428 Preston Street
Baltimore, MD 21202
6 issues/yr

Nutrition Weekly
Community Nutrition Institute
2001 South Street, NW
Washington, D.C. 20009
Weekly

Rapport
National Institute of Nutrition
210-1335 Carling Avenue
Ottawa, Ontario K1Z 8N8
613-725-1889
4 issues/yr

Tufts Diet and Nutrition Newsletter
Tufts Unversity, School of Nutrition
203 Harrison Avenue
Boston, MA 02111
12 issues/yr

APPENDIX K

DIETARY FINDINGS FROM HEALTH AND NUTRITION EXAMINATION SURVEY III DATA

Mean intake of selected nutrients consumed by males from 2 months to 80+ years of age in the United States, 1988-1991

NUTRIENTS	2 to 11 mo	1 to 2 yr	3 to 5 yr	6 to 11 yr	12 to 15 yr	16 to 19 yr	20 to 29 yr	30 to 39 yr	40 to 49 yr	50 to 59 yr	60 to 69 yr	70 to 79 yr	80+ yr
Sample size	439	601	744	368	338	868	844	735	625	473	546	444	296
Energy (kcal)	903	1339	1663	2036	2578	3097	3025	2872	2545	2341	2110	1887	1776
Carbohydrate (g)	119	176	225	272	346	381	353	335	298	266	253	231	225
Energy from carbohydrate (%)	52.7	53.2	54.8	53.5	54	49.6	47.6	47.4	46.9	46.3	48.7	49.4	51.2
Protein (g)	27	50	59	71	89	111	110	106	96	93	84	74	69
Energy from protein (%)	11.8	15	14.3	14.2	14.2	14.4	14.6	15.1	15.6	16.1	16.4	16	16
Total fat (g)	37	51	62	78	97	120	116	113	98	95	80	73	67
Energy from fat (%)	36.9	33.5	32.8	33.9	33.1	34.6	34	34.6	33.9	35.7	33.3	33.8	33.3
Saturated fat (g)	16	21	24	29	36	44	41	39	33	31	27	25	23
Monounsaturated fat (g)	9	10	23	29	37	45	44	43	37	36	30	27	26
Polyunsaturated fat (g)	8	9	11	14	18	22	23	23	21	20	16	15	13
Cholesterol (mg)	79	186	196	234	293	372	395	375	338	322	312	267	257
Alcohol (g)	0	>0	>0	>0	>0	13	23	18	18	12	11	7	4
Calcium (mg)	784	852	894	1007	1138	1274	1075	1049	834	854	875	808	721
Phosphorus (mg)	658	975	1112	1274	1517	1825	1712	1686	1452	1418	1378	1230	1147
Iron (mg)	15.9	9.7	12.5	14.5	19.5	18.6	17.9	19.2	18.2	17.3	16.6	15.8	16.2
Zinc (mg)	6.2	7	8.4	10.4	14.9	16.2	15.2	16	13.8	14.4	13.1	12.1	10.7
Magnesium (mg)	125	189	219	243	291	340	351	375	349	343	326	300	276
Copper (mg)	0.8	0.7	0.9	1.1	1.3	1.6	1.6	1.7	1.6	1.5	1.4	1.3	1.2
Sodium (mg)	623	2031	2675	3138	4018	4783	4659	4445	3980	3640	3409	3142	2861
Potassium (mg)	1366	1962	2110	2361	2791	3208	3260	3451	3263	3240	3107	2898	2595
Vitamin A (IU)	5362	3820	4524	4844	6069	4962	6623	7782	7788	7047	8306	8104	7331
Vitamin A (RE)	950	700	860	931	1231	959	1026	1245	1231	1085	1306	1322	1209
Vitamin C (mg)	136	90	104	110	129	116	121	123	115	114	107	102	97
Thiamin (mg)	1.2	1.1	1.5	1.7	2.3	2.3	2.1	2.1	1.9	1.9	1.8	1.7	1.7
Riboflavin (mg)	1.7	1.7	1.9	2.2	2.8	2.8	2.5	2.5	2.2	2.2	2.2	2.1	2
Niacin (mg)	12.6	12.4	16.9	20.4	27.6	30.3	30.4	29.7	28.3	27.5	25.2	22.5	21.4
Vitamin B_6 (mg)	0.8	1.2	1.5	1.7	2.3	2.4	2.3	2.3	2.2	2.1	2.1	1.9	1.9
Vitamin B_{12} (g)	3.1	3.3	4	4.4	6.8	6.8	6.9	7.3	6.8	5.8	6.1	5.3	5.9
Carotene (RE)	375	234	270	283	323	307	534	588	595	534	675	568	513
Vitamin E (TE)	11	4.8	6	7	14.7	10.1	10.1	11.6	10	11.3	9.8	8.9	9.2
Folate (mg)	160	183	238	278	382	339	323	389	317	318	331	303	304
Fiber (g)	4.7	9	11.2	13.1	15.1	17.4	18.7	20	18	18.3	17.6	17.2	16.5

IU, International unit; *RE,* retinol equivalent; *TE,* tocopherol equivalent.

From National Center for Health Statistics: *Energy and macronutrient intakes of persons ages 2 months and older in the U.S.: 1988-1991,* Advanced data from Vital and Health Statistics, No 255, Hyattsville, Md, 1994; and National Center for Health Statistics: *Vitamin and mineral intakes of persons ages 2 months and older in the U.S.: 1988-1991,* Advanced data from Vital and Health Statistics (in press).

Mean intake of selected nutrients consumed by females from 2 months to 80+ years of age in the United States, 1988-1991

NUTRIENTS	2 to 11 mo	1 to 2 yr	3 to 5 yr	6 to 11 yr	12 to 15 yr	16 to 19 yr	20 to 29 yr	30 to 39 yr	40 to 49 yr	50 to 59 yr	60 to 69 yr	70 to 79 yr	80+ yr
Sample size	432	630	803	877	373	397	838	791	602	456	560	407	313
Energy (kcal)	850	1236	1516	1753	1838	1958	1957	1883	1764	1629	1578	1435	1329
Carbohydrate (g)	112	163	204	229	243	254	241	228	213	199	199	185	179
Energy from carbohydrate (%)	52.4	53	54.4	52.9	54.4	52.4	50	49.7	49	49.8	51.1	52.4	54.5
Protein (g)	25	45	54	63	62	67	69	70	67	64	64	58	52
Energy from protein (%)	11.2	14.9	14.3	14.5	13.5	14.1	14.5	15.3	15.8	16.1	16.6	16.6	15.9
Total fat (g)	35	47	57	68	72	77	75	75	70	63	59	53	47
Energy from fat (%)	37.6	34	33.1	34.2	33.7	34.4	34	34.2	34.9	33.8	32.8	32.3	31.3
Saturated fat (g)	15	19	22	25	26	27	26	26	24	21	20	18	16
Monounsaturated fat (g)	9	17	21	25	27	28	28	27	26	23	22	19	17
Polyunsaturated fat (g)	8	8	10	13	14	16	16	16	15	14	13	12	10
Cholesterol (mg)	78	174	192	215	202	210	244	249	235	222	210	193	174
Alcohol (g)	0	0	0	0	0	2	9	8	5	5	4	2	1
Calcium (mg)	732	817	815	867	796	822	778	753	685	651	711	636	626
Phosphorus (mg)	604	904	983	1132	1079	1152	1137	1130	1067	1018	1048	957	898
Iron (mg)	15.1	9.3	11.2	13	12.3	12.5	12.4	12.7	12.1	11.8	13	12.8	11.7
Zinc (mg)	5.9	6.4	7.6	9.5	9.5	9.6	9.7	9.6	9.4	9.5	9.7	8.7	7.8
Magnesium (mg)	114	174	197	218	206	230	240	261	251	253	257	244	220
Copper (mg)	0.8	0.6	0.8	1	1	1.1	1.1	1.2	1.1	1.1	1.1	1	0.9
Sodium (mg)	524	1838	2383	2852	2927	3087	3002	2977	2919	2575	2578	24.11	2248
Potassium (mg)	1258	1832	1968	2080	1984	2208	2260	2480	2388	2445	2547	2375	2221
Vitamin A (IU)	4850	3575	4017	4439	4014	5179	4626	6044	5594	6055	7495	7786	7129
Vitamin A (RE)	892	674	742	823	738	816	786	909	829	934	1097	1155	1083
Vitamins C (mg)	138	87	100	91	91	101	87	99	86	93	111	98	105
Thiamin (mg)	1.2	1	1.3	1.5	1.3	1.5	1.4	1.4	1.3	1.3	1.4	1.3	1.3
Riboflavin (mg)	1.6	1.6	1.7	1.9	1.7	1.7	1.7	1.6	1.6	1.5	1.7	1.6	1.6
Niacin (mg)	11.8	11.7	15.1	17.8	17.1	18.3	19.6	19.2	19.2	18.7	19.2	17.3	17
Vitamin B_6 (mg)	0.8	1.2	1.4	1.5	1.4	1.5	1.5	1.5	1.4	1.5	1.6	1.6	1.6
Vitamin B_{12} (g)	3	3	3.4	4.3	4.1	3.9	4	4.7	4	4.3	4.2	3.6	3.5
Carotene (RE)	319	208	245	275	255	400	328	481	454	465	592	613	546
Vitamin E (TE)	11.2	4.7	5.8	6.8	6.9	8.2	7.7	8.2	7.5	7.5	8.3	7.6	7.4
Folate (mg)	180	182	214	235	220	234	230	237	220	239	279	272	255
Fiber (g)	4.1	8	10.2	11.8	11.4	12.6	12.5	13.5	12.8	13.7	14.7	14.6	12.6

IU, International unit; *RE,* retinol equivalent; *TE,* tocopherol equivalent.

APPENDIX L

FOOD FREQUENCY QUESTIONNAIRE FOR CALCIUM INTAKE ESTIMATION

TALLY	SCORE	FOOD TYPE	SERVING SIZE	I EAT THIS FOOD EVERY WEEK (SERVINGS/WEEK)	EVERY DAY (SERVINGS/DAY)
	300	Milk—whole, 2%, skim	1 cup		
	150	Cheese food or spread	1 oz		
	150	Cheese sauce	¼ cup		
	150	American cheese	1 slice		
	150	Cottage cheese	1 cup		
	250	Ricotta cheese	1 oz		
	150	Blue cheese	½ cup		
	200	Natural cheese (except cream cheese), including cheddar, Swiss, mozzarella, etc.	1 oz		
	285	Buttermilk	1 cup		
	300	Yogurt, flavored or plain	1 cup		
	450	Fast food milkshake	12 oz		
	165	Cocoa, from mix	1 packet		
	330	Eggnog	1 cup		
	280	Chocolate milk	1 cup		
	250	Macaroni and cheese, cheese souffle, lasagna, quiche, cannelloni, pizza	1 serving		
	180	Cream soup or chowder with milk	1 cup		
	115	Almonds	⅓ cup		
	180	Broccoli	1 cup		
	85	Beet greens/spinach	½ cup		
	160	Baked beans	1 cup		
	100	Figs, dried	5		
	140	Scalloped potatoes	1 cup		
	150	Soybeans	1 cup		
	150	Tofu	½ cup		
	30	Bread, white or whole grain	1 slice		
	120	Waffle or pancake	1 large		
	50	Muffin, biscuit, cornbread	1 medium		
	40	Rolls, buns	½		
	225	Egg McMuffin	1		
	130	Fast food cheeseburger or hamburger	1		
	110	Enchilada or bean burrito	1		
	125	Creamed fish and meats	1 cup		
	130	Shellfish, cooked	4 oz		
	200	Canned salmon with bones	½ cup		
	200	Sardines, smelts, herring	½ cup		
	100	Fudgesicle	1		
	125	Custard pie	1 slice		
	175	Ice cream or ice milk	1 cup		
	190	Pudding with milk	½ cup		
	200	Frozen yogurt	1 cup		

From Musgrave KO and others: *J Am Diet Assoc* 89:1484, 1989.

GLOSSARY

A

α(1-4) linkage A specific type of chemical bond between carbon atoms 1 and 4 of neighboring monosaccharide units in a polysaccharide.

α(1-6) linkage A specific type of chemical bond between carbon atoms 1 and 6 of neighboring monosaccharide units in a polysaccharide.

α-amylase An enzyme in saliva that partially digests starch (also known as ptyalin).

α-carotene One of the common carotenoids found in plant foods, which can serve as precursors of vitamin A.

abruptio placentae Separation of normally positioned placenta from the uterine wall; may result in hemorrhage and death of the fetus and/or mother.

Acceptable Daily Intake (ADI) 1% of the No Observable Effect Level (NOEL) of a chemical in a food product that a person could safely consume every day of his or her life.

acesulfame-K An alternative sweetener marketed as Sunette.

acetyl CoA Acetyl coenzyme A, the acetylated form of coenzyme A that plays a central role in energy metabolism.

acid-forming foods Foods in which the acid-forming minerals (for example, Cl, P, S) predominate over the alkali-forming minerals (for example, Ca, K, Na, Mg).

acidic amino acids Amino acids that contain an acidic carboxyl group in their side chains.

acids Substances that release hydrogen ions; soluble acids produce solutions with a pH value less than 7.0.

acrodermatitis enteropatica A rare genetic disease in which zinc absorption is significantly impaired for reasons not yet known.

acrolein A pungent decomposition product of fats, generated from the glycerol component of fats and responsible for the coughing attacks that can be caused by the fumes released by burning fat.

actin A contractile protein found in muscle filaments.

active sites The regions on the surface of enzymes at which the reactions catalyzed by the enzymes occur.

active transport Transport of a substance against a concentration gradient powered by the release of cellular energy (often from the hydrolysis of ATP).

activity equivalent The amount of activity needed to use up the energy supplied by a food.

acyl carrier protein A cellular protein involved in the metabolism of fatty acids, during which it carries the acyl groups derived from fatty acids.

adenine (A) one of the organic bases in DNA and RNA.

adipocyte A fat-storing cell.

adrenaline An early name for the hormone epinephrine, which is secreted by the adrenal gland that stimulates metabolism in response to stress.

adult growth A form of growth involving positive nitrogen balance that occurs in some adults for no obvious reason.

adult rickets Another term for the disease osteomalacia.

aerobic Requiring the presence of air.

aflatoxins The most lethal naturally occurring mycotoxins. They are not destroyed by cooking or processing and can impair the immune system and cause cancer. They are produced by the mold *Aspergillus flavus,* which grows on peanuts, corn, and cottonseed, especially when these have been damaged during harvest and are stored in warm, humid conditions. Aflatoxin can also appear in the milk of cattle that have been fed moldy grain.

agar A gum derived from algae that is used in many foods as a jelling agent and fat stabilizer.

alcohol dehydrogenase An enzyme that catalyzes the first step in the metabolism of ethanol.

alcohols A group of organic chemicals characterized by possession of one or more hydroxyl (OH) groups.

aldehydes A group of organic chemicals possessing a carbonyl group whose carbon atom is bonded to at least one hydrogen atom.

aliphatic amino acids Amino acids that contain only carbon and/or hydrogen atoms in their side chains.

alkali-forming foods Foods in which the alkali-forming (base-forming) minerals predominate over the acid-forming minerals.

alkaline Having the properties of an alkali, including a pH value greater than 7.0.

alkaline phosphatase An enzyme that can release phosphate into the plasma from various phosphorus-containing compounds.

alkalis Substances that neutralize acids and dissolve in water to yield solutions with a pH greater than 7.0.

alkalosis Excessive alkali in the blood.

allergenic Able to cause an allergy.

alpha-globulin2 The protein, also called vitamin D binding protein, which binds to vitamin D in blood plasma and transports it throughout the body.

alveoli Term used for cells of the mammary gland that produce and secrete milk (but also used for the saclike endings of the air passages in the lungs).

amenorrhea The absence of menstruation.

amide-containing amino acids Amino acids that contain an amide group in their side chains.

amine A compound that contains the amino group ($-NH_2$).

amino acid pattern (or profile) The pattern and proportion of essential and nonessential amino acids in a protein.

amino acid score A measure of protein quality based on measurements of the actual amounts of individual amino acids in a food, or in the diet as a whole relative to the need for the amino acid.

amino acid sequence The sequence in which amino acids are linked together into the structure of a protein.

amino acids The molecules from which proteins are built, each protein being composed of a specific sequence of linked amino acids.

amino group A chemical group composed of a nitrogen atom bonded to two hydrogen atoms ($-NH_2$).

amino-terminus The end of a peptide or polypeptide (protein) chain that carries a free amino group.

aminopeptidases Protease enzymes that cleave the peptide bond at the amino-terminus of a protein chain.

amniotic fluid The fluid that surrounds and protects the fetus in the uterus.

amylopectins Forms of starch composed of linked branched chains of glucose units.

amylose A form of starch composed of glucose units joined into unbranched chains.

anabolic Related to and promoting anabolism, the portion of metabolism that involves the synthesis of body compounds and tissues.

anabolic hormones Hormones that increase the rate of synthesis of bodily compounds and tissues and include insulin, androgens, and growth hormone.

anabolic steroids Steroid drugs that can stimulate anabolic metabolism and the growth of muscles.

anabolism The branch of metabolism that synthesizes body compounds and promotes tissue growth.

anaerobic Not requiring the presence of air.

anemia A deficiency of red blood cells or a deficiency of hemoglobin, or both.

anions Negatively charged ions (which are attracted toward a positively charged anode).

anorexia Loss of appetite.

anorexia nervosa A behavioral eating disorder characterized by chronic refusal to eat, often related to an abnormal and obsessive fear of becoming obese.

antagonists Chemicals that counteract or prevent the effect of the substance they antagonize.

antibodies Defensive proteins produced by the immune system. They bind to specific antigens on foreign materials and assist in inactivating them or eliminating them from the body.

anticodon A set of three bases on a transfer RNA molecule, which allows the transfer RNA to bind to a specific codon on messenger RNA, and thereby bring a specific amino acid to the ribosome during protein synthesis.

antidiuretic hormone (ADH) A hormone secreted by the pituitary gland, which acts on the kidneys to cause a decrease in water excretion within urine.

antigens The chemical groups on foreign materials that elicit an immune response against them and to which defensive antibodies can become bound.

antineuritis factor Another name for thiamin, so called for its role in preventing the inflammation of nerves known as neuritis.

antioxidants Compounds that inhibit the oxidation of other substances by undergoing "sacrificial" oxidation.

antirachitic factor Another term for vitamin D, so called for its role in preventing rickets.

antiscorbutic Scurvy preventive.

antivitamins Antagonists of vitamins that are chemically related to vitamins. They cannot perform the biological functions of vitamins and interfere with the function of true vitamins.

apatite Calcium phosphate, which is one of the major minerals laid down in developing bone tissue.

apocarotenals Intermediates in a pathway by which β-carotene can be converted into retinoic acid, without the formation of retinol as an intermediate.

apolipoproteins The protein components of plasma lipoprotein particles.

appetite suppressants Foods and drugs intended to suppress the appetite.

ariboflavinosis Riboflavin deficiency.

aromatic amino acids Amino acids that contain an aromatic group in their side chains.

ascorbic acid Vitamin C.

aspartame An alternative sweetener composed of the amino acids phenylalanine and aspartic acid. Sold under the brand name NutraSweet.

atherosclerosis A thickening of artery walls caused by the growth of hard deposits containing lipids and other materials.

atherosclerotic plaques The lesions associated with atherosclerosis, consisting of thickenings of the artery walls resulting from the growth of hard deposits containing lipids and other materials.

athyroidectomy The removal of all or part of the thyroid gland.

atomic number The number of protons within an atom.

atoms The fundamental particles of chemistry. Each element listed in the periodic table of the elements is composed of only one kind of atom.

ATP (adenosine triphosphate) The compound that acts as the main short-term energy storage and energy transfer molecule in living things. It releases energy when hydrolyzed to ADP and phosphate. ATP is often described as the "energy currency" within cells.

avidin A glycoprotein in egg whites that binds to biotin and retains it within a complex that is too big to be absorbed and is unaffected by digestive enzymes. Because avidin is denatured by cooking, cooked egg whites pose no threat to biotin status.

B

β(1-4) linkage A specific type of chemical bond between carbon atoms 1 and 4 of neighboring monosaccharide units in a polysaccharide molecule.

β-carotene A vitamin A precursor, which can be cleaved to release two molecules of retinol.

β-cryptoxanthin One of the common carotenoids found in plant foods, which can serve as precursors of vitamin A.

β-oxidation The metabolic pathway by which fatty acids are oxidized.

bariatrics The branch of medicine concerned with weight control.

basal metabolic rate The energy required to sustain basal metabolism.

basal metabolism The basic essential metabolic processes required to keep the body alive and healthy and, where applicable, growing at an appropriate rate.

base pairs The pairs of complementary bases that can hold two nucleic acid strands together, such as the base pairs that hold double-helical DNA together.

base-forming foods Foods in which the base-forming (alkali-forming) minerals (for example, Ca, K, Na, Mg) predominate over the acid-forming minerals (for example, Cl, P, S).

bases Substances that release hydroxide ions and/or react with and neutralize acids. Soluble bases are also known as alkalis.

basic amino acids Amino acids that contain a basic group within their side chains.

Basic Four The "Basic Four" food groups plan recommended in 1956 by the United States Department of Agriculture (USDA), to replace the Basic Seven plan for dietary guidance.

Basic Seven The "Basic Seven" food groups plan, which was promoted, in 1943, for dietary guidance as part of the National Wartime Nutrition Program of the United States Department of Agriculture (USDA).

beikost Any solid food added to an infant's diet.

Benedict Roth respiration apparatus A closed-circuit system used for indirect calorimetry, in which the subject receives oxygen only from a measured source of oxygen-rich air, and exhales into a container in which the waste carbon dioxide and water are removed while the remaining oxygen and nitrogen are recirculated.

benzocaine A local anesthetic used in many diet gums and candies to numb the surface of the tongue and thus destroy or diminish the sense of taste, thereby reducing food intake.

beriberi The classic thiamin deficiency disorder characterized by muscle weakness, loss of appetite, nerve degeneration, and sometimes edema.

bile A solution made in the liver, stored in the gall bladder, and released into the small intestine where it aids lipid digestion.

bilirubin A chemical formed during the degradation of heme; it is transported to the liver and then excreted in bile.

binding sites Sites on the surface of a chemical, such as a protein, to which other specific chemicals can become bound.

binge eating An eating disorder characterized by eating more food than most people would eat in a given amount of time, and a feeling that what is being eaten and how much is being eaten is out of the control of the person doing the eating.

bioavailable The amount of a dietary nutrient that is absorbed and/or utilized by the body.

biochemistry The branch of science that studies how the chemicals of the body sustain all of the body's biological functions; the science of the chemistry of life.

biocytin A biologically active derivative of biotin in which biotin is chemically combined with the amino acid lysine.

biogerontology The study of the physiological and medical aspects of aging.

biological value (BV) A measure of protein quality based on the percentage of absorbed nitrogen that is retained by the body.

biologically active amines A class of amines with specific biological effects found in some foods, notably aged cheeses, red wine, chicken, liver, and pickled herring.

Bitot's spots Spots in the conjunctiva of the eye, which are the symptom of the first stage of xerophthalmia caused by vitamin A deficiency.

blacktongue A niacin deficiency condition found in dogs.

blood sugar Another name for glucose.

body mass index (BMI) A person's weight in kilograms divided by height in meters squared.

bolus A small ball of food formed after chewing in the mouth and thrown into the esophagus by the act of swallowing.

bomb calorimeter The instrument used to perform direct calorimetry to measure the energy content of a food.

bonds The forces that hold chemicals together.

bone G1a protein Another name for osteocalcin.

Bovine somatotropin (**bST,** also known as **bGH,** for "bovine growth hormone") A growth hormone of cows, which was approved in 1993 for administration to dairy cattle, increasing their milk production efficiency by as much as 20%.

bradycardia An abnormally slow heart rate.

bran The outer layers of grain.

brown fat Specialized fat deposits found at various sites in the upper body and believed to be capable of generating heat by oxidizing fats when energy intake exceeds energy needs.

buffers Chemicals that are able to resist changes in pH when dissolved in aqueous solutions; they tend to maintain pH levels even if small amounts of acids or alkalis are added to the solutions containing them.

bulking agents Substances that give a feeling of fullness when eaten.

butyric acid The saturated fatty acid containing four carbon atoms, so-named because it was first isolated from butter.

C

calciferol Another term for vitamin D.

calcification The deposition of calcium-containing mineral crystals within developing bone tissue; also known as mineralization or ossification.

calcitonin A protein hormone produced in the thyroid gland involved in regulating calcium and phosphate balance.

calcium balance studies Studies that compare calcium intake with calcium excretion through urine and feces.

calcium equilibrium The state in which calcium intake equals calcium excretion.

calcium pantothenate A synthetic derivative of pantothenic acid that is available in crystalline form and is the form of pantothenic acid used in most nutritional supplements.

calcium rigor Inappropriately high level of muscle contraction caused by excessive calcium in the blood plasma.

caliper An instrument used to measure skinfold thickness.

caloric density The energy content of a food per unit of volume or weight, usually expressed in kcal/dl, or kcal/g.

Calorie Term (with capital "C") sometimes used to denote 1000 calories or 1 kcal.

calorie A fundamental unit of energy, equal to 4.1855 joules; 1000 calories equals 1 kcal, which is sometimes designated as 1 Calorie (with a capital "C").

Campylobacter jejuni A bacterium that can contaminate food and a leading cause of bacterial gastroenteritis.

cancer Malignant cellular neoplasm (tumor growth) that invades surrounding tissues and often metastasizes (spreads) to other parts of the body.

Caprenin An unnatural fat containing longer-chain fatty acids than those found in normal food; used as a low-calorie substitute for natural fat because it is only partially absorbed.

carbohydrate loading A dietary and exercise regimen used by some athletes to increase the amount of glycogen stored in liver and muscle.

carbohydrates A class of nutrients containing carbon, hydrogen, and oxygen atoms; most are known as sugars, starches, or dietary fibers.

carbonyl group A chemical group composed of a carbon atom attached by a double bond to an oxygen atom within the structure of an organic compound.

carboxy-terminus The end of a peptide or polypeptide (protein) chain, which carries a free carboxyl group.

carboxyl group A chemical group within organic compounds that is composed of a carbon atom bonded to a hydroxyl group and also joined by a double bond to an oxygen atom (–COOH). This chemical group is acidic because a hydrogen ion is readily detached from it.

carboxylases Enzymes that transfer carboxyl groups (or carbon dioxide groups) between compounds.

carboxylic acids Organic acids that contain at least one carboxyl group (COOH).

carboxypeptidases Protease enzymes that cleave the peptide bond at the carboxy-terminus of a protein chain.

carcinogens Cancer-producing substances.

cardiac output A measure of the capacity of the heart to pump blood.

cardiac sphincter The muscle at the point where the esophagus joins the stomach, which controls the entry of food into the stomach.

caries Tooth decay caused by the production of acid in the mouth due to the action of bacteria on carbohydrate.

cariogenic Liable to cause tooth decay (dental caries).

carotenodermia Condition in which skin, mainly on palms and soles of feet, takes on yellow or orange color as a result of excess dietary carotene.

carotenoids A class of retinoids that can serve as precursors of vitamin A.

carrageenan A gum derived from algae that is used in many foods as a jelling agent and fat stabilizer.

casein proteins A class of proteins in milk that forms hard curds when precipated by enzyme or acid in the stomach.

catabolic Concerned with the branch of metabolism known as catabolism, which involves the breakdown of substances in the body, including the reactions that release energy from foods.

catabolic hormones Hormones that decrease the overall rate of synthesis of body compounds by accelerating their breakdown. They include thyroid hormones and adrenocortical hormones.

catabolism The branch of metabolism that involves the breakdown of compounds in the body, including the reactions that release energy from foods.

catalysts Substances, such as enzymes and mineral elements, that speed up specific chemical reactions while remaining unchanged in the process.

cations Positively charged ions (which would be attracted towards a negatively charged cathode).

cell membrane The lipid bilayer membrane surrounding the cell.

cells The individual living units of life, each bounded by a cell membrane and containing a nucleus and other organelles.

cellular immune response The branch of the immune system that is mediated by cell-to-cell interactions.

cellular retinoic acid binding protein (CRABP) An intracellular protein that binds to retinoic acid and helps to regulate its metabolism.

cellular retinol binding protein (CRBP) An intracellular protein that binds to retinol and regulates its metabolism.

cellulose A complex carbohydrate composed of glucose units linked together in a form that humans cannot digest.

central nervous system (CNS) The brain and spinal cord.

cerebral clock theory A theory of aging that suggests that the brain somehow monitors the rate of metabolism and controls the rate of aging accordingly. Thus some kind of cerebral "clock" would form a link between the "rate of living" and the rate of aging.

ceruloplasmin A multifunctional copper-containing protein that converts iron to its ferric (Fe^{3+}) form, in which it can bind to apoferritin.

cevitamic acid Vitamin C (although the alternative name *ascorbic acid* is more common).

chain length A term used to refer to the number of carbon atoms within a fatty acid chain.

cheilosis A condition in which cracks appear at the corners of the mouth and the lips become inflamed. It can be caused by riboflavin deficiency.

chelates Complexes of some compound complexed with another chemical, such as a mineral ion, bound by several different points of interaction within the chelate.

chloride shift The transfer of chloride ions into and out of red blood cells in a way that maintains the electrical neutrality of the cells.

chlorophyll A green pigment in plants that is the main compound involved in absorbing the energy of the sun during photosynthesis.

cholecalciferol (vitamin D_3) The naturally occurring form of vitamin D, the one produced in animals from 7-dehydro cholesterol in skin.

cholecystokinin A polypeptide hormone normally secreted in the small intestine in response to the presence of fat. It stimulates the pancreas and gallbladder to increase their secretion of digestive enzymes.

cholesterol A waxy lipid whose structure contains multiple rings of carbon atoms; one member of the group of lipids known as sterols.

cholestryamine A cholesterol-lowering drug that binds to cholesterol-containing bile acids in the gastrointestinal tract and prevents their reabsorption.

chylomicrons The lowest density lipoprotein particles, containing triglycerides, monoglycerides, and small amounts of cholesterol and phospholipids.

chyme The homogeneous mass in the stomach produced by the mixing together of food and gastric secretions.

chymotrypsin A protease involved in the digestion of proteins.

cilia Very fine hairlike structures protruding from the surface of many cells lining various internal regions of the body.

cis A term used to describe double bonds between carbon atoms that have hydrogen atoms (or other chemical groups) attached to the *same* side of the double bond.

citric acid cycle The metabolic pathway in which acetyl CoA units become metabolized to release energy; also known as the Kreb's cycle and the tricarboxylic acid cycle.

clenbuterol A veterinary drug, used in Europe to build up muscle mass and strength in livestock before exhibition. In the United States it is not approved even for use on animals, but some athletes use it in an attempt to build up their own muscle mass and strength.

clofibrate A cholesterol-lowering drug that decreases the secretion of very low density lipoprotein (VLDL) particles from the liver.

Clostridium botulinum A microbial contaminant of food that produces a deadly neurotoxin in a low acid oxygen-free (anaerobic) environment such as found in canned vegetables with a low acid content. It is also present in some honeys.

Clostridium perfingens A microbial contaminant of food generally found in meat and poultry. It causes abdominal pain and diarrhea 8 to 24 hours after consumption of an infected meal.

cobalamin Vitamin B_{12}.

cocarboxylase Another term for thiamin pyrophosphate (TPP).

Codex Alimentarius A United Nations food safety organization founded in 1982 that attempts to standardize food safety practices and regulations throughout the world.

codon A set of three bases in mRNA that encodes the incorporation of a specific amino acid into a protein chain (or acts as a "stop" signal during protein synthesis).

coefficient of digestibility A number between 1 and 0 indicating the proportion of an ingested nutrient that ultimately becomes available to the body's cells.

coenzyme A A coenzyme that plays a major role in energy metabolism, being interconverted between its free form and its acetylated derivative acetyl coenzyme A.

coenzyme Q The generic name for a range of lipidlike substances that are somewhat similar in chemical composition to both vitamin K and vitamin E. They are all members of the group of compounds known as ubiquinones. Coenzyme Q plays a role in the respiratory chain in which the energy released from nutrients is trapped within ATP.

coenzymes Chemical groups that bind to enzymes and assist in their acts of enzymic catalysis.

cofactors Chemicals required to assist the protein parts of enzymes to perform their acts of catalysis.

cold-induced thermogenesis Shivering and a temporary process of heat production (thermogenesis) induced by exposure of the body to cold.

colipase An enzyme, generated from procolipase, which combines with pancreatic lipase and emulsified lipid droplets to convert triglycerides into free fatty acids and monoglycerides.

collagen An important structural protein in the body; the main protein within tendons, ligaments, and the intercellular material that binds cells together.

colostrum The first fluid secreted by the breast during late pregnancy and the first few days after birth. It is rich in immune factors and protein.

complementation The practice of combining different incomplete proteins to create a meal that provides sufficient amounts of all the essential amino acids overall.

complete proteins Proteins that contain all of the essential amino acids in proportions capable of promoting growth when they are the only proteins in the diet.

complex carbohydrates Large polysaccharide molecules composed of many sugar units linked together.

compound A substance containing two or more elements chemically combined.

computerized tomography A complex imaging procedure based on the extent to which x-rays pass through regions of the body with differing densities.

condensation Class of chemical reaction in which chemical units become bonded together in a process accompanied by the release of water.

cone cells Light-sensitive cells in the retina of the eye involved in the perception of color vision.

conjugase An enzyme (also known as folate hydrolase) that catalyzes the removal of glutamic acid residues from polyglutamate forms of folate in the intestinal lumen.

conjunctival impression cytology A way of obtaining a sample of cells from the surface of the eye by bringing a piece of filter paper in brief contact with the conjunctiva of the eye and then removing the paper, along with some adhered cells, for staining and microscopic analysis.

converted rice Rice prepared by parboiling the rice kernels before polishing. During this process the nutrients normally concentrated in the outer husk are driven into the kernel, where they remain when the husk is removed. This produces a refined product that has been enriched with its own original nutrients.

cornea The outer transparent layer of the eye.

coronary heart disease Heart disease associated with obstruction of the coronary blood vessels that supply blood to the heart.

cotransporter A transmembrane carrier protein shared by two different transported substances (also known as a symport).

cretinism Dwarfism caused by hyposecretion of the thyroid gland.

critical periods Periods during organogenesis when the absence of certain nutrients can cause specific congenital abnormalities.

cruciferous vegetables Vegetables such as broccoli and other members of the cabbage family.

crude fiber What remains of dietary fiber after treatment with acid and alkali. It consists primarily of cellulose and lignin.

cyanogenic glycosides Chemicals found in several hundred plants including lima beans, cassava, apple seeds, apricot kernels, and several grains. They break down during digestion to yield hydrogen cyanide, a highly toxic chemical capable of causing neurological damage.

cyanosis A condition of blueness, particularly of the skin, due to inadequate oxygenation of the blood.

cyclamates A class of alternative sweeteners, now banned in the United States.

cytoplasm The fluid interior of the cell.

cytoskeleton A network of structural proteins within the cytoplasm of the cell.

D

D-sugars Sugars that are "right-handed" in the sense that they rotate a beam of polarized light to the right.

Daily Reference Values (DRVs) Term used by the U.S. Food and Drug Administration (FDA) to refer to the reference amount of macronutrients (carbohydrate, fat, and protein) and electrolytes (sodium and potassium) used as standards for labeling purposes.

Daily Value (DV) A term used by the US Food and Drug Administration (FDA) to describe the amount of a nutrient used as the standard for labeling purposes. DVs are comprised of two sets of standards: DRVs and RDIs.

dark adaptation The recovery of the eye's sensitivity to light after exposure to bright light, for which vitamin A is required.

dark adaptation test A test that measures the speed of recovery of vision in dim light, after a period of exposure to bright light.

deamination The removal of amino groups from a molecule such as an amino acid.

deciduous teeth The first set of teeth that erupt through the gums and are then lost between the ages of 5 and 10 years.

degree of unsaturation A term used to refer to the number of carbon-carbon double bonds within an unsaturated fatty acid.

dehydrated Suffering from excessive loss of water.

dehydroepiandrosterone A weight-reducing aid not approved by the FDA for human use. It is a breakdown product of a hormone normally excreted in the urine.

Delaney clause A clause that was part of a 1958 amendment to the Federal Food and Cosmetic Act of 1938, which states that "no food or color additive may be deemed safe that has been found to cause cancer when ingested by man or animals."

denaturation The loss of a protein's functional three-dimensional structure due to environmental influences such as temperature or pH.

dental fluorosis Brown staining of teeth due to excessive fluoride deposition in the teeth.

dentin The middle layer of a tooth.

5-deoxyadenosylcobalamin One of the three main forms in which vitamin B_{12} occurs in the body (also known as coenzyme vitamin B_{12}).

deoxypyridoxine A vitamin B_6 antagonist.

dermatitis Inflammation of the skin.

detoxified Converted by the body's metabolism into harmless compounds; usually occurs in the liver.

dextrans Polysaccharides produced by caries-forming bacteria, which stick to the tooth surface to form dental plaques.

dextrin A carbohydrate produced by the partial degradation of starch.

dextrose Another name for glucose.

diabetes mellitus A clinical condition in which plasma and urine glucose levels are abnormally high, usually as a result of insulin deficiency.

diacidic Containing two acidic groups.

diacylglycerol Another name for a diglyceride.

dibasic Containing two basic groups.

dicumarol An anticoagulant drug that is chemically similar to vitamin K and that stimulates the conversion of vitamin K to vitamin K oxide in the liver. The vitamin K oxide then interferes with the normal role of vitamin K in blood coagulation.

dietary fiber All carbohydrate-related substances in food that cannot be digested, and so must pass through the gastrointestinal tract and be excreted in feces. Dietary fiber is composed of indigestible plant-based materials.

Dietary Goals A set of dietary goals prepared by the USDA and DHHS; published in the official document, *Dietary Goals for the United States,* ed 3, 1990.

differentiation The process by which immature cells become specialized (differentiated) to perform some specific function.

digestion The breakdown of food materials mechanically (through chewing) and chemically (by the action of digestive enzymes) until it is in a form from which its nutrients can be absorbed from the gastrointestinal tract into the blood and lymph.

diglyceride A compound in which two fatty acid groups are esterified to the trialcohol glycerol.

dihydrochalcones Compounds derived from fruits such as oranges and grapefruits that are being developed as alternative sweeteners.

dipeptidases A class of enzymes that cleave dipeptides into their individual amino acids.

dipeptide A molecule composed of two amino acids bonded together.

direct calorimetry The direct measurement of the heat produced by some process, including the burning of food or the activity of an intact human body.

disaccharides Simple sugars, such as sucrose, that contain two linked monosaccharide sugar rings.

discretionary salt The salt each person adds to food, as opposed to the nondiscretionary salt that is present in the food when it is presented to them.

disulfide bridges Links between different parts of a protein chain, formed by a bond between two sulfur atoms.

diuretics Substances that cause an increase in the loss of water via the kidneys within urine.

diverticulosis A condition associated with a weakening of the wall of the intestine; usually caused by pressure from hard stools.

dizygotic twins Twins derived from two different zygotes ("non-identical twins").

DMF index A measure of tooth decay based on the number of decayed, missing, and filled teeth, without evaluating the extent of any decay.

DNA Deoxyribonucleic acid, the genetic material of the cell.

dopamine oxygenase An enzyme that catalyzes the oxidation of dopamine to form the neurotransmitter norepinephrine (noradrenaline).

double-helix The structure in which DNA occurs within cells, in the form of two individual DNA molecules wound around each other.

doubly-labeled water technique A method of indirectly measuring carbon dioxide gas production, and, therefore, energy release, by "labeling" some of the water in the body with the two stable isotopes: ^{2}H (deuterium) and ^{18}O.

dry (wasting) beriberi A form of beriberi in which there is a gradual loss of body tissue and the victim becomes thin and emaciated.

dual photon absorptiometry An analytical technique used to assess calcium status by focusing light on the body and measuring the extent to which the light is absorbed.

duodenum The first short section of the small intestine, corresponding to approximately the first 8 inches after the exit from the stomach.

dysmenorrhea A condition experienced during menstruation, characterized by cramps, headache, nausea, and/or diarrhea.

E

eclampsia A potentially fatal condition that can develop from preclampsia during latter part of pregnancy; characterized by convulsions and coma.

ectomorphic Body type associated with a tall, thin stature.

edema The accumulation of fluid within tissues, making them soft and spongy with a bloated appearance.

eicosanoids A range of body compounds based on a framework containing 20 carbon atoms, which includes important physiological regulators known as prostaglandins, prostacyclins, thromboxanes, and leukotrienes derived from arachidonic and linolenic acid.

elastase A protease enzyme involved in the digestion of proteins.

electrolytes Dissolved electrically charged particles, in other words, dissolved ions.

electron-transport chain The system of carrier molecules embedded in the inner membrane of mitochondria that permit the formation of ATP in the process of oxidative phosphorylation.

electrons The fundamental negatively charged particles within atoms.

element A substance containing only one kind of atom.

embryo An animal, including a human, in the early stages of its intrauterine development. In humans, the embryo stage occupies the first 8 weeks after conception.

embryonic period Another term for organogenesis, the period of intrauterine development during which the cells of the embryo begin to differentiate into distinct tissues and functional units, which later become organs, such as the heart, lungs, liver, etc.

emulsified A term used to describe a lipid that has been suspended in water by being broken into tiny droplets. This process is usually assisted by an emulsifying agent that coats the lipid droplets in a way that prevents them from coalescing.

emulsified fats Fats that have been broken into tiny droplets and suspended throughout water in the form of an emulsion.

emulsions A mixture of two normally immiscible materials in which one of the materials is suspended within the other in the form of tiny droplets. The emulsions of most relevance to nutrition contain lipid droplets suspended in water.

enamel The outer layer of a tooth.

endocrine gland A gland that secretes hormones.

endocrine malfunction theory A theory of aging that proposes that some malfunction of hormonal control is the cause of aging.

endocytosis A process by which materials are taken into a cell within a tiny vesicle formed by the budding inwards of a portion of the cell membrane.

endogenous Derived from inside the body.

endogenous fecal calcium Calcium excreted within feces that has been absorbed into the body and then released into the digestive tract within digestive secretions.

endomorphic Body type associated with a short, stocky stature.

endopeptidases Protease enzymes that cleave peptide bonds in the middle of protein chains rather than at the ends of the chains.

endoplasmic reticulum (ER) Network of tubules and vesicles in cell cytoplasm that contributes to cell protein manufacture (via attached ribosomes) and distribution.

endosperm The nutritive tissue that surrounds the embryo in grains.

energy The capacity of a body or a physical system for doing work. There are two fundamental forms of energy: kinetic energy (the energy of motion) and potential energy (the energy of position).

energy balance The state in which the total energy intake equals total energy needs.

energy density The energy content of a food per unit of volume or weight, usually quoted in kcal/dl, kcal/ml, or kcal/g.

energy intake/energy balance method A method of estimating total energy needs, based on comparison of total energy intake over several days with the amount of energy required for any observed change in body composition.

enrichment The addition of a nutrient to a processed food to replace losses of the nutrient that occurred during processing or to enhance its nutritive composition. Most commonly used in reference to cereal products.

enterotoxin A toxin produced in the gastrointestinal tract by a microorganism.

enzyme inhibitors Chemicals that can bind to specific enzymes and inhibit their activity.

enzyme-substrate complex The complex that forms when a substrate of an enzyme-catalyzed reaction binds to its binding site on the appropriate enzyme.

epiphysis A region at the end of a "long bone" that regulates the growth of the bone.

epithelial cells Cells forming a lining of some part of the body either internally (for example, lungs) or externally (skin).

ergocalciferol (vitamin D_2) The naturally occurring form of vitamin D produced in plants from ergosterol.

ergogenic Energy-producing; a term describing certain foods and nutrients that have developed reputations as energy-yielding foods that can enhance athletic performance.

ergot A dangerous mycotoxin produced by a fungus that grows on rye and other grains.

error theories of aging Theories of aging proposing that aging is caused by the steady accumulation of aberrant macromolecules due to errors in the normal operations of the cell.

erythrobic acid D-ascorbic acid, which is widely used as a preservative in processed meat.

erythroblasts Immature cells in the bone marrow that give rise to red blood cells (erythrocytes).

erythrocytes Red blood cells. They are red because they are packed with hemoglobin molecules, which transport oxygen around the body.

erythropoiesis The process of red blood cell formation that occurs in the bone marrow.

erythropoietin A protein that is a natural human hormone, which stimulates the production of red blood cells in the bone marrow.

erythropoietinogen The protein precursor of erythropoietin, a protein that stimulates the production of red blood cells in the bone marrow.

Escherichia coli 0157:H7 A common bacterial contaminant of food first identified in 1982 and since associated with major outbreaks of food poisoning and deaths due to consumption of meat not cooked to 160° F.

essential fatty acids Fatty acids that must be present in the diet to maintain health. They are linoleic acid and α-linolenic acid.

ester linkages The bonds that hold together the organic acid and alcohol components of an ester. In triglycerides, for example, three fatty acids are bonded to the glycerol moiety by ester linkages.

esterified cholesterol Compounds in which a cholesterol molecule is bonded to a fatty acid molecule by an ester linkage.

ethanol The alcohol found in alcoholic beverages.

evolution The process of genetic change powered by natural selection, which is believed to support the origin of species and the continuing genetic change of species.

exchange lists Lists indicating foods that contain comparable amounts of nutrients such as carbohydrate, lipid, and a comparable amount of energy.

exocytosis A process in which the contents of a vesicle within a cell are secreted out of the cell, when the membrane of the secretory vesicle fuses with the membrane of the cell.

exogenous Derived from outside the body.

exogenous fecal calcium Unabsorbed dietary calcium, which passes through the intestinal tract without entering the tissues of the body.

exopeptidases Protease enzymes that cleave the final peptide bonds of a polypeptide chain. They can be carboxypeptidases (acting at the carboxy-terminus) or aminopeptidases (acting at the amino terminus).

exophthalmic goiter Another term for hyperthyroidism (or Graves' disease) in which there is oversecretion of thyroid hormones and a resulting increase in metabolic rate.

extracellular Outside of cells.

extracellular fluid Fluid outside of cells.

extracellular water Water in the body outside the cells of the body.

extraction When applied to milled grain, the proportion of the original grain that remains after milling; the lower the extraction, the higher the proportion of the original grain that remains.

extravascular Outside the circulatory system and also outside the body's cells.

extrinsic factor Original name for vitamin B_{12}.

F

facilitated diffusion The diffusion of a substance across a membrane, assisted by the presence of a protein embedded in the membrane that either binds to the diffusing substance or forms a pore to assist its passage.

factor 11 and 11A An alternative name for lipoic acid.

factor U Early name for a nutritional factor whose active ingredient is now known to be folic acid (folate).

facultative thermogenesis The portion of the thermic effect of food that is not due to obligatory thermogenesis.

familial combined hyperlipidemia A genetically dominant condition associated with elevated levels of apolipoprotein B in the blood. Individuals with this condition are often treated with blood lipid-lowering drugs.

fasting glucose level The level of glucose in the blood after a period of fasting; normally about 90 mg glucose/dl blood.

fats Triglycerides that are solids at room temperature, although the term fat is widely used to mean all lipids.

fatty acids Organic acids found in lipids. Each one consists of a hydrocarbon chain with a methyl group at one end and a carboxyl group at the other end.

feces Waste material excreted through the anus.

feed additives Chemicals present in food because they have been added to the rations of animals used for human food.

fenfluramine An appetite suppressant that, in contrast to most others, does not stimulate the central nervous system. It does, however, have side effects including drowsiness, lethargy, and depression.

fermentation General term for changes brought about by the action of microorganisms on natural products. Alcoholic beverages are produced by the fermentation of natural sugars by yeasts.

ferritin A soluble cellular iron-storage protein also found in blood, each molecule of which can contain up the 4500 iron ions.

ferritin model A method of assessing iron status by taking measurements of the serum ferritin level, the red cell protoporphyrin level, and the transferrin saturation level.

fetal alcohol syndrome (FAS) A condition associated with congenital abnormalities in infants due to consumption of alcohol by the mother during pregnancy.

fetal growth curve A growth curve summarizing the increase in weight of the fetus as it develops throughout pregnancy.

fetus Unborn young, especially in the later stages of pregnancy. In humans, the fetal stage occupies the period between 8 weeks after conception and birth.

fiber Indigestible materials in food, largely of plant origin.

fibrin Fibrous components of a blood clot.

fibrinogen Plasma protein that polymerizes to form fibrin.

fibroblast A type of cell with an irregular shape found throughout connective tissue. It synthesizes and maintains collagen and mucopolysaccharides throughout connective tissue.

flavin adenine dinucleotide (FAD) A riboflavin-containing coenzyme that plays a major role in energy metabolism.

flavin mononucleotide (FMN) A riboflavin-containing coenzyme.

flavin monooxygenase system One of the major drug-detoxifying enzyme systems in the body.

flavoproteins Proteins that, in their active form, incorporate one of the flavin-containing coenzymes.

fluffy cellulose An indigestible carbohydrate made from nonwoody plants, which can be used as a noncaloric flour in low-calorie baked foods.

fluid balance The balance between the amount of water being taken into the body and the amount of water being excreted from the body (also known as water balance).

fluorapatite A crystalline compound in teeth that contains fluoride ions and is relatively resistant to acid.

folate Folic acid; a generic term for pteroylglutamic acid (PGA) and related chemicals with biological activity.

folate hydrolase An enzyme (also known as conjugase) that catalyzes the removal of glutamic acid residues from polyglutamate forms of folate in the intestinal lumen.

folate-binding proteins Proteins able to bind to folate found, for example, in milk.

force A physical agency capable of altering the state of rest or motion of a body. When an unbalanced force is applied to an object it undergoes acceleration.

foremilk The milk secreted first in any one nursing of an infant (session on the breast).

formiminoglutamic acid (FIGLU) A metabolite of the amino acid histidine, which is excreted in the urine of people suffering from folate deficiency.

fortification The addition of a nutrient to a food to increase its nutrient content to greater than natural levels.

fructose A monosaccharide sugar, also known as levulose or fruit sugar, which occurs in many fruits and berries and makes up one third of the sugar in honey.

fruitarian A class of vegetarians who only eat fruit and nuts and perhaps honey.

fumonisin B-1 A dangerous mycotoxin produced by a mold that grows on corn.

functional groups Specific chemical groups such as the hydroxyl group, the carbonyl group, etc.

functional iron That portion of the iron in the body that is actually performing some biochemical function, rather than being transported or held in stores.

G

galactogogues Medicinal or food substances believed to stimulate lactation.

galactose A monosaccharide sugar that is released during the digestive breakdown of lactose.

galactosemia Excessively high levels of galactose in the blood.

gamma hydroxybutyric acid A new drug that is being illegally marketed to athletes as a steroid substitute. It is claimed to stimulate the production of human growth hormone, which in turn promotes the development of muscles. It is also promoted as a "street drug" and as an aid to sleep.

gastric banding A surgical procedure in which a plastic collar is placed around the stomach to reduce the capacity of the stomach to hold food.

gastrointestinal motility The rate of movement of material through the gastrointestinal tract.

gastrointestinal tract (GI tract) The tube passing from the mouth to the anus, including the oral cavity, pharynx, esophagus, stomach, and intestines.

gastroplasty The surgical reduction of stomach size.

gelatin A mixture of animal proteins widely used as a jelling agent in foods.

gelatinase An enzyme found in the stomach that liquefies gelatin.

Generally Recognized as Safe (GRAS) A classification bestowed on food ingredients that have been used for many years without any adverse effects (e.g., salt, sugar, vinegar) by the U.S. Food and Drug Administration (FDA).

genes The individual functional sections of DNA that encode protein molecules or functional RNA molecules.

genetic engineering The process of purposely altering genes and/or moving genes between different organisms, usually of different species.

genetic information The base sequence of DNA, which determines the structures of the proteins or RNAs encoded by the genes within DNA.

genetic material Nucleic acid (DNA or RNA), which acts as a store of genetic information for an organism.

geriatrics The branch of medicine concerned with aging.

gerontology A discipline concerned with the psychological, sociological, economic, physiological, and medical aspects of aging.

gestation The time between conception and birth.

globin The protein components of hemoglobin and myoglobin.

glossitis Inflammation of the tongue.

glucogenic Able to be used for the synthesis of glucose (commonly applied to certain amino acids).

glucomannam A substance that comes from a Japanese root called konjac, is sold as an "Oriental weight loss secret," but does nothing more than create a sense of fullness.

gluconeogenesis A metabolic pathway that reverses the net effect of glycolysis to form glucose from simpler metabolites.

glucose The six-carbon monosaccharide that is the major carbohydrate found in blood and the main monosaccharide released by the digestion of other carbohydrates. Also known as dextrose.

glucosinolates Chemicals found primarily in foods of the cruciferous family (cabbage, Brussels sprouts, cauliflower, and turnips) that at high concentrations (seldom found in modern varieties of vegetables) can be metabolized to chemicals that promote goiter. At lower concentrations, however, they may protect against certain cancers, especially of the colon and rectum.

glutathione peroxidase (Gpx) A selenium-containing enzyme that catalyzes the breakdown of hydrogen peroxide and organic hydroperoxides. The activity of Gpx is used to assess a person's selenium status.

glutathione reductase An enzyme found in red blood cells that requires the coenzyme FAD. The activity of glutathione reductase is used to assess a person's riboflavin status.

glycemic index A value associated with different foods, indicating the relative rate at which consumption of the food leads to glucose appearing in the blood. White bread has been given a glycemic index of 100.

glycerol The simple trialcohol, which is a component of all triglycerides.

glycogen A complex carbohydrate composed of multiple units of glucose. It has a highly branched structure and is the storage form of carbohydrate for muscle and liver. Sometimes known as animal starch.

glycogen synthase An enzyme that catalyzes the synthesis of glycogen from glucose.

glycolysis The metabolic pathway that results in the breakdown of glucose into two pyruvate molecules (in aerobic glycolysis) or two lactate molecules (in anaerobic glycolysis).

glycoproteins Proteins that have been modified by the addition of sugar groups.

goitrogens Substances in foods that interfere with the absorption/utilization of iodine or the functioning of thyroid gland.

Good Manufacturing Practices (GMP) A set of guidelines for the food industry, which sets out standards for the design and construction of food processing plants and equipment to ensure that they are easy to clean and sanitize. They also set standards for employee hygiene, the treatment of water, cleaning and sanitizing procedures for plants and equipment, management of unavoidable pests, and many other aspects of food processing.

Graves' disease Another term for hyperthyroidism (or exophthalmic goiter) in which there is oversecretion of thyroid hormones and a resulting increase in metabolic rate.

ground substance A gelatinous mixture of protein and polysaccharides that forms part of the structure of bones.

growth An increase in size due to the formation of new cells and/or the enlargement of existing cells.

growth charts Charts indicating expected and actual rates of growth.

growth facilitator A substance that facilitates the growth of the body.

growth hormone releasers Substances, largely proteins, containing high levels of the amino acid arginine, which stimulate the secretion of growth hormone.

growth period The final 7 months of pregnancy, during which the tissues and organs formed during organogenesis continue to grow and mature until they are able to sustain the infant's life when it leaves the womb.

guar gum A gum derived from legumes and used as jelling agents in foods.

H

Hassle-Free Guide A food guide plan produced by the United States Department of Agriculture (USDA) in 1979.

Hazard Analysis and Critical Control Points (HACCP) System A food safety system based on the premise that if one starts with good quality food ingredients, monitors each processing step, identifies critical control points where hazards may occur, and keeps these critical points under control, then the finished product should be safe and of high quality.

heart rate monitoring method A method of estimating total energy needs by constantly monitoring the heart rate, relative to the subject's baseline.

heat denaturation The denaturation of protein molecules by heat.

heat energy Energy due to the overall motion of atoms, molecules, or ions.

heat of combustion The amount of heat energy released by burning a known amount of a particular food in a bomb calorimeter, usually quoted in kilocalories per gram.

heme The iron-containing chemical group found within hemoglobin and other heme-proteins.

heme iron Iron that is bound within a heme group, such as the iron within hemoglobin.

heme oxygenase An enzyme involved in the degradation of heme groups, causing iron to be released from the heme groups.

hemicellulose A dietary fiber containing xylose, galactose, glucose, and other monosaccharides bonded together.

hemochromatosis An iron-storage disease due to a genetic defect that causes affected individuals to absorb unusually large amounts of iron and store it in tissues that do not normally store iron.

hemodilution Dilution of the blood.

hemolysis The rupture of red blood cells, causing their contents to escape into the plasma. It can be caused by oxidative damage to the red blood cell membranes.

hemosiderin An insoluble iron protein storage complex of iron found in liver, spleen, and bone marrow.

hemosiderosis A condition characterized by excessive storage of iron in the liver; also known as siderosis.

hepatic (or portal) vein The main vein leading from the intestine to the liver.

heterocyclic amines A class of carcinogenic amines that are produced when some foods are cooked, especially if exposed to flames.

hexoses Monosaccharides that contain six carbon atoms.

hexuronic acid Vitamin C (although the alternative name ascorbic acid is more common).

high biological value A term used to describe the quality of proteins that contain all of the essential amino acids in proportions capable of promoting growth when they are the only proteins in the diet.

high density lipoproteins (HDL) Lipoprotein particles that transport cholesterol to the liver.

high fructose corn syrup (HFCS) A preparation high in fructose prepared by treating cornstarch and sucrose with enzymes.

highly unsaturated fatty acids (HUFA) Fatty acids containing five or six carbon-carbon double bonds.

hindmilk The milk secreted toward the end of nursing period (session of breast-feeding).

histidine load test A test used to detect folate deficiency by testing urine for formiminoglutamic acid (FIGLU) after administration of a large dose of histidine.

homeostasis failure theory A theory of aging that the underlying cause of aging is a failure of the many complex networks of homeostasis, which normally keep the body stable and able to respond to change appropriately.

homeostatic mechanisms Biochemical and physiological systems that tend to maintain appropriate stability within the body.

hormones Chemical messenger substances in the body that are released into the blood from one specific location and that bind to target tissues at other locations and elicit specific responses.

host resistance factors Factors in colostrum and mature human milk that confer some immunity from infection to the breast-fed infant. The greatest concentration of these factors is found in colostrum, but significant amounts are found in mature milk.

human calorimeter A small insulated room that operates on the same basic principles as the bomb calorimeter. The heat given off by the subject causes a change in the temperature of a heat reservoir, such as water, surrounding the chamber, allowing the amount of energy released to be easily calculated.

human chorionic gonadotrophin (hCG) A hormone secreted by the placenta. The presence of hCG in blood and urine of the mother is the first chemical indicator that pregnancy has begun.

human growth hormone A natural hormone involved in promoting growth. It is being used as a steroid substitute by some athletes in the hope that it will promote the growth of muscle tissue.

humoral immune response The branch of the immune system that is mediated by antibodies that are released into the blood.

hydrocarbons A category of organic chemicals composed solely of carbon and hydrogen atoms.

hydrogenation The addition of hydrogen to a compound, such as the hydrogenation process that converts carbon-carbon double bonds into single bonds and so reduces the degree of saturation of fatty acids.

hydrolysis The splitting apart of a chemical by reaction with water, such as the hydrolysis of proteins and carbohydrates during digestion.

hydrophilic "Water-loving"; used to refer to chemical groups that readily mix with water.

hydrophobic "Water-hating"; used to refer to chemical groups that do not readily mix with water.

hydrostatic pressure The force, due to the pumping of the heart, that pushes water out of the blood and into the intracellular space. It is opposed by the oncotic pressure due to osmosis drawing water back into the blood.

hydroxyapatite A compound composed of calcium and phosphate that is a component of bones and teeth.

hydroxycobalamin One of the three main forms in which vitamin B_{12} occurs in the body.

hydroxyl A chemical functional group composed of an oxygen atom bonded to an hydrogen atom; the characteristic chemical group of alcohols.

hydroxyl-containing amino acids Amino acids that contain an hydroxyl group in their side chains.

hydroxyphenyl retinamide A synthetic analog of vitamin A being tested for the treatment of acne and other skin disorders.

hypercalcemia An excess of calcium in the blood.

hypercholesterolemia An abnormally high level of cholesterol in the blood.

hyperemesis Severe and continued nausea.

hyperglycemia Too much glucose in the blood (a fasting blood glucose of more than 200 mg/dl is used to diagnose diabetes mellitus).

hyperkalemia High levels of potassium in the blood.

hyperlipidemia High levels of lipids in the blood due either to a high dietary intake of lipids or a range of inherited defects of lipid metabolism.

hypernatremia High levels of sodium in the blood.

hyperplasia A form of growth associated with an increase in the *number* of cells.

hyperplastic A term used to refer to tissues that have developed more cells than normal.

hyperplastic obesity Severe obesity associated with an increase in fat cell number.

hypertension High blood pressure.

hyperthyroidism A condition in which there is oversecretion of thyroid hormones by the thyroid gland, resulting in an increased metabolic rate (also known as Graves' disease or exophthalmic goiter).

hypertrophic obesity Obesity due to additional *growth* of individual fat cells.

hypertrophy A form of growth associated with an increase in the *size* of cells.

hypocalcemic tetany A convulsive state caused by an insufficient supply of calcium to the nerves and muscles.

hypoglycemia Low levels of glucose in the blood.

hypokalemia Low levels of potassium in the blood.

hyponatremia Low levels of sodium in the blood.

hypophosphatemia Low levels of phosphate in the blood.

hypothyroidism A condition in which insufficient amounts of thyroid hormones are produced.

hypovitaminosis A Too little vitamin A in the blood.

I

iatrogenic malnutrition Nutritional problems arising as a result of medical treatment.

IgG Designation of a major class of immunoglobulins.

IgM Designation of a major class of immunoglobulins.

ileocecal valve The valve at the juncture of the end of the small intestine and the beginning of the large intestine.

ileum The final and longest section of the small intestine, between the jejunum and the large intestine.

imino acid An amino acidlike molecule that contains the imino group rather than a free amino group. Proline is the only imino acid that occurs in proteins.

immune system malfunction theory A theory of aging that suggests that a steady deterioration of the immune system leads to the slow deterioration of the body that we call aging.

immunoglobulins The proteins that include all types of antibodies.

impaired iron status A condition in which iron status is below certain standards of adequacy.

implantation The stage during the first two weeks of gestation, when the fertilized ovum (fertilized egg cell) becomes embedded in the wall of the uterus.

incomplete proteins Proteins that lack or have limited amounts of one or more essential amino acids.

index of nutrient quality (INQ) A quantitative measure of the nutrient density of a food in terms of its kilocalorie content, defined as follows:

$$\text{INQ} = \frac{\text{\% of RDA of a nutrient provided by a food}}{\text{\% of energy requirement provided by the food}}$$

indirect calorimetry Indirect methods of measuring heat production, such as by measuring how much oxygen a person consumes and how much carbon dioxide a person expires, and then using these values to calculate how much energy is being released by the oxidation of the energy-yielding nutrients in the body.

indirect food additives Food additives added unintentionally during processing.

indispensable nitrogen The amount of nitrogen needed by the body to synthesize all of the nitrogen-containing substances it needs, including amino acids.

insensible perspiration The continual and unnoticed loss of water from the surface of the body.

insoluble fiber Fiber that, for the most part, does not dissolve in water and is not digested by the body or by bacteria in the gut. It includes cellulose, some hemicelluloses, and lignin.

insulin A hormone secreted by the pancreas which is necessary for glucose utilization in most tissues.

intercellular Between the cells of the body.

interesterification A process of breaking and remaking ester linkages, which can be used to randomize the positions occupied by the fatty acid groups of triglycerides.

interferon The generic name for a range of small proteins, produced by lymphocytes, which play a major role in defending the body against viral infection.

internal energy The energy held within chemicals due to the movement of their electrons (kinetic energy), and due to the way in which their negatively charged electrons and positively charged nuclei are arranged relative to one another (potential energy).

interstitial Another term for the intercellular fluid compartment.

intracellular Inside the cell.

intracellular fluid The fluid inside cells.

intrauterine growth retardation (IUGR) Growth retardation caused by undernutrition of a fetus while growing in the uterus.

intrauterine nutrition The nutrition of the fetus while it is in the uterus.

intravascular Within blood vessels.

intrinsic factor The mucoprotein molecule secreted by gastric mucosal cells and required for the absorption of vitamin B_{12} into the body.

iodine-deficiency disorders A wide range of disorders that affects growth and development due to iodine deficiency.

iodized salt Table salt to which iodide has been added as a means of preventing iodine deficiency.

ionic bonds Chemical bonds between charged particles (ions).

ionized Existing in the form of a charged ionic group.

ions Electrically charged chemical particles.

iron-deficiency anemia Anemia caused by iron deficiency.

irritable bowel syndrome A condition characterized by frequent bowel movements stimulated by excessive dietary fiber intake.

isocaloric A term used to describe different foods and diets that provide the same number of kilocalories.

J

jaw wiring The wiring together of a person's jaws to limit them to a liquid diet.

jejunoileal bypass A surgical procedure in which the beginning of the jejunum is connected directly to the terminal portion of the ileum. This reduces the length of the absorptive surface of the intestine by as much as 20 feet. It is intended to reduce the proportion of energy-yielding nutrients in the diet that are actually absorbed into the body.

jejunum The middle section of the small intestine, between the duodenum and the ileum.

joule The international standard (SI unit) of work, energy, and heat.

K

keratin A structural protein found in the outer layer of skin and in fingernails and hair.

keratomalacia Irreversible changes in the cornea of the eye associated with severe vitamin A deficiency, capable of causing blindness.

kernicterus A condition characterized by a high level of bilirubin in blood, which gives skin a yellow color and can cause brain damage.

Keshan disease A selenium deficiency condition that causes cardiomyopathy (disease of the heart muscle). It is most commonly found in children and women of child-bearing age in some parts of China.

ketogenic Able to be converted into ketones (commonly used to describe certain amino acids).

ketones Organic chemicals containing a carbonyl group whose carbon atom is bonded to two other carbon atoms.

ketosis The condition of having abnormally high levels of ketones in the blood.

kilocalories The standard unit of energy used in nutrition in the United States; the amount of heat required to raise temperature of 1 kg water 1°C from 15 to 16°C.

kinetic energy The energy things possess because they are moving.

kwashiorkor A form of protein-energy malnutrition that most commonly affects young children between the ages of 2 and 5 years.

L

L-sugars Sugars that are "left-handed" in the sense that they rotate a beam of polarized light to the left.

labile Easily degraded.

lactase An enzyme produced by the intestinal mucosal cells that catalyzes the conversion of dietary lactose into glucose and galactose.

lactase insufficiency The state of having low levels of the enzyme lactase, leading to intolerance of milk and milk products due to the inability to digest lactose.

***Lactobacillus bifidus* factor** A nitrogen-containing carbohydrate in colostrum and human milk that encourages the growth of the bacterium *Lactobacillus bifidus.*

***Lactobacillus casei* factor** Early designation of a nutritional factor whose active ingredient is folic acid (folate).

lactoferrin An iron-containing protein found in human milk.

lactoperoxidase An enzyme in colostrum and human milk that can kill the *Streptococcus* bacteria.

lactose The disaccharide sugar found in milk (also known as milk sugar) formed when a molecule of glucose combines with a molecule of galactose.

lactose intolerance Intolerance of the disaccharide lactose and, therefore, of milk and milk products, due to an insufficiency of the enzyme lactase.

large intestine The final portion of the gastrointestinal tract between the small intestine and the anus.

lateral hypothalamic feeding center A center in the brain involved in regulating the consumption of food.

law of conservation of energy The physical law that energy cannot be created or destroyed, but simply transferred.

LDL receptor A receptor protein on the surface of liver cells that binds to low density lipoprotein (LDL) before its entry into cells.

lecithin:retinol acyltransferase (LRAT) An enzyme in liver cells known to catalyze the esterification of retinol to produce retinyl esters.

lecithins Phospholipids in which the nitrogen-containing vitamin-like substance called choline is attached to a phosphate group that forms part of the phospholipid structure.

legumes Members of the family of plants known as the Leguminosae, including peas and beans.

Leineis disease A form of dermatitis that can occur in infants and may be caused by biotin deficiency.

let-down reflex Release of milk from mammary glands due to action of the hormone oxytocin released from the posterior pituitary in response to sucking by infant.

lignin An insoluble fiber made up of a multiringed alcohol (noncarbohydrate) structure.

limiting amino acid The amino acid within a protein that is present in the smallest amount relative to the amount required for growth.

lipases Enzymes that catalyze the breakdown of lipids.

lipectomy The surgical removal of excess fat.

lipid bilayer The basic structure of all cell membranes, composed of two layers of lipid molecules arranged "back to back."

lipid peroxidation The oxidative formation of peroxide derivatives of lipids.

lipids A class of nutrients containing much carbon and hydrogen, a little oxygen, and sometimes other atoms. Lipids dissolve in ether or benzene and include fats, oils, and cholesterol.

lipofuscin Brown pigment that accumulates within tissues during aging, derived from breakdown products of lipids.

lipoic acid An organic acid isolated from liver and yeast that is essential for the growth of several microorganisms. It has not yet been shown to be a dietary essential for humans or other mammals. It does participate in certain biochemical reactions, but the amounts required are probably readily synthesized by the body.

lipoprotein lipase An enzyme that plays a key role in breaking down chylomicrons and VLDL particles, releasing their fatty acids and other lipids for entry into tissue cells.

lipoproteins Particles found in the bloodstream containing a core of lipids surrounded by a shell of protein, phospholipid, and cholesterol.

liposuction The suctioning off of subcutaneous fat to reduce body fat stores.

Listeria monocytogenes A deadly food-borne pathogen. Because, it has the unusual ability to grow at temperatures as low as 4° C, it thrives at normal refrigeration temperatures. It also survives freezing temperatures and grows at a wide range of pH values from 4.4 to 9.8. It is also very heat resistant, with a temperature of at least 70° C for 2 minutes required to reduce its numbers to a minimum. It is especially virulent in pregnant women and their fetuses, the elderly, and the immunosuppressed.

long-chain fatty acids Fatty acids containing 16 or more carbon atoms.

lovastatin A cholesterol-lowering drug that inhibits 3-hydroxy-3-methylglutaryl CoA reductase, a key enzyme in the biosynthesis of cholesterol.

low birth-weight (LBW) babies Babies weighing less that 5.5 pounds (2500 g) at birth.

low density lipoproteins (LDL) Lipoprotein particles that are formed from VLDL particles. They transport cholesterol to the cells of the body.

low magnesium tetany Uncontrolled neuromuscular tremors followed by seizures, caused by low magnesium levels.

lubricant A substance that enables solid materials to slip readily over each other, such as the synovial fluid within joints.

lumen The interior of a region of the body, such as the interior of the gastrointestinal tract.

lutein One of the common carotenoids found in plant foods, which can serve as precursors of vitamin A.

luxus consumption The release of heat energy, probably through the activity of unproductive or "futile" metabolic cycles, which apparently can allow some people to consume excess kilocalories but not put on weight.

lycopene One of the common carotenoids found in plant foods, which can serve as precursors of vitamin A.

lymphocytes The white blood cells responsible for mediating most aspects of the immune system, giving it its ability to defend against a wide range of infectious microorganisms.

lysosomes Membrane-bound organelles within cells responsible for the degradation of foreign materials taken into the cells by endocytosis.

lysozyme An enzyme found in almost all body fluids that is able to attack and digest the cell walls of bacteria.

M

macrobiotic Based on the principle of balance between opposing "yin" and "yang" characteristics.

macroelements Another term for the macronutrient minerals.

macromolecules Large polymeric molecules, such as proteins, nucleic acids, and complex carbohydrates, which are formed by the joining together of many smaller chemical units.

macronutrient minerals Minerals present in the body at a concentration of more than 50 ppm or 0.005% of body weight.

macrophages Large defensive cells that engulf and digest microorganisms by phagocytosis. They also synthesize and release lysozyme, lactoferrin, and "complement" proteins.

maltose A disaccharide sugar formed when two molecule of glucose become linked together.

marasmus A wasting condition caused by a chronic lack of energy in the diet. Now classified as a form of protein-energy malnutrition.

mastication The physical action of chewing.

maternal tissues The additional tissue added to a mother's body during pregnancy, excluding the actual products of conception; namely the additional blood, extracellular fluid, uterine tissue, breast tissue, and fat that develops.

matrix Strong but flexible material within developing bones composed of collagen and ground substance.

mean corpuscular volume model A method of assessing iron status by measuring the average volume of blood cells, the red cell protoporphyrin level, and the transferrin saturation level.

medial hypothalamic satiety center A center in the brain involved in regulating the consumption of food.

medium-chain fatty acids Fatty acids containing between 10 and 14 carbon atoms.

megaloblastic anemia A form of anemia (also known as macrocytic anemia) characterized by large red blood cells that continue to grow because they do not lose their nucleus when they should.

menadione A synthetic form of vitamin K.

menaquinone-n The generic name for the menaquinones (forms of vitamin K found in animal tissues), with a number in place of the n used to specify a particular menaquinone on the basis of the number of isoprenyl groups in its side chain.

menaquinones Naturally occurring forms of vitamin K found in animal tissues and synthesized by bacteria.

menarche Time of onset of menstruation during puberty in females.

Menke's kinky hair syndrome An inherited condition associated with low serum copper and ceruloplasmin levels; characterized by slow growth, degeneration of brain tissue, hypothermia, seizures, defective arterial walls, depigmentation of skin and hair, and peculiarly stubby white hair (Pili Torti).

messenger RNA (mRNA) The RNA copy of a gene that moves to the cell cytoplasm to direct the manufacture of a protein molecule.

metabolic body size Body weight in kilograms raised to the power of ¾.

metabolic chamber A modified version of the respiration chamber in which the heat given off by the subject is measured using thermocouples and heat-exchange disks attached to the skin.

metabolism The entire biochemical activities of an organism.

metalloenzymes Enzymes that include metal ions as part of their structure.

metalloproteins Proteins that include metal ions or atoms as part of their functional structure.

metallothionein A small metalloprotein able to bind to a variety of cations (positive ions) with a charge of 2+; it is responsible for various aspects of the homeostasis and transport of mineral ions.

methyl group A portion of an organic molecule composed of a carbon atom bonded to three hydrogen atoms (CH_3).

methylcellulose An indigestible synthetic carbohydrate used in low calorie foods to provide bulk but not energy.

methylcobalamin One of the three main forms in which vitamin B_{12} occurs in the body.

5-methyltetrahydrofolate The main form in which folate is transported around the body.

micelles Tiny spherical aggregates of lipids and other substances that play an important role in the digestion and transport of lipids.

microcytic hypochromic anemia Anemia caused by iron deficiency and characterized by small erythrocytes with little hemoglobin.

microelements Another term for the micronutrient minerals.

micronutrient minerals Minerals that are present in the body at a concentration of less than 50 ppm or 0.005% of body weight.

microvilli Very small projections covering the surface of the villi in the inner wall of the intestine.

mineralization The deposition of mineral crystals containing much calcium within developing bone tissue; also known as calcification or ossification.

minerals Elements used in the body to promote chemical reactions and that help form body structures.

mitochondrion Organelle within the cell where the key processes of oxidative energy metabolism occur.

mixed triglyceride A triglyceride in which at least two of the fatty acid groups differ.

mixed-function oxidase system One of the major drug-detoxifying enzyme systems in the body.

modified adult phase The phase of breast-feeding when the majority of the infant's nutrients are provided by selected foods available from the family's normal diet.

modified starches Starches that have been purposely modified to give them new properties such as improved stability to acid and heat.

molds A category of fungi found almost everywhere in nature. Most fungi are harmless and some are beneficial, but a few harmful types are a threat to the safety of our food supply. Under certain environmental conditions, some molds produce poisonous substances called mycotoxins. Some mycotoxins are known carcinogens, and others have been implicated in birth defects.

molecules Chemical particles composed of two or more atoms bonded together by covalent bonds (i.e., by the sharing of electrons between the atoms involved).

monoacylglycerol Another name for a monoglyceride.

monoglyceride A compound in which one fatty acid group is esterified to the trialcohol glycerol.

monomers The chemical units that combine to form polymers; amino acids are the monomers of proteins, nucleotides are the monomers of nucleic acids, and monosaccharides are the monomers of polysaccharides.

monosaccharides Simple sugars, glucose, fructose, and galactose, each containing a single sugar ring.

monounsaturated fatty acids Fatty acids that contain only one carbon-carbon double bond.

monozygotic twins Twins derived from the one zygote ("identical twins").

mucopolysaccharides Substances containing protein and carbohydrate.

mucoproteins Proteins that have been modified by the addition of sugar groups.

mucosa Lining layers of cells within regions of the body, such as the gastric mucosa (lining the stomach) and the intestinal mucosa (lining the intestines).

multiparas Women who are having a second or subsequent child.

multisubunit proteins Proteins formed by the aggregation of several distinct protein molecules referred to as the "subunits" of the multisubunit protein.

muscle tone or tonus The state of slight contraction in which all muscles are maintained, even when apparently relaxed.

mutations Changes in the structure of DNA that can cause heritable changes in an organism's genetic make-up.

mycotoxins Toxins produced by fungi such as molds. Some mycotoxins are known carcinogens, and others have been implicated in birth defects.

myelin A lipoprotein substance found in the myelin sheath around many nerve fibers, which electrically insulates the fibers and speeds their transmission of impulses.

myoinositol One of the vitamin-like compounds. It is a six-carbon compound chemically related to glucose and is also known as muscle sugar.

myosin One of the fibrous proteins found in muscle; it is involved in muscular contraction.

myxedematous cretinism The form of severe iodine deficiency characterized by dwarfism with hypothyroidism.

N

National Health And Nutrition Examination Survey (NHANES) The major surveys providing information on dietary habits and health in the United States conducted every 10 years by The National Center for Health Statistics.

Nationwide Food Consumption Survey (NFCS) The major dietary surveys in the United States conducted every 10 years by the United States Department of Agriculture (USDA).

negative calcium balance The state in which calcium excretion exceeds calcium intake.

negative nitrogen balance The state in which a person is excreting more nitrogen than the amount taken in.

neonatal hemorrhaging Bleeding soon after birth.

neonatal The period immediately after birth.

net protein utilization (NPU) A measure of protein quality that is based on the percentage of ingested nitrogen that is retained by the body.

neurological cretinism A form of severe iodine deficiency characterized by mental deficiency and deaf mutism.

neuromotor coordination The coordination between the nerves and muscles that controls movement.

neurotransmitter A chemical that is released from the end of one nerve cell to travel across the gap (synapse) between one cell and the next, and then binds to the next nerve cell to either stimulate or inhibit its transmission of a nerve impulse. Neurotransmitters are the chemicals responsible for transmitting nerve signals between nerve cells.

neutral Chemically neither acidic nor alkaline; having a pH equal to or very close to 7.0.

neutral foods Foods that have little effect on pH because they contain a roughly equal balance of acid-forming and alkali-forming minerals.

neutron activation A procedure that uses neutron bombardment for formation of radioactive nitrogen (N^{15}) and then N^{15} detection for the measurement of total body nitrogen in the living body.

neutrons Electrically neutral subatomic particles found in the nuclei of atoms.

niacin equivalent (NE) Units used to express niacin content of a food. It represents preformed niacin plus tryptophan equivalents (60 mg tryptophan = 1 mg niacin).

niacytin A niacin-containing compound in wheat bran that cannot usually be utilized by the body and is simply excreted in urine.

nicotinamide adenine dinucleotide (NAD) A niacin-containing coenzyme that plays a major role in many aspects of metabolism.

nicotinamide One form of the vitamin niacin.

nicotinamide adenine dinucleotide phosphate (NADP) A niacin-containing coenzyme that plays a major role in many aspects of metabolism.

night blindness A condition in which the eye recovers very slowly from exposure to bright light, due to a deficiency of vitamin A.

nitrogen balance A measure of the relationship between the amount of nitrogen taken into the body and the amount excreted. If nitrogen intake exceeds nitrogen loss, a person is in positive nitrogen balance. If nitrogen loss exceeds intake a person is in negative nitrogen balance. If nitrogen intake equals nitrogen loss a person is in nitrogen equilibrium.

nitrogen cycle The chemical process by which nitrogen is constantly recycled between living things and the environment.

nitrogen equilibrium The state in which a person's nitrogen intake exactly equals nitrogen losses.

nitrogen-fixing bacteria Bacteria that can convert nitrogen molecules (N_2) in the air to ammonia (NH_3), which can then be incorporated into many other organic compounds.

nitrosamines A class of carcinogenic amines that are formed from nitrates and nitrites in foods, either during drying and cooking, or when the food is in the gastrointestinal tract.

No Observable Effect Level (NOEL) The highest dose of a chemical, such as a pesticide, at which no adverse effect is seen in animals.

non-heme iron Iron that is not bound within heme groups.

nonfunctional iron Iron in the body that is not performing a specific biochemical function, but is simply being transported or held in stores.

nonpolar A term applied to compounds with no asymmetrically arranged charges and which therefore do not mix well with water.

nucleic acids DNA and RNA, which serve as the genetic materials of life.

nucleus (of atom) The central structure within an atom, composed of protons and neutrons.

nucleus (of cell) The organelle within the cell that contains the cell chromosomes.

nursing bottle syndrome Tooth decay caused by the practice of offering infants a bottle at bedtime and allowing them to fall asleep with the bottle in their mouth. It is caused by the long-term presence of any sugar-containing fluid (whether formula or fruit juice) close to the teeth.

nursing phase The phase of breastfeeding when human milk or an appropriate formula is the sole source of nutrients.

NutraSweet The brand name for the artificial sweetener aspartame.

nutrient density That ratio obtained by dividing a food's contribution to the needs for a nutrient by its contribution to kilocalorie needs. When the contribution to nutrient needs exceeds the contribution to kilocalorie needs, the food is considered to have a favorable nutrient density for the nutrient concerned.

nutrients Chemicals in food that nourish the body by providing energy, building materials, and substances required to regulate and/or assist in the catalysis of biochemical reactions.

nystagmus Involuntary rapid eye movement.

O

Oatrim A carbohydrate-based gel used as a fat substitute, containing a mixture of oat starch and fiber.

obese Having a body mass index (BMI) greater that 31.1 for men and greater than 32.3 for women representing excess body fat.

obesity The state of overweight corresponding to a body mass index (BMI) greater that 31.1 for men and greater than 32.3 for women.

obligatory losses Losses of a nutrient from the body that cannot be avoided.

obligatory thermogenesis The unavoidable energy cost associated with absorption and transport of nutrients and the synthesis of protein, fat, and carbohydrate required for the renewal of body tissues and the storage of energy.

oils Triglycerides that are liquid at room temperature. Oils are often included in the general category of "fat," although technically fats are triglycerides that are solids at room temperature.

Olestra The brand name of a sucrose polyester fat substitute.

omega (ω) carbon The methyl carbon at the end of a fatty acid chain.

oncotic pressure The force of osmosis drawing water from the intracellular space into the blood. It is opposed by hydrostatic pressure caused by the pumping of the heart, which pushes water out of the blood and into the intracellular space.

open-circuit indirect calorimetry A method of indirect calorimetry in which room air is breathed in, and the exhaled carbon dioxide generated from it is collected and measured. Knowing the amount of carbon dioxide produced in a given time allows calculation of the amount of oxygen consumed to generate that carbon dioxide; thus the amount of energy released can be calculated.

opsin A protein produced by the breakdown of rhodopsin in the rods and cones of the retina. It is involved in a chemical reaction that initiates a nerve impulse that results in the interpretation of light energy as vision.

organ A group of tissues adapted to a specific function; examples are the heart, stomach, and liver.

organelles Components of cells that perform specific functions, such as the mitochondria, endoplasmic reticulum, and ribosomes.

organic compounds Carbon-containing compounds, usually derived from living things or produced by modifying or mimicking the carbon-containing compounds of living things.

organogenesis The period of intrauterine development during which the cells of the embryo begin to differentiate into distinct tissues and functional units, which later become organs, such as the heart, lungs, and liver.

orthomolecular therapy The use of vitamins in extremely large amounts to try to treat psychiatric problems.

osmosis The passive diffusion of water across a semipermeable membrane.

osmotic pressure A measure of the ability of a solution to draw water into it by osmosis.

ossification The deposition of mineral crystals within developing bone tissue; also known as calcification or mineralization.

osteocalcin A protein whose precise function is not known, but which is found in bone and is known to have calcium-binding properties. It is also known as bone Gla protein.

osteomalacia A disease characterized by defective bone formation that is not necessarily due to vitamin D deficiency. It is most prevalent, however, in regions of the world where cultural customs prevent women from exposing their skin to sunlight, or where women bear and nurse children continuously throughout their fertile years.

overweight Having a body mass index (BMI) greater than the 85th percentile values of the BMI distributions for men and women aged 20 to 29 years.

ovolactopollovegetarian A person who will eat poultry, in addition to the foods considered acceptable by ovolactovegetarians (plant-based foods, milk, cheese, and eggs).

ovolactovegetarian A vegetarian who will also eat foods derived from animals without slaughter, such as eggs, cheese, and milk.

oxalates Chemicals found in rhubarb, tea, cocoa, and spinach that are metabolic precursors of kidney stones and that also interfere with the absorption of calcium when taken in high amounts.

oxidation Chemical term for a wide range of reactions involving the loss of electrons, and/or the addition of oxygen, and/or the loss of hydrogen. Oxidation processes are coupled to reduction processes as parts of redox reactions.

oxidation/reduction Chemical term applied to reactions in which one reactant is oxidized while the other is reduced. Such reactions are also known as redox reactions.

oxidative phosphorylation The process within mitochondria in which energy released from the oxidation of food molecules is used to form the high energy phosphorylated compound ATP.

oxytocin A hormone secreted by the posterior pituitary gland that causes uterine contractions and milk let-down.

P

P/S ratio The ratio of polyunsaturated fatty acids to saturated fatty acids within the fat of a food.

pantothenol The alcohol derivative of pantothenic acid, which is widely used in cosmetics.

parathormone A hormone that affects calcium and phosphate balance by altering renal transport; also known as parathyroid hormone.

parathyroid hormone A hormone that affects calcium and phosphate balance by altering renal reabsorption also known as parathormone.

passive diffusion The free movement of materials with their concentration gradients from areas of high to low concentration.

passive immunity Any form of immunity that does not require the activation of an individual's own active immune defenses. The host resistance factors, including antibodies, in colostrum and breast milk bestow a form of passive immunity on a breast-fed infant.

patulin A dangerous mycotoxin and potential carcinogen produced by molds found in rotten apples.

pectin A natural polysaccharide with the ability to attract and hold water. It is widely used as a gelling agent in preserves.

pellagra A disease caused by niacin deficiency, characterized by inflammation of the skin, diarrhea, and eventual mental incapacity.

pentoses Monosaccharide sugars containing five carbon atoms.

pepsinogens The precursor forms of the pepsin enzymes.

pepsins A class of protease enzymes found in the stomach.

peptide bonds The chemical bonds that link amino acids into the structure of a protein chain.

peptidyl glycine alpha-amidating monooxygenase A copper-containing enzyme that catalyzes the α-amidation of the precursors of many peptide hormones and hormone-releasing factors.

perishable Susceptible to a decline in quality over time. A classification given to foods that are susceptible to the introduction and the growth of pathogens.

peristalsis The churning wavelike action caused by the contraction and relaxation of muscles in the walls of the gastrointestinal tract.

permissible tolerance levels Levels for over 300 pesticides in food and/or feed that the Environmental Protection Agency has set as permissible maximum levels.

pescovegetarian A person who will eat fish, but not any land-based animals.

pH A numerical measure of the acidity or alkalinity of a solution. pH values less than 7.0 are acidic, and pH values greater than 7.0 are alkaline. pH 7.0 is referred to as neutral pH. The pH value is technically the negative logarithm (to the base 10) of the hydrogen ion concentration.

phentermine An appetite suppressant that has been used successfully on patients with moderate hypertension and diabetes.

phenylketonuria (PKU) A hereditary condition that causes an inability to metabolize excess phenylalanine.

phenylpropanolamine The active ingredient in many cold remedies, which is considered a safe and effective appetite suppressant by the FDA.

phosphatases Enzymes that can release phosphate from various phosphorus-containing compounds.

phospholipids Lipids in which a phosphorus-containing group is esterified to one of the hydroxyl groups of a glycerol molecule.

phosphoproteins Proteins that have phosphorus-containing chemical groups attached to them.

photosynthesis The process within plants in which the energy of the sun powers the production of energy-yielding compounds such as glucose.

phyloquinone A naturally occurring form of vitamin K found in plant-based foods.

physiological fuel value The amount of energy actually *available* to the body from a given amount of nutrient.

phytic acid A constituent of plant fiber that binds to positive ions (e.g., Ca++, Fe++) and thus can inhibit the absorption of these ions from the gastrointestinal tract.

phytochemicals Chemicals present in plants.

phytosterols A group of sterol lipids found in plants.

pica The habit of eating nonfood items such as dirt, paint chips, laundry starch, library paste, ice cubes, or clay.

PIVKA Protein Induced by Vitamin K Absence or Antagonism: an abnormal form of prothrombin present in people with vitamin K deficiency (also known as PIVKA-II).

PIVKA-II An alternative term for PIVKA (Protein Induced by Vitamin K Absence or Antagonism), indicating that it is an abnormal form of factor II (prothrombin).

placenta The organ that anchors the developing fetus to the uterus and provides a "bridge" for the exchange of nutrients and waste products between the mother and fetus.

plaques Coatings of carbohydrate (dextrans) and bacteria on the surface of teeth, which are precursors to the formation of dental caries.

plasma lipoproteins A class of lipoprotein particles found in plasma, including chylomicrons, very low density lipoproteins (VLDL), low density lipoproteins (LDL), and high density lipoproteins (HDL). They are involved in the transport of lipids around the body.

plasma proteins Proteins found in the blood plasma.

polar A term applied to compounds containing charged groups that allow the compound to mix well with other polar compounds, such as water.

polycythemia An increase in the number of red blood cells.

polymers Large chemicals composed of many smaller monomer units linked together.

polypeptides Molecules composed of many amino acids bonded together by peptide bonds. Large polypeptides are known as proteins.

polysaccharides Complex carbohydrates composed of many sugar units bonded together; they include the polysaccharides starch, glycogen, and cellulose.

polyunsaturated fatty acids (PUFA) Fatty acids containing two or more carbon-carbon double bonds.

ponderel index The ratio of height (meters) to the cube root of weight (kg).

positive calcium balance The state in which calcium intake exceeds calcium excretion.

positive energy balance The state in which a person's intake of kilocalories is in excess of kilocalorie expenditure.

positive nitrogen balance The state in which a person's nitrogen intake exceeds their nitrogen losses.

post-transcriptional modifications Modifications made to messenger RNA molecules after they have been copied from DNA but before they are used in protein synthesis.

postprandial hypoglycemia Reactive hypoglycemia that occurs after consuming a meal that was high in carbohydrate, especially simple sugars.

potential energy The energy systems contain because of the *positions* of their parts.

practical allowances Term applied to dietary allowances set by FAO/WHO, which considers availability of a nutrient in the food supply world-wide as well as its physiological need.

prealbumin A plasma protein that binds to retinol binding protein and assists the transport of vitamin A and prevents vitamin A from being filtered from the blood in the kidneys.

precursor A usually biologically inactive chemical that is converted into some other chemical, which usually is biologically active and chemically related to the original chemical.

preeclampsia A syndrome of abnormal conditions in pregnancy of unknown cause; symptoms include hypertension, proteinurea, and edema. Also known as toxemia of pregnancy. It may progress to eclampsia (severe toxemia), which can cause death.

pregnancy-induced hypertension A form of hypertension (high blood pressure) occurring during and brought about by pregnancy.

premature infants Infants born before completing 37 weeks of gestation.

primary structure The amino acid sequence of a protein.

primiparas Women having their first child.

prior sanction additives Food additives that were approved by the FDA before the implementation of the Delaney clause, which states that an additive known to be carcinogenic at any level in any animal may not be approved. If the safety of such additives is questioned, the additives must be subjected to further review.

privo conservation A fall in the basal metabolic rate to between 20% and 30% less than normal predicted levels, which occurs after long periods when energy intake is less than requirements (prolonged caloric undernutrition).

procolipase A proenzyme secreted by the pancreas that becomes activated to colipase by the action of the pancreatic trypsin enzyme. The colipase then combines with pancreatic lipase and emulsified lipid droplets to convert triglycerides into free fatty acids and monoglycerides.

products of conception The fetus, the amniotic fluid, and the placenta.

proenzymes Inactive enzyme precursors that later become activated due to chemical modification.

programmed aging theories Theories of aging that suggest that cells are somehow genetically programmed to age and die at a specific time.

prolactin A hormone secreted by the anterior pituitary gland that stimulates the secretion of milk by the mammary glands.

proteases Enzymes that catalyze the degradation (breakdown) of proteins.

protective foods A term sometimes used to refer to foods that provide significant amounts of vitamins and minerals in addition to adequate calories and protein.

protein efficiency ratio (PER) A measure of protein quality that is based on the ratio of the weight gain in grams to the grams of protein ingested by young rats.

protein quality A measure of how closely the mixture of essential amino acids in a protein matches the body's need for these amino acids.

protein turnover The constant breaking down and resynthesis of protein within the body.

proteins A class of compounds composed of linked amino acids. They contain carbon, hydrogen, nitrogen, oxygen, and sometimes other atoms in specific configurations.

proteins of low biological value Proteins that lack or have limited amounts of one or more essential amino acids.

prothrombin A plasma protein that, when activated by one of the clotting factors, catalyzes the conversion of fibrinogen to fibrin as part of the clotting mechanism of the blood.

protogen An alternative name for lipoic acid.

protons The positively charged subatomic particles found within the nuclei of atoms.

provitamin D A generic term for precursors of vitamin D found in animals and plants.

provitamins Chemical precursors of vitamins.

proximate composition The approximate composition of a food, in terms of the percentages of carbohydrate, fat, protein, fiber, and water present in a typical sample of the food.

pseudoalbinism A loss of pigmentation in skin and hair caused by selenium deficiency.

pteric acid A key intermediate in the synthesis of pteroylglutamic acid (folate).

pteroylglutamic acid (PGA) The parent compound of the range of compounds known collectively as folic acid or folate.

ptyalin An enzyme in saliva that partially digests starch (also known as α-amylase).

puberty The period during which the reproductive organs become functionally active and secondary sexual characteristics appear.

pylorus A muscular opening that separates the stomach from the small intestine.

pyridoxal An aldehyde form of vitamin B_6.

pyridoxamine An amine form of vitamin B_6.

pyridoxine Vitamin B_6.

pyridoxine kinase An enzyme that catalyzes the phosphorylation of vitamin B_6 within cells and thus retains the vitamin within cells, because the phosphorylated form cannot readily cross the cell membrane.

pyridoxine oxidase An enzyme that catalyzes the conversion of pyridoxine phosphate and pyridoxamine phosphate into pyridoxal phosphate. This important enzyme in vitamin B_6 metabolism requires riboflavin for its activity, which explains the similarities between many symptoms of riboflavin deficiency and vitamin B_6 deficiency.

pyridoxol An alcohol form of vitamin B_6.

pyruvic acid The 3-carbon compound that is the end product of aerobic glycolysis. It passes into the mitochondrion for further degradation via the citric acid cycle.

pyruvic aldehyde A toxic product of carbohydrate metabolism that accumulates in thiamin deficiency.

pyruvic oxidation factor An alternative name for lipoic acid.

Q

quaternary structure The way in which the subunits of a multisubunit protein are arranged together in space.

quinones The group of chemicals to which all forms of vitamin K belong.

R

radiation-induced additives Food additives that are formed in food as the result of radiation and not purposely added to the food.

radioimmunoassay A general procedure for performing assays based on the binding of radioactively labeled antibodies to the specific substances being assayed for.

RAR-alpha One of the three main classes of retinoic acid receptor proteins in the nuclei of cells (RARs).

RAR-beta One of the three main classes of retinoic acid receptor proteins in the nuclei of cells (RARs).

RAR-gamma One of the three main classes of retinoic acid receptor proteins in the nuclei of cells (RARs).

RARs Retinoic acid receptor proteins found within the nuclei of cells, involved in the mechanisms by which retinoic acid can control gene activity and hence cell differentiation.

rate of living theory A theory of aging that suggests that the rate of aging is closely related to a person's basal metabolic rate. According to this theory, the higher the basal metabolic rate, the shorter the life span, and vice versa.

reactant A chemical that participates in a specific chemical reaction, becoming converted into or incorporated within the product(s) of the reaction.

reactive hypoglycemia A condition of hypoglycemia that occurs from time to time in almost everyone, sometimes following a meal high in simple sugars or if a person has waited too long between meals.

recombinant DNA technology Another term for genetic engineering: the process of purposely altering genes and/or moving genes between different organisms, usually of different species.

recommended dietary allowances (RDAs) Levels of intake of essential nutrients that, on the basis of scientific knowledge, are judged by the Food and Nutrition Board to be adequate to meet the known nutrient needs of practically all healthy people.

redox reactions Reactions in which one reactant is reduced while another reactant is oxidized.

reduction Chemical term for a wide range of reactions involving the gain of electrons and/or the loss of oxygen and/or the gain of hydrogen. Reduction processes are coupled to oxidation processes as parts of redox reactions.

reference daily intakes (RDIs) Term used by the U.S. Food and Drug Administration (FDA) in nutrient labeling to refer to standards for vitamins, minerals other than sodium and potassium, and protein for certain groups.

regulated food additives Food additives that have been found to be safe on the basis of rigorous screening by the FDA.

relative dose response The quantitative value obtained from a relative dose response test.

relative dose response test A test in which the change in the concentration of a vitamin in the blood is compared to the change after the administration of a known amount of the vitamin.

residues Used as a term to refer to the individual amino acids of proteins.

resistance threshold The level of a toxin or microbial infection beyond which the body's defensive system succumbs to illness.

respiration *Aerobic* respiration is a general term for the processes that result in the absorption, transport, and utilization of oxygen within an organism, accompanied by the release of energy. The term anaerobic respiration is sometimes applied to the release of energy from compounds by metabolic pathways that do not require oxygen.

respiration chamber A small insulated room that operates on the same basic principles as the bomb calorimeter. The heat given off by the subject causes a change in the temperature of a heat reservoir, such as water, surrounding the chamber. This allows the amount of energy released to be easily calculated.

respiratory gas exchange The measurement of oxygen gas consumed and/or carbon dioxide gas exhaled.

respiratory quotient (RQ) The ratio of carbon dioxide produced to oxygen consumed (i.e., CO_2 produced divided by O_2 consumed).

resting energy expenditure (REE) A combination of basal energy needs, plus the thermic effect of food, plus a small amount of energy needed to perform the most basic sedentary activities, such as sitting quietly.

resting metabolic rate The metabolic rate measured when the subject is resting, but was permitted to walk about (be "ambulatory") immediately before the measurement.

reticulocytes Immature red blood cells; they are released from the bone marrow into the blood where they lose their nuclei and become mature red blood cells.

retina The light-sensitive lining in the interior of the eye.

retinal Vitamin A in its aldehyde form.

retinoic acid Vitamin A in its carboxylic acid form.

retinoic acid response element (RARE) A nucleotide sequence to which retinoic acid receptor proteins (RARs) can bind and so influence the activity of specific genes.

retinoid binding proteins Various categories of proteins that bind to retinoids.

retinoid X receptors (RXR) Receptor proteins that bind to retinoids and that are structurally unrelated to the retinoic acid receptors (RARs).

retinoids Forms of preformed vitamin A.

retinol Vitamin A in its alcohol form.

retinol dehydrogenase An enzyme that catalyzes the dehydrogenation of retinol.

retinol equivalent (RE) A unit used for quantifying the vitamin A value of sources of vitamin A, with 1 RE defined as 3.3 International Units of vitamin A.

retinol-binding protein (RBP) The protein that binds to retinol and transports it in blood plasma.

retinoyl-beta-glucuronide A synthetic analog of vitamin A being tested for the treatment of acne and other skin disorders.

retinyl esters Members of the vitamin A family of compounds, produced when retinol combines with an organic acid, usually palmitic acid.

retinyl palmitate The predominant retinyl ester within food.

rhodopsin A purple pigment, also known as visual purple, involved in the conversion of light energy into nerve impulses in the retina of the eye.

ribose A pentose sugar that is part of or a precursor of several important body compounds including RNA, DNA, and riboflavin.

ribosomes Complexes of protein and RNA that act as the sites of protein synthesis within cells.

rickets A disease characterized by softening of the bones because of poor calcium deposition within them caused by lack of vitamin D activity in the body.

rickets-preventive factor Another term for vitamin D, so named for its role in preventing rickets.

RNA Ribonucleic acid.

RNA polymerase The enzyme that catalyzes the transcription of DNA into RNA.

rod cells Light-sensitive cells in the retina of the eye.

S

saccharin A white crystalline powder used as an alternative sweetener.

SALATRIM Tryglycerides with short- and long-chained fatty acids that are members of a family of reduced energy fats that provide only 5 kcal/g.

saliva The thin mucuslike fluid secreted by the salivary glands.

Salmonella enteritidis A common microbial contaminant of food that has been associated with the consumption of raw or partially cooked eggs or egg-containing foods, most of which have been stored at room temperature. The rate of infections due to this organism has been increasing steadily since the mid-1980s, possibly due to the importation of infected chicken.

salts Compounds formed when an acid and base react together and neutralize one another. Table "salt" (sodium chloride) is one common type of salt.

secondary structures Specific patterns of folding within a protein chain.

secretin A hormone secreted by duodenal cells that stimulates the pancreas to release its digestive secretions.

secretory IgA A class of immunoglobulins present in colostrum and breast milk that plays a major role in defending an infant against viruses, bacteria, and other pathogens and harmful food components in the first few days of life.

selenocysteine A modified selenium-containing form of the amino acid cysteine found in plants.

selenomethionine A modified selenium-containing form of the amino acid methionine found in plants.

selenoprotein P A selenium-containing protein that may function as a selenium transport protein in blood plasma.

selenosis Selenium poisoning, which can be caused by an excessive intake of selenium usually provided in supplements.

serotonin 5-Hydroxytryptamine, an important neurotransmitter.

severe overweight Having a body mass index (BMI) greater than or equal to the 95th percentile values of the BMI distributions for men and women aged 20 to 29 years.

shearing A process in which carbohydrates are mixed with water under high pressure, used in the manufacture of some carbohydrate-based fat substitutes.

shelf stable A classification given to foods that have been processed to destroy all preexisting microorganisms. They can be stored at room temperature and should contain no microbial infections unless the packaging has been damaged.

short-chain fatty acids Fatty acids containing less than 10 carbon atoms.

sickle cell anemia A genetic disease due to a mutation in the gene that codes for hemoglobin.

side chain or group Atoms attached to the central carbon atom or chain giving compounds (i.e., amino acids and proteins) their distinguishing characteristics.

siderosis A condition characterized by excessive storage of iron in the liver; also known as hemosiderosis.

silicosis Condition caused by an accumulation of silicon in lung tissue.

simple carbohydrates Sugars, including the monosaccharides and disaccharides.

simple obesity An old term for obesity, based on the fact that obesity is due to energy intake in excess of energy needs.

simple triglyceride A triglyceride in which all three fatty acid groups are identical.

Simplesse A protein-based fat substitute.

single photon absorptiometry Analytical technique used to assess calcium status by focusing light on the body and measuring the extent to which the light is absorbed.

sleeping metabolic rate The metabolic rate measured when the subject is asleep.

Slendid A pectin-based fat substitute.

small for gestation age (SGA) Having a lower birthweight than expected for the length of gestation.

solanine A toxic compound found near the green skin of some potatoes (where they have been exposed to the light) and in potato sprouts.

soluble fiber Fiber that absorbs water to form a gel.

solute load A measure of the total amount of dissolved substances (solutes) produced by metabolism or ingested and that must be excreted by the kidneys.

solvent A liquid in which other substances are dissolved such as water, the solvent in which most of the chemicals of life are dissolved.

sorbitol A derivative of glucose, formed when glucose is chemically reduced by the addition of one hydrogen atom.

specific dynamic effect of food The original name for what is now known as the thermic effect of food.

spirulina A protein powder produced from algae, which is sold as an appetite suppressant. It has a high content of the amino acid phenylalanine.

Splendor The brand name of the alternative sweetener sucralose.

spontaneous hypoglycemia A form of hypoglycemia characterized by chronically low blood glucose levels caused by the overproduction of insulin by the pancreas.

Standard of Identity If a food is produced according to a specific recipe on file with the U.S. Food and Drug Administration (FDA), the label does not have to list its ingredients. In that case, the manufacturer is using its Standard of Identity to avoid disclosing its ingredients.

Staphylococcus aureus A microbial contaminant of food that produces a toxin that causes illness within 2 to 6 hours after infection. The most commonly infected foods are custard, cheese, egg salads, milk, and cream-filled products.

starch A complex carbohydrate composed of many glucose units attached in a form the body can digest.

starch blockers Drugs that at one time were promoted as agents able to block the digestive breakdown of starch and thus reduce the number of kilocalories available for absorption.

starch granules Granules within cells composed of large numbers of starch molecules aggregated together. Granules from different types of plant can be distinguished by physical examination under the microscope.

steatorrhea A condition in which fatty stools are produced because of the inefficient absorption of fats from the gut.

Stellar A starch-based fat substitute.

steroid substitutes A variety of nonsteroid drugs and other substances that some athletes are using to try enhance athletic performance.

sterols A class of lipids whose structure includes multiple rings of carbon atoms, and which includes the important lipid cholesterol.

subatomic particles Electrons, protons, and neutrons; the three types of particles within atoms.

subcutaneous fat Deposits of fat directly beneath the skin.

substrates The chemical reactants that participate in and are catalyzed by an enzyme.

sucralose An alternative sweetener produced by the selective chlorination of sucrose and marketed under the brand name Splendor.

sucrose A disaccharide sugar (also known as table sugar) formed when a molecule of glucose combines with a molecule of fructose.

sucrose polyester A fat substitute made by combining the disaccharide sucrose with fatty acids, via ester linkages, to produce giant polyester molecules.

sulfur-containing amino acids Amino acids that contain a sulfur atom in their side chains.

Sunette The brand name for the alternative sweetener acesulfame-K.

superfortified cereals Cereals that have been fortified to contain vitamins at levels far greater than would be originally present.

superoxide dismutase (SOD) A copper-containing enzyme responsible for protecting the body against the toxic effects of oxygen by metabolizing the superoxide free radical.

symport A transmembrane carrier protein shared by two different transported substances (also known as a cotransporter).

synergistic A term used to refer to two substances each of which enhance the physiological effects of the other.

system A collection of organs that act together to sustain the body, such as the digestive system and the circulatory system.

T

table salt Sodium chloride.

tachycardia An abnormally rapid heart rate.

Talin An alternative sweetener.

taurine A sulfur-containing amino acid that has recently been identified as a possible dietary essential for infants because of its role in the development of the central nervous system.

tertiary structure The final folded structure of a protein molecule.

tetany Spasmodic and uncontrolled contraction of the muscles due to increased excitability of the nerves; caused, for example, by low calcium levels.

thaumatins Sweet proteins obtained from the West African plant *Thaumatococcus danicii*, which are being developed as alternative sweeteners.

thermic effect of food A process of increased energy expenditure and therefore heat release that inevitably occurs between 1 and 3 hours after a meal because of the stimulating effect of the nutrients of food on metabolism in general.

thermogenesis The generation of heat within the body by the action of metabolism.

thiamin diphosphate Another term for thiamin pyrophosphate (TPP).

thiamin hydrochloride The commercially produced form of thiamin, which is readily soluble in water and somewhat more stable than other forms.

thiamin pyrophosphate (TPP) The coenzyme formed when two phosphate groups are added to thiamin. This active coenzyme form of the vitamin has also been known as thiamin diphosphate and cocarboxylase.

thiaminase A thiamin-splitting enzyme found in some freshwater fish, a few saltwater fish and some shellfish such as clams, shrimps, and mussels, in addition to bracken ferns. Fortunately, thiaminase is a heat-labile enzyme that is readily destroyed by the heat of cooking; therefore it is only a cause for concern in diets containing significant amounts of raw fish.

thiocytin (thiotic acid) An alternative name for lipoic acid.

thrombin An enzyme that catalyzes the conversion of fibrinogen to fibrin during blood clotting.

thromboplastin An enzyme released from the cells of wounded tissue or from blood platelets, which converts prothrombin into thrombin as part of the blood clotting mechanism.

thromboses Blockages of blood vessels.

thyroglobulin A glycoprotein in the thyroid gland that binds to iodine and acts as an iodine storage protein.

thyroid-stimulating hormone (TSH) A hormone that stimulates the production and release of the thyroid hormones.

thyroxine (T_4) A thyroid hormone containing four atoms of iodine that stimulates cellular metabolism.

thyroxine-releasing factor (TRF) A factor released by the hypothalamus that stimulates the pituitary gland to release thyroid-stimulating hormone (TSH).

tissue A collection of cells of the same or very similar type.

tocopherol equivalents (TE) A unit for the measurement of the vitamin E content of food, with 1 TE corresponding to 1 mg of α-tocopherol (also known as 1 International Unit of α-tocopherol).

tocotrienols Four of the biologically active forms of vitamin E.

tolerance level The level of exposure to a chemical, such as a pesticide, which is deemed safe and without health risk.

toxemia of pregnancy Another name for preclampsia, a syndrome of abnormal conditions in pregnancy, of unknown cause; symptoms include hypertension, proteinurea, and edema. It may progress to eclampsia (severe toxemia), which can cause death.

trabeculae A porous region within the structure of a bone.

trace elements Another term for the micronutrient minerals.

tranquilizers Drugs intended to reduce anxiety.

trans A term used to describe double bonds between carbon atoms, which have hydrogen atoms (or other chemical groups) attached to *opposite* sides of the double bond.

transamination The transfer of amino groups between chemicals.

transcellular fluid Fluid in regions of the body that do not readily exchange water with the bulk of the extracellular fluid compartment, such as the inside of the eyeballs and joints.

transcobalamins I, II, and III The three proteins to which vitamin B_{12} can become bound for transport throughout the body.

transcription The production of a messenger RNA copy of a gene by the action of the enzyme RNA polymerase.

transfer RNA (tRNA) The form of RNA responsible for bringing the appropriate amino acids to the ribosome during protein synthesis.

transferrin A protein that transports iron in the blood.

transitional phase The phase of breast-feeding when other specially prepared foods are introduced alongside human milk or formula.

transketolase An enzyme involved in the metabolism of glucose via the hexose monophosphate shunt or pentose pathway. The coenzyme thiamine pyrophosphate (TPP) is required for transketolase to function.

translation The process by which the base sequence of mRNA directs the production of a specific protein molecule. Translation occurs on ribosomes.

transthyretin A plasma protein that binds to retinol-binding protein. It assists in the transport of vitamin A and prevents vitamin A from being filtered from the blood in the kidneys.

triacylglycerols Another name for triglycerides.

triesters Compounds containing three ester linkages. The triesters of relevance to nutrition are the triglycerides (triacylglycerols), which comprise the major component of dietary lipid.

triglycerides Molecules composed of three fatty acids esterified to the trialcohol glycerol.

triiodothyronine (T_3) A thyroid hormone that contains three atoms of iodine that stimulates cellular metabolism.

tripeptide A molecule composed of three amino acids bonded together.

trypsin A protease enzyme involved in the digestion of proteins.

tryptophan An aromatic amino acid; one of the amino acids found naturally in proteins.

tryptophan load test A test for vitamin B_6 deficiency based on the body's ability to metabolize a loading dose of tryptophan. Urine is analyzed for the presence of xanthurenic acid after administration of the tryptophan. The appearance of xanthurenic acid in the urine indicates vitamin B_6 deficiency.

Type I iodothyronine-5'-deiodinase (ID-1) A selenium-containing enzyme that converts T_4 to T_3.

U

ubiquinones The class of chemicals that includes all forms of coenzyme Q.

ultratrace elements Minerals with estimated dietary requirements usually less than 1 mg/day and minerals for which dietary essentiality has not been firmly established.

umbilical cord Flexible structure connecting the fetus to the placenta; contains umbilical arteries and vein.

unsaturated A chemical term applied to compounds that contain carbon-carbon double bonds.

urinary excretion threshold The level of consumption of a nutrient at which any additional consumption will lead to the additional amounts of the nutrient being excreted in urine.

uterine milk Secretions of the uterine glands that nourish the embryo before the placenta becomes established.

uterus The hollow muscular organ in which the embryo and then fetus develops until birth (also known as the womb).

V

vegan A strict vegetarian, who eats only foods of plant origin.

vegetarian A person who eats only foods of plant origin (although many people who call themselves vegetarians also eat some animal-based products such as milk, cheese, and eggs).

very low density lipoproteins (VLDL) The lipoprotein particles that initially leave the liver, carrying cholesterol and lipid.

vesicle A membrane-bound structure.

Vibrio vulnificus A microbial contaminant of food, which is a member of the genus known for cholera and gastroenteritis outbreaks caused by seafood. It is attracted to the chitin in the outer shell of lobster, crab, and shrimp. It causes septicemia, which results in death in over 50% of patients in 2 days.

villi Small projections on the surface of the circular folds in the intestine.

visual purple Another name for rhodopsin, the purple pigment involved in the conversion of light energy into nerve impulses in the retina of the eye.

vitamin A value A measure of the quantity of preformed vitamin A *plus* the amount of vitamin A available from vitamin A precursors in a food.

vitamin B_c Old name for a nutritional factor whose active ingredient is now known to be folic acid (folate).

vitamin D binding protein (DBP) The protein, also called alpha-globulin2, which binds to vitamin D in blood plasma and transports it throughout the body.

vitamin D-1-hydroxylase An enzyme in the kidney, which catalyzes the conversion of 25-hydroxyvitamin D to 1,25-dihydroxyvitamin D.

vitamin M Early name for a nutritional factor essential for monkeys whose active ingredient is now known to be folic acid (folate).

vitamins Organic compounds needed in very small amounts in the diet to help regulate and support chemical reactions in the body.

Von Ebner's glands Glands at the base of the tongue that secrete the enzyme, lingual lyase.

W

waist-to-hip ratio (WHR) The ratio of a person's waist circumference to hip circumference.

water The chemical solvent in which most of the processes of life occur.

water balance The balance between the amount of water being taken into the body and the amount of water being lost from the body (also known as fluid balance).

water intoxication Symptoms caused by overconsumption of water.

water of metabolism The water that is released in the body as an end product of metabolism.

Wernicke-Korsakoff syndrome The most common form of thiamin deficiency in developed countries, particularly in the United States. It is associated with alcohol abuse and causes symptoms ranging from mild confusion to coma.

wet (edematous) beriberi A form of beriberi in which the victim suffers from swelling of the limbs, usually starting at the feet and progressing upward through the body to cause difficulty in walking. The accumulation of fluid in heart muscle that leads to heart failure and death.

wheat germ The portion of a kernel of wheat containing its genetic material, a rich source of vitamin E.

whey proteins A class of proteins, including lactalbumin, that is found in liquid remaining after casein is precipitated by enzymes or acid.

white fat The main type of fat in the body, so called because its white appearance distinguishes it from the more specialized brown fat deposits.

Wilson's disease A hereditary condition associated with chronic copper toxicity due to a failure to excrete copper in bile.

Women, Infants, and Children (WIC) A federally funded program to improve the nutritional status of targeted women, infants, and children.

X

xerophthalmia A term for the advanced form of eye lesions resulting from vitamin A deficiency.

xerosis conjunctiva An intermediate stage of changes in the eye associated with vitamin A deficiency when blood vessels infiltrate the cornea of the eye.

xylitol An "alcohol sugar" derived from xylose, which can be used as an alternative sweetener in candies and gum.

xylose A pentose sugar that is produced commercially from cellulose and hemicellulose.

Y

yang Designation of strength associated with foods in macrobiotic diets.

***Yersinia enterocolitica* 0:3** The microbe that causes yersinosis, which has symptoms similar to appendicitis.

yersinosis The illness, with symptoms similar to appendicitis, caused by infection with *Yersinia enterocolitica* 0:3.

yin Designation of weakness associated with foods in macrobiotic diets.

Z

zeaxanthin One of the common carotenoids found in plant foods, which can serve as precursors of vitamin A.

Zen macrobiotic diet An extreme form of vegetarian diet based largely or exclusively on brown rice and involving a balance of "yin" and "yang" characteristics.

zero tolerance A standard that allows no detectable amounts of potentially harmful chemicals or agents in foods, drugs, or cosmetics.

zweibach A dry bread produced for use by infants, containing considerable amounts of the partially degraded form of starch known as dextrin.

zygote A fertilized egg cell.

CREDITS

Chapter 1 Opener, SuperStock, Inc.; unn. fig., p. 2, Hahn/Payne: Focus on health, ed. 2, 1994, Mosby; unn. fig., p. 7, PhotoDisc; unn. fig., p. 14, B. Bourne; unn. fig., p. 15, C. Schwent.

Chapter 2 Opener, K. Reid/FPG International; unn. fig., p. 26, UNICEF; Fig. 2-4, USDA; Fig. 2-5, Health and Welfare Canada, 1992, Ottawa, Canada; Fig. 2-7, USDA/DHHS: Home and garden bulletin 232, ed. 3, Washington DC, 1990; Fig. 2-8, Health and Welfare Canada: Nutrition recommendations for Canadians, 1992, Ottawa, Canada; Figs. 2-9 to 2-14, data from Willet WC: Science 264:532, 1994; unn. fig., p. 51, B. Bourne.

Overview 1 unn. fig., p. 62, *Portrait of the Artist and his Wife* by Master of Frankfurt, late 15th -early 16th century, Koninklijk Museaum voor Schone Kunsten, Antwerp, Belgium; Fig. OV1-1, Thibodeau/Patton: Anatomy & physiology, ed. 2, 1993, Mosby.

Chapter 3 Opener, Index Stock; unn. fig., p. 82, The Sugar Association; Fig. 3-6, redrawn from Glinsmann WH, Irasquin H, Park YK: J. Nutr. 116(Suppl.):S1, 1986; unn. fig., p. 86, PhotoDisc; unn. fig., p. 88, B. Bourne; Fig. 3-9, adapted from Gray: GM: N Engl J Med 292:1225, 1975; Figs. 3-12 to 3-14, Thibodeau/Patton: Anatomy & physiology, ed. 2, 1993, Mosby.

Chapter 4 Opener, National Cottonseed Products Association; unn. fig., p. 112, Saffola Quality Foods; Fig. 4-1, Thibodeau/Patton: Anatomy & physiology, ed. 2, 1993, Mosby; Fig. 4-2, Gottfried: Human biology, 1994, Mosby; Figs. 4-3 and 4-12, Wardlaw/Insel: Perspectives in nutrition, ed. 2, 1993, Mosby; Fig. 4-10, redrawn from Enig MG: Nutrition Research Newsletter 12:68, 1993; Fig. 4-16, data from Raper NR, Zizza C, Rourke J: Home economics research report 50, Washington DC, 1992, USDA; unn. fig., p. 137, PhotoDisc.

Chapter 5 Opener, C. Van Der Lende/Image Bank; Fig. 5-4, Thibodeau/Patton: Anatomy & physiology, ed. 2, 1993, Mosby; Fig. 5-7, redrawn from Munro HN, ed.: Mammalian protein metabolism, vol. IV, New York, 1970, Academic Press; Fig. 5-8, courtesy Dr. B. Shannon, The Pennsylvania State University; Fig. 5-10, adapted from Allison JB: Trans NY Acad Sci 25:295, 1963; Fig. 5-13, data from Raper NR, Zizza C, Rourke J: Home economics research report 50, Washingon DC, 1992, USDA; Fig. 5-14, courtesy Professor R. Hendricksen. In McLaren: Color atlas and text of diet-related disorders, 1992, Mosby.

Chapter 6 Opener, F. Chalfant/Image Bank; Fig. 6-1 Fig. 6-4, courtesy USDA, Beltsville, MD; photo by F.S. Witte; Fig. 6-5, courtesy Dr. V. Stallings, and J. Tomezsko, Children's Hospital of Philadelphia; Fig. 6-6, courtesy J.L. Loomis, no. 11, Human Performance Lab, The Pennsylvania State University; unn. fig., p. 204, B. Bourne; Fig. 6-7, Thibodeau/Patton: Anatomy & physiology, ed. 2, 1993, Mosby.

Chapter 7 Opener, C. Noble/Adventure Photo; Fig. 7-1, derived from National Research Council: Diet and health: implications for reducing chronic disease risk, Washington DC, 1989, National Academy of Sciences. In USDA/DHHS: Nutrition and your health: dietary guidelines for Americans, ed. 3, Washington DC, 1990, U.S. Government Printing Office; Fig. 7-2, data from National Health and Examination Survey (NHANES) II, 1976-1980; Figs. 7-3 and 7-9, redrawn from Bray GA: Am J Clin Nutr 55:488S, 1992; Figs. 7-4 to 7-6, courtesy J.L. Loomis, no. 11, Human Performance Lab, The Pennsylvania State University; Fig. 7-7 and unn. fig., p. 242, Hahn/Payne: Focus on health, ed. 2, 1994, Mosby; Fig. 7-11, redrawn from Bray GA: Nutr Rev 49:33, 1991; Fig. 7-12, redrawn from Bray GA: Nutr Today 28:13, 1993; unn. fig., p. 250, Payne/Hahn: Understanding your health, ed. 3, 1992.

Chapter 8 Opener, P. Turner/Image Bank; Figs. 8-4 (inset) and 8-8 (inset), PhotoDisc; Fig. 8-10 (inset), T. Eynon.

Overview 2 unn. fig., p. 290, *Wheatfield* by Robert Zund, 1855, Arthur Stoll Collection, Corseaux; unn. fig., p. 291, *Cascade de Pissevache* (detail) by Johann Jakob Biedermann, 1855, Kunstmuseaum, Winterthur.

Chapter 9 Opener, Eckhard Photography; Fig. 9-3, Thibodeau/Patton: Anatomy & physiology, ed. 2, 1993, Mosby; Fig. 9-7, redrawn from McBean LD, Speckmann EW: Nutritive value of dairy foods. In Wong DP, ed.: Fundamentals of dairy chemistry, New York, 1988, Van Nostrand Reinhold; Figs. 9-8, 9-12, and 9-14, data from Raper NR, Zizza C, Rourke J: Home economics research report 50, Washington DC, 1992, USDA; Fig. 9-9 (inset), PhotoDisc.

Chapter 10 Opener, A. Johnson/Image Bank; Figs. 10-6, 10-10, and 10-14, data from Raper NR, Zizza C, Rourke J: Home economics research report 50, Washington DC, 1992, USDA.

Overview 3 unn. fig., p. 382, *Oranges* by Richard Mouck.

Chapter 11 Opener, C. Rosenfeld/Image Bank; Fig. 11-3, The Upjohn Company; Figs. 11-5 and 11-6, redrawn from Ross AC: J Nutr 123:346, 1993; unn. fig., p. 405, California Fresh Carrot Advisory Board; Fig. 11-7, data from Raper NR, Zizza C, Rourke J: Home economics research report 50, Washington DC, 1992, USDA; Fig. 11-8 (inset), T. Eynon; Fig. 11-9, The Nutrition Foundation, Inc., NY, and American Foundation for Overseas Blindness, Inc., NY; Fig. 11-12, redrawn from DeLuca HD: Nutr Today 28:6, 1993; unn. fig., p. 422, Fig. 11-14 (inset), and unn. fig., p. 428, PhotoDisc.

Chapter 12 Opener, L. Rubin/Image Bank; unn. fig., p. 438, PhotoDisc; unn. fig., p. 454, Williams: Basic nutrition and diet therapy, ed. 10, 1995, Mosby; Figs. 12-5, 12-12, and 12-15, data from Raper NR, Zizza C, Rourke J: Home economics research report 50, Washington DC, 1992, USDA; Fig. 12-6 (inset), courtesy Coca Cola Foods, Houston, TX; Fig. 12-8, adapted from Herbert V, Das KC: Folic acid and vitamin B12. In Shils ME, Olson JE, Shike M, eds.: Modern nutrition in health and disease, ed. 8, Philadelphia, 1994, Lea & Febiger; Fig. 12-9, data from Raper NR, Zizza C, Rourke J: Home economics research report 50, Washington DC, 1992, USDA; Fig. 12-10, Herbert V, Das KC: Folic acid and vitamin B12. In Shils ME, Olson JA, Shike M: Modern nutrition in health and disease, Philadelphia, 1994, Lea & Febiger; Fig. 12-11, Herbert V: Vitamin B12. In Nutrition Review: Present knowledge in nutrition, ed. 5, Washington DC, 1984, The Nutrition Foundation; Fig. 12-13, Merrill AH, Burnham FS: Vitamin B6. In Brown M, ed.: Present knowledge in nutrition, ed. 6, Washington DC, 1990, International Life Sciences Institute.

Chapter 13 Opener, L. Rubin/Image Bank; Figs. 13-3, 13-6, and 13-8, data from Raper NR, Zizza C, Rourke J: Home economics research report 50, Washington DC, 1992, USDA; Fig. 13-4 (inset), PhotoDisc; unn. fig., p. 499, UNICEF; Fig. 13-9, McLaren DS: Color atlas and text of diet-related disorders, 1992, Mosby; Fig. 13-13, courtesy D.M. Mock, MD, PhD, University of Arkansas for Medical Sciences & Arkansas Children's Hospital, Little Rock, AR; Fig. 13-14 (inset), PhotoDisc.

Chapter 14 Opener, GS Chapman/Image Bank; Fig. 14-1, Wardlaw/Insel/Seyler: Contemporary nutrition, ed. 2, 1994, Mosby; Fig. 14-4, data from Hytten FE, Leitch S: The physiology of human pregnancy, ed. 2, Oxford, England, 1971, Blackwell Scientific Publications; Fig. 14-5, adapted from Hytten FE, Leitch S: The physiology of human pregnancy, ed. 2, Oxford, England, 1971, Blackwell Scientific Publications; unn. fig., p. 529 and Fig. 14-8 (inset), UNICEF.

Chapter 15 Opener, D. Sundberg/Image Bank; unn. fig., p. 544, Wong: Whaley & Wong's essentials of pediatric nursing, ed. 4, July 1994, Mosby; Fig. 15-1, data from Meyer HF: Clin Pediatr 76:708, 1968; Martinez GA, Kruger FW: Pediatrics 76:1004, 1985; Institute of medicine: Nutrition during lactation, Washington DC, 1991, National Academy Press; Fig. 15-2, data from Fomon SJ: Nutrition of normal infants, 1993, Mosby; unn. fig., p. 555, courtesy Ross Products Division, Abbott Laboratories; unn. fig., p. 561, copyright 1993 Gerber Products Co. Reprinted with permission. All rights reserved; Figs. 15-5 and 15-6, adapted from Hamill PVV et al.: Physical growth: National Center for Health Statistics percentiles, Am J Clin Nutr 32:607, 1979. Data from the Fels Research Institute, Wright State University School of Medicine, Yellow Springs, OH. Copyright 1980 Ross Laboratories.

Chapter 16 Opener, D. Sundberg/Image Bank; Fig. 16-1, based on National Research Council, Food and Nutrition Board: Recommended Dietary Allowances, ed. 10, Washington DC, 1989; unn. fig., p. 576, courtesy Washington Apple Commission; Fig. 16-2, data from National Health and Nutrition Examination (NHANES) III, 1988-1992; Figs. 16-3, 16-4, and 16-6, adapted from Hamill PVV et al.: Physical growth National Center for Health Statistics percentiles, Am J Clin Statistics, Hyattsville, MD. Copyright 1982 Ross Laboratories; unn. fig., p. 587, courtesy Washington State Fruit Commission.

Chapter 17 Opener, P. Miller/Image Bank; Fig. 17-1, courtesy USDA Human Nutrition Research Center on Aging at Tufts University; Fig. 17-2, data from DHHS: Normal human aging: the Baltimore longitudinal study of aging, NIH pub. no. 84-2450. Washington DC, U.S. Government Printing Office; Fig. 17-3, redrawn from Frontera WR: J Appl Physiol 71:644, 1991; unn. fig., p. 617, PhotoDisc.

Chapter 18 Opener, M. Romanelli/Image Bank; unn. fig., p. 626, B. Bourne.

Chapter 19 Opener, Eckhard Photography; Fig. 19-1, adapted from Purdue University Cooperative Extension Service pamphlet; unn. figs., pp. 650 and 654, PhotoDisc.

Appendixes Fig. A-8, Thibodeau/Patton: Anatomy & physiology, ed. 2, 1993, Mosby.

I N D E X

Page numbers in italics indicate illustrations; *t* indicates tables.

E

Body Height Standard Proposed in Dietary Guidelines for Americans: A, 1985; and B, 1990

A. Desirable Body Weight Ranges*		
	Weight without Clothes (lbs)	
Height without Shoes	Men	Women
4′10″		92-121
4′11″		95-124
5′0″		98-127
5′1″	105-134	101-130
5′2″	108-137	104-134
5′3″	111-141	107-138
5′4″	114-145	110-142
5′5″	117-149	114-146
5′6″	121-154	118-150
5′7″	125-159	122-154
5′8″	129-163	126-159
5′9″	133-167	130-164
5′10″	137-172	134-169
5′11″	141-177	
6′0″	145-182	
6′1″	149-187	
6′2″	153-192	
6′3″	157-197	

B. Suggested Weight for Adults		
	Weight without Clothes (lbs)	
Height without Shoes	19 to 34 Years	35 Years and Over
5′0″	97-128†	108-138
5′1″	101-132	111-143
5′2″	104-137	115-148
5′3″	107-141	119-152
5′4″	111-146	122-157
5′5″	114-150	126-162
5′6″	118-155	130-167
5′7″	121-160	134-172
5′8″	125-164	138-178
5′9″	129-169	142-183
5′10″	132-174	146-188
5′11″	136-179	151-194
6′0″	140-184	155-199
6′1″	144-189	159-205
6′2″	148-195	164-210
6′3″	152-200	168-216
6′4″	156-205	173-222
6′5″	160-211	177-228
6′6″	164-216	182-234

A From The Metropolitan Life Insurance Company: New weight standards for men and women, *Stat Bull N Y Metropol Life Ins* 40:1, 1959; and B From The National Research Council: *Diet and health,* Washington, DC, 1989, National Academy Press.

* For women 18 to 25 years old, subtract 1 lb for each year under 25 years.

† The higher weights in the ranges generally apply to men, who tend to have more muscle and bone; the lower weights more often apply to women, who have less muscle and bone.